**Clinical Pediatric Endocrinology**

# Clinical Pediatric Endocrinology

**Edited by**

## Charles G. D. Brook
MA MD FRCP FRCPCH
Emeritus Professor of Paediatric Endocrinology
University College London

## Peter C. Hindmarsh
Reader in Paediatric Endocrinology
University College London

The Middlesex Hospital
Mortimer Street
London

**Foreword by**

## Howard S. Jacobs
Emeritus Professor of Reproductive Endocrinology
University College London

**Fourth edition**

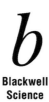

**Blackwell
Science**

© 2001 by
Blackwell Science Ltd
Editorial Offices:
Osney Mead, Oxford OX2 0EL
25 John Street, London WC1N 2BL
23 Ainslie Place, Edinburgh EH3 6AJ
350 Main Street, Malden
   MA 02148 5018, USA
54 University Street, Carlton
   Victoria 3053, Australia
10, rue Casimir Delavigne
   75006 Paris, France

Other Editorial Offices:
Blackwell Wissenschafts-Verlag GmbH
Kurfürstendamm 57
10707 Berlin, Germany

Blackwell Science KK
MG Kodenmacho Building
7–10 Kodenmacho Nihombashi
Chuo-ku, Tokyo 104, Japan

Iowa State University Press
A Blackwell Science Company
2121 S. State Avenue
Ames, Iowa 50014-8300, USA

First published 2001

Set by Graphicraft Limited, Hong Kong
Printed and bound in Great Britain
by MPG Books Ltd, Bodmin, Cornwall

The Blackwell Science logo is a
trade mark of Blackwell Science Ltd,
registered at the United Kingdom
Trade Marks Registry

A catalogue record for this title
is available from the British Library

ISBN 0-632-04774-7

Library of Congress
Cataloging-in-publication Data

Clinical pediatric endocrinology / edited by
Charles G. D. Brook, Peter C. Hindmarsh.—4th ed.
      p. ;   cm.
   Includes bibliographical references and index.
   ISBN 0-632-05148-5
   1. Pediatric endocrinology.   I. Brook, C. G. D.
(Charles Groves Darville)   II.  Hindmarsh,
P. C. (Peter C.)
   [DNLM:   1.  Endocrine Diseases—
Adolescence.   2. Endocrine Diseases—Child.
3. Endocrine Diseases—Infant.   4. Endocrine
Diseases—Physiopathology.   WS 330 C641
2000]
RJ 418 .C567 2000
618.92′4—dc21

                                          00-058501

DISTRIBUTORS

Marston Book Services Ltd
PO Box 269
Abingdon, Oxon OX14 4YN
(*Orders*: Tel:  01235 465500
           Fax: 01235 465555)

USA
Blackwell Science, Inc.
Commerce Place
350 Main Street
Malden, MA 02148 5018
(*Orders*: Tel:  800 759 6102
               781 388 8250
           Fax: 781 388 8255)

Canada
Login Brothers Book Company
324 Saulteaux Crescent
Winnipeg, Manitoba R3J 3T2
(*Orders*: Tel: 204 837 2987)

Australia
Blackwell Science Pty Ltd
54 University Street
Carlton, Victoria 3053
(*Orders*: Tel: 3 9347 0300
           Fax: 3 9347 5001)

For further information on
Blackwell Science, visit our website:
www.blackwell-science.com

# Contents

# List of contributors

**Professor Stephanie A. Amiel**
Department of Medicine
Guy's, King's & St Thomas' School of
    Medicine
King's College
London SE5 9RS
UK

**Dr A. Boneh**
Victorian Clinical Genetics Service
Royal Children's Hospital
Parkville
Melbourne 3052
Australia

**Dr Nicola Bridges**
Chelsea & Westminster Hospital
London SW1O 9NH
UK

**Professor C. G. D. Brook**
The Middlesex Hospital
Mortimer Street
London W1T 3AA
UK

**Professor Rosalind S. Brown**
Department of Pediatrics
University of Massachusetts Medical School
55 Lake Avenue North
Worcester, MA 01655
USA

**Dr C. R. Buchanan**
Department of Paediatrics
King's College Hospital
London SE5 9RS
UK

**Dr P. E. Clayton**
Senior Lecturer in Child Health
Royal Manchester Children's Hospital
Manchester M27 4HA
UK

**Miss Sarah Creighton**
Consultant Gynaecologist
University College London Hospital
London
UK

**Dr P. Dabadghao**
Department of Endocrinology and Diabetes
Royal Children's Hospital
Parkville
Melbourne 3052
Australia

**Dr M. T. Dattani**
Institute of Child Health
London WC1N 1EH
UK

**Professor S. Franks**
Institute of Reproductive and
    Developmental Biology
Imperial College School of Medicine
Hammersmith Hospital
London W12 0NN
UK

**Dr M. S. Gill**
MRC Research Fellow
Department of Medicine
Endocrine Sciences Research Group
University of Manchester
Manchester
UK

**Dr D. A. Heath**
Consultant Physician
Selly Oak Hospital
Raddlebarn Road
Birmingham B29 6JD
UK

**Dr P. C. Hindmarsh**
The Middlesex Hospital
Mortimer Street
London W1T 3AA
UK

**Professor R. L. Hintz**
Department of Pediatrics
Stanford University Medical Center
Stanford, CA 94305
USA

**Dr M. D. Kilby**
Reader in Fetal Medicine
Division of Reproductive Medicine and
    Child Health
University of Birmingham
Birmingham Women's Hospital
Birmingham B15 2TG
UK

**Dr J. C. P. Kingdom**
Maternal–Fetal Medicine Division
University of Toronto
Mount Sinai Hospital
Toronto M5G 1XS
Canada

**Mr T. R. Kurzawinski**
Pancreatic and Endocrine Surgery Unit
The Middlesex Hospital
London W1T 3AA
UK

**Professor E. R. Laws**
Department of Neurosurgery
University of Virginia Health System
PO Box 800212
Charlottesville, VA 22908
USA

**Dr N. J. Marshall**
Department of Molecular Pathology
UCL Medical School
London W1P 6DB
UK

**Dr D. R. Matthews**
Oxford Diabetes & Endocrinology Centre
The Radcliffe Infirmary
Oxford OX2 6HE
UK

**Professor Walter L. Miller**
Department of Pediatrics
University of California
San Francisco, CA 94143-0978
USA

**Professor P. D. E. Mouriquand**
Department of Paediatric Urology
Hospital Debrousse
Lyon Cedex 05
France

**Professor J. L. H. O'Riordan**
Emeritus Professor of Metabolic Medicine
University College London
The Middlesex Hospital
London W1T 3AA
UK

**Professor M. A. Preece**
Biochemistry, Endocrinology & Metabolism
   Unit
Institute of Child Health
University College London
London WC1N 1EH
UK

**Professor G. L. Robertson**
Center for Endocrinology, Metabolism, and
   Molecular Medicine
Northwestern University Medical School
Chicago, IL 60611-3008
USA

**Mr R. C. G. Russell**
Pancreatic and Endocrine Surgery Unit
The Middlesex Hospital
London W1T 3AA
UK

**Professor P. H. Saenger**
Department of Pediatrics
Division of Pediatric Endocrinology
Montefiore Medical Center
New York, NY 10467
USA

**Dr N. J. Shaw**
Consultant Endocrinologist
The Birmingham Children's Hospital
Birmingham B4 6NH
UK

**Dr Helen A. Spoudeas**
The Middlesex Hospital
London W1T 3AA
UK

**Professor D. M. Styne**
Department of Pediatrics
University of California Medical Center
Sacremento, CA 95817
USA

**Dr S. P. Taback**
Health Sciences Center
FE325-685 William Avenue
Winnipeg, Manitoba R3E OZ2
Canada

**Professor P. Vallance**
Centre for Clinical Pharmacology
The Rayne Institute
5 University Street
London WC1E 6JJ
UK

**Dr Angela Wade**
Paediatric Epidemiology & Biostatistics Unit
Institute of Child Health
University College London
London W9N 1EH
UK

**Dr G. L. Warne**
Associate Professor
Department of Endocrinology and Diabetes
Royal Children's Hospital
Parkville
Melbourne 3052
Australia

**Dr M. J. Wheeler**
Department of Chemical Pathology
St Thomas' Hospital
London SE1 7EH
UK

**Dr W. L. Whittle**
Department of Obstetrics & Gynecology
University of Toronto
Ontario M5G 1X5
Canada

**D. T. Wilcox**
Consultant Paediatric Urologist
Great Ormond Street Children's Hospital
London WC1N 3JH
UK

**Dr Diana F. Wood**
Department of Endocrinology
St Bartholomew's and the Royal London
   School of Medicine
The Royal London Hospital
London E1 1BB
UK

**Mr C. R. J. Woodhouse**
Reader in Adolescent Urology
Institute of Urology & Nephrology
London W1T 3AA
UK

# Foreword

Paediatric endocrinology holds a special fascination because it allows us to observe the contributions of endocrine control mechanisms to the infant's adaptation to birth and the child's transformation into an adult. Its intellectual challenges burgeon: the breadth of knowledge required of its practitioners encompasses, *inter alia*, molecular genetics (who could expect to care for a family with a child born with ambiguous genitalia without such understanding?) and statistical and clinical trials methodology, together with modern concepts of hormone secretion, metabolism and action. Diagnostic tests in paediatric endocrinology pose particular problems because of the changes in hormone secretion as children grow and mature. The extraordinary increase of information, the changing concepts of endocrine mechanisms of control and integration and the progress in therapeutics afforded by recombinant technology provide a continual challenge to physicians caring for children with endocrine disorders.

*Clinical Pediatric Endocrinology* provides both the aspiring paediatric endocrinologist and the experienced practitioner with an exemplary text. It opens with illuminating descriptions of how hormones interact with their target cells, of why the pulsatile nature of hormone secretion is important, of how hormones are measured and of how to use all this information to formulate an approach to endocrine investigation of children with suspected hormonal disorders. There follows a logical progression through endocrine physiology and the clinical results of endocrine dysfunction. Each section integrates normal function and pathology, to the advantage of our understanding of both. While there is a strong emphasis on modern concepts of molecular genetics, clinical wisdom is always apparent. The emphasis on the integration

of careful clinical observation with the natural history of growth and development is commendable because, as Professor Brook and Dr Hindmarsh remind us in Chapter 9, 'investigating normal children constitutes an assault'.

How is the clinician to cope with the rapid developments that are so much a feature of this subject? Two strategies are essential: a firm grounding in basic concepts of normal function and pathological processes is one and an organized approach to the framing of clinical questions is the other. The chapters describing the basis of valid clinical trials and developing an evidenced-based approach are therefore helpful contributions. Getting the diagnosis right and applying appropriate treatment are vital features throughout medicine, but are nowhere more important than in paediatric endocrinology: for these patients, the outcome of treatment remains for the rest of life. The implications become ever more clear when the child is managed by a team that, at the appropriate time, includes an adult endocrinologist. The seamless management that must be the aim of comprehensive patient care can only be achieved with knowledge and experience acquired in several disciplines, a theme that runs throughout the book.

Professor Brook and his colleagues have made a valuable contribution to the training and practice of paediatric endocrinology: compendious and informative, their book nonetheless makes exciting reading. While informed by the results of the latest ideas and technology, it is ultimately dedicated to excellence in patient care. I warmly recommend it.

Howard Jacobs
Emeritus Professor of Reproductive Endocrinology
Royal Free and University College, London Medical School
The Middlesex Hospital
London W1M 7AF
UK

# Preface to the Fourth Edition

Twenty years have passed since the first edition of this book was published, years in which the discipline of paediatric endocrinology has expanded greatly. Senior paediatric endocrinologists have contributed the forewords to the previous editions, and it is not by accident that the foreword to this edition is written by Dr Howard Jacobs, Professor of Reproductive Endocrinology at University College London and Consultant Physician at The Middlesex Hospital.

It is our firm belief that no paediatric endocrinology department should operate independently of its adult counterpart, and the friendship and collaboration that we have with Howard and our other colleagues in the adult disciplines at The Middlesex Hospital has been greatly appreciated. It has enabled us to provide at the London Centre for Paediatric Endocrinology a seamless service for patients from infancy, whom we see at Great Ormond Street Hospital for Children, to adolescence and adult life, when we manage them at The Middlesex Hospital.

This edition of *Clinical Pediatric Endocrinology* has again been rewritten from cover to cover. Many new colleagues have given generously of their time and expertise, as well as some old friends. Writing chapters for textbooks is not well rewarded, but the authors may have the satisfaction of knowing that their work is appreciated worldwide.

We considered that molecular biology, to which we paid special attention in the last edition, now merits a place in clinical practice. The newest section this time is about mechanisms of hormone action. The stalwart subjects have not been neglected and we hope that the book will retain its impact on clinical practice.

Once again, it is a pleasure to acknowledge the satisfaction of working with our friends at Blackwell Science (and those who work with them) to bring our book to publication.

C. G. D. Brook
P. C. Hindmarsh

# Preface to the First Edition

Endocrine problems are not uncommon in paediatric practice and are mostly, *faute de mieux*, rather badly managed by non-specialists. This is especially true in England, where paediatric specialities are relatively newly defined. The same is certainly less true of Europe as a whole and this book has its origins in the friendship of the European Society for Paediatric Endocrinology which has acted as a focus for the subject and which benefits greatly from its transatlantic corresponding members. If the book were to have a dedication, it would be to the health of the Society coupled with a toast to its American counterpart, the Lawson Wilkins Society.

I hope that the book will be of service to general paediatric departments and of help and interest to departments of (adult) endocrinology in their dealings with patients who are still growing. In a book of this size, there may well be sins of omission and commission and for these I alone can take responsibility and I apologize for them in advance. If any readers were to take the trouble to let me know about such sins for future reference, I would be very grateful.

In the completion of my editorial task I have been greatly assisted by Miss Lynette Napper and Mrs Sue Shorvon, my secretaries at The Middlesex Hospital, and by Mr Jony Russell and Mr Peter Saugman at Blackwell Scientific Publications. My co-authors and I thank them for assisting at the birth of our work.

C. G. D. Brook

# 1 Hormones and their target cells

**N. J. Marshall**

## Introduction

Hormones interact with target cells through specific receptors. Some of the characteristics of these receptors are summarized in Table 1.1. Clearly, a receptor must be readily accessible to its hormone, and thus the cellular location of the receptor reflects the chemical characteristics of its hormone. For example, water-soluble hormones, such as the pituitary-derived proteins and glycoproteins, are hydrophilic and cannot cross the lipid barrier presented by the cytoplasmic membrane. These therefore interact with receptors located on the cell surface. In contrast, lipid-soluble hormones, such as steroids and the thyroid hormones, bind to intracellular receptors located either in the cytosol or in the nucleus. The diversity of the different receptor groups is outlined in Fig. 1.1.

**Table 1.1.** Notable characteristics of hormone receptors

1. Hormones react with their receptors in a reversible manner. This can be described by the equation $H + R \rightleftharpoons HR$, where the position of equilibrium lies well to the right, i.e. hormones have high affinities for their receptors. The reversible nature of this reaction and the saturability of the system can be demonstrated with a series of classic ligand-binding experiments. Quantitative measurements of affinity constants and numbers of receptors per cell can be established by the application of the law of mass action. $K_d$ values range between pico- and nanomolar concentrations, which is appropriate for hormones as they circulate at these low concentrations.
2. Receptors exhibit high degrees of hormonal specificity.
3. The locations of receptors are appropriately tissue specific.
4. For some hormones, e.g. aldosterone, hormone specificity is crucially achieved by target tissue conversion.
5. Receptors for hormones fall into several discrete groups in terms of their structure and subcellular localization. These reflect the biochemical characteristics of their cognate hormones.
6. Receptors on cell surfaces trigger a wide range of intracellular signal transduction pathways. These also fall into several categories.

## Cell-surface receptors for hormones

There are two superfamilies of cell-surface receptors. The first is linked to tyrosine kinase and the second to G-proteins (Fig. 1.1). There is, however, an underlying structural unity in all cell-surface receptors. Each holoreceptor comprises three segments (Fig. 1.2).

**1** An extracellular component, otherwise known as the ectodomain, which binds the hormone with a high affinity. The N-terminal ectodomain is rich in glycosylation sites, but the functional significance of the attached oligosaccharide moieties is not known. The ectodomain is comparatively rich in cysteine residues, which form internal S–S bonds and repeated loops and are vital for the correct folding of this receptor region.

The ectodomain of receptors for some hormones can also be identified as a separate entity in the circulation. For example, the free ectodomain for growth hormone forms a circulating binding protein. The ectodomain of the thyroid-stimulating hormone (TSH) receptor can be cleaved relatively easily, and fragments in the circulation may be important for the so far unexplained induction of thyroid-stimulating antibodies that mimic TSH action as antireceptor autoantibodies.

**2** A membrane-spanning region, which varies in structure from a simple linear hydrophobic region to a more serpentine structure that crosses the membrane seven times. As might be expected, the membrane-spanning domain is rich in hydrophobic and non-charged amino acids. Approximately 25 of these are required to bridge the typical cytoplasmic membrane, which is 100 Å across. To do this they form an α-helix. The structure of the transmembrane domain can be much more complex than is shown in Fig. 1.2 (see Fig. 1.9).

**3** A cytosolic domain initiates the intracellular signalling cascade, which can itself be complex, with several branch points. Protein phosphorylation of sequences of proteins often plays an important role in signal transduction. The C-terminal cytoplasmic domain contains within its own structure, or links with, separate catalytic systems that

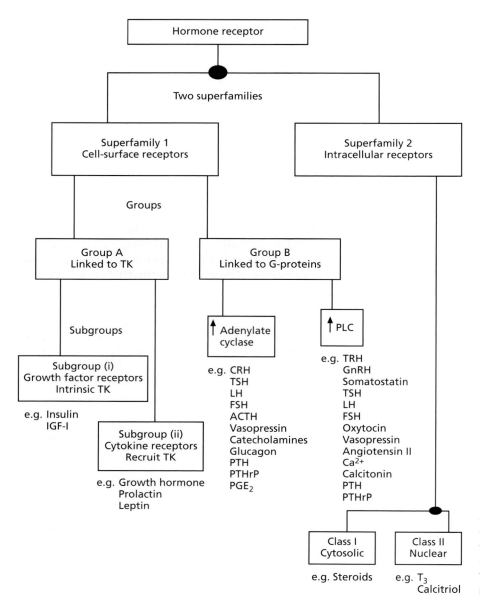

**Fig. 1.1.** A composite diagram showing the different classes of hormone receptors. Receptors for some hormones can occur in more than one type of class. For example, different types of PTH receptors link to different G-proteins, which then either couple to adenylate cyclase or phospholipase C (PLC). TK, tyrosine kinase.

initiate intracellular signals. Using recombinant technology, chimeric receptors have been formed by mixing and recombining segments of different receptors that fall within one of the receptor superfamilies. These demonstrate the functional independence of the three segments.

## Protein phosphorylation

The amino acids serine, threonine and tyrosine each carry a polar hydroxyl group (Fig. 1.3). These amino acids can be phosphorylated when a phosphate group is transferred from adenosine triphosphate (ATP) and substitutes for the polar hydroxyl group on the amino acid. This generates a co-valently bound phosphate (Fig. 1.4a). The energy transfer during this reaction leads to an activating conformational change of the phosphorylated protein. In many signalling pathways, the activated phosphorylated protein is then itself able to act as a protein kinase and phosphorylate the next protein in the sequence. In this way a phosphorylation cascade is generated which relays the intracellular signal along a pathway (Fig. 1.4b).

### Serine or threonine vs. tyrosine phosphorylation

Protein phosphorylation acts as a key molecular switch. The polar hydroxyl groups of serine and threonine are far more abundantly phosphorylated than those of tyrosine. Thus, phosphoserine and phosphothreonine residues account for the major fraction of the 10% of the proteins that are phosphorylated at any given time in a mammalian cell. Indeed, until

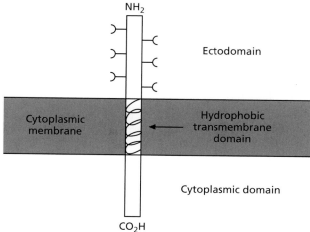

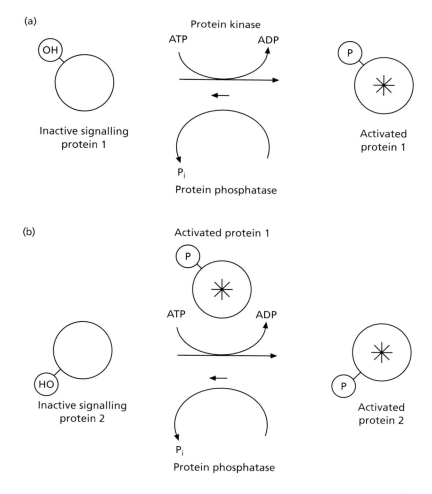

**Fig. 1.2.** Schematic representation of a membrane-spanning cell-surface receptor with three clearly identifiable domains: the ectodomain is bridged by a membrane-spanning component to the intracellular cytoplasmic domain. Each domain has characteristic structural features that reflect its location and function.

**Fig. 1.3.** The structures of the amino acids serine, threonine and tyrosine, which carry polar hydroxyl groups that can be phosphorylated.

1980, only phosphoserine and phosphothreonine had been identified as naturally occurring phosphoamino acids. Only about 0.1% of the phosphorylated proteins contain phospho-tyrosine residues. However, the relatively long side chain of phosphotyrosine, together with the unusual negative electron density of its aromatic ring (Fig. 1.3), makes tyrosine phosphorylation a particularly distinctive molecular switch. Tyrosine phosphorylation plays a particularly prominent role in signal transmission for hormones such as insulin and growth hormone.

**Fig. 1.4.** Protein phosphorylation and the generation of phosphorylation cascades. (a) Phosphorylation of protein 1 induces an activating conformational change due to the energetically favourable phosphorylation P of a hydroxyl group OH. (b) The initiation of a phosphorylation cascade. Phosphorylated protein 1 acts as a kinase and phosphorylates protein 2. The forward and backward reactions are catalysed by protein kinases and phosphatases respectively. There is a high degree of amino acid specificity so that serine/threonine kinases usually show essentially no cross-reactivity with tyrosine residues. Conversely, the kinases and phosphatases that react with tyrosine residues do not usually react with serine or threonine residues. The enzymes that are specific for either serine/threonine or tyrosine residues are inhibited by different compounds: this is used in their identification, as are antibodies capable of distinguishing the phosphoamino acids. The catalytic domain of tyrosyl phosphatases bears no resemblance to that of serine/threonine phosphatases or of the alkaline or acid phosphatases.

Phosphorylation of tyrosine not only activates the recipient protein but can also create important docking sites for subsequent protein–protein interactions. This is due to complementary conserved protein modules, known as SH2 and SH3 domains, on the docking proteins. These are approximately 100 amino acids long and contain a crucially positioned arginine (Arg-175), which facilitates binding to phosphotyrosine but not phosphoserine or phosphothreonine residues. The relatively long side chain of phosphotyrosine provides the appropriate length to dock into the grooves of the SH2/SH3 domains or the catalytic clefts of tyrosine phosphatases.

SH2/SH3 domains, with their highly distinctive molecular topologies, can be found in a diverse array of cytoplasmic signalling proteins. As detailed later, they are important for the docking of inactive, soluble tyrosine kinases to receptors that are anchored in the plasma membrane but which have been activated by hormone binding. These domains also play a passive role when they appear to link signalling proteins within a phosphorylation cascade. An appropriate analogy for this would be the use of adaptor plugs (or even transformers) when connecting electrical equipment.

## Cell-surface receptors and intracellular signalling

There are two major groups of cell-surface receptors linked to intracellular signals (Fig. 1.1). The first relies upon tyrosine kinase for the initiation of the downstream signals. The second major group is linked to G-proteins. This generates intracellular messages that activate pathways preferentially using serine or threonine kinases.

### Tyrosine kinase-linked cell-surface receptors

These have a relatively simple transmembrane segment and either have intrinsic tyrosine kinase activity located in the cytosolic domain or recruit tyrosine kinases subsequent to receptor activation by the binding of the hormone (Fig. 1.1).

*Receptors with integrated tyrosine kinase activity*
The most prominent member of this subgroup from an endocrine perspective is the receptor for insulin. However, these receptors typically bind ligands, such as epidermal growth factor (EGF) or fibroblast growth factor (FGF), that stimulate cell growth and proliferation and are therefore frequently referred to as growth factor receptors. The receptor for insulin-like growth factor I (IGF-I) is a member of this subgroup.

The fundamental structure of these receptors is depicted in Fig. 1.2. For ligands such as EGF and FGF, receptor occupancy is followed by dimerization of two adjacent monomeric receptors. Such dimerization of ligand-coupled receptors is a well-recognized phenomenon. This then leads to activation of the tyrosine kinase, which is integrated into the structure of the cytosolic domain. In contrast, the recep-

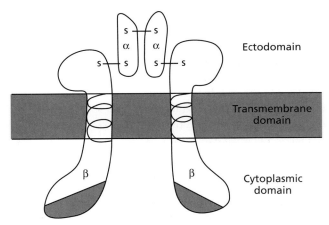

**Fig. 1.5.** Outline structure of the insulin receptor. The receptor is a heterotetrameric structure comprising two α- and two β-subunits as shown. Both subunits are derived from a single amino acid chain precursor. The molecular weight of the holoreceptor is ~ 400 kDa. One molecule of insulin binds to the ectodomain. The N-terminus of the first third of the β-subunit (193 amino acids) lies on the extracellular side of the membrane. The transmembrane domain consists of 23 hydrophobic amino acids organized in an α-helix, and the cytoplasmic domain (402 amino acids) accounts for approximately two-thirds of the β-subunit. The integrated tyrosine kinase domain is indicated by the hatched area of the cytoplasmic domain. The structure of the receptor for IGF-I, but not IGF-II, is similar to that of the insulin receptor. There is homology between both the insulin and the IGF-I receptors and the structure of IgG. The number of insulin receptors on insulin target cells is very variable (100–200 000), with adipocytes and hepatocytes expressing the highest numbers.

tors for both insulin and IGF-I pre-exist in their unoccupied state as preformed dimers (Fig. 1.5). However, again, occupancy of the ligand-binding pocket formed by the two α-subunits by one molecule of insulin or IGF-I results in activation of the tyrosine kinase integrated into the structure of the cytosolic domain.

*Signalling pathways activated by insulin*
The earliest response to insulin binding to its receptor is autophosphorylation of the cytosolic domain of the β-subunits themselves (Fig. 1.6). This initiates a complex series of response cascades that involve over 50 enzymes. The receptor's tyrosine kinase next phosphorylates a key substrate, namely insulin receptor substrate 1 or 2 (IRS-1 or -2). This phosphorylation is thought to be essential for almost all subsequent biological actions of insulin. IRS-1 is a 131-kDa protein that has 21 potential tyrosine phosphorylation sites, at least eight of which are phosphorylated by the activated insulin receptor.

Multiple phosphorylation of IRS-1 leads to the docking of several proteins with SH2 domains and the activation of divergent intracellular signalling pathways. For example, docking of the p85 subunit of phosphatidylinositol-3-kinase (PI3 kinase) leads to regulation of glucose transporter translocation. There is a superfamily of glucose transporters (GLUT1–4 and SGLT1). In the prime organs of insulin action, such as adipose tissue and skeletal or cardiac muscle, the predominant isoform is GLUT4. This is a 520-amino-acid protein that spans the membrane 12 times and catalyses glucose uptake into the cell. Insulin binding to its receptor leads to translocation of GLUT4 from intracellular vesicles to the cell membrane. After removal of bound insulin, the transporter returns to the intracellular pool. A branch point in this pathway leads to increased glycogen synthase activity, with consequent enhancement in glycogen synthesis together with increased gene expression for hexokinase-2 in these tissues. Reduced glycogen synthase and hexokinase-2 have been observed in muscle biopsies from non-insulin-dependent diabetes mellitus (NIDDM) patients. In addition, a reduction

in levels of IRS-1 and the p85 subunit of PI3 kinase has been reported for these subjects.

The mitogenic effects of insulin are signalled via an alternative pathway that diverges from phosphorylated IRS-1. Instead of binding to the SH2 domains of PI3 kinase, it docks with the SH2/SH3 domains of the growth factor receptor-bound protein 2 (Grb 2 protein). This adaptor protein links tyrosine-phosporylated receptors or cytoplasmic tyrosine kinases to regulators of small G-protein activity (Fig. 1.6). In this particular pathway, Grb 2 links IRS-1 to the GDP/GTP (guanosine diphosphate/guanosine triphosphate) exchange protein, Sos (son of sevenless protein). In turn, this brings the Sos–Grb2 complex into the proximity of the small G-protein, Ras, located as depicted in the plasma membrane (Fig. 1.6). This triggers Ras by the exchange of GTP for GDP.

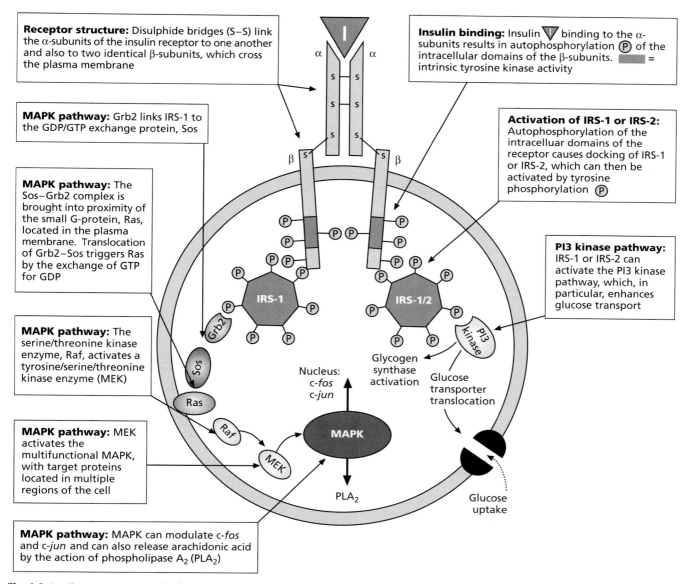

**Fig. 1.6.** Insulin receptor: an example of a receptor with intrinsic tyrosine kinase activity.

Ras activation stimulates a downstream cascade in which serine/threonine kinases, such as Raf, play an important role, with the latter activating a tyrosine/serine/threonine kinase (MEK), which subsequently activates a multifunctional serine/threonine kinase that is of central importance. This was originally named microtubule-associated protein kinase. However, in recognition of its broader role, it is now more commonly referred to as mitogen-activated protein kinase (MAPK). This kinase has target proteins located in multiple regions of the cell that are coupled to both cytoplasmic and nuclear responses. The latter lead to stimulation of gene expression, protein synthesis and cell growth.

### Defects in the insulin receptor/signalling pathways and consequent insulin resistance syndromes

Over 50 different mutations in the insulin receptor itself have been reported. There are three associated congenital syndromes of severe insulin resistance. These are, in ascending order of clinical severity, type A insulin resistance, Rabson–Mendenhall syndrome and leprechaunism/Donahue syndrome. As would be expected, all patients have impaired glucose metabolism together with raised insulin concentrations. Whereas patients with type A insulin resistance are usually not diagnosed until puberty, at the other end of the spectrum, namely leprechaunism, there is severe intrauterine growth retardation and the patients rarely survive beyond the first year of life. This extreme form of insulin resistance is considered to arise because of the absence of any functional insulin receptors. In contrast, Rabson–Mendenhall syndrome is probably the result of mutations that result in a severely defective but not totally inactive insulin receptor. Some patients with type A insulin resistance have mutations clustering in the tyrosine kinase domain of the receptor. However, two large studies have reported that the majority of type A patients have normal insulin receptors. These patients may harbour as yet unidentified mutations in any of the other critical insulin signalling molecules indicated in Fig. 1.6.

### Receptors that recruit tyrosine kinase activity

The best-known endocrine members of this second subgroup of this class of receptors are those for growth hormone (GH) and prolactin (PRL). These hormones, together with cytokines such as the interleukins and erythropoietin, share a common major structural feature in that they have four long α-helices arranged in an antiparallel fashion. As a consequence of these structural similarities, this subgroup is commonly referred to as the cytokine/haemopoietic receptor. There are at least 20 members, all of which share the basic receptor structure shown in Fig. 1.2. The ectodomain, which binds the ligand, is about 200 amino acids long and is the region of major homology. It has several conserved features and a characteristic ligand-binding pocket formed from two barrel-like modules. The cytoplasmic regions are variable in length and exhibit only limited similarities. However one

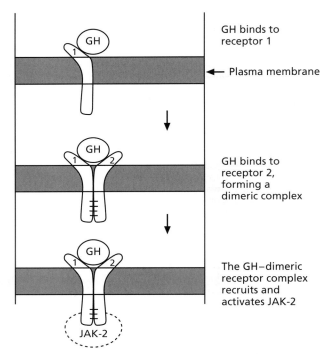

**Fig. 1.7.** Diagrammatic representation of GH binding to its cell-surface receptors and, via the formation of receptor dimers, subsequently recruiting Janus-associated kinase 2 (JAK-2). The two receptors depicted (1 and 2) have identical structures.

motif, which is found close to the membrane and is known as Box 1, is relatively highly conserved. This appears to be particularly important for the stimulation of mitogenic activity in the target cells.

### GH and PRL signalling pathways

The co-crystal structure of human GH with its receptor was analysed in 1992 and shown to be a ternary complex consisting of a single molecule of the hormone and two receptors. Parallel studies using mutational analysis of residues in the hormone revealed that each molecule of GH had two different sites, each of which could bind to the receptor. Moreover, this work demonstrated that the formation of the signal-transducing complex is sequential. Thus, after GH has bound to one molecule of receptor, this complex is associated with a second receptor molecule (Fig. 1.7). The dimerization of the cytoplasmic region in the ternary complex is particularly important for signal transduction. Such receptor homodimerization has also been reported for PRL and erythropoietin. However, further studies with cytokines have shown that this homodimerization model in fact applies to only a minority of cytokine receptors. The majority form heterodimers and oligomers with diverse cytoplasmic proteins.

### Tyrosine kinase recruitment

Although cytokine receptors themselves contain no identifiable enzymatic motifs that could function as tyrosine

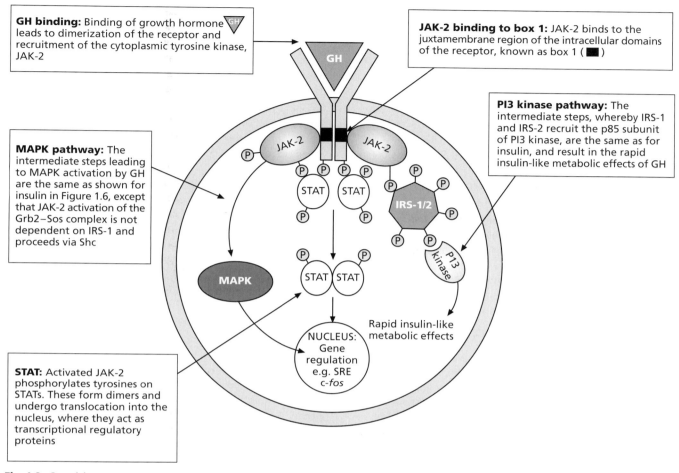

**GH binding:** Binding of growth hormone leads to dimerization of the receptor and recruitment of the cytoplasmic tyrosine kinase, JAK-2

**MAPK pathway:** The intermediate steps leading to MAPK activation by GH are the same as shown for insulin in Figure 1.6, except that JAK-2 activation of the Grb2–Sos complex is not dependent on IRS-1 and proceeds via Shc

**STAT:** Activated JAK-2 phosphorylates tyrosines on STATs. These form dimers and undergo translocation into the nucleus, where they act as transcriptional regulatory proteins

**JAK-2 binding to box 1:** JAK-2 binds to the juxtamembrane region of the intracellular domains of the receptor, known as box 1 ( ■ )

**PI3 kinase pathway:** The intermediate steps, whereby IRS-1 and IRS-2 recruit the p85 subunit of PI3 kinase, are the same as for insulin, and result in the rapid insulin-like metabolic effects of GH

NUCLEUS: Gene regulation e.g. SRE *c-fos*

Rapid insulin-like metabolic effects

**Fig. 1.8.** Growth hormone receptor: an example of a receptor that recruits tyrosine kinase activity.

kinases, it became apparent that cytokines such as interleukins 2 and 3, together with GH and PRL, rapidly induce tyrosine phosphorylation of proteins, including regions of the cytoplasmic domain itself. Within a few minutes of exposure of the target cells to the extracellular stimulators, tyrosine phosphorylation can be detected. Indeed, using cross-linking and immunoprecipitation techniques, it was deduced that tyrosine kinase was not only stimulated by GH occupancy of its receptor but that the kinase activity was also closely associated with the receptor. This kinase activity was identified as Janus-associated kinase 2 (JAK-2) (Fig. 1.8).

*Janus-associated kinases*
When first identified, the JAK family of kinases was 'orphan', as their regulators and functions were not then known; accordingly, they were first named JAK standing for 'just another kinase'. However, the four members of the family (JAK1-3 and Tyk-2) were eventually shown to contain a distinctive structural feature, two tandem kinase domains,

which were located at their carboxy termini. Because of this they were renamed Janus-associated kinases, after the Roman god Janus, who had two faces.

These cytosolic kinases are proteins of 120–135 kDa that are 40% identical. Kinase activity is due to a JH1 domain at the C-terminus, and there is a second JH2 domain, which, although similar to known kinases, lacks a motif for ATP binding: this may regulate JH1 activity. They are devoid of SH2/SH3 domains and the details of the mechanism by which they are recruited by the occupied cytokine receptors have yet to be established. GH and PRL receptors both recruit JAK-2, as does erythropoietin (Fig. 1.8), although there is some evidence that JAK-2 is constitutively associated with the PRL receptor. For GH and PRL receptors, a proline-rich docking site in the cytoplasmic domain, named Box 1, is key for JAK-2 association and subsequent activation. It has been suggested that the close association of the cytoplasmic domains of the dimerized receptors brings together the two JAK-2 molecules and that this allows cross-phosphorylation of each catalytic domain.

*STATs*

The major JAK substrates are, apart from themselves and the cytokine receptors, the so-called STAT proteins. These are latent transcription factor proteins, which contain 700–800 residues and share 30–40% identity. A crucial tyrosine residue is located in the carboxy terminus in a homologous position in all STAT proteins (residue 694), and phosphorylation of this is essential for STAT activation. STAT proteins have dual functions: *s*ignal *t*ransduction in the cytoplasm followed by *a*ctivation of *t*ranscription in the nucleus. The family members of STAT proteins have been named in the order of their identification. GH, PRL and erythropoietin induce tyrosine phosphorylation of STAT proteins 1, 3, 5a and 5b, but STAT 5 is probably the major axis of the JAK–STAT cascade. STAT phosphorylation is also an early response and can be detected within minutes of exposure of the target cells to these hormones.

SH2 domains on STAT proteins allow them to dock on crucially positioned phosphotyrosines on the cytokine receptors (Fig. 1.8). The STAT proteins are then themselves phosphorylated by the JAK proteins which have been recruited by the ligand-occupied receptors. Phosphorylated STAT proteins then dissociate from the occupied receptor–kinase complex and form dimers, to give homo- or heterodimers in the cytosol. Dimerization appears to be essential for their final translocation to the nucleus, where they activate immediate early response genes, which regulate proliferation, or more specific genes that determine the differentiation status of the target cell.

*Alternative pathways*

GH and PRL do not activate their target cells exclusively via the JAK–STAT pathway. As shown in Fig. 1.8, occupancy can also lead to stimulation of the MAPK and PI3 kinase pathways. This overlapping of signalling pathways for GH and insulin may account for the acute insulin-like effects of GH. In addition, GH and PRL have been reported to increase intracellular free calcium.

*Defects in the GH receptor/signalling pathways and consequent GH resistance syndromes*

Resistance to GH was first reported by Laron in 1966. Since then, severe resistance to GH characterized by grossly impaired growth despite normal or elevated GH levels in serum has been termed Laron syndrome. Molecular genetic investigations have shown that this disorder is mainly associated with mutations in the gene for the GH receptor (GHR). These can result in defective hormone binding to the ectodomain or reduced efficiency of dimerization of the receptor after hormone occupancy. It is an autosomal recessive disorder, and it is now appreciated that there is a range of phenotypic presentation.

As might be expected, exceptionally low levels of circulating IGF-I and its principal carrier protein, insulin-like growth factor binding protein 3, are also observed in Laron syndrome. Thus, the patients themselves form an *in vivo* bioassay for GH, suggesting either that the GH, which was present at a high concentration in the circulation, was bioinactive or that the receptor/signalling pathway was non-responsive. The finding that the administration of exogenous fully bioactive GH to Laron syndrome patients fails to elevate IGF-I levels supports the latter hypothesis. This was confirmed after the cloning of the gene for the GHR and the subsequent identification of multiple mutation sites in the gene in Laron patients.

The gene for the GHR contains 10 exons. In 1989, large deletions were detected in exons 3, 5 and 6 in two Laron syndrome patients. As exons 2–7 encode the signal peptide and the ectodomain of the GHR, and thus affect receptor binding, it was predictable that such large gene deletions at these loci would result in GH resistance.

The majority of defects reported since this early study have identified point mutations, i.e. the alteration of a single nucleotide in the DNA to another. Nonsense, missense, splice and frameshift mutations have now been reported in exons 4 and 7, which again affect the extracellular domain of the receptor for GH.

As previously mentioned, the ectodomain of the GHR can be identified in the circulation, where it forms a GH-binding protein (GHBP). Normal levels of GHBP, together with suspected Laron syndrome, would suggest that the defect was occurring after receptor binding. It is significant therefore that patients with normal GHBP levels typically exhibit a milder phenotype; in fact, 20–25% of Laron patients now fall into this category. For example, a missense mutation in the ectodomain that is not part of the GH binding site has been shown to result in the defective receptor dimerization despite unimpaired GH binding. Moreover, mutations in exons 8–10 are now being identified that affect the transmembrane or cytosolic domains, giving rise to inefficient or absent interactions with JAK-2 and consequently impaired intracellular signalling. On the other hand, Laron patients who have no apparent mutation in the gene coding for the GHR have now been identified. It is possible that their defect could be attributed to mutations in genes regulating downstream signalling. One case has now been reported of a patient with severe intrauterine growth retardation followed by postnatal growth failure, sensorineural deafness, GH resistance and mild mental retardation and in whom there appears to be a partial deletion in the gene coding for IGF-I. Clearly this would render the GH–IGF-I axis ineffective.

## G-protein-coupled receptors

*Receptor structure*

The second major group of cell-surface receptors consists of those which couple with G (guanine)-proteins associated with the inner surface of the cell membrane (G-protein-coupled

**Table 1.2.** Examples of G-protein-coupled receptors

| Hormone | Dominant G-protein α- subunit(s) |
| --- | --- |
| Thyrotrophin-releasing hormone | $G_q\alpha$ |
| Corticotrophin-releasing hormone | $G_s\alpha$ |
| Gonadotrophin-releasing hormone | $G_q\alpha$ |
| Somatostatin | $G_i\alpha/G_q\alpha$ |
| Thyroid-stimulating hormone | $G_s\alpha/G_q\alpha$ |
| Luteinizing hormone/human chorionic gonadotrophin | $G_s\alpha/G_q\alpha$ |
| Follicle-stimulating hormone | $G_s\alpha/G_q\alpha$ |
| Adrenocorticotrophic hormone | $G_s\alpha$ |
| Oxytocin | $G_q\alpha$ |
| Vasopressin | $G_s\alpha/G_q\alpha$ |
| Catecholamines | $G_s\alpha$ |
| Angiotensin II | $G_i\alpha/G_q\alpha$ |
| Glucagon | $G_s\alpha$ |
| Calcium | $G_q\alpha/G_i\alpha$ |
| Calcitonin | $G_s\alpha/G_i\alpha/G_q\alpha$ |
| Parathyroid hormone (PTH)/ PTH-related peptide (PTHrP) | $G_s\alpha/G_q\alpha$ |
| Prostaglandin $E_2$ | $G_s\alpha$ |

For somatostatin, vasopressin, angiotensin II, calcitonin and PTH/PTHrP different receptor subtypes determine α-subunit specificity, and there may be differential tissue distributions of these receptor subtypes. This phenomenon provides opportunities to develop selective therapeutic antagonists.

receptors, GPCRs) (Fig. 1.1). This leads to the generation of intracellular second messengers such as cyclic adenosine monophosphate (cAMP) and inositol 1,4,5-trisphosphate ($IP_3$). This is the largest of the cell-surface receptor groups, with over 140 members. Some are listed in Fig. 1.1 and in Table 1.2. Other extracellular receptors, including glutamate, thrombin, odourants and those responsible for the visual transduction of light, also act via GPCRs. Although the fundamental design of these receptors is as depicted in Fig. 1.2, the most striking structural difference from the tyrosine kinase-linked receptor group discussed under 'Tyrosine kinase-linked cell-surface receptors' lies in the transmembrane region. This takes the form of an elaborate serpentine membrane-spanning structure, which crosses the lipid bilayer of the plasma membrane seven times (Fig. 1.9a). The conserved hydrophobic transmembrane helices that make up this domain can be arranged to create a hydrophobic pore (Fig. 1.9b).

The size of the GPCR ranges from that for gonadotrophin-releasing hormone, with only 337 amino acid residues, to the largest, which is the calcium-sensing receptor, which has 1085 residues. The latter has an extended ectodomain (613 amino acids) which appears to bind $Ca^{2+}$ with a low affinity compared with the classic hormone receptors. This would be consistent with the higher concentration of $Ca^{2+}$ relative to that of hormones.

*Coupling to plasma membrane G-proteins*

G-proteins are key participants in cell activation by GPCRs. The linking G-proteins are the larger members of a super-family of regulatory proteins that function as molecular switches by binding and then hydrolysing GTP to GDP. The Ras protein (Fig. 1.6) is an example of the smaller membrane-associated G-proteins.

Hormone occupancy of a GPCR results in conformational changes in the receptor that are transmitted across the plasma membrane and so alter the extent and/or nature of receptor interaction with G-proteins. This is brought about by contacts between the intracellular loops and the C-terminal tail of the receptor and specific regions of the G-protein complex. This results in GTP exchange for GDP on the G-protein. The activated proteins then undergo major structural modifications and ultimately modulate the catalytic activity of adenylate cyclase or phospholipase C (PLC) within the membrane structure (Figs 1.10 and 1.11).

**The G-protein heterotrimeric complex in action**

In their resting state, the G-proteins exist as heterodimeric complexes with α-, β- and γ-subunits. The oligomer has a molecular weight of about 90 000, with the α-, β- and γ-subunits contributing approximately 45 000, 35 000 and 5000 respectively. In practice, the β- and γ-subunits associate with such a high affinity that the functional units are $G_\alpha$ and $G_{\beta\gamma}$ (Fig. 1.11). In the absence of a hormone-occupied and -activated receptor, these complexes form a 'G-protein pool' within the membrane.

After association of the G-protein complex with the occupied receptor, conformational changes in the α-subunit lead to an increased rate of dissociation of GDP, which is replaced by GTP. This guanine nucleotide exchange in turn causes the α-subunit to dissociate from the heterotrimeric complex. The liberated α-subunit, together with its activating GTP, then binds to a downstream catalytic unit, which is either adenylate cyclase or PLC (Fig. 1.10).

*G-subunits*

Although there are now known to be over 20 isoforms of the Gα-subunit, these may be grouped into four major subfamilies that have functional significance. These are $G_{s\alpha}$ and $G_{i\alpha}$, which activate or inhibit adenylate cyclase respectively, $G_{q\alpha}$, which activates PLC, and $G_{o\alpha}$, which activates ion channels (Fig. 1.10). A given receptor may interact with one or more of these family members, as listed in Table 1.2. Of those listed, more than half can be seen to interact with more than one Gα-subunit and thus moderate contrasting and sometimes apparently conflicting intracellular second-messenger

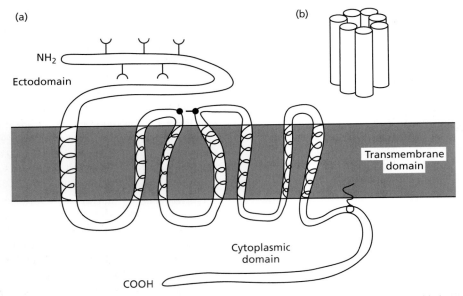

**Fig. 1.9.** A schematic representation of G-protein-coupled receptors (GPCRs) showing the seven transmembrane domains. (a) The structure is an elaborate variation of the three-segment design depicted in Fig. 1.2. The size of the N-terminal ectodomain is generally in proportion to the size of the cognate ligand, except that the $Ca^{2+}$ receptor has an unexpectedly large ectodomain. In the ectodomain, which obviously plays a key role in ligand binding, homology is lower than among the transmembrane and cytoplasmic domains. For example, for the thyroid-stimulating hormone, luteinizing hormone/chorionic gonadotrophin and follicle-stimulating hormone receptors, homology in the ectodomain is only 35–45%, but is far higher in the midregions. The ectodomain can be heavily glycosylated; this may contribute to as much as 40% of its mass. The ligand binding site is highly conformational, with several discontinuous elements contributing to the binding. The transmembrane domain has a characteristic heptahelical structure, most of which is embedded in the plasma membrane and provides a hydrophobic core. An intraloop disulphide bridge between the second and third extracellular loops may be formed by conserved cysteine residues, as shown. The cytoplasmic domain links the receptor to the signal-transducing G-proteins. For the β-adrenergic receptor it has been shown that specific regions in the third intracellular loop together with sections of the C-terminal tail are critical for G-protein coupling. A fourth intracellular loop may be formed by a cysteine residue in the C-terminal tail, which could be palmitoylated in some GPCRs. (b) Rearrangement of the seven transmembrane α-helices to form a hydrophobic pore.

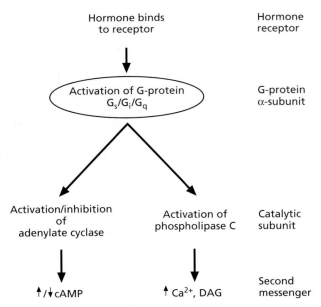

**Fig. 1.10.** The modulation of intracellular second messengers by hormonal activation of G-protein-linked cell-surface receptors. Note that, for a given hormone or extracellular modulator, the two pathways are not mutually exclusive and may interact. DAG, diacylglycerol.

systems. This receptor promiscuity can be attributed, among other things, to different receptor subtypes. In the case of calcitonin, these are differentially expressed at different stages of the cell cycle. On the other hand, the particular Gα-subunit selected for coupling may depend upon the concentration of the hormone. For example, TSH, calcitonin and LH/hCG (luteinizing hormone/human chorionic gonadotrophin) receptors activate adenylate cyclase at low concentrations, whereas with higher concentrations $G_{q\alpha}$ is recruited to activate PLC.

Structural studies, using chimeric Gα-subunits and mutagens or deletion of residues in the C-terminus of the Gα-subunit, emphasize the importance of this region in determining which Gα-subunit is recruited by an activated receptor. In fact, both the C-terminus and the N-terminus of Gα-subunits lie in close proximity to each other and face the plasma membrane, with its embedded Gβ/γ heterodimer, the receptor and the catalytic subunits. Anchorage to the membrane is provided by lipid modification of the C-terminal and N-terminal of Gα, among other structural features.

Selection is of course a two-way process, and complementary structural features on the cytoplasmic domain of the receptor also determine which Gα-subunit is coupled.

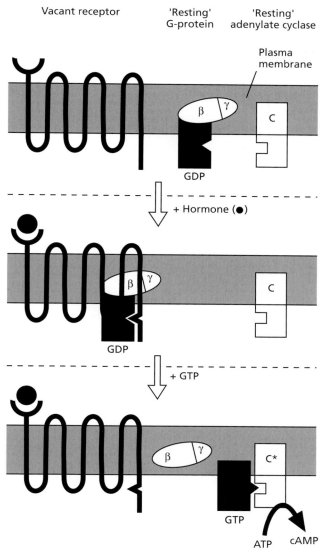

Vacant receptor    'Resting'       'Resting'
                   G-protein       adenylate cyclase

Plasma
membrane

β  γ

C

GDP

+ Hormone (●)

β  γ

C

GDP

+ GTP

β  γ

C*

GTP

ATP    cAMP

**Fig. 1.11.** A representation of G-protein-modulated activation of a membrane-bound enzyme such as adenylate cyclase. A hormone, e.g. adrenaline, binds to the extracellular region of the receptor. The third intracellular loop and the C-terminus of the receptor associates with a G-protein that has three subunits, α, β and γ. This leads to displacement of GDP by GTP and dissociation of the activated G-protein from the hormone–receptor complex. The α-subunit diffuses in the lipid bilayer and activates the catalytic subunit (C→C*), generating many molecules of cAMP.

The third intracellular loop and C-terminal tail have been shown to be crucial for the coupling of $G_s\alpha$-subunits to the β-adrenergic receptor or $G_{q\alpha}$ to the angiotensin II receptors. Moreover, progressive truncations of the C-terminal tail of PTH (parathyroid hormone) receptors resulted in a decrease in Gα-subunit selectivity. As might also be anticipated, using polypeptides corresponding to specific regions of the cytoplasmic domain of receptors, direct, receptorless activation of Gα has been observed. Conversely, polypeptides have been reported that will block receptor/Gα-subunit coupling

and thus selectively inhibit endogenous signal transduction pathways.

Gα-subunits can also function as a GTPase, which cleaves a phosphate from the GTP resulting in GαGDP. This endows the G-proteins with a mechanism for switching off their activation of the catalytic subunit. Hydrolysis of the GTP bound to Gα due to its intrinsic GTPase activity liberates the Gα-subunit from the catalyic subunit and allows reassociation of GαGDP with the Gβ/γ. This newly reformed heterotrimer then returns to the G-protein pool in the membrane. In this way an individual G-protein complex is recycled so that it can respond to further receptor occupation by ligand.

*G-protein and GPCR aberrations*
There are several examples of endocrinopathies that occur as a result of activating or inactivating mutations of G-proteins or receptors coupled to them. Pseudohypoparathyroidism (Albright's hereditary osteodystrophy) is associated with a loss of $G_{s\alpha}$ function, whereas McCune–Albright syndrome and some cases of acromegaly are linked to a gain in $G_{s\alpha}$ function and constitutive activation. The subsequent complex constellation of abnormalities can be explained in terms of trophic hormones that raise intracellular cAMP and drive the function and proliferation of different endocrine organs. On the other hand, nephrogenic diabetes insipidus can be the result of a mutation in the GPCR itself. Germline mutations in *Xq28*, coding for the V2 receptor, lead to a loss of receptor function so that circulating vasopressin, despite being very high, cannot increase urine concentration. Conversely, familial male precocious puberty (testotoxicosis), which is an autonomous form of endocrine hyperfunction, occurs as a result of germline activating missense mutations in the gene for the LH receptor. Thus, whereas GPCRs normally occur in a constrained, inhibited form, activating mutations presumably relieve crucial helix–helix interactions that are normally relieved only by hormone occupancy. Activating mutations in the transmembrane domain of the TSH receptor have been reported in 22 out of 28 toxic thyroid adenomas, and mutations in $G_{s\alpha}$ have been described in two autonomous thyroid nodules. In addition, resistance to TSH in three siblings has been attributed to mutations in the ectodomain of the TSH receptor.

*Intracellular second messengers*
*cAMP*
$G_{s\alpha}$ activates membrane-bound adenylate cyclase, which catalyses the conversion of ATP to the potent second messenger cAMP (Figs 1.10 and 1.11). This cyclic nucleotide in turn activates a cAMP-dependent protein kinase (PKA) that modulates multiple aspects of cell function.

There are least 10 isoforms of adenylate cyclase. Each has two sets of six membrane-spanning domains together with two cytoplasmic domains. They differ in particular in their interaction with negative regulators such as $G_{i\alpha}$ and Gβ/γ.

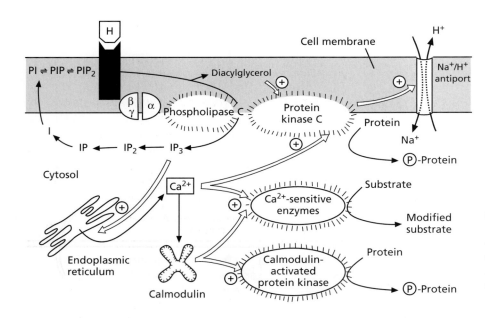

**Fig. 1.12.** Hormonal stimulation of phospholipid turnover and calcium metabolism within the cell. Some growth factors stimulate the sodium/hydrogen ion antiport to decrease intracellular H+ concentration and raise the pH, which can affect a variety of enzymes and intracellular reactions.

cAMP reacts with a repressive regulatory subunit on PKA, which then dissociates from the holoenzyme and unmasks a catalytic site that phophorylates serine and threonine residues. Thus $G_s\alpha$-subunits, via cAMP and PKAs regulate major metabolic pathways, including those for lipolysis, glycogenolysis and steroidogenesis (Table 1.2). PKA phosphorylates a transcription factor called CREB (*c*AMP *r*esponse *e*lement *b*inding protein). This is then translocated to the nucleus, where it binds to a short palindromic sequence in the promoter regions of cAMP-regulated genes referred to as CRE (*c*AMP *r*esponse *e*nhancer element) and thereby has a direct effect on gene transcription. This mechanism mediates the induction of genes for somatostatin.

The major signal terminating system is provided by a large family of phosphodiesterases (PDEs) which can be activated by a variety of systems, including direct PKA phosphorylation. PDEs rapidly hydrolyse cAMP to the inactive 5'-AMP and thereby close a feedback loop. In addition, cAMP-activated PKA, PKC and other more recently identified receptor kinases (GRKs) may phosphorylate serine and threonine residues in the intracellular loop and the C-terminal tail of GPCRs, which leads to receptor desensitization. An increase in a particular GRK, directed at the β-adrenergic receptor, has been reported in patients suffering from chronic heart failure.

*Diacylglycerol and* $Ca^{2+}$

More than 20 different extracellular regulators, including TRH (thyrotrophin-releasing hormone), GnRH (gonadotrophin-releasing hormone) and oxytocin, stimulate their target cells by GPCRs, which recruit G-proteins with the $G_q\alpha$-subunit (Table 1.2). The latter activates the membrane-associated PLC. This enzyme, which has three major isoforms (β, γ and δ), catalyses the reaction

$$PIP_2 = DAG + IP_3,$$

where $PIP_2$ is phosphatidylinositol 4,5-bisphosphate and DAG is diacylglycerol. $PIP_2$ is a minor membrane phospholipid, accounting for less than 1% of the total phospholipids in the plasma membrane. DAG and $IP_3$ (inositol phosphate) act as intracellular second messengers. DAG, together with a cofactor, phosphatidylserine, activates the cell membrane-associated PKC, whereas $IP_3$ is released into the cytosol, where it binds to calcium-mobilizing $IP_3$ receptor channels in the endoplasmic reticulum (Fig. 1.12). This causes a rapid 10-fold rise in cytosolic free $Ca^{2+}$, from a resting concentration of about 0.1 μM. $Ca^{2+}$ activates several $Ca^{2+}$-sensitive enzymes, including the protein kinase calmodulin and some isoforms of PKC. In fact, the name PKC was coined to reflect this $Ca^{2+}$ dependency. It also activates phospholipase $A_2$, which liberates arachidonate from phospholipids and thereby generates potent local tissue activators that are collectively known as eicosanoids. These include thromboxanes, leukotrienes, lipoxins and prostaglandins. Prostaglandins are well recognized paracrine and autocrine mediators and may amplify or prolong the responses to the original hormonal stimulus.

The rise in intracellular free $Ca^{2+}$ is of necessity only transient, and calcium mobilization is deactivated by several systems. For example, PLC-β can increase the rate of GTP hydrolysis from the $G_{q\alpha}$/GTP-activated complex, by acting as a GTPase-activating protein (GAP).

## Intracellular receptors for hormones

Steroid and thyroid hormones are not, in molecular terms, similar chemical structures, but nevertheless they bind to protein receptors that are members of a large superfamily of

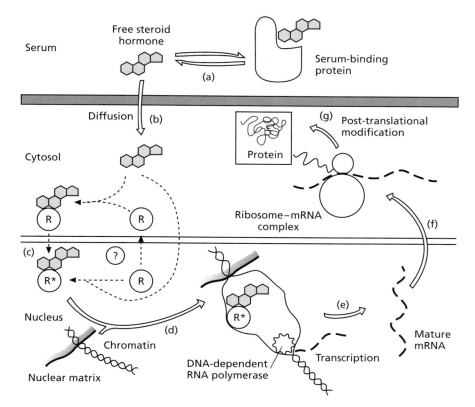

**Fig. 1.13.** Mechanism of steroid hormone action. Free steroid hormone in equilibrium with bound hormone (a) diffuses across the target-cell membrane (b) and binds to the steroid hormone receptor protein in the cytoplasm or in the cell nucleus. The hormone–receptor complex (c) interacts with chromatin and binds to a receptor site on the regulatory region of one DNA strand associated with a particular gene (d). This region is the hormone response element (HRE). The promoter region permits DNA-dependent RNA polymerase to start transcription to yield messenger RNA (e) which passes out of the nucleus (f) after post-transcriptional modification. Peptides are formed by translation of the message on ribosomes attached to the endoplasmic reticulum and modification of the proteins gives the final gene product (g).

intracellular receptors (Fig. 1.1), which are themselves structurally closely related. As these hormones are hydrophobic, they can diffuse across the plasma membrane of their target cells and so gain access to the intracellular receptors that are found in either the cytosol or the cell nucleus. These receptors function as hormone-regulated transcription factors (Fig. 1.13), controlling the expression of specific target genes by interaction with regions close to the gene promoters. Compared with the hormones that act via the rapidly responsive cell-surface receptor/second-messenger systems discussed above, the ultimate biological responses to steroid and thyroid hormones are sluggish. This is because they generate their responses via promotion of RNA (ribonucleic acid) and protein synthesis. There is therefore a characteristic lag period between the time of exposure of the target cell to the hormone and the onset of an *in vivo* biological response.

## The superfamily of receptors for steroid and thyroid hormones

There are more than 150 members of this superfamily of receptor proteins. The majority are at present orphan receptors, because no ligand has been identified for them, but the most important from an endocrine perspective are listed in Fig. 1.14. Each consists of a single polypeptide chain. Within this structure, three distinctive major modules can be identified. These are (a) a hormone-specific binding domain, which contains a region (AF2) responsible for hormone-dependent transcriptional activation at the C-terminus (the ligand binding site itself is a hydrophobic pocket); (b) a highly conserved DNA-binding domain; and (c) an N-terminal domain that is hypervariable both in length and in composition. For some receptors, the N-terminal domain appears to exert a transcriptional-activation function, because of a region referred to as AF1; this activation is not hormone dependent, i.e. it is constitutive. The modules function independently, as was demonstrated by the construction of hybrid or chimeric receptors in domain exchange experiments (Fig. 1.14).

The molecular weights of these receptors range from 46 kDa for the $T_3$ receptor to 100 kDa for the receptors for progesterone and mineralocorticoids. Notable regions of homology between the receptors, which can be as high as 60–90%, occur, indicating that they are related in evolution. It is speculated that the oncogene v-*erbA* or c-*erbA* may be their common ancestor. The superfamily is usually subdivided into two classes (Fig. 1.14) on the basis of their mode of action when activating transcription and the forms that they assume when they are unoccupied. All steroids act via class 1 receptors, whereas calcitriol, retinoic acid and $T_3$ utilize class II.

### The DNA-binding domain

This domain is characterized by the presence of two 'zinc fingers'. These are two polypeptide loops, each of which is

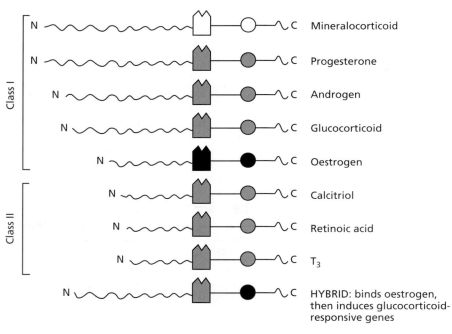

Key

⌂ : Highly conserved DNA-binding domain

◯ : Hydrophobic pocket which forms the hormone-binding domain

⌒C : Highly conserved amphipathic α-helix (AF2) at the C-terminus that exerts a powerful hormone-dependent transcriptional activation function

N ⌒ : The least conserved region. It exerts a transcriptional activation function (AF1) that is constitutive, i.e. does not depend upon hormone binding. The potency of this function varies greatly between the different receptors. It is high for glucocorticoid receptors but absent for calcitriol receptors

**Fig. 1.14.** The steroid–thyroid hormone receptor superfamily. Diagrammatic representation showing the relative sizes of these evolutionarily related proteins, which range in size from 395 to 984 amino acids.

10–20 amino acids long. A single zinc ion coordinates two cysteine and two histidine residues in each loop, and this stabilizes the structure. The two fingers are separated by approximately 12 amino acids. These distinctive fingers are obligatory for receptor interlocking with the target acceptor DNA in the hormone response element (HRE) and form the principal interface when this takes place.

For class I steroid receptors in their resting state, the zinc fingers are masked by the association of the receptor with a dimerized heat shock protein such as hsp 70, hsp 90 or others (Fig. 1.15). These high-molecular-weight complexes are partitioned between the cytosol and the nucleus with a steroid-specific distribution. For example, although 90% of the resting glucocorticoid receptors are cytosolic, those for the androgens are predominantly nuclear. When the receptors are associated with the hsp dimers, which obscures their zinc fingers, they cannot bind to nuclear DNA. Occupancy of the hormone binding site by a given steroid, however, leads to dissociation of the hsp dimer. This reveals the zinc fingers, and translocation to the nucleus then takes place

if required. The receptors themselves then dimerize and bind with four zinc fingers to a short region of DNA. The latter is referred to as the hormone response element (HRE) or, in the case of the T$_3$ receptor, the thyroid response element (TRE). Each zinc finger is thought to recognize a specific sequence of about five nucleotide pairs in the HRE. X-ray crystallographic analysis and protein nuclear magnetic resonance spectroscopy have been used to reveal the molecular details of zinc finger proteins interacting with the major groove of DNA.

Targeting of the hormone–receptor complex to the HRE acceptor is directed by remarkably few amino acids in the DNA-binding domain. These occur in a region called the P Box, which is located at the base of the first zinc finger. Alteration of just two amino acids in the zinc finger of the glucocorticoid receptor led to less stringent targeting so that the receptor could then bind to and activate oestrogen-responsive genes as well. Thus, with this receptor design, two sites on the receptor confer hormonal specificity: the hormone-binding site itself and the DNA-binding domain.

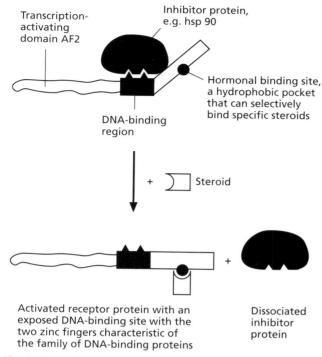

**Fig. 1.15.** Mechanism of activation of a steroid hormone receptor.

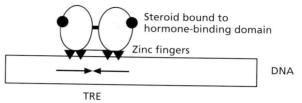

(a) Class I steroid receptors, which form homodimers

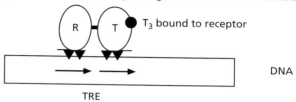

(b) Class II receptors (e.g. for $T_3$), which form heterodimers

**Fig. 1.16.** Receptor dimerization of ligand-occupied nuclear receptors. TRE, thyroid hormone response element; R, unoccupied retinoid X receptor, forms a heterodimer with the $T_3$ receptor.

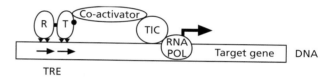

**Fig. 1.17.** Example of the mechanism of activation of transcription of a target gene by a ligand-occupied nuclear receptor such as that for $T_3$. TIC, transcriptor initiation complex; POL, polymerase.

Receptors for thyroid hormones are located exclusively in the nucleus. In their resting state they are already bound to the DNA and are activated by occupancy of the hormone-binding domain by thyroid hormones. This model also applies to receptors for calcitriol and retinoic acid, and these receptors are therefore grouped into a subclass, class II, within the superfamily (Fig. 1.14). $T_3$ receptors, which are constitutively nuclear, may inhibit or 'silence' basal gene transcription in the absence of the ligand. They may do this by recruiting a co-repressor protein that inhibits the activity of basal promoters but which dissociates from the receptor in the presence of $T_3$.

## Transcriptional activation

As outlined above, receptor dimerization is required before the ligand-occupied nuclear receptors can bind to their HRE. For class I steroid receptors, homodimers are formed that then bind to palindromically arranged heaxanucleotide half-sites (Fig. 1.16). In contrast, with a class II receptor, such as that for $T_3$, the receptor is usually bound to the acceptor DNA as a heterodimer with an unoccupied retinoid X receptor, although homodimeric interactions have also been reported.

The dimers are bound to the hormone response element (HRE), which is upstream from the target gene and its promoter region. DNA-dependent RNA polymerase action is controlled by the promoter region, and this in turn is subject to enhancing, or occasionally suppressive, influence by the dimerized hormone complex, bound to the HRE. Specific co-activator, or even co-repressor, proteins are recruited by the ligand-occupied dimerized receptors as shown in Fig. 1.17. These enhance or repress the function of the transcription–initiation complex that is assembled from a number of additional transcription factors together with RNA polymerase.

## Defective nuclear receptors

Since the isolation of the cDNA for nuclear receptors, extensive work has been undertaken to identify mutations in their genes that might then be associated with specific endocrinopathies. Table 1.3 attempts to summarize the progress that has been made, linking in many cases hormone resistance syndromes, which are characterized by reduction in target organ responsiveness to the circulating hormone, to identified defects. Mutations have been identified that lead to reduced ligand binding to the hormone-binding domain, impaired receptor dimerization and also a decrease in binding of the occupied receptor/dimer to the HRE.

| Receptor | Clinical effects | Molecular defects reported to date |
|---|---|---|
| Androgens (ARs) | Partial or complete androgen insensitivity syndromes | ↓Receptor number<br>↓Androgen binding<br>↓AR dimerization |
| | Kennedy syndrome | Expanded CAG repeat in N-terminus |
| | Breast cancer<br>Prostate cancer | ↓AR dimerization<br>↓AR responds to progesterone |
| Glucocorticoid | Generalized inherited glucocorticoid resistance | ↓Hormone binding<br>↓GR number<br>↓DNA binding |
| Oestrogen (ER) | Usually lethal Oestrogen resistance | ↓Hormone binding<br>↓DNA binding |
| $T_3$ (TR) | Resistance to thyroid hormone | ↓TRβ gene defects<br>↓$T_3$ binding |
| Calcitriol (VDR) | Calcitriol-resistant rickets | ↓VDR dimerization |

**Table 1.3.** Examples of underlying molecular defects and associated clinical effects of mutated nuclear receptors

## Target cell conversion of circulating hormones destined for nuclear receptors

There are several examples in which the target cell for hormones that act via nuclear receptors express a tissue-specific enzyme that locally converts a circulating hormone to a more potent metabolite. This then acts on the receptors with an increased affinity. For example, tissue-specific 5'-deiodinases convert thyroxine to $T_3$, 5α-reductase metabolizes testosterone to dihydrotestosterone and 1α-hydroxylase in the mitochondria of cells in the renal tubule converts 25-OH-vitamin D to calcitriol.

Conversely, in aldosterone-responsive cells in the kidney, an 11β-hydroxysteroid dehydrogenase (11β-HSD) converts cortisol to cortisone. This is important as cortisol, but not cortisone, binds to the mineralocorticoid receptor. As cortisol is present in the circulation at concentrations that are higher than those of aldosterone by 2–3 orders of magnitude, if not deactivated in this way it would cause inappropriate overactivation of the mineralocorticoid receptor. Because of the activity of this 11β-HSD, the receptor is therefore 'protected' from overstimulation. Deficiency or impaired function of this enzyme leads to the hypertension and hypokalaemia characteristic of the apparent mineralocorticoid excess (AME) syndrome.

## Summary

This chapter has outlined the major receptor-mediated pathways by which hormones regulate the function of their target cells. Our understanding of these systems has grown exponentially over the past few decades as the individual key participants have been identified. Inevitably, however, there are many molecular mechanisms that await elucidation and clinical conditions which have yet to be associated with defects in these complicated and diverse systems.

This review presents only the rudiments of the molecular grammar of the response systems. Given the large number of hormones and target tissues, the integrated system must of necessity be complex so that it may support the versatility of the *in vivo* situation. One complexity that has not been addressed is that of the extensive cross-talk between the individual pathways. For example, MAPK has been reported to phosphorylate serine residues in the N-terminal domain of the oestrogen receptor and thereby enhance its AF1 function, and STAT 5 has been shown to interact with glucocorticoid receptors.

# 2

# Hormone pulsatility

## D. R. Matthews and P. C. Hindmarsh

## Introduction

Rhythmic fluctuations occur at every level of Nature's organization. In the middle of the nineteenth century the constancy of the internal environment was pre-eminent in physiological thought. It was proposed that the main function of homeostasis was to protect the body from change in the external environment, and this principle demanded constancy of a variable function over a long period of time. The term was not meant to imply stagnation but rather that those critical systems within the body, such as blood oxygen, blood pH and body temperature, needed to be maintained within a narrow range.

As time progressed, concepts of homeostasis changed, influenced greatly by developments in control systems theory. The concept of allostasis has been applied to systems in which there is no clear physiological set point because the set point is fluid [1]. Allostasis refers to the ability to achieve stability through change. The advantage of allostatic systems is that they are more labile, allowing them to adjust to external and internal circumstances [2]. The allostatic-regulated systems and the homeostatic ones probably help maintain the internal milieu described originally by Claude Bernard (1865). Allostatic responses, within limits, may prove to be adaptive and protective, but when the system is activated for long periods of time or when the body is unable to control the situation they could become destructive. Feedback systems are examples of a protective system operating in this type of circumstance, whereas the persistent exposure to hormone levels, for example in Cushing syndrome, can be destructive to a number of target organ systems, e.g. bone demineralization.

Many hormones are secreted in pulses or have specific oscillatory activity. Oscillations have been described for insulin [3], growth hormone (GH) [4], cortisol [5] and the gonadotrophins [6]. The time course over which these regularly occurring cycles of hormone secretion take place is variable. Insulin has a dominant periodicity of 13 min, whereas GH pulses appear on average once every 3 h.

**Table 2.1.** Attributes of pulsatile systems

Mean concentration
Number of peaks
Frequency/periodicity
Regularity of peaks
Amplitude of peaks
Trough values
Shape of peaks
Rate of change of hormone concentrations
Frequency and/or amplitude modulation

In discussing methods of pulse analysis it is worth considering why we should analyse them. From a statistical point of view, a glance at an individual data series is enough to demonstrate the existence of oscillation. Where multiple data sets are available and when statements need to be made about group data, it becomes important to be able to extract attributes of pulsatility, which can then be pooled to provide a generic description. There are clinical reasons also for considering how to analyse hormone pulsatility. These relate to diagnosis and to the interpretation of therapeutic interventions in individuals and groups with similar pathophysiological problems. There are specific issues that need to be addressed in the assessment of pulsatility: these include the sampling interval to be used for the test under consideration, how the half-life of the hormone influences the choice of analytical method and what features of the pulsatile system might affect the results.

The techniques are numerous and the choice depends to a certain extent on the hypothesis that is being tested. For example, different techniques are appropriate if one wishes to examine the trend or the amplitude or the frequency of short-term oscillation. Table 2.1 summarizes the attributes of pulsatile systems that might be useful in understanding endocrine physiology and pathophysiology. It is the purpose of this chapter to describe some of the methodologies that assist in the analysis of pulsatile hormone secretion. Attention is also paid to the methods by which samples are collected and these observations have a generic use in the field of medicine. Consideration is also given to why endocrine systems employ episodic hormone secretion rather than a tonic signal.

## Why do hormones pulse?

The issue of hormone pulsatility and its biological significance needs to be discussed in the context of information transfer. The message that is passed between a source and its target comprises a quantitative component (a signal) and a qualitative component, which is equivalent to the concept of semantics in language. The classic view in biology focuses on the regulatory aspects of endocrine messengers and growth factors, coupled with analysis of various aspects of cell-to-cell communication. This may be a rather limited approach in its appreciation of communication. For example, in the endocrine system, transmission takes place over long time intervals and the distances covered are three to four orders of magnitude greater than in a system such as the nervous system. Signalling systems need to be broken down into their various components. The signal needs to be encoded at source, transmitted, received and decoded at the opposite end. Encoding increasing amounts of information at source, for example in the pituitary, can take place but an alternative but not exclusive approach is to increase the amount of information that can be safely sent.

Using the bloodstream as a channel of communication leads to a signalling process that takes place in a very noisy environment. Noise in the system can become a limiting factor. Increasing the channel's capacity can take place either by increasing the information content of a single message (monochemical transmission) or by using multiple messengers (plurichemical transmission).

Monochemical transmission strategies are the ones most often encountered in the endocrine system. The capacity of the channel is in proportion to the speed of transmission and the signal-to-noise ratio. Given the constant maximal channel capacity, this relationship predicts that, to receive transmission with as few errors as possible, one has to reduce the rate of transmission. The message could be coded either in digital (peptide present or absent) or analogue forms (amplitude and/or frequency modulation). The capacity of single peptides to increase the amount of information transferred is limited by the maximal rate of secretion of the peptide and the maximal capacity of the degradation mechanism. The situation can be improved slightly by decoding strategies that can retrieve additional information from the same molecule [7]. This is where different receptor subtypes may play an important role. Plurichemical transmission is rarely seen in the endocrine system.

## Signalling in a noisy environment

Although it is evident that endocrine signals should be reliable, it is less obvious that the precision of any individual signal will be limited by biological noise. Insulin may be secreted in response to a glycaemic stimulus but, as soon as the insulin is secreted into the circulation, it is subject to signal degradation by dilution, by binding to receptors on cells other than target cells and also by variable excretion. In addition, at the target organ itself, receptor number and affinity may change and intracellular degradation is variable.

Cellular down-regulation may at first sight seem to be a major nuisance in the signalling process. There are, however, aspects of down- and up-regulation that are advantageous and protective. In the case of insulin, there is a wide range of basal concentrations, determined in part by the degree of obesity of the individual. This raises the question of how the individual cells know whether the remainder of the body is thin or fat, resistant or sensitive. The only way they can know is from the signal itself. The cells that use a mean concentration as a state of resistance or sensitivity cannot, at the same time, use this signal to switch glucose uptake. In this situation, a change in concentration can be the signal and the message would be in the pulse and not in the mean background levels. In type 2 diabetes mellitus with high mean concentrations (indicating insensitivity) the lower pulse amplitude would generate less of a glucose-clearing effect [8].

## Maximizing signal efficiency

The endocrine system is a useful way of passing a message to millions of cells, but contained within this advantage is a grave inefficiency in that binding of the hormone may take place to cells where the hormone is not known to have a useful effect. For example, red blood cells can bind insulin without such a mechanism having any obvious action.

The practical advantage of pulsatile delivery is that high concentrations of hormone for short periods of time achieve greater end-organ responses identical to the same total concentration spread over a long period of time. Insulin is more efficient as a hypoglycaemic agent when delivered in pulses than as a steady-state infusion [9]. The reason for this is the nature of the dose–response curve for many receptor systems. At the lower end of a dose–response curve, moderate hormonal stimulation has little effect. Doubling the dose of hormone, but keeping the exposure time the same, will achieve more response than doubling the exposure time. However, if the dose chosen is close to the $EC_{50}$ concentration (achieving 50% of maximum response), a huge increase in efficiency of signalling will follow as operation will take place on the steepest part of the dose–response curve. Figure 2.1 illustrates the point: two doses of insulin of 5 units each will give rise to only 2 units of glucose uptake when the target organ is exposed to bursts 13 min apart. However, a 10-unit dose of

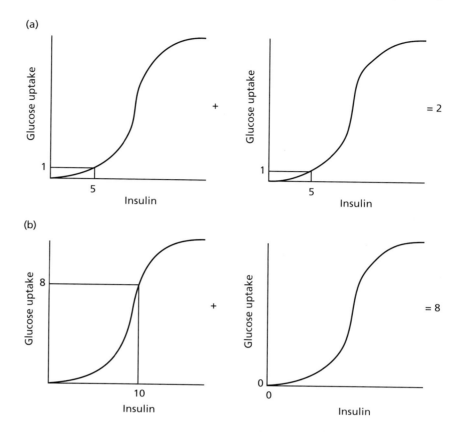

**Fig. 2.1.** Ten units of insulin administered as (a) two injections of 5 units each will generate only 2 units of glucose uptake, whereas (b) 10 units followed by zero will generate 8 units of glucose uptake.

insulin followed by no further administration of insulin will give an 8-unit increase simply because of the position in which the concentration operates on the dose–response curve.

Multiple small pulses are therefore inefficient in delivering the desired change because that sort of presentation is of continuing low-level activity. Likewise, at the other end of the dose–response curve, a non-physiological delivery of hormone in high constant doses is also ineffective in its ability to change signalling. Fine control is best achieved using doses around the $EC_{50}$, when only small increments are needed to induce change.

## Frequency and amplitude modulation

Classic thinking in endocrinology operates around the concept of concentration affecting a target organ and producing a single effect. As soon as pulsatility enters the equation, the system may signal by a variety of different mechanisms, for example amplitude modulation, frequency modulation or a combination of both. Frequency modulation is thought to be the domain of the nervous system and amplitude modulation classically occurs in the endocrine axes. What is now emerging is that no biological system uses pure amplitude or pure frequency modulation.

Both insulin and GH are highly pulsatile, and frequency domains in both can be demonstrated easily. Signalling changes are related predominately to amplitude but, because combinations of amplitude and frequency can alter the baseline, peaks and even the shape of a single pulse, other factors are important in terms of altering the receptor's response.

Feedback principles apply to many hormone systems and are best described in the glucose–insulin axis. Initially, the system appears easy to comprehend. Glucose rises, insulin rises to clear the glucose; glucose falls and insulin secretion falls. Things are not so straightforward! There are time lags: insulin is secreted by β-cells within minutes of glucose concentrations rising, but glucose takes a significant time to clear in the presence of hyperinsulinaemia. Although it takes about 15 min to observe the maximum rate of climb of glucose, it is about 45 min before euglycaemia occurs (Fig. 2.2) [10]. To make the situation worse, insulin continues to act for some time after glucose concentrations return to normal. With these time lags, a moment-to-moment relationship between glucose and insulin would be inappropriate.

Figure 2.2 illustrates how the system operates in a pulsatile mode. The elevation in blood glucose triggers insulin secretion, but not simply on the basis of the dose–response curve. Secretion is in the form of a finite package that gives rise to a pulse. The pancreas then becomes relatively quiescent for about 13 min. This time course is analogous to the time lag of 15 min for a maximum declination of glucose. Insulin secretion switches off for this time period [11] and secretion then

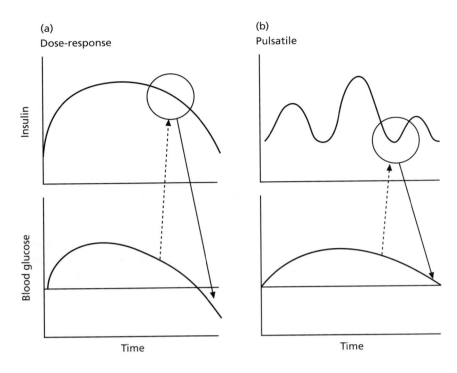

**Fig. 2.2.** (a) Insulin concentration (circled) responding to glucose level (dashed line) causes reactive hypoglycaemia. (b) Pulsatile secretion generates refractory periods (circle) making hypoglycaemia less likely.

recommences, depending on the new glucose level. In this situation, the total secretion will be less and glucose has an opportunity to react before the advent of the next pulse. Attainment of normoglycaemia, which is the aim of the exercise, is achieved in a more precise and controlled fashion.

## Constructing and analysing hormone profiles

### Collecting the data

Various methods have been devised to obtain hormone profiles. The first is to use discrete samples (such as 20-min sampling for 24 h); the second involves integrated sampling where blood is withdrawn continuously. The disadvantage of the discrete method is that identification of the true peak is highly dependent on how often samples are drawn. Although two or three concentrations may be well above the level of the previous two or three, the highest need not necessarily reflect the true height of the secretory burst, unless the time interval between the samples is very short. Knowledge of the half-life of the hormone under study can help to solve this problem.

The integrated sampling method has the advantage that no peak concentration can occur without this being reflected in the plasma collected; the disadvantage is that, unless the interval between samples is short, the peak concentration becomes rapidly diluted by the concentrations measured on the ascending and descending limbs of a pulse. Shorter profiles with more frequent sampling might circumvent this

problem but suffer from the problem that they could quite easily start after and finish before a hormone pulse, leading to a marked variation in the results obtained.

To define rhythm, sampling must take place over more than one cycle. It is important with any sampling technique also to consider the effect of the sampling interval on the possible results obtained. Inappropriately long sampling intervals can lead to spurious results and failure to detect the oscillation of a hormone concentration. A minimum of five or six samples per cycle is required to prevent the mismatching of infrequent sampling intervals to the predominant period of pulsatility that is being observed. This mismatching is known as aliaising and is illustrated in Fig. 2.3.

The sampling interval used determines the cycle frequency that can be detected. The lower the frequency of interest, the longer the time period over which measurements need to be taken; conversely, the higher the frequency, the more frequently observations must be made. A cautious approach needs to be taken with the latter statement. The observation of fast frequencies may be interesting from the secretory point of view, but it is probably of little relevance to the receptor if the clearance of the peptide is long [12].

### Analysis of profiles

The investigator needs to question whether any sophisticated analysis of a study is required. A single profile requires little analysis, since the graph contains all the information required. Where statements need to be made about populations or subpopulations or the changes within pathological states or

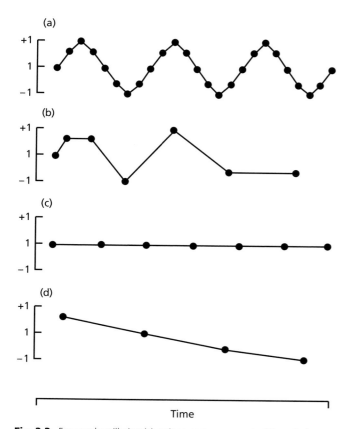

**Fig. 2.3.** For a real oscillation (a) an incorrect assessment of its period can be made using inappropriate sampling intervals (b, c and d).

following treatment intervention, more sophisticated techniques are required. The techniques for this fall under the general heading of 'time series analysis', which involves techniques for analysing regularly sampled data.

## Estimate of the mean concentration

Routine parametric statistics can be used to establish the mean and standard deviation of the data. Authors have often used the area under the curve. It is identical to the mean multiplied by the total duration of the sampling and conveys little more information. It is of value when the data are not sampled at regular intervals but, as already discussed, the analysis of such data leads to error.

## Pulse identification

Traditional methods of pulse analysis have used blinded scorers to identify peaks by inspection and to measure and count them for analysis. The exact criteria for pulse identification are difficult to define and the interassessor variation has not been defined. The aim of the method is easily understood but it is nonetheless largely subjective. Computer processing may allow rigid criteria of what constitutes a peak

and improved methodology to account for biological noise [13–16].

## Time series analysis

Several mathematical procedures can be applied to hormone profiles [17,18]. Two techniques used are autocorrelation and Fourier transformation. Autocorrelation (Fig. 2.4) is a technique for establishing whether there are regularly recurring waveforms (of any shape) within a data array. The method is independent of the shape of the wave and the start point of the profile. The end result is an estimate of period and an assessment of its significance.

If more than one frequency or rhythm is present in the time series, these underlying frequencies may be difficult to assess by inspection of the autocorrelation function because different frequencies can obscure each other. In this situation, as with any complex waveform, these can be deconvoluted into

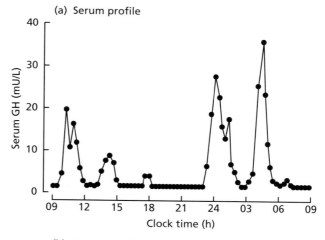

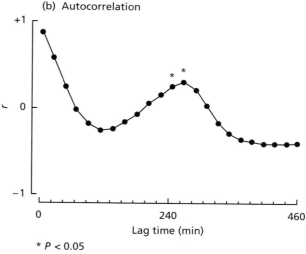

**Fig. 2.4.** Autocorrelation function (b) of serum growth hormone (GH) concentration profile (a) with a regular waveform (**) occurring at 240 min or 4 hourly. This can be cross-referenced with the actual data array.

a series of sinusoids. Amplitude and frequency components of the sinusoids can be dissected and this assessment is called Fourier transformation. The method is unbiased and remarkably robust. It allows groups of data to be compared and information to be provided on frequency, frequency modulation, amplitude and amplitude modulation.

### Deconvolution analysis

The concentration of a hormone measured at any point in time represents a balance between secretion from the gland of origin and clearance from the circulation. It is possible, from knowledge of hormone clearance or by making a priori assumptions about secretion, to work back from (deconvolute) the measured concentration [19,20]. The method is particularly useful for analysing hormone secretion and for understanding the physiology of that secretion. In addition, deconvolution analysis can be used to break down complex concentration waveforms into their secretory components.

### Baseline occupancy

Just as estimating peak amplitude and frequency is useful, some estimates of the trough values of hormone profiles may be needed to understand pathophysiological situations, e.g. acromegaly and Cushing syndrome. Trough analysis is more complex and, as a compromise, dwell-time at low concentrations has been used as a marker [21]. This method determines the proportion of time of the whole profile that is occupied at certain concentrations. For example, in the case of GH, the concentration at or below which the profile spent 5% of its time might be considered a marker of trough activity. Compared with deconvolution analysis, baseline occupancy (and for that matter any level one chooses) gives an estimate of end-organ/receptor exposure to the hormone.

### Chaos

The issue of regularity and chaos arises in complex data arrays where regularity is less obvious. Can the data be quantified and what are the implications? The traditional approach in biology is always to look for the simplest explanation. At first sight it seems inherently unlikely that biology is anything other than deterministic. Heart rate is controlled by natural pacemakers, which give rise to steady regular heart beats, but practical experience tells us that beats occasionally become dropped. In extremes, the rhythm becomes irregular, the change in timing of one beat making a bigger change in the next and so on. When this instability is persistent, it is termed chaos. At its extreme, in the case of heart rate, survival may be threatened. Is regularity then the preferred mode? The answer appears to be not quite: there have been a number of studies looking at heart rates in pathophysiological situations. In children who have had an aborted sudden infant death episode, for example, there is an association with greater heart rate regularity [22].

Oscillating systems have a high likelihood of becoming chaotic because they possess an element of feedback. The system will always opt to make something too large smaller and something too small larger. It is sometimes useful to determine at what level the factor will settle. Generally speaking, most people would aim to operate at something in the middle, neither too large nor too small. This is not true all the time, however.

The likelihood of chaos in endocrinology must be high. Isolated endocrine cells have their own inherent rhythm, and if an external rhythm with a different periodicity is imposed the ensuing hormone secretion will depend on the relationship between the two periods. In some instances, secretion will resume with some harmonic of the stimulus but, in others, random secretion will take place, giving irregular or chaotic patterns. The input and output of the control system in endocrinology can be measured and the two related. In addition, there is latency or lag within the system and, in theory, if the latency is altered (e.g. gain in the feedback loop increased), the system could become unstable and oscillate periodically. If the feedback system was made complex, periodic oscillations could ensue.

Attempts to measure these phenomena in endocrinology are in their infancy, although techniques have been devised for other areas of biology. Approximate entropy is such a measure that attempts to quantify regularity in data in conjunction with standard measures such as the mean and root mean squared. Entropy is a concept that addresses system randomness and predictability. The greater the entropy, the more the randomness and the less the system order. The models derived have been based on the Kolmogorov–Sinai entropy formula [23,24]. Modifications were required because this entropy formula needs no noise and infinite amounts of data. Approximate entropy measures the logarithmic likelihood that runs of patterns that are close remain close on the next incremental comparison. The higher the value, the more random the time series. The technique has been applied in a number of instances and, in the endocrine field, patients with osteoporosis have been shown to have a loss of chaotic oscillations in serum levels of parathyroid hormone [25].

Fractal analysis is an important area of chaos. Fractals are geometric shapes that are irregular but have the same degree of regularity on all sides. An object looks the same when examined from far or near. Sometimes parts of the object are exactly like the whole. Others are more random in nature, e.g. maps of coastlines. Measuring the coast of a country with ever-increasing precision means that its length becomes greater because ever smaller irregularities along the length need to be taken into account. For fractals, the counterparts of the familiar dimensions (0, 1, 2 and 3) are known as fractal dimensions. Mandelbrot [26] described an exponent of similarity termed the fractal dimension, and Katz and George [27]

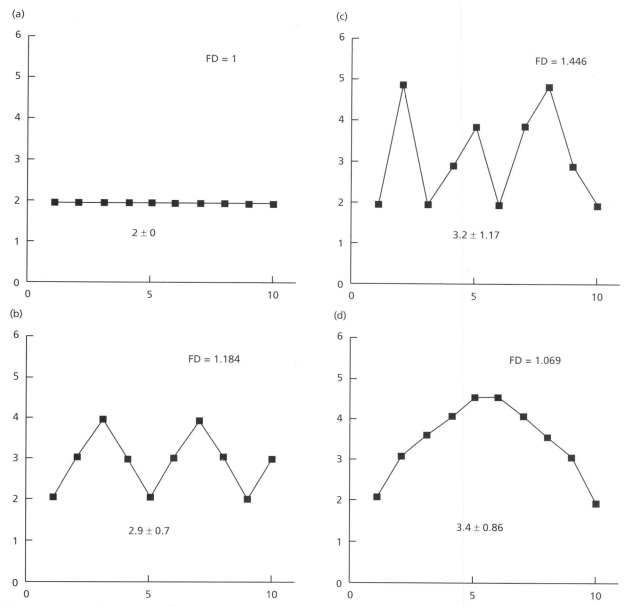

**Fig. 2.5.** Fractal analysis of (a) straight line, (b) two poles, (c) complex poles and (d) single pulse. Note fractal dimension (FD) is independent of the mean value and SD of the mean (figures under the data arrays).

described techniques to compute fractal dimensions from time series data.

Several algorithms exist to compute fractal dimensions (Fig. 2.5). The first point to note is that the technique is not strongly related to the mean and standard deviation that can be derived from a data array. A straight line has a fractal dimension equal to 1, as the next point is predicted from knowledge of the current situation. A single pulse has a fractal dimension close to 1, as there are points rising above each other (predictable) and falling below each other (predictable) but the points at the apex are less predictable, neither rising nor falling. More complex shapes have higher

fractal dimensions. This type of approach has been applied to a number of aspects of biology, e.g. blood flow [28] and heart rate analysis [29]. In the studies reported so far, a loss of complexity or a tendency to regularity might be construed as a sign of abnormality, as mentioned above.

## Clinical implications for hormone pulsatility

The analysis of hormone pulsatility in a clinical setting has been a relatively late addition to the clinician's armamentarium and one that has not achieved universal applicability.

This is largely because the techniques are not easily accessible. The construction of the time series is time-consuming and expensive, and the techniques emerged at a time when endocrine provocation tests or analysis of hormones in urine were well established and relatively simple to perform.

Many of the analytes measured in clinical endocrine practice do not exhibit a circadian rhythm or form a complex in the serum with binding proteins. Such situations assume that there are no long-term variations. Single samples would be unhelpful when the hormone in question is known to pulse, particularly when wide variations in pulse amplitude are to be expected, when a circadian or other long-term trend is present or if trough concentrations are low for considerable portions over a 24-h period. For example, the diagnosis of Cushing syndrome or acromegaly is predicated on establishing the presence of an inappropriate and persistent elevation of cortisol and GH concentrations respectively. It is not necessary for the elevation to be excessively high, because what appears to be more important is that there is no respite from persistent exposure to elevated levels – allostasis in operation. Basic principles tell the clinician that the chances of documenting the problem will be increased by increasing sample number. Simply taking a midnight and early morning cortisol sample limits the probability of confirming the presence of disease, particularly when the inherent variability in these parameters in the normal population is taken into account.

In the performance of diagnostic tests, the implications of a pulsatile system assume great importance. Efficiency, sensitivity and specificity are dependent to some extent on the repeatability and reproducibility of the tests. A pulsatile system influences both these facets in a number of ways. The majority of endocrine tests are conducted over short time courses, e.g. stimulation tests, and their results are often extrapolated to longer time frames. For example, GH provocation tests used to assess the GH secretory state in children are performed over a 2-h period and the results are then compared with height velocity measures obtained over long periods of time, often 1 year. That there is a relationship at all is surprising, that there are high false-positive and -negative results perhaps not. A further way in which hormone pulsatility may influence diagnostic tests is if the test itself (e.g. the stimulus applied) is influenced by oscillations within the system under study.

The GH response to insulin-induced hypoglycaemia, for example, is heavily influenced by the serum GH concentration at the commencement of the study. A number of investigators have demonstrated that the prevailing somatostatin tone, which is a determinant of the pulsatility of the hormone system, is an important factor in determining the magnitude of the response to any stimulus [30,31]. Many endocrine tests, particularly those derived for GH assessment, have been standardized in adults and conducted in the morning, a time of day when in adults there is little or no GH measurable in the circulation. This is acceptable for a normal individual but may not be for other situations.

Acromegaly is associated with a failure of glucose administration to suppress serum GH concentrations and a paradoxical rise in serum GH concentration after the administration of exogenous TRH (thyrotrophin-releasing hormone). A similar situation has been reported in tall pubertal children and in patients with anorexia nervosa, diabetes or chronic renal failure [32–35]. These conditions do not necessarily represent abnormalities in the GH axis, particularly when the timing of the test is viewed in the context of the wider data arrays. All these states are associated with GH hypersecretion. Careful analysis of longer data arrays reveals that such 'paradoxical' results can be predicted simply on the basis of the GH rhythm in these individuals rather than by any intrinsic abnormality in the regulation of GH secretion [34]. Figure 2.6 shows the GH response to a placebo or oral glucose load in a boy of tall stature.

In assessing the results of endocrine evaluation, it is generally assumed that when multiple samples are measured they are relatively constant, at least over short periods. A thyroxine measurement on one day should be the same or similar to one measured the next day or the next week. Although this may be generally true, it cannot be assumed. When important changes are postulated to be taking place, knowledge of inherent variability within the measurement

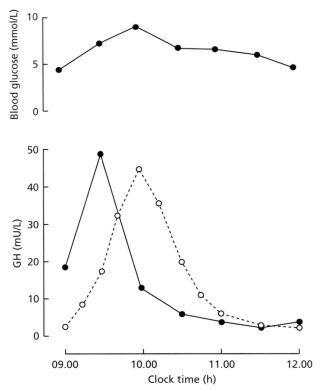

**Fig. 2.6.** Serum growth hormone (GH) concentrations in a boy of tall stature. ○, Spontaneous peak; ●, after oral glucose loading.

system is required. A number of studies are available to assist in this area. Generally speaking, group data are usually reproducible but problems can arise if it is assumed that oscillatory profiles are consistent from day to day [36].

## Therapeutic implications of hormone pulsatility

Despite the wide range of medications used by clinical endocrinologists, the principles derived from the analysis of hormone pulsatility have not been widely applied in therapeutic practice. The aim of hormone replacement is to mimic the physiological pattern of hormone secretion. Classic pharmacology dictates achieving a steady state, and this is what is required in terms of serum thyroxine levels in an individual. The same is not true for many of the pituitary hormones, such as GH or the gonadotrophins, for which a pulsatile mode of operation is the norm.

A more clear-cut situation arises for insulin. A beneficial effect in terms of blood glucose lowering comes from the administration of insulin in the physiological mode of presentation (i.e. pulsatile) compared with one given in continuous mode. This observation has been applied in the clinical setting to the management of diabetic ketoacidosis. Gone are the days of large-dose subcutaneous injections of insulin that led to high persisting circulating concentrations of insulin and subsequent down-regulation of the insulin receptor. This is not to say that giving insulin in a continuous infusion intravenously cannot be helpful, particularly if one wishes to avoid sudden sharp decrements in circulating glucose concentrations.

It is perhaps surprising that both growth and reproductive function can be achieved by subcutaneous administration of biosynthetic human GH or human chorionic gonadotrophin, despite the pulsatile manner of secretion of these hormones in physiology. The pharmacodynamics of such patterns of administration are vastly different from physiology but seem adequate. True, the system is pulsatile in the sense that the treatments may be given on a once-daily basis, but this scarcely matches physiology. It has to be remembered, however, that, although the end point we wish to observe (e.g. growth or ovulation) will be progressing satisfactorily, we do not know what other effects these agents may have when given in this fashion.

Within the normal menstrual cycle, for example, a wide range of pulse frequencies can be observed, ranging from 60 min in the follicular phase to 3 h during the luteal phase. Puberty can be induced with a similar wide range of pulse frequencies, implying a degree of 'redundancy' within the system [37]. Thus human chorionic gonadotrophin pulsatile treatment frequency is not critical. Redundancy may be wasteful, however: in the case of subcutaneous GH administration [38], growth itself seems dependent mainly on the upswing of the pulse so the additional exposure thereafter may not be necessary.

There are a number of studies that testify to the role of physiology in the maintenance of growth or ovarian function. Treatments with GnRH (gonadotrophin-releasing hormone) or GH-releasing hormone (GHRH) in a pulsatile fashion have been used by many groups to induce ovulation or to promote growth. Both regimens work effectively and efficiently considering the low doses of hypothalamic peptide required. When GHRH was given in a 3-hourly pulsatile manner during the night or over 24 h, growth acceleration was seen in a dose-dependent fashion. It was also more efficient on a dose-for-dose basis than when the peptide was given by a twice-daily regimen [39]. Similar growth rates can be achieved by continuous infusion of GHRH hormone, but here the dose needs to be significantly higher, almost 10-fold, in order to achieve a similar amount of GH release and growth rate [40].

## Conclusions

Pulsatility is a feature of endocrine systems and needs to be considered in the analysis of information derived from physiological and pathophysiological situations. Careful consideration needs to be given to how the information is collected, because false conclusions can easily be drawn as a result of an inappropriate choice of sampling intervals and sampling duration. A variety of methods are used to obtain samples, ranging from continuous withdrawal to intermittent sampling, and these techniques influence the types of information that can be derived from the study. Numerous methods of analysing the data series have been put forward, and each contributes to a different aspect of defining hormone pulsatility.

The choice of system of analysis is determined largely by the question that requires to be answered. A clear definition of the hypothesis to be tested is paramount before embarking on any study, whether of a physiological or a pathophysiological nature. There appear to be physiological advantages to pulsatile systems in endocrinology and understanding the perturbation of these systems is the key to understanding pathophysiological states.

Finally, the primary aim of endocrine therapeutics is to mimic as closely as is possible normal physiology, and consideration needs to be given to the physiology of the hormone system of interest in order to meet this fundamental component of clinical endocrine practice best.

## References

1 McEwen BS. Stress, adaption and disease. Allostasis and allostatic load. *Ann NY Acad Sci* 1998; 840: 33–44.

2 McEwen BS, Stellar E. Stress and the individual. Mechanisms leading to disease. *Arch Intern Med* 1993; 153: 2093–101.

3 Goodner CJ, Walike BC, Koerker DJ *et al*. Insulin, glucagon and glucose exhibit synchronous, sustained oscillations in fasting monkeys. *Science* 1977; 195: 177–9.

4 Honda Y, Takahashi K, Takahashi S *et al*. GH secretion during sleep in normal subjects. *J Clin Endocrinol Metab* 1969; 29: 20–9.

5 Krieger DT, Allen W. Relationship of bioassayable and immunoassayable plasma ACTH and cortisol concentrations in normal subjects and in patients with Cushing's disease. *J Clin Endocrinol Metab* 1975; 40: 675–87.

6 Clayton RN, Royston JP, Chapman J *et al*. Is changing hypothalamic activity important for the control of ovulation? *Br Med J* 1987; 295: 7–12.

7 Schofield PR, Shivers BD, Seeburg PH. The role of receptor subtype diversity in the CNS. *Trends Neurosci* 1990; 13: 8–11.

8 Lang DA, Matthews DR, Peto J, Turner RC. Cyclic oscillations of basal plasma glucose and insulin concentrations in human beings. *N Engl J Med* 1979; 301: 1023–7.

9 Matthews DR, Hermansen K, Connolly AA, *et al*. Greater in vivo than in vitro pulsatility of insulin secretion with synchronized insulin and somatostatin secretory pulses. *Endocrinology* 1987; 120: 2272–8.

10 Matthews DR. Physiological implications of pulsatile hormone secretion. *Ann NY Acad Sci* 1991; 618: 28–37.

11 Matthews DR. Insulin: the physiological basis of its administration. In: Radder JK, Lemkes HHPJ, Krans HMJ, eds. *Pathogenesis and Treatment of Diabetes Mellitus*. Dordrecht: Martinus-Nijhoff, 1986: 131–41.

12 Veldhuis JD, Evans WS, Rogol AD *et al*. Intensified rates of venous sampling unmask the presence of spontaneous high-frequency pulsation of luteinising hormone in man. *J Clin Endocrinol Metab* 1984; 59: 96–102.

13 Van Cauter E. Method for characterisation of 24 hour temporal variation of blood components. *Am J Physiol* 1979; 237: E255–64.

14 Santen RJ, Bardin CW. Episodic luteinising hormone secretion in man. Pulse analysis, clinical interpretation, physiological mechanisms. *J Clin Invest* 1973; 52: 2617–28.

15 Merriam GR, Wacher KW. Algorithms for the study of episodic hormone secretion. *Am J Physiol* 1982; 243: E31–8.

16 Veldhuis JD, Johnson ML. Cluster analysis: a simple versatile and robust algorithm for endocrine pulse detection. *Am J Physiol* 1986; 250: E486–93.

17 Chatfield C. *The Analysis of Time Series*, 3rd edn. London: Chapman & Hall, 1984.

18 Diggle PJ. *Time Series. A Biostatistical Introduction*. New York: Oxford University Press, 1990.

19 Turner RC, Grayburn JA, Newman GB, Nabarro JDN. Measurement of the insulin delivery rate in man. *J Clin Endocrinol Metab* 1971; 33: 279–86.

20 Veldhuis JD, Carlson ML. The pituitary gland secretes in bursts: appraising the nature of glandular secretory impulses by simultaneous multiple-parameter deconvolution of plasma hormone concentrations. *Proc Natl Acad Sci USA* 1987; 84: 7686–90.

21 Matthews DR, Hindmarsh PC, Pringle PJ, Brook CGD. A distribution method for analysing the baselines of pulsatile endocrine signals as exemplified by 24-hour growth hormone profiles. *Clin Endocrinol* 1991; 35: 245–52.

22 Pincus SM, Cummins TR, Haddad GG. Heart rate control in normal and aborted-SIDS infants. *Am J Physiol* 1993; 264: R638–46.

23 Pincus SM. Approximate entropy as a measure of system complexity. *Proc Natl Acad Sci USA* 1991; 88: 2297–301.

24 Pincus SM, Singer BH. Randomness and degree of irregularity. *Proc Natl Acad Sci USA* 1996; 93: 2083–8.

25 Prank K, Harms H, Dammig M, Brabant G, Mitschke F, Hesch R-F. Is there low dimensional chaos in pulsatile secretion of parathyroid hormone in normal human subjects? *Am J Physiol* 1994; 266: E653–8.

26 Mandelbrot BB. *The Fractal Geometry of Nature*. New York: Freeman, 1983.

27 Katz MJ, George EB. Fractals and the analysis of growth paths. *Bull Math Biol* 1985; 47: 273–86.

28 Glenny RW, Robertson HT. Fractal properties of pulmonary blood flow heterogeneity. *Appl Physiol* 1991; 70: 1024–30.

29 Yeragani VK, Srinivasan K, Wempati S, Pohl R, Balon R. Fractal dimension of heart rate time series in an effective measure of autonomic function. *J Appl Physiol* 1993; 75: 2429–38.

30 Devesa J, Lima L, Lois N, Lechjga MJ, Arche V, Tresguerres JAF. Reasons for the variability in growth hormone (GH) responses to GHRH challenge: the endogenous hypothalamic–somatotroph rhythm (HSR). *Clin Endocrinol* 1989; 125: 1387–94.

31 Suri D, Hindmarsh PC, Brain CE, Pringle PJ, Brook CGD. The interaction between clonidine and growth hormone releasing hormone in the stimulation of growth hormone secretion in man. *Clin Endocrinol* 1990; 33: 399–406.

32 Hindmarsh PC, Stanhope R, Kendall BE, Brook CGD. Tall stature. A clinical, endocrinological study. *Clin Endocrinol* 1986; 25: 223–31.

33 Maeda K, Kato Y, Yamaguchi N *et al*. Growth hormone release following thyrotrophin releasing hormone injection into patients with anorexia nervosa. *Acta Endocrinol* 1976; 81: 1–8.

34 Edge JA, Human DH, Matthews DR *et al*. Spontaneous growth hormone (GH) pulsatility is the major determinant of GH release after thyrotrophin-releasing hormone in adolescent diabetics. *Clin Endocrinol* 1989; 30: 397–404.

35 Gonzalez-Barcena D, Kastin AJ, Schalch DG *et al*. Responses to thyrotrophin releasing hormone in patients with renal failure and after infusion in normal men. *J Clin Endocrinol Metab* 1973; 35: 117–20.

36 Saini S, Hindmarsh PC, Matthews DR *et al*. Reproducibility of 24-hour serum GH profiles in man. *Clin Endocrinol* 1991; 34: 455–62.

37 Bridges NA, Hindmarsh PC, Matthews DR, Brook CGD. The effect of changing gonadotrophin-releasing hormone pulse frequency on puberty. *J Clin Endocrinol Metab* 1994; 79: 841–7.

38 Jorgensen JOL, Flyvbjerg A, Lauritzen T, Orskov H, Christiansen JS. Subcutaneous degradation of biosynthetic human growth hormone (GH) in GH deficient patients. *Acta Endocrinol* 1988; 118: 154–8.

39 Thorner MO, Rogol AD, Blizzard RM *et al*. Acceleration of growth rate in growth hormone-deficient children treated with human growth hormone-releasing hormone. *Pediatr Res* 1988; 24: 145–51.

40 Brain CE, Hindmarsh PC, Brook CGD. Continuous subcutaneous GHRH (1–29) NH2 promotes growth over 1 year in short slowly growing children. *Clin Endocrinol* 1990; 32: 153–63.

# 3 Hormone assays

## M. J. Wheeler

## Introduction

The concentration of hormones in biological fluids is remarkably small. For instance, the concentration of cortisol in serum is about one-millionth of the total protein concentration. Other commonly measured hormones are present in serum at a further 100 times smaller concentration, and in children some hormones are at an even lower concentration. Therefore, assays used to measure hormones must be exceptionally sensitive. Early assays were long, tedious and complex. Protein hormones, such as luteinizing hormone (LH) and follicle-stimulating hormone (FSH), were measured by bioassay using mice and rats, whereas steroids were commonly measured in urine with lengthy solvent extraction of large volumes of urine followed by paper chromatographic steps. Assays would take a whole week before results were obtained. Developments in the field of immunoassay have led to faster and more sensitive assays, so that, today, many hormones are easily detected in serum with results for many available in less than 30 min.

A constant challenge to the immunoassayist is one of specificity. The structures of steroid hormones are very similar, and it may be difficult to differentiate one steroid from another [1]. Protein hormones circulate in different forms, either as fragments with small pieces of protein removed, as subunits or as macromolecular forms [2,3]. The measurement of the biologically active form may be very difficult because more than one form of the hormone may bind to the hormone receptor. Many hormones, both proteins and steroids, circulate in blood bound to a binding protein, and decisions have to be made whether the total hormone or the non-protein-bound hormone is measured. If the non-protein-bound fraction is measured, the concentration may only be one-hundredth of the concentration of the total hormone (e.g. $T_4$, $T_3$, testosterone) [4,5].

Having developed an assay that is capable of measuring the hormone of interest in its clinically most relevant form,

**Table 3.1.** Physiological parameters associated with changes in hormone concentration

| Parameter | Hormones |
| --- | --- |
| Circadian rhythm | Growth hormone, adrenal steroids |
| Sleep | Growth hormone, prolactin |
| Puberty | LH, FSH, gonadal steroids, adrenal steroids |
| Stress and exercise | Growth hormone, cortisol, prolactin |
| Food | Insulin, glucagon |
| Age | Oestradiol, testosterone, SHBG, IGF-I, DHEAS |
| Sex | Oestradiol, testosterone |
| Menstrual cycle | LH, FSH, oestradiol, progesterone |
| Low and high body weight | Reproductive hormones |

SHBG, sex hormone-binding globulin; DHEAS, dehydroepiandrosterone sulphate.

interpretation of results is further complicated by physiological variables (Table 3.1). Some hormones demonstrate a marked circadian rhythm, which may develop during puberty, e.g. LH [6,7], and this has been examined as a possible diagnostic tool in the investigation of delayed puberty in children [8,9]. Many hormones, both steroids and proteins, are increased during times of stress, something which may confuse the interpretation of a result but again has been exploited clinically, e.g. the GH response to exercise in the investigation of GH deficiency in children [10]. Therefore, hormone assays must be highly sensitive and specific, and should show good reproducibility of results, so that changes during a dynamic test or over a period of time can be interpreted reliably.

Most hormones are measured in blood using immunoassay techniques but there is still a place for urine measurement, particularly in the investigation of enzyme disorders in steroid biosynthesis and in detecting synthetic steroids [11]. It has also been proposed that the measurement of growth hormone in urine is helpful in the investigation of growth hormone deficiency [12,13].

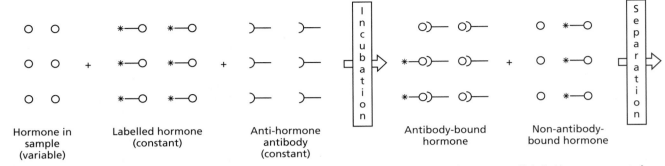

**Fig. 3.1.** A schematic representation of a competitive immunoassay. Hormone in the patient sample and a fixed amount of labelled hormone compete for a fixed, limited number of antibody binding sites. A variety of methods are used to separate antibody-bound hormone and unbound hormone. The amount of bound labelled hormone is then determined.

## Immunoassay methods

These methods may be divided into two main groups [14], competitive, or reagent-limited, assays and non-competitive, or reagent excess, assays. Examples of the former are radioassays, enzyme assays, fluoroassays and chemiluminescence assays, depending on whether a radioactive isotope, an enzyme or a chemical that will fluoresce or chemiluminesce is used as the 'label'. Competitive assays are most commonly used for the measurement of steroids and other very small molecules with only one epitope for antibody binding available (Fig. 3.1). The reagents are usually incubated for sufficient time to reach equilibrium. This can be enhanced by having the antibody in solution either dissolved or attached to a solid phase in suspension. One of the most common solid phases used today in the automated assays is magnetized particles of cellulose. Applying a simple magnetic force pulls the particles to the side or base of the reaction tube, allowing easy aspiration of the liquid phase and washing of the particles. Thorough washing of the particles results in a very low non-specific interference that increases the sensitivity of the assay. A labelled form of the hormone, which competes with endogenous hormone for a limited number of antibody binding sites, is used to generate the signal.

Immunometric assays (Fig. 3.2) use a labelled antibody for signal generation, and the most common format is the sandwich technique, which uses a second antibody as a capture antibody. This second antibody is bound to a solid phase and binds a proportion of the hormone in the serum. Reactions can be quite short because only enough hormone, sufficient to produce a detectable signal when the second antibody is attached, is required. The second antibody, to which is attached the signal-generating molecule, is added in excess so that it quickly binds to the captured hormone. The most common end point used today in both immunoassays and immunometric assays is chemiluminescence.

## Specificity

The ability to produce monoclonal antibodies [15,16] has led to increased specificity, particularly for peptide hormones. A monoclonal antibody recognizes a single epitope on a molecule. This may not be enough to provide absolute specificity as that epitope may also be present on circulating subunits and fragments of the same hormone or even a different hormone. Greater specificity is imbued by the use of a second monoclonal antibody that recognizes another unique epitope on the hormone. If the two monoclonal antibodies bind to epitopes at different ends of the molecule, then only the intact molecule will be captured and fragments and subunits are excluded. It may be that a subunit, e.g. β-subunit of human chorionic gonadotrophin (hCG), also has biological activity and by using two antibodies that bind to two different epitopes on the β-subunit the intact molecule and the β-subunit will be captured and measured.

Problems have arisen as a result of too great a specificity. In the late 1980s, two commercial assays were developed for LH that used a monoclonal antibody which bound to the linkage area of the α- and β-subunits [17]. It was subsequently shown [18] that in some normally menstruating women no LH was detected when these assays were used. Although inconvenient, such patients, who represented only about 2% of normal women, were easily identified because the LH was undetectable when the FSH was normal. More disturbing was the finding that in about 20% of normal women the LH concentration was about 50% of the true value. This was clinically unacceptable and the manufacturers had to redevelop their assays using different antibodies.

The ratios of the different isoforms of peptide hormones probably vary most during times of development and during increased secretion. As the various assays developed to measure a hormone use antibodies that recognize different epitopes of the hormone, they may also recognize the isoforms to differing amounts. This can result in quite large differences

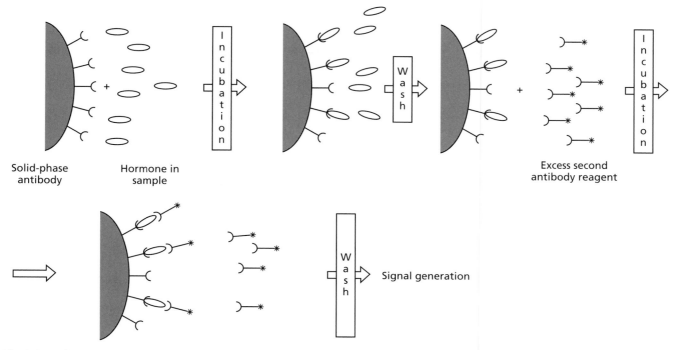

**Fig. 3.2.** A schematic representation of a sandwich-type immunometric assay. Hormone in the sample binds to a capture antibody, usually attached to a solid phase. Excess hormone is aspirated away and a second labelled antibody is added in excess. After a short incubation time excess labelled antibody is aspirated away. The amount of labelled antibody bound is then determined.

in the amount of hormone, detected by different methods, for the same sample [19]. Studies in my laboratory showed that, when LH was measured in the serum of prepubertal children using nine commercial kits, some kits could detect little LH, whereas others detected much greater concentrations [20]. When changing methods, a laboratory should carry out extensive comparative studies between the old and the new methods to establish how much the results from the two methods differ. Some differences may be specific to a particular population of patients, and therefore all age groups should be included in comparative studies.

## Hormone binding

Binding of a hormone to a specific binding protein may inhibit the measurement of the total concentration of the hormone. In this case, the hormone must be displaced from the protein before the immunoassay. It was common to carry out a solvent extraction of serum for the measurement of steroids. Over 95% of the steroid is commonly recovered in the extract with potentially cross-reacting conjugates remaining in the aqueous phase [21]. This is still the preferred procedure in some laboratories. Solvent extraction is not convenient for many laboratories, and other ways to displace hormones from their binding proteins have been developed. Large concentrations of another steroid or a substance that has minimal or no cross-reaction with the antibody but binds to the binding protein are added to the assay reagents to dis-

place the hormone from the binding proteins. For example, the addition of anilino naphthosulphonic acid to serum displaces thyroxine from thyroxine-binding globulin.

It is useful to understand several of the terms used by immunoassayists as they describe the features of an assay. Having this information helps in the interpretation of results and highlights the limitations that may exist.

## Definitions

### Cross-reaction

Cross-reaction describes the amount, in per cent terms, of an analyte similar to the one being measured that will be measured in an assay. For competitive assays, the cross-reaction is usually calculated from the analyte concentrations that bind 50% of the maximum tracer binding [22], but a similar principle can be applied to non-competitive assays (Fig. 3.3). For example, the antibody used in a cortisol assay may have a 30% cross-reaction with prednisolone. This means that, for a prednisolone concentration of 100 nmol/L, 30 nmol/L will be measured in the cortisol assay. In other words, in this situation the result for cortisol will be the cortisol concentration plus 30 nmol/L prednisolone. As prednisolone cross-reacts in all cortisol assays, it is misleading to measure cortisol in a patient treated with prednisolone using a routine cortisol assay.

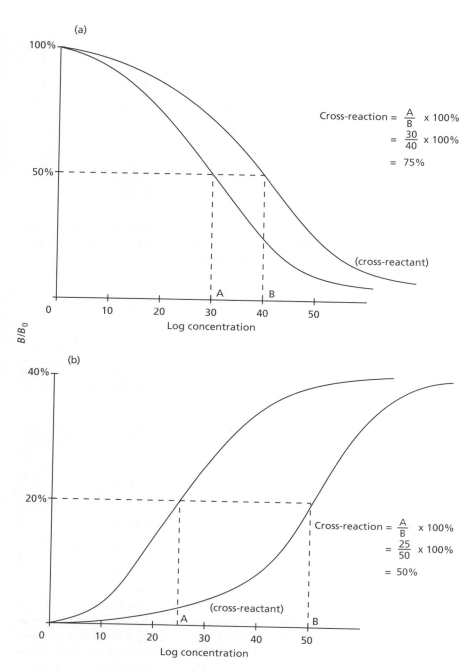

**Fig. 3.3.** Examples of the calculation of the cross-reaction of a substance with the antibody in (a) a competitive assay and (b) an immunometric assay. A and B refer to the concentrations at 50%.

The cross-reaction of an antibody must always be interpreted in the light of the circulating concentration of the cross-reactant. For instance, if the cortisol antibody had a cross-reaction of 30% with 11-deoxycortisol, this would be clinically insignificant in normal subjects as the highest concentration of 11-deoxycortisol in the serum is only about 18 nmol/L. The cross-reaction would become significant in cases of congenital adrenal hyperplasia because of an 11β-hydroxylase deficiency as concentrations of 11-deoxycortisol are usually well above 100 nmol/L. It would also be significant if cortisol was measured during a metyrapone test.

## Sensitivity

Sensitivity may now be described as either *analytical sensitivity* or *functional sensitivity*. Analytical sensitivity is the lowest concentration of analyte that is significantly different from zero and is usually the sensitivity quoted for an assay if the two terms are not used separately. There is no convention for calculating the analytical sensitivity and, although there has been debate over the correct calculation of sensitivity, its derivation has been described [23]. In many cases 20 replicate analyses of the zero standard are carried out and the standard

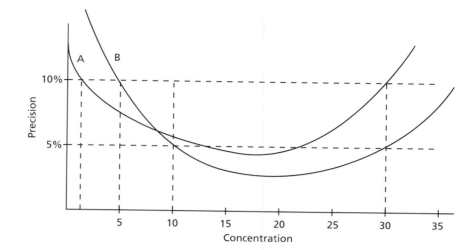

**Fig. 3.4.** The precision profiles for two methods A and B. Method A has a greater precision (<10%) at low concentrations whereas method B shows better precision than method A at higher concentrations. Choice of method would depend on the range of concentration to be encountered in clinical samples.

deviation (SD) of the response calculated. The concentration on the standard curve equivalent to either 2 SD or 2.5 SD from the zero response is taken as the sensitivity of the assay. Because of variation in the determination of analytical sensitivity and criticism of its usefulness [24], functional sensitivity based on the precision profile (described later) is more meaningful. The terms analytical and functional sensitivity were first used by Spencer [25,26] and applied to thyroid-stimulating hormone (TSH) assays. The functional sensitivity is defined as the lowest concentration at which the interassay precision is < 20% and can be determined from the between-assay precision profile (see below).

## Precision

Precision represents the reproducibility of the measurement of an analyte at different concentrations. Usually the intra-assay or within-assay precision (reproducibility of measurement in a single assay) and the interassay or between-assay precision (reproducibility of measurement between separate assays) are quoted for assays. Data quoted will represent best-case performance since usually it will be derived by one operator probably using one lot number of kit. Precision is affected by differences between operators, the lot numbers of kits, temperature and several other variables. Ekins [27] has shown that precision varies with analyte concentration so that a single figure for precision is not possible. After calculating the precision of an assay across a wide range of concentrations, the data are plotted to give a precision profile (Fig. 3.4). It is important to know the precision at different concentrations covered in any study since the error of measurement is less in a single assay than across several assays. The intra-assay precision will usually be better than the interassay precision. Therefore, specimens from studies examining changes in one individual on several occasions should be analysed in a single assay to improve the detection of small but important changes in concentration.

## Working range

The *working range* of an assay is derived from the precision profile and is the range of concentration over which the intra-assay precision is less than a chosen amount. Again, there is no convention for this, and for many years most assayists used a precision of < 10% to determine the working range [22]. Examination of Fig. 3.4 shows that, by using this convention, method A has a working range of 1 nmol/L to 30 nmol/L and method B a working range of 5 nmol/L to > 35 nmol/L. Therefore, method A shows greater sensitivity and is better suited to measure low concentrations. However, method B is superior to method A over the range 10–30 nmol/L as it achieves a precision of < 5%. It also shows better precision than method A at higher concentrations. The choice of method depends on several factors, which include the desired working range and precision. As many assays on the newer automated immunoassay analysers can achieve a precision of < 5% over much of the working range, it may be more informative now, when comparing methods, to quote the range of concentration over which a method has a precision of < 5% and < 10%. The working range using the between-assay or interassay precision profile is more meaningful for clinical purposes as it gives a better impression of the error of a result on different occasions over time. The functional sensitivity of an assay is the smallest concentration at which the interassay precision is less than 20% [26]. Often clinicians are uncertain whether observed changes on two or more occasions are due to assay error or reflect a significant clinical change. Knowing the interassay imprecision would help in the interpretation of results.

## Bias

Bias relates to the closeness of a result to a target value or the systematic error of measurement. This is probably of more concern to the assayist than to the clinician because, as long as reference ranges have been determined properly for the

**Table 3.2.** Situations which require separate reference ranges for the hormones affected

| Parameter | Hormones affected | Changes encountered |
|---|---|---|
| Neonate | 17-Hydroxyprogesterone<br>Testosterone in males | Rapid changes after delivery<br>Rises after first 2 weeks of life and then falls at about 8–10 weeks |
| Children | Reproductive hormones<br>Adrenal androgens<br>IGF-I | Low prepubertally and increase during puberty |
| Ageing adult | Gonadotrophins in women<br>IGF-I<br>DHEAS and DHEA<br>Testosterone in men<br>SHBG | Increase in postmenopausal women<br><br>Decrease with age<br><br>Increase as age increases |
| Menstrual cycle | Gonadotrophins<br>Oestradiol<br>Progesterone<br>Inhibins<br>17-Hydroxyprogesterone | Concentrations are different in the follicular, midcycle and luteal phases |
| Circadian rhythm | ACTH<br>Cortisol and other adrenal steroids<br>Testosterone in men | Higher levels in the morning than in afternoon and evening |
| Sleep | GH<br>Prolactin | Higher levels at night |
| Posture | Renin<br>Aldosterone | Increase in concentrations moving from supine to standing |

DHEA, dehydroepiandrosterone; DHEAS, dehydroepiandrosterone sulphate.

assay in use and no change in the assay occurs, the clinician can determine whether or not a patient has a 'normal' result.

## Reference range

The *reference range* or reference interval is the range of concentrations of an analyte found in a defined population with no apparent pathology. Laboratories may use the range quoted by a manufacturer if using a commercial kit, a range quoted in the literature or a range determined by analysing samples for a population using the laboratory assay. Establishing a reference range is not an easy task, and it is convenient if the manufacturer has data for men, women and children. For many hormones detailed age-related ranges are essential, e.g. insulin-like growth factor I (IGF-I). However, no consideration might have been given to ethnic origin, pubertal status, age, circadian rhythms or other parameters that could modify the data. Therefore, adopting a reference range produced by another institution should be done only after considering the likely peculiarities of the population(s) represented by the patients attending the home hospital or clinic. Commercial companies usually state that the reference range data are provided only as a guide, although some companies carry out detailed international studies to establish meaningful reference data for the users of their diagnostic kits.

Reference data for some populations, e.g. young children, or 24-h circadian rhythms may be very difficult to obtain, and ranges established by the company supplying the kit, or by another institute using the same method, may have to be adopted. A laboratory should avoid using a reference range established using either another method or from the literature. Clinicians can give invaluable help to laboratories trying to establish meaningful reference ranges by supplying blood from their patients and providing detailed clinical information.

The population used to establish a reference range should be clearly defined by sex, age range, time of day and time of menstrual cycle for women of reproductive age. As shown in Table 3.2, the concentration of a number of hormones changes throughout life and appropriate reference ranges should be available. In addition, the investigation of some diseases requires dynamic tests, and reference ranges for the response are also required.

## Other chemical methods used in hormone measurement

All hormones measured in blood routinely are measured by immunoassay techniques. Occasionally, a purification or separation step may be carried out before immunoassay, either to achieve greater specificity or to remove interferences. This may increase the turnaround time of results but is necessary to achieve reliable results. A few common examples are given.

## Adsorption

A commonly reported problem is the interference of immunoglobulins or heterophilic antibodies, particularly in assays using monoclonal antibodies. Patients with autoimmune disease may have rheumatoid factors that react with the antibodies in the assay. Other people may have antibodies in their blood to animal immunoglobulins (Igs) that will bind to the antibodies in the assay. Third, patients injected with monoclonal mouse IgG for radioimaging will often produce antibodies against mouse IgG, and these will bind to mouse monoclonal antibodies in the assay. Interference can be reduced by adding animal serum, such as mouse serum. The heterophilic antibodies, such as antimouse IgG antibodies, can also be adsorbed out of the serum by placing the serum in prepared tubes that have mouse IgG coated on to the inside of the tube. After a short incubation, the heterophilic antibody binds to the mouse IgG on the tube surface. With the interfering antibodies removed, the serum is removed and analysed by immunoassay.

## Solvent extraction

This was always used in the measurement of steroids and served three purposes: (a) it removed steroids from conjugates that might cross-react in the assay; (b) it displaced the steroid from binding proteins; and (c) it separated the steroids from protein interference. The common steroid assays can now be measured on automated immunoassay analysers without prior solvent extraction. The antibodies used are highly specific, and the steroids are usually displaced from the binding proteins by adding high concentrations of another steroid that does not cross-react in the assay. The displacing steroid (added in excess) binds to the binding protein and displaces the steroid of interest. For some assayists, solvent extraction is still the only way to measure steroids accurately and specifically, and to avoid interference from cross-reacting substances. Solvent extraction is carried out before immunoassay for rarer assays such as 5α-dihydrotestosterone, and it is essential for the measurement of steroids such as 17α-hydroxyprogesterone in the investigation of neonates because of cross-reacting steroids produced specifically at this time. Solvent extraction of steroids from serum is used before high-performance liquid chromatography (HPLC).

## High-performance liquid chromatography

This technique is used mostly in research studies of steroids but has also been used in clinical diagnosis to provide a profile of steroids in urine. Steroids are extracted from serum or urine with solvent. The solvent is dried down and redissolved in 'column solvent'. The extract is injected onto the HPLC column, with a pore size of typically 10, and is carried through the column by further solvent pumped at high pressure. The separation of different steroids depends on the type of column and solvent system used. This is a preparative technique since the concentration of steroids in serum and urine does not allow their detection by the ultraviolet (UV) detector of the HPLC system. The time from injection to elution of the steroids from the HPLC column is initially determined by running standard preparations. Fractions of eluate are then collected at specific times after each sample is injected onto the column. The eluate is dried down, reconstituted in assay buffer and the concentration of the steroid measured by immunoassay. The time of elution of each steroid is specific for the conditions used, but the consistent performance of the column is checked by adding a reference steroid at a high enough concentration to give a reading on the UV detector. It is a particularly useful technique when several steroids of the same family are to be measured [28]. This technique, commonly used for urine steroid profiling, has been replaced by gas chromatography–mass spectrometry (GC–MS).

## Mass spectrometry

In the past, mass spectrometry was confined to the measurement of small molecules such as the steroids. Typically, steroids were extracted from serum or urine with solvent and then separated in a gas–liquid chromatography system before analysis by mass spectrometry. Large molecules did not survive the desorption and ionization process. Instruments have been developed with milder desorption and ionization steps, allowing the analysis of large biomolecules. After ionization, the ions are separated and their mass spectrum determined. This spectrum gives what may be described as a fingerprint of the molecule. At the moment the main use of this technique in routine hormone analysis is in the measurement of urinary steroids [29,30], but it will undoubtedly have a much wider application in the future [31].

## Quality control

It is important to know that the results produced from one assay to another are consistent. Large changes in the bias of an assay can result from errors in reagent preparation, deterioration of reagents, pipetting errors, changes in temperature and several other variables. To ensure results are consistent, several quality control (QC) procedures may be followed. The standard procedure is to include QC samples. These are commonly commercially produced preparations, usually

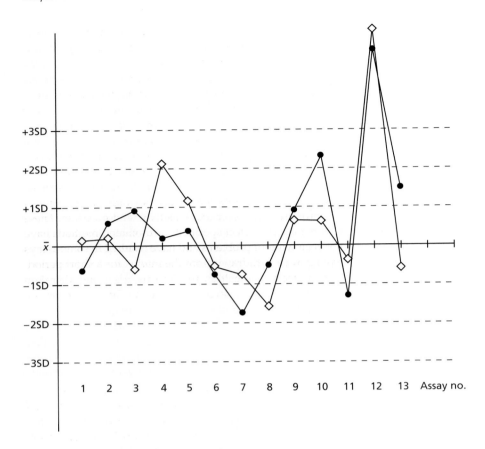

**Fig. 3.5.** A typical plot of a QC specimen run at the beginning (●) and at the end (◇) of the assay. Drift would be indicated by the latter having a constant bias to the former. Assay 12 should be rejected and the patient specimens reanalysed. There would be at least two, and often three, QCs of different concentrations run in every assay.

provided in lyophilized form, that are included in every assay. There has been much discussion over the number of QC specimens that should be analysed and the frequency of analysis. For manually prepared assays it is common to have QC specimens with low, medium and high concentrations. In an assay with only a few samples these may be analysed once only, whereas in assays with a large number of patient specimens the QC specimens may be analysed after every 20 or 30 specimens to monitor for a drift in results across the assay.

Automated assays show very good stability of the calibration curve during the working day and so allow a less frequent analysis of QC specimens. The current major analysers allow 'random access' analysis. This means that specimens can be put on the instrument in any order for whatever hormone and, as long as the reagents are loaded, the relevant hormones will be measured. Therefore, it is not possible to run the QC specimens after a certain number of analyses of a particular hormone.

A common approach is to run QC specimens at the beginning of the day to check that the machine is operating properly and that the calibration curve is giving the correct results. The QC specimens are then analysed again halfway through and at the end of the day. No matter what system is used, the results of the QC specimens must meet predetermined criteria. The most common approach is to plot the results on a

Shewart or Levy Jennings graph (Fig. 3.5). To set up this chart, the QC specimens should be analysed in 20 separate assays. The mean and standard deviation (SD) are calculated and plotted. The SD should reflect the interassay precision of the assay determined during the development of the assay or as stated by the manufacturer. Examining the QC plot will indicate whether the assay is acceptable. Assays may be rejected because the QCs indicate poor precision or show a constant unacceptable negative or positive bias. Where the changes are gross, the decision to reject an assay is easy. More commonly the QC results may be more borderline in acceptability.

In order to overcome the subjective assessment of QC data, Westgard *et al.* [32] developed a set of rules to help in the decision of whether to accept or to reject an assay. Clinicians do not have the time (or knowledge) to check whether the laboratories they use are maintaining acceptable standards. However, a high number of results that do not fit the clinical presentation should make the clinician suspicious that all may not be well with a particular assay.

In the UK, clinical laboratories must be accredited by a body known as Clinical Pathology Accreditation Ltd (CPA). One area that the inspectors examine is the QC procedures of the laboratory. In addition to internal QC specimens, clinical laboratories must also participate in external quality assessment (EQA) schemes. This is also a requirement of laboratory accreditation. The external quality assessment schemes themselves are accredited by CPA. Laboratories receive specimens at regular intervals from an EQA centre. These specimens must be analysed, along with clinical samples, within a specified time limit. The results are sent back to the EQA centre where they are processed along with the returns from all the other participating laboratories. The laboratory receives data that indicate the bias and imprecision of their methods. Limits are set for acceptable levels of these parameters and laboratories showing consistent unacceptable performance are referred to the Professional Advisory Panel of the relevant pathology discipline. It is also a requirement of accreditation that a laboratory must display their EQA performance data in the department.

The relevance of QC and quality assurance (QA) to the clinician is that the procedures should ensure assays of good quality that yield dependable patient results. Laboratories should be willing to share their performance data with clinicians so that they can understand the error in a result. The error will vary in the different analyte assays. For example, between-assay precision may be as low as 3–4% across the reference range for prolactin or cortisol but may be 8–9% for assays such as parathyroid hormone (PTH) and 11-deoxycortisol. A precision of 4% means that a result of 100 units/L could be from 92 units/L to 108 units/L using 2 SD limits of error and an error of 8% means the range of result would be from 84 units/L to 116 units/L. In the former case, a result of 100 units/L on one occasion and 113 units/L on another would suggest a significant increase but not in the latter case. The most important information of an assay for the clinician is the between-assay precision (representing 1 SD) as specimens are usually sent over a period of days, weeks or months. Within-assay precision is relevant to specimens sent from a dynamic test carried out on 1 day, e.g. insulin stress test, but in this situation large changes in hormone concentrations that are much greater than the precision of the assay are expected. As a rough guide, within-assay precision is usually about 1–2% less than between-assay imprecision, so that an assay with a between-assay precision of 5% will have a within-assay precision of 3–4%.

## Automation

One of the most significant changes in immunoassay technology has been the development of fully automated analysers [33,34]. These may enable one technician to provide the results for as many as 20 different analytes in a single day. Commercial competition has led companies to develop assays with much shorter incubation times and therefore quicker turnaround times. The cost of these automated assays may be several times the cost of an in-house assay using home-produced reagents, but this cost is often offset by a reduction in staff numbers. However, there may be a price to pay. Certain assays may not have the sensitivity required to address all clinical problems; other assays may suffer from severe interference effects or have inadequate specificity. With reduced numbers of staff, laboratories have been forced to automate more and more tests, but being able to put many tests on to a single analyser makes the organization of work much easier. This trend is predicted to continue over the next few years, but the development of more near-patient testing will provide a new challenge to laboratories.

Most assays have adequate performance, and assays on some of the newer analysers have outstanding precision. However, it is very difficult for a manufacturer to achieve the same excellent performance for all assays, and there is often a compromise between speed, sensitivity and precision. These factors may also affect specificity. Automated methods have not been without problems and have resulted in some assays having to be withdrawn from the market for a short period. Unexpectedly anomalous results can arise, and therefore clinicians should challenge a laboratory when results do not fit the clinical picture.

## Summary

It is the laboratory's responsibility to use methods for hormone measurement that are robust, sensitive, specific and suitable for clinical use. However, reduction in both the number of staff and the budget has driven the laboratory to use increasingly automated methods. This trend has restricted the choice of hormone assay, and in some cases a compromise has to be made, so that the performance characteristics of an assay may not be as good as the laboratory would like. Thus, there is a further responsibility of the laboratory to make clinicians aware of significant limitations of any assay. Nevertheless, use of hormone results and establishing reference ranges is a partnership between the laboratory and the clinician. Adequate clinical detail on result forms enable the laboratory to check whether hormone results are consistent with clinical expectations or not. Meetings between clinicians and laboratory personnel help both groups to understand each other's problems and give the clinician the opportunity to understand the limitations of the assays. At the same time, laboratories are able to develop strategies to meet clinical needs. As both groups' concern must be the needs of the patient, a partnership between the laboratory and clinician to achieve meaningful hormone results is an obvious outcome.

## References

1 Makin HLJ, Gower DB, Kirk DN. *Steroid Analysis*. London: Blackie Academic and Professional, 1995.
2 Leite V, Cosby H, Sobrinho LG, Fresnoza A, Santos MA, Friesen HG. Characterization of big, big prolactin in patients with hyperprolactinaemia. *Clin Endocrinol* 1992; 37: 365–72.

3 Phillips DJ, Albertson-Wikland K, Erikson K, Wide L. Changes in the isoforms of luteinizing hormone and follicle-stimulating hormone during puberty in normal children. *J Clin Endocrinol Metab* 1997; 82: 3103–6.

4 Larsen PR, Davies TF, Hay ID. The thyroid gland. In: Wilson JD, Foster DW, Kronenberg HM, Larsen PR, eds. *William's Textbook of Endocrinology*. Philadelphia: W.B. Saunders, 1998: 389–515.

5 Wheeler MJ. The determination of bio-available testosterone. *Ann Clin Biochem* 1995; 32: 345–57.

6 Boyar R, Finkelstein J, Roffwarg H, Kapen S, Weitzman E, Hellman L. Synchronization of augmented luteinizing hormone secretion with sleep during puberty. *N Engl J Med* 1972; 287: 582–6.

7 Apter D, Butzow TL, Laughlin GA, Yen SSC. Gonadotropin-releasing hormone pulse generator activity during pubertal transition in girls: pulsatile and diurnal patterns of circulating gonadotropin. *J Clin Endocrinol Metab* 1993; 76: 940–9.

8 Adlord P, Buzi F, Jones J, Stanhope R, Preece MA. Physiological growth hormone secretion during slow wave sleep in short prepubertal children. *Clin Endocrinol* 1987; 27: 355–6.

9 Tassoni P, Cacciani E, Cau M, Colli C, Tosi M, Zuchini S *et al.* Variability of growth hormone response to pharmacological and sleep tests performed twice in short children. *J Clin Endocrinol Metab* 1990; 71: 230–4.

10 Buckler JMH. Plasma growth hormone response to exercise as a diagnostic aid. *Arch Dis Child* 1973; 48: 565–7.

11 Wallace AM. Analytical support for the detection and treatment of congenital adrenal hyperplasia. *Ann Clin Biochem* 1995; 32: 9–27.

12 Skinner AM, Clayton PE, Price DA, Addison M, Soo A. Urinary growth hormone excretion in the assessment of children with disorders of growth. *Clin Endocrinol* 1993; 39: 201–6.

13 Hourd P, Edwards R. Current methods for the measurement of growth hormone in urine: a review. *Clin Endocrinol* 1994; 40: 155–70.

14 Davies, C. Introduction to the immunoassay principles. In: Wild D, ed. *The Immunoassay Handbook*, 2nd edn. London: Nature Publishing Group, 2001: 3–40.

15 Kohler G, Milstein C. Continuous cultures of fused cells secreting antibodies of predefined specificity. *Nature* 1975; 256: 495–7.

16 Kohler G, Milstein C. Derivation of specific antibody-producing tissue culture and tumour lines by cell fusion. *Eur J Immunol* 1976; 6: 511–9.

17 Pettersson K, Ding YQ, Huhtaniemi I. An immunologically anomalous luteinizing hormone variant in a healthy woman. *J Clin Endocrinol Metab* 1992; 74: 164–71.

18 Pettersson K, Ding YQ, Huhtaniemi I. Monoclonal antibody-based discrepancies between 2-site immunometric tests for lutropin. *Clin Chem* 1991; 37: 1745–8.

19 Celniker AC, Chen AB, Wert RM, Sherman BM. Variability in the quantitation of circulating growth hormone using commercial immunoassays. *J Clin Endocrinol Metab* 1989; 68: 469–76.

20 Wheeler MJ, D'Souza A, Horn AN. Evaluation of test kits for gonadotrophins. *Lancet* 1989; I: 616–17.

21 Wheeler MJ, Luther F. Development of testosterone assays for routine use. In: Hunter WM, Corrie JET, eds. *Immunoasssays for Clinical Chemistry*. Edinburgh: Churchill Livingstone, 1983: 113–16.

22 Davies C. Concepts. In: Wild D, eds. *The Immunoassay Handbook*. Basingstoke: The Macmillan Press, 1994: 83–115.

23 Rodbard D, De Munson PJ, Lean A. Improved curve fitting, parallelism, testing, characterization of sensitivity and specificity, validation, and optimisation for radioligand assays. In: *Radioimmunoassay and Related Procedures in Medicine*. Vienna: IAEA Vienna, 1978: 469–503.

24 Ekins RP. Immunoassay design and optimisation. In: Price CP, Newman DJ, eds. *Principles and Practice of Immunoassay*, 2nd edn. London: Macmillan Reference Ltd, 1997: 173–207.

25 Spencer CA. Thyroid profiling for the 1990s: Free T4 estimate or sensitive TSH measurement. *J Clin Immunol* 1989; 12: 82–9.

26 Nicoloff JT, Spencer CA. The use and misuse of sensitive thyrotropin assays. *J Clin Endocrinol Metab* 1990; 71: 553–8.

27 Ekins RP. General principles in hormone assay. In: Lorraine JA, Bell I, eds. *Hormone Assays and Their Clinical Application*, 4th edn. Edinburgh: Churchill Livingstone, 1976: 1–76.

28 Schoneshoffer M, Dulce HJ. Comparison of different high-performance liquid chromatography systems for the purification of adrenal and gonadal steroids prior to immunoassay. *J Chromatogr* 1979; 164: 17–26.

29 Honour JW. Steroid profiling. *Ann Clin Biochem* 1997; 43: 32–44.

30 Honour JW, Brook CGD. Clinical indication for the use of urinary steroid profiles in neonates and children. *Ann Clin Biochem* 1997; 43: 45–54.

31 Shackleton CHL. Mass spectrometry: application in steroid and peptide research. *Endocrine Rev* 1985; 6: 441–86.

32 Westgard JO, Barry PL, Hunt MR, Groth T. A multi-rule Shewart chart for quality control in clinical chemistry. *Clin Chem* 1981; 27: 493–501.

33 Day RG, Horschke WA, Hallahan M-T, Jackson T, Williams JS. System design solutions for high volume immunoassay analysis. *J Clin Ligand Assay* 1999; 22: 184–93.

34 Wheeler MJ. Automated immunoassay analyses. *Clin Biochem* 2001; 38 (in press).

# 4 Principles underlying endocrine tests

### P. C. Hindmarsh and C. G. D. Brook

## Introduction

There are a wide number of tests available for assessing endocrine function. A considerable amount of attention has been paid, rightly, to the underlying mechanisms assessed by the tests, how the samples should be collected and what type of measurement should be performed. Less attention has been paid, rightly, to the mathematical assumptions underlying the performance of diagnostic tests. The statistical theory behind many tests is in fact quite complex simply because the results do not follow an all-or-nothing law. Rather than being left with a clear-cut answer to the initial diagnostic question, the clinician is left with a series of probabilities as to whether or not the patient is likely to have the condition in question.

Clinical diagnosis identifies patient symptoms and signs that result from the underlying disorder. This can be achieved in a number of ways. First, by pattern recognition: we could say that the person looks so obviously panhypopituitary that there is no other likely explanation. Second, clinical algorithms can be applied to the problem. Figure 4.1 shows a possible approach to short stature. Finally, the gather-all approach could be used and all possible data collected. This is expensive and seldom productive, not least because no thought has gone into formulating a hypothesis about what actually was wrong. Most clinicians, however,

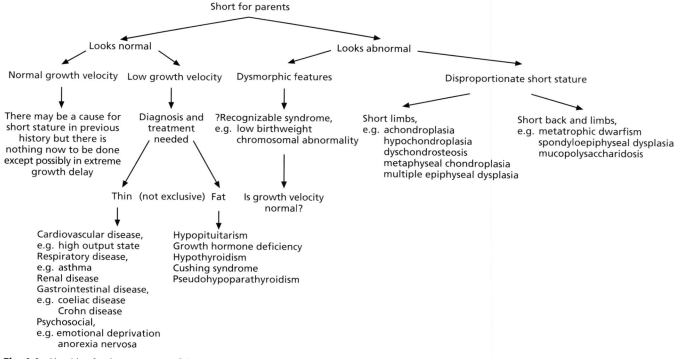

**Fig. 4.1.** Algorithm for the assessment of short stature.

settle for a list of potential diagnoses and use investigation to limit the length of the list.

It is possible to create an artificial gulf between what has gone on before the elucidation of symptoms and signs and what is about to happen, i.e. the performance of a test. This is unhelpful because the possibility of the presence of the disorder before testing has an important influence on the probability of the individual having the disorder after the completion of the test. This chapter reviews the principles underlying the diagnostic process using the paradigm of growth hormone (GH) testing in short children to elucidate the diagnosis of growth hormone deficiency (GHD).

## Clinical observations

Failure of physical growth is an important sign of systemic disease but also the hallmark of endocrine disease, because pituitary, thyroid, adrenal and gonadal hormones are all involved in the process. It is easy for an endocrinologist to concentrate on the results of investigations of the endocrine axis, but it is important to be clear that the categorization of an individual child depends on clinical evaluation and growth assessment. It does not depend, at least initially, on laboratory investigations, which should not be employed until and unless auxological data indicate them to be necessary. The diagnosis of GHD, for example, is largely by exclusion of other possible explanations for poor growth before accepting that the likely diagnosis is GHD [1]. This is important because, although growth in childhood is predominantly GH dependent [2,3], GH probably represents the final common pathway for the mediation of the growth process and is modulated by a number of other factors (Fig. 4.2).

It is likely that a child with a potential growth or endocrine disorder would undergo clinical examination and anthropometric assessment. The principles of the latter have been well described elsewhere [4–6]. The accuracy of the examination and precision of the anthropometry are crucial determinants for diagnosis [6]. Conventional approaches to growth disorders list features seen in association with certain conditions, but the power of clinical observation in determining the diagnosis is rarely discussed. Nor is the magnitude and cause of diagnostic error considered. Could a simple assessment of key clinical points improve diagnostic certainty to the point where testing is unhelpful? No test will help if the degree of uncertainty is high, and, equally, if the degree of certainty is high, why do the test?

## The evaluation of clinical points in the presentation of growth hormone deficiency

The characteristic clinical picture of GHD is of a short plump child with a round immature face. Birthweight is usually nor-

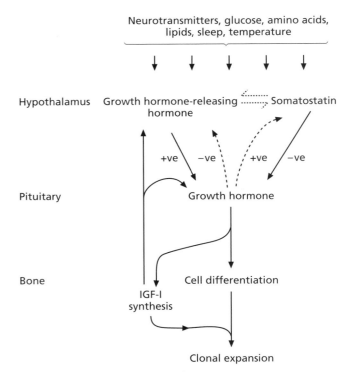

**Fig. 4.2.** The growth hormone cascade.

mal and poor growth is apparent from about 6 months of age (Fig 4.3) [7–9]. GHD may be isolated or associated with other pituitary hormone deficiencies. Small genitalia may point to associated gonadotrophin deficiency. Hypoglycaemia in the newborn period is often a feature of adrenocorticotrophic hormone (ACTH) deficiency. Prolonged neonatal jaundice raises the question of thyroxine (unconjugated) or cortisol (conjugated hyperbilirubinaemia) deficiency. Given these features, it might be possible on the basis of pattern recognition to ascribe the diagnosis of GHD to a patient with a high degree of certainty.

If, however, we simply restricted the assessment to obesity as a feature, we would rapidly run into problems. Testing the GH axis would yield a large number of individuals with a poor GH response, because obesity *per se* is associated with blunted GH responses to various stimuli [10,11]. What is demonstrated is the poor performance of obesity alone as a diagnostic criterion for GHD. Individuals who are growth hormone deficient are often obese, but the converse is clearly not the case.

What is required from the clinical standpoint is some assessment of the strength of various symptoms and signs in making the diagnosis of GHD. This might be achieved by introducing additional clinical information into the diagnostic model. At this juncture a note of caution needs to be sounded: little is known of the sensitivity and specificity of many of the clinical observations, either alone or in combination. The prevalence of many of the clinical features within

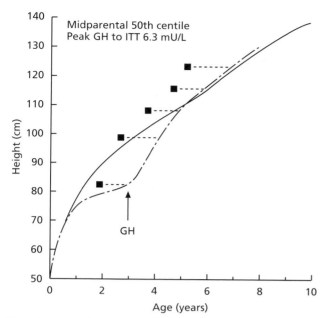

**Fig. 4.3.** Pattern of growth and response to treatment in severe idiopathic isolated GHD. Dashed line patient growth pattern. Solid line 50th centile for population height. Squares show bone age. ITT, insulin tolerance test.

the general population is unknown, which heightens the problem. Even the presence of specific features or combination of features will increase only slightly the likelihood of disease if they are relatively insensitive. However, as will be seen below, it is still possible for the clinicians to come out with the 'best estimate' for the probability that the individual has a particular condition or not. An understanding of the growth process (Chapter 8) is essential in this respect, as it will impact directly on the probability of disease presence.

Growth during the first year of life is largely dependent on nutrition, and poor growth during this time is most likely to be the result of nutritional or gastrointestinal problems [12]. The manifestation of GHD as a result of GH gene deletion is early and poor growth can be detected as early as the sixth month of postnatal life [7–9]. With advancing age, more GH has to be secreted to maintain concentrations of GH sufficient for growth, so idiopathic isolated pituitary GHD may present at any time. It is the degree of deficiency that dictates when the individual comes to medical attention, and the majority of cases of GHD in childhood, other than those secondary to cranial irradiation for leukaemia or brain tumours, could well be detected before the age of 5 years [13,14].

Assessing a child's growth by single or multiple measurements does not lead immediately to confirmation of the diagnosis because GH plays such a central role in the control of childhood growth [2,3]. There are many chronic illnesses in childhood that influence GH secretion, such as coeliac disease [15] and asthma, and the treatment of a number of chronic inflammatory diseases with exogenous glucocorticoids also influences growth, if not GH secretion [16].

Because of the multiple non-endocrine causes for poor growth, the clinician will tend to rule out the more common causes and then embark on a series of investigations to confirm or refute the hypothesis that the individual has GHD. The concept of testing a hypothesis reflects the need to account for the degrees of certainty or uncertainty of the underlying diagnosis. This is particularly important because techniques will now be described to evaluate and quantify the degree of certainty or uncertainty.

## Creating the environment for the test

Analysis of hormones in the circulation forms the backbone of endocrine practice. Such measures may use single samples or be derived from the measurement of multiple samples. Variations in hormone secretion take place on a day-to-day basis. The variations are not confined to short time intervals, as evidenced by the changes in gonadotrophins during the menstrual cycle. The majority of tests conducted in paediatric practice take place at a fixed time of the day. In the execution and interpretation of these tests, consideration needs to be given to the physiology of the hormone studied and the sampling interval chosen for the collection of blood samples. Finally, the test will only be as good as the framework within which the question is set.

## Hormone physiology

Many of the analytes measured in clinical endocrine practice do not have a circadian rhythm or are complexed in the serum to binding proteins. In such situations, it can be assumed that there are no long-term variations, although this may not always be the case (see Table 4.2). Cortisol, the gonadotrophins, GH and insulin are the best known of the hormones that pulse [17–20]. The implication of pulsatile secretion assumes great importance when assessing the performance of diagnostic tests [21]. Efficiency, sensitivity and specificity will all be dependent to some extent on the repeatability and reproducibility of the tests under study and the pulsatile system will influence both of these in a number of ways.

Most endocrine tests are conducted over short periods of time and their results are often extrapolated to longer time frames. For example, GH provocation tests used to assess the GH secretory state in children are performed over a 2-h period, and the results are then compared with height and growth velocity measurements obtained over a longer period of time, often 1 year. That there is a relationship is perhaps surprising; that there are high false-positive and false-negative rates, perhaps not. Hormone pulsatility may also influence diagnostic tests if the test itself (e.g. the stimulus applied) is influenced by oscillations within the system under study. It has been recognized for a long time that the GH

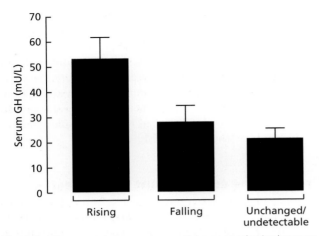

**Fig. 4.4.** GH response to exogenous growth hormone-releasing hormone depending upon whether pre-administration growth hormone levels are rising, falling or unchanged.

**Table 4.1.** Mean peak growth hormone response to insulin-induced hypoglycaemia with respect to peak and trough growth hormone concentrations in physiological profiles

|              | Low peaks | High peaks | Total |
|--------------|-----------|------------|-------|
| Low troughs  | 13.0      | 28.2       | 22.0  |
| High troughs | 7.6       | 21.4       | 13.9  |
| Total        | 9.8       | 25.1       |       |

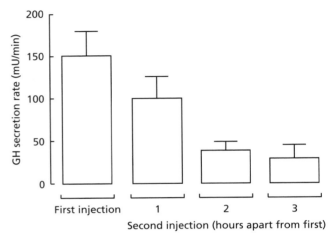

**Fig. 4.5.** Effect of differing time intervals on the growth hormone response to repeated growth hormone-releasing hormone administration.

response to insulin-induced hypoglycaemia is heavily influenced by the serum GH concentration measured at the commencement of the study. If it is measurable, a rise in GH in response to the hypoglycaemic stimulus is less likely [22].

Understanding hormone physiology is therefore essential both in defining the circadian rhythm in the variability of the hormone concentration under study and also in beginning to understand from the pattern of secretion what the underlying regulatory processes are. In the example quoted above of the GH response to insulin-induced hypoglycaemia, it is clear that the GH response at any point in time is going to be heavily dependent on the interplay between the hypothalamic regulatory proteins involved in GH release, namely GH-releasing hormone (GHRH) and somatostatin [23]. Figure 4.4 shows the effect of differing states of GH secretion before the application of a stimulus (GHRH) and how the response to the same exogenous stimulus varies. Subsequent studies have demonstrated that somatostatin, in particular, is a key determinant of the amount of GH released as a result of GHRH stimulation. Attempts have been made to take control of this variable [24] by pretreatment with somatostatin. GHRH combined with arginine is an alternative approach [25]. It was hoped that there would be advances in this area because of their potent GH-releasing qualities but they appear to suffer the same problems of reproducibility [26]. The importance of the trough concentration in determining GH responsivity and growth has also been demonstrated [27] (Table 4.1).

Other hormones and environmental factors also influence the amount of a hormone that may be released at any point in time. In the GH field, levels of thyroxine and cortisol, which directly alter gene transcription, influence the results obtained and these need to be controlled before undertaking a diagnostic study [28]. Similarly, the presence of high levels of glucose or free fatty acids may influence the response

obtained [29]. Alterations in sex steroid concentrations during puberty (or even during the course of the menstrual cycle) modify the gonadotrophin response to gonadotrophin-releasing hormone and the GH response to GHRH.

Endocrine systems are also subject to feedback from target tissues, and this is an issue not only in the interpretation of single provocation tests but also where second tests are performed in rapid succession to the first. This has been well documented in the growth hormone field, where a diminished response to GHRH can be observed if the second stimulus is applied 1, 2 or 3 h after the first [30] (Fig. 4.5). Cortisol responses to ACTH behave in a similar manner [31]. A gradual diminution in responsivity of the anterior pituitary can be documented with this type of approach. The implications of doing two tests on the same day, often following each other, are immense, because the cut-off that might be implied to determine normality or abnormality may not be the same for the second test as for the first, especially if the second stimulus is different from the first.

Many endocrine tests have been standardized in adults and conducted in the morning, a time of day when in the adult GH concentrations are low. This is acceptable for normal individuals but may not be for other situations. Acromegaly is associated with a failure of glucose administration to

**Table 4.2.** Within-individual coefficients of variation for pituitary hormones

|  | Coefficient of variation (1%) mean (range) |
| --- | --- |
| Mean 24-h serum GH concentration | 35 (9–58) |
| Mean 24-h serum LH concentration | 19 (5–29) |
| Serum IGF-I concentration | 21 (14–34) |
| Serum testosterone concentration | 13 (8–19) |

GH, growth hormone; IGF-I, insulin-like growth factor I; LH, luteinizing hormone.

suppress serum GH concentrations and a paradoxical rise in GH after the administration of exogenous thyrotrophin-releasing hormone (TRH). Similar situations have been reported in tall pubertal children and in patients with anorexia nervosa, diabetes mellitus or chronic renal failure [32–35], and the GH axis may well be normal. Results such as this can be predicted simply on the basis of the GH rhythm in these individuals rather than by defining any intrinsic abnormality in the regulation of GH secretion [34].

In assessing the results of endocrine evaluations, it is generally assumed that the single or multiple samples measured are relatively stable, at least over short periods. A thyroxine measurement on one day should be similar to one measured the next day or week. Although this may be generally true, it cannot be assumed. When important changes are postulated to be taking place, for example in a disease process, some knowledge of the inherent variability within the measurement system is required. In endocrine practice, we are well aware of the errors incurred in the measurement of hormones, and the between- and within-assay coefficients of variation greatly aid the interpretation of hormone measurements. In the short term, a number of studies have demonstrated variability within and between individuals in terms of endocrine tests [36–39]. Group data are usually reproducible but problems can arise if it is assumed that individual oscillatory profiles are consistent from day to day. Table 4.2 summarizes data relating to intraindividual coefficients of variation in 24-h hormone profiles measured over the course of 1 year [37]. These observations add an additional dimension to the comparison of studies obtained under one series of circumstances with a set obtained under another series of circumstances, particularly if they are separated by long periods of time.

Finally, it is clear from studies of acromegaly and Cushing disease, as well as physiological observations, that alterations in the exposure of target organs to the stimulating hormone greatly influences the end-organ response. Diagnosis of Cushing disease or acromegaly centres on establishing persistent elevation in cortisol or GH concentrations, but it is not necessary for this elevation to be great. More important is that there is no respite from persistent exposure to elevated levels.

From basic principles, analysis of hormone pulsatility tells the clinician that the chances of documenting the problem will be increased by increasing sample numbers. Taking a midnight and early-morning cortisol sample limits the probability of confirming the presence of disease, particularly when the variability in these parameters in the normal population is taken into account. A series of samples may be required.

### Sampling interval

The concept of generating false information by inappropriate sampling intervals is known as aliaising. The topic is covered in more detail in Chapter 2. Determining the correct sampling interval is part of the process involved in minimizing this problem. Knowledge of the half-life of the hormone is essential in order that a correct sampling interval can be created to obtain the required information. Using sampling intervals that are greater than the half-life of the hormone will lead to the potential for missing a response when it takes place and hence mislabelling the individual. Taking a large number of frequent samples will alleviate the problem, but this must be offset by the discomfort to the patient, the practicality and the expense. Sampling intervals need to be close to the half-life of the hormone under study but should not exceed it.

The sampling interval is also determined by the question. The use of the short Synacthen test with 30-min sampling is a reasonable approach for the assessment of the cortisol response to exogenous ACTH. To determine the response of cortisol precursors, such as 17-hydroxyprogesterone for the diagnosis of the heterozygous or homozygous state in congenital adrenal hyperplasia, 30-min sampling will not suffice. The 17-hydroxyprogesterone response occurs earlier than that of cortisol and might be missed by a 30-min sampling interval, except in the most extreme cases [38].

### Independent marker of stimulus application

In considering provocative tests, the situation may arise where no response is observed: a possible explanation is that the strength of the stimulus was insufficient to provoke hormone release. In such a situation, it is valuable to have an independent marker of stimulus application. In the insulin-induced hypoglycaemia test, this marker is glucose and the attainment of adequate hypoglycaemia. In the glucagon test, it may be the release of glucose. In other tests, there may be no independent markers so that doubt may be cast on the reliability of the non-response (e.g. of gonadotrophins to gonadotrophin-releasing hormone).

### How much stimulus to apply

Conventional endocrine tests use standard dosing schedules of the stimulus. These are usually adjusted for body size, but

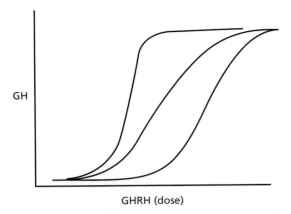

GH

GHRH (dose)

**Fig. 4.6.** Hypothetical dose–response curves to illustrate insensitivity, resetting and resistance.

all tend to generate a maximal response. This is reasonable if the investigator wishes to determine what is available under maximal stimulation (e.g. stress and cortisol release) but may not equate to the amount of hormone released to produce a target organ effect. Physiological studies of hormone release might be more meaningful than provocative studies. Rather than enter a debate in depth, it is probably more productive to consider what is actually required of the test in the first instance.

Maximal cortisol release can be achieved using doses of Synacthen, considerably less than that used in the standard Synacthen test [39,40]. The dose–response for cortisol is maximal to a concentration of ACTH at about 500–1000 ng per m$^2$ body surface area. This may detect more subtle forms of adrenal insufficiency [41]. Similarly, in the GH axis, GHRH tests are often used to show whether or not the gland is capable of releasing GH. However, more subtle questions might need to be asked, such as whether the gland has changed in its sensitivity to GHRH. A similar situation might be encountered in determining whether an individual has a degree of hormone insensitivity. Using the classic insulin-like growth factor I (IGF-I) generation test is unlikely to unravel subtleties in the target tissues. Figure 4.6 shows the dose–response curves that might be generated. A series of possible responses exist: there are those who are insensitive (reduced gradient of the dose–response curve), those that have reset their response (no change in gradient) but can still respond to a maximal stimulation and those who cannot, no matter how high the stimulus, achieve a maximal response (resistance).

### Is the test response reasonable?

Consideration needs to be given to the magnitude of the response to the stimulus. It is preferable that the response allows discrimination to be made between the normal and pathological situation. The response should be greater than the background hormone level in the unstimulated state. A

rise greater than three times the coefficient of variation of the assay at that concentration might be closer. Whatever is closer, the hormone levels should be easily measurable and responsible. Low but consistent responses seen in the heat (pyrogen) test are not helpful [42].

### Principles of diagnostic testing

The aim of any diagnostic test is to progress the clinical history and examination to the point where the care of the patient is altered. There is a vast and bewildering literature on GH testing, but the clinician can be guided by asking the questions detailed in Table 4.3.

Several of the points are considered further in this chapter, but the first two deserve special mention. First, it is unusual in endocrinology for there to be a diagnostic gold standard. The anterior pituitary is not accessible and molecular biology is not sufficiently advanced to give definitive answers. Care needs to be taken in ascribing the role of a gold standard. It may change with time but, more importantly, if it is infallible, no test, no matter how good, will ever surpass it. So, comparing the insulin tolerance test [ITT (the gold standard)] with 24-h profiles will always lead to the conclusion that the ITT is better; there could be no other conclusion [43]!

Second, the test must be well validated by application to large numbers of individuals with and without the condition. The temptation is to use the extremes but this may lead to a considerable overestimate of sensitivity and specificity [44] that may not be borne out in field studies [45,46].

### Normal ranges and cut-off values

Normal values in paediatric practice are the subject of many discussions. Performing many of the tests on normal children is unethical. Furthermore, standards would be needed for tall, normal and short children because their GH secretion differs [3]. In addition, both age and pubertal stage influence GH secretion [3] as does body composition [10,11]. Values for these would also have to be included.

The classic approach of defining normal data in terms of a Gaussian distribution does not come without hazard.

**Table 4.3.** Underlying principles of assessing tests

1. Has there been an independent blind comparison with the diagnostic 'gold standard'?
2. Was the test conducted in a wide range of patients with and without the condition?
3. Is the test reproducible?
4. What was the definition of normal in the test situation?
5. How might the test interact with others in a diagnostic sequence?
6. Does the test entail risk or reduce risk for the patient?

Endocrine testing rarely fits this distribution and, even if it did, it would imply that the lowest and highest 2.5% of values are abnormal and that all diseases have the same frequency – clearly unlikely. Creating upper and lower limits does not help either. It is more appropriate to identify a range of diagnostic test results beyond which the disorder of GHD is likely.

Most decisions on placing the value have been empirical rather than statistical. In practice, cut-off values could be chosen at an absolute extreme. If 100 short children were studied and GH sufficiency or deficiency was defined by a peak response of less than 5 mU/L, only 3–5% might have a response at this level. When testing the next 100 children, one or two normal individuals might have such a response. They will be outliers but they are important because the more patients studied, the greater the chance of finding outliers.

Moving the cut-off to more extreme values to exclude these patients restricts the population of treatable individuals. Relaxing the criteria interposes normal individuals into the diagnosis zone. Placing the cut-off is based partly on clinical judgement. As there is no disadvantage, apart from financial cost, in falsely labelling someone with GHD and treating them, a relaxed cut-off would be acceptable. A similar negotiation would be required in the consideration of other diagnostic tests in endocrinology. In the case of conditions such as acromegaly and Cushing disease we should probably err more on the side of caution, not least because of the nature of the treatments these conditions require.

## Specificity and sensitivity

Two principles operate when using diagnostic tests [21]. The first is that probability is a useful marker of diagnostic uncertainty. This is when the sensitivity (ability to detect a target disorder when present or true positive rate) and specificity (ability to identify correctly the absence of the disorder or true negative rate) become important. If both were 85%, 15% of patients with disease would have a negative result (false negative) and 15% without disease would have a positive result (false positive). Abnormal results would occur in patients with and without disease. Whatever the result, new information has been generated that may or may not influence decision-making. The second principle is that diagnostic tests should be obtained only when they can alter the management of the case, that is if the test result alters the probability of the disease. Sensitivity and specificity are important components of test performance, and Table 4.4 shows how they are calculated.

Sensitivity and specificity indicate how the test compares with the gold standard. But this is not quite what is required: in the clinical situation, it is more useful to know what a positive or negative test result means. Table 4.4 can yield more as it shows that 20 of 30 individuals (66%) with a positive test have GHD (positive predictive value) and 65 of 70 (93%) with

**Table 4.4.** Test results in 100 individuals with respect to a diagnosis of growth hormone (GH) insufficiency

| Test | GH insufficiency | | |
|------|---------|--------|-------|
| | Present | Absent | Total |
| Positive | 20 | 10 | 30 |
| Negative | 5 | 65 | 70 |
| Total | 25 | 75 | 100 |

Sensitivity = 20/25 = 80%.
Specificity = 65/75 = 87%.

a negative test do not (negative predictive value). The test can be used to generate these predictive values, which may or may not help strengthen the diagnosis.

Predictive values are easy to calculate but they are not constant and they change with the number of patients who have the target disorder. Applying the test to a different population from the one used to find the value in Table 4.4 might yield different results. For example, these results might have come from an endocrine service in which the prevalence of the condition would be expected to be higher than a community growth screening programme. If, in the latter, prevalence was 5% (probably less, given the data in the Utah Growth Study [47]) and the sensitivity and specificity were unchanged, then the positive predictive value would be 29% and the negative predictive value 99% – excellent for exclusion, but not for diagnosis.

## Pre- and post-test probability

The relationship between the probability of disease after the results of diagnostic tests are known (the post-test probability) and pre-test probability test of disease depends on the sensitivity and specificity of the test as shown in Fig. 4.7. There are two important points to note: the first is that the more certain the clinician is of the diagnosis before the test is performed, the less effect the confirmatory test has on the probability of disease. The obverse is also true. The second point is that tests will have major effects on the probability of disease in the intermediate zone. Testing is not likely to be beneficial if the pre-test probability is very high or low. This is one reason why screening for growth hormone secretory problems in short children on the basis of biochemical tests is unhelpful.

One problem that clinicians face is how to define the pre-test probability of the condition. Given the paucity of information on the prevalence of symptoms and signs associated with GHD in the general population, it is difficult at first sight to see how this can be achieved. There are a number of possible ways. The easiest is where a consensus is obtained from practising clinicians. This approach has been used in a

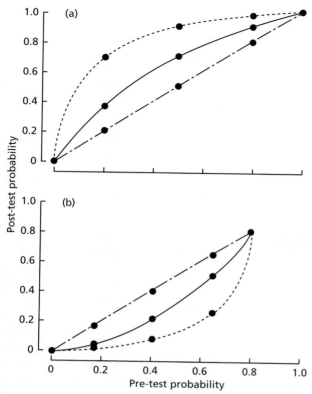

**Fig. 4.7.** The relation between pre-test and post-test probability of disease. The data were constructed using Bayes's theorem with a test sensitivity and specificity of either —, 70% or – – –, 90%. (a) The post-test probability if the test were positive; (b) the post-test probability if the test were negative. If the post-test probability were the same as the pre-test probability then the relation would be given by the 45° line.

**Table 4.5.** Growth hormone test results in situations of differing pre-test certainty

| Pre-test probability (%) | Post-test probability | |
|---|---|---|
| | Test positive | Test negative |
| 90 | 98 (+8) | 67 (−23) |
| 50 | 87 (+37) | 19 (−31) |
| 5 | 25 (+20) | 1 (−4) |

Change from pre-test probability in parenthesis.

was 5% (very certain that the patient does not have GHD) and the test is positive, all the result says is that the patient has a 1 in 4 chance of having the condition, so we would probably not treat. In the middle ground, certainty in either direction is dramatically improved.

## Multiple tests

Table 4.5 could have been made much larger by introducing the different pretreatment probabilities, as seen in Fig. 4.7. There comes a point, however, when post-test probability changes to a level where a decision has to be made to stop and either accept or reject the proposal that the condition is present. The decision to stop investigation and to treat or not depends on how convinced the clinician is of the diagnosis, the benefits and risks of the therapy and the potential yield and risks of further tests. There are two ways to assist this situation: conduct another test or use a more sophisticated analysis rather than a simple positive or negative.

This is problematic in the GH field because the methodology assumes that the results of the two tests are independent. The data about this are mixed. In normal individuals, undergoing repeat GHRH tests, dependence cannot be assumed [30]. Where repeat tests have been carried out in children, concordance was seen 50% of the time, a value close to that calculated for independent events using a test with a 70–85% efficiency. Another important issue is whether the test might change in individuals as they age. There is evidence that the clonidine test is less effective in releasing GH in young adults compared with that seen in children [48]. Whether the magnitude of the response to other stimuli can be assumed to remain unchanged is unknown.

Assuming that the two tests are carried out (on different days) and that they are dependent, the results could resemble Table 4.6. Here again, it has been assumed that the condition can be identified correctly by some other method. Results from these two tests can be combined and we can constrain the results so that both tests are positive and called positive; if both are negative or one or other is negative, then this is called negative (Table 4.7). The bottom of Table 4.7 shows the situation when both tests are negative.

slightly different manner in the area of clinical trials, in which case the issue is when to stop the clinical trial. Clinicians in this situation were asked before the study at what point they would accept that one treatment had a greater effect than another (e.g. 5%, 10% or 50% improvement). By obtaining this information it was possible to determine a pre-trial estimate of the level of improvement that would be required to convince sceptical clinicians compared with the enthusiasts for the study. Such a balance is useful and could be achieved in GHD by presenting a series of clinical scenarios to experienced clinicians and asking them to rate the probability that the individual will have GHD.

Clinicians are often faced with the situation where they feel really sure that the patient has the condition but the test does not confirm this. Table 4.5 analyses this concept. Here, specificity and sensitivity have been fixed and the effects on post-test probability are considered. In the situation of 90% pre-test probability that the patient is GH deficient, then, even if the test is negative in the individual, there is still a 67% probability (down 23%) that they have the condition, so treatment would still be justified. When the pre-test probability

**Table 4.6.** Results of applying two tests assessing growth hormone (GH) secretion (insulin-induced hypoglycaemia and clonidine) to patients with or without GH insufficiency

| | Insulin-induced hypoglycaemia | |
| --- | --- | --- |
| | Positive | Negative |
| Clonidine | | |
| Patients with GH insufficiency | | |
| Positive | 55 | 10 |
| Negative | 15 | 20 |
| Patients without GH insufficiency | | |
| Positive | 10 | 5 |
| Negative | 25 | 60 |

Replot on whether GH insufficiency present or absent and constraining both tests either to be positive or negative.

| | GH insufficiency | |
| --- | --- | --- |
| | Present | Absent |
| *Both tests positive for diagnosis | | |
| Both positive | 55 | 10 |
| One or both negative | 45 | 90 |
| Both tests negative to exclude | | |
| †Both positive | 80 | 40 |
| One or both negative | 20 | 60 |

*Sensitivity 55%; specificity 90%;
†Sensitivity 80%; specificity 60%.

**Table 4.7.** Information from Table 4.6 using different test combinations to define diagnosis

| | Growth hormone insufficiency | | |
| --- | --- | --- | --- |
| | Present | Absent | Cut-off |
| Both positive | 55 | 10 | Sensitivity 55% Specificity 90% |
| One positive | 25 | 30 | |
| Both negative | 20 | 60 | Sensitivity 80% Specificity 60% |

**Table 4.8.** Effect of applying different peak growth hormone (GH) cut-off values in response to insulin-induced hypoglycaemia for diagnosis of GH insufficiency

| GH concentrations (mU/L) | Efficiency (%) | Sensitivity (%) | Specificity (%) |
| --- | --- | --- | --- |
| 10 | 63 | 51 | 79 |
| 13.5 | 20 | 64 | 70 |
| 20 | 68 | 82 | 49 |

The assumption that both tests need to be positive maximizes specificity and avoids falsely labelling normal children, but it misses a lot of treatable individuals. Insisting that both tests are negative maximizes sensitivity, minimizes misdiagnoses but falsely labels a lot more normal children.

The construction of complex tables is largely an extension of these concepts but uses different levels of test result rather than having to rely on absolute cut-off values. Table 4.7 shows how the data from Table 4.6 can be used to produce three levels; we could demand that both tests are positive to give a sensitivity of 55% and a specificity of 90%, whereas both or only one is positive should give a sensitivity of 80% and a specificity of 60%. Table 4.8 gives an example of different cut-off values to define GH insufficiency/deficiency [49]. This would then serve as a base to allow post-test probability to be calculated to give an idea of how the diagnosis is changing.

More complex calculations can be used to produce probability ratios. These express the odds that a given level of diagnostic test result would be expected in a patient with GHD as opposed to one without this diagnosis. For a positive test, the likelihood ratio is sensitivity divided by (1—specificity). So, for Table 4.6, people with a positive GH test are 6.2 times as likely to come from patients with GH insufficiency/deficiency as from normal. The likelihood ratio for a negative test is the false-negative rate divided by specificity. This technique is independent of disease prevalence and can be applied at multiple cut-off levels. The most important value is that it allows for a sequence of tests to be created and a decision tree constructed. More details are given in Sackett *et al.* [50].

The concept of using complex tables such as these has not been used to any degree in endocrine practice. To illustrate the power of the approach further, an example from the gonadotrophin field can be worked [51]. LHRH and hCG (human chorionic gonadotrophin) tests were performed to try to differentiate hypogonadotrophic hypogonadism from delayed puberty. The authors concluded that sensitivity and specificity were good and that this combination of test was of value. There were problems with the data set: the individuals used to create the normal values were the same individuals who were used to evaluate the test. Further, although the authors discussed the issue of combining the tests, the combination was not tested in the formal manner described above. When this is done, different conclusions result. The tests are not so good for confirming the diagnosis of hypogonadotrophic hypogonadism; their strength lies in excluding the diagnosis.

One final area needs to be considered and this brings together the issue of two tests with pre-test probability. Several recent publications have suggested that individuals who were originally diagnosed with GHD do not appear to have the biochemical abnormality when the test is repeated later [52,53]. This has led to statements being made that these individuals are no longer GH insufficient, but a subtle mind shift has taken place. The clinicians have shifted subtly from wishing to make a diagnosis to one of excluding a diagnosis, without taking into account the laws of probability. Two issues are worth considering: the first is that the population studied during the second test is not the same as that during the first. Those studied during the first test, those thought unlikely to have the condition, have been excluded. If the absolutist approach were to be used, some of those not retested may have abnormal test results. A change of stance has taken place.

The second point also relates to some extent to the original diagnosis. It is worth rehearsing the scenario that has led to the second test. The child was initially evaluated because of concerns over short stature and poor growth. At that point a test was conducted because the clinician required an answer with which to rule in or rule out the diagnosis. Taking the situation depicted in Table 4.5, let us assume that the initial pre-test probability was 50% so that, having obtained a positive test, the post-test probability of the child having the condition rose to 87%. This value now forms the pre-test probability for the second test, not the 50:50 situation that the clinician faced before investigation. Information has been collected which influences the probability of the disease process being present. When the clinician comes to apply the second test, Table 4.5 shows that the post-test probability of the condition being present after the second test resides in the top line (98% of the test if the test is positive and 67% if the test is negative). It does not lie on the second line, which is the position that many clinicians have adopted by simply considering the second test not to be influenced by the acquisition of prior information.

The concept of acquisition of information during the course of evaluation is important. Clinical history and examination, along with the initial endocrinological investigation, changes the likelihood of disease being present. The situation does not stop at this point as additional information may be acquired such as that obtained from neuroimaging. For example, the presence of pituitary hypoplasia in a patient with GHD would significantly increase the likelihood of disease, whereas the clinician would be rightly sceptical of the GH test results in a situation where pituitary size is normal. This is because somatotroph mass makes up at least 50% of the size of the anterior pituitary. Neuroimaging may then be an important contributor to altering likelihood of disease, as would the growth response to intervention with GH therapy.

This is where the predictive models that have been derived [54,55] can be extremely important. If the response to inter-vention behaves along classic lines expected for severe GHD, this strengthens the likelihood that the individual has the condition. What is created is a huge decision tree whose branched structure represents all these pieces of information. The challenge to endocrinologists is to determine the strengths of the various components.

## Conclusions

Careful clinical assessments coupled with detailed anthropometric measurements are the keystone for the evaluation of any endocrinological disorder. The clinical features of endocrine disorders are not always pathognomonic. The presence of findings or a combination of findings that are specific but insensitive increase the likelihood of disease only slightly. In many situations in endocrine practice, there is no gold standard for diagnosis. In such a situation the application of probability to testing a hypothesis is essential. In the field of GH, the specificity and sensitivity of any of the tests of GH secretion are only 80%, so the clinician should expect false-positive and false-negative results. Careful consideration of test results in the light of probability theory needs to be made in order to maximize diagnostic certainty. The evaluation of an individual should not stop at the point that treatment is initiated, since ongoing information should be acquired from the response to GH therapy. Second tests of endocrine function need to be carefully constructed and interpreted in the light of probability theory. It is important at all stages to recognize that there are no absolutes and the clinician may operate effectively only when the likelihood of disease being present or absent is expressed in terms of probability.

## References

1 Milner RDG, Russell-Fraser T, Brook CGD *et al*. Experience with human growth hormone in Great Britain: the report of the MRC Working Party. *Clin Endocrinol* 1979; 11: 15–38.

2 Hindmarsh PC, Smith PJ, Brook CGD, Matthews DR. The relationship between height velocity and GH secretion in short prepubertal children. *Clin Endocrinol* 1987; 27: 581–91.

3 Albertsson-Wikland K, Rosberg S. Analysis of 24-hour growth hormone profiles in children: relation to growth. *J Clin Endocrinol Metab* 1988; 67: 493–500.

4 Tanner JM, Hiernaux J, Jarman S. Growth and physique studies. In: Weiner JS, Iounie JA, eds. *Human Biology: a Guide to Field Methods*. Oxford: Blackwell Scientific Publications, 1969.

5 Cameron N. *The Measurement of Human Growth*. London: Croom Helm, 1984.

6 Cox LA, Savage MD. Practical auxology: techniques of measurement and assessment of skeletal maturity. In: Kelnar CJH, Savage MD, Stirling HF, Saenger P, eds. *Growth Disorders: Pathophysiology and Treatment*. London: Chapman & Hall, 1998: 225–35.

7 Goossens M, Brauner R, Czernichow P, Duquesnoy P, Rappaport R. Isolated growth hormone deficiency Type 1A associated with a double deletion in the human growth hormone gene cluster. *J Clin Endocrinol Metab* 1986; 62: 712–16.

8 Wit JM, Van Unen H. Growth of infants with neonatal growth hormone deficiency. *Arch Dis Child* 1982; 67: 920–4.

9 Huet F, Carel J-C, Nivelon J-L, Chaussain J-L. Long term results of GH therapy in GH-deficient children treated before 1 year of age. *Eur J Endocrinol* 1999; 140: 29–34.

10 Rahim A, O'Niell P, Shalet SM. The effect of body composition on hecretin-induced growth hormone release in normal elderly subjects. *Clin Endocrinol* 1988; 49: 659–64.

11 Iranmanesh A, Lizaralde G, Veldhuis JD. Age and relative adiposity are specific negative determinants of the pregnancy and amplitude of growth hormone (GH) secretory bursts and the half-life of endogenous GH in healthy men. *J Clin Endocrinol Metab* 1991; 73: 1081–8.

12 Marcovitch H. Failure to thrive. *Br Med J* 1994; 308: 35–8.

13 Herber SM, Milner RDG. Growth hormone deficiency presenting under age 2 years. *Arch Dis Child* 1984; 59: 557–60.

14 Gluckman PD, Gunn A-J, Wray A. Congenital idiopathic growth hormone deficiency associated with early postnatal growth failure. *J Pediatr* 1992; 121: 920–3.

15 Vanderschuren-Lodeweyckx M, Wolter R, Mulla A *et al*. Plasma growth hormone in coeliac disease. *Acta Pediatr* 1973; 28: 349–57.

16 Crowley S, Hindmarsh PC, Matthews DR, Brook CGD. Growth and the growth hormone axis in prepubertal children with asthma. *J Pediatr* 1995; 126: 297–303.

17 Krieger DT, Allen W. Relationship of bioassayable and immunoassayable plasma ACTH and cortisol concentrations in normal subjects and in patients with Cushing's disease. *J Clin Endocrinol Metab* 1975; 40: 675–87.

18 Clayton RN, Royston JP, Chapman J *et al*. Is changing hypothalamic activity important for control of ovulation? *Br Med J* 1987; 295: 7–12.

19 Hunter WM, Friend JAR, Strong JA. The diurnal pattern of plasma growth hormone concentration in adults. *J Endocrinol* 1966; 34: 139–46.

20 Goodner CJ, Walike BC, Koerker DJ *et al*. Insulin, glucogen and glucose exhibit synchronous sustained oscillations in fasting monkeys. *Science* 1977; 195: 177–9.

21 Sox HC Jr. Probability theory in the use of diagnostic tests. *Ann Intern Med* 1986; 104: 60–6.

22 Youlton R, Kaplan SL, Grumbach MM. Growth and growth hormone. IV. Limitations of the growth hormone response to insulin and arginine in the assessment of growth hormone deficiency in children. *Pediatrics* 1969; 43: 989–1004.

23 Devesa J, Lima L, Lois N, Lechjga MJ, Arch V, Tresguerres JAF. Reasons for the variability in growth hormone (GH) responses to GHRH challenge: the endogenous hypothalamic–somatotroph rhythm (HSR). *Clin Endocrinol* 1989; 30: 367–77.

24 Tzanela M, Guyda H, Van Vliet G, Tannenbaum GS. Somatostatin pretreatment enhances growth hormone responsiveness to GH-releasing hormone: a potential new diagnostic approach to GH deficiency. *J Clin Endocrinol Metab* 1996; 81: 2487–94.

25 Bernasconi S, Volta C, Cozzini A *et al*. GH response to GHRH, insulin, clonidine and arginine after GHRH pretreatment in children. *Acta Endocrinol* 1992; 126: 105–8.

26 Massoud AF, Hindmarsh PC, Matthews DR, Brook CGD. The effect of repeated administration of hexarelin, a growth hormone releasing peptide, and growth hormone releasing hormone (GHRH) on growth hormone (GH) responsivity. *Clin Endocrinol* 1996; 44: 555–62.

27 Achermann JC, Brook CGD, Robinson ICAF, Matthews DR, Hindmarsh PC. Peak and trough growth hormone (GH) concentrations influence growth and serum like growth factor-1 (IGF-1) concentrations in short children. *Clin Endocrinol* 1999; 50: 301–8.

28 Pringle PJ, Stanhope R, Hindmarsh P, Brook CGD. Abnormal pubertal development in primary hypothyroidism. *Clin Endocrinol* 1988; 28: 479–86.

29 Cordido F, Fernandez T, Martinez T *et al*. Effect of acute pharmacological reduction of plasma free fatty acids on growth hormone (GH) releasing hormone-induced GH secretion in obese adults with and without hypopituitarism. *J Clin Endocrinol Metab* 1998; 4350–4.

30 Suri D, Hindmarsh PC, Matthews DR, Brain CE, Brook CGD. The pituitary gland is capable of responding to two successive doses of growth hormone releasing hormone (GHRH). *Clin Endocrinol* 1991; 34: 13–7.

31 Crowley S, Hindmarsh PC, Honour JW, Brook CGD. Reproducibility of the cortisol response to stimulation with a low dose of ACTH (1–24): the effect of basal cortisol levels and comparison of low-dose with high-dose secretory dynamics. *J Endocrinol* 1993; 136: 167–72.

32 Hindmarsh PC, Stanhope R, Kendall BE, Brook CGD. Tall stature. A clinical, endocrinological and radiological study. *Clin Endocrinol* 1976; 81: 1–8.

33 Maeda K, Kato Y, Yamaguchi N *et al*. Growth hormone release following thyrotrophin releasing hormone injection into patients with anorexia nervosa. *Acta Endocrinol* 1976; 81: 1–8.

34 Edge JA Human DH, Matthews DR *et al*. Spontaneous growth hormone (GH) pulsatility is the major determinant of the GH release after the thyrotrophin-releasing hormone in adolescent diabetics. *Clin Endocrinol* 1989; 30: 397–404.

35 Gonzalez-Barcena D, Kastin AJ, Schalch DG *et al*. Responses to thyrotrophin releasing hormone in patients with renal failure and after infusion in normal men. *J Clin Endocrinol Metab* 1973; 35: 117–20.

36 Donaldson DL, Holowell JG, Pan F, Gifford RA, Moore WV. Growth hormone secretion profiles: variation on consecutive nights. *J Paediatr* 1989; 115: 51–6.

37 Saini S, Hindmarsh PC, Matthews DR *et al*. Reproducibility of 24 h serum growth hormone profiles in man. *Clin Endocrinol* 1991; 34: 455–62.

38 Bridges NA, Hindmarsh PC, Pringle PJ, Honour JW, Brook CGD. Cortisol, androsteredine, dehydroepidrosterone sulphate and 17 hydroxyprogesterone responses to low dose of (1–24)ACTH. *J Clin Endocrinol Metab* 1998; 83: 3750–3.

39 Rasmuson S, Olsson T, Hagg E. A low dose ACTH test to assess the function of the hypothalamic–pituitary–adrenal axis. *Clin Endocrinol* 1996; 44: 151–6.

40 Zoelkers W. Comment on comparison of the low dose short synacthen test, the conventional dose short synacthen test and the insulin tolerance test for the assessment of the hypothalamic–pituitary–adrenal axis in patients with pituitary disease. *J Clin Endocrinol Metab* 1999; 84: 2973–4.

41 Agwu JC, Spoudeas H, Hindmarsh PC, Pringle PJ, Brook CGD. Tests of adrenal insufficiency. *Arch Dis Child* 1999; 80: 330–3.

42 Fisher S, Jorgensen JD, Orskov H, Christiansen JS. GH stimulation tests: evaluation of GH responses to heat test vs. insulin-tolerance test. *Eur J Endocrinol* 1998; 139: 605–10.

43 Rose SR, Ross JL, Uriarte M, Barnes KM, Cassorla FG, Cutler GB. The advantages of measuring stimulated as compared with spontaneous growth hormone levels in the diagnosis of growth hormone deficiency. *N Engl J Med* 1988; 319: 201–7.

44 Blum WF, Ranke MB, Kietzmann K, Gauggel E, Zeisel HJ, Bierich JR. A specific radioimmunoassay for the growth hormone (GH)-dependent somatomedin-binding protein: its use for diagnosis of GH deficiency. *J Clin Endocrinol Metab* 1990; 70: 1292–8.

45 Tillman V, Buckler JM, Kibirge MS *et al*. Biochemical tests in the diagnosis of childhood growth hormone deficiency. *J Clin Endocrinol Metab* 1997; 82: 531–5.

46 Mitchell H, Dattani MT, Nanduri V, Hindmarsh PC, Preece MA, Brook CGD. Failure of IGF-1 and IGFBP-3 to diagnose growth hormone insufficiency. *Arch Dis Child* 1999; 80: 443–7.

47 Lindsay R, Feldkamp M, Harris D, Robertson J, Rallison M. Utah Growth Study: growth standards and the prevalence of growth hormone deficiency. *J Paediatr* 1994; 125: 29–35.

48 Rahim A, Toogood A, Shalet SM. The assessment of growth hormone status in normal young adult males using a variety of provocative tests. *Clin Endocrinol* 1996; 45: 557–62.

49 Dattani MT, Pringle PJ, Hindmarsh PC, Brook CGD. What is a normal stimulated growth hormone concentration? *J Endocr* 1992; 133: 447–50.

50 Sackett DL, Haynes RB, Guyatt GH, Tugwell P. *Clinical Epidemiology: A Basic Science for Clinical Medicine*, 2nd edn. Boston, MA: Little-Brown, 1991: 144.

51 Dunkel L, Perheentupa J, Virtanen M, Maenpaa J. Gonadotropin-releasing hormone test and human chorionic gonadotropin deficiency in prepubertal boys. *J Paediatr* 1985; 107: 388–92.

52 Wacharasindhu S, Cotterill AM, Comacho-Hubner C, Besser GM, Savage MD. Normal growth hormone secretion in growth hormone insufficient children re-tested after completion of linear growth. *Clin Endocrinol* 1986; 45: 553–6.

53 Tauber M, Houlin P, Pienkowski C, Jouret B, Rochiccioli P. Growth hormone (GH) retesting and auxological data in 131 GH-deficient patients after completion of treatment. *J Clin Endocrinol Metab* 1997; 82: 352–6.

54 Tanner JM, Whitehouse RH, Hughes PC, Vince FP. Effects of human growth hormone treatment for 1–7 years on growth of 100 children with growth hormone deficiency, low birth weight, inherited smallness, Turner's syndrome and other complaints. *Arch Dis Child* 1971; 46: 745–82.

55 Ranke MB, Lindberg A. Approach to predicting the growth response during growth hormone treatment. *Acta Paediatr* 1996; 85 (Suppl.) (147): 64–65.

# 5 The placenta

## J. C. P. Kingdom, W. L. Whittle and M. D. Kilby

## Introduction

The birth of a healthy infant at term is dependent upon normal placental development. Conversely, disordered placentation is responsible for a wide range of pregnancy complications ranging from miscarriage (embryonic death), through second-trimester fetal death, to the classic third-trimester complications of pre-eclampsia, intrauterine growth restriction (IUGR) and abruption (premature placental separation [1]). Even in situations where standard obstetric outcomes (birthweight, cord blood gases and Apgar scores) are normal, a more subtle degree of placental dysfunction may, through the emerging concept of 'perinatal programming', lead to significant morbidity and disease in later life [2].

## Early events in placentation

Placentation begins with implantation of the blastocyst beneath the uterine epithelium 5 days after fertilization and differentiation into embryonic and extra-embryonic tissues, the latter forming the definitive chorioallantoic placenta. Important cell fate decisions are necessary in order that the placenta communicates with the mother, to prevent menstruation in the first instance [3]. The trophoblast compartment of the placenta proliferates and forms a syncytial 'shell' that surrounds the embryo, excluding maternal blood. Embryogenesis thus takes place in an environment that is significantly hypoxic relative to the well-perfused maternal decidua [4]; this may be designed to limit the possibility of oxidative stress during critical periods of embryonic development [5].

The proliferating mononuclear trophoblast includes a stem cell population that is capable of differentiating either as extravillous trophoblast, which invades the uterine stroma and maternal blood vessels, or as villous cytotrophoblast, which surrounds the floating and anchoring villi [6]. Villous development takes place in the entire shell around the embryo. However, as the conceptus grows rapidly and projects into the uterine cavity, those villi overlying the embryo regress through apoptosis to leave a layer of trophoblast cells known as the chorion laeve or smooth chorion. The chorion laeve fuses with the decidua of the uterine wall opposite that of the developing placental disc. Regulation of prostaglandin production by these membranes is a critical pathway for the initiation of labour.

Towards the end of the first trimester, when embryogenesis is completed, the trophoblast lineage consists of three cell types: an extravillous trophoblast in contact with maternal vessels, the villous trophoblast covering the floating villi in the intervillous space and the chorion laeve in contact with decidua and myometrium. Each of these trophoblast subtypes has distinct endocrine roles during fetal development and parturition.

## Extravillous trophoblast: development of the uteroplacental circulation

Extravillous trophoblast (EVT) surrounds the embryo, proliferating in response to a locally hypoxic environment within the maternal decidua. Proximal EVT forms anchoring columns as a result of its surface expression of integrins. More distally, the EVT separates and invades the uterine stroma because of a switch in integrin expression and local secretion of matrix proteins [7]. The predominant pathway of EVT invasion is stromal, although a small amount of EVT proliferates inside and thus occludes maternal vessels (spiral arterioles, venules and capillaries) [8,9]. A debate continues as to the onset of maternal blood flow inside the placenta [10,11].

The molecular control of EVT invasion is becoming clearer. The tips of first-trimester human placental villi can be explanted to study *in vitro* the effects of lowering oxygen tension upon EVT behaviour. Low oxygen tension (2% ambient oxygen tension) results in increased hypoxia-inducible factor 1 (HIF1) and transforming growth factor $\beta_3$ (TGF-$\beta_3$) expression and EVT proliferation, and antisense disruption of HIF1 or TGF-$\beta_3$ synthesis prevents hypoxia-induced EVT proliferation [12]. Proliferation studies show that only the proximal portion of the explanted tips progress through mitotic cell cycles [13]. The distal trophoblast retains S-phase markers because of endoreduplication to 8–16N complement of chromosomes.

A similar transition from mitotic to endoreduplication cell cycles occurs in the mouse placenta [14]; this process is controlled by transcription factors Mash2 and Hand1 [15] although transcriptional control of EVT differentiation has not yet been described in humans. Persistent mitosis in EVT is a feature of placental chorionic malignancy or gestational trophoblast disease [16]. The invasive nature of EVT breaches the maternal vasculature, bringing maternal blood into direct contact with the syncytiotrophoblast covering of the chorionic villi. The number of anatomical layers separating maternal and fetal blood is reduced to three (villous trophoblast, stroma and fetoplacental vascular endothelium). The resultant direct contact of maternal blood with the villous syncytiotrophoblast of the chorionic villi gives rise to the term haemochorial placentation.

In other primate species, placentation may be less invasive; for example, placentation is epithelio-chorial in sheep [17]. This difference may be important in translating endocrine knowledge for placental function from control of parturition in sheep to humans [18].

## Development of chorioallantoic placental villi

Human placental villi form in three stages, beginning 2 weeks after fertilization. Cytotrophoblast columns within the syncytium proliferate laterally as side branches known as *primary villi*. They are transformed into *secondary villi* by the central invasion of allantoic mesenchyme. Blood vessels form within this stroma, resulting in *tertiary villi*, and subsequently connect to the developing umbilical cord to establish the fetoplacental circulation. During the second trimester, the tertiary villi undergo extensive branching angiogenesis, transforming them into immature intermediate villi [19]. Fetal cardiac output and blood pressure rise, and Doppler studies of the umbilical arteries show a progressive rise in end-diastolic velocities [20]. Proximally, the immature intermediate villi differentiate into stem villi containing muscularized arterioles that lack innnervation by the autonomic nervous system [21]. Fetoplacental blood flow is therefore regulated by both the anatomical configuration of the vessels and the local endothelium–smooth muscle cell interactions [22].

Villous development throughout pregnancy is driven by three phases of vascular growth: vasculogenesis, branching angiogenesis and non-branching angiogenesis [23]. By 26–28 weeks of gestation, 10–16 generations of stem villi have formed. Subsequent development of the placenta then focuses on the peripheral gas and nutrient-exchanging structures in preparation for a rapid phase in fetal growth. To achieve this, immature intermediate villi transform into their mature counterparts, the mature intermediate villi, by stromal condensation [19]. In these structures, the longitudinal growth of capillaries exceeds that of the villi themselves, such that the villi stretch and capillary loops 'prolapse' laterally to form *terminal villi*. The active forward growth of the capillaries displaces cytotrophoblast and stroma, leaving only a thin layer of syncytiotrophoblast, the vasculo-syncytial membrane, separating maternal and fetal blood. The process of forming terminal villi occurs exponentially in the third trimester. It follows that this phase of placental growth is characterized by a predominance of non-branching angiogenesis in mature intermediate villi. By term, the surface area available for gas exchange in terminal villi reaches 13 m$^2$ [24] and their capillaries contain some 80 mL (25%) of total fetoplacental blood volume.

## Vascular development in chorionic villi

A number of growth factors and their receptors are expressed in the human placenta, the best-studied to date being the vascular endothelial growth factor (VEGF) family. In the human placenta, VEGF is expressed in villous (trophoblast and stromal Hofbauer cells) and maternal decidual cells during the first trimester. Circulating VEGF can be detected in maternal plasma at 6 weeks of gestation and rises to a peak at the end of the first trimester, in parallel with hCG [25]. Villous trophoblast VEGF expression appears to decline as pregnancy advances and has been confirmed by Western and Northern blotting studies [26]. *VEGF* transcription is induced under hypoxic conditions by HIF1, which has recently been described in the human placenta [12]. Secreted VEGF mediates its actions via two tyrosine kinase receptor isoforms, VEGF-R1 (flt-1) and VEGF-R2 (KDR).

VEGF-R2 binding by VEGF induces endothelial cell proliferation and thus angiogenesis, whereas binding to VEGF-R1 stimulates endothelial nitric oxide synthase (eNOS) and leads to inhibition of cytotrophoblast proliferation. VEGF induces branching angiogenesis *in vitro*, as demonstrated in the chick chorioallantoic membrane and avascular cornea assay. These data suggest that VEGF acting via VEGF-R2 may be responsible for the extensive branching angiogenesis found in the immature intermediate villi during the second trimester.

Placenta-like growth factor (PlGF) shares 53% sequence homology with VEGF. Synthesis appears localized to the villous and extravillous trophoblast, in contrast to VEGF. PlGF acts exclusively through the receptor VEGF-R1, although its angiogenic activity may be mediated in part by forming heterodimers with VEGF. The quality of angiogenesis induced by PlGF differs from VEGF in two ways. First, PlGF expression is stimulated by oxygen, which is opposite to VEGF; second, it appears to induce non-branching angiogenesis. Placental PlGF mRNA and protein levels both increase as gestation advances, which is in contrast to VEGF. This gradual shift in balance from the actions of VEGF to PlGF may explain the change in villous angiogenesis to the non-branching type necessary for the formation of terminal villi. VEGF-directed vasculogenesis and angiogenesis are modified during the process of placental villous differentiation as, for example, most of the peripheral capillaries in immature intermediate villi regress, whereas central capillaries transform into conductance vessels. Candidate genes for these processes include the angiopoietin and angiostatin families [23].

## Trophoblast deportation into the maternal circulation

The trophoblast compartment of the placental villi comprises a terminally differentiated syncytiotrophoblast layer, beneath which exists a discontinuous layer of proliferating cytotrophoblast. After cytotrophoblast division and syncytial fusion, DNA transcription and RNA translation largely cease [27]. Calculations from morphological studies indicate a 3 g/day excess of trophoblast loss in addition to that needed to cover growing villi [28]. This excess of trophoblast, typically shed as syncytial knots that have completed apoptosis, can be detected in the maternal circulation [29] and is filtered in the lungs.

Apoptosis is a physiological event in trophoblast biology; it may occur to excess in certain situations, such as intrauterine growth restriction [30], leading to a reduction in energy transport systems [31] that restricts nutrient transport and damages the protective barrier between mother and fetus. Trophoblast shed into the maternal circulation may be used for non-invasive prenatal diagnosis [32] and may incite graft-versus-host reactions in maternal skin in the third trimester, which manifests as pruritus and urticarial papules in pregnancy [33] and may explain the preponderance of systemic autoimmune diseases in women [34].

## Endocrine aspects of fetal growth

### Insulin-like growth factor family

The family of insulin-like growth factors (IGFs) participates in the development of the uteroplacental circulation and fetal growth [35,36]. IGF-I and IGF-II are secreted by the extravillous trophoblast. *In vitro* experiments indicate a role for IGF-II in promoting invasion in an autocrine manner [37]. The paracrine actions of locally synthesized IGF are controlled by the secretion of IGF-binding proteins, principally IGFBP-3, in the maternal decidua. The importance of IGF signalling to mammalian placentation has been elucidated from studies in mice [38]. IGF-I appears to increase the proliferation and migrating activity of proximal extravillous trophoblast (the ectoplacental cone), whereas IGF-II-promoted endoreduplication (resulting in terminally differentiated EVT) [39], sug-

gesting a cascade role for these proteins during trophoblast invasion.

The genetics of IGF signal regulation are interesting. Mouse and human IGF-II are imprinted, as only the male-derived allele is expressed in trophoblast [40]. By contrast, in mouse and most humans, IGF-R2 is maternally imprinted [41]. Gene-targeting studies demonstrate the positive influence of IGF-I, IGF-II and their receptors on fetal growth. However, in such a large family, a degree of genetic redundancy is likely and this is the case for IGFBP-2, as the null phenotype in mice shows no alteration in fetal growth factor [42].

Self-regulation of IGF-II has also been identified [43]. The IGF-II gene generates multiple mRNAs with different 5' untranslated regions (5' UTRs) termed IGF-II mRNA-binding proteins (IMPs) that are translated in a differential manner during development and suppress IGF-II translation. In mice, IMPs are produced in the placenta at day 12.5 and decline towards birth.

## Leptin

Leptin is the translated product of the obesity (*OB*) gene that confers satiety, thereby reducing food intake [44]. Circulating leptin concentrations increase in maternal blood during pregnancy and are elevated further in women with pre-eclampsia [45]. Maternal levels correlate with maternal but not neonatal anthropometric measures of fat storage [46]. Cord blood leptin correlates positively with birthweight and placental weight [46]. *In situ* hybridization studies indicate that leptin and its receptor are expressed in syncytiotrophoblast, and are increased in diabetic pregnancies [47]. Placental leptin may be involved in the pathogenesis of pre-eclampsia [48] and obesity is common among the mothers and offspring of pregnancies complicated by pre-eclampsia at term [49].

## Parturition

Activation of the fetal hypothalamo-pituitary-adrenal (HPA) axis is associated with birth in many species. The rise in fetal plasma glucocorticoid (GC) increases prostaglandin (PG) production, which in turn activates the myometrium, ripens the cervix and leads to active labour [50]. Prostaglandin production is indirectly influenced by GC production; in sheep, GC increases oestradiol production, whereas, in humans, GC increases corticotrophin-releasing hormone (CRH) production [51]. The role of the placenta in initiating labour in sheep is illustrated in Fig. 5.1.

After fetal HPA activation, PG production by the placenta is increased via up-regulation of the enzyme prostaglandin synthase type II (PGHS-II). This up-regulates placental P450c17 hydroxylase, thereby diverting pregnenolone to form oestrogen rather than progesterone. Oestrogen and oestradiol

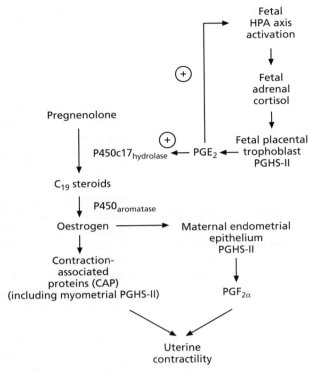

**Fig. 5.1.** Endocrine pathways in the initiation of labour in the sheep.

rise as progesterone falls, which explains the 'progesterone withdrawal' theory of labour.

In human parturition, activation of the fetal HPA axis is associated with labour, and the fetal membranes are thought to be the principal site of intrauterine PG production (Fig. 5.2). These membranes are composed of an amniotic epithelium, a mesenchymal layer and the chorionic laeve trophoblast layer. PGHS-II expression increases during labour in all three layers of the membranes [52] and, *in vitro*, GC increases amnion and chorion PG synthesis [53]. PG catabolism is regulated by prostaglandin dehydrogenase (PGDH), which is expressed in both the chorion layer of the fetal membranes and the villous syncytiotrophoblast [54].

Activities of this enzyme in cultured chorion trophoblast cells and explants are reduced in labour at term compared with non-labouring tissues [55]. Cortisol decreases PGDH activity to increase PG output by chorionic trophoblast cells *in vitro* [56]. The local bioavailability of cortisol in tissues is under the influence of 11β-hydroxysteroid dehydrogenase (11β-HSD) (Fig. 5.3), which interconverts active cortisol to inactive cortisone. Two major isoforms exist. Type 1, which is bi-directional, but generally acts as a reductase converting cortisone to cortisol, i.e. increasing local GC activity. 11β-HSD type II (11β-HSD-II) acts as a dehydrogenase, limiting local GC activity. The type II isoform is inducible and is expressed principally in kidney and placenta. Thus placental

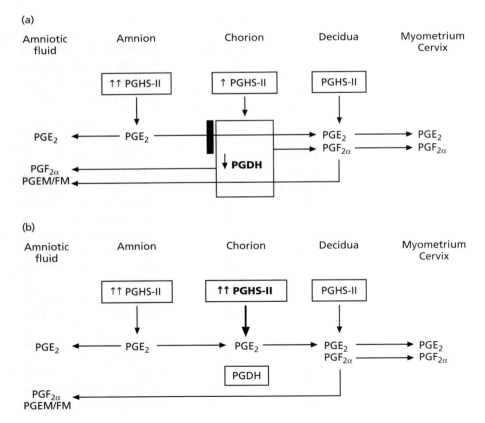

**Fig. 5.2.** Comparison of endocrine control of term (a) and preterm (b) labour in humans.

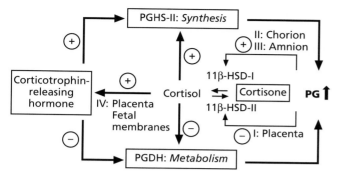

**Fig. 5.3.** Role of cortisol and corticotrophin-releasing hormone (CRH) in the regulation of prostaglandin production and labour in humans.

11β-HSD-II protects the fetus from high GC concentrations in the maternal compartment but in addition indirectly influences the activity of the fetal HPA axis. Increased 11β-HSD-II activity in syncytiotrophoblast towards term is induced by oestrogen [57], which reduces the negative influence on the fetal HPA axis resulting in fetal adrenal maturation.

PGs inhibit 11β-HSD-II activity [58]. Increased intrauterine PG production therefore decreases cortisol inactivation in the placenta, allowing more transplacental passage of maternal GC. A final factor influencing labour is corticotrophin-releasing factor (CRH), a hypothalamic peptide that is also produced in increasing quantities by the syncytiotrophoblast (Fig. 5.3). Placental CRH production increases in pregnancy [59] and CRH may induce relaxation of the lower uterine segment [60]. CRH promotes uteroplacental blood flow and increases PG production by differential effects upon PGDH and PGHS-II.

## Placental pathology

Placental pathology is extremely common; first trimester miscarriages with normal chromosomes (10%), pre-eclampsia (3%), preterm birth < 32 weeks of gestation (3%), premature placental separation (abruption) (1%) and intrauterine growth restriction (IUGR) (3%) together occur in 1 in 5 women [1]. Fetal lethality and IUGR are twice as common in males than in females [61] and umbilical artery Doppler studies are more frequently abnormal in males than in females [62]. These data suggest that genes controlling trophoblast function and placental development reside on the X chromosome.

Placental pathology may be multilayered. There may be developmental defect(s) in uterine artery transformation [7] or in chorionic villous development [63]. Chorionic villous development may be exaggerated by external influences such as altitude [64] or iron deficiency [65]. Maternal hypertension may perturb placental development through oxidative damage or thrombosis in the placenta, as may several systemic diseases. Drugs such as aspirin [66], vitamins C and E [67] or

heparin [68] may be used to try and preserve placental function in pregnancies at high risk for recurrent placental pathology.

## Intrauterine growth restriction

The more severe forms of IUGR that result in preterm delivery by caesarean section are associated with reduced fetoplacental blood flow (absent or even reversed end-diastolic flow velocities in the umbilical arteries) and chronic fetal hypoxia, increasing the risk of perinatal death, major morbidity and neurodevelopmental handicap in survivors [69]. Intensive ultrasound monitoring of fetal well-being, together with planned delivery by elective caesarean section, is necessary to prevent fetal death and reverse the associated severe pre-eclampsia that occurs in 40% of such cases [70]. Histological examination of placentas from these pregnancies shows a number of features of placental insufficiency, including placental infarction, widespread apoptosis of the syncytiotrophoblast, reduced development of gas-exchanging villi [63], and excessive oxidative stress in the vascular endothelium [71]. Damage to this placental barrier may be of relevance to fetal development because one important function of the trophoblast barrier is to exclude maternal corticosteroids from the developing fetus. Fetal brain development in IUGR may be perturbed by hypothyroidism and altered receptor expression within the fetoplacental unit [72].

## Pre-eclampsia

Pre-eclampsia is a multisystem disorder with onset after 20 weeks of gestation. It comprises hypertension, proteinuria and a variable degree of damage to the brain, liver and vascular systems [73]. The condition requires a placenta, but not a fetus, and reverses gradually after delivery.

Uteroplacental ischaemia is central to the pathogenesis of this condition [74] but the disease varies in its onset and severity and is influenced by racial origin, baseline blood pressure and body habitus. Pre-eclampsia at term is generally mild and associated with normal to increased birthweight [75]. More detailed studies indicate that pre-eclampsia at term is associated with placental hypertrophy, normal uterine Doppler blood flow and neonatal obesity [49]. By contrast, early-onset disease is more common in male fetuses, and is associated with abnormal uterine Doppler studies and significant IUGR [62].

The nature of placental hypertrophy in pre-eclampsia has not been established in cohort studies, but pathology series indicate a number of structural features, including cytotrophoblast proliferation, known as Tenney–Parker changes, which are suggestive of uteroplacental ischaemia [76]. Placental explants cultured under hypoxic conditions *in vitro* exhibit cytotrophoblast proliferation, although a concomitant reduction in syncytial fusion results in necrotic rather than apoptotic shedding [77]. As pre-eclampsia is characterized by an exaggerated systemic inflammatory response [78], a novel view of this disorder is that placental ischaemia shifts the balance of trophoblast shedding to necrotic material, thereby damaging the maternal vascular endothelium.

## Preterm labour: control of prostaglandin production

Preterm labour is multifactorial. By causing more than 70% of all preterm deliveries, it is clearly the major cause of perinatal morbidity and mortality. Some preterm labour is due to occult lower genital tract infection involving organisms of low pathogenic potential [79]. Preterm premature rupture of the membranes (PPROM) and preterm labour overlap but are normally considered distinct entities. From an endocrine perspective, the placenta and membranes produce contractile prostaglandins to effect delivery (Fig. 5.2); PGDH activity has been found to be reduced in the fetal membranes in some instances of preterm labour [80], whereas the activity of PGHS is increased.

Many aspects of placental endocrine function are disturbed in preterm labour and some may be detectable in maternal blood. Maternal CRH levels (Fig. 5.3) may be elevated before the onset of preterm labour [81]. Maternal plasma oestriol levels, which reflect activity of the fetal HPA axis, are increased in women before the development of idiopathic preterm labour, and prospective screening of maternal salivary oestriol identifies two-thirds of women destined to deliver preterm, although this is with a false-positive rate of 23% [82]. The consequences of increased fetal HPA activation include cervical ripening, and a prematurely short cervix identified by transvaginal ultrasound is highly predictive of extreme preterm birth [83]. Integration of maternal endocrinology and cervical ultrasound will probably improve our ability to predict the subset of women at greatest risk for preterm birth due to premature activation of the fetal HPA axis.

The expression of key enzymes regulating the production of PG by the placenta resides in the syncytiotrophoblast component of the villous trophoblast. As differentiation of the syncytial layer is intimately linked to the gradual switch from immature to mature villi, it follows that the ability of the placenta to trigger labour is related to villous differentiation. Placental villi from post-term pregnancies are relatively immature, while a significant proportion, perhaps one-third of placentas from 'unexplained' preterm labour patients, exhibit accelerated villous maturation [84]. The basis of this pathology is unknown and may just reflect a propensity for preterm birth to be triggered by placental thrombosis and uteroplacental ischaemia [85]. Alternatively, the explanation(s) for genetic, familial and recurrence risks for preterm birth could equally reside in the inheritance of genes influencing uterine contractility via their effects upon villous

differentiation. This concept of a placental clock is not new [86], but the idea that villous types vary in their ability to generate PG is, and deserves further study.

## Perinatal programming and the placenta

### Placental hypertrophy

The placenta is a plastic organ, capable of reacting to its external environment in order to achieve fetal survival. As it is highly vascular, and many vascular growth factor genes have hypoxia-sensitive promoters, the placenta can be viewed both as an oxygen-sensing and as an oxygen-transferring organ. Increased peripheral vascularization, and therefore increased placental weight, occur in several 'preplacental hypoxia' situations, such as iron-deficient anaemia [65] and high altitude [87]. Poor development of the uteroplacental circulation due to defective trophoblast invasion may likewise increase peripheral placental vascularization [76]. The placenta appears to alter its structure in response to the external environment even before embryogenesis is completed. Histological examination of first-trimester placentas from anaemic women shows gross alterations in the organization of fetal chorionic vessels [88]. These changes may affect right ventricular afterload during fetal life, as the placenta is perfused via the ductus arteriosus. Interestingly, anaemic rat pups have enlarged right ventricles [89]. These data provide a bench-to-bedside example of how one pathway of perinatal programming may be averted, namely to ensure women understand the importance of both iron and folate supplementation before conception [90].

### The placental cortisol barrier

Passage of maternal cortisol from mother to fetus is prevented by expression of the enzyme 11β-HSD-II in syncytiotrophoblast, such that a 3:1 gradient exists between the two circulations that converts the active steroid cortisol to cortisone [91–94]. Placental trophoblast 11β-HSD-II expression is severely reduced in villous placental tissues from pregnancies complicated by early-onset IUGR as a result of severe placental insufficiency [95] with a concomitant increase in fetal cortisol levels [94]. Fetal overexposure to cortisol may partly explain the inhibition of fetal growth associated with abnormal umbilical artery Doppler waveforms. In sheep experiments, administration of antenatal steroids results in IUGR [96], postnatal hypertension [97] and impaired glucose metabolism [98] similar to the syndrome X phenotype in adulthood [99]. An accumulating body of evidence illustrating the adverse effects of maternally administered steroids [100] is beginning to confine the use of repeated courses of antenatal steroid to randomized control trials.

Short-term exposure of the fetus at risk of preterm birth to maternal corticosteroids appears to be beneficial by accelerating lung differentiation [101]. However, the vast majority of fetuses at risk of preterm labour are in fact appropriately grown for gestational age. There is evidence that short-term steroids increase fetal oxygen consumption and lead to transient lactic acidosis in healthy sheep fetuses [102], and these effects may be manifest as alterations in fetal heart rate patterns, both in sheep and in humans [103]. Acute deterioration in fetal health leading to caesarean section has been noted anecdotally in preterm IUGR fetuses given steroids to assist lung maturation, suggesting that this subgroup does not tolerate steroids well. More recently, serial Doppler studies have been conducted to assess fetal well-being during steroid administration. Umbilical artery end-diastolic flow appears to reappear in severe IUGR, and although this has been interpreted as reassuring the waveforms show declining systolic function [104]. More studies are required to assess the risks and benefits of steroids in IUGR fetuses that have been chronically exposed to excessive maternal cortisol [100]. Many clinicians still offer multiple courses of steroids (betamethasone or dexamethasone) to women at risk of preterm delivery [105] but, in the light of long-term concerns [100], they should be confined to randomized control trials.

## Factors influencing placental weight

Epidemiological studies illustrate that the determinants of placental weight are more complex that mere oxygen supply. Smoking in excess of 10 cigarettes per day appears to increase placental weight [106]. The effects are sensed early by the placenta, as alterations in chorionic development can be detected early in the first trimester [107]. A recent cohort study of 1650 healthy pregnant Caucasian mothers found no effect of mild smoking upon placental weight, but pre-eclampsia was the predominant factor controlling fetal weight, conferring a 15–20% increase above that of normotensive controls (J. C. P. Kingdom, unpublished observation). As the majority of these pre-eclamptic pregnancies had normal uterine artery Doppler waveforms, it is unlikely that uteroplacental hypoxia was responsible for the excess placental weight; rather, excess placental weight appeared to correlate with intergenerational fat accumulation in the maternal lineage. Therefore, 'placental obesity' may be a female genetic trait, rather than a vascular response to chronic hypoxia. The concept of placental epidemiology has recently been reviewed [108].

## Future advances in placentology

One of the increasing frustrations in human placentology is the growing awareness that pathological processes begin very early in development. The observation of abnormal first trimester villous changes with anaemia [88] or smoking [107] are impressive snapshots of maldevelopment that cannot be further advanced through further human cross-sectional studies. Fortunately, we share the majority of our genome with other eutherian mammals, including rodents, which breed reliably, are experimentally accessible and permit the application of transgenic technology to understand the genetic basis of placental disorders [3]. Just as the study of endocrine pathways mediating labour in sheep has its limitations for understanding human preterm labour, so may the mouse have disadvantages in terms of understanding human placental pathology; however, the similarities are too great to be ignored.

By viewing placental development in terms of cell fate decisions and tissue morphogenesis, rather than by comparative anatomy, the potential of mouse transgenic research can be appreciated [109]. A growing array of genes is critical for development of the placenta. *Hand1* and *Mash2* are critical for invasive extravillous trophoblast development [15], while the first insights into genes critical for villous development have been realized with the discovery that *Gcm1* is necessary for labyrinthine (villous) morphogenesis [110]. Each of these genes is a trophoblast transcription factor. Since knockout studies of vascular growth factors, such as *Vegf*, produce early embryonic lethality [111], a growing body of evidence suggests that the trophoblast dominates placental development. For that reason, studies that address the functionality of trophoblast transcription factors are more likely to lead to the origins of early pregnancy loss and severe villous maldevelopment [63] than, for example, differences in vascular growth factor expression that may be merely induced environmentally [112].

Mouse placentology has recently taken on a new dimension with the advent of very high-frequency (40 MHz) ultrasound imaging. Dual (real-time and Doppler) capabilities now permit imaging of the placental and umbilical cord blood flow just 4 days after chorioallantoic fusion (Fig. 5.4) [113]. As in the human, we can now perform correlative studies of umbilical artery Doppler and placental development, the importance of which is to study heterozygous mutations (e.g. for *Gcm1*) and their interaction with the external environment.

## Conclusions

Until very recently, publications on other organs have exceeded those on the placenta 10- to 20-fold. Interest in perinatal programming, together with the wider application of technologies that permit imaging and transgenic experiments in mice, will accelerate interest in the placenta. Contemporary human offspring will form the first cohorts to participate in programming research, which will fall largely within the realm of paediatric endocrinology.

(a) (b)

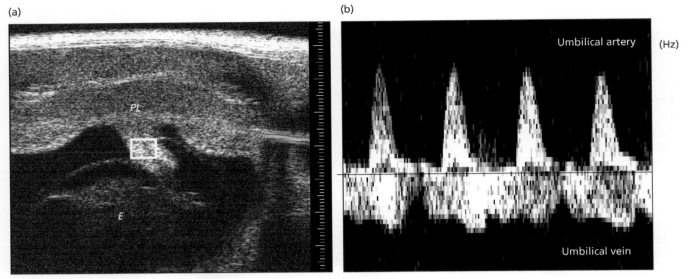

**Fig. 5.4.** Real-time (a) and pulsed Doppler (b) ultrasound of the mouse placenta at e11.5, 3 days after chorioallantoic fusion using a 40-MHz ultrasound biomicroscope (VisualSonics VS40) (18.5 days is full term). The rectangle shows the location of the pulsed Doppler sample volume on the umbilical cord that was used to obtain the velocity waveforms. Note minimal end-diastolic flow in the umbilical artery and pulsatile flow in the umbilical vein. In (a), the smallest increment on the scale is 100 µm. E, embryo; Pl, placenta (courtesy of Doctors Y. Q. Zhou, F. S. Foster and S. L. Adamson, unpublished observations).

## Acknowledgements

The authors are grateful to the many Granting Agencies that have supported their placental research including Medical Research Councils (UK and Canada); Action Research (UK); Tommy's Campaign (UK); Scottish Hospitals Endowment Research Trust (UK); West Midland Health Authority (UK); Canadian Institutes of Health Research (formerly Medical Research Council of Canada); Genesis Foundation, Department of Obstetrics & Gynecology, University of Toronto; and Physicians Services Incorporated Foundation of Ontario.

## References

1 Kingdom JCP, Jauniaux E, O'Brien PMS. The Placenta. *Basic Science and Clinical Practice*. London: RCOG Press, 2000.

2 O'Brien PMS, Wheeler T, Barker DJP, eds. *Fetal Programming: Influences on Development and Disease in Later Life*. London: RCOG Press, 2000.

3 Cross JC. Genetic insights into trophoblast differentiation and placental morphogenesis. *Semin Cell Dev Biol* 2000; 11: 105–13.

4 Rodesch F, Simon P, Donner C, Jauniaux E. Oxygen measurements in endometrial and trophoblastic tissues during early pregnancy. *Obstet Gynecol* 1992; 80: 283–5.

5 Watson AL, Palmer ME, Jauniaux E, Burton GJ. Variations in expression of copper/zinc superoxide dismutase in villous trophoblast of the human placenta with gestational age. *Placenta* 1997; 18: 295–9.

6 Tanaka S, Kunath T, Hadjantonakis AK, Nagy A, Rossant J. Promotion of trophoblast stem cell proliferation by FGF4. *Science* 1998; 282: 2072–5.

7 Lyall F, Kaufmann P. The uteroplacental circulation: extravillous trophoblast. In: Kingdom JCP, Baker PN, eds. *Intrauterine Growth Restriction: Aetiology and Management*. London: Springer, 2000: 85–130.

8 Aplin JD, Haigh T, Lacey H, Chen CP, Jones CJ. Tissue interactions in the control of trophoblast invasion. *J Reprod Fertil Suppl* 2000; 55: 57–64.

9 Lyall F, Bulmer JN, Kelly H, Duffie E, Robson SC. Human trophoblast invasion and spiral artery transformation: the role of nitric oxide. *Am J Pathol* 1999; 154: 1105–14.

10 Jaffe R, Jauniaux E, Hustin J. Maternal circulation in the first-trimester human placenta—myth or reality? *Am J Obstet Gynecol* 1997; 176: 695–705.

11 Simpson NA, Nimrod C, De Vermette R, Leblanc C, Fournier J. Sonographic evaluation of intervillous flow in early pregnancy: use of echo-enhancement agents. *Ultrasound Obstet Gynecol* 1998; 11: 204–8.

12 Caniggia I, Mostachfi H, Winter J *et al*. Hypoxia-inducible factor-1 mediates the biological effects of oxygen on human trophoblast differentiation through TGFbeta 3. *J Clin Invest* 2000; 105: 577–87.

13 Caniggia I, Lye SJ, Cross JC. Activin is a local regulator of human cytotrophoblast cell differentiation. *Endocrinology* 1997; 138: 3976–86.

14 Hattori N, Davies TC, Anson-Cartwright L, Cross JC. Periodic expression of the cyclin-dependent kinase inhibitor p57 (Kip2) in trophoblast giant cells defines a G2-like gap phase of the endocycle. *Mol Biol Cell* 2000; 11: 1037–45.

15 Scott IC, Anson-Cartwright L, Riley P, Reda D, Cross JC. The HAND1 basic helix–loop–helix transcription factor regulates

trophoblast differentiation via multiple mechanisms. *Mol Cell Biol* 2000; 2: 530–41.

16 Kim YT, Cho NH, Ko JH, Yang WI, Kim JW, Choi EK, Lee SH. Expression of cyclin E in placentas with hydropic change and gestational trophoblastic diseases: implications for the malignant transformation of trophoblasts. *Cancer* 2000; 89: 673–9.

17 Krebs C, Longo LD, Leiser R. Term ovine placental vasculature: comparison of sea level and high altitude conditions by corrosion cast and histomorphometry. *Placenta* 1997; 18: 43–51.

18 Norwitz ER, Robinson JN, Challis JR. The control of labor. *N Engl J Med* 1999; 34: 660–6.

19 Castellucci M, Scheper M, Scheffen I, Celona A, Kaufmann P. The development of the human placental villous tree. *Anat Embryol* 1990; 18: 117–28.

20 Hendricks SK, Sorensen TK, Wang KY, Bushnell JM, Seguin EM, Zingheim RW. Doppler umbilical artery waveform indices – normal values from fourteen to forty-two weeks. *Am J Obstet Gynecol* 1989; 161: 761–5.

21 Reilly RD, Russell PT. Neurohistochemical evidence supporting an absence of adrenergic and cholinergic innervation in the human placenta and umbilical cord. *Anat Rec* 1977; 188: 277–86.

22 Kingdom JC, Burrell SJ, Kaufmann P. Pathology and clinical implications of abnormal umbilical artery Doppler waveforms. *Ultrasound Obstet Gynecol* 1997; 9: 271–86.

23 Kaufmann P, Kingdom JCP. Development of the vascular system in the placenta. In: Risau W, Rudolph AM, eds. *Morphogenesis of Endothelium*. Amsterdam: Harwood Academic, 2000: 255–75.

24 Jackson MR, Mayhew TM, Boyd PA. Quantitative description of the elaboration and maturation of villi from 10 weeks of gestation to term. *Placenta* 1992; 13: 357–70.

25 Evans PW, Wheeler T, Anthony FW, Osmond C. A longitudinal study of maternal serum vascular endothelial growth factor in early pregnancy. *Hum Reprod* 1998; 13: 1057–62.

26 Cooper JC, Sharkey AM, Charnock-Jones DS, Palmer CR, Smith SK. VEGF mRNA levels in placentae from pregnancies complicated by pre-eclampsia. *Br J Obstet Gynaecol* 1996; 103: 1191–6.

27 Huppertz B, Frank HG, Reister F, Kingdom J, Korr H, Kaufmann P. Apoptosis cascade progresses during turnover of human trophoblast: analysis of villous cytotrophoblast and syncytial fragments in vitro. *Lab Invest* 1999; 79: 1687–702.

28 Huppertz B, Frank HG, Kingdom JC, Reister F, Kaufmann P. Villous cytotrophoblast regulation of the syncytial apoptotic cascade in the human placenta. *Histochem Cell Biol* 1998; 110: 495–508.

29 Johansen M, Redman CW, Wilkins T, Sargent IL. Trophoblast deportation in human pregnancy—its relevance for pre-eclampsia. *Placenta* 1999; 20: 531–9.

30 Smith SC, Baker PN, Symonds EM. Increased placental apoptosis in intrauterine growth restriction. *Am J Obstet Gynecol* 1997; 177: 1395–401.

31 Glazier JD, Cetin I, Perugino G *et al.* Association between the activity of the system A amino acid transporter in the microvillous plasma membrane of the human placenta and severity of fetal compromise in intrauterine growth restriction. *Pediatr Res* 1997; 42: 514–19.

32 Pertl B, Bianchi DW. First trimester prenatal diagnosis: fetal cells in the maternal circulation. *Semin Perinatol* 1999; 23: 393–402.

33 Aractingi S, Berkane N, Bertheau P *et al.* DNA in skin of polymorphic eruptions of pregnancy. *Lancet* 1998; 352: 1898–901.

34 Bianchi DW. Fetomaternal cell trafficking: a new cause of disease? *Am J Med Genet* 2000; 91: 22–8.

35 Westwood M. Role of insulin-like growth factor binding protein 1 in human pregnancy. *Rev Reprod* 1999; 4: 160–7.

36 Han VK, Carter AM. Spatial and temporal patterns of expression of messenger RNA for insulin-like growth factors and their binding proteins in the placenta of man and laboratory animals. *Placenta* 2000; 21: 289–305.

37 Aplin JD, Lacey H, Haigh T, Jones CJ, Chen CP, Westwood M. Growth factor–extracellular matrix synergy in the control of trophoblast invasion. *Biochem Soc Trans* 2000; 28: 199–202.

38 van Kleffens M, Groffen C, Lindenbergh-Kortleve DJ *et al.* The IGF system during fetal-placental development of the mouse. *Mol Cell Endocrinol* 1998; 140: 129–35.

39 Kanai-Azuma M, Kanai Y, Kurohmaru M, Sakai S, Hayashi Y. Insulin-like growth factor (IGF)-I stimulates proliferation and migration of mouse ectoplacental cone cells, while IGF-II transforms them into trophoblastic giant cells in vitro. *Biol Reprod* 1993; 48: 252–61.

40 Giannoukakis N, Deal C, Paquette J, Goodyer CG, Polychronakos C. Parental genomic imprinting of the human IGF2 gene. *Nature Genet* 1993; 4: 98–101.

41 Xu Y, Goodyer CG, Deal C, Polychronakos C. Functional polymorphism in the parental imprinting of the human IGF2R gene. *Biochem Biophys Res Commun* 1993; 197: 747–54.

42 Pintar JE, Schuller A, Cerro JA, Czick M, Grewal A, Green B. Genetic ablation of IGFBP-2 suggests functional redundancy in the IGFBP family. *Prog Growth Factor Res* 1995; 6: 437–45.

43 Nielsen J, Christiansen J, Lykke-Andersen J, Johnsen AH, Wewer UM, Nielsen FC. A family of insulin-like growth factor II mRNA-binding proteins represses translation in late development. *Mol Cell Biol* 1999; 19: 1262–70.

44 Rosenbaum M, Leibel RL. The role of leptin in human physiology. *N Engl J Med* 1999; 341: 913–15.

45 Teppa RJ, Ness RB, Crombleholme WR, Roberts JM. Free leptin is increased in normal pregnancy and further increased in preeclampsia. *Metabolism* 2000; 49: 1043–8.

46 Geary M, Pringle PJ, Persaud M *et al.* Leptin concentrations in maternal serum and cord blood: relationship to maternal anthropometry and fetal growth. *Br J Obstet Gynaecol* 1999; 106: 1054–60.

47 Persson B, Westgren M, Celsi G, Nord E, Ortqvist E. Leptin concentrations in cord blood in normal newborn infants and offspring of diabetic mothers. *Horm Metab Res* 1999; 31: 467–71.

48 Williams MA, Havel PJ, Schwartz MW *et al.* Pre-eclampsia disrupts the normal relationship between serum leptin concentrations and adiposity in pregnant women. *Paediatr Perinat Epidemiol* 1999; 13: 190–204.

49 Kingdom JCP, Geary M, Hindmarsh PC. Late-gestation preeclampsia results in perinatal obesity and increased placental weight [Abstract]. *J Soc Gynecol Invest* 2000; 7: 89A, 165.

50 Challis JR, Lye SJ, Gibb W. Prostaglandins and parturition. *Ann NY Acad Sci* 1997; 828: 254–67.

51 Whittle WL, Patel FA, Alfaidy N *et al.* Glucocorticoid regulation of human and ovine parturition: the relationship between fetal hypothalamic–pituitary–adrenal axis activation and intrauterine prostaglandin production. *Biol Reprod* 2001; 64: 1019–32.

52 Hirst JJ, Teixeira FJ, Zakar T, Olson DM. Prostaglandin endoperoxide-H synthase-1 and -2 messenger ribonucleic acid levels in

human amnion with spontaneous labor onset. *J Clin Endocrinol Metab* 1995; 80: 517–23.

53 Whittle WL, Gibb W, Challis JR. The characterization of human amnion epithelial and mesenchymal cells: the cellular expression, activity and glucocorticoid regulation of prostaglandin output. *Placenta* 2000; 21: 394–401.

54 Cheung PY, Walton JC, Tai HH, Riley SC, Challis JR. Immunocytochemical distribution and localization of 15-hydroxyprostaglandin dehydrogenase in human fetal membranes, decidua, and placenta. *Am J Obstet Gynecol* 1990; 163: 1445–9.

55 Pomini F, Patel FA, Mancuso S, Challis JR. Activity and expression of 15-hydroxyprostaglandin dehydrogenase in cultured chorionic trophoblast and villous trophoblast cells and in chorionic explants at term with and without spontaneous labor. *Am J Obstet Gynecol* 2000; 182: 221–6.

56 Patel FA, Clifton VL, Chwalisz K, Challis JR. Steroid regulation of prostaglandin dehydrogenase activity and expression in human term placenta and chorio-decidua in relation to labor. *J Clin Endocrinol Metab* 1999; 84: 291–9.

57 Pepe GJ, Babischkin JS, Burch MG, Leavitt MG, Albrecht ED. Developmental increase in expression of the messenger ribonucleic acid and protein levels of 11beta-hydroxysteroid dehydrogenase types 1 and 2 in the baboon placenta. *Endocrinology* 1996; 137: 5678–84.

58 Sun K, Yang K, Challis JR. Regulation of 11beta-hydroxysteroid dehydrogenase type 2 by progesterone, estrogen, and the cyclic adenosine 5′-monophosphate pathway in cultured human placental and chorionic trophoblasts. *Biol Reprod* 1998; 58: 1379–84.

59 Riley SC, Challis JR. Corticotrophin-releasing hormone production by the placenta and fetal membranes. *Placenta* 1991; 12: 105–19.

60 Grammatopoulos DK, Hillhouse EW. Role of corticotropin-releasing hormone in onset of labour. *Lancet* 1999; 354: 1546–9.

61 Mizuno R. The male/female ratio of fetal deaths and births in Japan. *Lancet* 2000; 356: 738–9.

62 Edwards A, Megens A, Peek M, Wallace EM. Sexual origins of placental dysfunction. *Lancet* 2000; 355: 203–4.

63 Krebs C, Macara LM, Leiser R, Bowman AW, Greer IA, Kingdom JC. Intrauterine growth restriction with absent end-diastolic flow velocity in the umbilical artery is associated with maldevelopment of the placental terminal villous tree. *Am J Obstet Gynecol* 1996; 175: 1534–42.

64 Mayhew TM, Burton GJ. Stereology and its impact on our understanding of human placental functional morphology. *Microsc Res Tech* 1997; 38: 195–205.

65 Hindmarsh PC, Geary MPP, Rodeck CH, Jackson MR, Kingdom JCP. Effect of early maternal iron stores on placental weight and structure. *Lancet* 2000; 356: 719–23.

66 Bower SJ, Harrington KF, Schuchter K, McGirr C, Campbell S. Prediction of pre-eclampsia by abnormal uterine Doppler ultrasound and modification by aspirin. *Br J Obstet Gynaecol* 1996; 103: 625–9.

67 Chappell LC, Seed PT, Briley AL, Kelly FJ, Lee R, Hunt BJ *et al.* Effect of antioxidants on the occurrence of pre-eclampsia in women at increased risk: a randomised trial. *Lancet* 1999; 354: 810–16.

68 Backos M, Rai R, Baxter N, Chilcott IT, Cohen H, Regan L. Pregnancy complications in women with recurrent miscarriage associated with antiphospholipid antibodies treated with low dose aspirin and heparin. *Br J Obstet Gynaecol* 1999; 106: 102–7.

69 Kingdom JCP, Smith GN. Diagnosis and management of IUGR. In: Kingdom JCP, Baker PN, eds. *Intrauterine Growth Restriction: Aetiology and Management.* London: Springer, 2000: 257–74.

70 Karsdorp VH, van Vugt JM, van Geijn HP *et al.* Clinical significance of absent or reversed end diastolic velocity waveforms in umbilical artery. *Lancet* 1994; 344: 1664–8.

71 Walsh SW, Vaughan JE, Wang Y, Roberts LJ. Placental isoprostane is significantly increased in preeclampsia. *FASEB J* 2000; 14: 1289–96.

72 Kilby MD, Verhaeg J, Gittoes N, Somerset DA, Clark PM, Franklyn JA. Circulating thyroid hormone concentrations and placental thyroid hormone receptor expression in normal human pregnancy and pregnancy complicated by intrauterine growth restriction (IUGR). *J Clin Endocrinol Metab* 1998; 83: 2964–71.

73 Roberts JM, Redman CW. Pre-eclampsia: more than pregnancy-induced hypertension. *Lancet* 1993; 341: 1447–51 [Erratum *Lancet* 1993; 342: 504].

74 Roberts JM, Hubel CA. Is oxidative stress the link in the two-stage model of pre-eclampsia? *Lancet* 1999; 354: 788–9.

75 Xiong X, Demianczuk NN, Buekens P, Saunders LD. Association of preeclampsia with high birth weight for age. *Am J Obstet Gynecol* 2000; 183: 148–55.

76 Kingdom JC, Kaufmann P. Oxygen and placental villous development: origins of fetal hypoxia. *Placenta* 1997; 18: 613–21.

77 Huppertz B, Kingdom JCP, Caniggia I *et al.* Oxygen modulates the balance between apoptosis and necrosis in human villous trophoblast [Abstract]. *Placenta* 1999; 20.

78 Redman CW, Sacks GP, Sargent IL. Preeclampsia: an excessive maternal inflammatory response to pregnancy. *Am J Obstet Gynecol* 1999; 180: 499–506.

79 Hillier SL, Martius J, Krohn M, Kiviat N, Holmes KK, Eschenbach DA. A case–control study of chorioamnionic infection and histologic chorioamnionitis in prematurity. *N Engl J Med* 1988; 319: 972–8.

80 van Meir CA, Matthews SG, Keirse MJ, Ramirez MM, Bocking A, Challis JR. 15-hydroxyprostaglandin dehydrogenase: implications in preterm labor with and without ascending infection. *J Clin Endocrinol Metab* 1997; 82: 969–76.

81 Korebrits C, Ramirez MM, Watson L, Brinkman E, Bocking AD, Challis JR. Maternal corticotropin-releasing hormone is increased with impending preterm birth. *J Clin Endocrinol Metab* 1998; 83: 1585–91.

82 Heine RP, McGregor JA, Dullien VK. Accuracy of salivary estriol testing compared to traditional risk factor assessment in predicting preterm birth. *Am J Obstet Gynecol* 1999; 180: S214–18.

83 Iams JD, Goldenberg RL, Meis PJ, Mercer BM, Moawad A, Das A *et al.* The length of the cervix and the risk of spontaneous premature delivery. *N Engl J Med* 1996; 334: 567–72.

84 Lettieri L, Vintzileos AM, Rodis JF, Albini SM, Salafia CM. Does 'idiopathic' preterm labor resulting in preterm birth exist? *Am J Obstet Gynecol* 1993; 168: 1480–5.

85 Gopel W, Kim D, Gortner L. Prothrombotic mutations as a risk factor for preterm birth. *Lancet* 1999; 353: 1411–12.

86 McLean M, Bisits A, Davies J, Woods R, Lowry P, Smith R. A placental clock controlling the length of human pregnancy. *Nature Med* 1995; 1: 460–3.

87 Mayhew TM, Jackson MR, Haas JD. Oxygen diffusive conductances of human placentae from term pregnancies at low and high altitudes. *Placenta* 1990; 11: 493–503.

88 Kadyrov M, Kosanke G, Kingdom J, Kaufmann P. Increased fetoplacental angiogenesis during first trimester in anaemic women. *Lancet* 1998; 352: 1747–9.

89 Crowe C, Dandekar P, Fox M, Dhingra K, Bennet L, Hanson MA. The effects of anaemia on heart, placenta and body weight, and blood pressure in fetal and neonatal rats. *J Physiol* 1995; 488: 515–19.

90 Trichopoulos D. Short-term and long-term effects of iron deficiency *in utero*. *Lancet* 2000; 356: 696.

91 Stewart PM, Murry BA, Mason JI. Type 2 11 beta-hydroxysteroid dehydrogenase in human fetal tissues. *J Clin Endocrinol Metab* 1994; 78: 1529–32.

92 Seckl JR, Benediktsson R, Lindsay RS, Brown RW. Placental 11 beta-hydroxysteroid dehydrogenase and the programming of hypertension. *J Steroid Biochem Mol Biol* 1995; 55: 447–55.

93 Sun K, Adamson SL, Yang K, Challis JR. Interconversion of cortisol and cortisone by 11beta-hydroxysteroid dehydrogenases type 1 and 2 in the perfused human placenta. *Placenta* 1999; 20: 13–9.

94 Kilby MD, Zhender D, Wood P, Holder R, Stewart PM. Amniotic fluid cortisol and cortisone concentrations and fetal growth in pregnancy. *Clin Endocrinol* 2001 (submitted).

95 Shams M, Kilby MD, Somerset DA *et al*. 11Beta-hydroxysteroid dehydrogenase type 2 in human pregnancy and reduced expression in intrauterine growth restriction. *Hum Reprod* 1998; 13: 799–804.

96 Sloboda DM, Newnham JP, Challis JR. Effects of repeated maternal betamethasone administration on growth and hypothalamic-pituitary-adrenal function of the ovine fetus at term. *J Endocrinol* 2000; 165: 79–91.

97 Dodic MCN, Wintour EM, Coghlan JP. An early prenatal exposure to excess glucocorticoid leads to hypertensive offspring in sheep. *Clin Sci* 1998; 94: 149–55.

98 Cox DB, Challis JRG, Fraser M. Placental development following maternal dexamethasone during early pregnancy [Abstract]. *J Soc Gynecol Invest* 1999; 6: 75A, 119.

99 Barker DJ, Hales CN, Fall CH, Osmond C, Phipps K, Clark PM. Type 2 (non-insulin-dependent) diabetes mellitus, hypertension and hyperlipidaemia (syndrome X): relation to reduced fetal growth. *Diabetologia* 1993; 36: 62–7.

100 Smith GN, Kingdom JC, Penning DH, Matthews SG. Antenatal corticosteroids: is more better? *Lancet* 2000; 355: 251–2.

101 Merrill JD, Ballard RA. Antenatal hormone therapy for fetal lung maturation. *Clin Perinatol* 1998; 25: 983–97.

102 Bennet L, Kozuma S, McGarrigle HH, Hanson MA. Temporal changes in fetal cardiovascular, behavioural, metabolic and endocrine responses to maternally administered dexamethasone in the late gestation fetal sheep. *Br J Obstet Gynaecol* 1999; 106: 331–9.

103 Henson G. Antenatal cortiscosteroids and heart rate variability. *Br J Obstet Gynaecol* 1997; 104: 1219–20.

104 Wallace EM, Baker LS. Effect of antenatal betamethasone administration on placental vascular resistance. *Lancet* 1999; 353: 1404–7.

105 Brocklehurst P, Gates S, McKenzie-McHarg K, Alfirevic Z, Chamberlain G. Are we prescribing multiple courses of antenatal corticosteroids? A survey of Practice in the UK. *Br J Obstet Gynaecol* 1999; 106: 977–9.

106 Williams LA, Evans SF, Newnham JP. Prospective cohort study of factors influencing the relative weights of the placenta and the newborn infant. *Br Med J* 1997; 314: 1864–8.

107 Jauniaux E, Burton GJ. The effect of smoking in pregnancy on early placental morphology. *Obstet Gynecol* 1992; 79: 645–8.

108 Hindmarsh PC. Placental epidemiology. In: Kingdom JCP, Jauniaux E, O'Brien PMS, eds. *The Placenta: Basic Science and Clinical Practice*. London: RCOG Press, 2000: 3–9.

109 Rinkenberger J, Werb Z. The labyrinthine placenta. *Nature Genet* 2000; 25: 248–50.

110 Anson-Cartwright L, Dawson K, Holmyard D, Fisher SJ, Lazzarini RA, Cross JC. The glial cells missing-1 protein is essential for branching morphogenesis in the chorioallantoic placenta. *Nature Genet* 2000; 25: 311–14.

111 Shalaby F, Rossant J, Yamaguchi TP, Gertsenstein M, Wu XF, Breitman ML, Schuh AC. Failure of blood-island formation and vasculogenesis in Flk-1-deficient mice. *Nature* 1995; 376: 62–6.

112 Khaliq A, Dunk C, Jiang J *et al*. Hypoxia down-regulates placenta growth factor whereas fetal growth restriction up-regulates placenta growth factor expression: molecular evidence for 'placental hyperoxia' in intrauterine growth restriction. *Lab Invest* 1999; 79: 151–70.

113 Aristizabal O, Christopher DA, Foster FS, Turnbull DH. 40-MHZ echocardiography scanner for cardiovascular assessment of mouse embryos. *Ultrasound Med Biol* 1998; 24: 1407–17.

# Physiology of sexual determination and differentiation

## P. H. Saenger

## Introduction

Sex determination and differentiation proceed in sequence. *Genetic sex* is determined at fertilization and determines the differentiation of the gonad; both testis- and ovary-determining genes have been elucidated. Differentiation of the gonads leads to the development of internal genital tracts and the external genitalia and hence the phenotypic sex during the first half of fetal life. The process is completed at puberty with the development of secondary sex characteristics. *Psychological sexual* (gender) identity is probably largely acquired postnatally by sociological influences on the developing personality. This postnatal process, together with prenatal hormonal influences (nature and nurture), moulds psychological sex.

Although the developmental events that occur subsequently in sex differentiation have long been known, the precise genetic, biochemical, endocrine and molecular mechanisms have been only partially elucidated. Careful evaluation of patients with a range of defects, from chromosome abnormalities to multifactorial conditions, coupled with studies in other mammals, particularly transgenic mice, have revealed new insights into the various mechanisms involved.

The testis-determining factor does not make up the entire Y chromosome but a region spanning only 14 kb on the short

arm [1] (Fig. 6.1). The gene for anti-Müllerian hormone (AMH) has been elucidated and reliable assays for its measurement have been developed [2–5]. The gene coding for the androgen receptor has been identified, furthering understanding of complete and partial androgen resistance syndromes [6–8]. This, coupled with the precise identification of the genetic defect that results in 5α-reductase deficiency, extends understanding of testosterone and dihydrotestosterone (DHT) action [9,10]. Finally, recent work shows that the female pathway is not simply a default pathway and that both *Wnt-4* and *Dax1* genes actively regulate female development [11,12].

The existence of common primordia for alternative pathways of sexual development is an ancient and widespread phenomenon in vertebrates. Structure and function of the testis and ovary are similar in many animals, suggesting that the pathways involved in building a testis or an ovary are conserved. Systems controlled primarily by temperature, hormones, gene dosage or dominant genes, depending on differing developmental circumstances of the animal, have evolved. Fish and other animals that live in water can rely on diffusion of chemical cues and presumably benefit from the ability to switch sex in adult life, depending on the optimal survival requirements of the group. Among lizards and turtles, instances of temperature-dependent and genotypic sex determination have been documented [13,14].

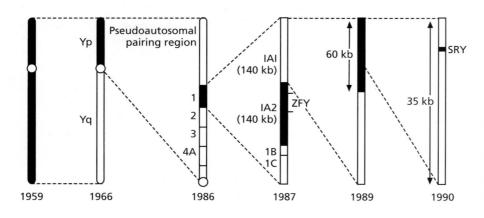

**Fig. 6.1.** Thirty-one years of hunting the testis-determining factor. The chromosome region thought to include the elusive factor is shaded. The search has narrowed from 30–50 million bases to less than 35 kb of *SRY*. Modified from McLaren [2].

Some evolutionary biologists suggest that the genetic switch on the mammalian Y chromosome has been super-imposed on older systems of sex determination that were primarily temperature or hormone based. Humans cannot, after all, rely on environmental cues for dimorphic development, either hormone or temperature based, because they develop within a temperature-controlled uterine environment bathed in maternal hormones [15].

The maternal hormone environment may explain why the fundamental developmental pathway in mammals is female. Jost [16] showed that surgical removal of the gonads during embryonic development of the rabbit resulted in development of female sexual characteristics, regardless of the chromosomal sex of the embryo. Hormones produced and exported by the developing testes are responsible for the differentiation of the male urogenital tract. Mainly because of Jost's experiments, the female development has often been referred to as the default pathway, but this is misleading because it would imply that the female pathway of sexual differentiation is not an active, genetically controlled process.

## Genetic sex: role of the sex-determining region of the human Y chromosome

The genetic sex is determined by whether the sperm contains a Y or an X chromosome [17]. The genetic male sex induces differentiation of the pluripotential primordial gonad into a testis. Complete female sexual differentiation occurs in the absence of male determinants [18–20] but female development is probably regulated by a specific genetic pathway as well.

The gonadal primordium common to both sexes is already visible in the 5-mm-long human embryo. The development of paired genital ridges shows some proliferation of the coelomic epithelium, and mesenchyme begins to differentiate into gonads at around the fourth week [21,22]. This development is heralded by the appearance of so-called sex cords. During this step, which is independent of genetic sex, the gonad is colonized by primordial germ cells that originate from the allantoid sac. When the cells have reached the gonadal primordium, they form the gonadal ridge with the existing epithelium. Subsequent differentiation into seminiferous tubules, which signals the first event of male differentiation, is initiated by a 'switch' mechanism brought on by a gene product of the Y chromosome.

In 1959 the Y chromosome was shown to be male determining in both mice and humans [17] so that 48,XXXY individuals are male and XO individuals are female [17,23,24]. An area on the short arm of the Y chromosome was identified as containing the testis-determining factor. At that stage, the H–Y antigen, a minor male-specific histocompatibility antigen, was widely believed to be the primary testis inducer [25], although it is actually located on the long arm of the Y chromosome [26] and appears to play more of a role in sper-matogenesis [27]. Attention was then directed to the area near the pairing and exchange (pseudoautosomal) region. This was termed zinc finger Y (ZFY) [28,29] but the demonstration of XX men without ZFY [30–32] ended its candidature [32,33].

By exploiting detailed maps of the sex-determining region of the human Y chromosome, the *SRY* gene was positionally cloned [33, 34]. Proof that it was indeed the male-determining factor required that expression of *SRY* in the fetal testis be confined to the somatic-supporting cell lineage, which is believed to be critical for testis determination, rather than to the germ cells [35]. In a now classic experiment, the laboratories of Goodfellow and Lovell-Badge [35,36] succeeded in fertilizing female XX eggs with the 14 kb *SRY* gene sequence and bred sex-reversed XX phenotypic male mice with gonads demonstrating testicular histology.

As might be predicted for a regulatory gene, *SRY* encodes a protein containing a DNA-binding motif and also shows a pattern for expression in the mouse that is entirely consistent with a role in testis determination. It is expressed for a short period in the somatic cells of the genital ridge (Fig. 6.2) [35,37], as shown by *in situ* hybridization, polymerase chain reaction and RNase protection techniques [37–39].

*SRY* in humans is a 14-kb single exon region adjacent to the pseudoautosomal region of the short arm of the Y chromosome (Fig. 6.1) [40]. Present in the 5′ flanking sequence are two tandem Sp1 recognition sites (Sp1 is a zinc finger transcription factor), which are likely to potentiate transcription. The protein contains an HMG (high mobility group) box centrally and almost all SRY mutations have occurred in the HMG box. The union of SRY with linear DNA induces a bend of about 80° and leads to a major conformational change in the DNA. Some of the mutations identified destabilize the protein, leading to more rapid degradation, whereas others alter the DNA contact sites, which precludes bending. Mutations in the SRY promoter sequence have also been described. Genes regulated by SRY include AMH and aromatase P450, but the effect on AMH appears to be mediated through an indirect interaction with an intermediate gene.

It is not clear at present how *SRY*, the 'switch', is turned on but it is clear that it is expressed in the critical period when gonadal differentiation takes place in the mouse. *SRY* is expressed only in the somatic cells of the genital ridge, not in the sperm cells [35], and *SRY* expression in adults is limited to the heads of the spermatids. The limited time of expression of *SRY* in the critical period is akin to the time-limited expression of other genes, such as homeobox genes and oncogenes, which are also expressed only at discrete stages of development [41]. Similarly, *SRY* is not the only gene causing testis determination, although it is the critical initial switch. Other genes on other chromosomes (possibly also regulated by *SRY*) play as yet unidentified functions in the completion of orderly sexual differentiation.

Although *SRY* as a typical transcription factor alone can promote testicular development in 46,XX males in the

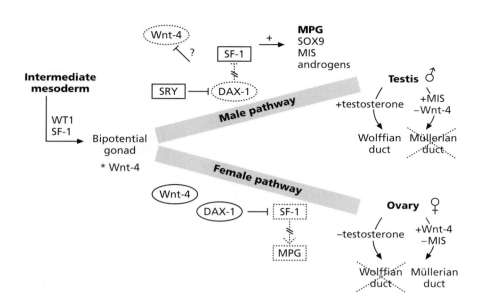

**Fig. 6.2.** Simplified genetic model for mammalian sex determination. In both sexes Wt1 and SF-1 are required for the formation of a bipotential gonad, in which the expression of *Wnt-4* is also sex-independent (*). In males, *Wnt-4* gene expression is inactivated after sex determination, and Y-chromosomal SRY suppresses DAX-1 function. As a result, *SF-1* remains active and male pathway genes (MPGs) are induced, which leads to testis differentiation. In females, *Wnt-4 and DAX-1* are active after sex differentiation, because of the absence of inhibiting genes such as *SRY*. DAX-1 represses SF-1 thus inhibiting the activation of MPGs, and this leads to the female phenotype. Testosterone production enables the further development of Wolffian ducts in males, whereas the Müllerian ducts degenerate in the absence of Wnt-4 and the presence of Müllerian inhibitory substance (MIS). The situation is the opposite in females, where the Müllerian ducts persist and the Wolffian ducts regress. Modified from Heikkilä *et al*. [55].

absence of any other Y-linked genes [35,42,43], sex reversal does not always occur, and *SRY*-negative males have been described. The most likely explanation is that the *SRY* transgene is sensitive to position effects [41]. It may be affected by adjacent DNA sequences and its new chromosomal location or by the spread of X inactivation curtailing *SRY* action. *SRY* initiates testis development through interaction with other genes [44], some of which have been involved in regulation; others will be downstream targets of *SRY*. In the *SRY*-negative male, a gain of function mutation downstream of *SRY* would explain male development. Because *SRY* is shown to be the only Y-linked gene required to bring about male development in the mouse, mutations in genes elsewhere in the genome could explain cases of male development in XX males lacking *SRY* and XY females where *SRY* is intact [41,45–47]. Neither overproduction nor duplication of *SRY* has any further effect on sex determination in males, as judged, for instance, by the analysis of XYY males [34,48,49].

Several other genes suspected of having roles in developmental decisions in the embryo (for example some homeobox-containing genes) also show expression in the adult testis. *SRY* could have one role in the embryo in testis determination and another, postnatally, in male germ cell development [34,47]. *SRY* mRNA expression in humans and in some other mammals occurs over a longer period than the approximate 40-h window of expression during mouse gonadogenesis. The gene is expressed in tissues other than those of the gonad and testis in marsupial, human and mouse, but no role has been ascribed to expression of *Sry/SRY* in other tissues. For example, in humans with mutations in *SRY*, no defects other than sex reversal have been described.

It is very likely that the interactions between the somatic

cell matrix and the penetrating germ cell are also important in gametogenesis. In the example of transgenic mice [35], the *SRY* germ cell acts as the switch-on gene in the XX gonadal ridge initiating the process of testicular differentiation. Since the gonadal ridge is always derived from somatic cells, this implies that *SRY* is not normally present in the germ cells in normal differentiation.

SRY and SOX proteins (see below) belong to HMG proteins that display site-specific DNA-binding properties [50]. They bind to the minor groove of the DNA helix. They recognize bent DNA and they bind linear DNA and induce a bend when they bind [44]. They function as local organizers of chromatin structure and thus play an architectural role in facilitating the assembly of nucleoprotein complexes at the target site [51].

## Other genes regulating gonadal sex

The development of the indifferent gonad from the mesenchyme is induced in the genital ridge under the control of autosomal genes acting as transcription factors (Table 6.1). These factors are generally also involved in the development of other organs, such as kidney, adrenal gland and urogenital systems. They act in genital ridge development before the dimorphic stage [52] but disruption of the Y-linked *SRY* and autosomal genes cannot account for all cases of XY sex reversal, which simply indicates that additional control networks remain to be identified.

### Wilms tumour gene 1

*WT1* is expressed early in urogenital ridge development

**Table 6.1.** Chromosomal localization of genes involved in gonadal determination and associated malformations in the event of genetic variation apart from gonadal dysgenesis

| Name | Chromosome location | Human disorder | Associated malformation |
|---|---|---|---|
| WT1 | 11p13 | Yes | Wilms' tumours, gonadoblastoma |
| | nephropathy, | | |
| LIM1 | 11p12–13 | No | – |
| SF-1 (FTZF1) | 9q33 | Yes | Adrenal insufficiency |
| SRY | Yp11.3 | Yes | None |
| DAX-1 | Xp21 | Yes | Duplication–sex reversal, mutation–adrenal insufficiency |
| SOX9 | 17q24.3–25.1 | Yes | Campomelic dysplasia |
| DMRTI/DRMT2 | 9p24.3 | Yes | Renal malformation, mental retardation |
| Wnt-4 | ? | No | – |

Modified from Hiort O (2000) *Horm Res* 53 (Suppl. 1): 38–24.

and its expression continues in the developing kidneys and gonads, becoming restricted to the Sertoli and granulosa cells in the latter [53]. *WT1* is probably critically involved in mesenchyme-to-epithelium transition.

In humans, *WT1* hemizygosity and deletions of 11p13 are associated with the WAGR syndrome (Wilms tumour, anitidia, genitourinary abnormalities and mental retardation). Exonic mutations in Denys–Drash syndrome and intronic mutations in Frasier syndrome leading to alternative splice products are associated with kidney abnormalities and ambiguous or female external genitalia in male patients. In WAGR, the appearances are more along the lines of undescended testes and hypospadias. The gonads are absent in *WT1* knockout mice and this causes the internal sex ducts and external genitalia to develop along the female pathway [54]. The role of the *WT1* gene in gonadal differentiation is not sex-specific, as gonadal dysgenesis also occurs in 46,XX individuals. This suggests its importance is in the formation of the bipotential gonad rather than testicular development. The genital abnormalities in Denys–Drash syndrome are not limited to 46,XY patients [55].

### Lhx9

The absence of the LIM homeobox gene *Lhx9* in the urogenital ridge results in failure of gonadal and renal formation in *Lhx9* knockout mice, so that the genetically male mice are phenotypically female. No human mutation has yet been described in this gene [55,56].

## Steroidogenic factor 1 (SF-1)

The role of SF-1 in gonadal formation is not yet clear [57]. SF-1, the product of the *FTZ1/F1* gene, is a nuclear receptor first expressed in urogenital ridges before their differentiation into the gonads and adrenals [58]. Its mRNA is also found in developing brain regions. Mice lacking SF-1 fail to develop gonads, adrenals and the ventromedial hypothalamus. It

activates AMH expression in Sertoli cells and regulates the expression of a number of enzymes needed for testosterone biosynthesis in Leydig cells [59].

SF-1 mutation caused sex reversal and adrenal failure in a 46,XY patient who was phenotypically female and had neonatal adrenal failure. Müllerian structures were normal, and the gonad contained immature tubules consistent with SRY being the primary testis-determining gene in mammals. The incomplete gonadal development observed suggests that SF-1 is necessary for subsequent male sexual differentiation [60].

SF-1 binds to a common DNA sequence in the promoters for P450scc,c11,c21,c17 and P450$_{aro}$. There must also be a cell-specific factor regulating the steroidogenic genes since P450c11 and P450c21 are expressed in adrenals but not in the gonad, whereas P450$_{aro}$ is expressed in gonads but not in the adrenals. SF-1 is expressed in both organs.

### SOX9

*SOX9* (SRY box related) is an autosomal *SRY*-related gene expressed in differentiating Sertoli cells. It is connected with chondrogenesis as an activator of the type II collagen gene, which is essential for formation of the extracellular matrix of cartilage. Deficiency of *SOX9* leads to male-to-female sex reversal and campomelic dysplasia [61–63]. *SOX9* duplication leads to autosomal XX sex reversal, so an extra dose of *SOX9* is sufficient to initiate testis differentiation in the absence of SRY. This is the first demonstration of XX sex reversal by an autosomal gene [64].

## Female development

### Dax1

In most of the cases described above, mutation of a gene led to male-to-female sex reversal, suggesting that female development is a default pathway relative to male development. This is an oversimplification because *Dax1* is a gene involved in adrenal as well as ovarian and testicular development [65,66]. It shares many properties with SF-1.

The gene is on the X chromosome and was termed *d*osage-sensitive sex reversal locus—*a*drenal hypoplasia congenita—*c*ritical region on the X-gene 1, also termed *Ahch*. The *Dax1* gene consists of two exons separated by a 3.4-kb intron. It is an orphan nuclear receptor with a typical ligand-binding domain but it does not have a typical zinc finger DNA-binding domain. Instead, its amino-terminal portion contains a novel domain in which several repeats of two putative zinc finger structures are found. *DAX-1* is expressed during ovarian development but suspended during testicular formation, implying a critical role of this gene in ovarian formation.

*DAX-1* is suppressed by *SRY* during testicular development (see Fig. 6.2). Overexpression causes male-to-female sex reversal. Humans carrying a mutation in the *DAX-1* gene have an X-linked recessive form of adrenal hypoplasia congenita, which includes hypogonadotrophic hypogonadism [65–69].

### Wnt-4

Recent studies of the *Wnt* gene family have identified *Wnt-4* signalling as a promoter of female development. Wnts are intercellular growth and differentiation factors and *Wnt-4* is expressed in the indifferent gonads of both sexes after the sex-specific differentiation brought on by other genes. It is down-regulated in the male gonad but maintained in the female. Unlike the sex-specific regulation of *Wnt-4* in the gonads, expression in the Müllerian ducts is sex dependent. It is also expressed in kidney mesenchyme and during pituitary gland development [11,70].

After sex determination triggered by *SRY*, the expressions of *DAX-1* and *Wnt-4* are suppressed in males, leading to prompt activation of downstream male pathway genes (MPGs). In females, absence of *SRY* allows *DAX-1* and *Wnt-4* to be expressed and MPGs are not activated. Investigations using *Wnt-4*-deficient mice indicate that the absence of gene function can lead to female-to-male sex reversal and thus development of the female pathway cannot just be a default process. The ovaries of mutant mice show a greater morphological resemblance to testes than to normal ovaries. Testosterone biosynthesis is activated in the gonads of female *Wnt-4*-deficient mice and, probably for this reason, the Wolffian ducts are stabilized and remain. On the other hand, Müllerian ducts are absent from both sexes in *Wnt-4* knockout mice. Oocytes degenerate in mutant ovaries before birth. *Wnt-4* appears to be required for formation of the Müllerian ducts and differentiation of the interstitial cell lineage and oocyte development. It may well be the gene necessary for the initiation of the female pathway in mammalian sex determination [55].

In addition to these genes of gonadal development, others are suspected of playing important roles as sexual regulators of testicular differentiation. Deletions of chromosomes 9p and 10q have been associated with sex reversal in 46,XY individuals, most of whom have mental retardation and craniofacial abnormalities [71]. The degree of genital ambiguity varies. Of special interest is a small region on chromosome 9p23–24 that harbours two genes of interest for testicular development both deleted in a hemizygous concomitant fashion in 46,XY sex reversal. These genes, named *DMRT1* and *DMRT2*, are related to proven sex-determining genes in other organisms and are solely expressed in the testes in humans [72].

Taken together, these findings suggest that *SRY* is the switch gene in the male but that the differentiation of the gonads into endocrine organs is controlled by different intrinsic gonadal or other factors. Furthermore, the mechanism that converts the gonads from autonomous endocrine tissue to gonadotrophin dependency is not understood.

## Gonadal differentiation and development

Gonadal development is apparent from about 5 weeks of gestation as a thickened area of the urogenital ridge. Until the 12-mm stage (approximately 42 days of gestation) the embryonic gonads of males and females are indistinguishable. Further proliferation takes place with epithelial projections (primary sex cords) growing into the mesenchyme defining two zones, the cortex and medulla.

By 42 days 300–700 primordial germ cells have seeded the undifferentiated gonads. They are the precursors of oogonia and spermatogonia. In the male under the influence of *SRY*, contact between these cells and somatic cells is made earlier than in the female gonadal ridge, at around 7–8 weeks of gestation [73]. The differentiation of the gonadal ridge into the testes by 43–50 days of gestation is a rapid phenomenon that contrasts with the slower and delayed development of the ovary, which will not become apparent until 140 days of gestation with the formation of granulosa cells. Leydig cells are apparent by about 60 days and differentiation of the male external genitalia occurs by 65–77 days of gestation [21,22,74–76].

*SRY* committing the gonad to male development may accelerate gonadal development in the male. Since testicular architecture and function is established early, male sex hormones are being produced before the male fetus becomes submerged in a sea of maternally derived oestrogen. The presence of testosterone and AMH counteracts the danger of the fetus becoming feminized [77–79], which is presumably why testes develop faster than ovaries in all mammalian species investigated [80].

The differentiation that follows testicular determination is a direct consequence of hormonal factors produced by the testes [20]. Although ovarian-determining genes have been documented in mice [11,55], it is not clear whether the ovary plays an active role in controlling subsequent steps of female gonadal development (Fig. 6.2).

In the mouse the gene for AMH is switched on exactly 1.5 days after *SRY* is switched off. AMH expression is controlled by *SRY* through a number of intermediate steps. The gene for AMH encodes a 506-amino-acid protein that shows marked homology with TGF-β (transforming growth factor β) and the β-chain of porcine inhibin and activin. The gene has been localized on the short arm of chromosome 19 [3,81]. AMH is secreted by fetal Sertoli cells and it is also secreted postnatally until 8–10 years of age and can be used clinically as a marker for the presence of Sertoli cells and hence the presence of testicular tissue [77, 81]. AMH is also secreted by follicular cells postnatally in the ovary. In the presence of functional testes, Müllerian ducts involute under the influence of AMH, which causes morphological cell death locally. These data suggest a potential paracrine/autocrine action of AMH in the gonad [5].

AMH action requires high concentrations, and active binding to a membrane receptor in the mesenchymal cells surrounding the Müllerian ducts is necessary. Both lack of AMH as well as insensitivity to this hormone has been described in human disease. In persistent Müllerian duct syndrome, 46,XY males are characterized by the presence of fallopian tubes and uterus. The external genitalia are male, and testicular function is otherwise normal. In AMH deficiency, mutations within the AMH gene have been demonstrated. Patients with persistent Müllerian ducts may have low, normal or even high AMH levels in serum. This can only be explained by an AMH receptor defect in some cases.

The type II AMH receptor, necessary for binding of ligand and exertion of AMH action, has been cloned, and functionally relevant mutations have been demonstrated in patients with persistent Müllerian duct syndrome. The AMH type II receptor gene has been localized on chromosome 12. The defect is inherited in an autosomal recessive fashion [82]. In Sertoli cells, the orphan nuclear receptor, steroidogenic factor 1 (*SF-1*), binding directly to the AMH gene promoter [83], may regulate the AMH gene, suggesting that *SF-1* plays a much broader role in gonadal development by regulating downstream target genes other than those involved in steroidogenesis [5]. A regulatory effect of *SRY* on AMH receptor expression has also been reported [84].

## Testes (Fig. 6.3 and Table 6.2)

Fetal testes, which are located near the kidney, begin their descent at the twelfth week of fetal age. They reach the inguinal region at midgestation and appear in the scrotum only during the last 12 weeks of gestation. The mechanical endocrine factors that guide this descent are still unclear but it is currently believed that the transabdominal descent is not androgen dependent. A role of AMH in descent has been implied, postulating a bihormonal theory (androgens *and* AMH) of testicular descent, but this is unproven at present [85,86].

Leydig cells formed from interstitial tissue (developing mesonephros) appear at about day 60. By the eighth postfertilization week, Leydig cells are actively secreting testosterone, and Sertoli cells, still immature, are secreting AMH. By 14–18 weeks of gestation, Leydig cells take up more than half the volume of the testes. This coincides with the peak concentration of testosterone in fetal serum [73,87,88]. The peak of Leydig cell development also follows peak placental human chorionic gonadotrophin (hCG) release. The fetal pituitary gland thus controls testicular development only in the second and third trimester.

After the eighteenth week, the number of Leydig cells decreases and by 27 weeks the seminiferous tubules are separated by a narrow interstitium containing a few Leydig cells. Fetal Leydig cells lack crystals of Reinke, which develop at the time of puberty [52].

Both male and female gonads have 3β-hydroxysteroid dehydrogenase enzyme (3β-HSD). Testes and ovaries acquire the capacity to secrete the characteristic hormones at the same stage of embryonic development but the activity of 3β-HSD is 50-fold greater in the fetal testes than in the ovary. Concomitant with the expression of the luteinizing hormone (LH) receptor and increasing androgen production, steroidogenic enzymes (P450scc, 3β-HSD and P450c17, all of which are essential for androgen biosynthesis) are expressed in the Leydig cells. The enzyme 17β-HSD, which converts androstenedione to testosterone, is expressed later [89,90]. Gonadotrophins are apparently not required for testosterone synthesis until later in embroygenesis [91].

hCG synthesized by the placenta provides potent LH activity during early embryonic and sexual differentiation [89]. LH receptors (LHRs) are present in the fetal testes from the twelfth week, and gonadotrophins may be necessary for initiation of testosterone synthesis. P450scc and P450c17 genes are expressed in fetal testes during the fourteenth and sixteenth week. Thereafter, as hCG concentrations decline, so do the mRNA levels for these steroidogenic enzymes, suggesting strongly that the expression of these genes is regulated by hCG [92]. Peak fetal serum testosterone concentrations are reached at 16 weeks of gestation and decline thereafter. Late testosterone-mediated events in male development, such as growth of the male external genitalia, are modulated directly by hormones from the pituitary gland. This explains the association of congenital hypopituitarism and microphallus [93]. At birth, cord blood testosterone levels are still somewhat higher in males than in females [93,94].

LHR mutations result both in loss and in gain of function, depending on their localization [95,96] (Fig. 6.4). Inactivating

(a)

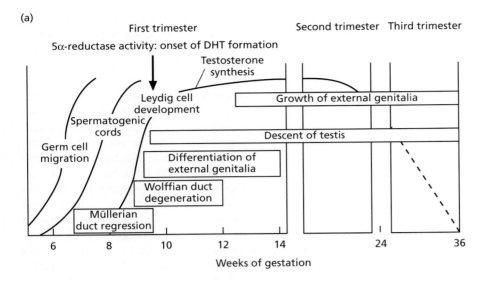

(b)

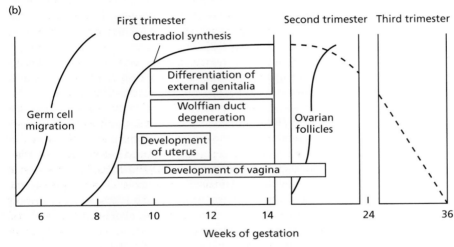

**Fig. 6.3.** Relationship between the differentiation of gonads and anatomical differentiation of human male (a) and female (b) embryos.

**Table 6.2.** Comparative features of fetal and neonatal gonadal function

| Testes | Ovary |
|---|---|
| Early histological definition | Prolonged monomorphic state |
| Several determining genes | One putative determining gene identified |
| Delayed germ cell maturation | Germ cells in early meiotic arrest |
| Early autonomous steroid secretion | No evidence of steroid secretion |
| LHR and steroid enzymes expressed | Delayed expression of LHR and aromatase |
| High fetal testicular testosterone content | Low ovarian oestradiol content |
| Prominent postnatal Leydig and Sertoli cells | Prominent postnatal follicles |
| High postnatal serum testosterone levels | Low postnatal serum oestradiol levels |

LHR, luteinizing hormone receptor.
Modified from Hughes IA *et al.* (1999) *Acta Paediatr Suppl.* 428: 23–30.

mutations of the LHR are associated with gonadotrophin unresponsiveness and lead to Leydig cell agenesis and subsequently to defective sexual differentiation. More often the result is a completely female phenotype, but incomplete virilization (isolated micropenis) due to partial receptor responsiveness with subnormal androgen synthesis has been described [97]. These mutations are typically located in the transmembrane domain of the receptor but mutations within

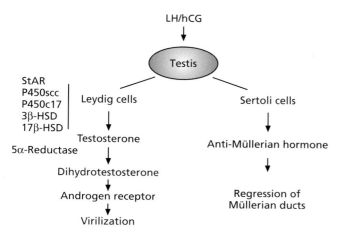

**Fig. 6.4.** Steps of male sexual differentiation. [Modified from Hiort O (2000) *Horm Res* 53 (Suppl. 1): 38–4.]

the extracellular domain have been reported to result in loss of function. These molecular abnormalities imply an active role of the LHR in Leydig cell growth and differentiation.

During the neonatal period there is a rapid five- to sixfold multiplication of Sertoli cells under trophic control of follicle-stimulating hormone (FSH). It is possible that the number of Sertoli cells acquired at this age is a determinant of the potential for spermatogenesis at puberty. More distinct evidence for the role of FSH in Sertoli cell development in humans is provided by decreased spermatogenesis and testis size in adult men with inactivating mutations of the FSH receptor gene. In response to treatment with recombinant FSH, testicular volume and inhibin levels increase in prepubertal boys with gonadotrophin deficiency [98,99].

The Leydig cell population becomes reactivated in the postnatal period under the influence of a transient increase in LH secretion from the pituitary. Both Leydig cell mass and testosterone levels peak at 3 months of age. The physiological relevance of this rise is unclear at present. However, the use of a gonadotrophin-releasing hormone (GnRH) antagonist to prevent the rise in testosterone in male rhesus monkeys delayed the subsequent onset of puberty [100].

## Ovary (Fig. 6.3 and Table 6.2)

The absence of testicular cords is the distinguishing feature of ovary formation. After their migration from the yolk sac, the primordial germ cells are engulfed by mesenchymal cells. By 12 weeks of gestation the transition of oogonia to oocytes is evident marking the true beginning of the ovary. Folliculogenesis starts at about 16 weeks of gestation. Stromal cells differentiate to form thecal cells, which develop the characteristics of steroid-secreting cells (like Leydig cells). The human fetal ovary is capable of converting androgens to oestrogens as early as the eighth week of fetal life. Fetal

ovarian P450scc and P450c17 gene expression is low, so production of all steroids is low including oestrogen. Aromatase activity is present at low levels. Expression of FSH and LH receptors is delayed [101] and AMH is not detectable.

Ovarian somatic cells appearing around the twentieth week form granulosa cells that encircle the oocytes to form single layers characteristic of primordial follicles. At the fifth month of fetal age the fetal ovary is developed. It contains initially approximately seven million germ cells. By birth, the number has fallen to two million and to 400 000 at puberty [102], of which only about 400 will undergo ovulation. Apoptosis is thought to be the mechanism underlying follicular atresia [52].

The ovary may lose its integrity and become a streak without germ cells when the process of oocyte formation is not normal. This may explain streak gonads in girls with Turner syndrome, who have normal ovaries in the second trimester but streak ovaries at birth or soon thereafter. A normal 46,XX karyotype is not necessary for induction of ovarian development, but normal meiosis may be necessary for preservation of normal oocyte numbers [103,104]. Although oestrogen formation does not appear to be essential for normal development of the female phenotype, oestrogen may play a role in the development of the ovary itself [105] (Fig. 6.4).

Inactivating mutations of the LH receptor in females cause amenorrhoea and anovulation, but no abnormality in sex differentiation or follicular development [106], which is indirect evidence for gonadotrophin-independent ovarian development in the fetus. Fetal gonadotrophin levels peak at 20 weeks in the female, and FSH levels are higher in the female [107]. Postnatally, no significant rise in androgens or oestrogens is seen. The ovary is more quiescent in fetal and neonatal life. The contrasting features of the fetal and neonatal testis and ovary are summarized in Table 6.2.

## Differentiation of internal and external genitalia (Fig. 6.5)

By the seventh week of intrauterine life, the fetus is equipped with the primordia of both male and female genital ducts. The Müllerian ducts, if allowed to persist, form the Fallopian ducts, the corpus of the uterus and the upper third of the vagina and cervix. The Wolffian ducts, on the other hand, have the potential for differentiating into epididymis, vas deferens, seminal vesicles and the ejaculatory ducts [105].

Before the ninth week of human development the urogenital tract is identical in both sexes. Two pairs of genital ducts give rise to the Wolffian and Müllerian ducts. Wolffian ducts, which are initially the excretory ducts of the mesonephros, become androgen dependent only when renal function of the definitive kidney has been initiated [108]. Wolffian ducts disappear in the absence of androgens. If androgens are present, the Wolffian ducts become stabilized and eventually become

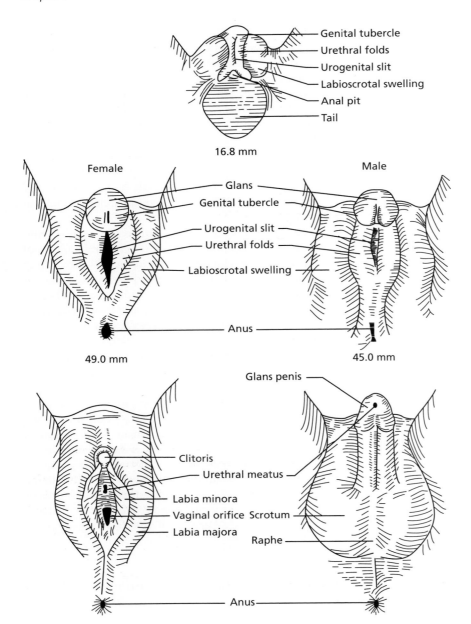

Female          Male

Glans
Genital tubercle
Urogenital slit
Urethral folds
Labioscrotal swelling

Anus

49.0 mm          45.0 mm

Genital tubercle
Urethral folds
Urogenital slit
Labioscrotal swelling
Anal pit
Tail

16.8 mm

Glans penis

Clitoris
Urethral meatus
Labia minora
Vaginal orifice   Scrotum
Labia majora

Raphe

Anus

**Fig. 6.5.** Differentiation of male and female external genitalia from indifferent primordia. Male development will occur only in the presence of androgenic stimulation during the first 12 fetal weeks. Measurements indicate fetal crown–rump length.

the vas deferens system (vasa deferentia, seminal vesicles and ejaculatory ducts). The anterior part of the Wolffian duct communicates with the seminiferous tubules, and the posterior part of each Wolffian duct forms the vas deferens and the seminal vesicle. In the female, Wolffian duct stabilization cannot be maintained by systemic testosterone administration. Therefore, Wolffian ducts are not maintained in virilized females, even when the virilizing agent reaches the fetus very early in pregnancy [71]. The Wolffian duct is apparently sensitive only to testosterone produced locally by the fetal testis [1]. Testosterone is the active hormone in Wolffian duct differentiation and stabilization. The onset of 5α-reductase activity, and thus formation of DHT, begins later [72], and the

Wolffian duct does not contain 5α-reductase activity at this stage.

## Steroids (Fig. 6.6)

The acute stimulation of steroid biosynthesis is mediated by the steroidogenic acute regulatory protein (StAR), which is an active transporter of cholesterol through the inner mitochondrial membrane, the site where steroids are synthesized [109]. Mutations within StAR lead to a severe lack of adrenal steroidogenesis as well as a lack of virilization in 46,XY individuals in lipoid congenital adrenal hyperplasia [110].

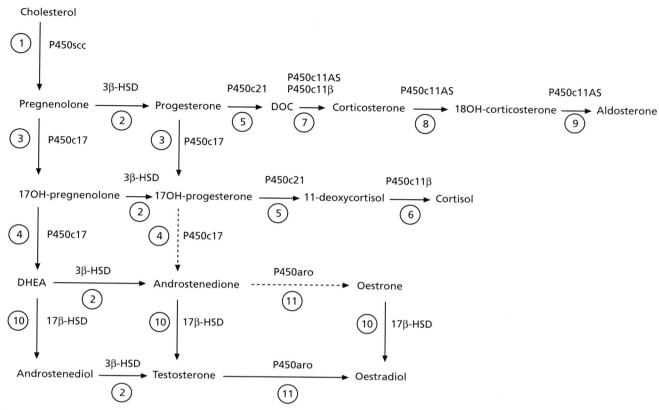

**Fig. 6.6.** Steroid scheme. Principal pathways of human adrenal steroid hormone synthesis. Other quantitatively and physiologically minor steroids also are produced. The chemical identities of the enzymes are shown by each reaction. Reaction 1: mitochondrial cytochrome P450scc mediates 20α-hydroxylation, 22-hydroxylation, and scission of the 20–20 carbon bond to convert cholesterol to pregnenolone. Reaction 2: 3β-HSD mediates 3β-hydroxysteroid dehydrogenase and isomerase activities. Reaction 3: in the adrenal fasciculata and reticularis, P450c17 catalyses the 17α-hydroxylation of pregnenolone to 17-hydroxypregnenolone and of progesterone to 17-hydroxyprogesterone. Reaction 4: the 17,20-lyase activity of P450c17 converts 17-hydroxypregnenolone to DHEA (dehydroepiandrosterone), but very little 17-hydroxyprogesterone is converted to Δ⁴ androstendione. Reaction 5: P450c21 catalyses the 21-hydroxylation of both progesterone and 17-hydroxyprogesterone. Reaction 6: P450c11β converts 11-deoxycortisol to cortisol. Reactions 7, 8 and 9: in the adrenal zona glomerulosa, DOC is converted to corticosterone, then to 18-hydroxycorticosterone and finally to aldosterone by P450c11AS. DOC also may be converted to corticosterone by P450c11β in the zona fasciculata. Reactions 10 and 11 are found principally in the testes and ovaries. Reaction 10: several isozymes of 17β-HSD, a short-chain dehydrogenase, mediate both 17-ketosteroid reductase and 17β-hydroxysteroid dehydrogenase activities, converting DHEA to androstenediol, androstenedione to testosterone and oestrone to oestradiol. Reaction 11: testosterone is converted to oestradiol by P450aro (aromatase). [From Miller WL (1988) Molecular biology of steroid hormone synthesis. *Endocr Rev* 9: 295–318; with permission.]

Because placental steroidogenesis is not StAR dependent, the fetus can survive to term. Cholesterol accumulates within testes and adrenals, further disrupting steroid biosynthesis by the non-StAR-dependent route(s). This is in contrast to the ovary, where there is little evidence of steroid formation in fetal life and in the first postnatal years; therefore, ovarian steroidogenesis is less impaired [110] (Table 6.2). As only single follicles are selected during the menstrual cycle, it is only in these that lipid accumulation occurs leading to anovulatory cycles.

Defects in the first enzymatic step, side-chain cleavage, have not been described in humans and, as it would affect also placental steroidogenesis, it could function as a lethal factor [111]. P450c17 is encoded by a single-copy gene on chromosome 10q24.3, and mutations can inhibit all functions

or, selectively, the 17/20-lyase, with only minimal inhibition of 17α-hydroxylase function [112,113]. The third enzyme is 3β-HSD, which exists in two isoforms that have been cloned. Both genes are localized on chromosome 1p13.1. In 3β-HSD deficiency mutations within the gene encoding for the type II enzyme have been found. 3β-HSD type II is predominantly expressed in adrenals and gonads; hence its blockade results in congenital adrenal hyperplasia and in defective virilization in males.

Although the enzymes listed above synthesize gluco- and mineralocorticoids and sex steroids, both 17β-HSD and 5α-reductase are restricted to androgen synthesis. At least five different isoenzymes of 17β-HSD exist. Only mutations in the type 3 enzymes have been demonstrated to be responsible for abnormal sex differentiation in patients with 17β-HSD deficiency [114,115]. Affected XY individuals have ambiguous genitalia but may virilize at puberty.

## Urogenital sinus and external genitalia: role of dihydrotestosterone (Figs 6.2 and 6.5)

The common anlagen are the genital tubercle, the urethral folds and the labioscrotal swelling. The paired urethral folds surround a urogenital groove. Masculinization begins in the male fetus by a lengthening of the anogenital distance. The labioscrotal swellings fuse in midline forming the scrotum. The urethral folds close and elongate forming the shaft of the penis and the cavernous urethra. The genital tubercle becomes the corpora cavernosa and the glans penis. Formation of the penis is complete at 12–14 weeks' gestation, and labioscrotal fusion cannot be achieved in female fetuses exposed to androgens after this time. Growth of the penis continues throughout gestation and is normally mediated by the pituitary gland-dependent Leydig cell stimulation of the fetal testis. The urogenital sinus increases in length and forms the prostatic and perineal urethra. At 12–14 weeks the penile urethra is formed [116,117].

Although testosterone is the androgen that differentiates the Wolffian duct, it acts only as a prohormone in other androgen-dependent tissues, notably the urogenital sinus and the external genitalia. In these tissues, testosterone is converted to the more potent 5α-DHT by a microsomal 5α-reductase. Thus testosterone and DHT play selective roles in embryogenesis. Both testosterone and DHT bind to the same high-affinity androgen receptor protein within the cells of androgen-dependent target areas [116]. The affinity of the androgen receptor is much greater for DHT than it is for testosterone (Fig. 6.7).

Testosterone enters the target cell by passive diffusion and either binds to the androgen receptor or is metabolized to DHT, which then binds to the same receptor. The androgen receptor complex binds to acceptor sites on nuclear chromatin and ultimately initiates transcription of mRNA, starting the complex metabolic processes of androgen action [118,119]. The gene for the androgen receptor has been cloned to the long arm of the X chromosome near the centromere [80].

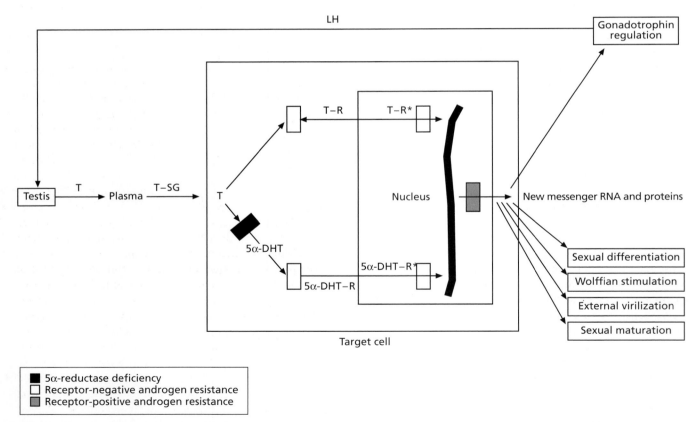

**Fig. 6.7.** Mechanism by which androgens act to virilize the male embryo. Three types of mutations are particularly informative in proving the clinical applicability of this model: 5α-reductase deficiency and receptor-positive and receptor-negative androgen resistance syndromes. DHT, dihydrotestosterone; LH, luteinizing hormone; R, high-affinity androgen receptor protein; R*, transformed androgen receptor exposing its DNA-binding domain; SG, sex hormone-binding globulin; T, testosterone.

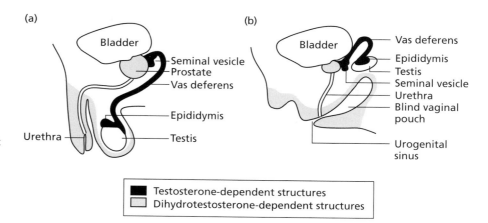

**Fig. 6.8.** (a) Suggested selective role of testosterone and DHT in normal male sexual differentiation. (b) Findings in males who cannot convert testosterone to DHT (5α-reductase deficiency). Testosterone-dependent structures are normal, although testes are not descended. DHT-dependent structures are not developed. Blind vaginal pouch is frequently present.

In the urogenital tubercle, high activity of 5α-reductase at the time of sex differentiation provides DHT for preferential binding to the androgen receptor. The reason that testosterone mediates some androgen effects and DHT mediates others is currently not clear, but it may involve subtle differences in the affinity of the receptor for the androgen, some aspect of the metabolism of testosterone, or both [116].

DHT develops the prostate, prostatic utricle, scrotum, penis with male-type urethra and the glans penis. On the other hand, increases in muscle mass and voice changes at puberty appear to be mediated by testosterone. Acne, beard growth, temporal hairline recession, body hair and prostatic growth, however, seem to be mediated by DHT, which also plays a negative feedback control of LH. The enzyme 5α-reductase is present in the urogenital sinus and external genitalia anlagen before masculinization (Fig. 6.8) [8,9,120,121].

## Androgen resistance

The binding of testosterone and DHT to the receptor complex has been hypothesized to result in a conformational change in the receptor, exposing its DNA-binding domain and enabling it to bind to the nuclear chromatin. The binding of androgen receptor complex to DNA initiates transcription of mRNA and ultimately translation into androgen-specific protein. In humans with complete androgen insensitivity, a number of binding abnormalities of the androgen receptor have been described. Absence of high-affinity binding has been demonstrated (receptor negative). Subjects with normal binding and absent androgen receptor complex binding to nuclear chromatin (receptor positive) have also been described. The androgen receptor (AR) gene belongs to the steroid receptor superfamily and is composed of eight exons, as well as an androgen- and a DNA-binding domain (Fig. 6.9). Various defects result in synthesis of abnormal androgen receptor. Mutations in the androgen-binding domain result in receptor-negative androgen insensitivity, whereas muta-

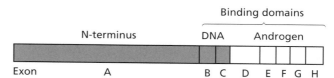

**Fig. 6.9.** Schematic presentation of androgen receptor. The amino-terminal portion is coded by exon A. Its role is probably modulatory. The DNA-binding domain is coded by exons B and C and the androgen-binding domain is encoded by exons D, E, F, G and H.

tions in the DNA-binding domain result in receptor-positive binding abnormalities to DNA [8]. Several groups were able to clone and sequence the gene for the human AR [6,7,122–126]. The gene has been mapped to Xq11–12 [127].

The general pattern of clinical symptoms observed in androgen insensitivity syndrome (AIS) patients results from a combination of defective androgen action in androgen-dependent target tissues, despite normal or even elevated testicular androgen secretion and the normal ability of the fetal testes to produce AMH. AIS patients show, therefore, defective masculinization of the external genitalia with defective Wolffian duct development in conjunction with usually absent Müllerian duct derivatives [128].

The partial androgen insensitivity syndrome is based on partial impairment of AR function. It results in a wide spectrum of external undervirilization or just abnormal sperm maturation within the testes [8,129]. More than 400 different mutations have been identified in AIS in the 10 years elapsed since cloning of the *AR* gene. Several obvious mutational hotspots exist. The most commonly seen alteration are missense mutations in the *AR* gene, which may result in AIS or partial AIS (PAIS). The gene is regulated by a number of co-activators and co-repressors, and many individuals with the phenotype display no mutation in the coding region for the actual receptor. Abnormalities in co-activators of the androgen receptor gene have been postulated.

Knowledge of predictors of the phenotype due to a specific

**Table 6.3.** Characterization of the two 5α-reductase isoenzymes

|  | Type 1 | Type 2 |
|---|---|---|
| Molecular weight | 29 000 | 29 000 |
| Number of amino acids | 292 | 254 |
| Optimum pH | Basic (8.0) | Acidic (6.0) |
| $K_m$ (μM) | 24 | 0.3 |
| Chromosomic location of gene | 5 | 2 |
| Body sites | Skin,* liver, adrenal, kidney | Skin,† prostate, epididymis, seminal vesicles, testes, liver |

$K_m$, enzymatic Michaelis–Menten constant.
*Hair follicles and distal sebaceous gland lobes.
†Hair follicles and duct of sebaceous glands.
Modified from Azziz R et al. (2000) *Endocrinol Rev* 21: 347–62.

genetic abnormality within the *AR* gene is limited. In a significant proportion of patients with a mutated *AR* gene, the genetic aberration has occurred after conception as an early somatic mutation [130,131]. This genetic pattern leads to a mosaicism, mutated and wild-type AR proteins, and hence to increased androgen sensitivity [130–132]. Whether alternative pathways of androgen action are significant in the determination of the male phenotype remains to be elucidated.

## 5α-Reductase deficiency

Two 5α-reductase genes have been cloned. These genes encode two different isoenzymes distinguishable on the basis of biochemical, pharmacological and genetic criteria. The type I isoenzyme is encoded on chromosome 5 and expressed in low levels in the prostate. High levels are present in scalp hair follicles. Type I isoenzyme is relatively insensitive to the 5α-reductase inhibitor finasteride. The type II isoenzyme encoded on chromosome 2 is expressed in high levels in the prostate and many other androgen-sensitive tissues. It is exquisitely sensitive to finasteride (Table 6.3) [9,120].

5α-Reductase deficiency has been the consequence of mutations in the type I gene in all cases studied. The type I isoenzyme is necessary for the reduction of androgens to inhibit excess formation of oestrogens, and thus mice lacking this enzyme fail to uphold normal pregnancies [133]. A specific role for 5α-reductase type I in male sex differentiation has not been shown. Molecular analysis indicates that the majority of patients with steroid 5α-reductase type II deficiency have various mutations. One genetic isolate in New Guinea has a deletion of the type II gene. Since only the type II gene is responsible for 5α-reduction of testosterone in genital skin, defects in the type I gene would not be expected to be associated with inadequate masculinization [10, 120].

No hormones are necessary for normal differentiation of female external genitalia. In the 8-week female fetus, the genital tubercle becomes the clitoris, the labioscrotal swelling, the labia majora and the urethral fold the labia minora. The labioscrotal swellings do not fuse, and the perineal anogenital distance does not increase [134,135]. Cavitation for vaginal development is first observed at 15 weeks and is complete at 18 weeks. In the male fetus, caudal growth of the rudimentary vaginal chord is inhibited, and canalization of this rudimentary structure yields the prostatic utricle, which opens just beneath the bladder neck between the orifices of the vasa deferentia [135].

## References

1 Rubin RT, Reinische JM, Haskett RF. Postnatal gonadal steroid effects on human behavior. *Science* 1981; 211: 1318–24.

2 McLaren A. What makes a man? *Nature* 1990; 346: 216–17.

3 Cohen-Haguenauer O, Picard JY, Mattei MG et al. Mapping of the gene for anti-Müllerian hormone to the short arm of human chromosome 19. *Cytogenet Cell Genet* 1987; 44: 2–6.

4 Donahoe PK, Care RL, MacLaughlin DT et al. Müllerian-inhibiting substance; gene structure and mechanism of action of a fetal repressor. *Rec Prog Horm Res* 1987; 43: 431–67.

5 Rey R. Endocrine, paracrine and cellular regulation of post-natal anti-Müllerian hormone secretion by Sertoli cells. *Trends Endocrinol Metab* 1999; 9: 271–6.

6 Chang C, Kokontis J, Liaso S. Structural analysis of complementary DNA and amino-acid sequences of human and rat androgen receptors. *Proc Natl Acad Sci USA* 1988; 85: 7211–15.

7 Lubahn DB, Joseph DR, Sullivan PM et al. Cloning of human androgen receptor complementary DNA and localization to the X chromosome. *Science* 1988; 240: 327–30.

8 Quigley CA, De Bellis A, Marschke KB et al. Androgen receptor defects: historical, clinical and molecular perspectives. *Endocr Rev* 1995; 16: 271–321.

9 Thigpen AE, Davis DL, Milatovich A et al. The molecular genetics of steroid 5α-reductase deficiency. *J Clin Invest* 1992; 90: 799–809.

10 Wilson JD, Griffin JE, Russell DW. Sterol 5α-reductase 2 deficiency. *Endocr Rev* 1993; 14: 577–94.

11 Vainio S, Heikkilä M, Kispert A et al. Female development in mammals is regulated by Wnt-4 signalling. *Nature* 1999; 397: 405–9.

12  Yu RN, Ho M, Saunders TL *et al.* Role of Ahch in gonadal development and gameto-genesis. *Nature Genet* 1998; 20: 353–7.

13  McCarrey JR, Abbott UK. Mechanisms of genetic sex determination, gonadal sex-determination and germ-cell development in animals. *Adv Genet* 1979; 20: 217–90.

14  Crews D. Temperature, steroids and sex determination. *J Endocrinol* 1994; 142: 1–8.

15  Capel B. Sex in the 90s: SRY and the switch to the male pathway. *Annu Rev Physiol* 1998; 60: 497–523.

16  Jost A. Recherches sur la différentiation sexuelle de l'embryo de lapin. *Arch Anat Microsc Morph Exp* 1947; 36: 271–315.

17  Whelsons WJ, Russell LB. The Y chromosome as a bearer of male determining factors in the mouse. *Proc Natl Acad Sci USA* 1959; 45: 560–6.

18  Mittwoch U. Do genes determine sex? *Nature* 1969; 22: 446–8.

19  Polani PE. Abnormal sex development in man. I. Anomalies of sex-determining mechanisms. In: Justin CR, Edwards RG, eds. *Mechanism of Sex Differentiation in Animals and Man.* London: Academic Press, 1981: 465–547.

20  Jost A, Vigier B, Prepin J, Perchellet JP. Studies on sex differentiation in mammals. *Rec Prog Horm Res* 1973; 29: 1–41.

21  Jirasek JE. Morphogenesis of the genital system in the human. *Birth Defects* 1977; 13: 13–19.

22  Jirasek JE. Principles of reproductive endocrinology. In: Simpson JL, eds. *Disorders of Sexual Differentiation.* New York: Academic Press, 1976: 52–111.

23  Ford CE, Jone KW, Polani PE *et al.* A sex chromosome anomaly in a case of gonadal dysgenesis (Turner's syndrome). *Lancet* 1959; 1: 711–13.

24  Jacobs PA, Strong JA. A case of human intersexuality having a possible XXY sex-determining mechanism. *Nature* 1959; 183: 302–3.

25  Wachtel SS, Ohno S. The immunogenetics of sexual development. *Prog Med Genet* 1979; 3: 109–42.

26  Simpson E, Chandler P, Goulmy E *et al.* Separation of the genetic loci for the H-Y antigen and for testis determination on human Y chromosome. *Nature* 1987; 326: 876–8.

27  Lau YFC, Chan K. The putative testis-determining factor and related genes are expressed as discrete sized transcripts in adult gonadal and somatic tissues. *Am J Hum Genet* 1990; 45: 942–52.

28  Page DC, Mosher R, Simpson EM *et al.* The sex-determining human Y chromosome encodes a finger protein. *Cell* 1987; 51: 1091–104.

29  Page DC, Brown LG, de la Chapelle A. Exchange of terminal portions of X and Y chromosomal short arms in human XX males. *Nature* 1987; 328: 437–40.

30  Palmer MS, Sinclair AH, Ellis NA *et al.* Genetic evidence that ZFY is not the testis-determining factor. *Nature* 1989; 342: 937–9.

31  Palmer MS, Berta P, Sinclair AH *et al.* Comparison of human ZRY and ZFY transcripts. *Genetics* 1990; 187: 1618–85.

32  Burgoyne PS. Thumbs down for the zinc finger? *Nature* 1989; 342: 860–2.

33  Sinclair AH, Berta P, Palmer MS *et al.* A gene from the human sex-determining region encodes a protein with homology to a conserved DNA binding motif. *Nature* 1990; 346: 240–4.

34  Gubbay J, Collignon J, Koopman P *et al.* A gene mapping to the sex-determining region of the mouse Y chromosome is a member of a novel family of embryonically expressed genes. *Nature* 1990; 346: 245–50.

35  Koopman P, Gubbay J, Vivian N *et al.* Male development of chromosomally female mice transgenic for SRY. *Nature* 1991; 351: 117–21.

36  Lovell-Badge R. Sex determining gene expression during embryogenesis. *Philos Trans R Soc London Series B* 1992; 335: 159–64.

37  Koopman P, Munsterberg A, Capel B *et al.* Expression of a candidate sex-determining gene during mouse testis determination. *Nature* 1990; 348: 450–2.

38  Jeske YWA, Bowles J, Greenfield A *et al.* Expression of a linear SRY transcript in the mouse genital ridge. *Nature Genet* 1995; 10: 480–2.

39  Hacker A, Capel B, Goodfellow P *et al.* Expression of SRY, the mouse sex-determining gene. *Development* 1995; 121: 1603–4.

40  Shapiro LJ. X and Y chromosome organization. The pseudoautosomal region. In: Rosenfeld R, Grumach M, eds. *Turner Syndrome.* New York: Marcel Dekker, 1990: 3–11.

41  Redline RW, Williams AJ, Patterson P *et al.* Human HOXU.E: a gene strongly expressed in the adult male and female urogenital tracts. *Genomics* 1992; 13: 425–30.

42  Hawkins JR, Koopman P, Berta P. Testis-determining factor and Y-linked sex reversal. *Curr Opin Genet Dev* 1991; 1: 30–4.

43  Jager RJ, Anvret M, Hall K *et al.* Human X female with a frame shift mutation in the candidate testes determining gene SRY. *Nature* 1990; 348: 452–3.

44  Ferrari S, Harley VR, Pontiggia H *et al.* SRY, like HMG1, recognizes sharp angles in DNA. *EMBO J* 1992; 11: 497–506.

45  Eccles MR, Wallis LJ, Fidler AE *et al.* Expression of the PAX 2 gene in human fetal kidney and Wilms tumor. *Cell Growth Differ* 1992; 3: 279–89.

46  Ohno S. Major sex-determining genes. New York: Springer-Verlag, 1979.

47  Wolgemuth DJ, Viviano CM, Gizang-Ginsberg F *et al.* Differential expression of the mouse homeobox-containing gene HOX-1.4 during male germ cell differentiation and embryonic development. *Proc Natl Acad Sci USA* 1987; 50: 5815–17.

48  Hawkins JR. Mutational analysis of SRY in XY females. *Hum Genet* 1993; 2: 347–50.

49  Jacobs PA, Brunton M, Melville MD. Aggressive behavior, mental sub-normality and the XYY male. *Nature* 1965; 208: 1351–2.

50  Harley VR, Jackson DI, Hextal PJ. DNA binding activity of recombinant SRY from normal males and XY females. *Science* 1992; 225: 453–6.

51  Grosschedl R, Giese K, Page DC. HMG domain proteins: architectural elements in the assembly of nucleoprotein structures. *Trends Genet* 1994; 10: 94–100.

52  Hughes IA, Coleman N, Faisal Ahmed S *et al.* Sexual dimorphism in the neonatal gonad. *Acta Pediatr Scand* 1999; 428: 23–30.

53  Pritchard-Jones K, Fleming S, Davidson D *et al.* The candidate Wilms' tumor gene is involved in genito urinary development. *Nature* 1990; 346: 194–7.

54  Kreidberg JA, Sariola H, Loring JM *et al.* WT-1 is required for early kidney development. *Cell* 1993; 74: 679–91.

55  Heikkilä M, Peltoketo H, Vainio S. Genetic regulation of female development – lessons from Wnt-4. In: Saenger P and Pasquino AM (eds). *Optimising Health Care for Turner Patients in the 21st Century.* Amsterdam: Elsevier Science, 2000: 29–41.

56  Birk OS, Casiano DE, Wassif CA *et al*. A dosage sensitive locus at chromosome Xp21 is involved in male to female sex reversal. *Nature Genet* 1994; 7: 497–501.

57  Parker RL, Schimmer BP. Steroidogenic factor 1: a key determinant of endocrine development and function. *Endocrinol Rev* 1997; 18: 361–77.

58  Okeda Y, Shen WH, Ingraham HA *et al*. Developmental expression of mouse steroidogenic factor-1, an essential regulator of steroid hydroxylase. *Mol Endocrinol* 1994; 8: 654–62.

59  Giulli G, Shen WH, Ingraham HA. The nuclear receptor SF-1 mediates sexually dimorphic expression of Müllerian inhibiting substance in vivo. *Development* 1997; 124: 1799–807.

60  Achermann JC, Ito M, Ito M, Hindmarsh PC, Jameson JL. A mutation in the gene encoding steroidogenic factor-1 causes XY sex reversal and adrenal failure in humans. *Nature Genet* 1999; 22: 125–6.

61  Moraisda Silva S, Hacker A, Harley V *et al*. SOX 9 expression during gonadal development implies a conserved role for the gene in testis differentiation in mammals and birds. *Nature Genet* 1996; 14: 62–8.

62  Kent J, Sheatley SC, Andrew JE. A male-specific role for SOX 9 in vertebrate sex determination. *Development* 1996; 122: 2813–22.

63  Kwok C, Weller PA, Ginoli S *et al*. Mutations in SOX 9 the gene responsible for Campromelic dysplasia and autosomal sex reversal. *Am J Hum Genet* 1995; 57: 1028–36.

64  Huang B, Wang S, Ning Y *et al*. Autosomal XX sex reversal caused by duplication of SOX 9. *Am J Med Genet* 1999; 87: 849–53.

65  Nachtigal MW, Hiokawa Y, Enyeart-Van Houten DL *et al*. Wilms' tumor and Dax-1 modulate the orphan nuclear receptor SF-1 in sex-specific gene-expression. *Cell* 1998; 93: 445–54.

66  Yu RN, Ho M, Saunders TL *et al*. Role of Ahch in gonadal development and gameto-genesis. *Nature Genet* 1998; 20: 353–7.

67  Swain A, Harvaez V, Burgoyne B *et al*. Dax-1 antagonizes SRY action in mammalian sex determination. *Nature* 1998; 391: 761–7.

68  Parker KL, Schimmer BP. Ahch and the feminine mystique. *Nature Genet* 1998; 20: 318–19.

69  Muscatelli F, Strom TM, Walker AP *et al*. Mutations in the Dax-1 gene give rise to both x-linked adrenal hypoplasia congenita and hypogonadotropic hypogonadism. *Nature* 1994; 372: 672–6.

70  Stark K, Vainio S, Vassileva G *et al*. Epithelial transformation of metanephric mesenchyme in the developing kidney regulated by Wnt-4. *Nature* 1994; 372: 679–83.

71  Pfeiffer RA, Rauch A, Trantmann U *et al*. Defective sexual development in an infant with 46,XY der(9)t (8;9) (q23.1; p23) mat. *Eur J Pediatr* 1999; 158: 213–16.

72  Raymond CS, Parker ED, Kettlewell JR *et al*. A region of human chromosome 9p required for testis development contains two genes related to known sexual regulators. *Hum Mol Genet* 1999; 8: 989–96.

73  George FW, Wilson JD. The regulation of androgen and estrogen formation in fetal gonads. *Ann Biol Anim Biochem Biophys* 1979; 19: 129–306.

74  Blyth B, Douchett JAV. Gonadal differentiation: a review of the physiological process and influencing factors based on recent experimental evidence. *J Urol* 1991; 145: 689–94.

75  Hastie ND. PAX in our time. *Curr Biol* 1992; 1: 324–44.

76  Francavilla S, Cordeschi G, Properzi G *et al*. Ultrastructure of fetal human gonad before sexual differentiation and during early testicular and ovarian development. *J Submicrosc Cytol Pathol* 1990; 22: 389–400.

77  Tran D, Meusy-Dessole N, Josso N. Anti-Müllerian hormone is a functional marker of foetal Sertoli cells. *Nature* 1977; 269: 411–12.

78  Sharpe RM, Skakkeback NE. Are oestrogens involved in falling sperm counts and disorders of the male reproductive tract? *Lancet* 1992; 1: 1392–4.

79  Charpentier G, Magre S. Masculinizing effect of testes on developing rat ovaries in organ culture. *Development* 1990; 110: 839–49.

80  Mittwoch U, Burgess AMC, Baker PJ. Male development in a sea of oestrogen. *Lancet* 1993; 2: 123–4.

81  Josso N. Pediatric applications of anti-Müllerian hormone research. *Horm Res* 1994; 43: 243–8.

82  Rey R, Picard JY. Embryology and endocrinology of genital development. *Baillière's Clin Endocrinol Metabolism* 1998; 12: 17–33.

83  Shen WH, Moore CC, Ikeda Y *et al*. Nuclear receptor steroidogenesis factor 1 regulate the Müllerian inhibiting substance gene: a link to the sex determination cascade. *Cell* 1994; 77: 651–61.

84  Hacq CM, King CY, Ukiyama E *et al*. Molecular basis of mammalian sexual determination: activation of Müllerian inhibiting substance gene expression by SRY. *Science* 1994; 266: 1494–500.

85  Saenger P, Reiter EO. Management of cryptorchidism. *Trends Endocrinol Metab* 1992; 3: 249–53.

86  Fentener van Vlissingen FM, Van Zoelen EJJ, Usem PJF *et al*. In vitro model of the first phase of testicular descent: identification of a low molecular weight factor from fetal testis involved in proliferation of gubernaculum testis cells and distinct from specified polypeptide growth factors and fetal gonadal hormones. *Endocrinology* 1988; 123: 2868–77.

87  Baker TG. A quantitative and cytological study of germ cells in human ovaries. *Proc R Soc London (Biol)* 1963; 158: 417–44.

88  George FW, Simpson ER, Milewich L *et al*. Studies on the regulation of the onset of steroid hormone biosynthesis in fetal rabbit gonads. *Endocrinology* 1979; 105: 1100–6.

89  Baillie AH, Ferguson MM, Hart DMK. Histochemical evidence of steroid metabolism in the human genital ridge. *J Clin Endocrinol Metab* 1966; 26: 738–41.

90  Lejeune H, Habert R, Saez JM. Origin, proliferation and differentiation of Leydig cells. *J Mol Endocrinol* 1998; 20: 1–25.

91  Clark SJ, Ellis N, Styne DM *et al*. Hormone ontogeny in the ovine fetus. XVII. Demonstration of pulsatile luteinizing hormone secretion by the fetal pituitary gland. *Endocrinology* 1984; 115: 1774–9.

92  Voutilainen R. Hormonal development in the fetal gonad. In: Sizonenko PC, Aubert ML, eds. *Developmental Endocrinol*. New York: Raven Press, 1990: 27–37.

93  Lovinger RD, Kaplan SL, Grumbach MM. Congenital hypopituitarism associated with neonatal hypoglycemia and microphallus: four cases secondary to hypothalamic hormone deficiencies. *J Pediatr* 1975; 87: 1171–81.

94  Forest MG. Physiological changes in circulating androgens. In: Forest MG, eds. *Androgens in Childhood Pediatric and Adolescent Endocrinology*, Vol. 19. Basle: Karger, 1989: 104–29.

95  Min KS, Liu X, Fabritz J *et al*. Mutations that induce constitutive activation and mutations that impair signal transduction modulate the basal and/or agonist-stimulated internalization of the lutropin/choriogonadotrophin receptor. *J Biol Chem* 1998; 273: 34911–19.

96  Therninen AM, Martens JW, Brunner HG. Activating and inactivating mutations in LH receptors. *Mol Cell Endocrinol* 1998; 145: 137–42.

97  Misrahi M, Bean I, Meduri G *et al*. Gonadotrophin receptors and the control of gonadal steroidogenesis, physiology and pathology. *Baillière's Clin Endocrinol Metab* 1998; 12: 35–66.

98  Tapanainen JS, Aittomäki K, Min J *et al*. Men homozygous for an inactivating mutation of the follicle-stimulating hormone (FSH) receptor gene present variable suppression of spermatogenesis and fertility. *Nature Genet* 1997; 15: 205–6.

99  Raino T, Toppari J, Perheentupa J *et al*. Treatment of prepubertal gonadotrophin-deficient boys with recombinant human follicle-stimulating hormone. *Lancet* 1997; 350: 263–4.

100  Mann DR, Akinbarni MA, Gould KG *et al*. Sexual maturation in male rhesus monkeys: importance of neonatal testosterone exposure and social rank. *J Endocrinol* 1998; 156: 493–501.

101  Sokka T, Hämälainen T, Huhtaniemi I. Functional LH receptor appears in the neonatal rat ovary after changes in the alternatively splicing pattern of the LH receptor mRNA. *Endocrinology* 1992; 130: 1738–40.

102  Pryse-Davies J, Dewhurst CJ. The development of the ovary and uterus in the fetus, newborn and infant: a morphological and enzyme histochemical study. *J Pathol* 1971; 103: 5–25.

103  Sinclair AH. The cloning of SRY. In: Wachtel S, eds. *Genetics of Sex Determination*, San Diego, CA: Academic Press, 1994: 23–41.

104  Held KR. Turner's syndrome and chromosome Y (editorial). *Lancet* 1993; 342: 128.

105  George FW, Wilson JD. Sex determination and differentiation. In: Knobel E, Neill JN, eds. *The Physiology of Reproduction*, 2nd edn. New York: Raven Press, 1994: 3–28.

106  Toledo SP, Brunner HG, Kraaij R *et al*. An inactivating mutation of the luteinizing hormone receptor causes amenorrhea in a 46,XX female. *J Clin Endocrinol Metab* 1996; 81: 3850–4.

107  Reyes FI, Boroditsky RS, Winter JSD *et al*. Studies on human sexual development: II. Fetal and maternal serum gonadotrophin and sex steroid concentration. *J Clin Endocrinol Metab* 1974; 28: 612–17.

108  Price D, Zaaijer HP, Ortiz E *et al*. Current views on embryonic sex differentiation in reptiles, birds and mammals. *Ann Zool* 1975; 1 (Suppl.): 173–95.

109  Saenger P. New developments in congenital lipoid adrenal hyperplasia. *Pediatr Clin N Am* 1997; 44: 397–421.

110  Bose HS, Sugawara T, Strauss JF III *et al*. The pathophysiology and genetics of congenital lipoid adrenal hyperplasia. *N Engl J Med* 1996; 335: 1870–8.

111  Lin D, Gitelman SE, Saenger P *et al*. Normal genes for the cholesterol side chain cleavage enzyme, P450scc, in congenital lipoid adrenal hyperplasia. *J Clin Invest* 1991; 88: 1955–62.

112  Biason-Lauber A, Leiberman E, Zachmann M. A single amino acid substitution in the putative redox partner-binding site of P450c17 as cause of isolated 17,20-lyase deficiency. *J Clin Endocrinol Metab* 1997; 82: 3807–12.

113  Geller DH, Auchus RJ, Mendonca BB *et al*. The genetic and functional basis of isolated 17,20-lyase deficiency. *Nature Genet* 1997; 17: 205.

114  Andersson S, Geissler WM, Wu L *et al*. Molecular genetics and pathophysiology of 17β-hydroxysteroid dehydrogenase 3 deficiency. *J Clin Endocrinol Metab* 1996; 81: 130–6.

115  Moghrabi N, Hughes IA, Dunaif A *et al*. Deleterious missense mutations and silent polymorphism in the human 17β-hydroxysteroid dehydrogenase 3 gene (HSD17β3). *J Clin Endocrinol Metab* 1998; 83: 285–60.

116  Wilson JD, Griffin JE, Leshin M *et al*. Role of gonadal hormones in development of sexual phenotypes. *Hum Genet* 1981; 58: 78–84.

117  Wilson JD. Testosterone uptake by the urogenital tract of the rabbit embryo. *Endocrinology* 1973; 92: 1192–9.

118  Griffin KD, Wilson JD. The androgen resistance syndromes: 5α-reductase deficiency, testicular feminization, and related disorders. In: Scriver C, Baudet A, Sly W *et al*. eds. *The Metabolic Basis of Inherited Disease*, 6th edn. New York: McGraw-Hill, 1989: 1919–44.

119  Migeon CJ, Wisniewski AB. Sexual differentiation: from genes to gender. *Horm Res* 1998; 50: 245–51.

120  Russell DW, Wilson JD. Steroid 5α-reductase: two genes, two enzymes. *Ann Rev Biochem* 1994; 63: 25–6.

121  Saenger P. Steroid 5α-reductase deficiency. In: Josso N, ed. *The Intersex Child*. Basle: Karger Publishers, 1981: 156–70.

122  McPhaul MJ, Marcelli M, Zoppi S *et al*. The spectrum of mutations in the androgenreceptor gene that causes androgen resistance. *J Clin Endocrinol Metab* 1993; 76: 17–23.

123  Marcelli M, Tilley WD, Wilson JE *et al*. A single nucleotide substitution introduces a premature termination codon into the androgen receptor gene of a patient with receptor-negative androgen resistance. *J Clin Invest* 1990; 85: 1522–8.

124  Marcelli M, Zoppi S, Grino PB *et al*. A mutation in the DNA-binding domain of the androgen receptor gene causes complete testicular feminization in a patient with receptor-positive androgen resistance. *J Clin Invest* 1991; 87: 1123–6.

125  Marcelli M, Zoppi S, Wilson CM *et al*. Amino acid substitutions in the hormone-binding domain of the human androgen receptor alter the stability of the hormone receptor complex. *J Clin Invest* 1994; 94: 1642–50.

126  Trapman J, Klaassen P, Kupier GGJM *et al*. Cloning, structure and expression of a cDNA encoding the human androgen receptor. *Biochem Biophys Res Commun* 1988; 145: 241–8.

127  Brown CJ, Goss SJ, Lubahn DB *et al*. Androgen receptor locus on the human X-chromosome: regional localization to qX11–12 and description of a DNA polymorphism. *Am J Hum Genet* 1989; 44: 264–9.

128  Migeon B, Brown TF, Axelman J *et al*. Studies of the locus for androgen receptor: localization on the human X chromosome and evidence for homology with the Tfm locus in the mouse. *Proc Natl Acad Sci USA* 1981; 78: 6339–43.

129  Sinnecker GHG, Hiort O, Nitsche EM *et al*. Functional assessment and clinical classification of androgen sensitivity in patients with mutations of the androgen receptor gene. *Eur J Pediatr* 1997; 156: 7–14.

130  Hiort O, Sinnecker GHG, Holterhus PM *et al*. Inherited and de novo androgen receptor gene mutations: Investigation of single-case families. *J Pediatr* 1998; 132: 939–43.

131 Holterhus PM, Wiebel J, Sinnecker GHG *et al*. Clinical and molecular spectrum of somatic mosaicism in androgen insensitivity syndrome. *Pediatr Res* 1999; 46: 684–90.

132 Brinkmann AO, Blok LJ, de Ruiter PE *et al*. Mechanisms of androgen receptor activation and function. *J Steroid Biochem Mol Biol* 1999; 69: 307–13.

133 Mahendroo MS, Cala KM, Landrum DP *et al*. Fetal death in mice lacking 5α-reductase type I caused by estrogen excess. *Mol Endocrinol* 1997; 11: 917–27.

134 O'Rahilly R. The development of the vagina in the human. *Birth Defects* 1977; 13: 123–36.

135 Ulfelder H, Robboy SJ. Embryonic development of the vagina. *Am J Obstet Gynecol* 1976; 126: 769–76.

# 7 Endocrinology of the newborn

### G. L. Warne, P. Dabadghao and A. Boneh

## Introduction

For every newborn infant, birth is both an end and a beginning. Birth represents the separation of the fetus from its placenta, ending transplacental nutrition and oxygenation. From that moment, enteral nutrition and oxygenation via the lungs must take over. The circulatory system has to change as the placental circulation is abruptly diverted to the lungs and the low fetal arterial blood pressure in late gestation rises to a high arterial blood pressure postnatally. The constantly warm and watery milieu of the intrauterine environment is replaced by one providing an array of new and ever-changing sensory experiences: sound, light, touch, pain, smell, taste and wide fluctuations in ambient temperature. Less obvious, but equally dramatic, structural and functional changes occur in other internal organs and systems of the body. A great deal of information has been accumulated about the ontogeny of changes in the endocrine system. Many advances have come from the comparatively new field of molecular embryology and, in the next decade, the human genome project is likely to uncover many genes involved in organogenesis and hormone synthesis. The great challenge after that will be to define their exact function and their interrelationships.

In this chapter, we discuss the genes known to be involved in the regulation of endocrine organogenesis, the ontogeny of the fetal endocrine system, the hormonal changes that occur in the newborn period, endocrine disorders that are encountered in the newborn and the management of these conditions. The management of ambiguous genitalia, however, has been omitted because it has been discussed in the preceding chapter.

## Embryology of the endocrine system

### The hypothalamus and pituitary (Table 7.1)

Possibly the first hormone to be made in the embryo is gonadotrophin-releasing hormone (GnRH), which is made in large quantities in the preimplantation embryo and stimulates the secretion of chorionic gonadotrophin (CG). CG stimulates maternal progesterone secretion by the ovaries, thus ensuring implantation of the embryo. Thus the embryo is, in terms of the hormones it makes, like a small hypothalamus.

### The anterior pituitary

As the embryo develops and the brain begins to form, the pituitary gland is first represented as an outpouching (Rathke's pouch) of the primitive pharyngeal stomadeum that fuses with an outpouching of the floor of the third ventricle between the fifth and seventh weeks. Over the subsequent 1–8 weeks, blood vessels and connective tissues grow caudally from the pars tuberalis in the developing brain to invade the pituitary and surround its stalk. The pituitary portal circulation is fully established by 12–17 weeks. The hypothalamic nuclei are identifiable at 15–18 weeks. The five distinct cell types in the mature anterior pituitary [secreting gonadotrophins, adrenocorticotrophic hormone (ACTH), growth hormone (GH), thyroid-stimulating hormone (TSH) and prolactin (PRL)] are all derived from a common pluripotent progenitor cell.

Cells secreting prolactin are seen first in the pituitary at 5 weeks, but GH- and ACTH-secreting cells are not seen until around 8–10 weeks. Luteinizing hormone-releasing hormone (LHRH) neurones migrate from the embryonic olfactory placode along the pathway of the nervus terminalis–vermonasal complex, reaching the hypothalamus by 9 weeks. A gene (KAL1) located at Xp22.3 that encodes a cadherin-like cell adhesion factor controls this migration. In cases of X-linked Kallmann syndrome (isolated gonadotrophin deficiency and either anosmia or hyposmia), mutations in KAL1 have been identified and shown to be associated with a failure of GnRH neuronal migration. GnRH can be detected in the fetal brain as early as 4.5 weeks but the hypothalamic pulse generator is not fully functional until 12 weeks.

Luteinizing hormone (LH) and follicle-stimulating hormone (FSH) secretion begins at 10 weeks, and there is a peak

**Table 7.1.** The pituitary

| | Age post conception (months) | | | | | |
|---|---|---|---|---|---|---|
| | 1 | 1.5–2 | 3 | 3.5–4 | 5 | 5–term |
| Morphology | Rathke's pouch visible | Pars tuberalis visible<br>By 8 weeks, connective tissue and blood vessels grow in anterior lobe and establish direct neurohormonal connection<br>GH- and ACTH-secreting cells seen | Characteristics of adult pituitary visible<br><br>Acidophil cells detectable | Basophils seen | Neurosecretory material demonstrable in posterior pituitary. Lactotrophs seen | |
| Prolactin | 5 weeks: prolactin synthesis starts gland content ↑ progressively after week 10 (serum levels low until week 26). Progressive ↑ in serum PRL from week 26 to term. Brain and hypothalamic control of PRL secretion matures from around 16 weeks. Amniotic fluid PRL is glycosylated. Fifty per cent originates from decidual cells | | | | | |
| ACTH | ACTH levels reached their peak at midgestation and are higher throughout gestation than in postnatal life. Levels fall at term | | | | | |
| GH | | GH synthesis and secretion begin around 8–10 weeks | Pituitary GH content ↑ from 1 nmol (10 weeks) to 45 nmol (16 weeks)<br>Fetal plasma GH 1–4 nmol/L first trimester | Plasma GH peaks at 6 nmol/L at midgestation and falls progressively in the second half of gestation to ≈ 1.5 nmol/L at term. By 3 months, mature responses occur to sleep, glucose and L-dopa | | |
| LH and FSH | | By 2.5 months, LHRH neurones are operative in the mediobasal hypothalamus | LHRH secretion is unrestrained between 3.5 and 5 months | > 5 months, negative feedback develops. Suppression of LHRH is more marked in the male fetus because of testosterone. At term, LHRH secretion is low | | |
| Genes expressed | *Pit1*<br>*Prop1*<br>*Hesex-1* | | | | | |

in fetal serum LH levels at 18–22 weeks. LH and FSH levels in cord blood are low but there is a surge of serum LH in the male about 30 min after birth. Female LH values remain low until maternal oestrogen has disappeared from the circulation and then rise. Testosterone levels in the male are higher than in the female 3–12 h after birth with a second peak at 30–60 days. LH and FSH levels remain relatively high throughout the first 6 months of life in boys and for 2–3 years in girls.

Pituitary TSH secretion is first seen at 10–12 weeks. Blood levels of TSH rise progressively and there is a fourfold rise between the second trimester and term. TSH becomes responsive to thyrotrophin-releasing hormone (TRH) in the third trimester. Immediately after birth, triggered either by cold stress or the cutting of the cord, there is a sharp increase in serum TSH secretion, which lasts 48 h.

Fetal GH levels are much higher than after birth because there is a paucity of GH receptors (GHRs) and also because the inhibitory somatostatin tone is low. Fetal serum insulin-like growth factor (IGF-I) levels are relatively low. Neverthe-

less, fetal growth is considered to be dependent upon IGF-I regulated in the fetus not by GH but by the glucose–insulin axis. The prenatal surge in serum cortisol leads to an induction of GHRs, and GH levels then begin to fall, declining further very soon after birth. Another factor inhibiting postnatal GH release is the rise in free fatty acid levels that follows the onset of non-shivering thermogenesis [1]. Growth hormone levels are higher in the newborn than in the older infant and child.

The *intermediate* lobe of the fetal pituitary is curiously large at midgestation, although its physiological role is unclear and it virtually disappears by term. The intermediate lobe synthesizes pro-opiomelanocortin (POMC), which is cleaved in the intermediate lobe to release α-MSH (α-malanocyte-stimulating hormone) and β-endorphin, and, in the anterior lobe, ACTH and β-lipotrophin.

The *posterior* lobe of the pituitary is a direct extension of neural tissue growing down from the diencephalon and is functional by 12 weeks. It contains arginine vasopressin (AVP), oxytocin and arginine vasotocin (AVT, a hormone precursor not found in the pituitary after birth). AVP levels are higher in stressed infants than in those who are not stressed. The neonatal kidney is capable of responding to AVP, although paucity of AVP receptors restricts the maximal urine osmolality to about 600 mosmol/kg.

## Genetic regulation of pituitary development

A number of genes involved in the differentiation and development of the pituitary have been identified in animal models with inherited forms of dwarfism (Snell, Ames) and in humans with developmental abnormalities of the pituitary [2]. These genes appear to be linked in a cascade of factors regulating the differentiation of specific tissues and cell types. *Pit1* was found to be the site of the mutation causing hypopituitarism in the Snell dwarf mouse, and subsequently its human homologue, *POU1F1*, was identified and mapped to chromosome 3p11. An inactivating mutation in *POU1F1* results in combined deficiencies in GH, TSH and PRL.

The Ames dwarf mouse, which has a phenotype similar to that of the Snell mouse, was shown to have a mutation in a gene called Prophet of Pit1 (*Prop1*). *Prop1* is on a different chromosome from *Pit1* but is necessary for *Pit1* expression. A mutation in *Prop1* results in the same hormonal deficiencies as would be expected for the inactivation of *Pit1* but, in addition, affected subjects have gonadotrophin deficiency. In humans, *PROP1* maps to 5q. There appear to be many more patients with congenital hypopituitarism who have *PROP1* mutations (32% of unrelated patients in one series [3]) than who have *POU1F1* mutations.

A linkage study of patients with familial septo-optic dysplasia (SOD) led to the discovery of mutations in *HESX1*, a homeobox gene expressed in the cranial end of the pharyngeal pouch destined to become Rathke's pouch, and in the diencephalon. It is regarded as the first gene to be expressed in the cascade of events leading to pituitary differentiation. The human gene maps to 3p21.2–p21.1. Another gene, *Nkx-2.1*, has been shown to regulate development of the ventral diencephalon in the mouse. Transgenic mice in which *Nkx-2.1* was knocked out failed to develop a pituitary gland. Less is known about other genes such as *P-Lim*, *ETS1* and *Brn4*, although they are all expressed during early forebrain development.

Two genes, *DAX-1* and *SF-1*, are expressed in the developing ventromedial hypothalamus (VMN), as well as in the developing gonad and adrenal cortex. *Sf-1* knockout mice have no gonads, adrenal glands or VMN. A human subject with sex reversal and adrenal failure has been shown to have a mutation in *SF-1* [4].

Leukaemia inhibitory factor (LIF) is expressed in the fetal and adult pituitary and plays a role in the differentiation of the corticotroph cell lineage by inducing expression of the POMC and ACTH genes [5]. Transgenic mice overexpressing LIF have deficiencies of GH and FSH associated with over-

secretion of ACTH and cortisol because of corticotroph hyperplasia [6].

## Congenital hypopituitarism

Mutations in known genes (*POU1F1*, *PROP1* or *HESX1*) account for a high proportion of cases of congenital hypopituitarism [3]. The combination of GH and cortisol deficiencies in infancy causes severe hypoglycaemia that usually responds only to replacement therapy with both hormones. TSH-based neonatal screening programmes fail to detect hypothyroidism due to TSH deficiency. Persistent jaundice in a newborn infant should prompt the measurement of serum thyroxine. Males with congenital hypopituitarism often have a very small penis [a feature of GH deficiency (GHD) and/or of gonadotrophin deficiency] and the testes may be undescended.

The diagnosis of congenital hypopituitarism is often not straightforward. Dynamic pituitary function testing is rarely performed in newborn infants. The normal range for GH is higher in neonates than later in childhood, and levels that are low for an infant under conditions of hypoglycaemia may be wrongly interpreted as normal. The combination of low cortisol, GH and thyroxine levels in an infant with hypoglycaemia and ketonuria strongly suggests hypopituitarism. This type of hypoglycaemia does not respond to glucagon because hepatic glycogen stores are low. Serum insulin levels will also be appropriately low. The optic discs may be hypoplastic and cranial ultrasound may show absence of the septum pellucidum in patients with SOD. In about half of all patients with congenital hypopituitarism, a magnetic resonance imaging (MRI) scan shows attenuation or interruption of the pituitary stalk, with or without associated corpus callosum defects. The risk of intellectual disability is higher if the patient has a defect in the corpus callosum.

## The thyroid (Tables 7.2 and 7.3)

The thyroid, like the pituitary, is derived from the primitive pharyngeal lining. At around 4 weeks, a thickening appears in the floor of the pharyngeal stomadeum and develops into a protrusion that moves down the neck, connected to the buccal cavity by the thyroglossal duct. As the thyroid anlage descends, it comes to rest against the fourth pharyngeal arch. The parathyroid glands, which are derived from the third and fourth pharyngeal arches, become embedded in the developing thyroid and parafollicular cells invade from the fifth pharyngeal arch. The thyroglossal duct atrophies and eventually disappears (although remnants may remain in the line of descent). Although the mature thyroid gland has two lobes, both develop from the same mass of thyroid cells. A small projection of thyroid tissue (the pyramidal lobe) may remain to represent the lower end of the thyroglossal duct.

The ability to synthesize thyroglobulin is acquired by 7 weeks and by 11 weeks the gland can concentrate iodine and

**Table 7.2.** The fetal thyroid

| | Gestation (months) | | | | | |
|---|---|---|---|---|---|---|
| | **1** | **2** | **2.5** | **3** | **3.5** | **4** |
| Morphology | Fusion of the thyroid diverticulum (endodermal epithelium in floor of pharynx) and ultimobranchial body (mesenchymal neural crest in the fourth pharyngeal pouch) to form thyroid anlage | Displaced caudally Thyroglossal duct degenerates | | Complex cord-like arrangements | Follicular arrangements devoid of colloid | Colloid-filled follicles |
| Biochemistry | Capacity to form thyroglobulin present | | TBG detectable in serum | Gland able to concentrate iodine and synthesize thyroxine | | Progressive increase in serum concentration of thyroxine Rate of $T_4$ metabolism to $rT_3$ and $T_3$ higher than postnatal rate |
| Genes expressed | *Hoxa3* *Pax8* *TTF1* (thyroid, lung) *TTF2* | | | | | |

**Table 7.3.** Ontogeny of the thyroid

| | Postnatal age | | | | |
|---|---|---|---|---|---|
| | **At birth** | **24 h** | **5 days** | **10 days** | **1 year** |
| Thyroid hormones | $T_4 \approx$ maternal TBG > maternal $T_3 <$ maternal $RT_3$, $T_3$ sulphate ↑↑ in cord blood | $T_4$ ↑ ('hyperthyroid' range) $T_3$ ↑↑ ('hyperthyroid' range) ↑ extrathyroidal conversion of $T_4$ to $T_3$ $rT_3$ ↑↑ | $rT_3$ normal | Decline in levels of $T_3$ and $T_4$ but still exceed adult values | $T_4$, $T_3$ levels equivalent to adult values |
| TSH | Surge begins half an hour after birth | Peak TSH level (mean ≈ 10.5 mU/L) | Mean level ≈ 3.6 mU/L | Basal concentration similar to that of older children | Basal concentration similar to that of older children |

synthesize thyroxine. Thyroxine-binding globulin (TBG), which is of hepatic origin, appears in the circulation at 10 weeks. The pituitary becomes capable of secreting TSH in the 10–12th week, and thereafter thyroid growth accelerates. Fetal serum TSH rises in the second trimester and remains higher than maternal levels to term. In the fetus, thyroxine is preferentially metabolized to reverse $T_3$ ($rT_3$), which is biologically inactive, rather than $T_3$. Immediately after birth, the metabolism of $T_4$ is switched to favour the production of $T_3$, rather than $rT_3$ [7].

The fetus receives negligible amounts of TSH from the maternal circulation, but maternal $T_4$ has to cross the placenta. If for any reason it does not, the brain does not develop normally. Because of this, cord blood levels of thyroxine in babies with congenital athyreosis are 30–50% of normal, rather than zero. Maternal thyroid autoantibodies are able to cross the placenta and can cause malfunction of the fetal thyroid.

Congenital hypothyroidism is due to athyreosis in 30–45% of cases, and ectopic dysgenesis of the gland (arrest in the line of normal descent) is the cause in another 40%. Genetic factors associated with athyreosis have been identified but, so far, none has been found in association with ectopic dysgenesis of the thyroid. In the mouse, three transcription factors (*Ttf1*, *Ttf2* and *Pax8*) have been identified and shown to be expressed during thyroid organogenesis [8]. An extensive search in Italian patients showed a *PAX8* mutation in a mother and son who both had congenital hypothyroidism, but no mutations could be found in either *TTF1* or *TTF2*. *PAX8* (2q12–2q14) is expressed in the developing excretory system and the thyroid. Its expression is necessary for the formation of follicular cells in the thyroid. In transgenic mice with no *Ttf1* (thyroid transcription factor 1) gene, neither follicular nor parafollicular cells form.

The cause of ectopic dysgenesis of the thyroid, which is the cause of congenital hypothyroidism in about 40% of cases, is still unknown. Of the remaining causes of congenital hypothyroidism, dyshormonogenesis accounts for the majority (10–15% of all cases). Unexpectedly few of these have proven to have mutations in the thyroid peroxidase (*TPO*) gene. In Pendred syndrome (goitrous hypothyroidism associated with a cochlear malformation causing hereditary nerve deafness), the *TPO* gene is normal but mutations are found in *PDS*, a gene located at 7q31 that encodes a 780-amino-acid protein called pendrin. Pendrin is closely related to a number of sulphate transporters. Thyroglobulin (TG) is heavily sulphated, and it is speculated that a mutation in *PDS* may somehow interfere with TG function by impairing post-translational sulphation. The role of pendrin in the cochlea has not been established. There is also some experimental evidence linking pendrin to the transport of chloride and iodide [9], but confirmation that pendrin is, in fact, a sulphate transporter is lacking.

## Hypothyroxinaemia

One child in 4000 in most communities with thyroid screening programmes has congenital hypothyroidism. The classically hypothyroid infant moves little, feeds slowly, is jaundiced, has supraorbital oedema, dry skin, constipation, a hoarse cry, enlargement of the tongue and an umbilical hernia. Closure of the posterior fontanelle is delayed and, on radiograph, the distal femoral epiphysis is absent. In addition, the serum TSH level is high. Infants born to mothers with autoimmune thyroid disease may be born with transient hypo- or hyperthyroidism due to transplacental passage of TSH receptor-blocking or receptor-stimulating IgG autoantibodies respectively.

Rarely, infants are born with hypothyroidism due to TSH deficiency and these will not be detected in a screening programme based on a TSH assay. Other pituitary deficiencies may be present (as, for example, in infants with mutations in *POU1F1*, *PROP1* or *HESX1*). Infants with combined GH and ACTH deficiencies, in addition to TSH deficiency, will have severe hypoglycaemia, and boys will have a micropenis. Cranial ultrasonography may show evidence of SOD or holoprosencephaly, or an MRI scan may show an ectopic pituitary bright spot, an attenuated or interrupted pituitary stalk and/or a defect in the corpus callosum.

Patients with X-linked thyroxine-binding globulin (TBG) deficiency must be differentiated from those with pituitary defects. TBG deficiency (1:2800 males) is nearly as common as congenital hypothyroidism. In the complete form, serum $T_4$ levels (both total $T_4$ and free $T_4$) are extremely low, but TSH is normal and the patient is clinically normal, requiring no treatment. Mutations have been identified in the TBG gene, which is located at Xp22.2.

The most difficult infants to assess are those who are premature (usually less than 30–32 weeks' gestational age), those who are sick and those whose serum $T_4$ is low with a normal TSH. It is unclear whether this hypothyroxinaemia is due, as Fisher and Polk [10] state, to 'a state of transient hypothalamic-pituitary TSH deficiency' or that the changes in thyroid function tests reflect the effects of various cytokines and circulating inhibitors. As well as $T_4$, serum TBG and $T_3$ levels are also low in a high proportion of preterm infants. The question of whether or not the hypothyroxinaemia of prematurity or neonatal illness should be treated with thyroid hormone is also a vexed one. Most trials [11] show no beneficial effect.

## Iodine deficiency and iodine excess

One-third of the world's population has iodine deficiency, and in iodine-deficient communities the incidence of congenital hypothyroidism with goitre is 32–80% [12]. Not all iodine-deficient hypothyroid infants are born with goitre: some have thyroid atrophy and these infants have been found to have circulating thyroid growth-inhibiting antibodies. The most severely impaired infants, those with severe neurological as well as cognitive deficits, were iodine deficient prenatally and the mother was herself hypothyroid because of iodine deficiency [13]. Intrauterine iodine deficiency can impair brain development without causing neonatal hypothyroidism. In this way, the average intelligence of entire populations can be impaired [14].

Infants exposed to iodine-containing surface disinfectants (such as those who have undergone heart surgery) are at great risk of developing transient hypothyroidism secondary to iodine intoxication. This is sufficiently common to make it mandatory to carry out routine thyroid function testing after exposure. In these infants, the thyroid scan shows increased uptake, contrary to what might be expected, and the gland is normally situated. In this situation, when there is good reason to suspect that excess iodine was responsible for the hypothyroidism, it is sufficient to give thyroxine replacement for a relatively short period (25–50 μg/day for 3 months), then gradually to reduce the dose while monitoring serum TSH levels weekly.

## The infant of a hyperthyroid mother

The development of Graves disease in a pregnant woman presents the obstetrician with a dilemma: whether to advocate surgical or medical treatment. Radioactive iodine would certainly not be considered because of its effects on the fetal thyroid gland. In general, medical treatment using antithyroid drugs would be first choice. Propylthiouracil and methimazole both readily cross the placenta and affect fetal thyroid function. The dose chosen should only reduce maternal thyroxine levels to the upper end of the normal range.

The fetus of a thyrotoxic mother may be exposed to a mixture of maternal autoantibodies, some of which are stimulatory whereas others are inhibitory. Maternal autoantibodies cross the placenta and as a result 1% of infants of thyrotoxic mothers are born with hyperthyroidism. Fetal hyperthyroidism can be detected prenatally as tachycardia or goitre large enough to be imaged with ultrasound. Intrauterine growth retardation is common. Early onset of labour and premature rupture of the membranes is much more likely to occur and there is an increased risk of fetal death *in utero*. The main clinical features of neonatal thyrotoxicosis are tachycardia, restlessness, failure to thrive and lid retraction. Goitre is almost always present. Tachycardia may progress to cardiac failure. Hyperthermia and muscular hypotonia may be seen. Treatment is with antithyroid drugs (carbimazole or propylthiouracil), with or without β-adrenergic blockade.

After birth, TSH receptor-stimulating and -inhibiting antibodies may disappear from the infant's circulation at different rates, and the thyroid may be stimulated at one stage, and inhibited at another. Neonatal thyrotoxicosis is usually transient, but if the infant is the source of the TSH receptor-stimulating antibodies the hyperthyroidism persists. A serious consequence of prolonged hyperthyroxinaemia is premature fusion of the cranial sutures, which may lead to microcephaly and intellectual disability. Not all types of neonatal thyrotoxicosis are antibody-mediated. A familial form of thyrotoxicosis has been described in association with an activating mutation of the TSH receptor gene [15]. In this condition, total thyroidectomy may be necessary.

## The parathyroid glands and parafollicular C cells of the thyroid

The parathyroid glands are derived from the third and fourth pharyngeal pouches and first become visible at the end of the first trimester (Table 7.4). The fifth pharyngeal pouch contributes the calcitonin-secreting parafollicular or C cells, which are contained within paired ultimobranchial bodies that are taken up into the thyroid gland. Calcitonin is believed to play a more important physiological role in the fetus than in postnatal life.

The parathyroid glands are functionally mature throughout the second and third trimesters. At term, however, immunoassayable PTH levels are usually low or undetectable, but high PTH bioactivity and high levels of calcitonin are found. During intrauterine development, an ATP-dependent placental calcium pump, believed to be regulated by parathyroid hormone-related protein (PTHrP), ensures that the fetal serum calcium is maintained at a higher level than that of the mother. Ovine fetal parathyroid glands contain high levels of PTHrP, and there are contributions of PTHrP from the placenta, amniotic membranes and fetal tissues [16]. Knockout mice with targeted disruption of the PTHrP gene have levels of ionized calcium significantly lower than in normal mice,

**Table 7.4.** Parathyroid hormone/calcium regulation

| First trimester | Second and third trimesters |
|---|---|
| Parathyroid glands and parafollicular cells identified at the end of the first trimester | Parathyroids functionally mature from start of second trimester |

although total serum calcium remains the same. These mice are born with skeletal abnormalities and do not survive [17]. Human neonates have detectable serum PTHrP levels, but the levels are not high enough to explain the high PTH bioactivity. The combination of high serum calcium and high levels of calcitonin promote the mineralization of bone in the fetus.

## Neonatal hypocalcaemia

Transient neonatal hypocalcaemia is very common in birth-asphyxiated neonates, in the infants of diabetic mothers, in the infants of mothers with hyperparathyroidism, and in premature infants. In each case, the hypocalcaemia is believed to be due to transient hypoparathyroidism. In the infant of a diabetic mother, the hypoparathyroidism may be secondary to hypomagnesaemia. In infants of hyperparathyroid mothers, the fetal parathyroids are suppressed by hypercalcaemia of maternal origin. Hypocalcaemia may be induced during exchange transfusion because of the presence of a chelating agent in the transfused blood.

Persistent neonatal hypocalcaemia is rare and may be associated with di George syndrome (hypoplasia of the thymus and parathyroids, with associated outflow defects in the heart). In this condition, 90% of patients have a 22q11 deletion. The hypocalcaemia usually resolves in early childhood. Persistent hypocalcaemia may also be due to an activating mutation in the extracellular calcium-sensing receptor gene [18,19].

Hypocalcaemia in infancy is associated with rapid eye blinking, jerking, tetany and convulsions. Treatment is with an intravenous infusion of calcium, 12 mmol/m$^2$ over 3 h, which usually elevates serum calcium by 0.5–1.0 mmol/L and during which cardiac monitoring is advisable. A single infusion may be sufficient in cases of transient hypocalcaemia. Refractory hypocalcaemia may be secondary to hypomagnesaemia. Persistent hypoparathyroidism is treated with calcitriol. Pseudohypoparathyroidism, in which there is resistance to the end-organ effects of parathyroid hormone, rarely causes neonatal hypocalcaemia.

## Neonatal hypercalcaemia

Hypercalcaemia is rarely encountered in neonates but may occur due to familial hypocalciuric hypercalcaemia (FHH). In this autosomal dominant disorder, an inactivating mutation disrupts the normal function of the extracellular calcium-sensing receptor in the parathyroid gland, altering its set point so that higher than usual levels of calcium are needed to suppress PTH secretion. The heterozygous form is benign, but the homozygous form results in severe neonatal hyperparathyroidism requiring surgery [20]. Another condition, idiopathic hypercalcaemia of infancy, is due to increased sensitivity to vitamin D. Hyperparathyroidism may occur, occasionally sporadically, but more often in association with one of the familial MEN (multiple endocrine neoplasia) syndromes.

## The adrenal glands

The human fetal adrenal cortex grows rapidly between the 10th and 15th weeks and, at around 12 weeks, the adrenal gland and the kidney are not very different in size (Table 7.5). At term, the fetal adrenals, weighing 8–10 g, are nearly as large as adult adrenals and they secrete 100–200 mg of steroid per day. The fetal adrenal has a very large inner zone occupying 70% of the volume and a much thinner permanent (or 'definitive') zone. The inner (fetal) zone secretes large amounts of the androgen precursors, dehydroepiandrosterone (DHEA) and DHEA sulphate (DHEAS), pregnenolone sulphate and a range of uniquely fetal $C_{19}$ steroids (particularly $\Delta^5,3\beta$-hydroxysteroids) that are converted to oestriol by the placenta. The measurement of maternal oestriol excretion during pregnancy is as much a test of the function of the fetal adrenal cortex as of the placenta.

The evidence in favour of ACTH being the principal regulator of growth in the fetal zone comes from *in vitro* experiments on cultured fetal adrenal cells. These experiments show that ACTH stimulates mitotic activity and that its mitogenic effects are mediated by growth factors. IGF-I, IGF-II, EGF (epidermal growth factor) and bFGF (basic fibroblast growth factor) stimulate cell proliferation, whereas activin and transforming growth factor (TGF)-$\beta$ are inhibitory [21]. It has also been observed, however, that ACTH levels in human fetal blood reach a peak at midgestation and are falling in the third trimester when the adrenal cortex is rapidly growing.

After birth, the adrenal gland weight rapidly decreases in the first 2 weeks and most of the change occurs in the fetal zone, which falls from 85% of total volume to 3%. There is, at this time, a marked expansion in fetal zone stroma (connective tissue and blood vessels) with haemorrhagic changes, as well as a great increase in the apoptotic index. A slower decline in fetal zone size continues after the first 2 weeks. Meanwhile, the subcapsular definitive zone expands and there is a centripetal migration of definitive zone cells into the degenerating fetal zone. The definitive layer undergoes further anatomical and functional zonation into the fasciculata-reticularis, which secretes cortisol and androgens, and the glomerulosa, which secretes aldosterone.

The dramatic changes that occur in the neonatal adrenal cortex remain unexplained. Indeed, the importance of the fetal zone itself is unclear. Infants born prematurely continue to excrete fetal zone products at a constant rate until they reach term, after which excretion of these products declines at a rate similar to that seen after birth at term. This suggests that the postnatal involution of the fetal zone is related to gestation rather than birth itself [22]. Infants with X-linked adrenal hypoplasia congenita (AHC) due to a mutation in the

**Table 7.5.** The adrenal gland

| | Weeks post conception | | |
| --- | --- | --- | --- |
| | 6–8 | 9 weeks onward | Term |
| Morphology | Adrenal cortex is derived from mesenchymal cells on the coelomic cavity lining arising adjacent to the urogenital ridge. Inner fetal zone visible. Outer definitive zone visible | Rapid growth of fetal adrenal gland. Between 9 and 12 weeks eosinophilic cells in the fetal zone become well-differentiated and capable of steroidogenesis | Term combined adrenal mass 8 g, 80% fetal zone |
| Genes expressed during adrenal morphogenesis | *SF-1*, *DAX-1*, genes encoding steroidogenic enzymes | | |
| Steroidogenesis | Expression of genes for the steroidogenic enzymes is independent of pituitary function. There is a paucity of 3β-HSD and relatively high steroid sulphatase activity. Major fetal steroids are DHEA, DHEAS, pregnenolone sulphate, several $\Delta^5$-steroids. Limited amounts of $\Delta^5$ 3-ketosteroids including cortisol and aldosterone | | |
| Aldosterone | Midgestation: low aldosterone levels unresponsive to secretogogues | | Term: fetal adrenal capable of secreting aldosterone but poor correlation between PRA and aldosterone in cord blood |

gene encoding the nuclear hormone receptor, DAX-1, have little or no permanent zone but the fetal zone is intact. They survive to term but are born with hyperpigmentation and rapidly lose salt and water because of adrenal insufficiency. In two cases treated by the author, parturition was delayed. It is well known that in sheep the fetal adrenal cortex controls parturition.

For some steroids, blood levels in the newborn are significantly affected by prematurity. Serum 17-hydroxyprogesterone values are higher in premature infants than those born at term, while levels of cortisol and aldosterone are lower, suggesting that prematurity is associated with lower levels of activity in 21-hydroxylase, 11β-hydroxylase and 18-hydroxylase [23]. Fetal serum cortisol levels rise from about 35 weeks of gestation. There is a poor correlation between plasma renin activity and serum aldosterone in cord blood.

## Congenital adrenal hyperplasia

The *CYP21B* gene, which encodes 21-hydroxylase (P450c21), is located on chromosome 6 so close to the gene encoding HLA (human leucocyte antigen) that, for the most part, inheritance of one implies inheritance of the other. Pedigree analysis can be performed on families into which a child with 21-hydroxylase deficiency has been born using the HLA haplotype of the fetus (determined in a chorionic villus or amniotic fluid sample) as a surrogate marker for its *CYP21B* status. This method is negated, however, by occasional recombination events that give rise to false results, and when one of the parental haplotypes is not expressed in the fetal sample. The most reliable way of establishing a prenatal diagnosis of congenital adrenal hyperplasia (CAH) is to prepare DNA from a chorionic villus sample and then perform a direct mutational analysis of *CYP21B* [24]. Even this, however, is not perfect because the match between genotype and phenotype is not as tight as might be expected [25]. The measurement of steroid levels in a 15-week amniotic fluid sample has become unfashionable, but this method of diagnosis does at least confirm the phenotype in a case of classic 21-hydroxylase deficiency.

## Neonatal screening for 21-hydroxylase deficiency congenital adrenal hyperplasia

Several million infants worldwide have now been screened at birth for CAH [26]. The argument for doing so is that most cases are detected by screening earlier than they would be detected clinically and that deaths due to undiagnosed adrenal crisis will be prevented. Screening is based on the measurement of 17-hydroxyprogesterone in dried blood spots collected onto filter paper. A cut-off level of 30 nmol/L is appropriate for samples collected after 48 h. It is not appropriate to use cord blood samples because levels of 17-hydroxyprogesterone are always high. False-positive diagnoses in premature infants are avoided by using reference levels

related to gestational age [27]. In a sample of 1.9 million newborn infants screened in Texas, the incidence of classic CAH was 1 in 16 008 and the ratio of salt wasting–simple virilizing forms was 2.7:1 [28]. False-negative screening results in cases of non-classic CAH have been reported. The applicability of this type of approach to different populations is not well documented. Assuming these ratios are correct then it would be expected also that affected females would be detected to a large extent by the presence of ambiguous genitalia. This would leave undetected males at risk of salt loss and simple virilizers or late onset. Detecting the former would be worthwhile but the latter would be questionable. Overall, therefore, answers still need to be provided about the actual societal benefit of this process.

## X-Linked adrenal hypoplasia congenita

A family history of congenital adrenal insufficiency confined to males suggests the diagnosis of X-linked AHC [29]. During gestation, maternal oestriol excretion will be extremely low because of lack of fetal adrenal precursors. Affected infants are born deeply pigmented, particularly of the lips, buccal mucosa, tongue, areolae and genitalia. Severe hypoglycaemia and lethargy due to glucocorticoid deficiency develop in the first hours or days of life, and, after a week or so, progressive salt wasting with vomiting, dehydration and an electrolyte disturbance (hyponatraemia and hyperkalaemia) worsens the situation. Death is inevitable if replacement therapy with hydrocortisone, salt and fludrocortisone is not started promptly. AHC is due to an inactivating mutation in *DAX-1*. This gene, located at the pseudoautosomal boundary on Xp, lies adjacent to the gene for steroid sulphatase and therefore some infants with AHC also have ichthyosis. *DAX-1* is also expressed in the ventromedial hypothalamus and this may explain why patients with AHC also have isolated gonadotrophin deficiency.

## Antenatal steroid treatment to prevent bronchopulmonary dysplasia of prematurity

Antenatal steroid therapy has been offered to women with premature onset of labour (< 32–34 weeks) since the early 1970s (Table 7.6). The aim of treatment is to reduce the risk of neonatal bronchopulmonary dysplasia (BPD). The usual course of treatment involves two injections of either betamethasone or dexamethasone given 24 h apart and then repeated courses at 7- to 10-day intervals (occasionally as many as 6–10 courses) may be given. A meta-analysis of the randomized trials, 1972–94 [30], and other reports showed a treatment-related reduction in the incidence of respiratory distress syndrome, bronchopulmonary dysplasia, intraventricular haemorrhage and mortality. Pituitary–adrenal responses to stimulation with CRH (corticotrophin-releasing hormone) were not affected by antenatal exposure to steroids

**Table 7.6.** Actions of glucocorticoids in the preterm human fetus

| | |
|---|---|
| Lung | Induces expression of surfactant proteins B and C |
| | Reduces interalveolar wall thickness |
| | Increases airspace volume and lung compliance |
| | Through induction of pulmonary β-adrenergic receptors, potentiates the clearance of lung liquid by catecholamines |
| Thyroid | Enhances conversion of $T_4$ to $T_3$ |
| Adrenal medulla | Stimulates phenylethanolamine-N-transferase, which catalyses the methylation of noradrenaline to adrenaline |
| Carbohydrate metabolism | Increases hepatic glycogen storage |
| | Stimulates glucose 6-phosphatase |
| Gastrointestinal tract | Stimulates differentiation of gastric epithelial cells |
| | Regulates the processing of lipoproteins in jejunal epithelium |
| Heart | Important effects on cardiac development |
| Other | Regulate the expression of the prolactin receptor (in sheep) |
| | Increases expression of GHR |

in very low birthweight preterm infants. A follow-up study of premature infants at the corrected age of 2 years showed a lower rate of neurological impairment in the group exposed antenatally to steroids than in a control group [31]. These results are more reassuring than the report showing that, in fetal rat brain, antenatal exposure to dexamethasone alters c-*fos* and the AP-1 family of nuclear transcription factors [32]. Other concerns about the safety of the treatment have been raised. In growth-retarded neonates born to mothers with pregnancy-associated hypertension, the risk of sepsis is increased by antenatal exposure to steroids [33]. In sheep, repeated courses of betamethasone given to the pregnant ewe resulted in significant fetal growth retardation that persisted to term [34].

### Postnatal steroid treatment of preterm infants

The practice of treating preterm (< 34 weeks) infants with steroids began in the 1980s. The aim of treatment in this instance is to reduce inflammation in the lungs, or sometimes it is to reduce laryngeal inflammation and swelling after intubation. Of the many regimens in use, the two most popular doses of dexamethasone (IV or oral) are 0.15 mg/day in 2–4 divided doses and 0.5 mg/kg/day. The duration of treatment ranges from < 1 to 6 weeks. Further variation exists in relation to the age of patients when they are started on treatment: here, the range is 4 to > 21 days.

The results of this treatment are starting to look disturbing. Although the treatment does reduce ventilator dependency and improve lung function, neurological function 1 year after a 42-day tapering course of dexamethasone was significantly worse than in an untreated control group of preterm infants. In the dexamethasone-treated group, 25% had cerebral palsy and 45% had abnormal neurological examination findings vs.

7% and 16%, respectively, in the untreated group [35]. Other side-effects include hypertrophic cardiomyopathy [36] and renal calcification. Furthermore, treatment did not reduce the risk of death [37].

### Prenatal dexamethasone treatment for suspected or confirmed 21-hydroxylase deficiency

If a couple have previously produced a child with 21-hydroxylase deficiency, the mother may elect to take dexamethasone in subsequent pregnancies with the aim of suppressing the fetal adrenal glands. In so doing, she would be hoping to prevent an affected female fetus from being born with ambiguous genitalia. This use of dexamethasone in antenatal treatment was first introduced by French workers in 1984. It has turned out to be of limited success: one-third of treated girls require no surgery, one-third have mild virilization and one-third still require surgery. To be effective, the treatment has to be started as early in the pregnancy as possible (6 weeks or less) and the dosage must be sufficient to suppress maternal oestriol excretion. Fetal sexing and prenatal diagnosis are undertaken by chorionic villus sampling at 10–12 weeks, which is well after treatment has been started. Treatment is stopped if the fetus is male or an unaffected female.

The dose of dexamethasone given to the mother is large: up to 20 µg/kg per day in three doses has been advocated. Weight gain, skin changes, a rise in blood pressure, emotional changes, cushingoid facial changes and alteration of glucose tolerance are all possible side-effects for the mother [38].

Little is known about long-term effects of antenatal exposure to dexamethasone for children with CAH or those who had treatment for part of the pregnancy but turned out to be unaffected. A Swedish study [39] found that three of six affected girls had serious long-term consequences and one-third of the unaffected children had some problem. Other studies have reported more optimistic results [40]. Antenatal dexamethasone treatment is not yet a standard therapy that any obstetrician or paediatrician should freely use before much more evaluation has taken place [41].

## The gonads and genitalia

The gonad is derived from the intermediate mesoderm, from which the bipotential genital ridge differentiates, and the dorsal endoderm of the yolk sac, from which germ cells migrate in the fourth and fifth weeks, reaching the connective tissues of the gonad at around 7 weeks. Until the appearance of testicular cords made up of Sertoli cells at 6 weeks, the fetal testis and ovary are indistinguishable. Leydig cells differentiate from migratory mesonephric stromal cells, which are attracted by as yet unknown signals believed to be produced in the male gonad. The gonad, adrenal and kidney all initially develop close together and, as the testes descend, they may carry rests of adrenocortical cells with them. Surgeons, who refer to them as 'golden granules', often see these. If these adrenal rests are subjected to prolonged ACTH stimulation, as in a patient with CAH who neglects to take his medications regularly, they may become hyperplastic and cause testicular enlargement sufficiently marked that a malignant tumour may be mistakenly diagnosed. In the mouse, a testicular hormone called Insl3 (insulin-like 3) [42], a member of the insulin-like family that is secreted by the Leydig cells, controls intra-abdominal testicular descent. Targeted disruption of the *Insl3* gene leads to maldevelopment of the gubernaculum and the result is bilateral cryptorchidism [43]. Insl3 is also secreted by theca cells of the postnatal ovary, and females homozygous for *Insl3* mutations are subfertile and have deregulation of the oestrous cycle. *INSL3* is found in the human genome.

### Development of the human ovary

The fetal ovary develops at a very different rate from the fetal testis. It differentiates weeks later than the testis and, whereas germ cells are seen in the testis by 7 weeks, oocytes are not seen in the ovary until the 11–12th week. The number of primordial follicles in both ovaries reaches a lifetime peak (6–7 million) at 20 weeks' gestation and it then declines so that, by term, only 2 million remain. The fetal ovary makes no Müllerian inhibitory substance (MIS) and very little oestrogen. It has no role to play in regulating sexual differentiation.

### Genes involved in sex determination

#### SRY: *the testis-determining gene*

A single gene called *SRY* controls the switch directing gonadal differentiation into the male pathway. Mutations in *SRY* account for 20% of cases of XY gonadal dysgenesis.

*SRY* is located within the Y-specific region adjacent to the boundary of the pseudoautosomal region [44] that undergoes pairing with a homologous region on the X chromosome at meiosis. Its single exon encodes a protein of 223 amino acids. The central 77 amino acids constitute the HMG (high-mobility group) box, which is shared by many other proteins, including SOX9. Binding of SRY to DNA occurs between the HMG box and recognition sequences in the DNA. *SRY* is an 'architectural transcription factor' because it bends DNA, bringing distant sequences into apposition, allowing them to interact. What these sequences might be is still unknown.

Three genes, *WT1*, *SF-1* and *SOX9*, are known to be expressed in the bipotential genital ridge during its differentiation from the intermediate mesoderm. *WT1*, the Wilms tumour-suppressor gene (located at 11p13) [45], is expressed in both the primitive kidney and the genital ridge. Its expression seems to relate particularly to the transition from mesenchyme to epithelium. *WT1* is a transcription factor with 10 exons and four zinc fingers that binds to an ERG1 consensus binding sequence. *SRY* is strongly activated by certain WT1 isoforms *in vitro*. The MIS (Müllerian inhibitory substance) gene is strongly repressed *in vitro* by the same set of WT1 isoforms, as is the androgen receptor (AR) gene promoter [46]. At present, the relevance of these findings to what happens *in vivo* in unknown. Germline mutations in *WT1* result in the Denys–Drash syndrome, in which both renal (either Wilms tumour or a progressive form of glomerulosclerosis, or both) and gonadal abnormalities (streak gonad with high neoplastic potential) coexist. Intronic mutations in WT1 alter the isoform ratio leading to sex reversal and glomerular damage – Frasier syndrome.

The nuclear hormone receptor, steroidogenic factor-1 (SF-1) [47], regulates the expression of the cytochrome P450 enzymes. It is expressed in the urogenital ridge prior to the differentiation of the gonad and is then expressed in the developing testis but not in the developing ovary. Homozygous male and female *SF-1* knockout mice develop neither adrenal glands nor gonads. In addition, they show impaired gonadotroph function and agenesis of the ventromedial hypothalamic nucleus. SF-1 also regulates the adrenocorticotrophin receptor, the steroidogenic acute regulatory protein (StAR) and, in the pituitary, the α-subunit of the glycoproteins. Certain oxysterols (particularly 25-hydroxycholesterol) show specific binding to SF-1 and stimulate SF-1-dependent transcription. There is evidence of a synergistic effect of WT1 and SF-1 on the expression of the Müllerian inhibitory substance (*MIS*) gene. A human mutation in *FTZF1*, the gene encoding SF-1, has been reported in a child with XY sex reversal and adrenal failure [4].

*SOX9* is another gene that is expressed in the genital ridge at a very early stage, and also in the skeleton. Mutations in *SOX9* result in *campomelic dysplasia*, a severe birth defect causing bowing of the long bones (SOX9 directly regulates the type II collagen gene) and sex reversal due to gonadal dysgenesis in 75% of XY individuals [48]. In the mouse, the male (XY) genital ridge produces high levels of *Sox9* mRNA but the female (XX) genital ridge does not. Expression is localized to Sertoli cells within the sex cords of the developing testis.

## DAX-1 *and* DMT1

*DAX-1*, located at Xp21, is a member of the nuclear receptor superfamily [49] and is expressed in steroidogenic tissues as well as in Sertoli cells, pituitary gonadotrophs and in the ventromedial hypothalamus. In the presence of a weak *SRY* gene, duplication of *DAX-1* causes XY sex reversal, whereas an inactivating mutation of *DAX-1* causes adrenal hypoplasia congenita (AHC). The physiological role of Dax1 is considered to be inhibitory to testis development through an anti-*Sry* effect. In Y-1 adrenocortical cells, DAX-1 inhibits steroidogenesis at multiple levels, including the rate-limiting step controlled by StAR (the steroidogenic acute regulatory protein).

The distal portion of 9p is a region implicated in human XY sex reversal. A gene called *DMT1* maps to that chromosomal region and is expressed only in testis. Its role in the regulation of testis differentiation has yet to be fully elucidated.

## The internal genital ducts

Before sexual differentiation, the fetus possesses a pair of Wolffian ducts and a pair of Müllerian ducts. Development of the Wolffian ducts is closely related to that of the kidney and urinary tract. The Wolffian ducts are not only precursors to the vasa deferentia, seminal vesicles and epididymis, but also to the ureters, which bud off from the lower ends of the Wolffian ducts near their point of fusion. Growth and development of each Wolffian duct is stimulated by the testosterone secreted by the ipsilateral fetal testis. Another testicular hormone, MIS, controls development of the Müllerian ducts. MIS is a protein secreted by the Sertoli cells. As its name indicates, it inhibits Müllerian duct development. The organs which develop from the Müllerian ducts – the uterus, the fallopian tubes and the upper part of the vagina – only form in the absence of MIS. Occasionally, phenotypic males are found to have a uterus and the cause of this persistent Müllerian duct syndrome is a mutation either in the *MIS* gene (50% of cases) or the gene encoding the MIS receptor.

## The external genitalia

In early embryonic life, the external genitalia of males and females look exactly the same. Testosterone and dihydrotestosterone cause the genital tubercle to grow and become the penis and induce fusion of the genital folds so that they enclose the penile urethra. In the absence of androgen, or the ability to fully respond to androgen, the genitalia remain female or are only partially masculinized. Genes important for normal development of the male genitalia include all of the genes needed for testicular development, those required for normal steroidogenesis and the secretion of MIS, the androgen receptor (*AR*) gene, and the gene encoding 5α-reductase2. Ambiguities of the genitalia are covered in Chapter 6.

## Hypoplasia of the penis ('micropenis')

The stretched length of the penis in a full-term infant should be more than 2.5 cm (–2 SD) [50]. The presence of underlying pathology (gonad, pituitary) should be suspected if the penile length is less than this. Micropenis is most likely to be due to either gonadotrophin deficiency or GHD. There are many other causes [51] including androgen insensitivity, Prader–Willi syndrome and Klinefelter syndrome.

It may be difficult to establish a precise aetiological diagnosis in infancy. If the infant also suffers from hypoglycaemia, jaundice, hypothyroxinaemia or has incomplete testicular descent, hypopituitarism will be suspected. A cranial ultrasound examination may show changes of septo-optic dysplasia. MRI may show evidence of an undescended posterior (often incorrectly termed ectopic) pituitary bright spot, an attenuated or interrupted pituitary stalk, or both. LHRH or glucagon stimulation tests may be considered. If there is a family history of anosmia and hypogonadism, Kallmann syndrome is the likely diagnosis.

Long-term outcome studies [51,52] show that men who had micropenis at birth may continue to have a small penis but that 75% have intercourse and are able to form satisfactory sexual relationships. In infants and children with hypogonadotrophic hypogonadism, testosterone treatment (testosterone esters 25 mg intramuscularly every 4 weeks for 3–6 doses) successfully increases penile length into the normal range.

## Undescended testes

In 3.4% of term male infants and a higher proportion of premature infants, one or both testes will be incompletely descended. At 1 year, 0.8% remain undescended. If the testes are palpable but have not descended fully by age 9–12 months, intervention (either a course of human chorionic gonadotrophin or surgical orchidopexy, or both) is indicated. Incomplete descent of the testes, while common, may indicate the presence of underlying gonadotrophin deficiency, especially when associated with micropenis. In mice, a mutation in the gene encoding Insl3 (Leydig insulin-like hormone) has been shown to cause bilateral cryptorchidism [42], but it is not yet known if the same explanation applies to human cryptorchidism. If neither testis is palpable, it is essential to investigate for anorchia. Serum FSH and LH will be grossly elevated. A pelvic ultrasound or MRI examination is occasionally helpful in locating intra-abdominal testes. Imaging will also detect any persisting Müllerian duct remnants, which would be present if there was a more fundamental disturbance of testicular development (as in gonadal dysgenesis or persistent Müllerian duct syndrome because of a *MIS* gene or receptor mutation). The diagnosis of Kallmann syndrome can readily be made later in childhood when olfactory testing becomes possible, or by carrying out a mutational analysis of the *KAL1* gene.

## The endocrine pancreas

Both the endocrine and the exocrine cells of the fetal pancreas are of endodermal origin and smooth muscle cells in the pancreas are of mesodermal origin [53]. This overturns earlier work suggesting a neural crest origin for the endocrine cells [54]. Endocrine cells are dispersed throughout the exocrine tissues by 20 weeks and the islets of Langerhans are clearly differentiated by 31 weeks (Table 7.7). Genes involved in pancreas development include:

**1** *PDX-1* (13q12.1; encodes a homeodomain protein that acts as an insulin gene transcription factor and is essential for early pancreatic development);

**2** *REG* (located at 2p12);

**3** *REGL* (also at 2p12);

**4** *PAX4* (required for normal β-cell and somatostatin cell formation); and

**5** *PAX6* (expressed early in pancreatic development, required for α-cell differentiation, and expressed in mature islet cells).

When the pancreatic islets first differentiate, each cell is capable of becoming *any* type of islet cell. In fact, while cells are in the multipotent stage, they co-express several hormones. Throughout fetal life, transcription levels of insulin

and amylin are lower in the fetal pancreas than in the adult, whereas the reverse is true of glucagon and somatostatin. The fetal pancreas is known to be relatively insensitive to glucose [a feature that has plagued attempts at curing insulin-dependent diabetes mellitus (IDDM) using fetal islet cell transplantation]. This is not because the islets lack glucose transporters 1 and 2 or glucokinase: expression of all three in fetal pancreas has been documented.

## Neonatal hypoglycaemia

Hypoglycaemia is more common in the neonatal period than in any other phase of life. Infants are more prone to hypoglycaemia than children or adults because their gluconeogenic enzyme systems are immature and they have lower hepatic glycogen stores. Those particularly at high risk are infants of diabetic mothers, infants born small for gestational age (especially when the mother had pregnancy-associated hypertension), infants with sepsis or birth asphyxia and very premature infants. In the high-risk group, 8.6% of infants have hypoglycaemia, and, of these, 11–50% are found to have a major neurological handicap on follow-up [55,56]. Cerebral imaging shows lesions in the occipital and parietal lobes and in the thalamus [57,58].

What is the level of hypoglycaemia at which action should be taken? According to studies in which blood glucose concentrations were correlated with measured sensory-evoked responses, anything below 2.6 mmol/L is abnormal in the sense that brain function is impaired [56]. The clinical features of neonatal hypoglycaemia are due to cerebral dysfunction: jitteriness, seizures and apnoea. These events may occur for the first time in apparently healthy neonates after they

**Table 7.7.** The endocrine pancreas: ontogeny

| | Age post conception | | | |
| --- | --- | --- | --- | --- |
| | **4 weeks** | **8–10 weeks** | **Midgestation to term** | **Term** |
| | Fetal pancreas visible | α- and β-cells recognizable. Insulin, glucagon, somatostatin, pancreatic polypeptide cells identified. α-Cells > β-cells | Initially, α-cells ≫ β-cells. α-Cells reach a peak | α- and β-cells equal in number |
| Insulin | | | At 14–24 weeks, β-cells are functional. Secretion of insulin is at a low level. Response to arginine and glucose remains poor until term | Fetal pancreatic cells are functionally immature at birth but rapidly mature in the early neonatal period. The blunted state of their responses may be the secondary result of the stable glucose levels of the fetus created and maintained by transplacental transfer |
| Glucagon | | | Levels are relatively high in midgestation and progressively increase | |
| Glycogen stores | | Fetal liver glycogen storage is regulated by glucocorticoids and placental lactogen | | |

have been discharged from hospital [59]. A distinction is made between transient and persistent (> 1 week) hypoglycaemia. In the first week of life, most neonatologists are content to maintain blood glucose levels using an intravenous infusion of glucose. If hypoglycaemia persists for more than 1 week, investigation is necessary. Hyperinsulinism is the most common cause of persistent, severe hypoglycaemia.

### Persistent hyperinsulinaemic hypoglycaemia of infancy

Persistent hyperinsulinaemic hypoglycaemia of infancy (PHHI) is suspected in an infant with severe hypoglycaemia who needs glucose infused at > 8 mg/kg/min to maintain euglycaemia and who has no ketonuria. The diagnosis is confirmed if there is an inappropriately high insulin–glucose ratio. Measurement of C-peptide is also useful as its clearance is slower than insulin.

Just over half (58%) of infants with this condition have diffuse β-cell hyperfunction and the remainder have focal adenomatous islet cell hyperplasia [60]. PHHI may be inherited as an autosomal recessive trait, and, in such families, the genetic defect is in the gene encoding the β-cell potassium ATP (KATP) channel. This channel has two components: the sulphonyl urea receptor (SUR1) and a $K^+$ inward rectifier subunit, KIR6.2. Mutations found in PHHI result in the loss of channel activity in the β-cells, resetting their resting membrane and causing a constitutive repolarization. Voltage-gated $Ca^{2+}$ channels then open spontaneously, allowing cytosolic calcium ion concentrations to rise sufficiently for there to be a continuous release of insulin [61]. In sporadic focal adenomatous islet cell hyperplasia, a somatic mutation has been found [62] confined to the focal areas of abnormality in the pancreas. In these areas, the maternal allele of the imprinted chromosomal region 11p15 is lost. This region contains *SUR1/KIR6.2*.

The initial management of PHHI is medical. Diazoxide is a specific KATP channel agonist in normal β-cells, making it an entirely appropriate drug to try in a condition caused by a mutation affecting the KATP channel. A dose of 10–15 mg/kg/day in divided doses is sufficient. Diazoxide induces reversible hypertrichosis of the forehead, cheeks, arms, legs and lower back. Occasionally it may cause fluid retention (some clinicians therefore routinely advocate the combination of diazoxide with a thiazide diuretic). In addition, the thiazides act synergistically with diazoxide in regulating potassium channel function. If it is successful in preventing hypoglycaemia, it can be used safely for years. Most patients with PHHI outgrow the need for diazoxide by age 8–10 years.

If diazoxide is not effective in preventing hypoglycaemia in a dose of up to 15 mg/kg/day, surgery will probably be needed. As a short-term means of maintaining euglycaemia while preparing a patient for surgery, octreotide (a long-acting form of somatostatin) may be tried. In a small number of cases, long-term octreotide treatment is effective [63].

Surgery is a difficult option, because adenomas are rare and therefore the surgeon must decide how much of the pancreas to remove. One group [60] has had good results using preoperative pancreatic catheterization and intraoperative histological studies. They were able to distinguish between cases of focal adenomatous islet cell hyperplasia and diffuse β-cell hyperfunction. Those with the former were subjected to partial pancreatectomy and those with the latter had near-total pancreatectomy. The long-term outcome was much better for those with the diagnosis of focal adenomatous islet cell hyperplasia. The other group had a high prevalence of recurrent hypoglycaemia or of diabetes, hyperglycaemia and malabsorption.

Patients with PHHI have been shown to have persistently abnormal carbohydrate metabolism after the disappearance of hypoglycaemia, even if they had no surgery [64]. This is not surprising, in light of the discovery of genetic mutations affecting β-cell function in PHHI.

### Increased glutamate dehydrogenase activity can cause hyperinsulinism and hyperammonaemia

A new disorder has been described in a group of infants and children with an unusual and familial combination of congenital hyperinsulinism and hyperammonaemia. They have been shown to have increased glutamate dehydrogenase activity due to an activating mutation in the mitochondrial glutamate dehydrogenase gene. This excessive activity oxidizes glutamate to α-ketoglutarate, which in turn stimulates both insulin secretion by the β-cells and urea production in the liver [65].

### Beckwith–Wiedemann syndrome

The clinical features of Beckwith–Wiedemann syndrome (BWS) are PHHI, macroglossia, omphalocoele, hepatosplenomegaly, renal and adrenal dysplasia predisposing to malignancy (Wilms tumour and adrenocortical carcinoma), hemihypertrophy, overgrowth of the external genitalia in both males and females, accelerated linear growth until age 4–6 years and grooved earlobes. Hepatic tumours also occur with increased frequency. BWS is a sporadic condition caused by a mutation in the *p57(KIP2)* gene located at 11p15.5 [66]. The overgrowth associated with BWS can now be explained. The mutation in *p57(KIP2)* prevents it from performing one of its normal functions, which is to suppress the maternally inherited *IGF2* gene [67]. The presence of *two* active alleles for *IGF2* results in overgrowth of the infant and child with BWS.

### Transient neonatal diabetes mellitus

Diabetes mellitus in the neonatal period is rare. Hyperglycaemia is detected when the infant fails to thrive or

**Table 7.8.** Clinical signs suggestive of a metabolic disease

| Age | Clinical signs | Possible diagnosis |
|---|---|---|
| Day 1 of life | Seizures | Persistent hyperinsulinaemia<br>Mitochondrial cytopathy |
| Neonatal period* | Vomiting, feeding refusal, changes in respiration, prolonged jaundice, lethargy or irritability, movement disorder, seizures, hypo/hypertonia, changes in the level of consciousness | Organic acidaemias<br>Non-ketotic hyperglycinaemia<br>Urea cycle defects<br>Fatty acid oxidation defects<br>Tyrosinaemia, galactosaemia<br>Mitochondrial cytopathy |

*Symptoms should be considered in relation to the child's age (in days), fasting, food intake (i.e. specific sugars, protein, fat) and changes in diet.

becomes dehydrated. In most cases, the diabetes is transient, persisting for less than 12 months, but there is an increased risk for the development of type 2 diabetes later in life. An imprinted gene for transient neonatal diabetes has been localized to a 5.4-Mb region on chromosome 6q [68]. Antibodies to islet cell antigens and to insulin are invariably absent. Neonatal diabetes is also sometimes associated with pancreatic hypoplasia.

Assuming that the pancreas is morphologically normal on ultrasound, the treatment of neonatal diabetes mellitus would normally be with insulin. The standard soluble insulin preparations may need to be diluted to permit the very small doses needed. Oral sulphonylurea agents have been successfully tried in a few cases.

### The infant of a diabetic mother

Poorly controlled maternal diabetes is associated with an increased risk of spontaneous abortion, fetal malformation and fetal macrosomia [69]. The maternal blood glucose level during labour is inversely related to the blood glucose level in the neonate. This is because maternal hyperglycaemia induces hyperinsulinism and β-cell hyperplasia in the infant. Infants of diabetic mothers are prone to polycythaemia, renal vein thrombosis, hypocalcaemia, respiratory distress syndrome, jaundice, persistent fetal circulation, cardiomyopathy, congenital heart disease and malformations of other organ systems.

#### *Hypoglycaemia due to metabolic conditions*
Neonatal hypoglycaemia is not only due to hyperinsulinism but may be a prominent feature in a number of metabolic diseases. The presenting symptoms of metabolic diseases are non-specific (Table 7.8).

### Physical examination

Some findings on physical examination may be suggestive of a metabolic disease. These are summarized in Table 7.9.

**Table 7.9.** Clinical features suggestive of a metabolic disorder

| General appearance | Dysmorphism |
|---|---|
| Skin | Rash<br>Odour<br>Hyperkeratosis<br>Signs of chronic scratching |
| Head and neck | Craniomegaly<br>Dysmorphism<br>Bulging fontanelle<br>Abnormal eye movement |
| Chest | Signs of lung disease |
| Heart | Cardiomegaly<br>Signs of cardiac failure |
| Abdomen | Hepato ± splenomegaly<br>Signs of liver disease |
| Genitalia | Ambiguous genitalia |
| Skeleton | Signs of rickets<br>Bone or joint pain, contractures<br>Abnormal spine posturing/vertebral disease |
| Muscles | Muscle mass, wasting |
| Neurological | Muscle strength, tone<br>Sensation<br>Reflexes (tendon and archaic).<br>Movement disorders<br>Ataxia |

### Laboratory investigations

Blood, urine and cerebrospinal fluid (CSF) samples collected at the time of presentation may be diagnostic and are invaluable. Always attempt to collect these samples *before* commencing treatment, but do not delay treatment in crisis situations.

There are three initial questions to be answered:

**Table 7.10.** Investigation of a suspected metabolic disorder

|  | First-line tests | Second-line tests |
|---|---|---|
| Blood | Acid/base<br>Electrolytes<br>Glucose<br>Ammonia<br>Lactate<br>Acylcarnitines | Complete blood count<br>Plasma amino acids<br>Pyruvate<br>FA/ketones (specify: β-hydroxybutyrate and acetoacetate)<br>Liver transaminases<br>Urea, creatinine, calcium, phosphate<br>Uric acid<br>Cholesterol<br>Freeze additional plasma for further testing |
| Urine | pH, glucose, ketones, protein<br>Reducing substances<br>Organic acids | Freeze additional urine for further testing |
| CSF | Glucose, protein, lactate | Freeze additional CSF for further testing (amino acids, neurotransmitters, etc.) |

**Table 7.11.** Interpretation of laboratory results

| Metabolic condition | pH | Glucose | Ketones | Ammonia |
|---|---|---|---|---|
| Urea cycle defects | Normal or ↑ | Normal | Normal | ↑↑ |
| Organic acidaemias | ↓ | ↑, Normal or ↓ | Normal or ↑ | ↑ |
| Ketolysis defects | Normal or ↓ | Normal or ↑ | ↑↑ | Normal |
| FA oxidation defects | Normal or ↓ | Normal or ↓ | Normal or ↓ | Normal or ↑ |
| Hyperinsulinaemia | Normal | ↓↓ | Normal | Normal or ↑ |

1 Is there acidosis? Is it of metabolic origin?
2 Is there hyper- or hypoketonaemia?
3 Is there hyperammonaemia?

The tests in Table 7.10 should be carried out to answer these questions and the results need to be carefully interpreted (Table 7.11). In addition to these tests, brain computerized tomography (CT) or magnetic resonance imaging (MRI) and abdominal ultrasonographic examination may be helpful in the diagnostic process.

## How the premature infant is different from the full-term infant

Premature infants are more prone to hypoglycaemia because of immaturity in gluconeogenic and other enzyme systems, and because they have low stores of hepatic glycogen. They have less subcutaneous fat than term infants and may therefore have lower levels of $T_3$ because the conversion of $T_4$ to $T_3$ takes place in fat. The postnatal persistence of the fetal zone of the adrenal cortex is reflected in higher levels of 17-hydroxyprogesterone and lower levels of cortisol and aldosterone than in the term infant. Fetal steroids are detectable in the urine for longer than in the term infant. Because the lungs have had a shorter exposure to cortisol during intrauterine life, and because of the prematurity in lung development itself, surfactant induction is incomplete, alveolar fluid is cleared less efficiently and the premature infant is more prone to hyaline membrane disease and asphyxia. In addition, persistence of the fetal circulation is more likely to occur. Asphyxia increases the risk of neonatal hypocalcaemia, which is usually due to transient hypoparathyroidism. Calcium absorption from the gut is relatively poor in preterm infants and neither breast milk nor formula contain enough calcium to match intrauterine accretion rates. Oral calcium and phosphorus supplementation may be needed to prevent rickets and pathological fractures. In preterm infants, serum GH levels are higher and IGF-I levels lower than in full-term infants.

When assessing the results of endocrine tests carried out on a newborn infant, one should remember that women in premature labour are often treated with high doses of glucocorticoids to try to accelerate pulmonary maturation in the fetus. Depending on the duration of the treatment, this induces fetal adrenal suppression to a variable degree.

## The growth-restricted infant

Intrauterine growth restriction (IUGR) may result from poor intrauterine nutrition, or it may be the result of an underlying fetal disorder, such as infection, a chromosomal abnormality, a malformation or any one of a number of possible causes. The child with IUGR is prone to all of the disorders seen in the premature infant, except that the lungs tend to be more mature. Infants with IUGR who are well in the first weeks of life generally show complete catch-up to their birth centiles by 3 months, but those with significant illness tend not to do so well. The obstetric and perinatal issues surrounding IUGR are covered in more detail in Chapter 6 [70].

## Two dysmorphic syndromes that are recognizable in the newborn

### Turner syndrome

If Turner syndrome is recognized in the newborn, it is usually because the infant has one or more of the following features:
• lymphoedema of the hands and/or feet (sometimes of a single digit);
• cardiac failure or hypertension due to coarctation of the aorta or other cardiac malformation;
• redundant skin at the back of the neck or a cystic hygroma.

Closer inspection may then reveal facial features consistent with Turner syndrome (epicanthic folds, down-turned angles of the mouth, differences in the shape of the pinna) and fingernails that are hypoplastic, soft and turned up at the ends. The genitalia should, by definition, be female. Birth length is likely to be at the lower end of the normal range, or less.

Chromosome analysis will confirm the diagnosis. A small proportion of infants with the above features will be shown to have mosaicism in which a Y chromosome is present. The significance of this is that it greatly increases the chance that malignancy will develop in the gonad and therefore the gonads will need to be removed. The presence of an XY cell line would also increase the need for surveillance of renal function and urinary protein content to detect the changes of Drash syndrome. Other useful investigations in the neonatal period would be serum FSH and LH (grossly elevated levels are indicative of gonadal dysgenesis), an echocardiogram and renal ultrasound.

### Prader–Willi syndrome

Since the advent of DNA testing for Prader–Willi syndrome (PWS), the neonatal features of PWS – extreme floppiness and inability to suck – have been more frequently recognized for what they are, and the diagnosis is being made much earlier than in the past. In males, the penis is usually small and one or both testes may be small and/or undescended. The facial features of PWS are subtle and difficult to recognize in a neonate.

PWS is associated with either a deletion of the paternal allele at 15q11–13 or a duplication of the maternal allele at this locus. Early diagnosis makes accurate counselling possible, and dietary measures to prevent the development of obesity can be introduced. In some centres, GH treatment is advocated on the grounds that it may prevent growth retardation while at the same time improving the ratio of lean–fat body mass. Short-term, uncontrolled studies provide support for this hypothesis and adverse effects have not been seen. Whether or not GH treatment provides long-term benefit in children with PWS is still unknown.

## References

1 Gluckman P, Sizonenko S, Bassett N. The transition from fetus to neonate – an endocrine perspective. *Acta Paediatr* 1999; 88 (Suppl. 428): 7–11.
2 Zeitler P, Pickett C. Molecular aspects of pituitary development. In: Handwerger S, ed. *Molecular and Cellular Pediatric Endocrinology*. Totowa, NJ: Humana Press, 1999: 231–51.
3 Deladoey J, Fluck C, Buyukgebiz A *et al.* 'Hot spot' in the PROP1 gene responsible for combined pituitary hormone deficiency. *J Clin Endocrinol Metab* 1999; 84: 1645–50.
4 Achermann J, Ito M, Ito M, Hindmarsh P, Jameson J. A mutation in the gene encoding steroidogenic factor-1 causes XY sex reversal and adrenal failure in humans. *Nature Genet* 1999; 22: 125–6.
5 Ray R, Ren S, Melmed S. Leukemia inhibitory factor regulates proopiomelanocortin transcription. *Ann NY Acad Sci* 1998; 840: 162–73.
6 Yano H, Readhead C, Nakashima M, Ren S, Melmed S. Pituitary-directed leukemia inhibitory factor transgene causes Cushing's syndrome: neuro-immune-endocrine modulation of pituitary development. *Mol Endocrinol* 1998; 12: 1708–20.
7 Santini F, Chiovato L, Ghirri P *et al.* Serum iodothyronines in the human fetus and the newborn: evidence for an important role of placenta in fetal thyroid hormone biosynthesis. *J Clin Endocrinol Metab* 1999; 84: 493–8.
8 Grüters A, Krude H, Biebermann H, Liesenkotter L, Schoneberg T, Gudermann T. Alterations of neonatal thyroid function. *Acta Paediatr Suppl* 1999; 88 (Suppl. 428): 17–22.
9 Scott D, Wang R, Kreman T, Sheffield V, Karniski L. The Pendred syndrome gene encodes a chloride-iodide transport protein. *Nature Genet* 1999; 21: 440–3.
10 Fisher D, Polk D. Development of the thyroid. *Baillière's Clin Endocrinol Metabolism* 1989; 3: 627–57.
11 LaFranchi S. Thyroid function in the preterm infant. *Thyroid* 1999; 9: 71–8.
12 Sullivan K, May W, Nordenberg D, Houston R, Maberly G. Use of thyroid stimulating hormone testing in newborns to identify iodine deficiency. *J Nutr* 1997; 127: 55–8.
13 Haddow J, Palomaki G, Allan W *et al.* Maternal thyroid deficiency during pregnancy and subsequent neurophysiological development of the child. *N Engl J Med* 1999; 341: 549–55.
14 Boyages S, Halpern J, Maberly G *et al.* Endemic cretinism: possible role for thyroid autoimmunity. *Lancet* 1989; 2: 529–32.
15 Zimmermann D. Fetal and neonatal hyperthyroidism. *Thyroid* 1999; 9: 727–33.
16 Curtis N, Thomas R, Gillespie M, King R, Rice G, Wlodek M. Parathyroid hormone-related protein (PTHrP) mRNA splicing

and parathyroid hormone/PTHrP receptor mRNA expression in human placenta and fetal membranes. *J Mol Endocrinol* 1998; 21 (2): 225–34.

17 Kronenberg H, Lanske B, Kovacs C *et al.* Functional analysis of the PTH/PTHrP network of ligands and receptors. *Rec Prog Horm Res* 1998; 53: 283–301.

18 Okazaki R, Chikatsu N, Nakatsu M *et al.* A novel activating mutation in calcium-sensing receptor gene associated with a family of autosomal dominant hypocalcemia. *J Clin Endocrinol Metab* 1999; 84: 363–6.

19 Thakker R. Disorders of the calcium-sensing receptor. *Biochim Biophys Acta* 1998; 1448 (2): 166–70.

20 Pollak M, Seidman C, Brown E. Three inherited disorders of calcium sensing. *Medicine* 1996; 75 (3): 115–23.

21 Midgley P, Russell K, Oates N, Howlonia P, Shaw J, Honour J. Adrenal function in preterm infants: ACTH may not be the sole regulator of the fetal zone. *Pediatr Res* 1998; 44: 887–93.

22 Midgley P, Russell K, Oates N, Shaw J, Honour J. Activity of the adrenal fetal zone in preterm infants continues to term. *Endocrinol Res* 1996; 22: 729–33.

23 Nomura S. Immature adrenal steroidogenesis in preterm infants. *Early Hum Dev* 1997; 49 (3): 225–33.

24 Wedell A. An update on the molecular genetics of congenital adrenal hyperplasia: diagnostic and therapeutic aspects. *J Pediatr Endocrinol Metab* 1998; 11: 581–9.

25 Chin D, Speiser P, Imperato-McGinley J *et al.* Study of a kindred with classic congenital adrenal hyperplasia: diagnostic challenge due to phenotypic variance. *J Clin Endocrinol Metab* 1998; 83: 1940–5.

26 Pang S, Shook M. Current status of neonatal screening for congenital adrenal hyperplasia. *Curr Opin Pediatr* 1997; 9: 419–23.

27 Papendieck LGD, Prieto L, Chiesa A, Bengolea S, Bergada C. Congenital adrenal hyperplasia and early newborn screening: 17 alpha-hydroxyprogesterone (17 alpha-OHP) during the first days of life. *J Med Screen* 1998; 5: 24–6.

28 Therrell B, Berenbaum S, Manter-Kapanke V *et al.* Results of screening 1.9 million Texas newborns for 21-hydroxylase-deficient congenital adrenal hyperplasia. *Pediatrics* 1998; 101 (Part 1): 583–90.

29 Reutens A, Achermann J, Ito M *et al.* Clinical and functional effects of mutations in the DAX-1 gene in patients with adrenal hypoplasia congenita. *J Clin Endocrinol Metab* 1999; 84 (2): 504–11.

30 Crowley P. Antenatal corticosteroid therapy: a meta-analysis of the randomized trials, 1972 to 94. *Am J Obstet Gynecol* 1995; 173: 322–35.

31 Salokorpi T, Sajaniemi N, Rajantie I *et al.* Neurodevelopment until the adjusted age of 2 years in extremely low birth weight infants after early intervention – a case control study. *Pediatr Rehabil* 1998; 2 (4): 157–63.

32 Slotkin T, Zhang J, McCook E, Seidler F. Glucocorticoid administration alters nuclear transcription factors in fetal rat brain: implications for the use of antenatal steroids. *Brain Res Dev Brain Res* 1998; 111: 11–24.

33 Elimian A, Verma U, Canterino J, Shah J, Visintainer P, Tejani N. Effectiveness of antenatal steroids in obstetric subgroups. *Obstet Gynecol* 1999; 93 (2): 174–9.

34 Jobe A, Newnham J, Willet K, Sly P, Ikegami M. Fetal versus maternal and gestational age effects of repetitive antenatal glucocorticoids. *Pediatrics* 1998; 102: 1116–25.

35 O'Shea T, Kothadia J, Klinepeter K *et al.* Randomized placebo-controlled trial of a 42-day tapering course of dexamethasone to reduce the duration of ventilator dependency in very low birth weight infants: outcome of study participants at 1-year adjusted age. *Pediatrics* 1999; 104 (1, Part 1): 15–21.

36 Miranda-Mallea J, Perz-Verdu J, Gasco-Lacalle B, Saez-Palacios J, Fernandez-Gilino G, Izquierdo-Macian I. Hypertrophic cardiomyopathy in preterm infants treated with dexamethasone. *Eur J Pediatr* 1997; 156 (5): 394–6.

37 Kothadia J, O'Shea T, Roberts D, Auringer S, 3rd RW, Dillard R. Randomized placebo-controlled trial of a 42-day tapering course of dexamethasone to reduce the duration of ventilator dependency in very low birth weight infants. *Pediatrics* 1999; 104 (1, Part; 1): 22–7.

38 Pang S, Clark A, Freeman L *et al.* Maternal side effects of prenatal dexamethasone therapy for fetal congenital adrenal hyperplasia. *J Clin Endocrinol Metab* 1992; 75: 249–53.

39 Lajic S, Wedell A, Bui T, Ritzen E, Holst M. Long-term follow-up of prenatally treated children with congenital adrenal hyperplasia. *J Clin Endocrinol Metab* 1998; 83: 3872–80.

40 Carlson A, Obeid J, Kanellopoulou N, Wilson R, New M. Congenital adrenal hyperplasia: update on prenatal diagnosis and treatment. *J Steroid Biochem Mol Biol* 1999; 69 (1–6): 19–29.

41 Miller W. Dexamethasone treatment of congenital adrenal hyperplasia in utero: an experimental therapy of unproven safety. *J Urol* 1999; 162: 537–40.

42 Nef S, Parada L. Cryptorchidism in mice mutant for Insl3. *Nature Genet* 1999; 22: 295–9.

43 Zimmermann S, Steding G, Emmen J *et al.* Targeted disruption of the Insl3 gene causes bilateral cryptorchidism. *Mol Endocrinol* 1999; 13: 681–91.

44 Graves J, Wakefield M, Toder R. The origin and evolution of the pseudoautosomal regions of human sex chromosomes. *Hum Mol Genet* 1998; 7: 1991–6.

45 Little M, Wells C. A clinical overview of *WT1* gene mutations. *Hum Mutat* 1997; 9: 209–25.

46 Shimamura R, Fraizer G, Trapman J, Lau Y, Saunders G. The Wilms' tumour gene WT1 can regulate genes involved in sex differentiation and differentiation: SRY, Mullerian-inhibiting substance, and the androgen receptor. *Clin Cancer Res* 1997; 3: 2571–80.

47 Bertherat J. The nuclear receptor steroidogenic factor-1 (SF-1) is no longer an orphan. *Eur J Endocrinol* 1998; 138: 32–3.

48 Foster J. Mutations in SOX9 cause both autosomal sex reversal and campomelic dysplasia. *Acta Paediatr Jpn* 1996; 38: 405–11.

49 Zanaria E, Muscatelli F, Bardoni B *et al.* An unusual member of the nuclear hormone superfamily responsible for X-linked adrenal hypoplasia congenita. *Nature* 1994; 372: 635–41.

50 Tuladhar R, Davis P, Batch J, Doyle L. Establishment of a normal range of penile length in preterm infants. *J Pediatr Child Health* 1998; 34: 471–3.

51 Bin-Abbas B, Conte F, Grumbach M, Kaplan S. Congenital hypogonadotropic hypogonadism and micropenis: effect of testosterone treatment on adult penile size where sex reversal is not indicated. *J Pediatr* 1999; 134: 579–83.

52 Woodhouse C. Sexual function in boys born with extrophy, meningomyelocoele, and micropenis. *Urology* 1998; 52: 3–11.

53 Percival A, Slack J. Analysis of pancreatic development using a cell lineage label. *Exp Cell Res* 1999; 247: 123–32.

54 Andrew A, Kramer B, Rawdon B. The origin of gut and pancreatic neuroendocrine (APUD) cells – the last word? *J Pathol* 1998; 186: 117–18.

55 Yamaguchi K, Mishina J, Mitsuishi C, Takamura T, Nishida H. Follow-up study of neonatal hypoglycaemia. *Acta Paediatr Jpn* 1997; 39 (Suppl. 1): S51–3.

56 Sinclair J. Approaches to the definition of neonatal hypoglycemia. *Acta Paediatr Jpn* 1997; 39 (Suppl. 1): S17–20.

57 Barkovich A, Ali F, Rowley H, Bass N. Imaging patterns of neonatal hypoglycemia. *Am J Neuroradiol* 1998; 19: 523–8.

58 Kinnala A, Riakalainen H, Lapinleumu H, Parkkola R, Kormano M, Kero P. Cerebral magnetic resonance imaging and ultrasonographic findings after neonatal hypoglycemia. *Pediatrics* 1999; 103 (Part 1): 724–9.

59 Moore A, Perlman M. Symptomatic hypoglycemia in otherwise healthy, breastfed term newborns. *Pediatrics* 1999; 103 (Part 1): 837–9.

60 Lonlay-Debeney PD, Poggi-Travert F, Fournet J *et al.* Clinical features of 52 neonates with hyperinsulinism. *N Engl J Med* 1999; 340: 1169–75.

61 Aguilar-Bryan LJBJ. Molecular biology of adenosine triphosphate-sensitive potassium channels. *Endocrinol Rev* 1999; 20 (2): 101–35.

62 Fournet J, Verkarre V, de Lonlay P *et al.* Loss of imprinted genes and paternal SUR1 mutations lead to hyperinsulinism in focal adenomatous hyperplasia. *Ann Endocrinol* 1998; 59: 485–91.

63 Thornton P, Alter C, Katz L, Baker L, Stanley C. Short- and long-term use of octreotide in the treatment of congenital hyperinsulinism. *J Pediatr* 1993; 123: 637–43.

64 Stanley C, Lieu Y, Hsu B *et al.* Hyperinsulinism and hyperammonemia in infants with regulatory mutations of the glutamate dehydrogenase gene. *N Engl J Med* 1999; 338: 1352–7.

65 Liebowitz G, GlaSeries B, Higazi A, Salameh M, Cerasi E, Landau H. Hyperinsulinemic hypoglycemia of infancy (nesidioblastosis) in clinical remission: high incidence of diabetes mellitus and persistent beta-cell dysfunction at long-tern follow-up. *J Clin Endocrinol Metab* 1995; 80 (2): 386–92.

66 Zhang P, Liegeois N, Wong C *et al.* Altered cell differentiation and proliferation in mice lacking p57KIP2 indicates a role in Beckwith–Wiedemann syndrome. *Nature* 1997; 387: 151–8.

67 Weksberg R, Shen D, Fei Y, Song Q, Squire J. Disruption of insulin-like growth factor 2 imprinting in Beckwith–Wiedemann syndrome. *Nature Genet* 1993; 5 (2): 143–50.

68 Gardner R, Mungall A, Durham I *et al.* Localisation of a gene for transient neonatal diabetes mellitus to an 18.72 cR3000 (approximately 5.4 Mb) interval on chromosome 6q. *J Med Genet* 1999; 36 (3): 192–6.

69 Rey E, Atti C, Bonin A. The effects of first-trimester diabetes control on the incidence of macrosomia. *Am J Obstet Gynecol* 1999; 181: 202–6.

70 Kingdom JCP, Smith G. Diagnosis and management of IUGR. In: Kingdom J, Baker P, eds. *Intrauterine Growth Restriction – Aetiology and Management*. London: Springer, 2000: 257–70.

# 8  Normal growth and its endocrine control

**P. E. Clayton and M. S. Gill**

## Introduction

Growth can be defined as an increase in size by accretion of tissue. It is observed in the whole organism, in body regions, in organ systems or in the cellular environment. Growth is dependent on cellular hyperplasia (an increase in cell number), hypertrophy (an increase in cell size) and apoptosis (programmed cell death). Hyperplasia and apoptosis are genetically regulated to limit the size of an organ or body. The speed and success of growth in the whole organism will depend on the relative rates of these three cellular events. Their correct coordination will allow a fertilized egg to develop into a mature adult, whereas their disruption may generate variable degrees of whole-body or regional growth failure.

The control of the growth process is related to many complex interacting factors, including internal cues such as genotype, external factors such as nutrition and environment, and internal signalling systems such as hormones and growth factors. Tissue growth may not end with the completion of whole-body growth. Some cells retain their ability to proliferate, most notably the liver and endocrine tissues. Other cells can be renewed but remain terminally differentiated, such as blood and epidermal cells, whereas other cells, like those in the nervous system, have a limited capacity to regenerate. In addition whole-body growth is not a smooth symmetrical event: there is marked variation in organ and regional growth through childhood and adolescence (Fig. 8.1). Thus, the time at which an organ system is vulnerable to adverse events will vary.

How these events are brought together to generate the diverse pattern of normal human growth will be presented in this chapter, with the issue of clinical recognition of normal growth and development highlighted. Although this chapter deals with normality, lessons learnt from murine strains, transgenically modified to under- or overexpress growth genes, as well as natural human gene mutations, will be used to illustrate key factors required for successful human growth.

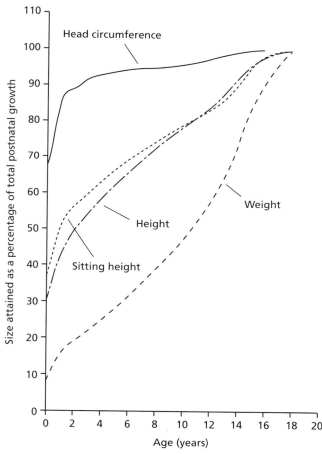

**Fig. 8.1.** Growth in different parts of the body in boys [data derived from Freeman *et al.* [15], head circumference (Tanner, 1978) and sitting height/subischial leg length (Tanner–Whitehouse, 1978) charts].

## Stages of growth

There are four stages of growth [fetal, infant (I), childhood (C) and pubertal (P)] to be considered. The growth trajectory of the last three stages can be represented mathematically by the

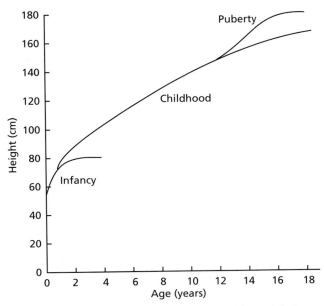

**Fig. 8.2.** The infancy–childhood–puberty (ICP) model of growth for boys. Data shown are the mean height values (cm) for age (from Karlberg *et al.* [1,2]).

**Table 8.1.** Requirements for normal human growth

Absence of chronic disease
Emotional stability, secure family environment
Adequate nutrition
Normal hormone actions
Absence of defects impairing cellular/bone growth

'ICP-growth model' (Fig. 8.2) [1,2]. Growth during the first 3 years of extrauterine life results from a combination of a rapidly decelerating infancy component and a slowly decelerating childhood component. The latter dominates the mid-childhood years but is altered at adolescence by the pubertal contribution, which is modelled on a sigmoid curve.

Throughout the growing years, it is useful to consider the attributes required for normal growth (Table 8.1). Chronic illness is a potent cause of growth failure because of the effects of the disease on dividing cells and its secondary effects on nutrition. It is for this reason that growth monitoring is such an essential component of child health surveillance and that auxological assessment should be undertaken whenever a child attends hospital. A secure caring environment is a vital prerequisite for normal growth: emotional deprivation is a potent cause of dramatic growth failure. An adequate nutritional intake must be taken but energy requirements for normal growth are modest. Total daily energy expenditure (TEE) is based on four components: (1) basal metabolic rate, accounting for 55–60% of TEE; (2) thermic effect of food, accounting for 10%; (3) energy expended in activity, which is highly variable and accounts for approximately 25% of TEE; and (4) energy required for growth. The last one, which will vary according to growth rate, makes the smallest contribution to TEE. Thus food/energy intake, which would normally match TEE, must be severely restricted to cause growth failure. It is also essential that cells have the capacity to divide and respond to hormonal and growth factor influences. This is amply demonstrated in conditions where there is a fundamental abnormality in cell growth, such as a mutation in fibroblast growth factor-3 receptor resulting in achondroplasia or in those infants with intrauterine growth restriction who fail to catch-up postnatally (e.g. Russell–Silver syndrome).

## The fetus

During the first trimester, tissue patterns and organ systems are established. During weeks 1–3, the three germ layers (ectoderm, mesoderm and endoderm) are formed within the embryonic disc, and in weeks 4–8 there is rapid growth and differentiation to form all the major organ systems in the body. In the second trimester, the fetus undergoes major cellular hyperplasia, and in the third trimester organ systems mature in preparation for extrauterine life. Changes in crown–rump and crown–heel length and weight through gestation are illustrated in Fig. 8.3. During weeks 4–12, crown–rump growth velocity equates to 33 cm per annum, from 12 to 24 weeks to 62 cm per annum and from 24 weeks to term to 48 cm per annum. Growth velocity is therefore maximal in the second trimester. Weight gain over the same intervals, extrapolated to kilograms per annum, shows a different pattern with modest gains during weeks 4–12 (0.1 kg/year) followed by 2.7 kg/year in weeks 12–24, escalating in the last 16 weeks to 8.7 kg/year. Maximal weight gain is therefore achieved in the third trimester, although there is a declining weight velocity in the last weeks of pregnancy (Fig. 8.3).

The orchestration of this combination of rapid cell division and differentiation as well as morphogenesis is dependent, in part, on a class of developmental genes belonging to the homeobox family [3]. The homeobox (a 180-basepair DNA sequence, encoding a 60-amino-acid homeodomain) was originally discovered in the genome of the fruit fly *Drosophila*, but it is present in all multicellular organisms. Homeobox-containing genes encode for proteins that include a homeodomain and bind DNA, thereby controlling gene expression and hence cell differentiation and organ development. Class I *Hox* homeobox genes are involved in patterning embryonic structures such as the axial skeleton, the limbs, digestive and genital tracts, and in craniofacial and nervous system development. Abnormalities in human homeobox genes usually give rise to specific organ malformation, but there are also genes that have a wider impact on whole-body growth (Table 8.2).

Throughout gestation, fetal growth is constrained by maternal factors and placental function, but is coordinated by

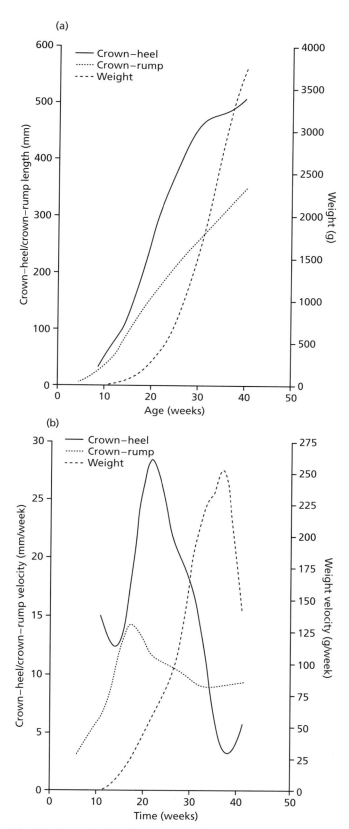

**Fig. 8.3.** Crown–heel length, crown–rump length and weight (a) and velocity (b) of the fetus from 4 weeks' gestation (data taken from References 7 and 49).

**Table 8.2.** Examples of homeobox gene mutations causing human growth/developmental disorders [3,26,27].

| | |
|---|---|
| *PAX6* | Aniridia; Peter's anomaly (defect of anterior chamber of the eye); anophthalmia |
| *MSX1* | Craniosynostosis |
| *SHOX* | Short stature in Turner syndrome; rare cause of *idiopathic* short stature; Leri–Weill dyschondrosteosis |
| *HESX1* | Familial septo-optic dysplasia |
| *PIT1* | Combined GH, TSH and prolactin deficiencies |
| *PROP1* | Congenital hypopituitarism |

GH, growth hormone; TSH, thyroid-stimulating hormone.

growth factors [4]. These can act locally in a paracrine manner [produced in one site to act on adjacent tissue, e.g. insulin-like growth factor I (IGF-I) and IGF-II, fibroblast growth factor, epidermal growth factor, transforming growth factors α and β] or as endocrine hormones (produced in one site and moving to a separate site for action, e.g. insulin). Nutrition, passing from the mother to the fetus, plays a rate-limiting role. Placental transport of nutrients and metabolites can occur by three mechanisms: (1) simple diffusion, where transfer is limited by blood flow through the placenta and placental surface area (e.g. oxygen, carbon dioxide, urea); (2) carrier-mediated facilitated diffusion down a concentration gradient and therefore not requiring energy (e.g. glucose and lactate); and (3) active transport using carrier proteins and energy (e.g. amino acids). Factors that control nutrient transport are not fully characterized, but growth hormone (GH) and IGF-I acting on the maternal and/or fetal sides of the placenta have been shown to alter diffusion capacity and lactate uptake in the sheep model [5].

Understanding factors that can control fetal growth has assumed increasing importance as epidemiological studies have firmly established links between intrauterine and early extrauterine growth restriction (I/EUGR) and the risk of developing health problems in later life [6]. These include hypertension, cardio- and cerebrovascular disease, insulin resistance and non-insulin-dependent diabetes mellitus. The link between early growth and later disease is postulated to occur through programming, where an insult (e.g. maternal undernutrition) at a critical period in fetal development leads to a permanent deleterious metabolic alteration that renders an individual prone to specific disease later in life. Hormones and growth factors are potential targets for programming. Evidence is accumulating that insulin and the GH–IGF axis are modified in those born with IUGR. Exactly how these changes translate into disease is not yet defined.

## The infant

During the first year, infants grow rapidly in length, but at a sharply decelerating rate (Fig. 8.4). A similar pattern is observed

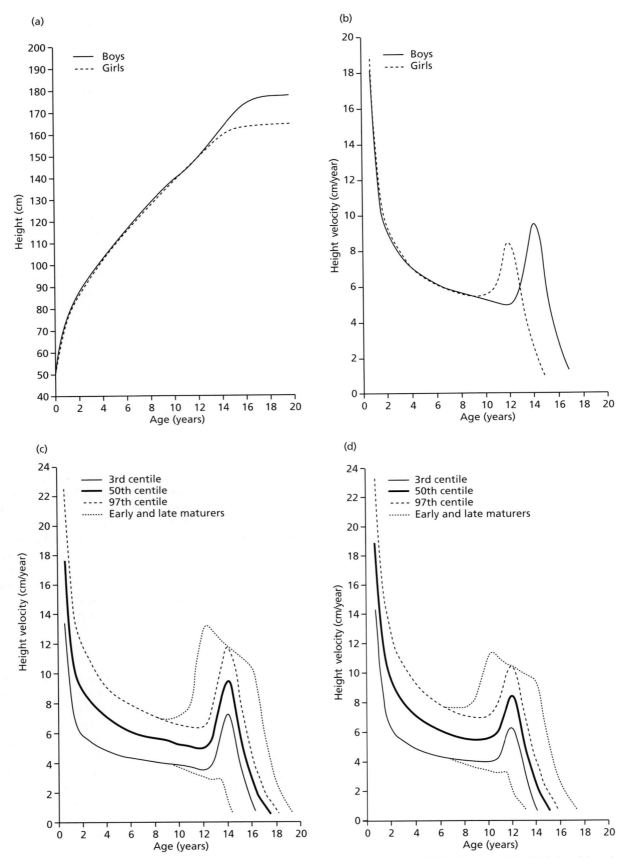

**Fig. 8.4.** Height (a) and mean height velocity (b) for boys and girls according to age (from Freeman *et al.* [15] and Tanner *et al.* [17]). Timing of the pubertal growth spurt for early and late maturers in boys (c) and girls (d) [from Tanner–Whitehouse growth velocity charts (1976)].

**Table 8.3.** Summary of the phenotypes associated with inactivation/overexpression of genes within the GH–IGF axis [38,46,47].

| Genotype | Birth weight (% normal) | Phenotype at birth | Postnatal growth | Adult weight (% normal) | Adult phenoptype |
|---|---|---|---|---|---|
| 1. GH(+) | 100 | Normal | Increased from 3 weeks, when IGF-I levels increased | 200 | Organomegaly, increased skeletal growth, IGF-I levels 2- to 3-fold higher |
| 2. GH(–) | 100 | Normal | Reduced from 3 weeks | 60 | Hypoplastic liver |
| 3. IGF-I(+) | 100 | Normal | Increased from 4 weeks | 130 | Organomegaly, no increase in skeletal size, IGF-I levels 1.5-fold higher |
| 4. GH(–)/IGF-I(+) | 100 | Normal | Normal | 100 | Increased brain size |
| 5. IGF-I(–) Total | 60 | Small | 95% die, survivors have reduced growth rate | 30 | Delayed/incomplete sexual development |
| Hepatic | 100 | Normal | Normal | 100 | Normal |
| 6. IGF-II(–) | 60 | Small, placental hypoplasia | Normal growth rate | 60 | Small, normal proportions |
| 7. IGF-I R(–) | 45 | Postnatal death, no respiration | NA | NA | NA |
| 8. IGF-I(–)/IGF-II(–) | 30 | Postnatal death, no respiration, placental hypoplasia | NA | NA | NA |
| 9. IGF-I R(–)/IGF-I(–) | 45 | Postnatal death, no respiration | NA | NA | NA |
| 10. IGF-I R(–)/IGF-II(–) | 30 | Postnatal death, no respiration, placental hypoplasia | NA | NA | NA |
| 11. IGF-II(+) | 160 | Large, disproportionate organ overgrowth, postnatal death | NA | NA | NA |
| 12. IGF-II R(–) | 135 | Organomegaly, most die perinatally, some survive | NA | NA | NA |

for weight gain. It has been postulated that nutritional input is the principal regulator of growth over this period with minimal contribution from GH. However, data from both humans and transgenic animal models suggest that the hormones and receptors within the GH–IGF axis do play a part in this early phase of growth (Table 8.3). Nevertheless, it is during this period that alterations in dietary intake are likely to have the greatest impact on growth performance. Early obesity in an otherwise normal infant is more likely to lead to tall stature than obesity developing later in childhood.

The correlation between length and weight and mean parental size at birth is poor, reflecting the dominant influence of the intrauterine environment over the genotype [7]. Once this effect is removed, a period of 'catch-up' or 'catch-down' growth during the first 2 years commonly occurs while the infant establishes its own growth channel. Catch-up growth starts soon after birth and is completed over 6–18 months, whereas catch-down growth commences between 3 and 6 months and is completed by 9–20 months. By 2 years of age, this process has increased the correlation between length and one parent's height to an $r$-value of 0.5, and length and midparental height to an $r$-value of 0.7–0.8. Likewise, the correlation between an individual's birth length and his/her adult height has an $r$-value of only 0.3, but, by 3 years of age, the correlation between height and final height has increased markedly to $r = 0.8$.

Although growth charts give the impression that growth is linear, this is far from the true pattern of growth. Most studies that have examined short-term growth (day to day, week to week) agree that it is non-linear (saltatory) [8], although there is dispute over its exact form. One model proposes that all infant growth occurs in short intense bursts over 24 h, separated by long periods of growth *stasis* [9]. The question of how day-to-day activity within the GH–IGF axis might generate such an infant growth trajectory has not been addressed.

## The child

By 4 years of age, average growth velocity has declined to 7 cm/year and thereafter declines steadily until adolescence, the prepubertal nadir in average velocity being 5–5.5 cm/year (Fig. 8.4). On an individual basis, however, there is the well-recognized mid-childhood growth spurt. In addition, if an individual is measured throughout childhood, oscillations in growth velocity of variable amplitude are observed, which occur within a period of approximately 2 years (Fig. 8.5) [10]. Seasonal variation in growth rate is also well described [8]. Thus, the whole process of normal growth requires variability controlled by inherent, presumably genetic, mechanisms as well as by external influences.

Childhood is the period during which GH, in addition to thyroid hormone, is thought to be the major determinant

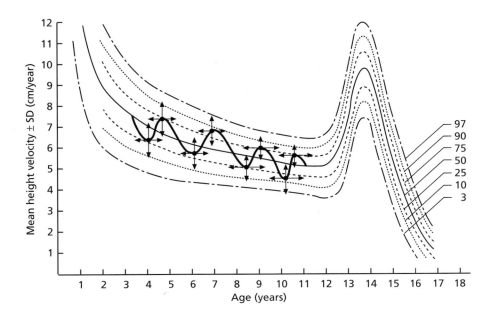

**Fig. 8.5.** Oscillations of growth velocity in the Edinburgh Growth Study (from Butler *et al.* [10]). The horizontal and vertical arrows represent the range of timing and amplitude, respectively, for each growth spurt.

of growth. It is therefore the time when dysfunction in the GH axis may be recognized. In the ICP model, the childhood component is first recognized at 6 months of age, but becomes predominant over the waning infancy component by 3 years. In the Swedish study, in which this model was devised, it was possible to detect an abrupt change in growth velocity as the childhood component was initiated in 76% of the subjects [2]. This was thought to represent the time at which GH became active. There is, however, abundant evidence that the GH axis is active in the fetus, and thus the increasing influence of GH in this early period of childhood growth is likely to be gradual rather than an 'on–off' phenomenon.

When growth in childhood is observed short term, it is, as in infancy, a non-linear process. One model is of growth spurts with intervening periods of very slow or absent growth (Fig. 8.6) [11]. Weight changes appear to show a reciprocal relationship with the height changes, in that growth stasis is accompanied by weight gain while growth spurts coincide with weight stasis. An understanding of how this pattern of short-term height and weight gain relates to the GH–IGF axis is an important objective for understanding exactly how height gain is achieved.

Over this period, there is relatively little difference in height between boys and girls (Figs 8.4 and 8.7). In addition, body composition, as measured by DEXA (dual-energy X-ray absorptiometry) scanning, shows similar amounts of fat and fat-free mass in the two sexes prepubertally [12]. Nevertheless, girls do have some subtle differences in maturation, demonstrating skeletal maturity at birth that is 3–6 weeks ahead of that seen in boys, and there is a 2-year advance by the onset of puberty.

## Puberty

In physical terms, puberty may be defined as the transition from the prepubertal state through the development of secondary sexual characteristics to the achievement of adult stature. There is marked sexual dimorphism in the timing of these events (Fig. 8.8) [13]. There is also wide variation in pubertal timing within each sex. The later onset of pubertal growth in boys gives them an additional 2 years of prepubertal growth compared with the girls. The height gained in this time (8–10 cm), in addition to the greater amplitude of pubertal growth in boys (3–5 cm more than the female growth spurt), gives rise to the 12.5-cm difference in adult height between the sexes.

It is during this phase that the issue of growth tempo becomes obvious. Constitutional delay of growth and puberty (CDGP) is common and can be considered a variant of normal. The condition can be associated with chronic disease, for example atopy, but more usually occurs in isolation, often with a family history. Pubertal development commences late and the growth spurt is blunted. Although CDGP may present in the pubertal years, some children may have shown slow growth much earlier in childhood. The corollary of these conditions is tall stature and early puberty. The earlier puberty is, the greater is the magnitude of pubertal growth. The net result is that both early and late maturers should achieve a comparable height (Fig. 8.7). The genes that contribute to this variation in physical development have not yet been characterized.

During puberty, marked changes in body composition occur. Using skin-fold thickness to derive fat mass (FM), fat-free mass (FFM) and percentage body fat (%BF), boys gain

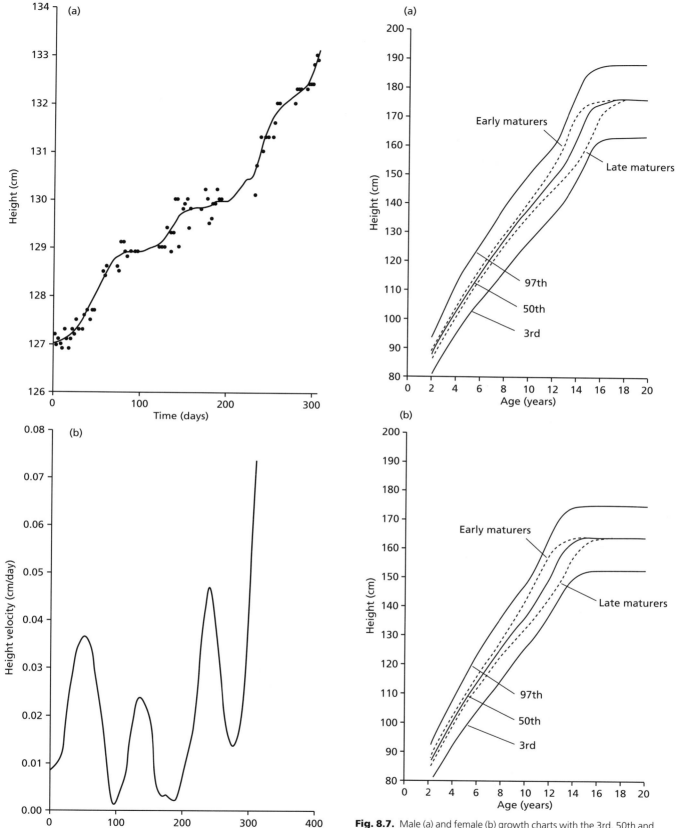

**Fig. 8.6.** (a) Growth curve for a child measured three times a week over 1 year. ●, Original measurements; ———, indicates the line of best fit derived by non-linear regression. (b) Height velocity curve for the same child (from Thalange *et al.* [11]).

**Fig. 8.7.** Male (a) and female (b) growth charts with the 3rd, 50th and 97th centiles for height indicated in solid lines. The dashed lines represent the 10th and 90th centiles for tempo (i.e. 10th, late maturers; 90th, early maturers (from Tanner and Buckler [50]).

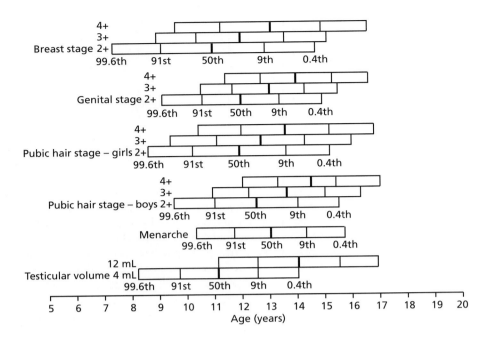

**Fig. 8.8.** Comparison of the timing of stages of puberty in boys and girls (data taken from Child Growth Foundation 1996 growth charts).

approximately 30 kg in weight over puberty (from 12 to 18 years), 82% being accounted for by FFM, whereas girls gain approximately 18.5 kg, only 68% being FFM. However, there are relatively small changes in %BF – 1.7% in boys and 3% in girls [14]. If data on FM and FFM are derived from DEXA scanning, a similar change in FFM is reported over male puberty, but only 50% of weight gained by girls was due to FFM [12]. This illustrates the difficulties in estimating body composition.

## Clinical recognition of normal growth

The ability to quantify growth over time against well-constructed reference standards is the cornerstone of auxological assessment. The variations in normal growth outlined above mean that observation needs to be undertaken over a year (or even longer) in order to define a problem. The tools required for this assessment are relatively simple and include growth charts (for height, weight, sitting height and sub-ischial leg length, body mass index, height velocity and head circumference), standards for pubertal timing (usually included on growth charts), non-dominant wrist radiographs for the assessment of bone age and an orchidometer for the measurement of testicular volume (see Chapter 9).

### Height and weight

Height should be plotted on a growth chart on which the measured heights of the biological parents have been entered [15]. The point at which parental height is plotted is sex dependent: if the index case is male, the father's height and

the mother's height + 5 inches/12.5 cm will be plotted, the reverse for a girl. Midparental height is defined as the midpoint between these (corrected) heights, and the target range is 3.5 inches/8.75 cm either side of this point. If it is considered that a major secular trend in height has occurred between the child's generation and that of the parents, 3 cm can be added to the midparental height. If the child's height falls outside the target range, a growth disorder may be present. There may of course still be an abnormality of growth when the height is within the target range, if the midparental height or one parent's height falls outside the lower centile. In these cases an autosomal dominant growth disorder may be present.

One further way to express height (and any other auxological data), which controls for age and sex, is to derive a standard deviation score (SDS). This requires knowledge of the mean and standard deviation of height at all ages in each sex, and is calculated as:

SDS = (observed height – mean height for age and sex) ÷
standard deviation for that age and sex.

Normal values would be expected to fall between ± 2 SDS in 95% of cases.

Weight is considered an important parameter in the assessment of infant well-being, in the phase of life where nutrition has such an important impact on the growth process. In childhood, weight measurements (ideally taken on calibrated electronic scales) are usually taken coincident with the height. They should be plotted on a chart, and their relation to height can be assessed by calculating the body mass index [defined as weight (kg) ÷ height$^2$ (m$^2$)], which can be plotted on a centile chart [16].

## Growth velocity

A single height measurement plotted in relation to parental heights gives useful information, but does not reflect the dynamic nature of growth. For this, serial height measurements should be taken. Height velocity (cm/year) is then calculated as the amount grown in centimetres divided by the time interval between measurements in years [17]. In order to maintain a position close to a given height centile, velocity should not fall below the twenty-fifth or above the seventy-fifth centile in successive years. Even in experienced hands, the technical error of measurement is of the order of 0.15 cm. If velocity is based on measurements taken at short intervals, such as 3 months, errors in the height will be magnified four times when extrapolating to an annual growth rate. If this is combined with the non-linearity of growth, an accurate perspective of growth is difficult to obtain. It is therefore paramount that growth should be monitored over 12 months. Even then, the cycles of growth through the prepubertal years could lead to a false impression about growth performance. Measurement over longer periods may be required. The probability that growth velocity over 2 successive years will be inadequate becomes increasingly small. The theoretical chance of annual growth velocities in a normal child being below the twenty-fifth centile over 2 years (assuming that the velocity in each year is independent) would be $0.25 \times 0.25 = 6.25\%$ and below the tenth centile would be 1%.

Assessment of growth velocity around puberty is complicated by the degree of physical development and the timing of the pubertal growth spurt. It is this variation that gives rise to the wide peak of height velocity on growth charts (Fig. 8.4) and prevents the calculation of height velocity SD scores.

## Bone age (see Chapter 9)

Bone maturation can be directly observed by visualization of epiphyseal growth plates on radiographs. In normal children there is an orderly development of the epiphyseal centres in growing bones. It has therefore been possible to generate standards for bone maturation in each sex throughout childhood and adolescence [18]. Bone age has evolved as a measure that quantifies physical maturation [19]. Diagnostic information is not obtained from the bone age and assessment may be difficult or impossible in certain circumstances, such as some skeletal dysplasias or in children exposed to long-term immunosuppressive steroid treatment.

## Puberty

There is marked variation in the timing of events within normal puberty (Fig. 8.8) [13]. It is therefore most important to compare an individual's development with population standards in order to define normality but, once puberty is initiated, the sequence of development should be ordered and completed within the appropriate time frame. Failure to progress as well as failure to enter puberty could indicate abnormality. The pubertal growth spurt starts early in puberty in girls but later in boys (Fig. 8.8), but in both sexes the magnitude of the spurt is inversely related to the age at peak height velocity.

## Secular trends

Changes in growth and development (either positive or negative) occur in a population from one generation to the next. For anthropometric measurements, such changes have mostly been positive and have been linked to improvements in nutrition and economic conditions [20]. A secular trend therefore can be considered as a barometer of a nation's health and considerable changes have been documented in many countries over the last 200 years. One dramatic example of this was the increase in height of Japanese boys between 1950 and 1960, which peaked at an increment of 8 cm in height per decade at age 14 years. There is evidence that the secular trend in adult height is diminishing, particularly in Norway and Sweden. Presently rates throughout the world vary from 0.3 cm to 3.0 cm per decade. As there is no apparent secular trend in birth size, increases in stature develop soon after birth and probably within the first 2 years. For Europe and the USA, between 1880 and 1980 stature has altered by 1.5 cm/decade in children, 2.5 cm/decade in adolescence and 1 cm/decade in adulthood.

These trends can be more prominent in certain sections of a population. The secular trend in growth and maturation tends to be more pronounced in those from low socioeconomic groups, those with poorly educated parents and those from rural areas. The effect of this is to raise the lower height centiles and to reduce the variability in the timing of puberty. Over time this can obviously have implications to the clinician whose task is to assess whether a child is showing normal development or not. It is important therefore for growth reference standards to be updated.

## The endocrine control of growth

The principal hormones influencing growth are GH and the IGFs but many other hormones contribute, such as thyroxine, adrenal androgens, sex steroids, glucocorticoids, vitamin D, leptin and insulin, often channelled through interaction with the GH–IGF axis.

## Growth hormone

### Hypothalamic control of GH secretion

GH is secreted from the anterior pituitary into the circulation

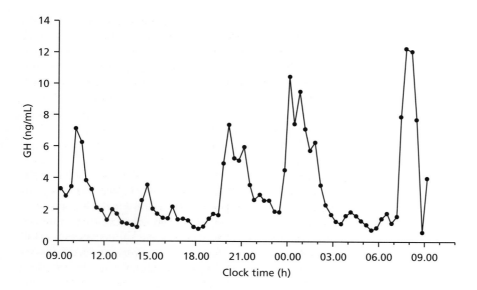

**Fig. 8.9.** Changes in the serum concentration of growth hormone (GH) (ng/mL) over 24 h with samples measured at 20-min intervals.

in discrete pulses every 3–4 h, with very low concentrations of GH present between pulses (Fig. 8.9). This pattern of GH secretion is determined primarily by the interaction between the hypothalamic peptides growth hormone-releasing hormone (GHRH) and somatostatin (SS) [21]. The amplitude of the GH peak is determined by GHRH, which stimulates the pituitary somatotrophs to increase both the secretion of stored GH and GH gene transcription. SS tone determines the trough levels of GH by inhibiting GHRH release from the hypothalamus and GH secretion from the pituitary. Withdrawal of SS is the most important factor in determining the time of a pulse, as GH pulsatility is maintained under constant infusion of GHRH.

A dwarf mouse model [the *little* (*lit/lit*) mouse] illustrates the importance of GHRH in the production of GH secretion. These animals have identifiable pituitary somatotrophs but they contain only 10% of the normal GH content, in addition to having reduced levels of GH mRNA. The somatotrophs of the *little* mouse are resistant to GHRH stimulation, suggesting a problem in GHRH signalling. GHRH binds to a specific cell-surface receptor, which interacts with intracellular G-proteins to stimulate the production of cyclic adenosine monophosphate (cAMP) and transmit an intracellular signal. Sequencing of the GHRH receptor in the *little* mouse demonstrated an inactivating mutation in the extracellular domain of the receptor that prevents GHRH binding [22]. Mutations in the GHRH receptor, which cause severe GH deficiency (GHD) in humans, have now been identified. A nonsense mutation in exon 3, resulting in a premature stop codon, has been found in three small, unrelated kindreds from the Indian subcontinent, and a novel splice-site mutation has been found in a large, consanguineous kindred from Brazil [23].

Studies involving synthetic GH-releasing peptides (GHRPs), such as the hexapeptide GHRP-6, have led to the identifica-

tion of a third pathway that interacts with GHRH and SS to elicit GH release from the pituitary [24]. GHRH and GHRP in combination had a synergistic effect on GH release, indicating that separate receptors for each ligand were likely to be present. This led to the recognition of the GH secretagogue (GHS) pathway. The GHS receptor, like the GHRH receptor, is a G-protein-coupled receptor, which is expressed both in the hypothalamus and in the pituitary. The endogenous ligand for this receptor has been isolated – ghrelin. Ghrelin was isolated in the stomach and is an octynylated peptide that has the properties predicted from the synthetic GHS studies. The classic GHRH–SS model of GH release (Fig. 8.10) will now need to be reworked to include ghrelin [51].

Ghrelin is localized also in the hypothalamus. This suggests that the more important role for these agents is through interactions with GHRH. Administration of GHRP-6 alone to patients with a hypothalamo-pituitary disconnection does not increase GH secretion, and the synergistic elevation of GH is absent when GHRP is given in combination with GHRH. There is also evidence that, in addition to its direct effects on the pituitary, synthetic GHS induce GHRH release from GHRH-secreting neurones but they do not appear to exhibit any inhibition of SS release. Thus, according to the model in Fig. 8.10, GH pulses occur as a result of hypothalamic stimulation of the pituitary by both GHRH and ghrelin, whereas the timing of the GH pulse is determined by SS withdrawal [24].

### Pituitary control of GH secretion

The human GH gene forms part of a cluster of five similar genes found on the long arm of chromosome 17 [21]. Within this gene cluster are two genes for GH isohormones (*GH-N* and *GH-V*), two genes for placental lactogen and a single gene encoding a placental lactogen-like protein. The main

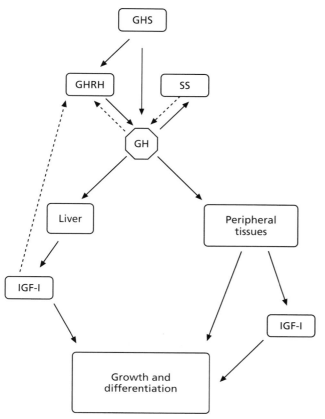

**Fig. 8.10.** Schematic representation of the GH–IGF (growth hormone–insulin-like growth factor) axis. GH is released from the pituitary under the dual regulation of growth hormone-releasing hormone (GHRH) and somatostatin (SS), with additional control coming from the influence of the GH secretagogue (GHS). GH then acts either on the liver or on the peripheral tissues to stimulate the production of IGF-I, which along with GH itself mediates growth and differentiation.

form of GH found in the circulation comes from the *GH-N* (or normal) gene, which is expressed primarily in the pituitary. The full-length transcript from the *GH-N* gene encodes a 191-amino-acid, 22-kDa protein that makes up 85–90% of pituitary GH, whereas alternative splicing of the mRNA transcripts generates a 20-kDa species that lacks amino acids 32–46 and accounts for the remaining 5–15%. Deletion of the *GH-N* gene in humans leads to severe postnatal growth failure. Treatment with GH generates a short-lived growth response due to the development of anti-GH antibodies.

Within the promoter of the *GH-N* gene are binding sites for the homeobox transcription factor Pit1, which determine pituitary-specific expression of GH. Pit1 is also essential for normal pituitary development. It is one of a number of homeodomain gene products required for pituitary organogenesis [25]. The pituitary gland is formed during the second month of development in the human, when Rathke's pouch grows upwards from the roof of the stomadeum and meets the infundibulum growing downwards from the diencephalon. The infundibulum goes on to form the pituitary stalk and posterior pituitary while Rathke's pouch differentiates into the specific cell lineages comprising the anterior pituitary. The homeodomain factors, which are responsible for this, are expressed in a distinct spatial and temporal fashion. Much of the knowledge regarding pattern of expression of these proteins has been gained from mouse studies. Initial organ determination occurs at embryonic day (e) 8.5. This stage is characterized by the expression of three homeodomain genes *Rpx/Hesx1*, *P-OTX* and *P-Lim* within Rathke's pouch in all regions that contain precursors for the five anterior pituitary cell types (somatotrope, lactotrope, thyrotrope, gonadotrope and corticotrope). *Rpx/Hesx1* expression decreases at e14.5 coincident with the emergence of the somatotrope, lactotrope and thyrotrope cell lineages. Although the specific targets of *Rpx/Hesx1* remain unknown, mice lacking this gene exhibit anterior central nervous system (CNS) defects and pituitary dysplasia. In contrast to *Rpx/Hesx1*, expression of *P-OTX* and *P-Lim* persists throughout pituitary development and activates gene transcription of all the pituitary hormones.

*Pit1* is required for the development, proliferation and differentiation of GH-, prolactin- and thyroid-stimulating hormone (TSH)-secreting cells. These lineages, however, are initiated by the appearance at e10.5 of another homeodomain transcription factor *Prophet of Pit1* (*Prop1*, so-called because its expression occurs in advance of *Pit1*). *Prop1* expression is maximal at e12.0, in the regions where *Pit1* is first expressed, and is not found in any other tissue or in the mature pituitary. *Pit1* gene expression begins on e14.5, coincident with the decline in *Prop1*. The Ames and Snell dwarf mice serve as illustrations of the key roles that *Prop1* and *Pit1* play in pituitary development. Both strains of mice are growth retarded and have combined GH, prolactin and TSH deficiencies and hypoplastic pituitaries, indicative of failure of *Pit1* cell lineages. The Ames dwarf mouse has an inactivating mutation in *Prop1*, which prevents activation of *Pit1* gene expression and therefore results in the absence of *Pit1*-dependent cells. In contrast, the Snell mouse has detectable *Pit1* gene expression but has no somatotropes, lactotropes or thyrotropes because of a point mutation in the DNA-binding domain of *Pit1*, which renders it inactive. The determination of the corticotrope, rostral tip thyrotrope and gonadotrope cell lineages occurs early in pituitary development between e8.5 and e11.5, preceding expression of *Pit1* but requiring *Prop1*.

These studies indicate that there are a number of other points in the GH axis upstream of the GH gene itself that may cause postnatal growth failure when inactivated. The human homologue of *Rpx/Hesx1* has been implicated in familial septo-optic dysplasia, a rare condition characterized by optic nerve hypoplasia, absent septum pellucidum and corpus callosum, pituitary hypoplasia and hypopituitarism [26]. In addition, mutations in *Pit1* cause GH, TSH and prolactin deficiencies, whereas defects in *Prop1* have been demonstrated in cases of combined pituitary hormone deficiency [27].

## Other factors influencing GH secretion

There are a considerable number of other factors that influence GH secretion acting directly on the pituitary via stimulation of GHRH, inhibition of SS or a combination of both. These include neuropeptides (e.g. galanin, opioids), metabolites (e.g. glucose, free fatty acids), hormones (e.g. oestrogen, testosterone), physical exercise and sleep [21]. GH itself and its downstream effector, IGF-I, are both capable of regulating secretion via negative feedback mediated by somatostatin. IGF-I probably also acts on the pituitary directly. Central administration of GH in rats fails to suppress endogenous GH secretion in the presence of antisera to SS, whereas cells that contain SS mRNA also express GHR mRNA. *In vitro* studies of rat hypothalamic tissue have demonstrated a dose-dependent increase in SS release in response to IGF-I treatment, whereas administration of recombinant IGF-I to normal men suppresses endogenous GH secretion by up to 85%.

A negative relationship exists between body mass index, a marker of body fatness, and GH secretion in normal prepubertal children as well as in obese children. The fact that GH secretion increases after weight loss or fasting suggests that diminished GH is a result of obesity rather than a cause. However, the signal by which adiposity effects the reduction in GH secretion is not known. Hyperinsulinaemia in obese subjects has been proposed as an alternative mechanism for the reduction in GH secretion. Insulin and IGF-I concentrations in obese children are either normal or elevated, despite the reduction in GH levels. Such subjects exhibit normal or increased growth. The hyperinsulinaemia may stimulate increased IGF-I, which stimulates growth but also suppresses GH secretion by negative feedback.

## GH in the circulation

Growth hormone can be detected in the fetal pituitary from around 8 weeks of gestation and in the serum from 10 weeks, before the complete maturation of the hypothalamo-pituitary axis [28]. Serum levels of GH rise to very high levels, peaking around 24 weeks, then decline through to birth and fall further after the first 2 weeks of postnatal life. The high concentrations of GH throughout gestation are a reflection of the time taken for the neuroendocrine control of GH secretion to develop. In early gestation, GH release from the pituitary is uncontrolled. The decrease in GH after 24 weeks is then associated with the development of the inhibitory mechanisms governing GH release.

Few data exist on the longitudinal changes in GH secretion with age in prepubertal children, but cross-sectional data suggest that GH pulse amplitude increases with age [29]. This has been confirmed by studies using urinary GH measurement as a surrogate for pituitary GH that show a gradual increase in GH through the prepubertal years [30]. The most profound changes in GH secretion occur through the pubertal years with a marked increase in the amplitude of GH pulses [29]. Both androgens and oestrogens increase GH secretion during puberty, although the androgen effect is mediated through the oestrogen receptor by aromatization of testosterone to oestrogen. Maximal levels of GH secretion coincide with the timing of peak height velocity in both sexes and thereafter secretion declines into adulthood.

In prepubertal and pubertal children, episodic GH release from the pituitary generates a serum concentration profile consisting of large peaks of GH, lasting 1–2 h separated by periods of low basal secretion (Fig. 8.9). The pattern of GH secretion is important in generating the diversity of actions mediated by GH. In rodents the sexual dimorphism in GH secretion parallels differences in growth rates [31]. Male rats secrete GH in discrete pulses separated by low trough levels and grow at a faster rate than female rats, who exhibit high basal GH levels and less pulsatility. In addition, pulsatile infusion of GH in GH-deficient rats stimulates growth whereas continuous infusion is associated with its metabolic actions. This sexual dimorphism in GH secretion is also evident in humans [32]. Average daily GH output is greater in women than in men, a difference that disappears when corrected for oestrogen concentrations. There are also differences in the profile of 24-h GH secretion between the sexes: in men there are small pulses in daylight hours with large nocturnal pulses, but in women there is less diurnal variation but more frequent pulses. Furthermore, there are associations between the peak and trough attributes of 24-h GH secretion and different end points of GH action: trough concentrations of GH are correlated with body composition and metabolic parameters, whereas peak concentrations correlate with IGF-I production [33].

The pattern of GH in the circulation is further complicated by the presence of GH-binding proteins (GHBPs) [34]. Two forms have been identified that bind GH with either low or high affinity. The low-affinity GHBP remains uncharacterized but accounts for 10–15% of GH binding in the circulation and may bind 20-kDa GH preferentially. The high-affinity GHBP is a 61-kDa glycosylated protein representing a solubilized form of the extracellular region of the GH receptor (GHR) that binds both the 20-kDa and 22-kDa forms of GH. The physiological significance of GH circulating in a high-molecular-weight complex with GHBP is unclear, but one consequence is an increase in the plasma half-life of GH from ~ 20 min to several hours. Studies *in vivo* of co-administration of GHBP and GH to hypophysectomized and GH-deficient rats have shown that the effects of GH on weight gain and bone growth are potentiated by the presence of GHBP [35]. A similar role in humans has not yet been demonstrated.

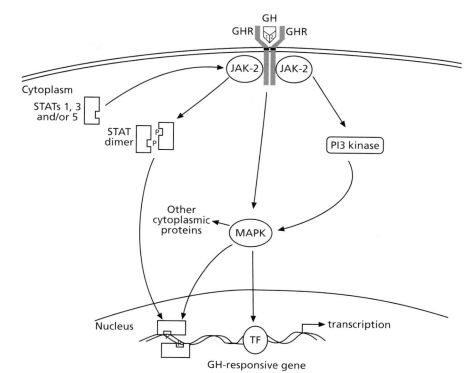

**Fig. 8.11.** Schematic representation of the action of GH at the cellular level. A single molecule of growth hormone (GH) binds to two GH receptors (GHRs) followed by the recruitment and activation of a receptor-associated tyrosine kinase (JAK-2). The GH signal can be transmitted to the nucleus through the STAT (signal transducers and activators of transcription) pathway or via the MAPK (mitogen-activated protein kinase) pathway either directly or via PI3 kinase (phosphatidylinositol-3-kinase) with the net result of activating transcription factors (TFs) that act on GH-responsive genes.

## Cellular actions of GH

GH exerts its effects on target tissues by binding to a specific GHR that is expressed in a variety of tissues, in particular the liver [36]. Figure 8.11 shows a simplified scheme for the transduction of GH signals at the cellular level. A single molecule of GH binds sequentially to two GHRs, the process of dimerization being critical to the activation of intracellular signal transduction. GH contains two different regions, site 1 and site 2, which interact with the extracellular domains of the two GHRs. Binding of GH at site 1 to a single GHR is followed by recruitment of a second GHR that interacts at site 2 to form the GHR–dimer complex. The GHR contains no intrinsic tyrosine kinase activity but upon activation by GH is phosphorylated by a receptor-associated tyrosine kinase, JAK-2, a member of a family of tyrosine kinases, which are involved in signal transduction by cytokine receptors. Activation of JAK-2 by GHR dimerization results in JAK-2 autophosphorylation, GHR phosphorylation and the initiation of phosphorylation cascades. GH signal transduction can proceed through a number of pathways, of which the MAPK (mitogen-activated protein kinase) pathway, the STAT (signal transducers and activators of transcription) pathway and the PI3 kinase (phosphatidylinositol 3-OH-kinase) pathway are the best characterized (see Chapter 1).

The net result of GH signal transduction is the activation of genes involved in mediating the effects of GH. The exact roles of the individual signalling pathways used by GH are not known, but there is some evidence that different pathways may be activated in different cell types or alternatively may be used differentially according to the diversity of GH actions. An example of this is the activation of early response genes encoding transcription factors involved in cell growth and differentiation, such as c-*jun* and c-*fos*. Activation of c-*fos* in the 3T3-F442A adipocyte cell line induces expression of a number of genes involved in adipocyte differentiation, whereas activation of c-*myc* stimulates cell proliferation [36]. An important target of GH is the IGF-I gene, whose product mediates many, if not all, of its growth-promoting actions *in vivo*.

Abnormalities in the GHR and its signal transduction pathway cause GH insensitivity (GHI) and postnatal growth failure. GHI is a heterogeneous disorder, characterized by high circulating levels of GH, low serum IGF-I and IGFBP-3 concentrations and normal, low or even high levels of GHBP. The majority of individuals with GHI have mutations in the GHR that prevent GH signal transduction. However, in some cases of GHBP-positive GHI, where no receptor abnormalities can be found, postreceptor defects have been postulated. The elevated concentration of circulating GH in this disorder is a consequence of the failure of negative feedback by GH on its own secretion, and IGF-I and IGFBP-3 are low because of the inability of GH to stimulate their production [37].

## Insulin-like growth factors and their binding proteins

IGF-I and IGF-II are single-chain polypeptide hormones with structural homology to proinsulin and are expressed in multiple organs and tissues under both endocrine and tissue-specific autocrine and/or paracrine regulation. Both are important in fetal growth and development but only IGF-I appears to be critical for postnatal growth. This may be because IGF-II does not appear to be regulated by GH, which is the primary determinant of circulating IGF-I concentrations in postnatal life. IGFs in the circulation bind to the IGFBPs, a family of distinct but structurally homologous proteins that share the ability to bind both IGFs with high affinity. The IGFs are present in the circulation at concentrations approximately 1000 times that of insulin, and one major role of the IGFBPs is to prevent the potential insulin-like activity of IGFs [38]. Nearly all IGF in the circulation will be associated with a binding protein. The IGFBPs extend the half-life of the IGFs within the vascular space, thus creating a circulating reservoir of IGF activity, and provide a transport mechanism regulating movement of IGFs across the capillary walls. They also play a role in controlling IGF distribution to specific cell types or receptor subtypes, thus modulating the paracrine effects of IGFs.

### IGF-I gene expression

IGF-I gene expression is complex with cell-type and regional differences in expression. The IGF-I gene is composed of six exons that undergo alternative splicing to generate four different mRNA transcripts, each containing four of the six exons (Fig. 8.12). Exons 1 and 2 each contain distinct promoter regions and 5′ non-coding sequences. They each

encode a portion of the signal peptide. The terminal region of the signal peptide and the sequence for the mature IGF-I peptide are found in exons 3 and 4. The latter also codes for the proximal part of the C-terminal E-domain peptides, which are cleaved during prohormone processing into Ea and Eb peptides. Exon 5 encodes the remainder of the Eb peptide and exon 6 the Ea peptide. Both exons also contain a 3′ untranslated region and polyadenylation sites. mRNA transcripts containing exons 1, 3, 4 and 6 are termed IGF 1A and exons 1, 3, 4 and 5 are termed IGF 1B (class 1 transcripts). Similarly transcripts containing exons 2, 3, 4 and 6 are termed IGF 1A′ and exons 2, 3, 4 and 5 IGF 1B′ (class 2 transcripts). Class 2 transcripts show greater GH dependency than class 1. Additional diversity in the mRNA transcripts is generated from heterogeneous transcription initiation sites in each promoter, differential polyadenylation and variable mRNA stability. The physiological significance of this differential expression of IGF-I mRNA transcripts, particularly as they all encode an identical mature protein, remains to be determined although there is some evidence that it may target IGF-I to an endocrine vs. paracrine and/or autocrine role [39].

### Cellular actions of IGFs

Two distinct receptors for the IGFs have been identified: the type I or IGF-I receptor, which is homologous to the insulin receptor, and the type II or IGF-II receptor, also known as the mannose-6-phosphate receptor [38]. The mitogenic actions of IGF-I and IGF-II are mediated almost entirely through the IGF-I receptor using a signal transduction cascade similar to that used by insulin. In contrast with IGF-I, little is known about the interactions and consequences of IGF-II binding to its receptor, the mannose-6-phosphate receptor. This receptor is so-called because of its ability to bind to mannose-

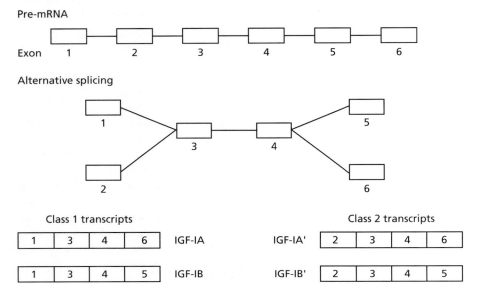

**Fig. 8.12.** IGF-I gene expression. The IGF-I gene is composed of six exons that undergo alternative splicing to generate two classes of IGF-I mRNA transcripts. Exons 1 and 2 encode the signal peptides and exons 3 and 4 code for the mature peptide. Exons 5 and 6 contain the sequence for different carboxy-terminal peptide extensions which are cleaved during prohormone processing.

6-phosphate groups on glycoproteins. On the cell surface the receptor binds extracellular glycoproteins before endocytosis and is also found in the Golgi apparatus in the cytoplasm, where it functions to translocate lysosomal enzymes to the endosomes. One postulated role for the receptor is to internalize IGF-II for degradation within the lysosomes, as IGF-II binding is enhanced when mannose-6-phosphate is associated with the receptor. Furthermore, IGF-II does not appear to mediate any of its biological effects through this receptor, acting instead through the IGF-I receptor.

### Insulin-like growth factor binding proteins

The common feature of the IGFBPs, as mentioned above, is their ability to bind IGFs with high affinity, which in general terms is of similar magnitude as the affinity of the type I and II IGF receptors for IGFs [38]. IGFBP-1 and -2 contain an RGD (Arg–Gly–Asp) amino acid motif that is involved in binding to the extracellular matrix, in particular to integrins, and may provide a mechanism by which IGFBPs mediate capillary transport of IGFs. Similarly IGFBP-3 and -4 can also bind to the cell surface but through glycosaminoglycan binding sites. An important feature of IGFBPs is that the binding affinity of IGF-I and IGF-II for a given IGFBP may differ: IGFBP-1, -3 and -4 bind both IGF-I and IGF-II with equal affinity whereas IGFBP-2, -5 and -6 have higher affinity for IGF-II.

IGFBP-3 is the major IGFBP in the circulation accounting for most of the IGF-I binding capacity and, like IGF-I, is strongly GH dependent. The main site of IGFBP-3 production is in the liver under GH control, although it is also expressed in most peripheral tissues. When bound to IGF-I, IGFBP-3 associates with another GH-dependent protein, the acid labile subunit (ALS), to form a ternary complex of 150 kDa molecular weight. In general, the molar concentration of IGFBP-3 in the circulation is equal to the sum of both IGF-I and IGF-II, reflecting the role of IGFBP-3 as the major carrier of IGF. ALS is present in a molar excess, indicating that virtually all IGFBP-3 and IGF exist in the form of the ternary complex.

IGFBP-1 is the only IGFBP whose serum concentrations are not stable during the day, owing to its acute regulation by insulin. It is for this reason that IGFBP-1 is implicated in the maintenance of glucose homeostasis by inhibiting the insulin-like effects of IGFs. IGFBP-2 is the second most abundant IGFBP in the serum, where it binds IGF-II preferentially. Little is known about the physiological role of IGFBP-2 in humans. IGFBP-4 is the major IGFBP produced by bone cells and has been detected in the medium of cultured osteoblasts and fibroblasts. The major role of IGFBP-4 is thought to be regulation of bone formation and resorption, where it inhibits IGF-induced bone formation. IGFBP-5 is the major binding protein stored in bone and, in contrast to IGFBP-4, potentiates IGF-induced bone cell proliferation. Finally IGFBP-6 is found in serum and cerebrospinal fluid and binds IGF-II preferentially.

## Control of growth

### Physiological actions of GH and IGF-I on bone growth

The major role of GH during growth and development is to promote longitudinal bone growth. Two hypotheses have been generated to explain the mode of action of GH in generating a growth response. The somatomedin hypothesis proposes that GH mediates its effects on its target tissues via stimulation of hepatic IGF-I production, which in turn acts as a classic endocrine hormone (Fig. 8.13a). The alternative hypothesis, the dual effector theory, is based on the premise that growth is a result of the differentiation of precursor cells followed by clonal expansion. According to this hypothesis, GH directly promotes the differentiation of cells and the development of IGF-I responsiveness. Clonal expansion of these differentiated cells is then mediated by local production of IGF-I in response to GH (Fig. 8.13b) [40]. Although there

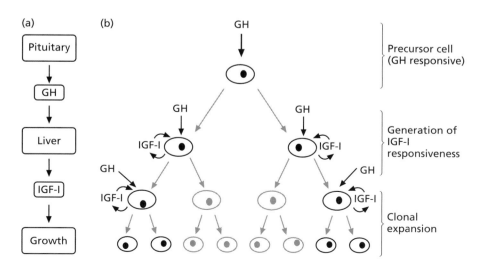

**Fig. 8.13.** The somatomedin hypothesis (a) and dual-effector theory (b) of growth hormone (GH) action. IGF-I, insulin-like growth factor I.

remains a great deal of debate about which of these hypotheses holds true *in vivo*, it is clear that both GH and IGF-I have independent and overlapping effects on bone growth.

The epiphyseal growth plate consists of prechondrocyte germinal cells that differentiate into a layer of proliferating chondrocytes and then undergo hypertrophy and ossification. Evidence against the somatomedin hypothesis came from studies in which GH was injected directly into rat tibial growth plate and was found to stimulate bone growth at the site of entry. Subsequent studies suggested that GH and IGF-I act on cells at different stages of maturation, with GH acting on progenitor cells and IGF-I on stimulated cells at later stages of development. These observations formed the basis of the dual effector theory of GH action, which has been found to hold true in other sites such as adipose tissue. Further evidence for this direct effect of GH on bone growth came from *in vivo* binding studies, which demonstrated that GH bound only at the germinal cell layer and not the proliferative or hypertrophic layers. In addition, when IGF-I was locally administered to bone in hypophysectomized rats there was only modest growth compared with the effect of GH. This was thought to be because the mitogenic effects of IGF-I can only be directed at differentiated cells in the proliferative layer, IGF-I being unable to recruit progenitor cells from the germinal layer. In addition, selective knockout of IGF-I in the liver does not alter growth of the animal (see below).

Comparison of the growth-promoting effects of systemic administration of GH and IGF-I in hypophysectomized rats has shown that both agents increase body weight, longitudinal bone growth, cell proliferation and cell productivity. However, GH was always more effective than IGF-I. The difference in efficacy of these two agents on whole-body growth is thought to be due to their respective effects on the generation of IGFBPs. Treatment with GH causes an elevation of the 150-kDa ternary complex containing ALS, IGFBP-3 and IGF-I, whereas IGF-I administration is accompanied by a rise only in the 50-kDa complex containing IGF-I and IGFBP-3. The 150-kDa complex is more stable in the circulation and thus the reservoir of IGF in the circulation can be maintained over a longer period of time. Furthermore, GH may stimulate local production of IGF-I, which can act in an autocrine and/or paracrine manner, whereas the mitogenic effects of administration of IGF-I rely upon its translocation to the tissues. Optimal growth relies upon adequate GH secretion, a stable circulating pool of IGF-I in addition to paracrine and/or autocrine actions of IGF-I and GH in peripheral tissues [40].

### Fetus and infant

Fetal growth is generally considered to be GH independent and primarily determined by nutrition, IGFs and other growth factors. According to the ICP model, GH-dependent growth does not begin until the transition from infant growth to the childhood phase towards the end of the first year of life [2]. However, there is some evidence that GH may play a role in fetal development. GHRs that are capable of binding GH are detectable in many tissues from 15 weeks of gestation, and circulating GH levels are high during midgestation [28]. A reduction in birth size has been observed in infants with congenital GHD, accompanied by progressive growth failure in the first year of life. However, the relatively normal birth size of subjects with less severe GHD has been proposed to be a result of a compensatory stimulation of GHRs by GH variants such as placental lactogen or prolactin. To date, it remains unclear exactly what role GH plays in fetal growth and development.

Concentrations of the IGFs and IGFBPs in fetal cord sera at birth have been found to reflect infant size. Thus, IGF-I, IGF-II and IGFBP-3 were significantly reduced and IGFBP-1 significantly elevated in intrauterine growth-restricted babies compared with those of average size for gestational age (AGA). In babies born large for gestational age, IGF-I, insulin and IGFBP-3 were increased and IGFBP-1 reduced compared with AGA babies. In addition, at birth IGF-I levels are higher in term than in preterm infants [41]. All these observations point to a role for the IGF axis in the growth and development of the human fetus.

The recent discovery of a patient with a homozygous partial IGF-I gene deletion has provided further insights into the role of IGF-I in human development. In this child exons 4 and 5 of the IGF-I gene were absent, generating an IGF-I transcript containing exon 3 spliced directly onto exon 6, which if translated would be expected to generate a peptide of 25 amino acids from exon 3 with a nonsense addition of eight residues. The features of this child included severe intrauterine growth restriction, which persisted after birth, as well as mirocephaly and sensorineural deafness, indicating a role for IGF-I in CNS development. IGF-I levels were undetectable by radioimmunoassay while GH levels were high, supporting the role of IGF-I in regulating GH secretion by negative feedback [42].

### Childhood

The primary determinant of growth during childhood is GH. Although it is clear that GH administration to GH-deficient children promotes growth, the way in which GH mediates growth in normal children is less clear. The main approach to this question has been to examine changes in components of the GH–IGF axis in cross-sectional studies of both normal and short children and relate this to stature and growth. GH secretion itself increases through the mid-childhood years, mainly due to increases in GH pulse amplitude with no change in pulse frequency [29]. Furthermore, the sum of GH pulse amplitudes over a 24-h period does correlate with growth rate but in an asymptotic manner (Fig. 8.14) [43]. Low GH secretion is associated with poor growth as expected, but a wide range of GH secretion can occur in children growing

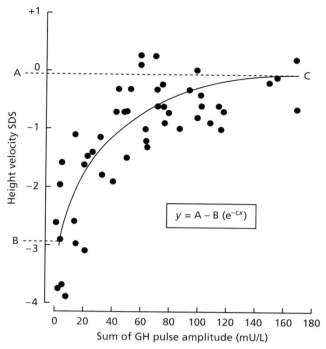

**Fig. 8.14.** Relationship between GH secretion and growth velocity expressed as a standard deviation score (SDS) (from Hindmarsh *et al.* [43] ).

at a normal rate. This means that once an adequate level of GH secretion has been attained additional factors must be responsible for variation in growth rates between individuals. One such factor may be individual differences in GH sensitivity, i.e. the degree to which IGF-I and other GH-dependent peptides are elevated in response to GH. During the prepubertal years IGF-I and IGFBP-3 increase with age and are positively related to GH secretion. Both IGF-I and IGFBP-3 are positively correlated with height standard deviation score, and serum IGF-I levels correlate with height velocity in the following year [44]. However, for any given level of GH secretion there is considerable interindividual variation in IGF-I levels that may be generated by differences in GH pulsatility. It has been suggested that circulating IGF-I concentrations correlate better with peak than with basal GH levels, and thus the manner in which GH is presented to responsive tissues may be of critical importance to the growth process.

## Puberty

The most marked changes in growth in childhood occur after the onset of puberty and are accompanied by corresponding changes in the GH–IGF axis. Growth in puberty is determined by both GH and sex steroids, with each contributing ~ 50% to the gain in height. The sex difference in attainment of peak height velocity is mirrored by the times at which maximal GH secretion occurs. In addition to augmentation of GH

release, oestrogen is important for skeletal maturation and fusion of the epiphyses. This has been exemplified by the description of an adult male with a deleterious mutation in the oestrogen receptor. In this subject, statural growth had continued into adulthood because of incomplete epiphyseal closure associated with decreased bone mineralization [45].

Serum concentrations of IGF-I and IGFBP-3 also exhibit alterations during puberty. IGF-I concentrations increase markedly through puberty, reaching peak values approximately 1 year later in boys than in girls and at least 2 years later than average peak height velocity. IGFBP-3 levels increase modestly during puberty, peaking earlier in girls than in boys and declining thereafter. However, IGF-I levels increase to a greater extent than IGFBP-3, leading to an increased level of 'free' or non-complexed IGF-I. This may have enhanced biological activity [44].

## Insights from transgenic and gene-targeted animal models

The most compelling evidence for the roles of the IGFs and their receptors in normal fetal development has been gained through a series of elegant genetic studies in mice using gene-targeting and transgenic technology (Table 8.3) [38,46]. These studies began in the early 1980s with the transgenic approach, in which specific genes coupled to a promoter construct were introduced into germline cells, leading to animals that overexpress the gene of interest. The first example was a mouse model in which the human GH gene was coupled to the mouse metallothionein-I promoter, leading to increased levels of circulating GH. These animals were of normal birthweight but increased postnatal growth became evident from approximately 3 weeks of age, the time at which IGF-I levels began to increase. By adulthood the transgenic mice were twice the weight of their wild-type littermates but also exhibited signs of organomegaly.

In parallel, a mouse model of GHD was generated whereby circulating GH was ablated by coupling the rat GH gene to diphtheria toxin. In agreement with the overexpression studies, growth failure was not evident until 3 weeks postnatally and adult mice were only 60% of normal wild-type littermates. These studies provided support for the somatomedin hypothesis in that the growth-promoting effects of GH were only manifest at the time when IGF-I came under the control of GH. Increased postnatal growth was also demonstrated in IGF-I transgenic animals, although growth was not as dramatically increased as in the GH model. Circulating concentrations of IGF-I were only elevated 1.5-fold. Crossing of GH(–) with IGF-I(+) mice provided a clear demonstration that IGF-I overexpression can mediate long bone growth in the absence of GH, as these double transgenic mice were identical in size to their normal littermates. An additional feature of this strain, however, was the presence of increased brain size, indicating IGF-I-specific effects on organ growth.

The above experiments demonstrated the role of GH and IGF-I in postnatal growth, but targeted disruption of the IGF system has provided insights into fetal growth. To date, the prevailing dogma has been that IGF-I was involved in post-natal growth and IGF-II was responsible for growth *in utero*. Accordingly, mice deficient in the IGF-II gene were found to be 60% of the size of wild-type littermates at birth with no effect on postnatal growth, such that the size ratio between the IGF-II-deficient and wild-type mice remained identical. However, mice with an IGF-I gene knockout exhibited a sim-ilar prenatal growth deficit to IGF-II(–) mice, and further-more only 5% of animals survived after birth. Those mice which survived suffered postnatal growth restriction leading to animals 30% the size of normal littermates.

More recently, using a tissue-specific method of gene targeting, animals have been engineered that are unable to produce IGF-I in the liver but maintain peripheral tissue gene expression [47]. Hepatic IGF-I is the main source of cir-culating IGF-I concentrations and is thought to constitute 'endocrine' IGF-I. Thus the somatomedin hypothesis would predict that these animals would show an identical pheno-type to the complete knockouts. However, fetal and postnatal growth is not different from wild-type littermates, implying that, in the absence of endocrine IGF-I, paracrine and/or autocrine production of IGF-I in the peripheral tissues can generate normal growth and development.

When the type I IGF receptor was targeted for knockout, fetal growth restriction was more severe than in either the IGF-I or the IGF-II single deletants, with birthweight being 45% of the wild type, indicating some functional redundancy between the IGFs. None of these mice was viable. It is well recognized that both IGF-I and IGF-II mediate their actions through the type I receptor, but the increased severity of growth restriction in the receptor knockout suggested that IGF-I can compensate to some degree for the absence of IGF-II and vice versa. After the studies of single gene knockouts came the engineering of combinatorial knockouts in which single knockout lines were crossed to give double knockouts. Animals lacking both IGF-I and IGF-II were not viable post-natally, with affected animals 30% of normal size at birth. A combined IGF-I and type I receptor mutant generated an identical phenotype to that of the type I receptor knockout alone, indicating that all IGF-I actions are mediated through the type I receptor. In contrast, deletion of IGF-II and the type I receptor together resulted in the same phenotype as the IGF-I/IGF-II knockout with birthweights of affected animals 30% of the wild type. These findings further complicate this area by implying the presence of an as yet unidentified receptor through which IGF-II mediates at least some of its growth-promoting actions.

The type II IGF/mannose-6-phosphate receptor can be excluded from this role, as mice in whom this receptor is inactivated exhibit overgrowth *in utero* and postnatal death, with birthweights 135% of the wild type. These mice have phenotypic features of Beckwith–Wiedemann syndrome, a human condition with disproportionate organ overgrowth. Overexpression of IGF-II in transgenic models also leads to overgrowth and postnatal death. It is of note that both the IGF-II receptor and IGF-II undergo genomic imprinting: the type II receptor is only expressed from the maternal gene and promotes small infant size, whereas IGF-II is expressed from the paternal allele and leads to increased infant size. This is thought to be an evolutionary strategy in which the opposing functions of the two genes are balanced.

## Integration of endocrine signals into whole-body growth

Human growth occurs on average over 16 years in girls and 18 years in boys, and during that time is a non-linear process with week-to-week, seasonal and year-to-year variation. Most studies of GH–IGF hormone output have been under-taken in subjects that have a growth disorder on 1 day of that child's growing life, then related to a short period of their current growth. In these circumstances relationships between growth rate, stature and hormone output have been found. It has been less easy to relate growth rate and GH output in normal children. In those studies that have collected longi-tudinal measurements of the GH–IGF axis, it has become clear that there is considerable variation in hormone levels from day to day, week to week and month to month – coefficients of variation for serum IGF-I 40%, for urinary GH and urinary IGF-I 55% and 37% respectively. In fact, in nor-mal children, significant rhythms in urinary GH excretion, used as a surrogate of integrated serum GH concentrations, have been identified over these intervals [48]. These data suggest that, just as the pulsatile pattern of serum GH within 24 h affects the actions of GH, so the pattern in which GH is released over time is likely to be an important factor in generating normal growth.

## Conclusion

An understanding of the normal mechanisms of growth is essential to the recognition of a disorder. A period of observa-tion, often over a year or more, may be required to ensure that abnormal growth is distinguished from normality. If dis-ordered growth is present, then an explanation should be sought by considering whether an abnormality in any of the factors listed in Table 8.1 is present. Investigation of hormone output and action may be required. The GH–IGF axis is particularly important to assess, so that GHD, a readily treat-able condition, can be identified. However, it is important to appreciate that the dynamic relationship between GH and IGF-I is not straightforward and hence the diagnosis of an abnormality must be undertaken with great care.

Molecular biology is helping the understanding of the

genes and genetic events that underlie normal and disordered human growth. New growth disorders are being recognized (e.g. IGF-I gene deletion), and the aetiology of well-characterized disease (e.g. congenital hypopituitarism) is being defined. Modification of gene expression by stem cell or targeted knockout continues to be a useful approach to understanding the precise role of GH, the IGFs and their receptors in growth.

Knowledge of precisely how the actions of growth hormones are translated into non-linear growth remains poor. More complete knowledge here may help devise strategies to treat more growth-disordered children more effectively.

## References

1 Karlberg J, Fryer JG, Engstrom I, Karlberg P. Analysis of linear growth using a mathematical model. II. From 3 to 21 years of age. *Acta Paediatr Scand* (Suppl.) 1987; 337: 12–29.

2 Karlberg J, Engstrom I, Karlberg P, Fryer JG. Analysis of linear growth using a mathematical model. I. From birth to three years. *Acta Paediatr Scand* 1987; 76: 478–88.

3 Mark M, Rijli FM, Chambon P. Homeobox genes in embryogenesis and pathogenesis. *Pediatr Res* 1997; 42: 421–9.

4 de Pablo F, Scott LA, Roth J. Insulin and insulin-like growth factor I in early development: peptides, receptors and biological events. *Endocrinol Rev* 1990; 11: 558–77.

5 Gluckman PD. Clinical review 68: the endocrine regulation of fetal growth in late gestation: the role of insulin-like growth factors. *J Clin Endocrinol Metab* 1995; 80: 1047–50.

6 Barker DJP. *Mother, Babies and Disease in Later Life*. London: BMJ Publishing, 1994.

7 Tanner JM. *Foetus into Man: Physical Growth from Conception to Maturity*, 2nd edn. Cambridge, MA: Harvard University Press, 1978.

8 Hermanussen M. The analysis of short-term growth. *Horm Res* 1998; 49: 53–64.

9 Lampl M, Veldhuis JD, Johnson ML. Saltation and stasis: a model of human growth. *Science* 1992; 258: 801–3.

10 Butler GE, McKie M, Ratcliffe SG. The cyclical nature of prepubertal growth. *Ann Hum Biol* 1990; 17: 177–98.

11 Thalange NK, Foster PJ, Gill MS, Price DA, Clayton PE. Model of normal pre-pubertal growth. *Arch Dis Child* 1996; 75: 427–31.

12 Rico H, Revilla M, Villa LF, Hernandez ER, Alvarez-de BM, Villa M. Body composition in children and Tanner's stages: a study with dual-energy x-ray absorptiometry. *Metabolism* 1993; 42: 967–70.

13 Tanner JM, Whitehouse RH. Clinical longitudinal standards for height, weight, height velocity, weight velocity, and stages of puberty. *Arch Dis Child* 1976; 51: 170–9.

14 Buckler JMH. *A Reference Manual of Growth and Development* Oxford: Blackwell Scientific Publications, 1979.

15 Freeman JV, Cole TJ, Chinn S, Jones PR, White EM, Preece MA. Cross sectional stature and weight reference curves for the UK, 1990. *Arch Dis Child* 1995; 73: 17–24.

16 Cole TJ, Freeman JV, Preece MA. Body mass index reference curves for the UK, 1990. *Arch Dis Child* 1995; 73: 25–9.

17 Tanner JM, Whitehouse RH, Takaishi M. Standards from birth to maturity for height, weight, height velocity, and weight velocity: British children, 1965. *Arch Dis Child* 1966; 41: 454–71.

18 Greulich WW, Pyle ST. *Radiographic Atlas of Skeletal Development of Hand and Wrist*. Stanford, CA: Stanford University Press, 1959.

19 Bayley N, Pinneau SR. Tables predicting adult height from skeletal age revised for use with the Greulich-Pyle hand standards. *J Pediatr* 1952; 40: 423–41.

20 Hauspie RC, Vercauteren M, Susanne C. Secular changes in growth and maturation: an update. *Acta Paediatr Suppl* 1997; 423: 20–7.

21 Strobl JS, Thomas MJ. Human growth hormone. *Pharmacol Rev* 1994; 46: 1–34.

22 Lin SC, Lin CR, Gukovsky I, Lusis AJ, Sawchenko PE, Rosenfeld MG. Molecular basis of the little mouse phenotype and implications for cell type-specific growth. *Nature* 1993; 364: 208–13.

23 Salvatori R, Hayashida CY, Aguiar-Oliveira MH *et al.* Familial dwarfism due to a novel mutation of the growth hormone-releasing hormone receptor gene. *J Clin Endocrinol Metab* 1999; 84: 917–23.

24 Smith RG, Vander PL, Howard AD *et al.* Peptidomimetic regulation of growth hormone secretion. *Endocrinol Rev* 1997; 18: 621–45.

25 Parks JS, Adess ME, Brown MR. Genes regulating hypothalamic and pituitary development. *Acta Paediatr Suppl* 1997; 423: 28–32.

26 Dattani MT, Martinez BJ, Thomas PQ *et al.* Mutations in the homeobox gene HESX1/Hesx1 associated with septo-optic dysplasia in human and mouse. *Nature Genet* 1998; 19: 125–33.

27 Rotwein P. Human growth disorders: molecular genetics of the growth hormone-insulin-like growth factor I axis. *Acta Paediatr Scand* 1999; 88: 148–51.

28 Gluckman PD, Grumbach MM, Kaplan SL. The neuroendocrine regulation and function of growth hormone and prolactin in the mammalian fetus. *Endocrinol Rev* 1981; 2: 363–95.

29 Hindmarsh PC, Matthews DR, Brook CG. Growth hormone secretion in children determined by time series analysis. *Clin Endocrinol* 1988; 29: 35–44.

30 Skinner AM, Price DA, Addison GM, Clayton PE, Mackay RI, Soo A, Mui CY. The influence of age, size, pubertal status and renal factors on urinary growth hormone excretion in normal children and adolescents. *Growth Reg* 1992; 2: 156–60.

31 Gevers EF, Wit JM, Robinson IC. Growth, growth hormone (GH)-binding protein, and GHRs are differentially regulated by peak and trough components of the GH secretory pattern in the rat. *Endocrinology* 1996; 137: 1013–18.

32 Jaffe CA, Ocampo LB, Guo W *et al.* Regulatory mechanisms of growth hormone secretion are sexually dimorphic. *J Clin Invest* 1998; 102: 153–64.

33 Hindmarsh PC, Fall CH, Pringle PJ, Osmond C, Brook CG. Peak and trough growth hormone concentrations have different associations with the insulin-like growth factor axis, body composition, and metabolic parameters. *J Clin Endocrinol Metab* 1997; 82: 2172–6.

34 Baumann G. Growth hormone heterogeneity: genes, isohormones, variants, and binding proteins. *Endocrinol Rev* 1991; 12: 424–49.

35 Clark RG, Mortensen DL, Carlsson LM *et al.* Recombinant human growth hormone (GH)-binding protein enhances the growth-promoting activity of human GH in the rat. *Endocrinology* 1996; 137: 4308–15.

36 Carter SC, Schwartz J, Smit LS. Molecular mechanism of growth hormone action. *Annu Rev Physiol* 1996; 58: 187–207.

37 Clayton PE, Freeth JS, Whatmore AJ, Ayling RM, Norman MR, Silva CM. Signal transduction defects in growth hormone insensitivity. *Acta Paediatr Suppl* 1999; 88: 174–8.

38 Jones JI, Clemmons DR. Insulin-like growth factors and their binding proteins: biological actions. *Endocr Rev* 1995; 16: 3–34.

39 Phillips LS, Pao CI, Villafuerte BC. Molecular regulation of insulin-like growth factor-I and its principal binding protein, IGFBP-3. *Prog Nucleic Acid Res Mol Biol* 1998; 60: 195–265.

40 Ohlsson C, Bengtsson BA, Isaksson OG, Andreassen TT, Slootweg MC. Growth hormone and bone. *Endocrinol Rev* 1998; 19: 55–79.

41 Giudice LCZF, Gargosky SE, Dsupin BA *et al.* Insulin-like growth factors and their binding proteins in the term and preterm human fetus and neonate with normal and extremes of intrauterine growth. *J Clin Endocrinol Metab* 1995; 80: 1548–55.

42 Woods KA, Camacho HC, Savage MO, Clark AJ. Intrauterine growth retardation and postnatal growth failure associated with deletion of the insulin-like growth factor I gene. *N Engl J Med* 1996; 335: 1363–7.

43 Hindmarsh P, Smith PJ, Brook CG, Matthews DR. The relationship between height velocity and growth hormone secretion in short pre-pubertal children. *Clin Endocrinol* 1987; 27: 581–91.

44 Juul A, Dalgaard P, Blum WF *et al.* Serum levels of insulin-like growth factor (IGF)-binding protein-3 (IGFBP-3) in healthy infants, children, and adolescents: the relation to IGF-I, IGF-II, IGFBP-1, IGFBP-2, age, sex, body mass index, and pubertal maturation. *J Clin Endocrinol Metab* 1995; 80: 2534–42.

45 Smith EP, Boyd J, Frank GR *et al.* Estrogen resistance caused by a mutation in the estrogen-receptor gene in a man. *N Engl J Med* 1994; 331: 1056–61.

46 Wood TL. Gene-targeting and transgenic approaches to IGF and IGF binding protein function. *Am J Physiol* 1995; 269: E613–E622.

47 Yakar S, Liu J-L, Stannard B *et al.* Normal growth and development in the absence of hepatic insulin-like growth factor I. *Proc Natl Acad Sci USA* 1999; 96: 7324–9.

48 Thalange NK, Gill MS, Gill L *et al.* Infradian rhythms in urinary growth hormone excretion. *J Clin Endocrinol Metab* 1996; 81: 100–6.

49 Arey LB. *Developmental Anatomy*, 7th edn. Philadelphia: W.B. Saunders, 1966.

50 Tanner JM, Buckler JM. Revision and update of Tanner–Whitehouse clinical longitudinal charts for height and weight. *Eur J Pediatr* 1997; 156: 248–9.

51 Kojima N, Hosoda K, Date Y *et al.* Ghrelin is a growth hormone-releasing acetylated peptide from stomach. *Nature* 1999; 402: 656–60.

# 9 Growth assessment
## Purpose and interpretation

**C. G. D. Brook and P. C. Hindmarsh**

## Introduction

Measurement is the basis of growth assessment and growth assessment is the basis of the practice of clinical paediatric endocrinology. Measurements made accurately and precisely and interpreted correctly are more specific and more sensitive than analyses of single hormone concentrations in children. This is especially true of hormones that are secreted in a pulsatile fashion or with circadian or longer rhythms.

Anthropometric measurements are not difficult to perform. They do, however, like all measurements, require attention to detail in order to minimize error, and they should be treated in exactly the same way as making measurements in a laboratory. These should be presented as coefficients of variation in terms both of repeated measurements of characteristics of a subject on the same day and of a measure of reproducibility on subsequent visits. Generally speaking, where clinical decisions are to be made on such measurements then coefficients of variation for anthropometric measurements of less than 0.1% are required. As will become clear, even this stringent criterion leaves plenty of room for error.

The reason for this stress on precision is because single measurements of growth are very much less helpful than repeated ones over a period of time. Since the errors of measurement are cumulative on each occasion, measurements carried out by different people using different techniques on different occasions lead to considerable difficulties in accurately assessing rates of growth. For this reason, many of the measurements regularly made in paediatric clinics are of little use in growth assessment beyond gaining an overall impression, whereas attention to detail would render them an invaluable record of child health, and point to whether or not a diagnosis of a growth disorder is required. Table 9.1 shows a matrix for the measurements of stature and shows how easy it is to build up cumulative errors especially when measurements are made over short periods of time.

The issue of accuracy relates to how well the measuring device measures what it says it does. In other words, a fixed

**Table 9.1.** Effect of coefficients of variation (SD/mean × 100) of a measurer on likely errors in measurement

| Height (cm) | Potential error in measurement (mm) | | |
| --- | --- | --- | --- |
| | **CV = 0.2%** | **CV = 0.1%** | **CV = 0.05%** |
| 80 | 3.2 | 1.6 | 0.8 |
| 100 | 4.0 | 2.0 | 1.0 |
| 120 | 4.8 | 2.4 | 1.2 |
| 140 | 5.6 | 2.8 | 1.4 |
| 160 | 6.4 | 3.2 | 1.6 |

length should be the same no matter how or when it is measured. Calibration of instruments essentially deals with this problem. The final component of measurement error is dependability. In a sense this relates to precision and is separated to remind everyone that differences in height can result from non-endocrine/nutrition factors, such as the change in height during the day as a result of spinal column compression due to standing against gravity.

## Quality control measures

Additional measures can be used to describe errors in measurement. The technical error of measurement (TEM) is obtained by carrying out a number of repeat measurements on the same subject either by the same observer or by two or more observers. Differences can then be entered into the following equation:

$$\text{TEM} = \sqrt{(\Sigma D^2)/2N}$$

where $D$ is the difference between measurements and $N$ is the number of individuals measured. The units are the same as the units of measurement.

Reliability or the coefficient of reliability can be estimated from the equation:

$$R = 1 - [(TEM)^2 / (SD)^2]$$

where SD is the total intersubject variance for the study including measurement error. *R* ranges from 0 to 1. This value is useful for comparing different anthropometric measures and for estimating sample size in anthropometric studies.

A long-term assessment of measurement quality needs to be instigated in the clinic. This should take the same form as that used for tracking of the quality of laboratory measurements. This can be presented graphically with the identification of levels of error that are acceptable, and the identification of those that need to be flagged for future review and those that need to be addressed immediately. This system is particularly useful where multiple measurers are used, for example in multicentre clinical trials. Unfortunately, unlike laboratory quality control systems, where standards can be issued to the participating laboratories for evaluation, the same cannot be done for children! As a compromise, measurements should be made 'blind' and in triplicate on a series of children of different heights selected from the clinic population at regular intervals of 6 months.

## Height

For children under 2 years of age, supine length should be measured (Fig. 9.1). This requires the combined efforts of two persons and the holding of the head in the Frankfurt plane (with the tragus vertically below the outer canthus of the eye) by pressure under the mastoid processes of the skull is particularly important. Reliable crown–heel and crown–rump lengths are easily obtainable and, although repeatability may be more difficult to attain than in older children, rates of growth under the age of 2 years are so rapid that errors are balanced by the size of the increments in length.

Over the age of 2, standing measurements are required and a stadiometer should be used for this purpose (Fig. 9.2). In

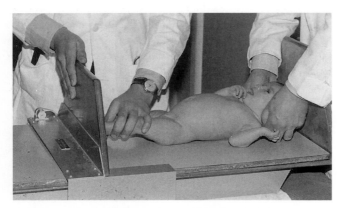

**Fig. 9.1.** Measurement of supine length. (Reproduced with permission from Brook CGD (1982) *Growth Assessment in Childhood and Adolescence*. Oxford: Blackwell Scientific Publications.)

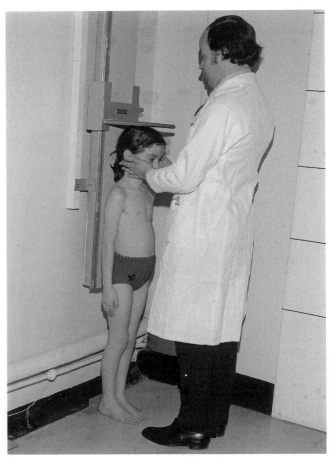

**Fig. 9.2.** Measurement of standing height using a stadiometer. (Reproduced with permission from Brook CGD (1982) *Growth Assessment in Childhood and Adolescence*. Oxford: Blackwell Scientific Publications.)

measuring stature, the standard position of the skull should be used routinely and, in all instances, gentle traction is applied to eliminate postural changes. Whether stretching is essential or not is debatable, but what it ensures is that care is given to the correct positioning of the child before measurement. Length changes as the day goes on but, as most children will be measured in clinics that occur at the same time of day on each occasion, the diurnal variation of stature is not of great clinical significance.

In the practice of paediatric endocrinology, the measurement of upper- and lower-body segments can be of considerable help. The use of span or pubis-to-ground measurements is not recommended because of the difficulty in making them precise. Measurements of sitting height (Fig. 9.3) and of crown–rump length in infants are preferred.

Most of the anthropometric instruments used in clinical practice have digital counter displays. These counters greatly reduce observer instrument errors, but they do mean that there is no direct reading of each measurement. At the beginning of the clinic therefore the accuracy of the machine

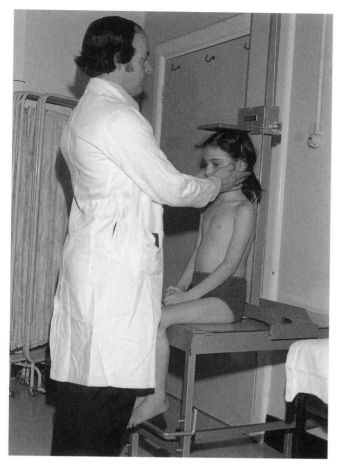

**Fig. 9.3.** Measurement of sitting height. (Reproduced with permission from Brook CGD (1982) *Growth Assessment in Childhood and Adolescence*. Oxford: Blackwell Scientific Publications.)

counter must be checked by using either a minimum reading counter, which is available on some instruments, or by the use of a standard length on others.

The purpose of measuring height is usually to assess growth velocity; in order to do this, a period of time sufficient for the expected increment of stature to exceed the combined errors of the two measurements on the two occasions must be allowed. Thus, height velocities in babies can be computed over weeks, whereas a prepubertal 14-year-old boy may need to be watched for a whole year to determine whether his growth velocity is normal. Since the computation of time in months is difficult, practitioners are urged always to use decimal dates and ages (Table 9.2).

## Weight

Measurements of weight can be useful as surrogate markers for growth when the latter is very rapid. Thus, in the newborn nursery, measurements of weight are a valuable indicator of

good health. The older a child becomes, the less value can be placed on weight or even on weight change over a period of time. To be of any use, measurements of weight have to be recorded accurately on proper equipment, and beam scales are the only acceptable instrument for use in this respect. Particular attention needs to be drawn to the fact that children between the ages of 2 and 10 years gain only about 17 kg, a velocity of less than 2 kg per year. Compared with height, the variations in weight during the day are enormous because of water balance, and when this is taken in conjunction with the use of inaccurately sprung weighing scales the undesirability of using weight as an estimate of children's growth becomes immediately apparent.

## Assessment of nutrition

Body composition can be measured by impedance, by the estimation of total body water, by radiograph, by computerized tomography, by magnetic resonance imaging and by many other physical and chemical methods. In clinical practice skinfold thicknesses are easy to measure. They are much more helpful than the computation of body mass indices in childhood, they are easy to perform and can be converted to estimates of total body fat [1].

Skinfold thicknesses are measured by picking up a fold of skin and subcutaneous fat in a standard position, usually over the mid-point of the triceps muscles and under the scapula at 45° to the spine. The jaws of the skinfold calliper are applied, and the needle of the dial of the instrument falls rapidly and then, suddenly, very slowly. The measurement of skinfold thickness should be recorded at that moment (Fig. 9.4). By convention, the left side of the body is always used for anthropometric measurements but, if the child has an obvious deformity, such as a hemiplegia, it is better to use the other side. In babies it is worth measuring both sides of the body and taking the average value for skinfold thicknesses [2].

The use of circumferential measurements is a variation in the assessment of nutrition. Such measures offer a less pure assessment of fatness since a circumferential measurement of a limb includes not only fat but also bone and muscle. This can be helpful in particular instances, such as in the clinical management of eating disorders over a period of time. They are the only way of assessing head growth and the accurate measurement of head circumference is useful in child developmental assessment. As is so often the case, the equipment provided for making circumferential measurements is inadequate: the use of linen, plastic or paper tape measures makes the value of longitudinal measurements much less satisfactory than the use of a proper tape that has sufficient length at the end to make the reading of the circumference easy and is thin enough not to slide about. All these instruments are available from Holtain Limited, Crosswell, Crymych, Dyfed, SA41 3UF, Wales.

| | 1 Jan | 2 Feb | 3 Mar | 4 Apr | 5 May | 6 Jun | 7 Jul | 8 Aug | 9 Sep | 10 Oct | 11 Nov | 12 Dec |
|---|---|---|---|---|---|---|---|---|---|---|---|---|
| 1 | 000 | 085 | 162 | 247 | 329 | 414 | 496 | 581 | 666 | 748 | 833 | 915 |
| 2 | 003 | 088 | 164 | 249 | 332 | 416 | 499 | 584 | 668 | 751 | 836 | 918 |
| 3 | 005 | 090 | 167 | 252 | 334 | 419 | 501 | 586 | 671 | 753 | 838 | 921 |
| 4 | 008 | 093 | 170 | 255 | 337 | 422 | 504 | 589 | 674 | 756 | 841 | 923 |
| 5 | 011 | 096 | 173 | 258 | 340 | 425 | 507 | 592 | 677 | 759 | 844 | 926 |
| 6 | 014 | 099 | 175 | 260 | 342 | 427 | 510 | 595 | 679 | 762 | 847 | 929 |
| 7 | 016 | 101 | 178 | 263 | 345 | 430 | 512 | 597 | 682 | 764 | 849 | 932 |
| 8 | 019 | 104 | 181 | 266 | 348 | 433 | 515 | 600 | 685 | 767 | 852 | 934 |
| 9 | 022 | 107 | 184 | 268 | 351 | 436 | 518 | 603 | 688 | 770 | 855 | 937 |
| 10 | 025 | 110 | 186 | 271 | 353 | 438 | 521 | 605 | 690 | 773 | 858 | 940 |
| 11 | 027 | 112 | 189 | 274 | 356 | 441 | 523 | 608 | 693 | 775 | 860 | 942 |
| 12 | 030 | 115 | 192 | 277 | 359 | 444 | 526 | 611 | 696 | 778 | 863 | 945 |
| 13 | 033 | 118 | 195 | 279 | 362 | 447 | 529 | 614 | 699 | 781 | 866 | 948 |
| 14 | 036 | 121 | 197 | 282 | 364 | 449 | 532 | 616 | 701 | 784 | 868 | 951 |
| 15 | 038 | 123 | 200 | 285 | 367 | 452 | 534 | 619 | 704 | 786 | 871 | 953 |
| 16 | 041 | 126 | 203 | 288 | 370 | 455 | 537 | 622 | 707 | 789 | 874 | 956 |
| 17 | 044 | 129 | 205 | 290 | 373 | 458 | 540 | 625 | 710 | 792 | 877 | 959 |
| 18 | 047 | 132 | 208 | 293 | 375 | 460 | 542 | 627 | 712 | 795 | 879 | 962 |
| 19 | 049 | 134 | 211 | 296 | 378 | 463 | 545 | 630 | 715 | 797 | 882 | 964 |
| 20 | 052 | 137 | 214 | 299 | 381 | 466 | 548 | 633 | 718 | 800 | 885 | 967 |
| 21 | 055 | 140 | 216 | 301 | 384 | 468 | 551 | 636 | 721 | 803 | 888 | 970 |
| 22 | 058 | 142 | 219 | 304 | 386 | 471 | 553 | 638 | 723 | 805 | 890 | 973 |
| 23 | 060 | 145 | 222 | 307 | 389 | 474 | 556 | 641 | 726 | 808 | 893 | 975 |
| 24 | 063 | 148 | 225 | 310 | 392 | 477 | 559 | 644 | 729 | 811 | 896 | 978 |
| 25 | 066 | 151 | 227 | 312 | 395 | 479 | 562 | 647 | 731 | 814 | 899 | 981 |
| 26 | 068 | 153 | 230 | 315 | 397 | 482 | 564 | 649 | 734 | 816 | 901 | 984 |
| 27 | 071 | 156 | 233 | 318 | 400 | 485 | 567 | 652 | 737 | 819 | 904 | 986 |
| 28 | 074 | 159 | 236 | 321 | 403 | 488 | 570 | 655 | 740 | 822 | 907 | 989 |
| 29 | 077 | | 238 | 323 | 405 | 490 | 573 | 658 | 742 | 825 | 910 | 992 |
| 30 | 079 | | 241 | 326 | 408 | 493 | 575 | 660 | 745 | 827 | 912 | 995 |
| 31 | 082 | | 244 | | 411 | | 578 | 663 | | 830 | | 997 |

**Table 9.2.** Decimals of a year. If the date today is 8 August 2001 (2001.600) and the child was born on 19 April 1997 (1997.296), his age is 4.304 years

Reproduced with permission from Brook CGD (1982) *Growth Assessment in Childhood and Adolescence.* Oxford: Blackwell Scientific Publications.

## Standards

In an ideal world, growth standards would be available for local populations adjusted for ethnic origin and socio-economic circumstances. In practice these are not available, but the situation is far from disastrous because estimates of growth rate are largely independent of growth attained and standards for velocities of height, weight, head circumference, skinfold thicknesses, etc. are generally applicable. A most useful compendium of reference standard charts has been assembled by Buckler [3].

It is worth pointing out the difference between standards and reference charts. To construct a standard we would need a population, or a sample of that population, who were normal, i.e. no evidence of illness or other factors known to influence growth. Acquiring such a population is difficult, time-consuming and expensive. Reference values are also constructed from a population, usually consisting of a large sample size, and including persons with and without illness. Owing to the large sample size chosen, it generally depicts what is happening in the normal population but technically it is not a standard. This difference is not usually an issue but it could be in certain circumstances. Body mass i    : (BMI) charts are one area. If BMI is used as a proxy measure for obesity and if obesity is associated with increased cardiovascular mortality and morbidity then we need good charts to help detect the condition early and to monitor intervention. In this situation a standard chart would be required not a reference one as it would include the obese population.

Standards or reference charts are usually presented in terms of centiles, which describe the variation of a characteristic

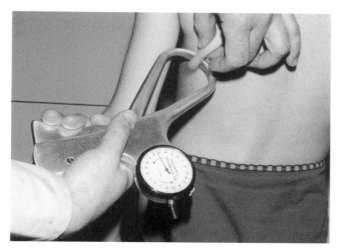

**Fig. 9.4.** Measurement of subscapular skinfold thickness. (Reproduced with permission from Brook CGD (1982) *Growth Assessment in Childhood and Adolescence*. Oxford: Blackwell Scientific Publications.)

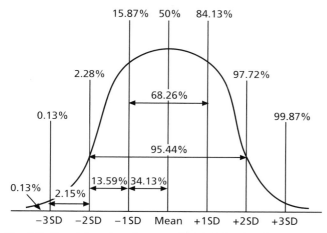

**Fig. 9.5.** The relation of centiles to standard deviations in a characteristic normally distributed. (Reproduced with permission from Brook CGD (1982) *Growth Assessment in Childhood and Adolescence*. Oxford: Blackwell Scientific Publications.)

in a population. Where such a characteristic is distributed in a normal (Gaussian) fashion, centile values correspond to standard deviations in the populations. Thus, 68% of the population has a height within one standard deviation on either side of the mean and one standard deviation corresponds to the 16th and 84th centiles. Similar figures apply to other measurements (Fig. 9.5).

It is important to remember that the distribution of a characteristic in a population does not have to be assumed before making a centile chart. Most data are accumulated either on a one off basis on many children of different ages (cross-sectional data) or by measuring the same children repeatedly as they grow (longitudinal data). As long as samples are large, the difference in practice is relatively

less important. For example, the 1990 UK Height Reference Charts are cross-sectional in nature but describe the pubertal growth spurt (longitudinal event) very well because of the large sample size. Since longitudinal growth studies take many years to complete, there are few of them. Most standards include data of both types and are properly called mixed longitudinal.

## Bone age and height prediction

The assessment of skeletal maturity provides a guide to the amount of growth that has already taken place compared with the amount of growth that is to come. It plays a part in the general assessment of maturity but it is a bad guide to the onset of puberty and of little help in making a diagnosis. Assessments of skeletal maturity are generally performed too freely and too frequently, and conclusions are drawn on them that are rarely warranted in clinical terms. It often comes as a surprise to practitioners to learn, for example, that the events of puberty are not more closely allied to estimates of skeletal maturity than they are to chronological age, except for menarche, which is fairly closely tied to a skeletal maturity of 13 years [4].

There are two main methods of estimating bone age and three systems that can be used for the prediction of mature height. The first and most widely used methods uses the *Atlas of Skeletal Development* by Greulich and Pyle [5]. In this method the development of each epiphyseal centre in the hand and wrist is compared with a series of standard pictures chosen to be typical for boys and girls of different ages. By comparing the radial epiphysis with the standards and noting the age with which its appearance most closely corresponds followed by similar comparisons of the ulnar, first metacarpal epiphyses and so on throughout the bones of the hand and wrist, an average bone age can be calculated. This is laborious but it gives accurate and reproducible results. The tables of Bayley and Pinneau [6,7] indicate the proportion of growth that has passed at any one bone age. These tables can be used to predict mature adult height from a measurement of stature taken with the chronological age and bone age measured by the Greulich and Pyle method. They are robust for individuals with considerably advanced or retarded bone ages in comparison with chronological age and are therefore useful in pathological situations [8].

The difficulty with the Greulich and Pyle method is that in routine clinical practice there can be a temptation to compare the whole radiograph with whole-hand standards. This is often the case when skeletal assessment is performed by a radiologist who is not interested in fine interpretation. Such practice can be identified by the style of a report that is of no help in growth assessment. Examples of such suspect reports follow. 'Bone age normal for chronological age'. Since two standard deviations of bone age cover approximately

18 months on either side of chronological age, this does not help much. 'The bone age corresponds most closely to the female standard of 7 years and 10 months'. This is not much help either because two standard deviations on either side of 7 years and 10 months reported for girls cover 40 months. 'Between 8 years and 10 months and 10 years'. A height prediction for a tall girl age 8 with a height of 145 cm based on this would lead to mean height predictions between 185 and 175 cm, not even allowing for the errors in prediction. This would hardly help in the decision whether or not treatment was needed to limit ultimate stature.

The second main method in use for the assessment of skeletal maturity is the one described by Tanner *et al.* [9]. In this method each bone has to be compared in turn with a series of radiographic standards and a textual description of bone maturation. A sex-specific score is allotted to each stage. The scores are added and compared with standards for age and sex yielding an exact reading of skeletal maturity. Although this sounds laborious, it takes about 45 seconds if the scores are added on a pocket calculator, and the results can be used in predictive equations provided in the same text. Coefficient of variation within and between observers using this method should be considerably less than 2%.

The third method of predicting adult height is that of Roche *et al.* [10]. Here recumbent length, nude weight, mid-parental stature and a Greulich and Pyle bone age are used to predict adult stature; clearly the first two criteria provide some problems for an adolescent clinic. Adjustment from standing height and weight in underclothes are probably permissible. Since this method has built in the problems of estimating bone age by the atlas method, it is probably not a good alternative to the Tanner one.

All these methods used correctly give reproducible results but, not surprisingly considering how they were designed, the newer height prediction tables of Tanner and of Roche are superior to that of Bayley and Pinneau for projecting final height in normal children. This includes tall normal children [8] but, for subjects with growth disorders and endocrine conditions, the older and simpler tables of Bayley and Pinneau give more accurate results.

## Pubertal status

This is assessed according to the criteria described by Tanner [11] and the criteria are as follows.

### Boys: genitalia development (Fig. 9.6)

Stage 1  Preadolescent: testes, scrotum and penis are of about the same size and proportion as in early childhood.
Stage 2  Enlargement of scrotum and testes. Skin of scrotum reddens and changes in texture. Little or no enlargement of penis at this stage.
Stage 3  Enlargement of the penis, which occurs at first mainly in length. Further growth of testes and scrotum.
Stage 4  Increased size of penis with growth in breadth and development of glans. Testes and scrotum larger; scrotal skin darkened.
Stage 5  Genitalia adult size and shape.

### Girls: breast development (Fig. 9.7)

Stage 1  Preadolescent elevation of papilla only.
Stage 2  Breast bud stage: elevation of breast papilla as small mound. Enlargement of areolar diameter.
Stage 3  Further enlargement and elevation of breast and areola, with no separation of their contours.
Stage 4  Projection of areola and papilla to form a secondary mound above the level of the breast.
Stage 5  Mature stage: projection of papilla only, due to recession of the areola to the general contour of the breast.

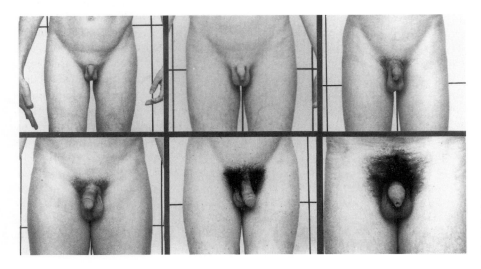

**Fig. 9.6.** Tanner stages of male genital and pubic hair development. (Reproduced with permission from Styne DM (1995) *Clinical Paediatric Endocrinology,* 3rd edn. Oxford: Blackwell Science.)

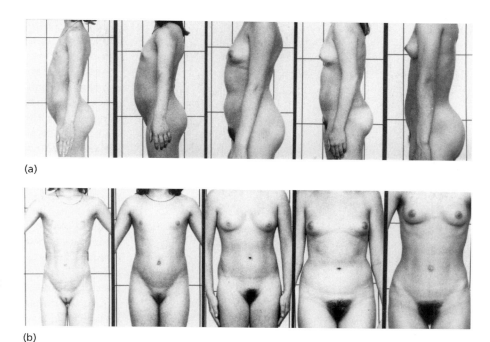

(a)

(b)

**Fig. 9.7.** Tanner stages of breast (a) and pubic hair (b) development. (Reproduced with permission from Styne DM (1995) *Clinical Paediatric Endocrinology*, 3rd edn. Oxford: Blackwell Science.)

## Both sexes: pubic hair (Figs 9.6 and 9.7)

Stage 1 Preadolescent: the vellus over the pubes is not further developed than that over the abdominal wall, i.e. no pubic hair.

Stage 2 Sparse growth of long, slightly pigmented downy hair, straight or slightly curled, chiefly at the base or along the labia.

Stage 3 Considerably darker, coarser and more curled. The hair spreads sparsely over the junction of the pubes.

Stage 4 Hair now adult in type, but the area covered is still considerably smaller than in the adult. No spread to the medial surface of the thighs.

Stage 5 Adult in quantity and type with distribution of the horizontal (or classically feminine pattern). Spread to medial surface of thighs but not up linea alba or elsewhere above the base of the inverse triangle.

Stage 6 Spread of pubic hair up linea alba.

## Both sexes: axillary hair

Stage 1 Preadolescent: no axillary hair.
Stage 2 Scanty growth of slightly pigmented hair.
Stage 3 Hair adult in quantity and quality.

Testicular size should be recorded as testicular volume. This is easily assessed by comparison with standard ovoids and the Prader orchidometer (Fig. 9.8a) is an indispensable aid to this purpose. The testes are palpated by one hand and the orchidometer is held in the other. Standards are available against which testicular volume can be compared [12] (Fig. 9.8b).

Under no circumstances should these ratings be lumped together in an overall stage of puberty, because each depends on upon different endocrinological events and each therefore has its own significance. A standard rating for a boy might read G (genitalia) 3, PH (pubic hair) 3, Ax (axillary hair) 2, 8/10 (mL for testicular volume in the right and left testes, respectively, the figures being written while the examiner looks at the scrotum). Pubic hair growth reflects both adrenal and testicular androgens; genital growth and axillary hair reflect testicular testosterone secretion and testicular volume gonadotrophins [luteinizing hormone (LH) to a volume of about 8 mL and with follicle-stimulating hormone (FSH) to adult size].

For a girl a recording of pubertal stage might be B (breasts) 4, PH (pubic hair) 4, Ax (axillary hair) 2, and then some designation of whether or not menarche has occurred. Breast development is a reflection of ovarian oestradiol secretion, although gonadotrophins may play a part because the breast development of a girl with puberty induced for hypogonadotrophic hypogonadism is cosmetically much less satisfactory than that seen in her hypergonadotrophic counterpart. Menarche indicates negative feedback on gonadotrophins. Pubic and axillary hair result from adrenal androgen secretion, probably facilitated by oestradiol because Turner girls get some pubic hair spontaneously, but it increases greatly when oestrogen replacement treatment is introduced.

The importance of correct assessment of puberty cannot be overemphasized. Where stages are seriously discrepant (separated by more than one Tanner stage) or testicular volumes inappropriate for the rest of the stages of puberty, there is nearly always pathology to be uncovered.

(a)

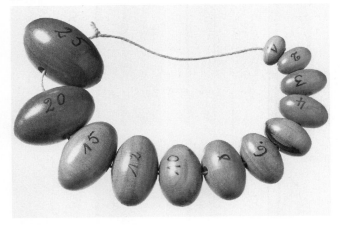

(b)

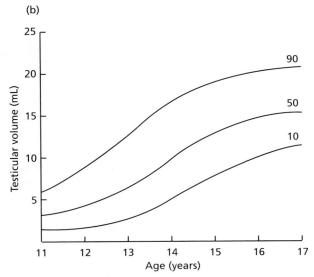

**Fig. 9.8.** (a) Prader orchidometer and (b) centiles for testicular size [12]. (Reproduced with permission from Styne DM (1995) *Clinical Paediatric Endocrinology*, 3rd edn. Oxford: Blackwell Science.)

## Conclusion

Measurements are made routinely of height, sitting height, weight, triceps and subscapular skinfold thickness, head circumference and puberty ratings.

On the first attendance, the heights of both parents should be measured. The value, if either of the heights is reported, is greatly reduced because of the tendency to report an idealized height of the spouse. In general, fathers underestimate the mother's stature and mothers overestimate the father's.

Birth data on the child and siblings should be gathered, together with the measurement of the heights of siblings where possible. It is customary to ask about parental entry into puberty, usually as the age of the maternal menarche. When the result accords with the physician's presumption,

there is satisfaction all round but the contrary is not unusual, so the value of this question is doubtful except in a social context.

Assessment of skeletal maturity may be helpful on this occasion, but only in terms of predicting the long-term outcome. It is not helpful for determining whether there is anything wrong with the child or what the diagnosis might be.

Decimal age should be calculated, and the data either plotted on the appropriate charts or calculated as standard deviation scores (*z*-scores, SDS). The parental height centile positions should also be entered on the growth chart to give an idea of whether or not the child is near to expected height for age for the family. If a boy's chart is being used, the mother's centile position will be plotted after adding 12.6 cm to her measured height. The father's height is entered directly. If a girl's chart is being used, the mother's height is entered directly but the father's height must be adjusted by the subtraction of 12.6 cm to ascertain his centile position.

At a subsequent visit, the routine measurements will be repeated and it will be possible on this occasion to calculate the height velocity using the two decimal ages to calculate the time interval and the two height measurements to calculate the gain. The result should either be plotted on a chart or the SDS calculated. Note that there is no point in relating height velocity to bone age – at least not unless there is a bone age increment and a height velocity related to the increment, and even then it has a suspect status. Why should they be related?

It is not possible to calculate height velocity SDS or plot the values over the age of 10 years in a girl or 11 years in a boy because of the effect of puberty on the standards. In the individual case, relating the velocity to the assessment of puberty is highly relevant.

With this knowledge it will be possible to sort out most disorders of growth in children, to monitor effects of treatment and to point the necessity for further investigation or, more importantly, to indicate normality. When results are normal, further investigation is wrong: investigating normal children constitutes an assault.

## References

1 Brook CGD. Determination of body composition of children from skinfold measurements. *Arch Dis Child* 1971; 46: 182–4.

2 Whitelaw AGL. Influence of maternal obesity in subcutaneous fat in the newborn. *Br Med J* 1976; 1: 985–6.

3 Buckler JMHA. *A Reference Manual of Growth and Development*, 2nd edn. Oxford: Blackwell Science, 1997.

4 Marshall WA. Interrelationships of skeletal maturation, sexual development and somatic growth in man. *Ann Hum Biol* 1974; 1: 29–40.

5 Greulich WW, Pyle SI. *Radiographic Atlas of Skeletal Development of Hand and Wrist*. Stanford, CA: Stanford University Press, 1959.

6 Bayley N, Pinneau R. Table for predicting adult height from skeletal age revised for use with the Greulich–Pyle hand standards.

*J Pediatr* 1952; 40: 423–41 (published erratum appears in *J Pediatr* 1953; 41: 371).

7 Post EM, Richman RA. A condensed table for predicting adult stature. *J Pediatr* 1981; 98: 440–2.

8 Zachmann M, Sobradillo B, Frank M, Frisch H, Prader A. Bayley–Pinneau. Roche–Wainer–Thissen and Tanner Height predictions in normal children and in patients with various pathologic conditions. *J Pediatr* 1978; 93: 429–55.

9 Tanner JM, Whitehouse RH, Cameron N, Marshall WA, Healy MJR, Goldstein H. *Assessment of Skeletal Maturity and Prediction of Adult Height (TW2 Method)*, 2nd edn. London: Academic Press, 1983.

10 Roche AF, Wainer WAI, Thissen D. The RWT method for the prediction of adult stature. *Pediatrics* 1975; 56: 1027–33.

11 Tanner JM. *Growth at Adolescence*, 2nd edn. Oxford: Blackwell Scientific Publications, 1962.

12 Zachmann M, Prader A, Kind HP, Hafliger H, Budliger H. Testicular volume during adolescence. *Helv Pediatr Acta* 1974; 29: 61–72.

# 10 Management of disorders of size

R. L. Hintz

## Control of growth: overview of disorders of size

One of the most frequent problems faced by paediatric endocrinologists is a disorder of the size or shape of the patient. Although everyone can observe a large amount of variability in the human population, many parents and their children want to conform to an idealized standard. This has led to many referrals to paediatric endocrinology clinics.

The control of growth is complex, involving many hormonal and non-hormonal components (Fig. 10.1). Many of the hormones are controlled via the hypothalamo-pituitary axis [1]. Thus, the secretion of growth hormone (GH), which leads to the secretion of insulin-like growth factors (IGFs), is under the control of hypothalamic neuropeptide hormones known as GH-releasing hormone (GHRH) and somatostatin. The secretion of thyrotrophin-simulating hormone (TSH), follicle-stimulating hormone (FSH), luteinizing hormone (LH) and adrenocorticotrophic hormone (ACTH), all of which play major roles in the control of growth, are themselves under the control of hypothalamic neurohormones. In addition, the secretion of insulin, which is not directly under pituitary control, also plays an important role in the control of cellular growth [2].

Many non-hormonal factors play major roles in the control of growth. Foremost among these is nutrition, as without substrate no cell could grow or divide. There are also underlying genetic factors, which determine potential for growth not only for the whole organism but also for each organ and tissue. In addition, there are a host of tissue growth hormones, such as epidermal growth hormone (EGF) and nerve growth hormone (NGF), the roles of which are only beginning to be understood in the overall control of growth [3]. The interaction of these hormonal and non-hormonal hormones leads to normal growth and development; abnormalities lead to growth disorders. A thorough understanding of the hormones controlling growth is crucial for a rational approach to the diagnosis and management of disorders of size.

## Growth hormone

GH is a 191-amino-acid-long polypeptide secreted by the somatotropes of the anterior pituitary gland. Neurohormones control these cells through the hypophysial portal system, and both a positive effector of GH secretion and an inhibitor of GH secretion exist [4]. Present data indicate that GHRH is responsible for the synthesis of GH secretion, seen mainly during the night-time hours and in response to meals and exercise, whereas the inhibitor of GH secretion, somatostatin, appears to be responsible for the pulsatile nature of GH secretion. There is a third hypothalamic neurohormone that is not yet completely characterized, the GH-releasing peptide (GHRP).

Two major forms of GH are synthesized, stored and secreted by the somatotropes [5]. The most abundant (approximately 90%) is the 22-kDa molecular weight form. In addition, there is an alternative splicing of the GH mRNA, which leads to a minor 20-kDa form of GH the physiological role of which is unknown.

GH secretion, like that of many other polypeptide hormones, is pulsatile [6]. In addition, GH has a striking

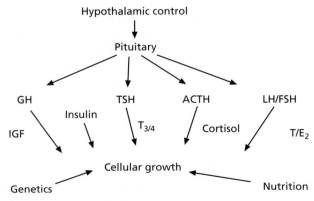

**Fig. 10.1.** Control of cellular growth.

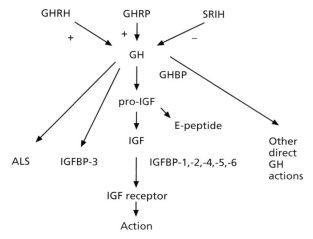

**Fig. 10.2.** The chain of GH action.

predilection for secretion in association with sleep. A large number of brain centres and neurotransmitters have been implicated in the control of GH. There is also evidence that one of the GH-stimulated peptides, IGF-I, plays an important feedback role at the level of both the hypothalamus and the somatotropes on the secretion of GH [7].

The secretion of GH leads to a complex chain of events (Fig. 10.2), which leads ultimately to the stimulation of growth at the endocrine level. After GH is released into the blood stream, a large proportion binds to a specific GH-binding protein (GHBP) [8]. It is now clear that this represents the extracellular portion of the GH receptor (GHR) site. Like many receptors for polypeptide hormones, the receptor site for GH consists of three polypeptide domains: an extracellular domain, which contains all of the three-dimensional structure necessary for the recognition of the hormone; a transmembrane domain, which is highly hydrophobic; and, finally, an intracellular domain, which contains the three-dimensional structure that leads to the biological action within the cell. In humans, it appears that there is a proteolytic cleavage of the extracellular domain of the GHR that leads to a soluble, circulating polypeptide which plays a major role in protein binding of GH in the serum. The exact biological role of this binding protein is unclear; however, it does serve as a useful index to the level of GHRs in the body. GHRs are widely distributed throughout tissues in the body, and it is the binding of the GH ligand to these GHRs that leads to the biological events within the cells themselves. Of the many direct biological events that are ascribed to GH action, one of the most important is control of the production of IGF-I.

## Insulin-like growth factor

IGF mRNA is widely distributed throughout the body and is under GH control, not only in the liver, as would have been predicted by the original somatomedin hypothesis, but in other tissues as well [9]. IGFs circulate bound tightly to proteins known as IGF-binding proteins (IGFBPs). In normal circumstances, there is little or no circulating free IGF-I or IGF-II polypeptides. Six distinct but homologous IGFBPs are known and at least four IGFBP-related proteins. By far the most abundant form of IGFBP in normal serum is IGFBP-3, a glycosylated protein of approximately 40 kDa molecular weight. The combined IGF-peptide/IGFBP-3 complex binds to yet another protein known as the acid labile subunit (ALS) to form a 150-kDa, three-subunit protein complex that is the major circulating form of the IGFs. In most circumstances this 150-kDa complex contains more than 90% of the total IGF in the serum.

A smaller proportion of the IGFs in serum circulate bound to the other forms of IGFBP (-1, -2, -4, -5, and -6). These IGFBPs are major components in certain bodily fluids, for example IGFBP-1 in amniotic fluid, IGFBP-2 in joint fluid and IGFBP-5 in cerebrospinal fluid. The biological purpose of this complex system for controlling the amount and distribution of IGF in the serum and extracellular fluid spaces is unclear. However, it does result in prolonging the circulating time of IGFs in plasma, and may play a major role in modulating the delivery of the IGF peptides to the receptor sites on cells.

Just as there is more than one form of IGF, there is more than one form of IGF-like receptor found on the surface of cells [10]. The type 1 IGF receptor has the strongest affinity for IGF-I and a less strong binding of IGF-II and insulin. This receptor resembles the insulin receptor in its subunit construction and amino acid sequence, and appears to have been derived from the insulin receptor during evolution.

The type 2 receptor has its highest affinity for IGF-II and somewhat less affinity for IGF-I. Unlike the situation with the type 1 or the insulin receptor, the type 2 IGF receptor has little affinity for insulin itself. The molecular corollary of this observation has been that there is no structural relationship between the type 2 receptor and either the type 1 receptor or the insulin receptor. Rather, the type 2 receptor appears to be a bifunctional receptor with ligand specificity for both IGF peptides and for mannose 6-phosphate. The role of the type 2 receptor in the control of growth is controversial.

Most of the biological actions of GH on the control of growth appear to be subserved by the chain of action initiated by GH. This leads to the production of IGF-I and its delivery to the IGF type 1 receptor sites in the tissues (Fig. 10.2). It is this chain of action that has been most clearly linked to the anabolic and growth-promoting events which we associate with GH in the whole organism. Any abnormality in this complex chain of events can lead to growth failure.

## Thyroid hormone

Thyroid hormone plays an important role in the control of growth. Like the GH–IGF axis, there is a hypothalamic mechanism of control, with the neurohormone thyrotrophin-stimulating hormone (TRH) being secreted by specialized neurones into the hypophyseal portal system leading to the release of the pituitary hormone TSH [11].

TSH leads to the production and release of the thyroid hormones ($T_4$ and $T_3$). Like the IGFs, they are bound almost totally to plasma proteins that control their half-life and tissue delivery. The thyroid hormone receptor site, which is widely distributed throughout cells in the body, subserves thyroid hormone action. This receptor site is located intracellularly, similar to that of steroid hormones, and the ligand–$T_3$ complex binds to chromatin and DNA to initiate mRNA synthesis.

Without thyroid hormone action through its receptor sites, GH and IGFs are unable to stimulate anabolic and growth responses. Furthermore, there is a close interaction of thyroid hormone with GH secretion [12]. In the presence of hypothyroidism, GH secretion from the pituitary gland is decreased in response to both pharmacological and physiological stimulation. Therefore, the normality of thyroid hormone secretion must be proven before any attempt is made to assess GH secretion.

## Oestrogens and androgens

Oestrogens and androgens are secreted in low concentrations after the fetal and perinatal periods of life until there is an increase in LH and FSH before the onset of puberty [13]. Both influence the secretion of GH. The increase in GH secretion at the time of puberty plays a major part in the pubertal growth spurt. Direct end-organ effects of both androgens and oestrogens have been demonstrated in a variety of experimental systems. In addition to the direct and indirect roles that androgens and oestrogens play in the stimulation of growth, oestrogens play the major role in the maturation of bones and the ultimate disappearance of the epiphyseal centres, the event that results in the cessation of linear growth.

Like the thyroid hormones, the sex hormones appear to act by diffusing into the cell and binding to specific receptor sites of the steroid/TSH category. The binding of androgens and oestrogens initiates changes in the three-dimensional structure, which allows the interaction of these activated receptors with chromatin and the chromosomal DNA. This leads to the production of specific mRNA and secretion of specific proteins leading to the biological action observed. The evaluation of sex hormone secretion plays an important part in the evaluation of disorders of size, particularly in the peripubertal period.

## Adrenal androgens

Adrenal androgens have an adjunctive role in the events of puberty and act in concert with androgens from the testes and ovary to lead to growth stimulation by direct and indi-

rect means and to maturation of the bones [14]. Adrenal glucocorticoids have a bimodal action in the control of growth. A minimal level is necessary for cells to function, grow and divide. On the other hand, many observations have shown that even a slight excess of glucocorticoids makes cells in the body unresponsive to the other hormonal growth-stimulating agents reviewed above [15], and to marked slowing of linear growth.

## Non-humoral factors

Other non-humoral factors also control growth. Without adequate food, and therefore without adequate substrates for cells, no effective growth can occur. This is clearly seen in kwashiorkor and marasmus [16] but is also manifested in many more subtle clinical disorders in nutrition. Genetics also plays an important role in determining the growth potential in the gorilla, the human and the chimpanzee. On a more subtle level, it is clear that the differences in stature among humans depend to a large extent upon differing genetic constitutions. To date, our best, but relatively crude, way of determining these underlying genetic hormones is parental and familial heights [17].

Tissue growth factors, such as fibroblast growth factor (FGF), play a critical though largely unknown role in the control of growth of the organism [3]. This is best illustrated by achondroplasia, which is caused by a defect in the gene for the FGF receptor [18]. Further work will be necessary to relate these individual growth factors to clinical disorders of growth. Finally, the role of systemic disease in the growth of children and adolescents cannot be overemphasized. Even in the presence of normal hormonal, nutritional and genetic hormones, underlying systemic disease such as inflammatory bowel disease can interfere with growth potential [19]. The existence of short stature in a patient is an important clue to the physician as to the underlying condition of the patient.

## Short stature

The accuracy of determining height depends on using adequate equipment and a careful technique by trained personnel. Short stature is usually defined as a height less than –2 SD (standard deviations) for age or less than the third centile (–1.88 SD) for age compared with standards based on an appropriate sample of a normal population. The definition of short stature is arbitrary, and other cut-off points have been used. The absolute height at which a child can be considered to have short stature varies considerably depending on the reference population.

This is a particular problem in multiethnic societies as children from ethnic and family backgrounds that lead to relatively short adult stature may still be compared with native children who are destined to be taller because of their

**Table 10.1.** Causes of short stature

Non-pathological short stature
    Constitutional delay
    Familial
    Nutritional

GH related causes
    GHD
    GH resistance syndrome (Laron syndrome).

Hypothyroidism

Sex hormone-related causes
    Delayed puberty
    Hypogonadotrophic hypogonadism (Kallmann syndrome).

Glucocorticoid excess
    Cushing disease
    Pharmacological administration

Genetic causes
    Chromosomal
        Turner syndrome (XO and variants).
        Down syndrome (21 trisomy).
    Syndromes
        Pseudohypoparathyroidism
        Prader–Willi syndrome
        Laurence–Moon–Biedl syndrome
        Skeletal dysplasias
        Miscellaneous (Russel–Silver, Seckel, etc.)

genetic background. The population cross-sectional definition of short stature may also be at variance with the background of an individual's family. An individual on the 10th centile can be perceived to be short by the family if the parents are tall. To determine the significance of this, midparental height (MPH), alternatively known as target height, should be calculated with the 10th to 90th centile range being determined using the following formulae:

For boys: MPH = [father's height + (mother's height + 13) ]/
        $2 \pm 7.5$ cm

For girls: MPH = [father's height – 13 + (mother's height) ]/
        $2 \pm 6$ cm

If the individual falls outside this range, a reason should be sought. Standards may be helpful to assess a child's height in relation to the height of the parents [20]. As might be expected from the multiplicity of control mechanisms for growth, there are many causes of short stature (Table 10.1).

The majority of short children do not have underlying hormonal or genetic disease. One study of short children in Scotland ($n = 449$) found only 24% of them to have an organic cause [21]. Eight per cent had GH deficiency (GHD), giving a prevalence of 1/4000. An even lower frequency of pathology has been suggested [22].

Children with significant short stature without a definite organic cause have been referred to as having 'normal variant' or idiopathic short stature (ISS). Many come from short families and might be classified as familial short stature. Others are from average-sized families and have delayed bone ages and so could be classified as having constitutional delay of growth. The reality in clinical practice is that many short children have a combination of these features, and subcategorization of normal variant short stature is not helpful.

Hidden within the large number of normal children are some who have clinically important disorders for which the physician must search. As a group, children with ISS have lower mean secretion of GH and lower mean concentrations of circulating IGF-I than age-matched control subjects. This has led to the suggestion that some of them have subtle abnormalities in GH secretion and/or action and may benefit from treatment with GH [23].

Nutritional disorders, including maternal deprivation, anorexia and bulimia, can certainly lead to children being short for their age. Psychosocial deprivation and chronic disease (e.g. coeliac disease, inflammatory bowel disease), as well as diseases of the kidneys and chest, and blood disorders (e.g. thalassaemia), can also present as short stature, and the physician dealing with growth disorders must be alert to the possible presence of these problems. Many children born small for gestational age (SGA) fail to have adequate catch-up growth and remain small throughout childhood. Of SGA infants, 40% show catch-up growth to the normal range before 6 months of age [24], and a further 25% catch up before 3 years of age. Another 20% catch up after 3 years, and approximately 15% show no catch-up growth. The last two groups never achieve their genetic potential. The growth patterns of low birthweight, preterm infants differ from those born SGA. Catch-up growth for length is found during the first postnatal year but during the next 2 years no further catch-up occurs [25], and size at 3 years is directly related to size at birth. Children with low birth length represent 20% of the population of short teenagers at age 18 [26].

Clinical abnormalities of GH secretion or action cause short stature. In GHD, there is a disorder either of hypothalamic control of GH secretion or an inability of the pituitary itself to secrete GH [27]. The consequences of classic GHD are reflected not only in low concentrations of circulating GH, as assessed by both physiological and pharmacological stimulation, but also in extremely low concentrations of IGF-I and a consequent decrease in the growth rate. These children respond to GH treatment with a marked increase in growth rate.

An interesting disorder of the chain of GH action is Laron syndrome (also known as GH-insensitivity syndrome). This disorder, originally described in Ashkenazi Jews, is ethnically and geographically more widely distributed [28]. Laron syndrome is a group of genetic disorders of the GHR that make the GHR unable to bind GH. This results in an increase in circulating GH concentrations (due to lack of IGF feedback), a decrease in the level of circulating GHBP derived from the GHR, markedly decreased concentrations of IGF-I and extremely poor growth rates. Children with Laron syndrome respond to treatment with synthetic IGF-I with an increased rate of growth, thus validating the somatomedin hypothesis [29]. It is possible that more subtle abnormalities of the GHBP or GHR underlie the cause of some undiagnosed cases of poor growth [30].

Any degree of hypothyroidism leads to a decrease in growth rate, and eventually short stature [31]. There is a remarkable increase in growth rate after thyroid therapy is instituted. Some patients with severe hypothyroidism present with a form of precocious puberty in which there is premature activation of gonadotrophins apparently associated with the high concentrations of TRH secretion by the hypothalamus. Treatment of hypothyroidism can lead to a rapid onset of central puberty, leading to an accelerated advance in skeletal maturity that may compromise the final height.

Short stature due to inadequate sex hormone secretion is commonly seen in boys with delayed puberty and sometimes in girls. Treatment with short courses of androgen has been used in boys with severely delayed puberty [32]. The delay in puberty is usually physiological, but can also be associated with hypogonadotrophic hypogonadism in both boys and girls. A relatively common form of hypogonadotrophic hypogonadism in both boys and girls is Kallmann syndrome, in which the hypogonadotrophic hypogonadism is associated with anosmia [33]. These patients can be treated with androgens or oestrogens as appropriate.

Short stature can be associated with hypersecretion of glucocorticoids caused by an increase in ACTH secretion (Cushing disease) [34], or the hypersecretion of glucocorticoids by a functioning adrenal tumour or by exogenous administration of glucocorticoids. These patients need to be treated by the control of their excess glucocorticoid secretion. Although by far the most common cause of glucocorticoid excess leading to growth failure is in association with the treatment of steroid-responsive diseases such as asthma or renal disorders with pharmacological doses of glucocorticoids, the obvious manoeuvre of decreasing or stopping the glucocorticoid therapy may in practice be very difficult to accomplish because of exacerbation of the underlying disease state.

The most common genetic disorder leading to short stature is Turner syndrome [35]. The mechanism of the short stature is not clear, but it is not GH-related. These girls are born short and have poor growth rates during childhood, which leads to a progressive decrease in height compared with their peers. They fail to enter puberty because of the ovarian failure associated with Turner syndrome, and thus achieve very short adult stature with an average final height of approximately 4' 7" (140 cm). The use of GH treatment has had some success in increasing growth rates and final height in girls with Turner syndrome [36]. Although the majority of these children have delayed puberty, one-fifth develop secondary sex characteristics and even menstruate. Thus, it cannot be too strongly recommended that any physician dealing with a girl who is pathologically short with no other established diagnosis should *always* obtain chromosomes, irrespective of the presence or absence of secondary sex characteristics.

Other genetic causes of short stature include Russell–Silver syndrome, Noonan syndrome, pseudohypoparathyroidism, Aarskog syndrome, Sprintzen syndrome, Down syndrome, Laurence–Moon–Biedl syndrome, Weaver syndrome, Prader–Willi syndrome and skeletal dysplasias.

## Management of short stature

Children who have growth failure over a significant period of time develop short stature. As most short children are normal, the approach to short stature must be a careful balance designed not to miss a pathology disorder without overevaluation (Fig. 10.3). The key to the initial evaluation of short stature is the history and determination of the auxological parameters.

The history should include the birth history and past growth of the child, family history of height and development, any evidence for systemic disease and a careful inquiry into the child's nutrition. The physical examination should be focused on evidence of systemic disease or malnutrition, and anomalies suggestive of chromosomal disease.

The relative proportions of the spine and leg length (by measuring sitting height) can provide important clues to the presence of a specific syndrome or genetic abnormality. Children with height greater than –2 SD below the average for age and/or a height velocity appropriate for age are probably normal. If the child has *significant short stature* and/or a decreased growth rate (a height below –2.5 SD for age, and/or a height velocity less than –1 SD for age) and no evidence of hypothyroidism, systemic disease or malnutrition, an abnormality of the GH–IGF axis should be considered.

Because of the profound influence of thyroid hormone on the GH axis, it is important that any hypothyroidism be diagnosed and adequately treated before testing for GHD is carried out. Many people have found that IGF-I and IGFBP-3 concentrations are valuable screening tests for inadequate GH secretion in childhood with specificities above 70% [37], although this is not universally agreed [38]. Values of IGF-I above –1 SD for age in children effectively exclude GHD, and values of IGF-I and IGFBP-3 below –2 SDS strongly suggest an abnormality of GH secretion or action.

The physician must consider other causes of low IGF-I concentrations in addition to GHD, such as malnutrition and chronic disease, before the diagnosis of GHD is made. If IGF-I or IGFBP-3 concentrations are *higher* than –1 SD below the mean for age, GH–IGF axis dysfunction is unlikely. Non-

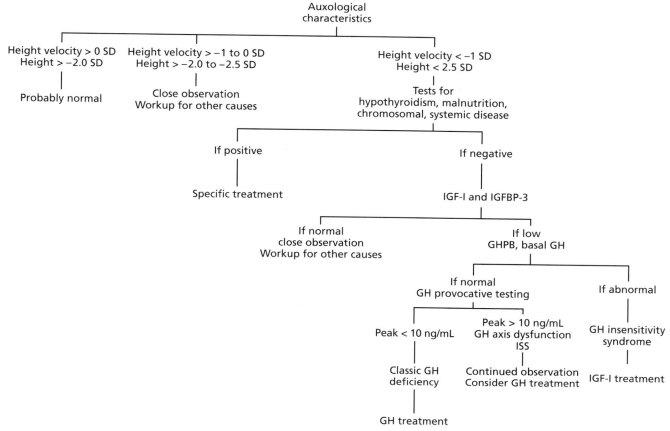

**Fig. 10.3.** Diagnostic approach to short stature.

hormonal causes of short stature should be reconsidered, and the child should be followed to determine the rate of growth. If IGF-I or IGFBP-3 is *lower* than –1 SD below the mean for age, GH–IGF axis dysfunction is likely, and further investigation of the GH–IGF axis is indicated. This may include the measurement of GHBP, basal GH, IGF-II, IGFBP-2, GH provocative testing or GH secretion studies to further document the abnormality in the GH–IGF axis.

If basal GH is elevated or GHBP is less than 2 SD below the mean, the patient has GH-insensitivity syndrome (GHIS). This includes Laron syndrome and variants, which are due to abnormalities of the GHR. Treatment with IGF-I is likely to be effective. The physician must be aware of other causes of the combination of high basal GH and low GHBP, which include malnutrition and chronic disease.

Children with a height between –2 and –2.5 SD and/or a height velocity between –1 and 0 SD for age should be carefully observed and may require further testing. If the history and physical examination are unable to assure the physician of the child's normality, initial laboratory investigation can include an assessment of thyroid and renal function [$T_4$, TSH, BUN (blood urea nitrogen) or creatinine], a screen for the presence of chronic inflammatory disease [ESR (erythrocyte sedimentation rate) or other], a $CO_2$ to assess the possibility of renal tubular acidosis, a complete blood count (CBC), and others as indicated. Determining bone age may also be useful in the evaluation of the short child, but only for height prediction purposes. Karyotypes should be performed in females with otherwise unexplained significant short stature and in males with significant anomalies.

In cases where short stature seems likely to be associated with an abnormality of GH secretion, provocative testing of GH may be of value. It should be carried out only after careful evaluation has revealed a clinical picture consistent with GHD. Provocative GH testing in children uses many standardized protocols. A peak value of GH in two provocative tests below 10 ng/mL in a polyclonal GH RIA (radioimmunoassay) (or equivalent lower value in two-site GH assays) is consistent with GHD in a child. Sex hormone priming may be needed in cases of constitutional delay of growth and puberty to distinguish this normal variant from GHD.

If the GH peak is less than 10 ng/mL in a polyclonal RIA or an equivalent lower value in a two-site GH assay, the diagnosis of classic GHD is made. It is important to use a GH assay that has been well validated and standardized, and that the variability in GH assays, testing and normal responses must be recognized. There are many potential pitfalls in the interpretation of provocative testing of GH secretion, and both false positives and negatives are frequent [39].

Once the diagnosis of classic GHD is established, a thorough evaluation for other pituitary hormone deficiencies and magnetic resonance imagining (MRI) of the head should be carried out to establish the cause and degree of hypothalamic or pituitary disease. GH treatment is clearly indicated in these cases. If the GH peak on provocative testing is greater than 10, the diagnosis is unclear. Some possibilities include GH insufficiency, idiopathic short stature, partial GH insensitivity and malnutrition. Careful clinical follow-up is indicated, and GH treatment may be considered if the growth rate is persistently low and no other cause of growth failure is found.

The approved indications for GH treatment are for children with significant short stature due to inadequate GH secretion, for adults with GHD and associated changes in body composition, energy level, strength and metabolism, for children with Turner syndrome and poor growth, and chronic renal failure with a poor growth rate. Turner patients can be treated with GH without the necessity of testing GH secretion. Children with poor growth as a result of chronic renal failure can also be treated with GH without the necessity of testing of GH secretion.

A child with GH secretion not consistent with the diagnosis of classic GHD but with significant short stature and persistently low growth rate for age may still be considered for a trial of GH treatment, especially if there is a history of hypothalamo-pituitary disease or cranial irradiation [23].

## Tall stature

Children and adolescents with height more than 2 SD or above the 97th centile are considered tall. There are many causes (Table 10.2), but most tall children are normal and come from tall families or genetic groups. As a group, they may have higher rates of GH secretion and higher concentrations of IGF-I [40]. These findings suggest that at least one of the reasons underlying tall stature is a genetically determined increase in GH secretion and/or action. Another common cause is overnutrition (especially in infancy), leading to exogenous obesity. Studies of obesity in childhood have demonstrated that almost all of the patients are above the 50th percentile of height for age, irrespective of their genetic background, and a high proportion of them are above the 97th percentile of height for age. Owing to neuroendocrine reasons that are not fully defined, these obese children have relatively low secretion of GH, as determined both by physiological and pharmacological stimulation [41].

There are well-documented instances of pituitary tumours with excess GH secretion leading to tall stature, including the famous Alton Giant [42]. These tumours are exceedingly rare.

**Table 10.2.** Causes of tall stature

Non-pathological tall stature
  Genetic/familial
  Obesity

Pituitary gigantism

Hyperthyroidism

Sex hormone-related causes
  Precocious puberty
  Hypogonadotrophic hypogonadism

Adrenal hormone-related causes
  Precocious adrenarche
  Adrenogenital syndrome
  Adrenal tumours

Genetic causes of tall stature
  Disorder of sex chromosomes
    Kleinfelter syndrome (XXY)
    Extra Y (XYY, XYYY, etc.)
  Genetic syndromes
    Marfan syndrome
    Homocystinuria
    Cerebral gigantism (Sotos syndrome)
    Weaver syndrome

It is important to exclude this possibility in rapidly growing children, and a serum level of IGF-I is probably an adequate screen for pituitary secretion of excess GH.

Hyperthyroidism is associated with tall stature in childhood [42]. These patients may grow rapidly under the influence of high concentrations of thyroid hormone, but their epiphyseal centres also mature faster so that they finish their growth prematurely.

Precocious puberty is well known to be associated with relatively tall stature [43], and it is the best clinical illustration of the role of sex hormone secretion in growth. Delayed puberty as a result of hypogonadotrophic gonadotrophism, oestrogen receptor deficiency, aromatase deficiency or Kallmann syndrome can be also associated with tall stature late in childhood or in early adult life. The explanation is that although these children grow relatively slowly during the time that other children their age are undergoing their pubertal growth spurt, they continue to grow long after the majority of children have reached the end of puberty and can eventually attain a tall stature. In fact, even children with physiological delayed puberty can end up tall for their age, as illustrated by the growth data on the eighteenth-century German poet Schiller [44].

Adrenal causes of tall stature are common. Children with precocious adrenarche, in which there is an increased secretion of adrenal androgens early in childhood associated with the other events in puberty, can have rapid growth rates and develop clinically significant tall stature. Children with congenital adrenal hyperplasia can present with tall stature along with signs of adrenal stimulation and the early development of secondary sex characteristics [45]. This syndrome of early development and relatively tall stature for age can also be seen with functioning adrenal tumours, leading to androgen secretion. Patients with tall stature as a result of hypersecretion of androgens fuse their epiphyses early and have short or low-normal adult height.

The genetic influence on the non-pathological causes of tall stature, including familial and ethnic group related, have already been discussed. In addition, Klinefelter syndrome (XXY karyotype) as well as genetic males with extra Y chromosomes (XYY, XYYY, etc.) can also present with tall stature [46]. Marfan syndrome and homocystinuria, and cerebral gigantism (Sotos syndrome), are also relatively common genetic syndromes that are associated with tall stature [47].

## Management of tall stature

Just as is true of the other disorders of body size, the majority of tall children are normal. Thus, the family history is very important in these cases. As most cases are not pathological but related to genetic hormones, an important first step is to determine the target height expected for the child from the height of the parents (Fig. 10.4). This target range can be used to reassure the parents and child in many instances. In most cases the issue uppermost in the minds of the parents and to a

certain extent the child is not so much the height at the moment of consultation but a concern about what the ultimate stature of the child will be. Thus, it is important to make predictions of adult height that have some validity. The Bailey–Pinneau tables are the best method for predicting adult height in patients with tall stature. The physical examination can provide important clues that alert the physician to the potential presence of a pathological condition. Normally the arm span should not exceed the child's height by more than 5 cm.

For the standards for sitting height and the upper-to-lower ratios (where the length of the upper and lower body segments are measured from the pubic symphysis) the physician should consult nomograms. Most very tall normal individuals have long extremities, although they do not exceed the normal range. The presence of a truly eunichoid habitus with disproportionately long limbs should lead to further evaluation of a possible pathological condition. The failure of normal pubertal development with closure of the epiphyses of the long bones can lead to disproportionately long limbs. This can be due to gonadal failure, but other causes of an abnormal puberty need to be considered. Patients with aromatase deficiency or oestrogen receptor mutations have much delayed bone maturation and continue to grow into their third decade of life. They do not have tall stature during childhood, but tall stature can be seen in the late teenage years and beyond.

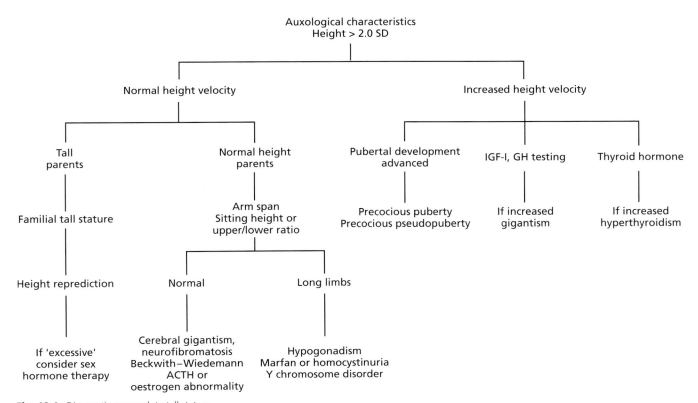

**Fig. 10.4.** Diagnostic approach to tall stature.

Klinefelter syndrome (47,XYY karyotype) and individuals with karyotypes XYY and XXYY may present with tall stature even before puberty, and manifest disproportionate long extremities before and during puberty. Klinefelter syndrome is the most common abnormality of sex chromosomes in postnatal life with an incidence of 1 out of 600 live births, but it presents only rarely to the paediatric endocrinologist because most of the children have growth patterns in childhood and adolescence within the broad range of normal.

Marfan syndrome (arachnodactyly) may also present with tall stature and relatively long extremities. The impression of long extremities in these patients is magnified by their poor muscular mass and arachnodactyly. It is now known that Marfan syndrome is caused by fibrin deficiency. It is an autosomal dominant disorder, but has quite variable penetrance so that not all patients are diagnosed. It is therefore important to carefully examine the parents and siblings for signs of the disorder. Marfan syndrome is also manifested by eye and heart abnormalities, and requires continuous follow-up by a cardiologist. A near phenocopy of Marfan syndrome is homocystinuria. The physical habitus of patients with homocystinuria is strikingly similar to Marfan syndrome, but the abnormalities of the eye are distinct. Homocystinuria can be diagnosed by a simple urinary nitroprusside test.

A record of the child's growth in previous years is extremely important in evaluating these children. Accelerated growth is observed in cerebral gigantism (Sotos syndrome) only in the first 2 years of life, followed by normal growth rate and normal final height. The facial features of these patients may resemble acromegaly and mental retardation is variable. Beckwith–Wiedemann syndrome results from overexpression of IGF-I in fetal life. These babies are big at birth with organomegaly, and they frequently have omphalocoele and hypoglycaemia. They may continue to grow rapidly during the first year of life but thereafter have a normal growth rate.

Other rare causes of tall stature are associated with endocrine abnormalities. Patients with isolated glucocorticoid deficiency due to partially inactivating mutations of the ACTH receptor are tall in childhood, and their bone age (BA) is advanced. Neurofibromatosis may be associated with unexplained tall stature or with optic glioma and gigantism in the absence of a pituitary adenoma. True pituitary gigantism as a result of increased GH secretion is extremely rare. It may be due to a GH-secreting pituitary adenoma or to a GHRH-secreting pancreatic carcinoma. IGF-I concentrations are almost always more than 2 SD above the mean for age level, and this serves as a reasonable screening test for true gigantism. Serum GH cannot be suppressed by a glucose load or TRH. In selected cases where the diagnosis is unclear, a GH profile at 20-min intervals over at least 8 h may be necessary and should show no return to nadir serum GH of less than 2 μg/L. Cranial MRI will usually be diagnostic of a pituitary lesion, and an abdominal CT (computerized tomography) should demonstrate the pancreatic carcinoma in those

unusual cases with GHRH secretion as a cause of increased GH secretion and gigantism. Growth acceleration may also be seen in prolonged untreated patients with hyperthyroidism. In these cases the bone age is advanced and the symptoms and signs of hyperthyroidism are present.

## Therapy

The decision about growth-reducing therapy has to be made by the patient and her/his parents in collaboration with the medical care team. The medical information presented by the physician should address current knowledge of the physical and mental benefits and the risks of the two options, tall stature or sex steroid therapy. The efficacy of therapy after puberty has commenced is doubtful, whereas the cautious induction of early puberty is bound to limit the final height in the same way as does natural precocious puberty.

## The overweight child

There has been a spectacular increase in the percentage of overweight children in Western societies in the past decades [48]. The reasons for this increase are multiple, but changes in diet and activity patterns are paramount. The amount of fat in the diet of children has increased considerably in the past few decades, at least partly linked to the growth of the fast food industry. The reasons for the decrease in physical activity in children certainly relate to the increase in time spent watching television [49] and the disappearance of physical education programmes from many schools. The net result is that children on the average are taking in more calories and expending fewer calories, with the natural result being an increase in the average adiposity.

The increase in adiposity in children is also mirrored by a great increase in the average adiposity of adults. As there is a high correlation of obese children becoming obese adults, an increase in adiposity in childhood is the harbinger of the even greater public health problem of adult obesity, with all of its accompanying health problems [50].

Many methods have been used to quantify obesity. Of the sophisticated tools available, careful measurement of height and weight are among the most useful and accurate. One of the most useful has been the body mass index (BMI) [51]. The BMI is calculated as the weight in kilograms divided by the height in meters squared (BMI = weight/height$^2$). The normal adult values for BMI are 19–22 kg/m$^2$ but it is important to use age-related standards in children.

Weight may also be expressed as a percentage of the ideal weight for age and height, and there are standard tables available for this calculation. Obesity can be defined according to the per cent overweight above the ideal weight for height, with greater than 120% of ideal body weight being considered mild obesity, and greater than 130% of ideal body weight being defined as severe obesity. Although both of these numbers provide a relatively convenient way to estimate relative adiposity, they both suffer from the fact that they do not really always reflect adiposity. An athletic youngster with relatively increased muscle mass can easily have a BMI and percentage of ideal body weight that suggest obesity, but not have any increase in body fat. Therefore, other methods have been developed to attempt to measure body adiposity more directly.

These methods include skinfold thickness [52], bioelectric impedance [53], underwater weighing and the use of imaging techniques such as ultrasound, CT and MRI [54]. All of these methods have certain weaknesses. The use of skinfold thickness requires an operator experienced at using skinfold callipers in a reproducible way. Bioelectric impedance, while relatively easy to perform, does not always reflect adiposity accurately and requires an electronic instrument not available in many clinics. Underwater weighing does give an accurate assessment of body density, but requires equipment that is not readily available to the physician in practice. Ultrasound, CT and MRI can directly visualize body fat and distinguish it from other body compartments and therefore might be considered the state of the art. However, they all require specialized equipment and are too expensive to be anything but research tools.

The primary control of body fat is the balance between dietary intake and energy expenditure. In normal circumstances the amount of body fat is tightly regulated by a control of appetite and satiety by hypothalamic centres. Recent work has delineated the existence of a feedback hormone secreted from adipose tissue, known as leptin, which plays a role in the hypothalamic control of appetite [55]. Although disorders of leptin are the primary cause of human obesity in only very rare instances, it can be hoped that further research in this area will lead to a better understanding of the control of satiety, and may even result in useful new therapies.

There are a variety of well-known risk hormones for the development of obesity in childhood. It has been estimated [56] that 40% of obesity is due to genetic factors [57]. This may reflect inherited difference in the feedback control of appetite or metabolism so that when exposed to an environment in which calories and fat intake are not limited the subject will become obese. Some of these as yet undefined genetic factors may have had survival value earlier in evolution when recurrent famine was common, but in modern affluent societies they can lead to severe overweight and its associated health problems. It is unclear how much familial risk is due to genetics and how much is due to environmental influences such as family dietary and activity patterns.

By far the most common cause of obesity in childhood is environmentally determined obesity ('simple obesity'). The most important clinical clue that this is the diagnosis is the presence of above-average stature. Almost all of the children with simple obesity have a height above the 50th percentile

for age, and the majority of them have a height above the 75th percentile for age. Thus, the measurement of a child's stature at a single stroke eliminates essentially all of the pathological causes of obesity if it is above average. In addition these children frequently have a family history of overweight. They may have a slightly advanced BA and as a group have a relatively early onset of puberty. Psychological disturbances are commonly present. It is difficult or impossible to determine whether the psychological disturbance is the primary cause of the obesity, or is a secondary consequence of the obesity. Obese children are frequently treated differently by their peers and adults. The metabolic effects accompanying the development of severe obesity include hyperinsulinaemia and glucose intolerance, hyperlipidaemia, hypertension, coronary heart diseases, sleep apnoea, and hirsutism.

If an obese child is of below-average stature, particularly if there is evidence of a decreased growth rate, the pathological causes of obesity must be considered [58]. Endocrine causes are present in a small minority of obese children, but they are important for several reasons. First of all, they are eminently diagnosable and treatable. They are also important because many parents, and referring physicians, are looking for an explanation other than simple obesity and will not be satisfied unless they feel that these potential endocrine causes of overweight are addressed in a serious way. The endocrine causes of obesity are hypothyroidism, steroid excess and GHD.

In hypothyroidism obesity is due to decreased energy expenditure. In addition to the well-known abnormalities of TSH and thyroxine, a markedly low BA may be found.

Steroid excess can be due either to exogenous administration or to an increase in endogenous production. Even a small excess of steroids above physiological concentrations can cause obesity in childhood. In most cases, the administration of exogenous glucocorticoids is linked to a disease state and is immediately obvious from the medical history. The rarer endogenous causes of steroid excess, Cushing disease and the even more unusual cases of excess production of adrenocorticotrophin homologues or glucocorticoid steroids from a tumour, can be much more difficult to diagnose. In childhood, severe obesity is relatively uncommon in Cushing disease, and the hallmarks of the syndrome are a decrease in growth rate, hypertension, plethora, mild to moderate obesity of predominately central distribution and striae. The presence of a 'buffalo hump' is not particularly helpful in the paediatric age group. The biochemical abnormalities in Cushing syndrome in childhood may be relatively subtle and open to conflicting interpretations. A 24-h urine free cortisol may be the most sensitive single screening test. The determination of a serum cortisol, especially at a time when it is normally low, and Cortrosyn stimulation tests also play important roles in the approach to the diagnosis of Cushing disease. Specific aetiology is further diagnosed by low- and high-dose dexamethasone suppression tests and by imaging studies.

GHD can also present with obesity. Growth retardation and mild truncal obesity may be the only presenting signs of GHD. In more severe cases the syndrome is more complete. With GH therapy there is a decrease in fat mass because of the lipolytic effect of GH, and the obesity subsides rapidly.

All of these endocrine causes of short obesity share the concomitant presence of a low growth rate, and almost always a stature below the average for age. Therefore, the vast majority of children with obesity can be confidently said not to have any endocrine disease as a cause of their short stature. However, in the unusual cases in which it appears that an endocrine disorder may be the root cause of obesity, it must be borne in mind that obesity itself can cause abnormalities of endocrine physiology.

These endocrine consequences include low serum GH, high GHBP and normal IGF-I and IGFBP-3. The cortisol secretion rate is increased, as are urinary 17-hydroxycorticosteroids and 17-hydroxyketosteroids, but serum cortisol is normal. In the male, serum testosterone is decreased and oestrogen increased, and in the female both oestrogen and androgen are increased. Insulin resistance is frequently present. All of these secondary endocrine effects of obesity must be kept in mind when interpreting the results of any endocrine testing.

As the major control mechanisms of appetite and satiety reside in the hypothalamus, it is not surprising that a wide variety of central nervous system (CNS) tumours, malformation and damage can result in abnormal weight gain. In many cases these diagnoses are obvious from the medical history or the presence of compulsive eating or lack of satiety. However, in some cases the hypothalamic disturbance is masked and needs to be investigated specifically. There are other cases, such as pseudohypoparathyroidism or Prader–Willi syndrome, in which the root cause of obesity is felt to be a hypothalamic disorder but the nature of the lesion has not been defined. One can also obtain a history of birth or casualty trauma of the hypothalamus. Hypothalamic tumours may lead to uncontrollable appetite. Any time a hypothalamic lesion is suspected an MRI is indicated.

There are a variety of syndromes that frequently have obesity as one of their common presenting features (Table 10.3). Some have chromosomal defects as their aetiology. Perhaps the most common of these to present to a paediatric endocrinologist is Prader–Willi syndrome. This syndrome has been associated with abnormalities of chromosome 15 [59]. Typically there is hypotonia in infancy, which can be severe enough to come to the attention of a neurologist. The onset of obesity is usually at 1–4 years of age. These patients frequently have small chubby hands and feet, and hypogonadism. Undescended testes and a small penis are frequently seen in the male. They may also have mild to moderate mental retardation. Now that there are specific chromosomal methods available to diagnose this syndrome, it has become clear that there is actually a wide variation in the clinical presentation of this

**Table 10.3.** Causes of obesity

Environmentally determined obesity (simple obesity)

Pathological disturbances as a cause of obesity
  Endocrine
    Hypothyroidism
    GHD
    Steroid excess
  Hypothalamic disturbances
    CNS tumours and damage
    Pseudohypoparathyroidism
  Syndromes as a cause of obesity
    Chromosomal defects
      Prader–Willi
      Klinefelter
      Down
    Genetic defects
      Laurence–Moon–Biedl

disorder. Therefore, the physician dealing with obese children must have a high index of suspicion for disorders of chromosome 15. Other chromosomal disorders that can be associated with overweight include Turner syndrome, Klinefelter syndrome and Down syndrome.

A large number of additional genetic causes of overweight in childhood have been described. Alstrom syndrome is an autosomal recessive disease. These children have the onset of obesity at 2–5 years of age. Like Prader–Willi syndrome, the males may have hypogonadism. However, they have normal growth and mental development, and no chromosomal abnormality has been demonstrated. Laurence–Moon–Biedl syndrome is also an autosomal recessive disorder. The onset of obesity is at 1–2 years of age and stature may be normal or short. Polydactyly, retinitis pigmentosa with early night blindness and hypogonadism are usually present. Mild renal failure and a defect in urinary concentration may be present. Carpenter syndrome is an autosomal recessive disorder characterized by facial and limb dysmorphism with normal growth and mild mental retardation. Patients with Cohen syndrome have a history of hypotonia, like Prader–Willi syndrome, but their onset of obesity is at mid-childhood. They have narrow hands and feet with characteristic faces. Beckwith–Wiedemann syndrome presents in infancy with macrosomia, visceromegaly, neonatal hyperinsulinaemic hypoglycaemia. They may have postnatal gigantism and increased subcutaneous fat, and an increased muscle mass, including macroglossia. These patients have an increased incidence of malignancies, especially Wilms tumour, and must be under long-term surveillance because of this. This interesting syndrome is caused by problems with the imprinting of the IGF-II gene.

The discovery of leptin as at least one component of the feedback loop from adipocytes to the hypothalamic control of appetite generated hope that this hormone might explain a significant number of patients with severe obesity and perhaps even be a new therapeutic agent [55]. Serum leptin is positively correlated with the degree of obesity; however, leptin deficiency in humans is very rare, and attempts to treat simple obesity with synthetic leptin have not had impressive results.

Probably the most frequent syndrome associated with obesity in childhood is polycystic ovarian disease (PCO) and its variants. These patients represent an extension of what is now called 'syndrome X' or 'metabolic syndrome' in adults [60]. The hallmarks of this disorder are obesity, insulin resistance and hypertension. Signs of hyperandrogenism and acanthosis nigricans are frequently present. In the females with this disorder there are frequently menstrual irregularities and high concentrations of LH. There may be an association between the development of metabolic syndrome and small for gestational age birth, although this point is still disputed.

## An approach to diagnosis and management

The physician evaluating overweight children should realize that the majority do not have a pathological cause of their problem. The first step in the diagnostic approach to overweight is the measurement of height, and the determination of how the child's height compares with age-related standards (Fig. 10.5). If the child's height is above the 50% for age, one can argue that no other test needs to done, unless there

are other unusual features in the history or physical examination. This overweight child will need to be enrolled in a therapeutic programme that includes environmental manipulation and behavioural modification.

Other diagnostic clues may be found in the physical examination. There are two major distinct patterns of fat distribution seen. Feminine (or gynoid) distribution is predominantly peripheral or lower-body obesity. Masculine (or android) distribution is obesity predominantly of the central parts of the body including the abdomen. A central pattern of adiposity is associated with an increased risk for cardiovascular morbidity and can be found in Cushing syndrome. The presence of hirsutism suggests either a disorder of steroid production or PCO. The finding of acanthosis nigricans is correlated with the presence of insulin resistance. In PCO the onset of obesity is in late prepuberty or puberty. The presence of menstrual disorders, hirsutism and acne increase the suspicion of PCO. Any significant decrease in the degree of obesity will ameliorate virilization. Glucose intolerance develops in patients with obesity, and more so when acanthosis nigricans is present, and often leads to the onset of type II diabetes mellitus. Familial obesity can be related to known genetic diseases, unknown genetic hormones, the family eating habits or a combination of all of them. The success rate of weight reduction is lower in familial obesity.

Another set of causes of pathological obesity is drugs. Several phenothiazines, antidepressants, valproate and carbamazepine and glucocorticoids (at doses above replacement) all increase body weight.

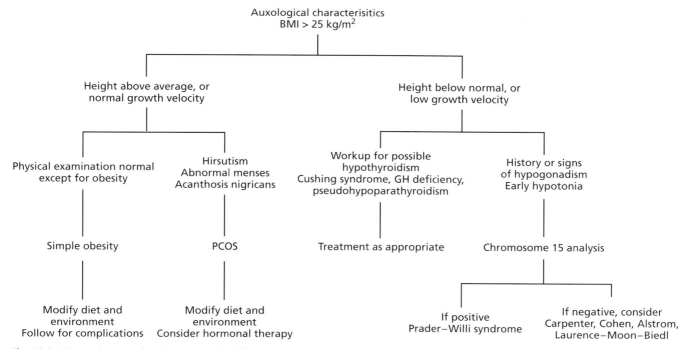

**Fig. 10.5.** Diagnostic approach to the overweight child. PCOS, polycystic ovary syndrome.

Obesity with growth retardation may occasionally be the presenting sign of craniopharyngioma. However, more commonly, morbid obesity develops after the partial or complete removal of the craniopharyngioma. Many of these children develop massive obesity postoperatively and frequently have normal growth despite GHD. Whether this growth without the apparent presence of GH is due to hyperinsulinaemia, hyperprolactinaemia, the maintenance of normal IGF-I concentrations in these patients or a combination of all of these hormones is unclear [61].

## The underweight child

A child who has a weight less than 70% of the average for age or a BMI of less than 17 kg/m² can be regarded as underweight. As is true of other disorders of size in childhood, the physician must keep in mind that many of these children do not have a pathological state. The causes of underweight in children are outlined in Table 10.4. There is no doubt that the most common cause worldwide is malnutrition. This is an important public health and political problem, although not one whose therapy is within the purview of the paediatrician and endocrinologist.

Thin children are usually part of a familial, ethnic or cultural picture. The exact balance that genetics and culturally determined nutritional patterns play is unclear. Such cases rarely come to the attention of an endocrinologist, either because the family recognizes this as a familial pattern or because of the attitude common in industrialized societies that 'you can never be too rich or too thin' [62]. The responsibility of the physician is to ensure that no element of malnutrition is present and that there is no pathological cause. A careful history, including nutritional attitudes and food intake, family history, feeding practices and bowel habits can usually determine such a cause.

Gastrointestinal disease is probably the most common cause of underweight not due to abnormalities of nutrition.

**Table 10.4.** Causes of underweight

---

Malnutrition

The 'normal thin' child
  'You can never be too rich or too thin'

Gastrointestinal disease

Eating disorders
  Anorexia nervosa
  Bulimia

Athletic syndromes

Endocrine disorders

---

Frequently, but not always, there is a history of gas, abdominal cramping, frequent bowel movements or abnormal stools to alert the physician to the presence of these disorders. However, frequently these signs are not present and the child presents with only a slow growth rate and short stature, with or without underweight. For this reason, many paediatric endocrinologists screen for the presence of coeliac disease with antiendomysial antibodies, and inflammatory bowel disease with a sedimentation rate as part of their routine evaluation of the underweight child. In selected instances, referral to a gastroenterologist for evaluation is indicated.

Eating disorders are common. In Western society, the incidence of both anorexia nervosa and bulimia is increasing [63]. The very nature of these disorders means that patients go to great lengths to hide their disease from their parents and friends, to the extent of prevaricating about their food intake and habits. These disorders must be searched for carefully in cases of underweight, especially in adolescent girls. Careful questioning about body image and attitudes towards food will usually lead to an indication that an eating disorder may be present. Discussion with the parents and children about their attitudes towards food and body shape are also frequently revealing. Referral of these cases to a specialist in eating disorders and their treatment should be strongly considered if there is a reasonable suspicion that an eating disorder might be present.

Another frequent cause of underweight in the adolescent is what has been called athletic syndromes [64]. In these cases, the underlying cause of underweight is poor nutrition, but it is done deliberately in association with a strong motivation to succeed in some athletic endeavour. This is frequently associated with gymnastics and ballet, whose participants often hold a strong opinion that thin is better, or wrestling, where there is pressure to achieve the lowest practicable weight class for competition. These children are frequently more open about their food habits than those with eating disorders, but treatment is frequently complex and requires an understanding approach and the involvement of other health professionals, the coaches and the parents. The physician's responsibility is to ensure that appropriate evaluation and treatment are available, and that no other cause of underweight is present.

Endocrine disorders can present with underweight, although they are probably the rarest causes. Addison disease can present with weight loss: usually the history of vomiting, weakness and increasing pigmentation is obtained. Hyperthyroidism can also present as a wasting disease and may not always have other obvious clinical features.

## Management

The diagnostic approach to the underweight child is outlined in Fig. 10.6. The important first step is to determine

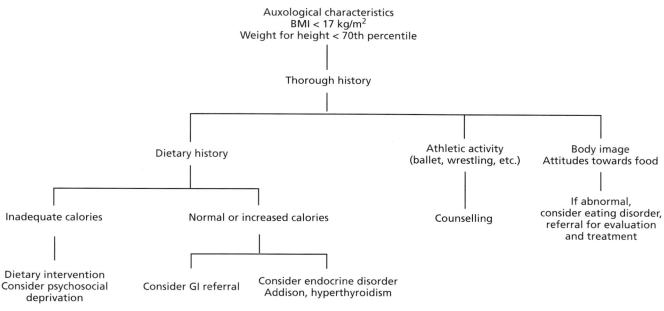

**Fig. 10.6.** Diagnostic approach to the underweight child.

whether the child is in fact abnormally thin. If so, the focus must be on careful evaluation of the dietary intake. This requires a thorough history, focused especially on the type and quantity of food, the attitudes towards food and body image of the patient and parent, and any history of disturbance of bowel function or gastrointestinal distress. It is also important to determine whether the child is engaged in an activity in which thinness is considered an advantage, such as ballet, gymnastics or wrestling. Any indication of a gastrointestinal disorder or eating disorder should lead to an immediate referral to a specialist in the appropriate area. Only in the rare instance where the history or physical examination warrant should endocrine investigation be undertaken.

## Summary and conclusion

The physician dealing with paediatric problems should always be alert to abnormalities in growth as an important clue to the underlying health of the patient. Advances in the understanding of the control of growth have led not only to better understanding but also to better diagnosis and therapy of growth disorders. Many growth disorders are associated with disorders of pubertal development and therefore may present to the clinician dealing with paediatric and adolescent gynaecological problems. A thorough understanding of the hormones controlling growth should allow the clinician to approach the diagnosis and management of disorders of growth in a logical and efficient manner.

## References

1 Lechan RM. Neuroendocrinology of pituitary hormone regulation. *Endocrinol Metab Clin N Am* 1987; 16: 475–501.
2 Van Assche FA, Holemans K, Aerts L. Fetal growth and consequences for later life. *J Perinat Med* 1998; 26: 337–46.
3 Hintz RL. Growth hormones. *Curr Opin Pediat* 1990; 2: 786–93.
4 Reichlin S. Neuroendocrinology. In: Wilson JD, Foster DW, eds. *Williams Textbook of Endocrinology*, 9th edn. Philadelphia: W. B. Saunders, 1998: 165–248.
5 Baumann G. GH heterogeneity: genes, isohormones, variants, and binding proteins. *Endocrinol Rev* 1991; 12: 424–49.
6 Muller EE, Locatelli V, Cocchi D. Neuroendocrine control of GH secretion. *Physiol Rev* 1999; 79: 511–607.
7 Chapman IM, Hartman ML, Pezzoli SS *et al*. Effect of aging on the sensitivity of GH secretion to insulin-like growth hormone-I negative feedback. *J Clin Endocrinol Metabolism* 1997; 82: 2996–3004.
8 Spencer SA, Leung DW, Godowski PJ, Hammonds RG, Waters MJ, Wood WI. GH receptor and binding protein. *Recent Prog Horm Res* 1990; 46: 1652–81.
9 Hintz RL. The somatomedin hypothesis of GH Action. In: Kostyo J, Goodman HM, eds. *A Handbook of Physiology: Section 7: the Endocrine System*: Vol. V. *Hormonal Control of Growth*. New York: Oxford University Press, 1999: 481–500.
10 Rechler MM, Nissley SP. Insulin-like growth hormone (IGF)/somatomedin receptor subtypes: structure, function, and relationships to insulin receptors and IGF carrier proteins. *Horm Res* 1986; 24: 152–9.
11 Morley JE. Neuroendocrine control of thyrotropin secretion. *Endocr Rev* 1981; 2: 396–436.

12 Giustina A, Wehrenberg WB. Influence of thyroid hormones on the regulation of GH secretion. *Eur J Endocrinol* 1995; 133: 646–53.

13 August GP, Grombach MM, Kaplan SL. Hormonal changes in puberty. III. Correlation of plasma testosterone, LH, FSH, testicular size and bone age with male pubertal development. *J Clin Endocrinol Metab* 1972; 34: 319–26.

14 Tanner JM. Growth and endocrinology of the adolescent. In: Gardner L, ed. *Endocrine and Genetic Disease of Childhood*, 2nd edn. Philadelphia: W. B. Saunders, 1975: 14–64.

15 Robyn JA, Koch CA, Montalto J, Yong A, Warne GL, Batch JA. Cushing's syndrome in childhood and adolescence. *J Paediatr Child Health* 1997; 33: 522–7.

16 Hintz RL, Suskind R, Amatayakul K, Leitzmann C, Olson RE. Somatomedin and GH in children with protein calorie malnutrition. *J Pediatr* 1978; 92: 153–6.

17 Tanner JM, Goldstein H, Whitehouse RH. Standards for children's height at ages 2–9 years allowing for height of parents. *Arch Dis Child* 1970; 45: 755–62.

18 Horton WA. Fibroblast growth hormone receptor 3 and the human chondrodysplasias. *Curr Opin Pediatr* 1997; 9: 437–42.

19 Savage MO, Beattie RM, Camacho-Hubner C, Walker-Smith JA, Sanderson IR. Growth in Crohn's disease. *Acta Paediatr Suppl* 1999; 88: 89–92.

20 Tanner JM, Goldstein H, Whitehouse RH. Standards for children's height at ages 2–9 years allowing for height of parents. *Arch Dis Child* 1970; 45: 755–62.

21 Vimpani GV, Vimpani AF, Lidgard GP, Cameron EHD, Farqhuar JW. Prevalence of severe GH deficiency. *Br Med J* 1977; 2: 427–30.

22 Parkn JM. Incidence of GH deficiency. *Arch Dis Child* 1974; 49: 904–5.

23 Hintz RL, Attie KM, Baptista J, Roche A. Effect of GH treatment on adult height of children with idiopathic short stature. Genentech Collaborative Group. *N Engl J Med* 1999; 340: 502–7.

24 Paz I, Seidman DS, Danon YL, Laor A, Stevenson DK, Gale R. Are children born small for gestational age at increased risk of short stature? *Am J Dis Child* 1993; 147: 337–9.

25 Sung I, Vohr B, Oh W. Growth and neurodevelopmental outcome of very low birth weight infants with intrauterine growth retardation: comparison with control subjects matched by birth weight and gestational age. *J Pediatr* 1993; 123: 618–24.

26 Karlberg J, Albertsson-Wikland K. Spontaneous growth and final height in SGA infants. *Pediatr Res* 1993; 33: 5.

27 Hintz RL. GH Deficiency. In: Kelnar CJH, Savage MO, Stirling HF, Saenger P, eds. *Growth Disorders: Pathophysiology, Treatment*. London: Chapman & Hall Medical, 1998.

28 Fielder PJ, Guevara-Aguirre J, Rosenbloom AL, Carlsson L, Hintz RL, Rosenfeld RG. Expression of serum insulin-like growth hormones, IGF binding proteins, and the GH-binding protein in heterozygote relatives of Ecuadorian GH-receptor deficiency patients. *J Clin Endocrinol Metab* 1992; 74: 743–50.

29 Ranke MB, Savage MO, Chatelain PG, Preece MA, Rosenfeld RG, Wilton P. Long-term treatment of GH insensitivity syndrome with IGF-I. Results of the European Multicentre Study. The Working Group on GH Insensitivity Syndromes. *Horm Res* 1999; 51: 128–34.

30 Goddard AD, Dowd P, Chernausek S *et al.* Partial growth-hormone insensitivity: the role of growth-hormone receptor mutations in idiopathic short stature. *J Pediatr* 1997; 131: S51–5.

31 Rivkees SA, Bode HH, Crawford JD. Long-term growth in juvenile acquired hypothyroidism: the failure to achieve normal stature. *N Engl J Med* 1988; 318: 599–602.

32 Wilson DM, Kei J, Hintz RL, Rosenfeld RG. Effects of testosterone enanthate treatment for pubertal delay. *Am J Dis Child* 1988; 142: 96–9.

33 Seminara SB, Hayes FJ, Crowley WF Jr. Gonadotropin-releasing hormone deficiency in the human (idiopathic hypogonadotropic hypogonadism and Kallmann's syndrome): pathophysiological and genetic considerations. *Endocr Rev* 1998; 19: 521–39.

34 Newell-Price J, Trainer P, Besser M, Grossman A. The diagnosis and differential diagnosis of Cushing's syndrome and pseudo-Cushing's states. *Endocr Rev* 1998; 19: 647–72.

35 Ranke MB, Pfluger H, Rosendahl W *et al.* Turner syndrome: spontaneous growth in 150 cases and review of the literature. *Eur J Paediatr* 1983; 141: 81–8.

36 Hintz RL, Attie KM, Compton PG, Rosenfeld RG. Multihormonal studies of GH treatment of Turner syndrome: The Genentech National Cooperative Growth Study. In: Albertsson-Wikland K, Lippe B, eds. *Turner Syndrome in a Life-Span Perspective*. Amsterdam: Elsevier, 1995: 167–73.

37 Hintz RL. The role of auxologic and growth hormone measurements in the diagnosis of GH deficiency. *Pediatrics* 1998; 102: 524–6.

38 Mitchell H, Dattani MT, Nanduri V, Hindmarsh PC, Preece MA, Brook CG. Failure of IGF-I and IGFBP-3 to diagnose GH insufficiency. *Arch Dis Child* 1999; 80: 443–7.

39 Rosenfeld RG, Albertsson-Wikland K, Cassorla F *et al.* Diagnostic controversy: the diagnosis of childhood GH deficiency revisited. *J Clin Endocrinol Metab* 1995; 80: 1532–40.

40 Albertsson-Wikland K, Rosberg S. Analysis of 24-hour GH profiles in childhood: relation to growth. *J Clin Endocrinol Metab* 1988; 67: 493–500.

41 Veldhuis JD, Iranmanexh A, Ho KK *et al.* Dual defects in pulsatile GH secretion and clearance subserve the hyposomatotropism of obesity in man. *J Clin Endocrinol Metab* 1991; 72: 51–9.

42 Wong GW, Lai J, Cheng PS. Growth in childhood thyrotoxicosis. *Eur J Pediatr* 1999; 158: 776–9.

43 Neely EK, Hintz RL, Parker B, Bachrach LK, Cohen P, Olney R, Wilson DW. Two year results of treatment with depot leuprolide acetate therapy for central precocious puberty. *J Pediatr* 1992; 121: 634–40.

44 Tanner JM. *A History of the Study of Human Growth*. Cambridge: Cambridge University Press, 1981: 106–12.

45 New MI, Newfield RS. Congenital adrenal hyperplasia. *Curr Ther Endocrinol Metab* 1997; 6: 179–87.

46 Robinson A, Lubs HA, Bergsma D. Summary of clinical findings: profiles of children with 47,XXY, 47,XYY, and 47,XXX karyotypes. *Birth Defects* 1982; 18: 1–5.

47 Sotos JF. Overgrowth. Section VI. Genetic syndromes and other disorders associated with overgrowth. *Clin Pediatr* 1997; 36: 157–70.

48 Fredriks AM, van Buuren S, Wit JM, Verloove-Vanhorick SP. Body index measurements in 1996–7 compared with 1980. *Arch Dis Child* 1996; 2000 (82): 107–12.

49 Robinson TN. Reducing children's television viewing to prevent obesity: a randomized controlled trial. *J Am Med Assoc* 1999; 282: 1561–7.

50 Parsons RJ, Power C, Logan S, Summmerbell CD. *Int J Obes Relat Metab Disord* 1999; 23 (Suppl. 8): S1–107.

51 Roland-Cachera M-F, Cole TJ, Sempe M, Tichet J, Rossignol C, Charraud A. Body mass index variations: centile from birth to 87 years. *Eur J Clin Nutr* 1991; 45: 13–21.

52 Brook CGD. Determination of body composition in children from skinfold measurements. *Arch Dis Child* 1971; 48: 725–8.

53 Duerenberg P, Van der Kooy K, Leenan R, Schouten FJM. Body impedance is largely dependent on the intra- and extra-cellular water distribution. *Eur J Clin Nutr* 1989; 43: 845–55.

54 van der Kooy K, Seidell JC. Techniques for the measurement of visceral fat: a practical guide. *Int J Obes* 1993; 17: 187–96.

55 Roemmich JN, Rogol AD. Role of leptin during childhood growth and development. *Endocrinol Metab Clin North Am* 1999; 28: 749–64.

56 Bouchard C. Genetic aspects of human obesity. In: Bjorntorp P, Brodoff BN, eds. *Obesity*. Philadelphia: JB Lippincott, 1992: 343–51.

57 Fogelholm M, Nuutinen O, Pasanen M, Myohanen E, Saatela T. Parent–child relationship of physical activity patterns and obesity. *Int J Obes Relat Metab Disord* 1999; 23: 1262–8.

58 Borjeson M. Overweight children. *Acta Paediatr Scand* 1962; 51 (Suppl. 132): 1–76.

59 Hall JG. Genomic imprinting and its clinical implications. *N Engl J Med* 1992; 326: 827–9.

60 Vanhala M. Childhood weight and metabolic syndrome in adults. *Ann Med* 1999; 31: 236–9.

61 Tiulpakov AN, Mazerkina NA, Brook CG, Hindmarsh PC, Peterkova VA, Gorelyshev SK. Growth in children with cranio-pharyngioma following surgery. *Clin Endocrinol* 1998; 49: 733–8.

62 Wang MC, Ho TF, Anderson JN, Sabry ZI. Reference for thinness in Singapore – a newly industrialized society. *Singapore Med J* 1999; 40: 502–7.

63 Rizvi SL, Stice E, Agras WS. Natural history of disordered eating attitudes and behaviors over a 6-year period. *Int J Eat Disord* 1999; 26: 406–13.

64 Dale KS, Landers DM. Weight control in wrestling: eating disorders or disordered eating? *Med Sci Sports Exerc* 1999; 31: 1382–9.

# 11 The physiology of puberty

## D. M. Styne

## Introduction

The physical and psychological changes of puberty occur because of orderly, sequential changes in endocrine activity. Far from being a *de novo* event in the second decade of life, puberty is a recapitulation of endocrine activity of the fetal and neonate period [1]. Puberty is restrained by the central nervous system during the juvenile pause until the age dictated by genetics for secondary sexual development in that individual.

## Secular trends in puberty

The age of puberty in girls today is earlier than in past centuries, as demonstrated by the decrease in the age of menarche in industrialized European countries and in the USA of 2–3 months per decade over the past 100–150 years (Fig. 11.1) [2]. This trend ceased in the USA in girls born after

1940, probably because of the improvement and stability in socioeconomic conditions, nutritional status and states of health. A survey by the United States National Center for Health Statistics noted the age of menarche in the USA at 12.8 years in 1974 [3,4], and a recent cross-sectional survey in the USA supports this age for this decade. This contrasts with cultures in which the standard of living has changed little and where no trend towards earlier menarche has been documented [5]. Curiously, in Bologna, Italy, the secular trend towards earlier menarche ceased and there is now a trend towards increasing age of menarche, which is postulated to be due to extended psychological stress and possibly increased physical activity [6].

The age of puberty in boys is less well defined and documented than the age of menarche. However, the influence of socioeconomic conditions on the age of male puberty is reflected in the age of voice breaking in the Leipzig chorus of J. S. Bach during the War of Austrian Succession. The boys ceased to function as boy sopranos at a later age in the more stressful war-time years compared with the earlier age of

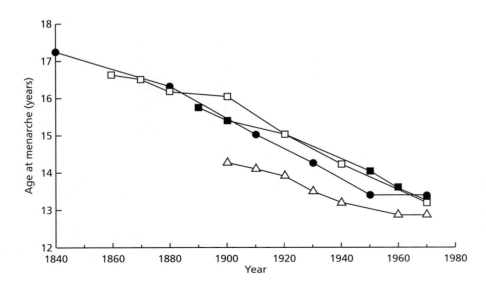

**Fig. 11.1.** Changes in age at menarche, 1840–1978 (redrawn and modified from data in Tanner and Eveleth [157]). Note the decrease of approximately 3 months per decade over the last 150 years and the plateau after 1950–60 in Norway and the USA. □, Finland; ●, Norway; △, USA; ■, Sweden.

voice change (and presumably earlier pubertal development) in times of peace [7]. Further evidence for a later age of puberty in past centuries is provided by the age that boys stopped growing; adult height was not reached until after the age of 20 during the last two centuries compared with 17 years at present [8].

The interaction of nutritional status and puberty is extremely important in areas of the world where the food supply is suboptimal. Delayed puberty is a feature of chronic disease and malnutrition; strenuous physical activity in girls can delay puberty, especially when associated with thin habitus [9]. Moderate obesity is associated with earlier menarche and constitutionally advanced physical development; in contrast, pathological obesity is associated with delayed menarche [10]. Inactive, bedridden children with developmental delay reach menarche at an earlier age and at lower body fat than do similarly delayed children who are more active [11].

Genetic factors play an important role in the onset of puberty, as illustrated by the similar age of menarche between members of an ethnic population; in the USA, African American girls have a mean age of menarche at 12.2 years, whereas Caucasians have an average age of menarche of 12.9 years [5]. The ethnic differences in the age of secondary sexual development remains even if the effects of social or economic factors are eliminated. Further evidence for the genetic influence is the concordance of the age of menarche between mother–daughter pairs. Thus, when socioeconomic and environmental factors lead to optimal nutrition, general health and infant care, the age of onset of puberty in normal children is mainly determined by genetic factors [12].

## Physical changes of puberty

The physical changes in individuals are defined by objective descriptions of the stages of maturation of secondary sexual characteristics [13–16]. These are denoted as Tanner stages or sexual maturation stages. In an attempt to avoid embarrassment of examinations, self-assessment by asking the subject to compare their development with standard drawings of pubertal development may be invoked. Unfortunately, the reproducibility or agreement of self-assessment with physical examinations by physicians is low according to several studies, and physical examination is essential for accurate assessment of puberty [17]. This is even more important in cases where the subject has an aberrant body image, such as in anorexia nervosa [18].

### Female

Many factors contribute to breast formation including growth hormone (GH), insulin-like growth factor I (IGF-I) and insulin but, in terms of development at puberty, the breast is primarily controlled by oestrogen secreted by the ovaries (Figs 11.2 and 11.3). Breast development may be unilateral for several months, which may cause unfounded concern to girls or parents. Indeed, surgical biopsies have been performed inappropriately on girls in whom it was not appreciated that asymmetrical development is normal. Changes in the diameter of the papilla of the nipple are linked to stages of pubertal development, as is the shape and, to some degree, the size of the breast [19]. Nipple papilla diameter does not increase much during pubic hair stage (PH) 1–3 or breast stage (B) 1–3 (diameter 3–4 mm), but it does increase after stage B3, providing an objective method of differentiating stage 4 from 5 (final diameter approximately 9 mm) (Table 11.1). Even though the growth of pubic and axillary hair is mainly under the influence of androgens secreted by the adrenal gland, the stage of breast development is usually equal to the stage of pubic hair development in normal girls (Fig. 11.2). However, since different endocrine organs control

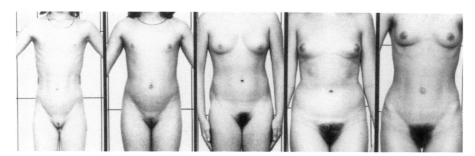

**Fig. 11.2.** Stages of female pubic hair development, modified from Marshall and Tanner [13], Reynolds and Wines [16] and Dupertuis *et al.* [15]. Stage 1: preadolescent; the vellus over the area is not further developed than that over the anterior abdominal wall, i.e. no pubic hair. Stage 2: sparse growth of long, slightly pigmented, downy hair, straight or only slightly curled, appearing chiefly along the labia. This stage is difficult to see on photographs. Stage 3: hair is considerably darker, coarser and curlier. The hair spreads sparsely over the junction of the labia. Stage 4: hair is now adult in type, but the area covered by it is still considerably smaller than in most adults. There is no spread to the medial surface of the thighs. Stage 5: hair is adult in quantity and type, distributed as an inverse triangle of the classic feminine pattern. The spread is to the medial surface of the thighs but not up the linea alba or elsewhere above the base of the inverse triangle.

**Table 11.1.** Nipple diameter vs. breast (B) and pubic hair (PH) stages: comparison of longitudinal and cross-sectional data*

| Stage | Nipple size (mm) | |
|---|---|---|
| | Cross-sectional data | Longitudinal data |
| B1 | 2.89 (0.81) | 3.0 (0.77) |
| B2 | 3.28 (0.89) | 3.37 (0.96) |
| B3 | 4.07 (1.32) | 4.72 (1.40)† |
| B4 | 7.74 (1.64)† | 7.25 (1.46)† |
| B5 | 9.94 (1.38)† | 9.41 (1.45)† |
| PH1 | 2.95 (1.02) | 3.14 (1.31) |
| PH2 | 3.32 (0.91) | 3.69 (1.34) |
| PH3 | 4.11 (1.54) | 4.44 (1.17)† |
| PH4 | 7.15 (1.81)† | 6.54 (1.47)† |
| PH5 | 9.66 (1.59)† | 8.98 (1.56)† |

*Results are means ± SD (in parentheses).
†Significantly different from previous stage, $P < 0.05$. From Rohn [19].

these two processes, the stages of each phenomenon should be classified separately. Although rarely evident in individuals, increase in height velocity rather than breast development is actually the first sign of puberty in girls (Fig. 11.4).

## Ovarian development in puberty

Oogonia arise from the primordial germ cells in the wall of the yolk sac near the caudal end of the embryo. By the sixth month of fetal life, the cells have migrated to the genital ridge and progressed through sufficient mitoses to reach a complement of 6–7 million oogonia [20], which represents the maximal number of primordial follicles the individual will have throughout life. Meiosis begins but is not completed as the nucleus and chromosomes persist in prophase to mark the conversion of the oogonia to primary oocytes. Primordial follicles are composed of the primary oocyte surrounded by

a single layer of spindle-shaped cells, which will develop into granulosa cells, and a basal lamina, which will be the boundary of the theca cells later in development. Because of apoptosis, there are 2–4 million primordial follicles left at birth but only 400 000 remain at menarche [21].

At the time of the first ovulation the first meiotic metaphase converts the primary oocyte into the secondary oocyte, which is extruded into the fallopian tubes [22]. The ovum does not form until the time of sperm penetration, when the second polar body is eliminated. The ovum contains a haploid set of chromosomes to join with the haploid set of chromosomes of the sperm. Although some follicles in the fetus and child progress to the large antral stage, all developing follicles undergo atresia before puberty, and few large follicles develop in the child. However, the presence of more than six follicles with a diameter of more than 4 mm indicates the presence of pulsatile gonadotrophin secretion and may be seen in normal prepubertal girls, in pubertal girls before menarche and in patients recovering from anorexia nervosa. This 'multicystic' appearance is considered characteristic of a phase of mainly nocturnal pulsatile gonadotrophin secretion before positive feedback (Fig. 11.5) [23]. Standards for ovarian and uterine size and shape are available for normal girls and those with Turner syndrome [24–26]. The uterus lies in a craniocaudal direction in childhood without the adult flexion. The myometrium enlarges during early puberty, thereby enlarging the corpus leading to the adult corpus-to-cervix ratio. The cervix develops its adult shape and size just before menarche, and the cervical canal enlarges.

As discussed below, ovulatory periods may develop well before secondary sexual development is complete in the pubertal girl. It is clearly important to realize that girls who appear immature can be fertile.

## Other changes in females

The vagina lengthens early in female puberty and continues to elongate at least until menarche. The mucosa of the vulva

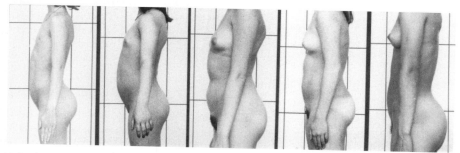

**Fig. 11.3.** Stages of breast development, modified from Marshall and Tanner [13] and Reynolds and Wines [16]. Stage 1: preadolescent; elevation of papilla only. Stage 2: breast bud stage; elevation of breast and papilla as a small mound, enlargement of areolar diameter. This can be quite subtle. Stage 3: further enlargement of breast and areola, with no separation of their contours. Stage 4: projection of areola and papilla to form a secondary mound above the level of the breast. Stage 5: mature stage; projection of papilla only, resulting from recession of the areola to the general contour of the breast.

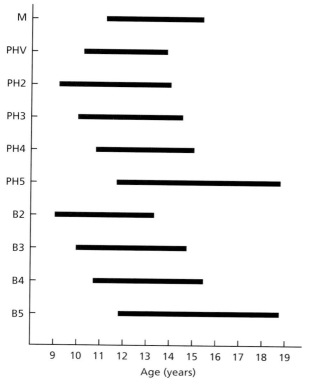

**Fig. 11.4.** The range of attainment of various stages of puberty in Western European females. M, menarche; PHV, peak height velocity; PH2–5, pubic hair stages; B2–5, breast stages (data from Marshall and Tanner [14] and Van Wieringen *et al.* [158]). These ages do not strictly correspond to US girls, who reach the stages at younger ages (see text).

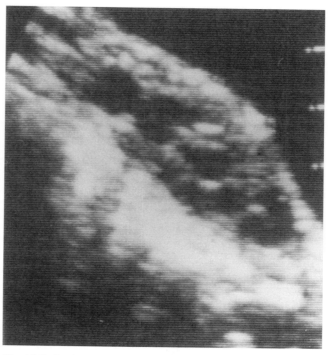

**Fig. 11.5.** Ovarian ultrasound image from a normal prepubertal 8.8-year-old girl. The ovary has a multicystic morphology (more than six cysts of >4 mm in diameter). The bladder is the dark area above and 1-cm markers are shown (from Stanhope *et al.* [23]).

and vagina become softer and thicker, and the hymen thickens with enlargement of the hymenal orifice at puberty [27]. Mucosal changes of the vagina are demonstrable, but the acquisition of a sample of vaginal secretion for clinical diagnosis is rarely indicated, and may be physically or psychologically traumatic to a child. The analysis of a urocytogram is an easier method of collection of a sample of vaginal surface cells found in a voided urine sample, but this interpretation is rarely performed today and laboratories have little experience in the analysis of the procedure [28]. Before menarche there are about 10% superficial cells in the population of the cells of the vaginal mucosa and, with oestrogen stimulation, the layer becomes thicker and the cells have an increase in glycogen content. Just before menarche the cells are mostly adult-type cornified cells. Observation of the vagina in the months before menarche reveals a dulling of the mucosa from the reddish tint of prepuberty to a pinkish colouration. Because of oestrogen stimulation the epithelial glands begin to produce a clear mucoid secretion that forms threads when dry, similar to the pattern found in the adult female at the middle of the menstrual cycle. The vaginal fluid becomes acidic with the progression of puberty, whereas prepubertal secretions are alkaline or neutral.

The mons pubis develops more fat and enlarges with puberty. The labia become larger and the surfaces develop fine wrinkles. The clitoris enlarges slightly with normal puberty, but noticeable virilization indicates a pathological process.

## Male

The growth of the penis and genitalia in the male usually correlates with pubic hair development, since both features are under androgen control. However, for the most accurate assessment the stages of pubic hair development and of genital development should be determined independently since, for example, pubic hair growth without testicular enlargement suggests an adrenal rather than a gonadal source of androgens (Fig. 11.6) [29].

Growth of the testes is usually the first sign of puberty in the male (Fig. 11.7). A useful method of assessing testicular volume utilizes the Prader orchidometer, a string of ellipsoids of known volume, which are compared with the size of the testes of the subject (Fig. 11.8 and Table 11.2) [30]. In general, when the longitudinal measurement of a testis is greater than 2.5 cm excluding the epididymus or if testicular volume exceeds 4 mL by comparison with the Prader orchidometer, pubertal testicular enlargement has begun. Most of the

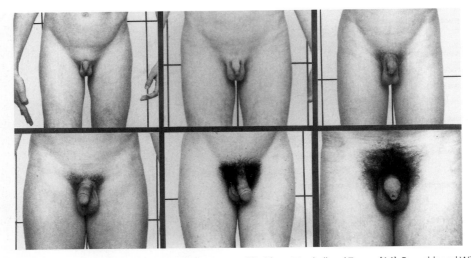

**Fig. 11.6.** Stages of male genital development and pubic hair development, modified from Marshall and Tanner [14], Reynolds and Wines [16] and Dupertuis *et al.* [15]. Genital. Stage 1: preadolescent; testes, scrotum and penis are about the same size and proportion as in early childhood. Stage 2: the scrotum and testes have enlarged; there is a change in the texture and also some reddening of the scrotal skin. The testes are longer than 2.5 cm in longest diameter and reach 4 mL of volume. Stage 3: growth of the penis has occurred, at first mainly in length but with some increase in breadth; there is further growth of the testes and scrotum. Stage 4: the penis is further enlarged in length and breadth with development of the glans. The testes and scrotum are further enlarged. The scrotal skin has further darkened. Stage 5: genitalia are adult in size and shape. No further enlargement takes place after stage 5 is reached. Pubic hair. Stage 1: preadolescent; the vellus over the area is not further developed than that over the abdominal wall, i.e. no pubic hair. Stage 2: sparse growth of long, slightly pigmented, downy hair, straight or slightly curled, appearing chiefly at the base of the penis. This stage can be quite subtle. Stage 3: hair is considerably darker, coarser and curlier, and spreads sparsely over the junction of the pubes. Stage 4: hair is now adult in type, but the area it covers is still considerably smaller than in most adults. There is no spread to the medial surface of the thighs. Stage 5: Hair is adult in quantity and type, distributed as an inverse triangle. The spread is to the medial surface of the thighs but not up the linea alba or elsewhere above the base of the inverse triangle. Stage 6: most men will have further spread of the pubic hair.

increase is due to enlargement of the Sertoli cells rather than the Leydig cells; in familial Leydig and germ cell maturation (testotoxicosis), the testes remain relatively small compared with the remarkable growth of the phallus and pubic hair, for the Leydig cells rather than the Sertoli cells are enlarged. Stage 2A is proposed as a useful classification when testicular volume exceeds 3 mL: further pubertal progression is noted in 82% of boys within 6 months after reaching this stage [31].

The prepubertal testes consist mainly of Sertoli cells, but the adult testes are mostly composed of germ cells in the seminiferous tubules. The seminiferous tubules enlarge during puberty and form tight occlusive junctions leading to the development of the blood–testicular junction [32]. Leydig cells are present in small numbers in prepuberty, although the interstitial tissue is mainly composed of mesenchymal tissue. At puberty the Leydig cells become more apparent.

Spermatogenesis can be detected histologically between 11 and 15 years of age, and sperm is found in early-morning urine samples by a mean of 13.3 years of age (spermarche) [33]. Ejaculation occurs by a mean of 13.5 years without consistent relationship to testicular volume, pubic hair development or phallic enlargement [34]. Although adult morphology, motility and concentration of sperm is not found

until the bone age advances to 17 years [35,36], it is important to realize that immature-appearing boys can be fertile.

The voice changes in boys during puberty are due to lengthening of the vocal chords and enlargement of the larynx, cricothyroid cartilage and laryngeal muscles [37]. It 'breaks' at a mean of 13.9 years and the adult voice is present in Swedish adolescents by 15 years [38], i.e. between stages 3 and 4 of puberty [39].

Facial hair begins to develop on the corners of the upper lips and the upper cheeks at approximately 15 years. It spreads to the midline of the lower lip and cheek by 16 years and ultimately to the sides and the lower border of the chin at or after pubic hair and genital stage 5. The jaw becomes more prominent, as does the nose, during pubertal development. All of the changes in facial appearance and voice clearly continue after secondary sexual development has been completed, as simple observation and hearing will confirm.

### Gynaecomastia

Breast enlargement occurs to some degree in 39–75% of boys, usually during the first stages of puberty [40,41]. This appears because of an increase in oestrogen before testos-

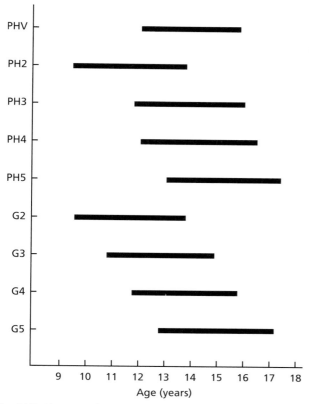

**Fig. 11.7.** The range of attainment of various stages of puberty in Western European males. PHV, peak height velocity; PH2–5, pubic hair stages; G2–5, genital stages (data from Marshall and Tanner [14] and Van Wieringen *et al.* [158]). These ages do not strictly correspond to those of US boys, who reach the stages at younger mean ages.

(a)

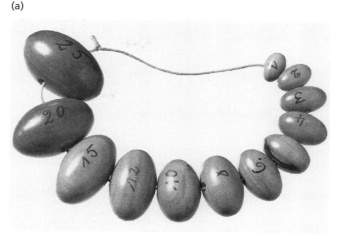

(b)

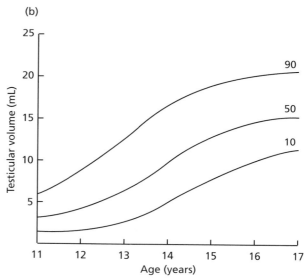

**Fig. 11.8.** (a) The Prader orchidometer. The numbers noted on the ellipsoids indicate the volume in millilitres. These devices are available in plastic or wood. (b) 10th, 50th and 90th centiles of testicular size in boys at different ages (redrawn from Zachmann *et al.* [30]).

terone concentrations reach levels to oppose the oestrogen. In most cases the tissue regresses within 2 years, but occasionally in normal boys, often obese boys, and frequently in pathological conditions, such as Klinefelter syndrome or partial androgen resistance, where the effective amount of testosterone is reduced, gynaecomastia remains permanent. Surgery, usually through a peri-areolar incision is the only method of therapy at present, although non-aromatizable androgens or aromatase inhibitors are under study as potential treatments.

### Other changes of puberty in boys and girls

Other features of growth during puberty include widening of the shoulders in boys and widening of the hips in girls. The growth of the spine increases the upper to lower segment ratio until the adult value is reached. Axillary hair is found in 93% of African American girls and 63% of Caucasian girls by 12 years [5]; boys develop axillary hair at a mean of 14 years. Acne vulgaris is found at a mean age of 12.2 years in boys, although it may the first sign of puberty in girls [42,43].

### Skeletal maturity

Although no diagnosis is made by determination of bone age, support for a suspected diagnosis may be offered. Further, bone age assessment will allow the prediction of final height. Bone age in some respects reflects more closely the physiological stage of the patient than chronological age; normal variations in the tempo of development or diseases that affect pubertal development may cause laboratory values to be abnormal for chronological age but remain appropriate for bone age. Bone age is usually determined in the USA by the Greulich and Pyle *Atlas* [44], whereas the Tanner–Whitehouse method [45] is used more frequently by paediatric endocrinologists in Europe. It does not matter which method is used

**Table 11.2.** Correlation of testicular volume with stage of pubertal development

| | Pubertal stage | | | | |
|---|---|---|---|---|---|
| | 1 | 2 | 3 | 4 | 5 |
| TVI* | 1.8 | 4.5 | 8.2 | 10.5 | – |
| Volume (cm³)† | 2.5 | 3.4 | 9.1 | 11.8 | 14 |
| Volume (cm³)‡ | 1.8 | 4.2 | 10.0 | 11.0 | 15 |
| Volume (cm³)§ | 1.8 | 5.0 | 9.5 | 12.5 | 17 |

*Testicular volume index calculated by (length × width of right testis and length × width of left testis)/2 (data from Burr *et al.* [161] and August *et al.* [162]).
†Volume estimated by comparison with ellipsoid of known volume (orchidometer) that is equal to or smaller than the testes (data from Zachmann *et al.* [30]).
‡Volume by comparison with orchidometer (data from Waaler *et al.* [163]).
§Measurement with calipers and average volume of both testes calculated by 0.52 × longitudinal axis × transverse axis (data from Waaler *et al.* [163]).

as long as it is used by an experienced observer with a high degree of reproducibility. Estimations performed infrequently by radiologists may be very misleading.

## Bone mineral density

The most important phases of bone accretion occur during infancy and puberty. In the teenage years, girls reach peak mineralization between 14 and 16 years, whereas boys reach a later peak at 17.5 years [46,47] (Fig. 11.9). Both peaks come after peak height velocity has been reached in either sex. There is an important influence of genetics since decreased bone mass is familial; this is the case even before puberty [48]. Exercise in the prepubertal phase is important in assuring appropriate bone mass [49,50]. Patients with delay in puberty for any reason will have a significant decrease in bone accretion [51,52]. Unfortunately, excessive exercise will itself delay puberty, so there are limits to the beneficial effects of exercise. The ultimate form of this phenomenon is the combination of exercise-induced amenorrhoea, premature osteoporosis and disordered eating, known as the female athlete triad [53]. Calcium absorption is increased and bone turnover decreased in girls with Turner syndrome treated with oestrogen, demonstrating the importance of gonadal steroids in bone maturation [54]. Bone mass may increase with sex steroid replacement. Children with precocious puberty tend to have increased bone accretion but treatment with a gonadotrophin-releasing hormone (GnRH) agonist will lower this and result ultimately in bone density values below normal. Unfortunately, in the USA, only a minority of adolescents receive the recommended daily allowance of calcium, and it

is feared that an epidemic of osteopenia or even osteoporosis will follow in a few decades time. However, studies in Europe have not found a strong correlation between calcium intake and bone mineral density (BMD) during puberty or young adulthood, suggesting that the normal age of puberty is the most significant factor in achieving peak bone mineralization [55,56]. It seems prudent nonetheless to ensure adequate calcium intake in patients with delayed or absent puberty or to ensure that they are treated with the GnRH agonists.

## Body composition

Percentages of lean body mass, skeletal mass and body fat are equal between prepubertal boys and girls, but as boys go through puberty total body bone mass and fat-free mass continue to increase, whereas in girls only body fat and fat-free mass increase [57]. The increase in lean body mass starts at 6 years in girls and 9.5 years in boys and is the earliest change in body composition of puberty [58]. At maturity, men have 1.5 times the lean body mass and almost 1.5 times the skeletal mass of women, whereas women have twice as much body fat as men. The hips normally enlarge during puberty in girls but the waist does not in the absence of progressive increasing obesity; this leads to a decreased waist–hip ratio [59].

There is a disturbing worldwide increase in the prevalence of overweight and obesity. The USA leads the way, with a prevalence of 11% for obesity (BMI > 95th percentile) and 22% for overweight (BMI > 85th centile) in teenagers, which represents a doubling of the prevalence of obesity in the last 10 years [60]. Other countries have similar trends and, even in those in which malnutrition was found in the majority of citizens in the past, obesity is replacing undernutrition when the food supply increases.

## Growth in puberty

The puberty growth spurt encompasses the most rapid phase of growth after the neonatal period and follows the decreasing growth rate of the late childhood phase. It begins in girls before the onset of secondary sexual characteristics, but only the most careful observation reveals this earliest stage of the phenomenon [61]. The growth spurt of boys starts on average 2 years after that in girls; in the USA, take off for the growth spurt is 9 years in girls and 11 years in boys with peak height velocity (PHV) at a mean of 13.5 years in boys and 11.5 years in girls [62]. These ages correspond to breast stage 2–3 in girls and genitalia stage 3–4 in boys, with 5 for completion in 95% of boys [13,61,63,64].

The mean difference in adult height between men and women of 12.5 cm is due mainly to the taller stature of boys at the onset of the pubertal growth spurt and also to the

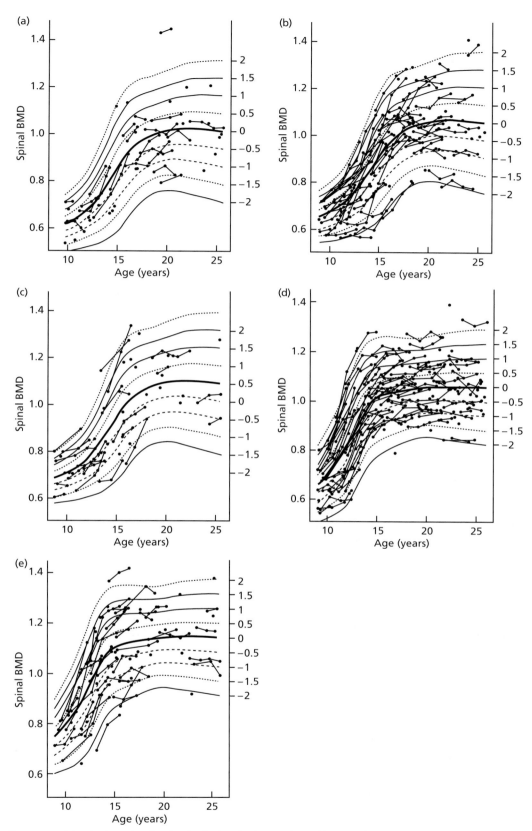

**Fig. 11.9.** Spinal bone mineral density determined in a longitudinal study of 423 males and females of various ethnic groups demonstrating the increase during puberty [46]. (a) Hispanic male; (b) Asian/White male; (c) Black male; (d) non-Black female; (e) Black female.

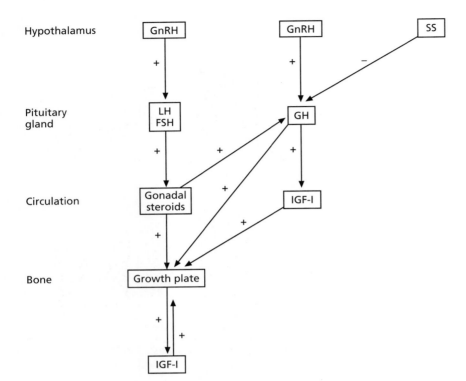

Hypothalamus

Pituitary gland

Circulation

Bone

**Fig. 11.10.** Interaction of the major growth-promoting hormones during the pubertal growth spurt. +, Positive influences; –, inhibitory influences. IGF-I measured in the circulation is secreted by the liver and other tissues (endocrine action). Sex steroids and growth hormone (GH) exert stimulatory effects upon the production of IGF-I arising in bone and cartilage, which exerts effects upon the cells of origin (autocrine action) and upon neighbouring cells (paracrine action) (redrawn from data in Attie *et al.* [65]). FSH, follicle-stimulating hormone; GnRH, gonadotrophin-releasing hormone; LH, luteinizing hormone; SS, somatostatin. It is now known that it is oestradiol that stimulates the increased secretion of growth hormone and which causes terminal differentiation of the epiphyses.

increased height gained during the pubertal growth spurt in boys compared with girls [64]. A girl who has experienced menarche usually has no more than 2.5% of her growth remaining since menarche closely accords to a bone age of 13 years, the only event of puberty more closely related to skeletal than chronological age. A postmenarcheal girl has 5–7.5 cm of growth remaining before adult height is reached, although the range of postmenarcheal growth extends to 11 cm.

The puberty growth spurt is mediated by many endocrine influences. Sex steroids exert a direct effect upon the growing cartilage and an indirect effect of increasing GH secretion, which itself increases growth (Fig. 11.10) [65]. Patients lacking sex steroids because of hypothalamo-pituitary disorders or gonadal disease have no puberty growth spurt. Increasing sex steroid production at puberty stimulates increased amplitude (but not increased frequency) of spontaneous growth hormone secretion [66]. Peak stimulated growth hormone secretion increases during puberty in comparison with stimulated growth hormone concentrations in the prepubertal child; indeed, prepubertal children may have sufficiently low growth hormone responses to stimuli that an incorrect diagnosis of growth hormone deficiency might be inferred [67]. The increased growth hormone of puberty in turn stimulates increased production of IGF-I. Thus, pubertal growth is accompanied not only by higher serum sex steroid concentrations but also by increased episodic secretion of GH and increased serum concentrations of IGF-I (Fig. 11.11) [68].

Oestrogen, either from the ovary or aromatized from testicular testosterone, is the factor that mediates the increased GH response during puberty [69]. A prepubertal child given an androgen that can be aromatized to oestrogen, such as testosterone, will have augmented GH secretion. If an androgen such as dihydrotestosterone, which cannot be aromatized to oestrogen, is administered there is no increase in GH secretion. Likewise, if an oestrogen-blocking agent such as tamoxifen is administered to a pubertal subject, GH secretion will fall [70]. GH-deficient children and those with GH insensitivity do not have a pubertal growth spurt. Thyroid hormone is necessary in sufficient amounts to allow the pubertal growth spurt to proceed. The rapid growth rate is accompanied by an increase in markers of bone turnover such as serum alkaline phosphatase, serum bone alkaline phosphatase, osteocalcin, Gla protein and the amino-terminal propeptide of type III procollagen; thus normal adult values of these proteins are lower than concentrations found in puberty [71,72].

Plasma IGF-I rises during normal puberty with girls having an earlier rise than boys [73]. IGF-I rises in precocious puberty as well due to increased sex steroid secretion, but values decrease with GnRH agonist treatment [68]. IGF-I is decreased for chronological age in delayed puberty, and a mistaken diagnosis of GH deficiency may be suggested; if IGF-I values are interpreted by bone age such errors should not occur.

Oestrogen has a biphasic effect on growth; in small amounts it stimulates growth whereas in large amounts it causes cessation of growth [74,75]. Oestrogen plays a major

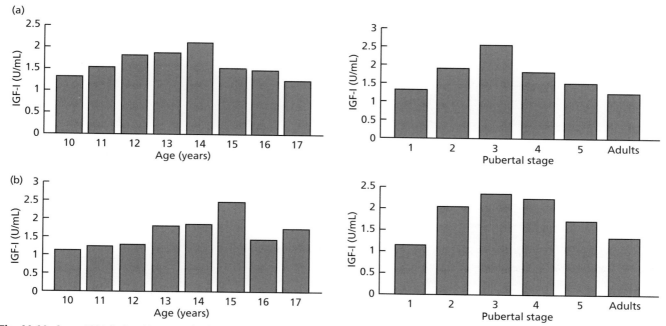

**Fig. 11.11.** Serum IGF-I displayed by age and pubertal stage in (a) females and (b) males. The peak of serum IGF-I found during puberty is evident (redrawn from data in Grumbach and Styne [1]).

role in the final stages of epiphyseal fusion. Patients who cannot make or respond to oestrogens are informative about the importance of oestrogen in the fusion of epiphyses. Patients with either oestrogen receptor deficiency or aromatase deficiency have tall stature, continued growth into the third decade as a result of lack of fusion of the epiphyses of the long bones, increased bone turnover, reduced BMD, osteoporosis and absence of a pubertal growth spurt [76]. Thus, oestrogen, not androgen as previously presumed, is the factor that fuses the epiphyses of the long bones and causes cessation of statural growth. This fact suggests new areas of treatment for short stature including aromatase inhibitors, which might allow continued time for growth before epiphyseal fusion [77].

Patients with Turner syndrome are characteristically short. Although they lack oestrogen owing to ovarian failure, it is the lack of the homeobox gene, *SHOX*, at the pseudoautosomal locus of the X chromosome, which accounts for the extreme short stature [78].

## Limits of normal pubertal development

The upper and lower bounds of the age of onset of puberty should be set 2.5 SD above and below the mean. Comprehensive studies of British and Swiss children indicate a similarity in the age of attainment of most stages of pubertal development, except for menarche (Tables 11.3 and 11.4) [63,79]. Previous data from the USA were limited (the surveys started at ages too old to note the onset of puberty in a large propor-

tion of the population) but suggested a similarity between the European and US data, except that US children reached the stages of puberty 6 months earlier than European children did [80,81]. A study carried out in medical offices by specially trained paediatricians studying 17 070 girls brought in for routine visits recently provided new data about the age of onset of puberty in girls in the USA [5].

This study revealed that 3% of white US girls reach stage 2 breast development by 6 years of age and 5% by 7 years, whereas 6.4% of black girls had stage 2 breast development by 6 years and 15.4% by 7 years. This was not a population sampled longitudinally as was available in Europe and the study has been criticized because the girls visited the doctors' offices randomly but for a reason (possibly illness) rather than being studied in a standardized random basis, but it is the largest study available in the USA. The data redefine the age of diagnosis of precocious puberty in US children: secondary sexual development starting before 6 years in black girls and before 7 years in white girls is precocious.

There is no indication that girls today start puberty at an age earlier than during the last several decades, so the data do not support a secular trend. Nine years is still taken as the lower bound of normal pubertal development in males. However, the most recent government surveys do suggest a tendency towards earlier puberty in boys in the USA. The implications of these recent data on the age of puberty in the USA on the evaluation of European children are not clear at present.

| Stage | British girls* | | Swiss girls† | | US girls‡ | |
|---|---|---|---|---|---|---|
| | Mean (years) | SD | Mean (years) | SD | Mean (years) | SD |
| Breast stage 2 | 11.50 | 1.10 | 10.9 | 1.2 | 11.2 | 0.7 |
| Pubic hair stage 2 | 11.64 | 1.21 | 10.4 | 1.2 | 11.0 | 0.5 |
| Peak height velocity | 12.14 | 0.88 | 12.2 | 1.0 | | |
| Breast stage 3 | 12.15 | 1.09 | 12.2 | 1.2 | 12.0 | 1.0 |
| Pubic hair stage 3 | 12.36 | 1.10 | 12.2 | 1.2 | 11.8 | 1.0 |
| Pubic hair stage 4 | 12.95 | 1.06 | 13.0 | 1.1 | 12.4 | 0.8 |
| Breast stage 4 | 13.11 | 1.15 | 13.2 | 0.9 | 12.4 | 0.9 |
| Menarche 1 | 13.47 | 1.12 | 13.4 | 1.1 | | |
| Pubic hair stage 5 | 14.41 | 1.21 | 14.0 | 1.3 | 13.1 | |
| Breast stage 5 | 15.33 | 1.74 | 14.0 | 1.2 | | |

**Table 11.3.** Age at stage of puberty in girls

*Determined in a prospective study of sequential photographs by Marshall and Tanner [13].
†Determined in a prospective longitudinal study of physical examinations as part of the First Zurich Longitudinal Study of Growth and Development (reported by Largo and Prader [63].
‡Mean age of menarche in the US is 12.8 years, with white girls at 12.9 years and black girls at 12.2 years. Determined in a prospective longitudinal study in Ohio (from Roche *et al.* [164].

| Stage | British boys* | | Swiss boys† | | US boys‡ | |
|---|---|---|---|---|---|---|
| | Mean (years) | SD | Mean (years) | SD | Mean (years) | SD |
| Genitalia stage 2 | 11.64 | 1.07 | 11.2 | 1.5 | 11.2 | 0.7 |
| Genitalia stage 3 | 12.85 | 1.04 | 12.9 | 1.2 | 12.1 | 0.8 |
| Pubic hair stage 2 | 13.44 | 1.09 | 12.2 | 1.5 | 11.2 | 0.8 |
| Genitalia stage 4 | 13.77 | 1.02 | 13.8 | 1.1 | 13.5 | 0.7 |
| Pubic hair stage 3 | 13.90 | 1.04 | 13.5 | 1.2 | 12.1 | 1.0 |
| Peak height velocity | 14.06 | 0.92 | 13.9 | 0.8 | | |
| Pubic hair stage 4 | 14.36 | 1.08 | 14.2 | 1.1 | 13.4 | 0.9 |
| Genitalia stage 5 | 14.92 | 1.10 | 14.7 | 1.1 | 14.3 | 1.1 |
| Pubic hair stage 5 | 15.18 | 1.07 | 14.9 | 1.0 | 14.3 | 0.8 |

**Table 11.4.** Age at stage of puberty in boys

*Determined in a prospective study of sequential photographs by Marshall and Tanner [14].
†Determined in a prospective longitudinal study of physical examinations as part of the First Zurich Longitudinal Study of Growth and Development (reported by Largo & Prader [63]).
‡Determined in a prospective longitudinal study in Ohio (from Roche *et al.* [164]).

The age of menarche in the USA is 12.8 years and has not varied since the last government study published in 1973 [3]. White girls experience menarche later (12.9 years) than African American girls (12.3 years) but this approximately half-year difference is less than the 1-year difference between the age of onset of puberty between the ethnic groups [5].

The upper bounds of normal pubertal development have not changed. Boys should enter the early stages of puberty by 13.5 years (14 years is usually used for convenience) and girls by 13 years to avoid the label of delayed puberty. Puberty does not often occur spontaneously after 18 years of age. English girls complete secondary sexual development in a mean of 4.2 years, but the range is 1.5–6.0 years; the mean for boys is 3.5 years, with a range of 2.0–4.5 years [13,14].

## Endocrine changes of puberty
(Figs 11.12 and 11.13)

### Hypothalamic GnRH

GnRH is a 10-amino-acid peptide produced from a larger 69-amino-acid prohormone precursor. The gene coding for GnRH is located on chromosome 8 [82]. Neurones producing GnRH originate in the primitive olfactory placode early in the development of mammals and then migrate to the medial basal hypothalamus [83,84]. The control of this migration is related to a gene in the Xp22.3 locus of the X chromosome, the *KAL* gene. The absence of the *KAL* gene causes Kallman

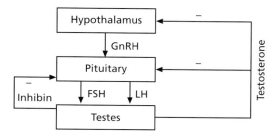

**Fig. 11.12.** Schematic representation of the hypothalamo-pituitary-testicular axis with stimulatory and inhibitory influences demonstrated.

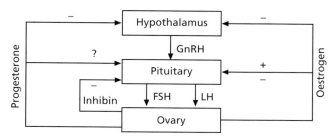

**Fig. 11.13.** Schematic representation of the hypothalamo-pituitary-ovarian axis with stimulatory and inhibitory influences demonstrated.

syndrome, a decrease or lack of gonadotrophin secretion together with hyposmia due to disordered development of the olfactory bulb [85,86]. The gene product of *KAL*, ANOSMIN-1, is postulated to be an extracellular matrix component with antiprotease activity and adhesion function. Abnormalities of the *KAL* gene disrupt the terminal navigation of the early olfactory axons or directly affect the initial steps of olfactory bulb differentiation [87,88].

Some of the genes responsible for hypothalamic function that are linked to disease are known. The *DAX-1* (dosage-sensitive sex reversal and adrenal hypoplasia congenita on the X chromosome, gene 1) gene is altered in adrenal hypoplasia congenita, which is associated with hypogonadotrophic hypogonadism [89,90]. Hypogonadotrophic hypogonadism appears to occur only in conjunction with adrenal hypofunction; new evidence indicates that a separate defect in spermatogenesis occurs and that affected patients are resistant to GnRH stimulation [91,92].

Abnormalities of the *PROP1* gene at 5q cause absence or extremely low values of luteinizing hormone (LH) and follicle-stimulating hormone (FSH), and puberty is absent or, if it begins, fails to progress [93]. Abnormalities of the *Pit1* gene at 3p11 lead to deficient growth hormone and prolactin but do not appear directly to affect GnRH, although puberty may be late, as is frequently the case in growth hormone-deficient children [94].

GnRH is released in episodic boluses into the hypothalamo-pituitary portal system. Its half-life is only 2–4 min and

the daily metabolic clearance is 800 L/m$^2$ [95]. The frequency of episodic release varies with development, sex and the stage of the menstrual period. A variation of the frequency of secretion of GnRH changes the amount of LH and FSH released, and, due to their differing half lives, the serum levels of each. Sole replacement of GnRH in GnRH-deficient hypogonadal patients will restore the release of both LH and FSH in appropriate amounts to allow fertility. This supports the theory that this single hypothalamic factor controls both LH and FSH [86]. Inhibin is a potent suppressor of FSH secretion and also affects the balance of LH and FSH.

GnRH is localized mainly in the hypothalamus in adults but is also found in the hippocampus, cingulate cortex and the olfactory bulb [96]. There is no discrete nucleus that contains all of the GnRH neurones. Gonadotrophins are normally released into the blood stream in a pulsatile manner because of the pulsatile nature of GnRH secretion (Fig. 11.14). Episodic secretion appears to be an intrinsic property of the hypothalamic neurones that produce and secrete the stimulatory peptide GnRH; culture of immortalized hypothalamic cells demonstrate pulsatile GnRH secretion from individual cells [97,98]. This GnRH pulse generator, which is the basis of the central nervous system (CNS) control of puberty and reproductive function, is affected by biogenic amine neurotransmitters, peptidergic neuromodulators, neuroexcitatory amino acids and neural pathways; adrenaline and noradrenaline increase GnRH release whereas dopamine, serotonin and opioids decrease GnRH release (reviewed in [1]). Testosterone and progesterone inhibit GnRH pulse frequency. The decrease in gonadotrophin secretion during childhood before the onset of puberty, the juvenile pause, appears to be mediated by the CNS. Gamma-amino butyric acid (GABA) is probably the major cause of the suppression of GnRH secretion that occurs physiologically during the juvenile pause of mid-childhood [99]. Damage to the CNS due to increased intracranial pressure or tumour may release the inhibition and bring about premature pubertal development [1].

Isolation of the arcuate nucleus of the mediobasal hypothalamus from the rest of the brain does not stop menstruation in monkeys, although its ablation does. Pulsatile administration of GnRH to monkeys with ablated arcuate nuclei can restore pulsatile gonadotrophin secretion and varying the frequency of administration will change the ratio of LH to FSH [100]. This suggests that the arcuate nucleus is a locus of control of GnRH secretion and emphasizes the importance of the pulsatile administration of GnRH to the pituitary gland.

GnRH stimulates the production and secretion of LH and FSH from the gonadotrophs. GnRH affects gonadotrophs by binding to cell-surface receptors [101,102], which triggers increased intracellular calcium concentration and phosphorylation of protein kinase C in a manner similar to other peptide receptor mechanisms. There appear to be readily

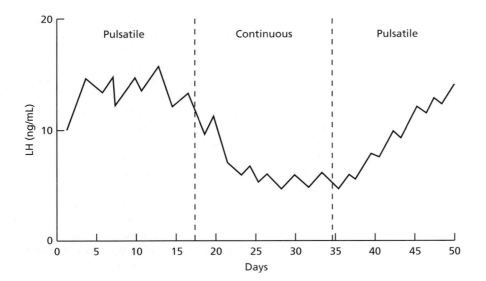

**Fig. 11.14.** Effect of pulsatile administration of GnRH on LH levels in contrast to continuous infusion of GnRH in adult oophorectomized rhesus monkeys in which gonadotrophin secretion has been abolished by lesions that ablated the medial basal hypothalamic GnRH pulse generator. There is suppression by the same dose per time period when administered by continuous infusion rather than by pulses in the same animals and resumption of episodic secretion of LH and FSH with the resumption of pulsatile administration of GnRH (redrawn from data in Belchetz *et al.* [100]).

releasable pools of LH that lead to a rise in serum LH within minutes after a bolus of GnRH, as well as other pools of LH which take longer to mobilize. Although episodic stimulation by GnRH increases gonadotrophin secretion, continuous infusion of GnRH decreases LH and FSH secretion and down-regulates the pituitary receptors for GnRH (Fig. 11.14). A decrease in the number of GnRH receptors occurs first and a decrease in the action of the occupied receptors upon the gonadotrophs follows. This phenomenon is utilized in the treatment of central precocious puberty. Oestrogens increase and androgens decrease GnRH receptors. These alterations in GnRH receptors have an important role in regulating gonadotroph function. There are receptors for GnRH on gonads, but there is no evidence that these receptors are of physiological importance in human beings.

## Pituitary gonadotrophins

FSH and LH are glycoproteins composed of two subunits, an α-subunit, which is identical for all the pituitary glycoproteins, and distinct β-subunits, which confer specificity upon each. The β-subunits have 115 amino acids with two carbohydrate side chains. Human chorionic gonadotrophin (hCG) produced by the placenta is almost identical in structure to LH (except for an additional 32 amino acids and additional carbohydrate groups) and causes all the biological effects. The LH β-subunit gene is on chromosome 19q13.32, close to the gene for β-hCG, and the FSH gene is at 11p13 (reviewed in [103]). There are rare cases of mutations in the β-subunit of gonadotrophin molecules that cause pathological effects: a single case of an inactivating mutation of β-LH caused absence of Leydig cells and lack of puberty, whereas two cases of inactivating mutations of β-FSH led to lack of follicular maturation and amenorrhoea and in two males azoospermia [104,105].

The same gonadotroph cell produces both LH and FSH. The gonadotrophs are spread throughout the anterior pituitary gland and abut upon the capillary basement membranes to allow access to the systemic circulation. Inactive gonadotroph cells that are not stimulated, e.g. as a result of disease affecting GnRH secretion, are small in diameter, whereas the gonadotroph cells of castrated individuals or those with absence of gonads such as in Turner syndrome, which are stimulated by large amounts of GnRH, are large in diameter and demonstrate prominent rough endoplasmic reticulum (RER) [106].

Serum gonadotrophin concentrations change during the progression of pubertal development (Table 11.5). Because of the episodic nature of gonadotrophin secretion, a single gonadotrophin determination will not reveal all about the secretory dynamics of these hormones. However, newer third-generation assays are sufficiently sensitive to indicate the onset of puberty in single basal unstimulated samples; this technique is replacing the GnRH stimulation test in many applications. Biological assays (using cells in culture responsive to the gonadotrophins) reveal patterns of secretion different from when gonadotrophins are measured by immunological assays (Fig. 11.15) [107]. The cause of the difference between these two methods of detection is related to glycosylation of the molecules.

GnRH must stimulate gonadotrophin release before any other factors can affect gonadotrophin secretion. However, in the presence of GnRH stimulation, sex steroids and gonadal peptides can change gonadotrophin secretion. Negative-feedback inhibition is manifest when sex steroids decrease pituitary LH and FSH secretion at the hypothalamic and pituitary levels. This is demonstrated in individuals with gonadal dysgenesis, who cannot secrete oestrogen and who have very high concentrations of LH and FSH during infancy and puberty, a time in which normal children suppress

**Table 11.5.** Serum gonadotrophins, gonadal and adrenal steroids in stages of pubertal development in (a) girls and (b) boys. Values are taken from standards of Quest Diagnostics with permission.

(a) Girls

| Tanner stage | LH (IU/L) | FSH (IU/L) | Oestradiol (pg/mL) | DHEAS (µg/dL) |
|---|---|---|---|---|
| 1 | 0.01–0.21 | 0.50–2.41 | 5–10 | 5–125 |
| 2 | 0.27–4.21 | 1.73–4.68 | 5–115 | 15–150 |
| 3 | 0.17–4.12 | 2.53–7.04 | 5–180 | 20–535 |
| 4 | 0.72–15.01 | 1.26–7.37 | 25–345 | 35–485 |
| 5 | 0.30–29.38 | 1.02–9.24 | 25–410 | 25–530 |

(b) Boys

| Tanner stage | LH (IU/L) | FSH (IU/L) | Testosterone (µg/dL) | DHEAS (µg/dL) |
|---|---|---|---|---|
| 1 | 0.02–0.42 | 0.22–1.92 | 2–23 | 5–265 |
| 2 | 0.26–4.84 | 0.72–4.60 | 5–70 | 13–380 |
| 3 | 0.64–3.74 | 1.24–10.37 | 15–280 | 60–505 |
| 4 | 0.55–7.15 | 1.70–10.35 | 105–545 | 65–560 |
| 5 | 1.54–7.00 | 1.54–7.00 | 265–800 | 165–500 |

DHEAS, dehydroepiandrosterone sulphate; FSH, follicle-stimulating hormone; LH, luteinizing hormone.

gonadotrophins with their active gonadal secretion of sex steroids [108] (Fig. 11.17). The protein inhibin, a product of both ovary and testes, and follistatin, an ovarian product, also exert potent direct inhibitory effects upon FSH secretion at the pituitary level. Progesterone slows the LH pulse frequency.

Oestradiol will decrease gonadotrophin secretion at lower levels but at higher levels will cause positive feedback and, in the right circumstances, cause the midcyle LH surge that leads to ovulation. Positive feedback may be demonstrated at midpuberty in female subjects. Rising serum oestrogen secretion primes the gonadotrophs to produce LH until, at a critical stage at the middle of the menstrual period, a large surge of LH is released, causing ovulation [109]. Several steps must prepare the hypothalamo-pituitary-gonadal axis for positive feedback, including an adequate pool of LH to release and priming of the ovary to produce adequate oestrogen. This delicate preparation is a reason that so few of the initial periods of puberty are ovulatory.

## Sex steroids

The Leydig cells of the testes synthesize testosterone through a series of enzymatic conversions for which cholesterol is the precursor. When LH binds to Leydig cell membrane receptors, the ligand–receptor complex stimulates membrane-bound

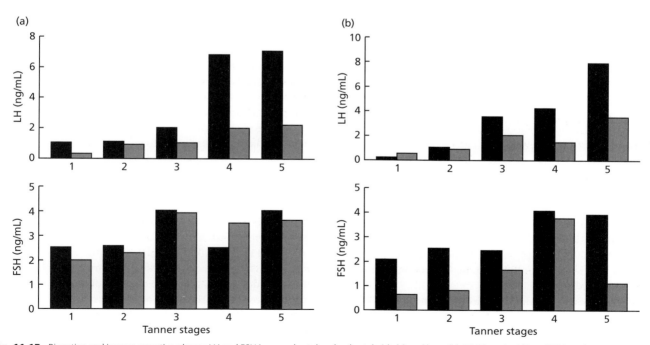

**Fig. 11.15.** Bioactive and immunoreactive plasma LH and FSH in prepubertal and pubertal girls (a) and boys (b). ■, Bioactive LH and FSH; and □, immunoreactive LH and FSH. The concentration of LH is expressed as nanograms per millilitre and that of FSH as nanograms per millilitre (hFSH 1–3) (redrawn from data in Reiter *et al.* [159] and Beitins and Padmanabhan [107]). Bioactive LH in boys and girls and bioactive FSH in boys is present in greater concentrations than are immunoactive LH and FSH during puberty.

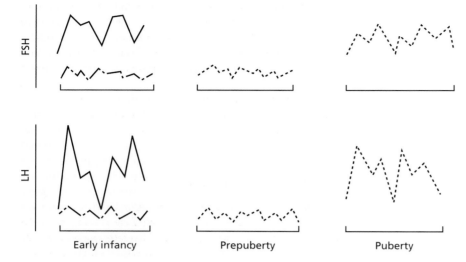

**Fig. 11.16.** Schematic diagram of the change in the pattern of pulsatile FSH and LH secretion in early infancy, childhood and puberty. There is a pronounced sex difference in amplitude between the male and female infant. After infancy the activity of gonadotrophin secretion diminishes during the juvenile pause which lasts for almost a decade (modified from Grumback and Kaplan [142]). ——, Female; – – – –, male; - - - -, male and female.

adenyl cyclase to increase cyclic adenosine monophosphate (cAMP), which then stimulates protein kinase. This causes the stimulation of the conversion of cholesterol to pregnenolone by P450scc (side-chain cleavage enzyme), the first step in the production of testosterone (reviewed in [110]). After exposure to LH, the number of receptors for LH and the postreceptor pathway decrease their responsiveness to LH for at least 24 h. This explains the clinical finding of resistance to LH after daily injections of LH compared with every-other-day injections of LH. When assessing the response of testes to LH, hCG or LH must be administered at 2- to 3-day intervals to eliminate such down-regulation.

When testosterone is secreted into the circulation, it is bound to sex hormone-binding globulin (SHBG) [111,112]. The remaining free testosterone is the active moiety. At the target cell, testosterone dissociates from the binding protein, diffuses into the cell and may be converted by $5\alpha$-reductase 2 (a surface enzyme located on the sexual skin and elsewhere and coded by a gene on chromosome 2 [113]) to dihydrotestosterone or converted to oestrogen by aromatase (CPY19 [114]). Testosterone or dihydrotestosterone attaches to androgen receptors that are encoded by a gene on the q arm of the X chromosome (Xq11–q12) [115]. Either sex steroid attaches to a nuclear receptor, which changes in conformation by the act of binding. The testosterone–receptor complex then attaches to the steroid-responsive region of genomic DNA. Transcription and translation occur by the androgen effect, which leads to protein production (reviewed in [110]).

The effects of testosterone are different from those of dihydrotestosterone: a fetus without dihydrotestosterone will not virilize fully. The androgen receptor has a greater affinity for dihydrotestosterone than for testosterone. Testosterone will suppress LH secretion, maintain Wolffian ducts and produce the male body habitus, whereas dihydrotestosterone is mostly responsible for the virilization of the external genitalia

and for much of the secondary sexual characteristics of puberty including phallic growth, prostate enlargement, androgen-induced hair loss and beard growth. Androgens exert other effects in the body: testosterone promotes muscle development, stimulates enzymatic activity in the liver and stimulates haemoglobin synthesis. Androgens must be converted to oestrogen to stimulate bone maturation at the epiphyseal plate [116].

FSH binds to specific receptors on the cell surface of Sertoli cells and causes a sequence of events that culminates in increased protein kinase in a manner similar to the stimulatory effect of LH on Leydig cells. However, FSH causes an increase in the mass of seminiferous tubules, and in an undefined way it supports the development of sperm. A boy with an hCG-secreting tumour will have Leydig cell stimulation without the FSH effect and without seminiferous tubule stimulation: the result will be virilization without much testicular enlargement.

Oestrogen is produced mainly by the follicle cells of the ovary, utilizing the same initial steps as testosterone production with a final aromatization process (reviewed in [117]). In the female, LH binds to membrane receptors of ovarian cells and stimulates the activity of adenyl cyclase to produce cAMP, which stimulates the production of the low-density lipoprotein (LDL) receptor to increase binding and uptake of LDL-cholesterol and the formation of cholesterol esters (reviewed in [117]). LH stimulates the rate-limiting enzyme P450scc, which converts cholesterol to pregnenolone, initiating steroidogenesis. After the onset of ovulation, LH exerts major effects upon the theca of the ovary. FSH binds to its own cell-surface receptors on the glomerulosa cells and stimulates the conversion of testosterone to oestrogen.

The main active oestrogen in humans is oestradiol. Oestrogens circulate bound to SHBG and follow the same general pattern of action at the cell level as described for testosterone. Oestradiol produces effects upon the breast and uterus and affects the distribution of adipose tissue and bone. Low concentrations of oestradiol are difficult to measure in standard assays. New experimental bioassays for oestrogen are sensitive enough to differentiate between boys and girls in prepuberty, between prepuberty and puberty in girls and between normal girls and those with premature thelarche, who secrete only a small amount of oestrogen above age-matched control subjects [118–120].

## Testosterone-binding globulin

Less than 2% of circulating testosterone is free and active; the rest is bound to testosterone-binding globulin (TeBG) [121]. TeBG consists of heterogeneous monomers, each of which binds one molecule of androgen. Androgen decreases TeBG and oestrogen stimulates TeBG formation. Thus, with the secretion of testosterone in male puberty and the resulting decrease in TeBG causing an increase in free testosterone, there is a magnification of the androgen effect during puberty. In pubertal girls, TeBG rises with oestrogen secretion, binding available androgens and decreasing the overall androgen effect.

## Prolactin

Prolactin, GH and human chorionic somatomammotropin are derived from a common ancestor and share amino acid homologies. Prolactin contains 199 amino acids with three disulphide bonds; the gene is on chromosome 6 [122]. Lactotrophs of the anterior pituitary gland produce prolactin and are suppressed by prolactin-inhibitory factor (dopamine) in the basal state. Thus, hypothalamic disease may destroy prolactin-inhibitory factor leading to increased prolactin secretion, or pituitary disease may destroy the lactotrophs leading to decreased prolactin secretion; prolactin thus serves an important role in differential diagnosis, even if its role is limited in the non-pregnant individual. Prolactin rises in girls during pubertal development, but there is no change in prolactin concentrations during male puberty [123]. Prolactinomas secrete an increased amount of prolactin in the basal state or after thyroid-releasing hormone (TRH) stimulation.

## Inhibin

Inhibin is a heterodimeric glycoprotein member of the transforming growth factor β (TGF-β) family produced by the Sertoli cells in the male and by the ovarian granuloma cells and the placenta in the female [124]. Inhibin suppresses FSH secretion from the pituitary gland and provides another explanation for different serum concentrations of LH and FSH with only one hypothalamic peptide (GnRH) stimulating them. Activin is a subunit of inhibin and has the opposite effect, stimulating the secretion of FSH from the pituitary gland. Originally measured decades ago by bioassay, immunoassays are now available to detect inhibin concentrations. Inhibin B secretion rises in early puberty in both boys and girls and then levels off [125]. The infant male has values of inhibin B higher than those achieved in adult males for the first 1–1.5 years after birth, further indicating the activity of the testes during this early period [126,127]. Absence of inhibin due to gonadal failure causes a greater rise in serum FSH than LH in pubertal-aged and adult subjects.

## Anti-Müllerian hormone

Anti-Müllerian hormone (AMH) belongs to the same TGF-β family as inhibin and is produced from the Sertoli cells of the fetal testes and the granulosa cells of the fetal ovary [128,129]. In normal males, AMH is high in the fetus and newborn but decreases thereafter with a further drop at puberty. Patients with dysgenetic testes have decreased serum AMH whereas values are elevated in males with Sertoli cell tumours or females with granulosa cell tumours. AMH assays might be used to differentiate a child with congenital anorchia who has no testicular tissue from one with undescended testes who has testicular tissue that can produce AMH. Girls have low levels of AMH in the newborn period.

## Prostate-specific antigen

Prostate-specific antigen (PSA) rises early in puberty from undetectable concentrations in most prepubertal boys [130]. This change appears closely related to rising androgen concentrations.

## Growth hormone

GH is a single-chain 191-amino-acid protein with two disulphide bonds, which is most prevalent in the 22-kDa forms. GH is released in pulses but concentrations remain low for much of the day in normal and GH-deficient patients alike; it appears to be the ability to release substantial peaks of GH that differentiates the two. GH secretion increases at the time of puberty apparently from stimulation by increased secretion of sex steroids [66]. The amplitude of GH secretory bursts rises with puberty, although the frequency of secretory peaks does not change. Children with delayed puberty lack this rise that is characteristic of puberty, and their peak values may even approximate the concentrations of GH seen in GH deficiency. Thus the diagnosis of GH secretion becomes problematic in delayed puberty. Remarkably, the GH response to administration of GH-stimulating hexapeptides increases in puberty, just as the response to administration of GH-releasing hormone rises in puberty, even though the two GH stimulatory factors work through different receptors [131].

## Insulin-like growth factors

The structure of the insulin-like growth factors (IGFs) resembles proinsulin with A and B chains connected by a disulphide bond. IGF-I is sensitive to GH secretion as well as nutritional factors, although malnutrition will lower IGF-I in spite of elevated serum GH, and obesity will maintain normal serum concentrations of IGF-I even though GH secretion is suppressed. Serum IGF-I concentrations are normally low at birth but rise throughout childhood until approximately the time of the pubertal growth spurt, when a several-fold increase in serum IGF-I concentration occurs [68]. Serum values of IGF-I then fall to the adult range (Fig. 11.10). The rise in serum IGF-I concentrations at puberty is caused by several factors, including increased secretion of GH [65], and a direct effect of sex steroid secretion causing increased production of IGF-I from the cartilage independent of changes in GH (Fig. 11.10).

## Leptin

Leptin is a hormone produced in the adipose cells that suppresses appetite by attaching to its receptor in the hypothalamus [132]. Leptin plays a major role in puberty in mice and rats as a genetically leptin-deficient mouse (ob/ob) will not start puberty; however, leptin replacement will remedy the situation and leptin administration will push an immature but normal mouse through puberty. One of the few leptin-deficient human beings at 9 years of age had a bone age of 13 years but no significant gonadotrophin pulses and no evidence of pubertal development; this indicated a gonadotrophin-deficient state, as in the ob/ob mouse. With leptin treatment gonadotrophin peaks appeared and suggested that puberty would also appear [133]. These data and others suggested that leptin might be the elusive factor that triggers the onset of puberty.

There is a younger age of puberty and menarche in obese children and leptin seemed a likely candidate to account for this phenomenon. However, leptin increases in girls during puberty in synchrony with the increase in fat mass, whereas leptin decreases in puberty in boys with a decrease in fat mass and increase in fat-free mass; leptin varies with body composition only [134,135]. Thus, in otherwise normal adolescents there is no convincing evidence that leptin triggers pubertal development. Leptin appears permissive of puberty but not the cause of its onset or progression.

## Ontogeny of endocrine pubertal development
(Fig. 11.16)

The midgestation human fetus exhibits endocrine activity that is quite similar to the changes of puberty. The fetal hypothalamus contains GnRH-containing neurones by 14 weeks of gestation, and the fetal pituitary gland contains LH and FSH by 20 weeks [136]. The hypothalamo-pituitary portal system develops by 20 weeks of gestation, allowing hypothalamic GnRH to reach the pituitary gonadotrophs. Stimulation by GnRH causes gonadotrophin secretion to rise to extremely high values at midgestation, with a decrease thereafter. Initially, unrestrained GnRH secretion by the hypothalamus comes under restraint from the CNS by midgestation and, probably also to some degree, from increased circulating sex steroid concentrations, which exert a restraining effect upon gonadotrophin secretion until after birth.

At term, gonadotrophin concentrations are lower than midgestation but still relatively high. Elevated serum testosterone concentrations emanating from the fetal testes during the later half of gestation demonstrate the bioactivity of the fetal gonadotrophins; fetal testosterone secretion early in pregnancy is caused by placental hCG stimulation. Gonadotrophin values rise once again in an intermittent pattern after birth with episodic peaks noted up to 2–4 years after birth [137]. These peaks can confuse the diagnosis of precocious puberty during this period after birth because it is hard to differentiate normal postnatal gonadotrophin peaks from those caused by precocious puberty. Oestrogen and testosterone from the infantile gonads also rise episodically during this period but mean serum values of gonadotrophins and sex steroids during infancy remain much lower than found in the fetus and the pubertal subject, but higher than those found during the juvenile pause of approximately 4–9 years of age. Because sex steroids suppress gonadotrophin secretion to a significant degree during the first years after birth, agonadal patients such as those with Turner syndrome exhibit high (castrate) values of serum gonadotrophins (Fig. 11.17) [108]. Remarkably, girls with Turner syndrome have the same pattern of pulsatile gonadotrophin secretion as normal girls, but with higher amplitudes of the pulses [138].

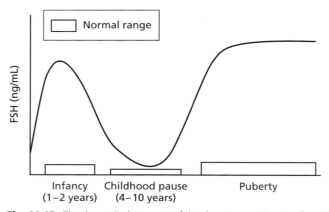

**Fig. 11.17.** The change in the pattern of the plasma concentration of FSH with age in patients with Turner syndrome compared with normal girls (redrawn from data in Conte *et al.* [108]). The pattern in Turner syndrome is qualitatively the same as in normal girls but quantitatively higher.

During the juvenile pause, gonadotrophin concentrations and gonadal activity remain at a low level of activity, restrained by the CNS. Even in children without gonadal function, such as those with Turner syndrome, serum gonadotrophin concentrations are low, demonstrating that the presence of the gonads is not necessary to suppress gonadotrophin secretion during the childhood pause. Pituitary gonadotrophin secretion may be low during the juvenile pause, but supersensitive assays now demonstrate pulsatile gonadotrophin secretion at the same frequency as noted during puberty, but at decreased amplitude [139,140]. Thus the major change of puberty may involve the amount of gonadotrophin secreted, but not the timing of the pulses [141]. Likewise, testosterone and oestrogen are measurable in the infant circulation in sensitive assays, demonstrating low but definite activity of the infantile gonads.

Certain clinical situations demonstrate the presence of the CNS restraint characteristic of the juvenile pause. Hydrocephalus, subarachnoid cysts or posterior hypothalamic tumours may destroy the restraining loci of the CNS and allow central precocious puberty to progress as early as the first postnatal year. When some of these conditions are reversed, such as by the removal of the cyst or shunting of the hydrocephalus, puberty will cease (Fig. 11.18) [142].

Central precocious puberty may also occur because of a hamartoma of the tuber cinereum [143]. This mass of heterotopic hypothalamic tissue contains GnRH neurones and may secrete pulsatile GnRH during childhood in a spontaneous manner that is not under the control of the normal CNS restraining mechanism. Thus gonadotrophins rise and sex steroids are elaborated and secreted. The hamartoma is not a neoplasm and does not enlarge. Hamartomas of the tuber cinerium are generally thought to cause precocious puberty by GnRH secretory activity rather than by mass; however, two examples of hamartomas of the tuber cinerium causing central precocious puberty contained no GnRH but rather TGF-α, which itself can stimulate GnRH secretion [144].

During the peripubertal period, before physical changes, gonadotrophin secretion rises first at night [145] (Fig. 11.19). Sequential sampling demonstrates a rise in sex steroid secretion during the late night/early morning, which follows by hours the peaks of gonadotrophins demonstrating the biological chain of events. Early-morning serum testosterone values are higher just before the onset of secondary sexual development; this phenomenon is exploited as a method of predicting the onset of puberty in individual boys. Girls also have circadian variation in testosterone production with higher values once puberty starts than prepubertal girls; the levels in prepuberty correlate with dehydroepiandrosterone sulphate (DHEAS) secretion, suggesting an adrenal origin of the testosterone, whereas in puberty the origin of the testosterone appears to be the ovaries [146]. As puberty progresses, the secretion of gonadotrophins and sex steroids occurs more during the day, until no circadian rhythm remains.

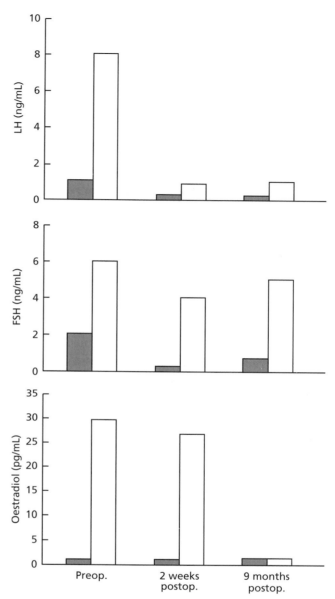

**Fig. 11.18.** The change in gonadotrophin and oestradiol secretion before and after removal of a subarachnoid cyst in a 3-year-old girl with central precocious puberty. □, Response to administration of 100 μg GnRH to test secretory activity; ■, basal values (redrawn from data in Grumbach and Kaplan [142]).

During the peripubertal period there is also a change in the response of pituitary gonadotrophs to exogenous GnRH administration [147]. The pattern of LH release increases, so that the adult pattern of response to GnRH is achieved during puberty. The release of FSH shows no such change with development, although female subjects have more FSH release than male subjects at all developmental stages.

The change in LH secretion after exogenous GnRH administration is used as an indication of a change in endogenous

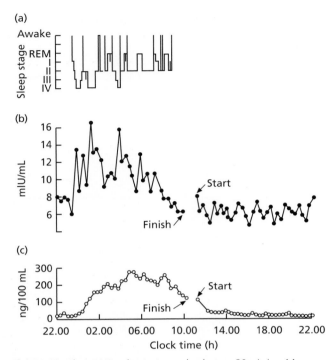

**Fig. 11.19.** Plasma LH and testosterone levels every 20 min in a 14-year-old boy in pubertal stage 2. The histogram displaying sleep stage sequence is depicted above the period of nocturnal sleep. (a) Sleep stages are rapid eye movement (REM) with stages I–IV shown by depth of line graph. (b) Plasma LH (●) is expressed as mIU/mL. (c) Plasma testosterone (○) is expressed as ng/100 mL (from Boyar *et al.* [160]).

GnRH release with pubertal development; the GnRH stimulation test is invoked to differentiate disorders of puberty, and puberty can be artificially induced by GnRH treatment. If GnRH is administered in low-dose boluses at 60- to 120-min intervals for 5 days, a prepubertal subject or one with hypothalamic deficiency of GnRH will convert gonadotrophin release and sex steroid secretion to a pubertal pattern of peaking LH values every 60–120 min [148]. Thus the pituitary response 'matures' with exogenous GnRH administration, suggesting that increasing endogenous GnRH secretion induces puberty normally in the same way. Patients with gonadotrophin deficiency can be treated with episodic GnRH boluses administered by a miniature programmable pump to induce secondary sexual development, menses and ovulation or spermatogenesis; pregnancies are regularly induced in gonadotrophin-deficient women by these methods [149].

Since gonadotrophin secretion is episodic, individual serum samples did not demonstrate a clear pattern of change with puberty when older radioimmunoassays were used. New ultrasensitive assays can differentiate basal gonadotrophin concentrations in a subject in the prepubertal stage from a pubertal subject. Sex steroids are less variable than gonadotrophin concentrations during pubertal development and show a general stepwise increase with each stage of puberty. Thus, sex steroid determinations may serve a diagnostic purpose complementary to the measurement of gonadotrophin concentrations in the assessment of puberty.

## Positive feedback and the menstrual cycle

Positive feedback might be considered the ultimate developmental stage of hypothalamo-pituitary-gonadal reproductive development in girls; positive feedback develops in females at approximately midpuberty [109]. By this process a rising concentration of oestrogen greater than 200–300 pg/mL persisting for more than 48 h [150] triggers the release of a bolus of LH from the pituitary gonadotrophs, which stimulates ovulation about 12 h later. This positive feedback effect of oestrogen is in contrast to negative feedback, whereby lower concentrations of oestradiol suppress GnRH secretion; positive feedback cannot occur unless negative feedback precedes it. Oestradiol also increases pituitary gland sensitivity to GnRH, which, in addition to an increase in GnRH pulse frequency, increases LH secretion. Thus a follicle must be of adequate size to produce adequate oestrogen to exert the positive feedback effect, the pituitary gland must have sufficient readily releasable LH to effect a surge of LH release, and the hypothalamus must be able to secrete adequate GnRH to cause the stimulation of pituitary release.

These conditions do not develop until well into the pubertal process. The increase in oestrogen also suppresses FSH to allow, in the presence of LH, luteinization of the follicle. There is a reawakening of interest in intraovarian processes that play an important role in the menstrual cycle. There is the aforementioned endocrine activity through proteins and sex steroids elaborated in the ovary, but paracrine and other local effects of factors, including proteolytic enzymes (collagenase and plasmin) and prostaglandins E and F and hydroxyeicosotetranoic acid ethyl esters, are of importance in the normal menstrual cycle and ovulation [151,152].

The menstrual cycle is divided into the initial follicular phase up to the midcycle oestradiol and LH peaks and the luteal phase thereafter. The increased oestrogen secretion of midpuberty at the end of the follicular phase stimulates the growth of the endometrium. However, the decreased oestrogen and progesterone at the end of the luteal phase during the decline of the corpus luteum leaves the hyperplastic endometrium without endocrine support. This leads to necrosis of the endometrium and the menstrual flow commences. The first 2 years of menses are anovulatory in 55–90% of cycles. Not until 5 years after menarche are 80% ovulatory [153,154].

## Adrenarche

The adrenal androgens, dehydroepiandrosterone and androstenedione, produced by the zona reticularis, rise 2 or more years before gonadotrophins and sex steroids rise [155]. This process of adrenarche begins by 6–8 years of age in normal subjects, and continues until late puberty (Table 11.5).

The control of the increased activity of the adrenal gland at the time of secondary sexual development remains an enigma [156]. In the absence of adrenocorticotrophic hormone (ACTH), no change in the minimal secretion of these androgens occurs, but there is no change in ACTH secretion at adrenarche that can explain adrenarche, and ACTH appears to be necessary but not sufficient. Adrenarche occurs years before a rise in gonadotrophin secretion occurs, eliminating gonadotrophins as the cause of adrenarche. Alternatively, there may be another pituitary hormone, as yet undiscovered, that triggers the process of adrenarche. There may be an internal adrenal mechanism related to the changing milieu of adrenal cortical enzymes that changes the mix of steroid precursors and products in the adrenal gland which causes adrenarche.

The presence or absence of adrenarche does not seem to influence the onset of puberty. Patients with Addison disease, who have no adrenal function, experience puberty at an appropriate age and children with premature adrenarche also enter gonadarche at a normal age. Thus adrenarche is usually temporally coordinated with gonadarche in the pubertal process of normal individuals, but appears not to play an important role in the progression of gonadarche.

# References

1 Grumbach MM, Styne DM. Puberty. Ontogeny, neuroendocrinology, physiology, and disorders. In: Wilson JD, Foster DW, Kronenberg MD, Larsen PR, eds. *William's Textbook of Endocrinology*, 9th edn. Philadelphia: W. B. Saunders Company, 1998: 1509–625.

2 Tanner JM. The trend toward earlier menarche in London, Oslo, Copenhagen, the Netherlands and Hungary. *Nature* 1973; 243: 95.

3 MacMahon B. Age at menarche. In: *National Health Survey*. DHEW Publication No. (HRA) 74–1615, Series 11, No. 133. Washington, DC: Department of Health Education and Welfare, 1973.

4 Zacharias L, Rand M, Wurtman R. A prospective study of sexual development in American girls: the statistics of menarche. *Obstet Gynecol Surv* 1976; 31: 325–37.

5 Herman-Giddens ME, Slora EJ, Wasserman RC *et al.* Secondary sexual characteristics and menses in young girls seen in office practice: a study from the Pediatric Research in Office Settings network. *Pediatrics* 1997; 99: 505–12.

6 Veronesi FM, Gueresi P. Trend in menarcheal age and socioeconomic influence in Bologna (northern Italy). *Ann Hum Biol* 1994; 21: 187–96.

7 Daw SF. Age of boys' puberty in Leipzig, 1727–49, as indicated by voice breaking in J.S. Bach's choir members. *Hum Biol* 1970; 42: 87–9.

8 Tanner JM. *A History of the Study of Human Growth*. Cambridge: Cambridge University Press, 1981: 286–98.

9 Warren MP. The effects of exercise on pubertal progression and reproductive function in girls. *J Clin Endocrinol Metab* 1980; 51: 1150–7.

10 Hartz AJ, Barboriak PN, Wong A. The association of obesity with infertility and related menstrual abnormalities in women. *Int J Obes* 1979; 3: 57–73.

11 Osler DC, Crawford JD. Examination of the hypothesis of a critical weight at menarche in ambulatory and bedridden mentally retarded girls. *Pediatrics* 1973; 51: 674–9.

12 Zacharias L, Wurtman RJ. Age at menarche. *N Engl J Med* 1969; 280: 868–75.

13 Marshall WA, Tanner JM. Variations in pattern of pubertal changes in girls. *Arch Dis Child* 1969; 44: 291–303.

14 Marshall WA, Tanner JM. Variations in the pattern of pubertal changes in boys. *Arch Dis Child* 1970; 45: 13–23.

15 Dupertuis CW, Atkinson WB, Elftman H. Sex differences in pubic hair distribution. *Hum Biol* 1945; 17: 137–42.

16 Reynolds EL, Wines JV. Individualized differences in physical changes associated with adolescence in girls. *Am J Dis Child* 1948; 75: 329–50.

17 Hergenroeder AC, Hill RB, Wong WW, Sangi-Haghpeykar H, Taylor W. Validity of self-assessment of pubertal maturation in African American and European American adolescents [see comments]. *J Adolescent Health* 1999; 24: 201–5.

18 Hick KM, Katzman DK. Self-assessment of sexual maturation in adolescent females with anorexia nervosa [see comments]. *J Adolescent Health* 1999; 24: 206–11.

19 Rohn RD. Nipple (papilla) development in puberty: longitudinal observations in girls. *Pediatrics* 1987; 79: 745–7.

20 Peters H, Byskov AG, Grinsted J. Follicular growth in fetal and prepubertal ovaries of humans and other primates. *Clin Endocrinol Metab* 1978; 7: 469–85.

21 Baker TG. A quantitative and cytological study of germ cells in human ovaries. *Proc R Soc London B Biol Sci* 1999; 158: 417–33.

22 Ross GT. Follicular development: the life cycle of the follicle and puberty. In: Grumbach MM, Sizonenko PC, Aubert MI, eds. *Control of the Onset of Puberty*. Baltimore: Williams & Wilkins, 1990: 376–86.

23 Stanhope R, Adams J, Jacobs HS *et al.* Ovarian ultrasound assessment in normal children, idiopathic precocious puberty, and during low dose pulsatile gonadotrophin releasing hormone treatment of hypogonadotrophic hypogonadism. *Arch Dis Child* 1985; 60: 116–19.

24 Salardi S, Orsini LF, Cacciari E *et al.* Pelvic ultrasonography in girls with precocious puberty, congenital adrenal hyperplasia, obesity, or hirsutism. *J Pediatr* 1988; 112: 880–7.

25 Bridges NA, Cooke A, Healy MJ, Hindmarsh PC, Brook CG. Standards for ovarian volume in childhood and puberty. *Fertil Steril* 1993; 60: 456–60.

26 Haber HP, Ranke MB. Pelvic ultrasonography in Turner syndrome: standards for uterine and ovarian volume. *J Ultrasound Med* 1999; 18: 271–6.

27 Wheeler MD. Physical changes of puberty. *Endocrinol Metab Clin N Am* 1991; 20: 1–14.

28 Collett-Solberg PR, Grumbach MM. A simplified procedure for evaluating estrogenic effects and the sex chromatin pattern in exfoliated cells in urine: studies in premature thelarche and gynecomastia of adolescence. *J Pediatr* 1965; 66: 883–90.

29 Reynolds EL, Wines JV. Physical changes associated with adolescence in boys. *Am J Dis Child* 1951; 82: 529–47.

30 Zachmann M, Prader A, Kind HP, Hafliger H, Budliger H. Testicular volume during adolescence. Cross-sectional and longitudinal studies. *Helv Paediatr Acta* 1974; 29: 61–72.

31 Biro FM, Lucky AW, Huster GA, Morrison JA. Pubertal staging in boys. *J Pediatr* 1995: 127: 100–2 [published erratum appears in *J Pediatr* 1995; 127: 674].

32 Gondos B, Kogan SJ. Testicular development during puberty. In: Grumbach MM, Sizonenko PC, Aubert ML *et al*. eds. *Control of the Onset of Puberty*. Baltimore: Williams and Wilkins, 1990: 387–402.

33 Nielsen CT, Skakkebaek NE, Richardson DW *et al*. Onset of the release of spermatozoa (spermarche) in boys in relation to age, testicular growth, pubic hair, and height. *J Clin Endocrinol Metab* 1986; 62: 532–5.

34 Laron Z, Arad J, Gurewitz R, Grunebaum M, Dickerman Z. Age at first conscious ejaculation: a milestone in male puberty. *Helv Paediatr Acta* 1980; 35: 13–20.

35 Janczewski Z, Bablok L. Semen characteristics in pubertal boys. III. Semen quality and somatosexual development. *Arch Androl* 1985; 15: 213–18.

36 Janczewski Z, Bablok L. Semen characteristics in pubertal boys. II. Semen quality in relation to bone age. *Arch Androl* 1985; 15: 207–11.

37 Peschel ER, Peschel RE. Medical insights into the castrati in opera. *Am Sci* 1987; 75: 578–83.

38 Karlberg P, Taranger J. The somatic development of children in a Swedish urban community. *Acta Paediatr Scand* 1976; 258 (Suppl.): 1–148.

39 Harries M, Hawkins S, Hacking J, Hughes I. Changes in the male voice at puberty: vocal fold length and its relationship to the fundamental frequency of the voice. *J Laryngol Otol* 1998; 112: 451–4.

40 Carlson SE. Gynecomastia. *N Engl J Med* 1980; 404: 795–9.

41 Nuttall FQ. Gynecomastia as a physical finding in normal men. *J Clin Endocrinol Metab* 1979; 48: 338–40.

42 Lucky AW, Biro FM, Huster GA, Morrison JA, Elder N. Acne vulgaris in early adolescent boys. Correlations with pubertal maturation and age. *Arch Dermatol* 1991; 127: 210–16.

43 Lucky AW, Biro FM, Huster GA, Leach AD, Morrison JA, Ratterman J. Acne vulgaris in premenarchal girls. An early sign of puberty associated with rising levels of dehydroepiandrosterone. *Arch Dermatol* 1994; 130: 308–14.

44 Greulich WS, Pyle SI. *Radiographic Atlas of Skeletal Development of the Hand and Wrist*. Stanford, CA: Stanford University Press, 1959.

45 Tanner JM, Whitehouse RH, Marshall WA *et al*. *Assessment of Skeletal Maturity and Prediction of Adult Height: TW 2 Method*. New York: Academic Press, 1975.

46 Bachrach LK, Hastie T, Wang M *et al*. Bone mineral acquisition in healthy Asian, Hispanic, Black and Caucasian youth: a longitudinal study. *J Clin Endocrinol Metab* 1999; 84: 4702–12.

47 Magarey AM, Boulton TJ, Chatterton BE, Schultz C, Nordin BE, Cockington RA. Bone growth from 11 to 17 years: relationship to growth, gender and changes with pubertal status including timing of menarche. *Acta Paediatrica* 1999; 88: 139–46.

48 Ferrari S, Rizzoli R, Slosman D, Bonjour JP. Familial resemblance for bone mineral mass is expressed before puberty. *J Clin Endocrinol Metabolism* 1998; 83: 358–61.

49 Barr SI, McKay HA. Nutrition, exercise, and bone status in youth. *Int J Sport Nutr* 1998; 8: 124–42.

50 Bass S, Pearce G, Bradney M, Hendrich E, Delmas PD, Harding A, Seeman E. Exercise before puberty may confer residual benefits in bone density in adulthood: studies in active prepubertal and retired female gymnasts. *J Bone Mineral Res* 1998; 13: 500–7.

51 Finkelstein JS, Klibanski A, Neer RM. A longitudinal evaluation of bone mineral density in adult men with histories of delayed puberty. *J Clin Endocrinol Metab* 1996; 81: 1152–5.

52 Hergenroeder AC. Bone mineralization, hypothalamic amenorrhea, and sex steroid therapy in female adolescents and young adults. *J Pediatr* 1995; 126: 683–9.

53 De Craee C. Sex steroid metabolism and menstrual irregularities in the exercising female. A review. *Sports Med* 1998; 25: 369–406.

54 Mauras N, Vieira NE, Yergey AL. Estrogen therapy enhances calcium absorption and retention and diminishes bone turnover in young girls with Turner's syndrome: a calcium kinetic study. *Metabolism: Clin Exp* 1997; 46: 908–13.

55 Maggiolini M, Bonofiglio D, Giorno A *et al*. The effect of dietary calcium intake on bone mineral density in healthy adolescent girls and young women in southern Italy. *Int J Epidemiol* 1999; 28: 479–84.

56 Kardinaal AF, Ando S, Charles P *et al*. Dietary calcium and bone density in adolescent girls and young women in Europe. *J Bone Mineral Res* 1999; 14: 583–92.

57 Rico H, Revilla M, Villa LF, Hernandez ER, Alvarez de Buergo M, Villa M. Body composition in children and Tanner's stages: a study with dual-energy x-ray absorptiometry. *Metabolism* 1993; 42: 967–70.

58 Cheek DB. Body composition, hormones, nutrition and adolescent growth. In: Grumbach MM, Grave GD, Mayer FE eds. *Control of the Onset of Puberty*. New York: John Wiley & Sons, 1974: 424–47.

59 Hammer LD, Wilson DM, Litt IF *et al*. Impact of pubertal development on body fat distribution among white, Hispanic, and Asian female adolescents. *J Pediatr* 1991; 118: 975–80.

60 Troiano RP, Flegal KM, Kuczmarski RJ, Campbell SM, Johnson CL. Overweight prevalence and trends for children and adolescents. The National Health and Nutrition Examination Surveys. 1963–91. *Arch Pediatr Adolesc Med* 1995; 149: 1085–91.

61 Tanner JM, Whitehouse RH, Marubini E, Resele LF. The adolescent growth spurt of boys and girls of the Harpenden growth study. *Ann Hum Biol* 1976; 3: 109–26.

62 Abbassi V. Growth and normal puberty. *Pediatrics* 1998; 102: 507–11.

63 Largo RH, Prader A. Pubertal development in Swiss girls. *Helv Paediatr Acta* 1983; 38: 229–43.

64 Largo RH, Gasser TH, Prader A. Analysis of the adolescent growth spurt using smoothing spline functions. *Ann Hum Biol* 1978; 5: 421–34.

65 Attie KM, Ramirez NR, Conte FA, Kaplan SL, Grumbach MM. The pubertal growth spurt in eight patients with true precocious puberty and growth hormone deficiency: evidence for a direct role of sex steroids. *J Clin Endocrinol Metab* 1990; 71: 975–83.

66 Martha PM Jr, Rogol AD, Veldhuis JD. Alterations in the pulsatile properties of circulating growth hormone concentrations during puberty in boys. *J Clin Endocrinol Metab* 1989; 69: 563–70.

67  Marin G, Domene HM, Barnes KM, Blackwell BJ, Cassorla FG, Cutler GBJ. The effects of estrogen priming and puberty on the growth hormone response to standardized treadmill exercise and arginine–insulin in normal girls and boys. *J Clin Endocrinol Metab* 1994; 79: 537–41.

68  Harris DA, Van Vliet G, Egli CA *et al.* Somatomedin-C in normal puberty and in true precocious puberty before and after treatment with a potent luteinizing hormone-releasing hormone agonist. *J Clin Endocrinol Metab* 1985; 61: 152–9.

69  Veldhuis JD, Metzger DL, Martha PMJ *et al.* Estrogen and testosterone, but not a nonaromatizable androgen, direct network integration of the hypothalamo-somatotrope (growth hormone)-insulin-like growth factor I axis in the human: evidence from pubertal pathophysiology and sex-steroid hormone replacement. *J Clin Endocrinol Metab* 1997; 82: 3414–20.

70  Metzger DL, Kerrigan JR. Estrogen receptor blockade with tamoxifen diminishes growth hormone secretion in boys: evidence for a stimulatory role of endogenous estrogens during male adolescence. *J Clin Endocrinol Metab* 1994; 79: 513–18.

71  Calvo MS, Eyre DR, Gundberg CM. Molecular basis and clinical application of biologic markers of bone turnover. *Endocr Rev* 1996; 17: 333–68.

72  Sorva R, Anttila R, Siimes MA, Sorva A, Tahtela R, Turpeinen M. Serum markers of collagen metabolism and serum osteocalcin in relation to pubertal development in 57 boys at 14 years of age. *Pediatr Res* 1997; 42: 528–32.

73  Styne DM, Harris DA, Egli CA *et al.* Treatment of true precocious puberty with a potent luteinizing hormone-releasing factor agonist: effect on growth, sexual maturation, pelvic sonography, and the hypothalamic-pituitary-gonadal axis. *J Clin Endocrinol Metab* 1985; 61: 142–51.

74  Ross JL, Cassorla FG, Skerda MC *et al.* A preliminary study of the effect of estrogen dose on growth in Turner's syndrome. *N Engl J Med* 1984; 309: 1104–6.

75  Svan H, Ritzen EM, Hall K, Johansson L. Estrogen treatment of tall girls; dose dependency of effects on subsequent growth and IGF-I levels in blood. *Acta Paediatr Scand* 1999; 80: 328–32.

76  Grumbach MM, Auchus RJ. Estrogen: consequences and implication of human mutations in synthesis and action. *J Clin Endocrinol Metab* 1999; 84: 4677–443.

77  Cutler GBJ. The role of estrogen in bone growth and maturation during childhood and adolescence. *J Steroid Biochem Mol Biol* 1997; 61: 141–4.

78  Rao E, Weiss B, Fukami M *et al.* Pseudoautosomal deletions encompassing a novel homeobox gene cause growth failure in idiopathic short stature and Turner syndrome [see comments]. *Nature Genet* 1997; 16: 54–63.

79  Largo RH, Prader A. Pubertal development in Swiss boys. *Helv Paediatr Acta* 1983; 38: 211–28.

80  Harlan WR, Harlan EA, Grillo GP. Secondary sex characteristics of girls 12–17 years of age: the U.S. Health Examination Survey. *J Pediatr* 1980; 96: 1074–8.

81  Harlan WR, Grillo GP, Cornoni-Huntley J, Leaverton PE. Secondary sex characteristics of boys 12–17 years of age: the U.S. Health Examination Survey. *J Pediatr* 1979; 95: 293–7.

82  Adelman JP, Mason AJ, Hayflick JS *et al.* Isolation of the gene and hypothalamic cDNA for the common precursor of gonadotropin-releasing hormone and prolactin release-inhibiting factor in human and rat. *Proc Natl Acad Sci USA* 1986; 83: 179–83.

83  Schwanzel-Fukada M, Jorgensen KL, Bergen HT *et al.* Biology of normal luteinizing hormone-releasing hormone neurons during and after their migration from olfactory placode. *Endocr Rev* 1992; 13: 623–34.

84  Schwanzel-Fukuda M. Origin and migration of luteinizing hormone-releasing hormone neurons in mammals. *Microsc Res Technical* 1999; 44: 2–10.

85  Hall JE. Physiologic and genetic insights into the pathophysiology and management of hypogonadotropic hypogonadism. *Ann Endocrinol* 1999; 60: 93–101.

86  Seminara SB, Hayes FJ, Crowley WFJ. Gonadotropin-releasing hormone deficiency in the human (idiopathic hypogonadotropic hypogonadism and Kallmann's syndrome): pathophysiological and genetic considerations. *Endocr Rev* 1999; 19: 521–39.

87  Hardelin JP, Petit C. A molecular approach to the pathophysiology of the X chromosome-linked Kallmann's syndrome. *Baillière's Clin Endocrinol Metab* 1995; 9: 489–507.

88  Hardelin JP, Julliard AK, Moniot B *et al.* Anosmin-1 is a regionally restricted component of basement membranes and interstitial matrices during organogenesis: implications for the developmental anomalies of X chromosome-linked Kallmann syndrome. *Dev Dyn* 1999; 215: 26–44.

89  Muscatelli F, Strom TM, Walker AP *et al.* Mutations in the DAX-1 gene give rise to both X-linked adrenal hypoplasia congenita and hypogonadotropic hypogonadism. *Nature* 1994; 372: 672–6.

90  Zanarla E, Muscatelli F, Bardoni B *et al.* An unusual member of the nuclear hormone receptor superfamily responsible for X-linked adrenal hypoplasia congenita. *Nature* 1994; 372: 635–41.

91  Achermann JC, Wen-xia G, Kotlar J *et al.* Mutational analysis of DAX1 in patients with hypogonadotropic hypogonadism or pubertal delay. *J Clin Endocrinol Metab* 1999; 84: 4497–500.

92  Seminara SB, Achermann JC, Genel M, Jameson JL, Crowley WFJ. X-linked adrenal hypoplasia congenita: a mutation in DAX1 expands the phenotypic spectrum in males and females. *J Clin Endocrinol Metab* 1999; 84: 4509.

93  Wu W, Cogan JD, Pfeaffle RW *et al.* Mutations in PROP1 cause familial combined pituitary hormone deficiency. *Nature Genet* 1998; 18: 147–9.

94  Holl RW, Pfeaffle R, Kim C, Sorgo W, Teller WM, Heimann G. Combined pituitary deficiencies of growth hormone, thyroid stimulating hormone and prolactin due to Pit-1 gene mutation: a case report. *Eur J Pediatr* 1997; 156: 835–7.

95  Huseman CA, Kelch RP. Gonadotropin responses and metabolism of synthetic gonadotropin-releasing hormone (GnRH) during constant infusion of GnRH in men and boys with delayed adolescence. *J Clin Endocrinol Metab* 1999; 47: 1331.

96  Hsueh AJW, Jones BC. Extra pituitary actions of gonadotropin-releasing hormone. *Endocr Rev* 1981; 2: 437–61.

97  Wetsel WC, Valenca MM, Merchenthaler I *et al.* Intrinsic pulsatile secretory activity of immortalized luteinizing hormone-releasing hormone-secreting neurons. *Proc Natl Acad Sci USA* 1992; 89: 4149–53.

98  Mellon PL, Windle JJ, Goldsmith PC *et al.* Immortalization of hypothalamic GnRH neurons by genetically targeted tumorigenesis. *Neuron* 1990; 5: 1–10.

99  Mitsushima D, Hei DL, Terasawa E. Gamma-aminobutyric acid is an inhibitory neurotransmitter restricting the release of luteinizing hormone-releasing hormone before the onset of puberty. *Proc Natl Acad Sci USA* 1994; 91: 395–9.

100 Belchetz PE, Plant TM, Nakai Y, Keogh EJ, Knobil E. Hypophyseal responses to continuous and intermittent delivery of hypothalamic gonadotropin-releasing hormone. *Science* 1978; 202: 631–3.

101 Hazum E, Conn PM. Molecular mechanism of gonadotropin releasing hormone (GnRH) action. I. The GnRH receptor. *Endocr Rev* 1988; 9: 379–86.

102 Huckle W, Conn PM. Molecular mechanisms of gonadotropin releasing hormone action. II. The effector system. *Endocr Rev* 1988; 9: 387–95.

103 Thorner MO, Vance ML, Laws ER Jr, Horvath E, Kovacs K. The anterior pituitary. In: Wilson JD, Foster DW, Kroneberg HM, Larsen PR eds. *William's Textbook of Endocrinology*. Philadelphia: W. B. Saunders, 1998: 249–340.

104 Huhtaniemi I, Jiang M, Nilsson C, Pettersson K. Mutations and polymorphisms in gonadotropin genes. *Mol Cell Endocrinol* 1999; 151: 89–94.

105 Layman LC. Mutations in human gonadotropin genes and their physiologic significance in puberty and reproduction. *Fertil Steril* 1999; 71: 201–18.

106 Kovacs K, Horvath E. Gonadotrophs following removal of the ovaries: a fine structural study of human pituitary glands. *Endokrinologie* 1975; 66: 1–8.

107 Beitins IZ, Padmanabhan V. Bioactivity of gonadotropins. *Endocrinol Metab Clin N Am* 1991; 20: 85–120.

108 Conte FA, Grumbach MM, Kaplan SL, Reiter EO. Correlation of luteinizing hormone-releasing factor-induced luteinizing hormone and follicle-stimulating hormone release from infancy to 19 years with the changing pattern of gonadotropin secretion in agonadal patients: relation to the restraint of puberty. *J Clin Endocrinol Metab* 1980; 50: 163–8.

109 Reiter EO, Kulin HE, Hamwood SM. The absence of positive feedback between estrogen and luteinizing hormone in sexually immature girls. *Pediatr Res* 1974; 8: 740–5.

110 Griffin JE, Wilson JD. Disorders of the testes and the male reproductive tract. In: Wilson JD, Foster DL, Kronenberg MD, Larsen PR eds. *William's Textbook of Endocrinology*, 9th edn. Philadelphia: W. B. Saunders, 1998: 819–75.

111 Bartsch W, Horst HJ, Derwahl DM. Interrelationships between sex hormone-binding globulin and 17 beta-estradiol, testosterone, 5 alpha-dihydrotestosterone, thyroxine, and triiodothyronine in prepubertal and pubertal girls. *J Clin Endocrinol Metab* 1980; 50: 1053–6.

112 Horst HJ, Bartsch W, Dirksen-Thiedens I. Plasma testosterone, sex hormone binding globulin binding capacity and per cent binding of testosterone and 5alpha-dihydrotestosterone in prepubertal, pubertal and adult males. *J Clin Endocrinol Metab* 1977; 45: 522–7.

113 Russel DW, Wilson JD. Steroid 5 a hydroxylase; two genes/two enzymes. *Annu Rev Med* 1994; 63: 25–61.

114 Mahendroo MS, Mendelson CR, Simpson ER. Tissue specific and hormonally controlled alternative promoters regulate aromatase cyotchrome P450 gene expression in human adipose tissue. *J Biol Chem* 1993; 268: 19463–70.

115 Lubahn DR, Joseph DR, Sar M *et al.* The human androgen receptor: complementary dexoribonucleic acid cloning, sequence analysis and gene expression in prostate. *Mol Endocrinol* 1988; 2: 1265–75.

116 Smith EP, Boyd J, Frank GR *et al.* Estrogen resistance caused by a mutation by the estrogen-receptor in a man. *N Engl J Med* 1994; 331: 1056–61.

117 Carr BR. Disorders of the ovaries and female reproductive tract. In: Wilson JD, Foster DW, Kronenberg MD, Larsen PR eds. *William's Textbook of Endocrinology*, 9th edn. Philadelphia: W. B. Saunders, 1999: 751–817.

118 Klein KO, Baron J, Colli MJ, McDonnell DP, Cutler GBJ. Estrogen levels in childhood determined by an ultrasensitive recombinant cell bioassay. *J Clin Invest* 1994; 94: 2475–80.

119 Klein KO, Baron J, Barnes KM, Pescovitz OH, Cutler GJ. Use of an ultrasensitive recombinant cell bioassay to determine estrogen levels in girls with precocious puberty treated with a luteinizing hormone-releasing hormone agonist. *J Clin Endocrinol Metab* 1998; 83: 2387–9.

120 Klein KO, Mericq V, Brown-Dawson JM, Larmore KA, Cabezas P, Cortinez A. Estrogen levels in girls with premature thelarche compared with normal prepubertal girls as determined by an ultrasensitive recombinant cell bioassay. *J Pediatr* 1999; 134: 190–2.

121 Dunn JF, Nisula BC, Rodbard. D. Transport of steroid hormones: binding of 21 endogenous steroids to both testosterone-binding globulin and corticosteroid-binding globulin in human plasma. *J Clin Endocrinol Metab* 1991; 9(53): 58–68.

122 Owerbach D, Rutter WJ, Cooke NE *et al.* The prolactin gene is located on chromosome 6 in humans. *Science* 1981; 212: 815–16.

123 Aubert ML, Sizonenko PC, Kaplan SL *et al.* The ontogenesis of human prolactin from fetal life to puberty. In: Crosignani PG, Robyn C eds. *Prolactin and Human Reproduction*. New York: Academic Press, 1977: 9–20.

124 Vale W, Bilezikjian LM, Rivier C. Reproductive and other roles of inhibins and activins. In: Knobil E, Neil JD eds. *Physiology of Reproduction*, 2nd edn. New York: Raven Press, 1994: 1861–78.

125 Andersson A-M, Juul A, Petersen JH *et al.* Serum inhibin B in healthy pubertal and adolescent boys: relation to age, stage of puberty and FSH, LH, testosterone, and estradiol levels. *J Clin Endocrinol* 1997; 82: 3976–81.

126 Andersson AM, Toppari J, Haavisto AM *et al.* Longitudinal reproductive hormone profiles in infants: peak of inhibin B levels in infant boys exceeds levels in adult men. *J Clin Endocrinol* 1998; 83: 675–81.

127 Byrd W, Bennett MJ, Carr BR, Dong Y, Wians F, Rainey W. Regulation of biologically active dimeric inhibin A and B from infancy to adulthood in the male. *J Clin Endocrinol Metab* 1998; 83: 2849–54.

128 Josso N, Legeai L, Forest MG, Chaussain JL, Brauner R. An enzyme linked immunoassay for anti-mullerian hormone: a new tool for the evaluation of testicular function in infants and children. *J Clin Endocrinol Metab* 1990; 70: 23–7.

129 Hudson PL, Dougas I, Donahoe PK *et al.* An immunoassay to detect human mullerian inhibiting substance in males and females during normal development. *J Clin Endocrinol Metab* 1990; 70: 16–22.

130 Kim MR, Gupta MK, Travers SH, Rogers DG, Van Lente F, Faiman C. Serum prostate specific antigen, sex hormone binding globulin and free androgen index as markers of pubertal development in boys. *Clin Endocrinol* 1999; 50: 203–10.

131 Loche S, Cambiaso P, Carta D *et al.* The growth hormone-releasing activity of hexarelin, a new synthetic hexapeptide, in

short normal and obese children and in hypopituitary subjects. *J Clin Endocrinol Metab* 1995; 80: 674–8.

132 Van Gaal LF, Wauters MA, Mertens IL, De Considine RV, Leeuw IH. Clinical endocrinology of human leptin. *Int J Obes Relat Metab Disord* 1999; 23: 29–36.

133 Farooqi IS, Jebb SA, Langmack G *et al.* Brief report: effects of recombinant leptin therapy in a child with congenital leptin deficiency. *N Engl J Med* 1999; 341: 879–84.

134 Ahmed ML, Ong KK, Morrell DJ *et al.* Longitudinal study of leptin concentrations during puberty: sex differences and relationship to changes in body composition. *J Clin Endocrinol Metab* 1999; 84: 899–905.

135 Arslanian S, Suprasongsin C, Kalhan SC, Drash AL, Brna R, Janosky JE. Plasma leptin in children: relationship to puberty, gender, body composition, insulin sensitivity, and energy expenditure. *Metabolism: Clin Exp* 1998; 47: 309–12.

136 Gluckman PD, Grumbach MM, Kaplan SL. The neuroendocrine regulation and function of growth hormone and prolactin in the mammalian fetus. *Endocr Rev* 1981; 2: 363–95.

137 Forest MG. Pituitary gonadotropin and sex steroid secretion during the first two years of life. In: Grumbach MM, Sizonenko PC, Aubert AU eds. *Control of the Onset of Puberty*. Baltimore: Williams & Wilkins, 1990: 451–78.

138 Nathwani NC, Hindmarsh PC, Massarano AA, Brook CGD. Gonadotrophin pulsatility in girls with the Turner syndrome: modulation by exogenous sex steroids. *Clin Endocrinol* 1998; 49: 107–13138.

139 Goji K, Tanikaze S. Comparison between spontaneous gonadotropin concentration profiles and gonadotropin response to low-dose gonadotropin-releasing hormone in prepubertal and early pubertal boys and patients with hypogonadotropic hypogonadism: assessment by using ultrasensitive, time-resolved immunofluorometric assay. *Pediatr Res* 1992; 31: 535–9.

140 Dunkel L, Alfthan H, Stenman U *et al.* Gonadal control of pulsatile secretion of luteinizing hormone and follicle-stimulating hormone in prepubertal boys evaluated by ultrasensitive time-resolved immunofluorometric assays. *J Clin Endocrinol Metab* 1990; 70: 107–14.

141 Mitamura R, Yano K, Suzuki N, Ito Y, Makita Y, Okuno A. Diurnal rhythms of luteinizing hormone, follicle-stimulating hormone, and testosterone secretion before the onset of male puberty. *J Clin Endocrinol Metab* 1999; 84: 29–37.

142 Grumbach MM, Kaplan SL. The neuroendocrinology of human puberty: an ontogenetic perspective. In: Grumbach MM, Sizonenko PC, Aubert ML eds. *Control of the Onset of Puberty*. Baltimore: Williams & Wilkins, 1990: 1–68.

143 Judge DM, Kulin HE, Santen R *et al.* Hypothalamic hamartoma: a source of luteinizing-hormone-releasing factor in precocious puberty. *N Engl J Med* 1977; 296: 7–10.

144 Jung H, Carmel P, Schwartz MS *et al.* Some hypothalamic hamartomas contain transforming growth factor a, a puberty-inducing growth factor, not luteinizing hormone releasing hormone neurons. *J Clin Endocrinol Metab* 1999; 84: 4695–701.

145 Boyar R, Finkelstein J, Roffwarg H, Kapen S, Weitzman E, Hellman L. Synchronization of augmented luteinizing hormone secretion with sleep during puberty. *N Engl J Med* 1972; 287: 582–6.

146 Ankarberg C, Norjavaara E. Diurnal rhythm of testosterone secretion before and throughout puberty in healthy girls: correlation with 17beta-estradiol and dehydroepiandrosterone sulfate. *J Clin Endocrinol Metab* 1999; 84: 975–84.

147 Roth JC, Grumbach MM, Kaplan SL. Effect of synthetic luteinizing hormone-releasing factor on serum testosterone and gonadotropins in prepubertal, pubertal, and adult males. *J Clin Endocrinol Metab* 1973; 37: 680–6.

148 Corley KP, Valk TW, Kelch RP *et al.* Estimation of GnRH pulse amplitude during pubertal development. *Pediatr Res* 1981; 15: 157–62.

149 Chryssikopoulos A, Gregoriou O, Papadias C, Loghis C. Gonadotropin ovulation induction and pregnancies in women with Kallmann's syndrome. *Gynecol Endocrinol* 1998; 12: 103–8.

150 Filicori M, Butler JP, Crowley WFJ. Neuroendocrine regulation of the corpus luteum in the human. *J Clin Invest* 1999; 73: 1638–47.

151 Tsafiri A, Chun SY. Ovulation. In: Adashi EY, Rock JA, Rosenwaks Z eds. *Reproductive Endocrinology, Surgery and Technology*. Philadelphia: Lippincott-Raven, 1996: 236–49.

152 Chabbert B, Djakoure C, Maitre SC, Bouchard P. Regulation of the human menstrual cycle. *Front Neuroendocrinol* 1998; 19: 151–86.

153 Apter D, Vihko R. Serum pregnenolone, progesterone, 17-hydroxyprogesterone, testosterone and 5 alpha-dihydrotestosterone during female puberty. *J Clin Endocrinol Metab* 1977; 45: 1039–48.

154 Lemarchand-Beraud T, Zufferey MM, Reymond M. Maturation of the hypothalamo-pituitary ovarian axis in adolescent girls. *J Clin Endocrinol Metab* 1982; 54: 241–6.

155 Grumbach MM, Richards GE, Conte FA *et al.* Clinical disorders of adrenal function and puberty: an assessment of the role of the adrenal cortex in normal and abnormal puberty in man and evidence for an ACTH-like pituitary adrenal androgen stimulating hormone. In: James VHT, Serio M, Giusti G *et al.* eds. *The Endocrine Function of the Human Adrenal Cortex, Serono Symposium*. New York: Academic Press, 1977: 583–612.

156 Ghizzoni L, Mastorakos G, Vottero A. Adrenal hyperandrogenism in children. *J Clin Endocrinol Metab* 1999; 84: 4431–5.

157 Tanner JM, Eveleth PB. Onset of puberty. In: Bierich JR ed. *Puberty: Biologic and Social Components*. Leiden: HE Stenfert Kroese Publishers, 1975: 256.

158 Van Wieringen JD, Wafelbakker F, Verbrugge HP. Growth Diagrams 1965 Netherlands. *Second National Survey on 0–24 Year Olds. Netherlands Institute for Preventative Medicine TNO*. Gröningen: Wolters-Noordhoof Publishing 1971.

159 Reiter EO, Beitins IZ, Ostrea T, Gutai JP. Bioassayable luteinizing hormone during childhood and adolescence and in patients with delayed pubertal development. *J Clin Endocrinol Metab* 1982; 54: 155–61.

160 Boyar RM, Rosenfeld RS, Kapen S, Finkelstein JW, Roffwarg HP, Weitzman ED, Hellman L. Human puberty. Simultaneous augmented secretion of luteinizing hormone and testosterone during sleep. *J Clin Invest* 1974; 54: 609–18.

161 Burr IM, Sizonenko PC, Kaplan SL, Grumbach MM. Hormonal changes in puberty. I. Correlation of serum luteinizing hormone and follicle stimulating hormone with stages of puberty, testicular size, and bone age in normal boys. *Pediatr Res* 1970; 4: 25–35.

162 August GP, Grumbach MM, Kaplan SL. Hormonal changes in puberty. 3. Correlation of plasma testosterone, LH, FSH, testicular size, and bone age with male pubertal development. *J Clin Endocrinol Metab* 1972; 34: 319–26.

163 Waaler PE, Thorsen T, Stoa KF *et al*. Studies in normal male puberty. *Acta Paediatr Scand* 1974 (Suppl. 249): 1–36.

164 Roche AF, Wellens R, Attie KM, Siervogel RM. The timing of sexual maturation in a group of US white youths. *J Ped Endocrinol Metab*, 1995; 8: 11–8.

165 Fisher DA. *Endocrinology Test Selection and Interpretation*, 2nd edn. San Juan Capistrano: Quest Diagnostics, 1996: 1–333.

# 12  Disorders of puberty

**Nicola Bridges**

## Introduction

Maturation within the hypothalamus controls the timing of onset of puberty. The succession of endocrine changes that occur with pubertal development are relatively fixed and result in a consistent pattern of physical changes. Most abnormalities relate to abnormal timing of puberty (too early or too late) or loss of the normal pattern of physical changes (loss of consonance).

Disorders of puberty can be divided into:
• Sexual precocity. This can involve all the endocrine and physical changes of puberty (centrally mediated precocious puberty) or the appearance of secondary sexual characteristics in a sequence different from that of normal puberty.
• Pubertal delay and pubertal arrest. Delay in the appearance of secondary sexual characteristics may occur in an individual with normal endocrinology who ultimately attains normal sexual development or in a patient with a permanent defect. Arrest of development once puberty has commenced is rare but usually indicates the onset of an underlying illness.
• Disorders developing during puberty. The clinical features of polycystic ovarian disease often present in puberty. In boys, gynaecomastia is a normal feature of puberty and can present as a cosmetic problem.

## Sexual precocity

The terminology used to define sexual precocity can be confusing and individual patients may not fit into a given diagnostic category. In this chapter the term 'sexual precocity' is used for any secondary sexual characteristic appearing too early and the term 'precocious puberty' is limited to centrally mediated sexual precocity where the endocrine and physical features are exactly the same as in normal puberty. Some authors use the term 'pseudopuberty' for development that is not consonant.

Sexual precocity is conventionally defined as any secondary sexual characteristic occurring before 8 years in a girl and 9 years in a boy. There has been a secular trend in the age of normal puberty and this convention has been questioned because an increasing proportion of entirely normal children develop before these ages [1], although no new limits have been defined.

The source of the sex steroids and the rate of progression of physical signs are the important factors in guiding investigation and management. The potential sources of sex steroids in sexual precocity are:
• Gonads. In most situations gonadal steroids are secreted in response to pituitary gonadotrophin stimulation. The exceptions to this are rare cases of autonomous sex steroid secretion and very rare cases of tumours secreting gonadotrophins.
• Adrenal gland. After birth the fetal zone of the adrenal regresses and adrenal androgen secretion remains at a low level until mid-childhood when adrenarche supervenes, with an increased secretion of dehydroepiandrosterone sulphate (DHEAS) and androstenedione. The physiological levels of adrenal androgens usually have no physical effect but can stimulate growth of pubic and axillary hair and apocrine sweat. Adrenal tumours or adrenal enzyme defects (such as 21-hydroxylase deficiency) result in supraphysiological levels of adrenal androgens, which can manifest as severe hirsutism, genital growth or clitoromegaly, deepening of the voice or rapid growth and bone age advance.
• Tumours secreting sex steroids.
• Exogenous steroids.

## Causes of sexual precocity

### Gonadal steroids

#### Central precocious puberty in girls

Pituitary gonadotrophins stimulate gonadal activity in girls resulting in central precocious puberty, premature thelarche and slowly progressing variants of precocious puberty.

(a)

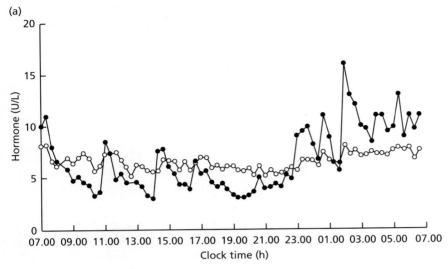

(b)

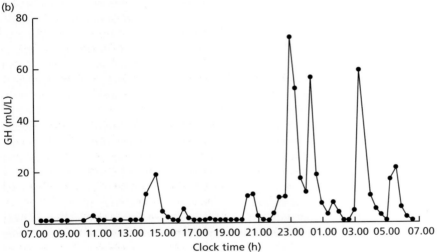

**Fig. 12.1.** Twenty-four-hour profile using 20-min sampling of (a) LH and FSH and (b) GH in a 5-year-old girl with central precocious puberty. The pattern of gonadotrophin and GH secretion is the same as in normally timed puberty. ●, LH; ○, FSH.

Centrally mediated precocious puberty is much more common in girls than in boys [2]. The endocrine and physical events occur in the same pattern and at the same pace as normally timed puberty (i.e. are consonant) – breast development followed by pubic hair growth, with normal pubertal growth and advancing bone age (Fig. 12.1). Pubertal development of the ovaries and the uterus can be seen at ultrasound [3]. The pattern of pituitary hormone secretion is the same as in a normally timed puberty. In most girls there is no central nervous system (CNS) defect, and magnetic resonance imaging (MRI) demonstrates a normal (pubertal) pituitary and hypothalamic area [4,5].

A small proportion of girls presenting with central precocious puberty have an underlying CNS lesion, although these lesions are not necessarily associated with the hypothalamus and pituitary (Table 12.1). Central precocious puberty is rarely the presenting sign of the CNS lesion [2] in girls, but

**Table 12.1.** CNS lesions associated with central precocious puberty

Tumours
  Chiasmatic/hypothalamic glioma [6]
  Pineal tumours and cysts
  Astrocytoma
  Ependymoma
  Pituitary adenoma

Other CNS lesions
  After CNS surgery or irradiation [7]
  Hydrocephalus (even if the period of raised intracranial pressure was brief [8]).
  Neurofibromatosis (in association with CNS pathology [9,10]).
  Post trauma
  Septo-optic dysplasia
  After meningitis/encephalitis
  Hypothalamic hamartoma

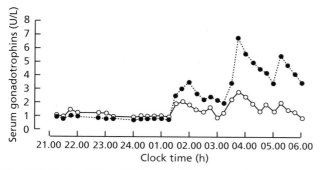

**Fig. 12.2.** Profile of LH and FSH in a girl with premature thelarche. There is overnight gonadotrophin pulsatility, with FSH predominating. Concentrations of LH and FSH are much lower than seen in precocious puberty. ●, FSH; ○, LH.

symptoms and signs of raised intracranial pressure must be carefully excluded.

Central precocious puberty and early puberty are common in otherwise healthy girls adopted from developing countries [11]. There is also evidence that central precocious puberty is more common in girls who have been sexually abused [12]. There are a number of dysmorphic syndromes where central precocious puberty is one of the features, for example Kabuki makeup syndrome [13].

In girls who present with breast development alone and no progression in puberty (premature thelarche), the underlying endocrine feature is a dominance in pulsatile follicle-stimulating hormone (FSH) secretion, which stimulates low concentrations of oestrogen secretion [14] (Fig. 12.2). This is different from the pattern seen in true puberty, where luteinizing hormone (LH) predominates [15]. Onset is typically in the first few years of life, breast development may be one sided and there may be a history of fluctuation in breast size. There is no change in height velocity or bone age advancement. Some authors have reported an increase in small ovarian cysts visualized at ultrasound [16].

A smaller group of girls present with clinical features somewhere between true central precocious puberty and premature thelarche. There is some advance in the physical signs of puberty which may be accompanied by increased growth velocity and bone age advance but not at the same pace as seen in normal puberty. This is called thelarche variant or slowly progressing variant of central precocious puberty [17–19]. The endocrine features are also on a spectrum between those of central precocious puberty and premature thelarche [17]. This means that a girl presenting with a short history of breast development alone may have premature thelarche or may progress through puberty slowly or rapidly, and the diagnosis may become clear only with follow-up [20].

## Central precocious puberty in boys

There appears to be no male equivalent to premature thelarche or slowly progressing variations of precocious puberty. Central precocious puberty in boys is much rarer than in girls and is almost invariably secondary to central lesions [2] (see Table 12.1). Idiopathic central precocious puberty in boys is either extremely rare or may not exist at all. For this reason all boys presenting with central precocious puberty must have cerebral imaging (preferably MRI).

## Gonadotrophin-independent sexual precocity

In McCune–Albright syndrome and testotoxicosis, pubertal levels of sex steroids are secreted by the gonads without gonadotrophin stimulation. The pattern of physical development is not necessarily the same as in normal puberty, because the pattern of endocrine changes seen is not the same (typically menstruation may occur at an inappropriately early stage of breast development). Some individuals have endocrine features of gonadotrophin-independent sexual precocity but do not appear to have either disorder and it has been suggested that the cellular abnormality of McCune–Albright syndrome may occur only in the gonadal tissue. In McCune–Albright syndrome, sexual precocity is associated with polyostotic fibrous dysplasia of bone and patches of skin pigmentation with a characteristic serrated edge (Fig. 12.3). Girls may have large ovarian cysts at ultrasound. Testotoxicosis is dominantly inherited and there may be a family history of sexual precocity in boys (girls with the defect are unaffected).

McCune–Albright syndrome and testotoxicosis are caused by abnormal function of the LH receptor [21]. In testotoxicosis there are mutations of the transmembrane domain of the LH receptor [22,23], the region important in interaction with the G-protein, which is the 'second messenger' of the receptor. In McCune–Albright, there is a mutation in the α-subunit of the G-protein itself [24]. The G-protein activates the cyclic adenosine monophosphate (cAMP) cascade within

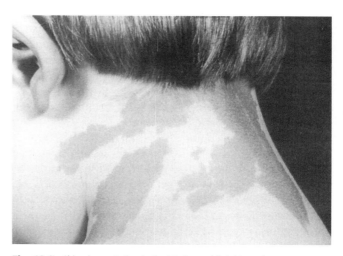

**Fig. 12.3.** Skin pigmentation in the McCune–Albright syndrome.

the cell, which initiates the cellular response to LH. Both abnormalities result in unlimited activation of the response, causing continued sex steroid secretion without gonadotrophin binding to the receptor.

Individuals with McCune–Albright syndrome are thought to be mosaic for the mutation, which is thought to occur during embryonic development in a somatic cell line. The expression of the abnormality in every cell is probably not compatible with life. McCune–Albright syndrome has been described in one of monozygotic twins [25]. The G-protein is shared by some other peptide hormone receptors, and other endocrine systems can be involved in McCune–Albright syndrome [26,27]. The presentation of the condition probably depends on the cell lines affected.

### Autonomous ovarian cysts

Ovarian cysts can secrete oestrogen in an autonomous manner and cause vaginal bleeding and breast development. Serum oestradiol concentration is elevated with low (suppressed) LH and FSH. Most ovarian cysts resolve spontaneously without surgery. A proportion of girls have recurrent cysts and some of these turn out to have McCune–Albright syndrome [28]. The differential diagnosis of isolated prepubertal vaginal bleeding includes hypothyroidism (see below), trauma, foreign body, tumours and sexual abuse.

### Hypothyroidism

In untreated hypothyroidism an elevation in FSH (Fig. 12.2) accompanies the elevated thyroid-stimulating hormone (TSH) [29]. Girls with untreated hypothyroidism may present with breast development or with vaginal bleeding. Ultrasound may demonstrate ovarian cysts [30]. The FSH falls to normal when the condition is treated.

### Tumours secreting gonadotrophin-releasing hormone or gonadotrophins

Hypothalamic hamartomas are benign intracranial tumours that present with centrally mediated precocious puberty and are associated with a typical pattern of epilepsy (gelastic seizures [31]). There is evidence that the sexual precocity is mediated by gonadotrophin-releasing hormone (GnRH) secretion from the tumour, at least in some cases [32,33].

Most patients presenting with sexual precocity as a result of gonadotrophin secretion from tumours are boys (although it has been reported in girls [34]), and most gonadotrophin-secreting tumours secrete human chorionic gonadotrophin (hCG). hCG secretion may be associated with secretion of other tumour markers such as α fetoprotein and pregnancy-specific glycoprotein. Secretion of LH by tumours has been reported [35]. The majority of hCG-secreting tumours are intracranial and include germ cell tumours [36] and

teratomas [37]. hCG secretion has also been described in hepatoblastoma [38,39] and in teratomas, some of which are associated with Klinefelter syndrome [40–42]. Gonadotrophin-secreting adenomas of the pituitary have been described in children [43].

## Adrenal steroids

### Premature adrenarche or premature pubarche

The physical features that can appear at adrenarche, pubic and axillary hair and the appearance of apocrine sweat, are called premature adrenarche or pubarche. There may be a small increase in height velocity and an advance in bone age. It is not clear why some children and not others develop physical changes at adrenarche. Studies using adrenocorticotrophic hormone (ACTH) stimulation have suggested an increased incidence of mild abnormalities of adrenal enzyme activity in these children [44], although there is no evidence that endogenous steroid concentrations are abnormal. Low birthweight has been suggested as a possible aetiological factor [45]. Endogenous puberty occurs at a normal time and final height is within the expected range for parents [46].

There is considerable racial variation, with premature adrenarche more common in children with origins in the Middle East, Eastern Europe and Africa. Children of Afro-Caribbean origin can have more exaggerated features of premature adrenarche, presenting with significant increases in bone age and height velocity. In a proportion of children, the distinction between premature adrenarche and serious adrenal pathology cannot be made on clinical grounds alone, and these children need investigation.

### Adrenal tumours

Adrenal cortical tumours can secrete androgens alone or androgens and cortisol and may present as Cushing syndrome [47]. Clitoromegaly, very rapid growth or bone age advance, extreme hirsutism or deepening of the voice are not likely to be caused by physiological concentrations of adrenal androgens. Distinguishing benign from malignant tumours is not always possible on histology but larger tumours are usually malignant [48]. Feminizing adrenal tumours have been described but are extremely rare [49].

### Congenital adrenal hyperplasia

Boys with congenital adrenal hyperplasia (21-hydroxylase or 11β-hydroxylase deficiency) who have not developed salt loss in the neonatal period may present in infancy or early childhood because of elevated androgen levels. Genital and pubic hair growth occurs without testicular enlargement. Height velocity and muscle bulk are increased. Bone age is advanced and adult height may be compromised.

Precocious puberty is a recognized complication of congenital adrenal hyperplasia. Elevated androgen levels, resulting from late diagnosis or poor compliance with medication, can act to 'mature' the hypothalamus and provoke early development. Pubertal development does not stop when the congenital adrenal hyperplasia is adequately treated and the final height can be significantly compromised [50,51].

## Tumours secreting sex steroids

As well as the adrenals, sex steroid-secreting tumours can occur in the gonads, or, rarely, elsewhere [52,53]. Most tumours secrete androgens [54], although feminizing tumours have been reported [55].

## Exogenous sources of sex steroids

A few cases of sexual precocity have been reported as a result of inadvertent contact with sex steroid-containing creams [56]. Although it has been suggested, there is no evidence that sex steroids in the environment or in foods can cause sexual precocity [57].

## Assessment and investigation of sexual precocity

Clinical assessment must include height and weight and a record of Tanner pubertal stages. Bone age assessment is of value if there is an increase in height velocity or concern over adult height. Other investigations should depend on the likely source of the sex steroids.

## Gonadal steroids

Clinical assessment will indicate if the development is consonant. Breast development in a girl or testicular enlargement in a boy suggest gonadal sex steroid secretion (except in a few very rare disorders). As discussed above, all boys must have cerebral imaging. In girls without neurological signs, the chances of finding a lesion are low [2]. Although there is considerable variation in practice, most clinicians are selective and do not perform MRI on all girls with central precocious puberty.

In girls the most useful assessment may be follow-up to determine the pace of development. Pelvic ultrasound may be of value in two situations. In puberty there is an increase in ovarian volume with an increase in follicle size and number, and a change in the shape of the uterus from tubular to pear shaped, with the appearance of an endometrial lining (Fig. 12.4) [3,58]. The same change is to be expected in central precocious puberty but not in premature thelarche. Pelvic ultrasound can provide some information about whether a girl will menstruate soon. This requires an endometrium of

about 5 mm, and although ultrasound is not helpful in predicting the time of menarche at that stage, it is highly unlikely that a girl will menstruate with a thin endometrium.

In centrally mediated puberty, sex steroid, LH and FSH levels remain low during the day until midpuberty and are always secreted in a pulsatile manner, so 'one-off' assays may not be helpful or easy to interpret. In premature thelarche low levels of oestradiol secretion have been detected using ultra-sensitive assays but not using standard assay methods [14]. In central precocious puberty the response to GnRH stimulation is the same as in normal puberty, with LH predominating. In gonadotrophin-independent puberty, the response to GnRH is flat, because of feedback suppression by elevated sex steroid concentrations. In McCune–Albright syndrome a radioisotope bone scan may be of value in detecting polyostotic fibrous dysplasia of bone.

## Adrenal steroids

Serum adrenal androgen levels are not helpful in confirming a diagnosis of premature adrenarche, but are likely (but not certain) to be elevated in adrenal tumours [47]. The urine steroid profile is likely to detect an adrenal tumour [59]. 17-Hydroxyprogesterone is likely to be elevated in 21-hydroxylase deficiency but the diagnosis may require ACTH-stimulated samples.

## Assessment of the need for treatment

Medical treatment can arrest the progress of puberty in central precocious puberty and gonadotrophin-independent sexual precocity. The consideration of instigating treatment may involve the discussion of loss of height prediction and the social or behavioural problems that puberty entails. For most children with sexual precocity the condition is not pathological and no treatment is required. In girls who appear to have central precocious puberty, careful assessment of the pace of progress is important before treatment, because this will demonstrate a proportion with slowly progressing variants of precocious puberty who would not benefit from treatment [18].

Children with central precocious puberty may appear much older than their true age and this can cause problems at school and socially. Pubertal levels of sex steroids in young children can provoke difficult behaviour. There are practical problems in dealing with periods in very young girls, and this may be more of a concern in girls with developmental delay or severe physical disabilities. In central precocious puberty the pubertal growth spurt occurs in the same way as in normally timed puberty. There is an increase in height velocity, and many present with tall stature. There is a rapid advance in bone age into the pubertal age range accompanied by a fall in predicted adult height (Fig. 12.5).

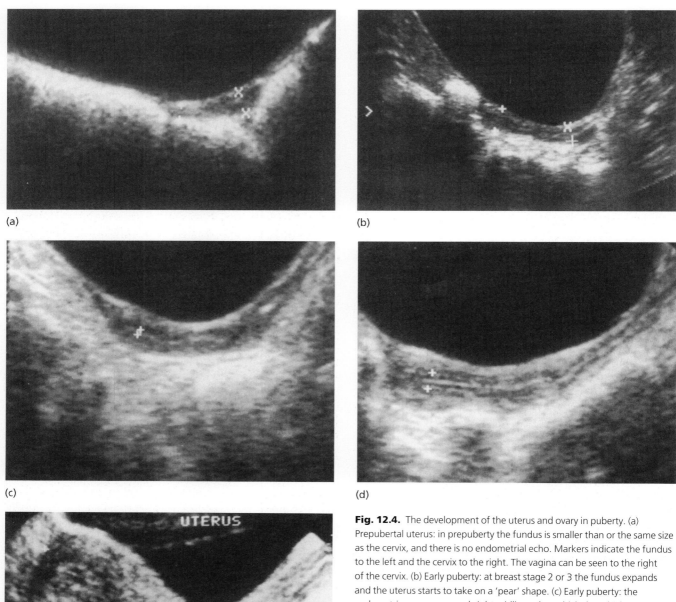

**Fig. 12.4.** The development of the uterus and ovary in puberty. (a) Prepubertal uterus: in prepuberty the fundus is smaller than or the same size as the cervix, and there is no endometrial echo. Markers indicate the fundus to the left and the cervix to the right. The vagina can be seen to the right of the cervix. (b) Early puberty: at breast stage 2 or 3 the fundus expands and the uterus starts to take on a 'pear' shape. (c) Early puberty: the endometrium appears as a bright midline echo, which then thickens. (d) Late puberty: menstruation does not occur until the endometrium is at least 5 mm thick. (e) Adult uterus: further growth occurs after menstruation until the uterus is of adult dimensions. (f) Prepubertal ovary: the ovary increases in volume throughout childhood. Small follicles are usually visible; the majority are 4 mm in diameter or less, although larger follicles are occasionally seen. (g) Multicystic ovary: in the years before puberty increasing gonadotrophin secretion stimulates an increase in ovarian volume and the growth of multiple larger follicles. (h) Midpuberty: larger follicles appear as gonadotrophin and oestrogen levels increase. (i) A dominant follicle: ovulatory cycles may not start for some time after menarche.

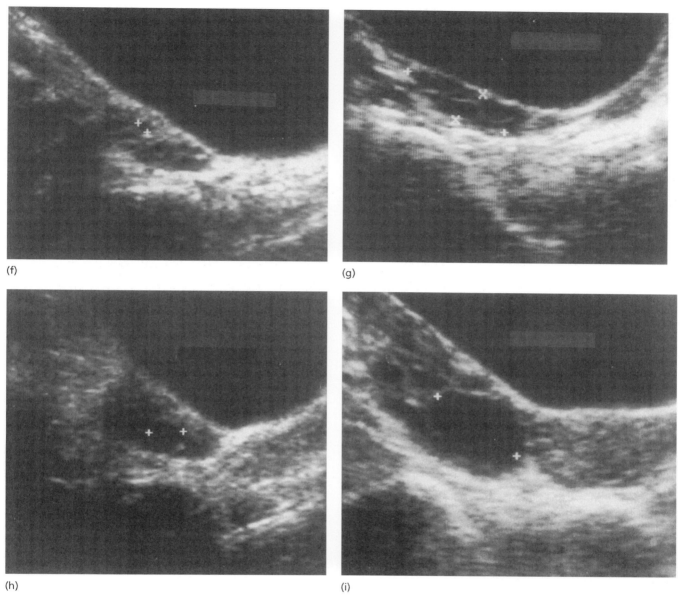

(f)

(g)

(h)

(i)

**Fig. 12.4.** Continued.

The height increment during the pubertal growth spurt is increased by its early occurrence, but final height is reduced because insufficient childhood growth has occurred before it starts. A similar loss of adult height occurs in gonadotrophin-independent sexual precocity or in any situation where there are pubertal concentrations of sex steroids.

Only a small proportion of children with precocious puberty benefit from treatment. The need for intervention should be assessed on an individual basis. The very youngest children clearly need treatment for the reasons discussed, but potential gains may be much more marginal in older subjects.

Treatment with depot injections or drugs requiring regular hospital reviews has a significant psychological impact and in many cases may not be worth any potential gain. Social and behavioural problems are not necessarily resolved by treatment, and many girls of normal intelligence can deal with having periods. Treatment cannot be justified on the grounds of height alone if the final height will be within the normal range, as is the case with many children with central precocious puberty (see below). Whether strict adherence to the concept of attaining genetic height potential is justified is unclear.

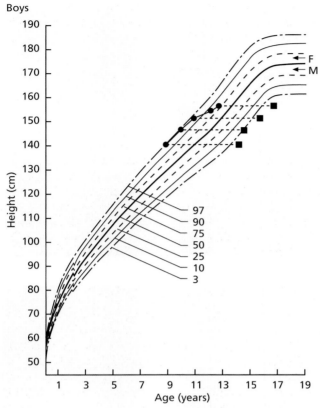

**Fig. 12.5.** Growth chart for a boy with untreated central precocious puberty. The boy presented at 8 years of age with centrally mediated precocious puberty secondary to a hypothalamic hamartoma, with a testicular volume of 8 mL. Rapid growth and bone age advance resulted in a diminishing height prediction. F, Father's height centile; M, mother's height centile; ■, bone age.

## Therapies available

GnRH analogues are the first choice of treatment in central precocious puberty because they have fewer side-effects than cyproterone acetate. Nasal preparations, daily subcutaneous injections and depot injections (monthly or 3 monthly [60]) have been used, with depot treatments probably the most convenient. GnRH analogues suppress gonadotrophin and sex steroid secretion and halt the progress of puberty; there may be regression of physical signs. There is a rise in sex steroid and gonadotrophin secretion at the start of treatment, before suppression occurs, and cyproterone acetate may be used to prevent a rapid advance in puberty at this point. There is a theoretical risk of loss of bone mineral density with treatment but no evidence that this is clinically significant [61,62].

Cyproterone acetate is an antiandrogen (i.e. it has action in blocking androgen receptors) with some progestagenic properties. Cyproterone is less effective than GnRH analogues in suppressing pubertal progress, but pubic and axillary hair regress in girls. It is used in treating McCune–Albright syndrome and testotoxicosis (where GnRH analogues are ineffective). Tiredness is a common side-effect and there is a risk of significant adrenal suppression [63]. Liver disease has been reported in a child with cirrhosis treated with cyproterone in large doses [64].

Testolactone and spironolactone are aromatase inhibitors and have been used in a number of trials treating McCune–Albright syndrome and testotoxicosis [65,66]. They have proved effective in halting progress. Flutamide (an anti-androgen) and ketoconazole (which inhibits steroid biosynthesis [67,68]) have not been widely used because of significant side-effects. There have been individual case reports of the use of tamoxifen but no larger studies [69].

## Growth and final height with and without treatment

For the reasons discussed above, final height is reduced in central precocious puberty and gonadotrophin-independent sexual precocity. Final height is normal in premature thelarche [70] and premature adrenarche [46]. Short stature has been reported as a feature in follow-up studies of untreated individuals with central precocious puberty [71], testotoxicosis [72] and McCune–Albright syndrome [73]. However, studies reporting the final height of untreated individuals indicate that most individuals with central precocious puberty have a final height within the normal range [74–76].

Treatment to arrest pubertal progress results in a reduction in sex steroid secretion and this in turn reduces the secretion of GH associated with the pubertal growth spurt [77]. This means that growth velocity falls with treatment and this is most marked for those with advanced bone ages. This reduction in height velocity limits the potential for treatment to 'restore lost height' [78].

Most studies of final height in central precocious puberty after treatment with GnRH analogues have demonstrated a small increase compared with the height prediction at the start of treatment [79–81]. There is no evidence of increased final height over height prediction with cyproterone acetate treatment [82,83]. The increment in final height is greater in the younger subjects [84], and there is no evidence of any height benefit for girls with 'early' but not precocious puberty [85]. There is no evidence of a benefit to the final height in girls with slowly progressing variants of precocious puberty [86].

The results of studies using GnRH analogues are dependent on height predictions based on bone age. These have limitations because they are derived from data gathered in normal children and are less accurate in pathological situations, including central precocious puberty [87]. Bayley–Pinneau predictions are more reliable in this situation than Tanner–Whitehouse [75].

There is no evidence of the best time to stop treatment with GnRH analogues. It is logical to stop once the subject has reached a normal age for the onset of puberty, and this is supported by the fact that studies using GnRH analogues to arrest puberty within the normal age range have not demonstrated an increase in final height [85,88]. Growth after stopping treatment is limited because these individuals have completed a proportion of their pubertal growth before treatment has started and there is an apparent loss of height prediction between the end of treatment and the final height in some studies [80,81].

A number of groups have examined the effect of adding GH treatment to GnRH analogues. This approach is supported by the results of using a combination of GH and GnRH analogues in GH-insufficient individuals [89,90]. Growth velocity is increased by treatment with a concomitant increase in height prediction. There are limited data on final height that suggest an improvement.

## Long-term outcome of sexual precocity

For most individuals, the problem is self-limiting with normal reproductive function. There is no evidence that early menarche results in early menopause. Impaired fertility has been reported in McCune–Albright syndrome where the abnormal pattern of activation continues into adult life [93]. There is an increased risk of obesity after central precocious puberty, which seems to be unrelated to treatment [94]. Normal menstrual function and fertility has been reported after stopping treatment with GnRH analogues [95,96]. Loss of bone density has been reported during treatment with GnRH analogues, but there is no evidence that this results in permanent loss of bone density [61,62]. The follow-up (at age 17.5 years) of a group of girls with precocious puberty demonstrated no significant long-term psychological consequences [97].

Follow-up of girls with premature adrenarche has demonstrated an increased prevalence of ovarian hyperandrogenism and polycystic ovarian disease [98,99]. Increased prevalence of polycystic ovarian disease has been reported in a few studies after central precocious puberty, but other studies using ultrasound follow-up have not confirmed this [58,100].

## Pubertal delay and pubertal failure

The majority of those who present with delayed puberty are boys. There may be concern because of delay in the physical changes of puberty or because of short stature. Most do not have any underlying defect and develop in time (constitutional delay). Spontaneous development can occasionally be very delayed indeed [101]. Assessment is aimed at detecting those with gonadal failure, those who are likely to have a permanent central defect and those with a cause for constitutional delay (usually a chronic illness). Treatment may be of benefit even if there is no underlying cause.

## Causes of gonadal failure

Radiotherapy and chemotherapy can result in gonadal failure in both sexes [102,103]. Turner syndrome is the commonest cause of gonadal failure in girls, although many girls with Turner syndrome are diagnosed well before pubertal age because of typical features or short stature. Gonadal failure in females is also associated with XY gonadal dysgenesis, auto-immune ovarian failure (which may be associated with a multiple autoimmune polyendocrinopathy syndrome) [104,105] and galactosaemia [106]. In boys gonadal failure can be caused by developmental defects such as anorchia or undescended testes or can follow torsion, infection or trauma.

### Central defects causing pubertal failure

Pituitary or hypothalamic damage (tumours, trauma, radiotherapy) can result in loss of gonadotrophin secretion. Gonadotrophin deficiency may be associated with multiple pituitary hormone defects in developmental defects of the pituitary. Isolated gonadotrophin deficiency can be associated with anosmia in Kallman syndrome (where the defect is in the GnRH-secreting neurones [21,107]), with adrenal failure in X-linked adrenal hypoplasia [108,109] and with X-linked ichthyosis [110,111]. Haemochromatosis associated with transfusion can result in permanent gonadotrophin deficiency [112].

### Disorders associated with constitutional delay and pubertal arrest

Pubertal delay is typically seen in chronic diseases such as asthma [113] (where the role of inhaled steroids remains uncertain), eczema, cystic fibrosis and inflammatory bowel disease [114–116].

Pubertal progress can halt with the development of a significant illness such as inflammatory bowel disease or malignancy, and pubertal arrest requires much more intensive investigation than delay. The onset of anorexia nervosa can result in pubertal delay or halt progress in puberty. Even when a normal eating pattern has been restored and weight returned to normal, normal activation of the hypothalamo-pituitary-gonadal axis can be delayed.

Pubertal delay in girls is associated with a range of activities where intense exercise is combined with the need for a very slim physique, such as ballet dancers, gymnasts and long-distance runners [117]. A study of young female ballet dancers demonstrated that pubertal delay was common, with many dancers reaching menarche only when resting because of injury. The same delay does not occur in children who have similar stress, such as child musicians [118,119]. Increased risk of pubertal delay and menstrual irregularity has been reported for adolescent females in a range of other sports [120,121]. Pubertal delay followed by amenorrhoea during intensive training in young athletes results in a significant risk of osteoporosis [122,123]. Bone density may improve in those who stop intensive training [124].

## Assessment and investigation

All patients presenting with delay of puberty should have height and Tanner pubertal stages recorded. Bone age with height prediction is indicated if there is short stature. Further investigation is indicated if there is a risk factor for gonadal failure, if any feature may be related to organic disease or if the clinical picture is of pubertal arrest rather than delay. The further the subjects are away from the normal age range for puberty, the more likely they are to have an organic cause for delay.

Turner syndrome should be considered in girls who are short compared with their parents, even if there are signs of puberty. In gonadal failure, lack of feedback suppression results in a rapid rise in gonadotrophin concentrations from 8 or 9 years of age, when gonadotrophin secretion starts to increase before normal puberty (Fig. 12.6). The LH and FSH concentrations in a single sample may be so high that they confirm the diagnosis. The gonadotrophin response to GnRH stimulation is exaggerated in gonadal failure.

Subjects at risk of a central defect should have an MRI scan of their hypothalamus and pituitary. Gonadotrophin pulsatility occurs mainly at night until midpuberty, so individual samples for LH and FSH are likely to be low (except in gonadal failure) and are of no value in predicting the future progress of puberty. GnRH testing has been studied extensively in pubertal delay, but may not clarify whether an individual will progress in puberty eventually or has a permanent defect [125,126]. Overnight sampling may demonstrate gonadotrophin pulsatility but will not predict future development in those with very low gonadotrophin levels. In girls a pelvic ultrasound may be reassuring that all is normal but has limited value in predicting future development.

## Treatment of pubertal delay and pubertal failure

Individuals with pubertal delay can experience significant problems: they may be bullied, excluded from social and sporting activities or find themselves treated as much younger than they are [127,128]. Many present because they are already experiencing difficulties and are keen to have treatment. Treatment in appropriate doses does not impair adult height and no long-term consequences have been reported [129]. There is no evidence of a cut-off age after which treatment should be offered, but there is certainly no advantage in waiting long periods in the hope of spontaneous puberty starting. For individuals with a demonstrated lesion who are not going to develop in puberty, induction of puberty should be planned to keep pace with the child's peers.

Oxandrolone is an anabolic steroid with weak androgenic action. An oral dose of 2.5 mg daily for 3 months will result in acceleration in height velocity [130]. There is no effect on pubertal development and this dose will not advance bone age or compromise the final height because it cannot be aromatized. The effect is most satisfactory for boys who have some signs of puberty (e.g. 6- to 8-mL testicular volume) but who have yet to reach their pubertal growth spurt, because the acceleration in height velocity then continues into the endogenous pubertal growth spurt. The dose can be repeated for a further 3 months if required. Oxandrolone can also be used in females but in much smaller doses.

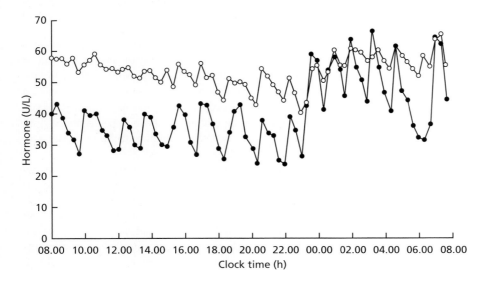

**Fig. 12.6.** Twenty-four-hour profile of gonadotrophin secretion in ovarian failure – a girl who had radiotherapy treatment for a pelvic sarcoma. Without sex steroid feedback, FSH and LH are secreted with a rapid pulse frequency and concentrations are elevated. ●, LH; ○, FSH.

Treatment with low-dose sex steroids is indicated for boys and girls who are prepubertal or in boys who are concerned about pubertal development as well as height. In boys 50 mg of testosterone esters every 4–6 weeks and in girls 2–5 µg of ethinyloestradiol can be given for 3–6 months. In many cases a short course of treatment is sufficient and can be stopped because the subject is satisfied with the results or because it has triggered endogenous pubertal development. If treatment is continued, the aim is gradually to increase the sex steroid dose to complete development over 2–3 years. In boys testosterone esters should be given in 6-month steps: 50 mg every 4 weeks, then 100 mg every 4 weeks, then 100 mg every 3 weeks and then 100 mg every 2 weeks (Fig. 12.7). A higher dose may be needed to give adult testosterone concentrations, and testosterone implants or patches may be suitable for maintaining adult concentrations of testosterone in those with a permanent defect.

In girls a daily dose of 5 µg, then 10 µg, then 15 µg and then 20 µg of oral ethinyloestradiol should be given in 6-month steps. A progestogen should be added in when a dose of 15 µg of ethinyloestradiol is reached, if there is a vaginal bleed or if the endometrium is thicker than 5 mm on ultrasound. For example, 30 µg of levonorgestrol daily (or equivalent non-$C_{19}$ progestogen) may be given for days 14–21.

Although this is frequently a cause of concern, there is no evidence that exogenous sex steroid treatment results in behaviour disturbance [131]. Pulsatile subcutaneous GnRH has been used successfully to induce puberty, with a pattern of administration designed to mimic normal puberty. This treatment has the advantage of being more physiological but is much more demanding for the subject and is rarely used outside clinical studies [132].

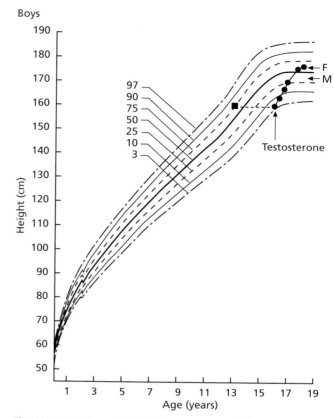

**Fig. 12.7.** Induction of puberty with testosterone. This boy presented with no signs of puberty at 16 years of age and was treated with testosterone. Virilization and a normal pubertal growth spurt were induced. His testicular volume did not progress to greater than 6 mL, and testosterone levels fell when the treatment was stopped. The diagnosis was hypogonadotrophic hypogonadism. F, Father's height centile; M, mother's height centile; ■, bone age.

## Long-term outcome

Most subjects with pubertal delay have spontaneous puberty and achieve normal final height. Although more childhood growth has occurred before the onset of the pubertal growth spurt, the magnitude of the growth spurt decreases as the subject gets older and thus there is no height advantage in delayed puberty, and the final height may in fact be reduced relative to target height for the parents [133,134].

Those with permanent defects must be followed to ensure that they are on sufficient sex steroid replacement: in women to give regular periods and maintain bone mass, and in men to give adult testosterone concentrations to maintain normal libido and regular shaving. Men with anorchia may want silicone implants to improve appearance. It is important to clarify any potential problems with fertility as previous discussions may have been forgotten or taken place when the individual was very young.

There is evidence that delayed puberty may result in permanent loss of bone mass, although this is not confirmed in all studies [135–137]. Late treatment and inadequate sex steroid dosage may result in increased long-term fracture risk. For female athletes and dancers there is an increased incidence of amenorrhoea and oligomenorrhoea after menarche, resulting in reduced bone mineral density and increased fracture risk [138].

## Gynaecomastia

Many normal boys develop gynaecomastia in midpuberty. Peripheral conversion of testosterone to oestrogen is thought to be responsible for this development, which is mild and resolves with time in most cases. Boys may present because of the cosmetic appearance or because of breast tenderness. Slightly overweight (but otherwise endocrinologically normal) boys experience the most severe problems, although severe gynaecomastia can be related to Klinefelter syndrome. There is no evidence that medical therapy is helpful in pubertal gynaecomastia, although a number of therapies have been tried in adult men with this condition [139]. A proportion will have problems severe enough to warrant surgery (liposuction or subareolar mastectomy).

## References

1  Kaplowitz PB, Oberfeld SE. Re-examination of the age limit for defining when puberty is precocious in girls in the United States: implications for evaluation and treatment. *Pediatrics* 1999; 104: 936–41.

2  Bridges NA, Christopher JA, Hindmarsh PC, Brook CGD. Sexual precocity: sex incidence and aetiology. *Arch Dis Child* 1994; 70: 116–18.

3  Jensen AB, Brocks V, Holm K, Laursen E, Muller J. Central precocious puberty in girls: internal genitalia before, during and after treatment with long acting gonadotropin releasing hormone analogues. *J Pediatr* 1998; 132: 105–18.

4  Robben SG, Oostdijk W, Drop SL, Tanghe HL, Vielvoye GJ, Meradji M. Idiopathic isosexual central precocious puberty: magnetic resonance findings in 30 patients. *Br J Radiol* 1995; 68: 34–8.

5  Koernreich L, Horev G, Blaser S, Danema D, Kauli R, Grunebaum M. Central precocious puberty; evaluation by neuroimaging. *Pediatr Radiol* 1995; 25: 7–11.

6  Collet Solberg PF, Sernyak H, Satin Smith M, Katz LL, Sutton L, Molloy P, Moshang T. Endocrine outcome in long term survivors of low grade hypothalamic/chiasmatic glioma. *Clin Endocrinol* 1997; 47: 79–85.

7  Ogilvy Stuart AL, Clayton PE, Shalet SM. Cranial irradiation and early puberty. *J Clin Endocrinol Metab* 1994; 78: 1282–6.

8  Lopponon T, Saukkonen AL, Serlo W, Tapanainen P, Ruokonen A, Knip M. Accelerated pubertal development in patients with shunted hydrocephalus. *Arch Dis Child* 1996; 74: 490–6.

9  Carmi D, Shohat M, Metzker A, Dickerman Z. Growth puberty and endocrine functions in patients with sporadic or familial neurofibromatosis type 1: a longitudinal study. *Pediatrics* 1999; 103: 1257–62.

10  Listernick R, Charrow J, Gutmann DH. Intracranial gliomas in neurofibromatosis type 1. *Am J Med Genet* 1999; 89: 38–44.

11  Virdis R, Street M, Zampolli M *et al.* Precocious puberty in girls adopted from developing countries. *Arch Dis Child* 1998; 78: 152–4.

12  Herman ME, Giddens AD, Sandler NE, Freidman NE. Sexual precocity in girls: an association with sexual abuse? *Am J Dis Child* 1988; 142: 431–3.

13  Kuroki Y, Katsumata N, Eguchi T, Fukishima Y, Suwa S, Kajii T. Precocious puberty in Kabuki Makeup syndrome. *J Pediatr* 1987; 110: 750–2.

14  Klein KO, Meriq V, Brown Dawson JM, Larmore KA, Cabezas P, Cortinez A. Estrogen levels in girls with premature thelarche compared with normal prepubertal girls as determined by an ultrasensitive recombinant cell bioassay. *J Pediatr* 1999; 134: 190–2.

15  Stanhope R, Abdulwahid NA, Adams J, Brook CGD. Studies of gonadotrophin pulsatility and pelvic ultrasound examinations distinguish between isolated premature thelarche and central precocious puberty. *Eur J Pediatr* 1986; 145: 190–4.

16  Freedman SM, Krietzer PM, Elkovitz SS, Saberman N, Leonidas JC. Ovarian microcysts in girls with isolated premature thelarche. *Pediatrics* 1993; 122: 246–9.

17  Stanhope R, Brook CGD. Thelarche variant: a new syndrome of precocious sexual development? *Acta Endocrinol* 1990; 123: 481–6.

18  Palmert MR, Malin HV, Boepple PA. Unsustained or slowly progressive puberty in young girls: initial presentation and long term follow up of 20 untreated patients. *J Clin Endocrinol Metab* 1999; 84: 415–23.

19  Fontoura M, Brauner R, Prevot C, Rappaport R. Precocious puberty in girls: early diagnosis of a slowly progressing variant. *Arch Dis Child* 1989; 64: 1170–6.

20  Pasquino AM, Pucarelli I, Passeri F, Segni M, Mancini MA, Municchi G. Progression of premature thelarche to central precocious puberty. *J Pediatr* 1995; 126: 11–14.

21  DiMeglio LA, Pescovitz OH. Disorders of puberty: inactivating and activating molecular mutations. *J Pediatr* 1997; 131 (Suppl.): 8S–12S.

22  Gromoll J, Partsch C-J, Simoni M *et al.* A mutation in the first transmembrane domain of the lutropin receptor causes male precocious puberty. *J Clin Endocr Metab* 1998; 83: 476–80.

23  Kremer H, Martens JWM, van Reen M *et al.* A limited repertoire of mutations of the luteinizing hormone (LH) receptor gene in familial and sporadic patients with male LH-independent precocious puberty. *J Clin Endocrinol Metab,* 1999; 84: 1136–40.

24  Weinstein LS, Shenker A, Gejman PV, Merino MJ, Friedman E, Spiegel AM. Activating mutations of the stimulatory G-protein in McCune–Albright syndrome. *N Engl J Med* 1991; 325: 1688–95.

25  Endo M, Yamada Y, Matsua N, Niikawa N. Monozygotic twins discordant for signs of McCune–Albright syndrome. *Am J Med Genet* 1991; 41: 216–20.

26  Kirk JMW, Brain CE, Carson DJ, Hyde JC, Grant DB. Cushing's syndrome caused by nodular adrenal hyperplasia in children with McCune–Albright syndrome. *J Pediatr* 1999; 134: 789–92.

27  Yoshimoto M, Nakayama M, Baba T *et al.* A case of neonatal McCune–Albright syndrome with Cushing syndrome and hyperthyroidism. *Acta Paediat Scand* 1991; 80: 984–7.

28  Rodruigez Macias KA, Thibaud E, Houang M, Duflos C, Bedjord C, Rappaport R. Follow up of precocious pseudopuberty associated with isolated ovarian follicular cysts 1999; 81: 53–6.

29  Pringle PJ, Stanhope R, Hindmarsh PC, Brook CGD. Abnormal pubertal development in primary hypothyroidism. *Clin Endocrinol* 1988; 28: 479–86.

30  Chen CH, Tiu CM, Chou YH, Cen WY, Hwang B, Niu DM. Congenital hypothyroidism with multiple ovarian cysts. *Eur J Pediatr* 1999; 158: 851–2.

31  Striano S, Meo R, Bilo L *et al.* Gelastic epilepsy: symptomatic and cryptogenic causes. *Epilepsia* 1999; 40: 294–302.

32  Uriarte MM, Klein KO, Barnes KM, Pescovitz OH, Loriaux DL, Cutler GB. Gonadotrophin and prolactin secretory dynamics in girls with normal puberty, idiopathic precocious puberty and precocious puberty due to hypothalamic hamartoma. *Clin Endocrinol* 1998; 49: 363–8.

33  Jung H, Carmel P, Scwartz MS, Witkin JW, Bentele KH, Westphal M *et al.* Some hypothalamic hamartomas contain transforming growth factor alpha, a puberty inducing growth factor, but not luteinising hormone releasing hormone neurons. *J Clin Endocrinol Metab* 1999; 84: 4695–701.

34  Kitanaka C, Matsutani M, Sora S, Kitanaka S, Tanae A, Hibi I. Precocious puberty in a girls with an HCG secreting immature teratoma. Case Report. *J Neurosurg* 1994; 81: 601–4.

35 Romer TE, Sachnowska K, Savage MO *et al.* Luteinising hormone secreting adrenal tumour as a cause of precocious puberty. *Clin Endocrinol* 1998; 48: 367–72.

36 Cho DY, Wang YC, Ho WL. Primary intrasellar mixed germ cell tumour with precocious puberty and diabetes insipidus. *Childs Nervous System* 1997; 13: 42–6.

37 Cohen AR, Wilson JA, Sadeghi-Nejad A. Gonadotrophin secreting pineal teratoma causing precocious puberty. *Neurosurgery* 1991; 28: 597–602.

38 Hermann A, White PF, Reily CA, Ritchey AK, Flye MW, Barwick KW. Hepatoblastoma presenting as isosexual precocity. The clinical importance of histologic and serologic parameters. *J Clin Gastroenterol* 1987; 9: 105–10.

39 Beach R, Bettts P, Radford M, Milward Sadler H. Production of human chorionic gonadotrophin by a hepatoblastoma resulting in precocious puberty. *J Clin Pathol* 1984; 37: 734–7.

40 Root AW, Bongiovanni AM, Eberlein WR. A testicular interstitial cell stimulating gonadotrophin in a child with hepatoblastoma and sexual precocity. *J Clin Endocrinol Metab* 1968; 28: 1317–22.

41 Derenoncourt AN, Castro Magana M, Jones KL. Mediastinal teratoma and precocious puberty in a boy with mosaic Kleinefelter syndrome. *Am J Med Genet* 1995; 55: 38–42.

42 Leschek EW, Doppman JL, Pass HI, Cutler GB. Localisation by venous sampling of occult chorionic gonadaotropin secreting tumor in a boy with mosaic Kleinefelter's syndrome and precocious puberty. *J Clin Endocrinol Metab* 1996; 81: 3825–8.

43 Ambrosi B, Bassetti M, Ferrario R, Medri G, Giannattasio G, Faglia G. Precocious puberty in a boy with a PRL-, LH- and FSH-secreting pituitary tumour: hormonal and immunocytochemical studies. *Acta Endocrinol* 1990; 122: 569–76.

44 Del Balzo P, Borrelli P, Cambiaso P, Danielli E, Cappa M. Adrenal steroidogenic defects in children with precocious pubarche. *Horm Res* 1992; 37: 180–4.

45 Ibanez L, Potau N, Fracois I, de Zegher F. Precocious pubarche hyperinsulinism and ovarian hyperandrogenism in girls: relation to reduced fetal growth. *J Clin Endocrinol Metab* 1998; 3558–62.

46 Ibanez L, Virdis R, Potau N *et al.* Natural history of premature pubarche: an auxological study. *J Clin Endocrinol Metab* 1992; 74: 254–7.

47 Wolther OD, Cameron FJ, Scheimberg I *et al.* Androgen secreting adrenocortical tumours. *Arch Dis Child* 1999; 80: 46–50.

48 Federici S, Galli G, Ceccarelli P *et al.* Adrenocortical tumours in children: a report of 12 cases. *Eur J Pediatr Surg* 1994; 4: 21–5.

49 Goto T, Murakami O, Sato F, Haraguchi M, Yokoyama K, Sasano H. Oestrogen producing adrenocortical adenoma: clinical, biochemical and immunohistochemical studies. *Clin Endocrinol* 1996; 45: 643–8.

50 Pescovitz OH, Comite F, Cassorla F *et al.* True precocious puberty complicating congenital adrenal hyperplasia: treatment with a LHRH analogue. *J Clin Endocrinol Metab* 1984; 58: 857–61.

51 Merke DP, Keil MF, Jones JV, Fields J, Hill S, Cutler GB. Flutamide, testolactone, and reduced hydrocortisone dose maintain normal growth velocity and bone maturation despite elevated androgen levels in children with congenital adrenal hyperplasia. *J Clin Endocrinol Metab* 2000; 85: 1114–20.

52 Masiakos PT, Flynn CE, Donahoe PK. Masculinising and feminisng syndromes caused by functioning tumors. *Semin Pediatr Surg* 1997; 6: 147–55.

53 Galifer RB, Sultan C, Margueritte G, Barneon G. Testosterone producing hepatoblastoma in a 3 year old boy with precocious puberty. *J Pediatr Surg* 1985; 20: 713–14.

54 Dittrich K, Gyorke Z, Sulyok E, Tunnessen WW. Picture of the month. *Arch Pediatr Adolesc Med* 1996; 150: 1215–19.

55 Dengg K, Fink FM, Heitger A, Tabarelli M, Kreczy A, Glatzl J, Berger H. Precocious puberty due to a lipid cell tumour of the ovary. *Eur J Pediatr* 1993; 152: 12–14.

56 Yu MY, Panyasavatsu N, Elder D, D'ercole JA. Sexual development in a two year old boy induced by topical exposure to testosterone. *Pediatrics* 1999; 104: 249.

57 Saenz de Rodruiguez CA, Bongiovanni AM, Conde de Borrego L. An epidemic of precocious development in Puerto Rican children. *J Pediatr* 1985; 107: 393–6.

58 Bridges NA, Cooke A, Healy MJR, Hindmarsh PC, Brook CGD. Ovaries in sexual precocity. *Clin Endocrinol* 1995; 42: 135–40.

59 Honour JA, Price DA, Taylor NF, Marsden HB, Grant DB. Steroid biochemistry of virilising adrenal tumours in childhood. *Eur J Pediatr* 1984; 142: 165–9.

60 Paterson WF, McNeill E, Donaldson MDC, Reid S, Hollman AS. Efficacy of Zoladex LA (goserelin) in the treatment of girls with central precocious puberty. *Arch Dis Child* 1998; 79: 323–7.

61 Heger S, Partsch CJ, Sippell WG. Long term outcome after depot gonadotropin releasing hormone agonist treatment of central precocious puberty: final height, body proportions, body composition, bone mineral density and reproductive function. *J Clin Endocrinol Metab* 1999; 84: 4583–90.

62 Boot AM, De Muink Keizer Schrama S, Pols HA, Krenning EP, Drop SL. Bone mineral density and body composition before and during treatment with gonadotrophin releasing hormone agonist in children with central precocious and early puberty. *J Clin Endocrinol Metab* 1998; 83: 370–3.

63 Savage DCL, Swift PGF. Effect of cyproterone acetate on adrenocortical function in children with precocious puberty. *Arch Dis Child* 1981; 56: 218–22.

64 Garty BZ, Dinari G, Gellvan A, Kauli R. Cirrhosis in a child with hypothalamic syndrome and central precocious puberty treated with cyproterone. *Eur J Pediatrics* 1999; 158: 367–70.

65 Laue L, Kenigsberg D, Pescovitz OH, Hench KD, Barnes KM, Loriaux DL *et al.* Treatment of familial male precocious puberty with spironolactone and testolactone. *N Engl J Med* 1989; 320: 496–502.

66 Leschek EW, Jones J, Barnes KM, Hil SC, Cutler GB. Six year results of spironolactone and testolactone treatment of familial male limited precocious puberty with addition of deslorelin after central puberty onset. *J Clin Endocrinol Metab* 1999; 84: 175–8.

67 Sonino N. The use of ketoconazole as an inhibitor of steroid production. *N Engl J Med* 1987; 317: 812–18.

68 Syed FA, Chalew SA. Ketoconazole treatment of gonadotropin independent precocious puberty in girls with McCune Albright syndrome: a preliminary report. *J Pediatr Endocrinol Metab* 1999; 12: 81–3.

69 Eugster EA, Shankar R, Feezle LK, Pescovitz OH. Tamoxifen treatment of progressive precocious puberty in a patient with McCune Albright syndrome. *J Pediatr Endocrinol Metab* 1999; 12: 681–6.

70 Salardi S, Cacciari E, Mainetti B, Manzzanti L, Pirazzoli P. Outcome of premature thelarche: relation to puberty and final height. *Arch Dis Child* 1998; 79: 173–4.

71 Murram D, Dewhust J, Grant DG. Precocious puberty: a follow up study. *Arch Dis Child* 1984; 59: 77–8.

72 Bertelloni S, Baroncelli GI, Lala R *et al.* Long term outcome of male limited gonadotrophin independent precocious puberty. *Horm Res* 1997; 48: 235–9.

73 Lee PA, Van Dop C, Midgeon CJ. McCune Albright syndrome: long term follow up. *J Am Med Assoc* 1986; 256: 2980–4.

74 Sigurjonsdottir TJ, Hayles AB. Precocious puberty. A report of 96 cases. *Am J Dis Child* 1968; 115: 309–21.

75 Bar A, Lindner B, Sobel EH, Saenger P, Martino Nardi J. Bayley Pinneau method of height prediction in girls with central precocious puberty: correlation with adult height. *J Pediatr* 1995; 126: 955–8.

76 Kauli R, Galatzer A, Kornreich L, Lazar L, Pertzelan A, Laron Z. Final height of girls with central precocious puberty untreated versus treated with cyproterone acetate or GnRH analogue. *Horm Res* 1997; 47: 54–61.

77 Ross JL, Pescovitz OH, Barnes K, Loriaux DL, Cutler GB. Growth hormone secretory dynamics in children with precocious puberty. *J Pediatr* 1987; 110: 369–72.

78 Arrigo T, Cisternino M, Galluzzi F *et al.* Analysis of the factors affecting auxological response to GnRH agonist treatment and final height outcome in girls with idiopathic central precocious puberty. *Eur J Endocrinol* 1999; 141: 140–4.

79 Paul D, Conte F, Grumbach MM, Kaplan SL. Long term effects of gonadotropin releasing hormone agonist therapy on final and near final height in 26 children with true precocious puberty treated at median age of less than 5 years. *J Clin Endocrinol Metab* 1995; 80: 546–51.

80 Carel JC, Roger M, Ispas S *et al.* Final height after long term treatment with triptorelin slow release for central precocious puberty: importance of statural growth after interruption of treatment. *J Clin Endocrinol Metab* 1999; 84: 1973–8.

81 Oostdijk W, Rikken B, Schreuder S *et al.* Final height in central precocious puberty after long term treatment with a slow release GnRH agonist. *Arch Dis Child* 1996; 75: 292–7.

82 Werder EA, Murset G, Zachmann M, Brook CGD, Prader A. Treatment of precocious puberty with cyproterone acetate. *Pediatr Res* 1974; 8: 248–56.

83 Sorgo W, Kiraly E, Homoki J *et al.* The effects of cyproterone acetate on statural growth in children with precocious puberty. *Acta Endocrinol* 1987; 115: 44–56.

84 Kletter GB, Kelch RP. Effects of gonadotropin releasing hormone analog therapy on adult stature in precocious puberty. *J Clin Endocrinol Metab* 1994; 79: 331–4.

85 Cassio A, Cacciari E, Balsamo A, Bal M, Tassinari D. Randomised trial of LHRH analogue treatment on final height in girls with onset of puberty aged 7.5–8 5 years. *Arch Dis Child* 1999; 81: 329–32.

86 Brauner R, Adan L, Malandry F, Zantleifer D. Adult height in girls with idiopathic true precocious puberty. *J Clin Endocrinol Metab* 1994; 79: 415–20.

87 Zachmann M, Sobradillo B, Frank M, Frisch H, Prader A. Bayley Pinneau, Roche Wainer Thissen, and Tanner height predictions in normal children and in patients with various pathological conditions. *J Pediatr* 1978; 93: 749–55.

88 Bouvattier C, Coste J, Rodrigue D *et al.* Lack of effect of GnRH agonists on final height in girls with advanced puberty: a randomised long term pilot study. *J Clin Endocrinol Metab* 1999; 84: 3575–8.

89 Adan L, Souberbielle JM, Zucker JM, Pierre Kahn A, Kalifa C, Brauner R. Adult height in 24 patients treated for growth hormone deficiency and early puberty. *J Clin Endocrinol Metab* 1996; 82: 229–33.

90 Cara JF, Krieter ML, Rosenfield RL. Height prognosis of children with true precocious puberty and growth hormone deficiency: effect of combination therapy with gonadotrophin releasing hormone analog and growth hormone. *J Pediatr* 1992; 120: 709–15.

91 Pasquino AM, Pucarelli I, Segni M, Matrunola M, Cerrone F. Adult height in girls with central precocious puberty treated with gonadotrophin releasing hormone analogues and growth hormone. *J Clin Endocrinol Metab* 1999; 84: 449–52.

92 Kohn B, Julius JR, Blethen SL. Combined use of growth hormone and gonadotrophin releasing hormone analogues: the national cooperative study experience. *Pediatrics* 1999; 104: 1014–17.

93 Boepple PA, Frisch LS, Weirman ME, Hoffman WH, Crowley WF. The natural history of autonomous gonadal function adrenarche and central puberty in gonadotrophin independent precocious puberty. *J Clin Endocrinol Metab* 1992; 75: 1550–5.

94 Palmert MR, Mansfield MJ, Crowley WF, Crigler JF, Crawford JD, Boepple PA. Is obesity an outcome of gonadotrophin releasing hormone agonist administration? Analysis of growth and body composition in 110 patients with central precocious puberty. *J Clin Endocrinol Metab* 1999; 84: 4480–8.

95 Jay N, Mansfield MJ, Blizzard RM *et al.* Ovulation and menstrual function of adolescent girls with central precocious puberty after therapy with gonadotrophin releasing hormone agonists. *J Clin Endocrinol Metab* 1992; 75: 890–4.

96 Feuillan PP, Jones JV, Barnes K, Oerter Klein K, Cutler GB. Reproductive axis after discontinuation of gonadotrophin releasing hormone analog treatment of girls with precocious puberty: long term follow up comparing girls with hypothalamic hamartoma to those with idiopathic precocious puberty. *J Clin Endocrinol Metab* 1999; 84: 44–9.

97 Ehrhart AA, Meyer Bahlberg HFL, Bell JJ. Idiopathic precocious puberty in girls: psychiatric follow up in adolescence. *J Am Acad Child Psychiatry* 1984; 23: 23–33.

98 Ibanez L, Potau N, Zampolli M, Street M, Carrascosa A. Girls diagnosed with premature pubarche show an exaggerated ovarian androgen synthesis from the early stages of puberty: evidence from gonadotrophin releasing hormone agonist testing. *Fertil Steril* 1997; 67: 849–55.

99 Banerjee S, Raghavan S, Wasserman E, Linder BL, Saenger P, DiMartino Nardi J. Hormonal findings in African American and Caribbean Hispanic girls with premature adrenarche: implications for polycystic ovarian syndrome. *Pediatrics* 1998; 102: 629.

100 Lazar L, Kauli R, Bruchis C, Nordenberg J, Galatzer A, Pertzelan A. Early polycystic ovary like syndrome in girls with central precocious puberty and exaggerated adrenal response. *Eur J Pediatr* 1995; 133: 403–6.

101 Quinton R, Cheow HK, Tymms DJ, Bouloux PM, Wu FC, Jacobs HS. Kallman's syndrome: is it always for life? *Clin Endocrinol* 1999; 50: 481–5.

102 Vaidya SJ, Atra A, Bahl S *et al.* Autologous bone marrow transplantation for childhood acute lymphoblastic leukaemia in second remission – long-term follow-up. *Bone Marrow Transplant* 2000; 25: 599–603.

103 Bakker B, Massa GG, Oostdijk W, Van Weel Sipman MH, Vossen JM, Wit JM. Pubertal development and growth after total-body

irradiation and bone marrow transplantation for haematological malignancies. *Eur J Pediatr* 2000; 159: 31–7.

104 Betterle C, Greggio NA, Volpato M. Autoimmune polyglandular syndrome type 1. *J Clin Endocrinol Metab* 1998; 83: 1049–55.

105 Hoek A, Schoemaker J, Drexhage HA. Premature ovarian failure and ovarian autoimmunity. *Endocr Rev* 1997; 18: 107–34.

106 Fraser IS, Russell P, Greco S, Robertson DM. Resistant ovary syndrome and premature ovarian failure in young women with galactosaemia. *Clin Reprod Fertil* 1986; 4: 133–8.

107 Rugliari EI, Ballabio A. Kallman syndrome: from genetics to neurobiology. *J Am Med Assoc* 1993; 270: 2713–16.

108 Hay ID, Smail PJ, Forsythe CC. Familial cytomegalic adrenocortical hypoplasia- an X-linked syndrome of pubertal failure. *Arch Dis Child* 1981; 56: 715–21.

109 Muscatelli F, Strom TM, Walker AP *et al*. Mutations in the DAX 1 gene give rise to both X linked adrenal hypoplasia congenita and hypogonadotrophic hypogonadism. *Nature* 1994; 372: 672–6.

110 Hernandez Martin A, Gonzalez Sarmiento R, De-Unamuno P. X-linked ichthyosis: an update. *Br J Dermatol* 1999; 141: 617–27.

111 Maya Nunez G, Torres L, Ulloa-Aguirre A *et al*. An atypical contiguous gene syndrome: molecular studies in a family with X-linked Kallmann's syndrome and X-linked ichthyosis. *Clin Endocrinol* 1999; 50: 157–62.

112 Oerter KE, Kamp GA, Munson PJ, Nienhaus AW, Cassorla FG, Manasco PK. Multiple hormone deficiencies in children with hemochromatosis. *J Clin Endocrinol Metab* 1993; 76: 357–61.

113 Merkus PJ, van Essen Zandvliet EE, Duiverman EJ, van Houwelingen HC, Kerrebijn KF, Quanjer PH. Long-term effect of inhaled corticosteroids on growth rate in adolescents with asthma. *Pediatrics* 1993; 91: 1121–6.

114 Brain CE, Savage MO. Growth and puberty in chronic inflammatory bowel disease. *Bailliere's Clin Gastroenterol* 1994; 8: 83–100.

115 Patel L, Clayton PE, Addison GM, Price DA, David TJ. Linear growth in prepubertal children with atopic dermatitis. *Arch Dis Child* 1998; 79: 169–72.

116 Johanesson M, Gottleib C, Hjelte L. Delayed puberty in girls with cystic fibrosis despite good clinical status. *Pediatrics* 1997; 99: 29–34.

117 Georgopoulos N, Markou K, Theodoropoulou A *et al*. Growth and pubertal development in elite female rhythmic gymnasts. *J Clin Endocrinol Metab* 1999; 84: 4525–30.

118 Warren MP. The effects of exercise on pubertal progression and reproductive function in girls. *J Clin Endocrinol Metab* 1980; 51: 1150–7.

119 Warren MP. Amenorrhea in endurance runners. *J Clin Endocrinol Metab* 1992; 75: 1393–7.

120 Constantini NW, Warren MP. Menstrual dysfunction in swimmers – a distinct entity. *J Clin Endocrinol Metab* 1995; 80: 2740–4.

121 Ronkainen H, Pakarinene A, Kauppila A. Pubertal and menstrual disorders of female runners, skiers and volleyball players. *Gynaecol Obstet Invest* 1984; 18: 183–9.

122 Gidwani GP. Amenorrhea in the athlete. *Adolescent Med* 1999; 10: 275–90.

123 Warren MP, Stiehl AL. Exercise and female adolescents: effects on the reproductive and skeletal systems. *J Am Med Women's Assoc* 1999; 54: 115–20.

124 Lindholm C, Hagenfeldt K, Ringertz H. Bone mineral content of young female former gymnasts. *Acta Paediatr* 1995; 84: 1109–12.

125 Lanes R, Gunczler P, Osuna JA. Effectiveness and limitations of the use of the gonadotropin-releasing hormone agonist leuprolide acetate in the diagnosis of delayed puberty in males. *Horm Res* 1997; 48: 1–4.

126 Ghai K, Cara JF, Rosenfield RL. Gonadotropin releasing hormone agonist (nafarelin) test to differentiate gonadotropin deficiency from constitutionally delayed puberty in teen-age boys – a clinical research center study. *J Clin Endocrinol Metab* 1995; 80: 2980–6.

127 Houchin LD, Rogol AD. Androgen replacement in children with constitutional delay of puberty: the case for aggressive therapy. *Bailliere's Clin Endocrinol Metab* 1998; 12: 427–40.

128 Saenger P, Sandberg DE. Delayed puberty: when to wake the bugler. *J Pediatr* 1998; 13: 724–6.

129 Arrigo T, Cisternino M, Luca De F *et al*. Final height outcome in both untreated and testosterone-treated boys with constitutional delay of growth and puberty. *J Pediatr Endocrinol Metab* 1996; 9: 511–17.

130 Buyukgebiz A, Hindmarsh PC, Brook CGD. Treatment of constitutional delay of growth and puberty with oxandrolone compared with growth hormone. *Arch Dis Child* 1990; 65: 448–52.

131 Susman EJ, Finkelstein JW, Chinchilli VM, Schwab J, Liben LS, D'arcangelo M *et al*. The effect of sex steroid replacement therapy on behaviour problems and moods in adolescents with delayed puberty. *J Pediatr* 1998; 133: 521–5.

132 Stanhope R, Brook CGD, Pringle PJ, Adams J, Jacobs HS. Induction of puberty by pulsatile GnRH. *Lancet* 1987; 2: 522–55.

133 Bourguignon J-P and the Belgian Study Group for Paediatric Endocrinology. Variations in duration of pubertal growth: a mechanism compensating for differences in timing of puberty and minimising their effects on final height. *Acta Paediatr Scand* 1988; 347 (Suppl.): 16–24.

134 Crowne EC, Shalet SM, Wallace WHB, Eminson DM, Price DA. Final height in girls with untreated constitutional delay of puberty. *Eur J Pediatr* 1991; 150: 708–12.

135 Finkelstein JS, Neer RM, Biller BM, Crawford JD, Klibanski A. Osteopenia in men with a history of delayed puberty. *N Engl J Med* 1992; 326: 600–4.

136 Finkelstein JS, Klibanski A, Neer RM. A longitudinal evaluation of bone mineral density in adult men with histories of delayed puberty. *J Clin Endocrinol Metab* 1996; 81: 1152–5.

137 Bertelloni S, Baroncelli GI, Ferdeghini M, Perri G, Saggese G. Normal volume tric bone mineral density and bone turnover in young men with histories of constitutional delay of puberty. *J Clin Endocrinol Metab* 1998; 83: 4280–3.

138 Keay N, Fogelman I, Blake G. Bone mineral density in professional female dancers. *Br J Sports Med* 1997; 31: 143–7.

139 Ting AC, Chow LW, Leung YF. Comparison of tamoxifen with danazol in the management of idiopathic gynecomastia. *Am Surg* 2000; 66: 38–40.

# 13 Reproductive endocrinology

**Diana F. Wood and S. Franks**

## Introduction

Disorders of the reproductive system are uncommon in childhood and adolescence, but their profound implications for future life mean that proper recognition and treatment is important. We present an outline of gonadal differentiation and development and the important physiological changes occurring in childhood and adolescence. The most important disorders of reproductive function that present in young patients are reviewed, with particular emphasis on the long-term sequelae for adult life.

## Gonadal development

### Fetal development

Gonadal function involves production of gametes and synthesis of the hormones that determine sexual development and reproductive function. The two functions are closely related and both are controlled by the hypothalamo-pituitary axis. In addition, a range of other endocrine, paracrine and autocrine factors that modulate gonadotrophin action and regulate cellular differentiation and replication influences ovarian and testicular activity. Coordination of these factors is necessary for normal development of the reproductive system in both sexes.

Genetic sex is determined at the time of conception and is the first component of a series of events leading to completion of the sexual phenotype. Normal development of the bipotential gonad is followed by gonadal differentiation into testes or ovaries, a process that begins at the seventh week of intrauterine life. Primary sexual differentiation describes the series of events leading to embryonic development of the internal and external genitalia. Secondary sexual differentiation, the response of multiple organs to sex hormone action, produces the full male or female phenotype and is concluded at the time of puberty. The development of the bipotential gonad and subsequent gonadal differentiation are complex (see Chapter 16 and [1,2]).

Differentiation of the testis occurs by the end of the seventh week of gestation and requires the formation of cords of somatic cells destined to become Sertoli cells. Primordial germ cells migrate from the yolk sac, become embedded in these seminiferous cords and mature during fetal development, changing from primitive spermatogonia into premeiotic spermatocytes at the time of birth. Sertoli cells immediately begin to secrete anti-Müllerian hormone (AMH), responsible for repression of the Müllerian ducts [3]. Development of the Wolffian duct system, which is necessary for the complete masculine phenotype, is dependent upon adequate testosterone production by fetal Leydig cells. These cells are apparent by the eighth week of gestation and possess luteinizing hormone (LH) receptors before the existence of functioning anterior pituitary tissue. Fetal LH receptors bind human chorionic gonadotrophin (hCG) at high affinity so that testosterone production is initially under the influence of placental hCG and regulated by fetal gonadotrophins only in the latter part of pregnancy [4]. Fetal testosterone production is detectable at 10 weeks and maximal at about 14–16 weeks of gestation.

During fetal life the testes descend from the retroperitoneal space into the scrotal sac, which itself develops from the gubernaculum within the abdominal cavity. The process of descent appears to be gonadotrophin dependent, is mediated by androgens and requires a number of other neural and hormonal inputs, including AMH [5]. About 5% of full-term and a higher percentage of premature male babies are born with cryptorchidism, although over half of these correct spontaneously by 1 year of age [6].

The ovary develops from the bipotential gonad and contains germ cells derived from the yolk sac and somatic cells derived from coelomic epithelium, mesenchyme and the mesonephros. Germ cell replication continues in the fetal ovary up until the fifth month of gestation when a maximum of six to seven million oogonia is reached [7]. Primary oocyte division is arrested in the diplotene phase, meiosis not being completed until many years later at the onset of ovulation. Oocytes arrested in meiosis become surrounded by a layer of primitive granulosa cells to form primordial follicles, a process that continues into the sixth month of postnatal life. Oocytes not incorporated into follicles undergo atresia, and this follicular growth and atresia continues throughout life [8]. By contrast to fetal testes, human fetal ovaries do not contain binding sites for LH or hCG although follicle-stimulating hormone (FSH) receptors appear towards the end of intrauterine life [9], and full follicular maturation depends upon cyclical gonadotrophin secretion in postpubertal life (reviewed in [10]).

## Clinical implications

Abnormalities of fetal gonadal development have profound implications for sexual differentiation and pubertal development and ultimately for fertility and psychosexual health. Recent identification of mutations in a number of important genes that direct the process of sexual differentiation help to clarify some disorders of gonadal dysgenesis and sexual ambiguity presenting in childhood and adolescence. These include mutations in the Wilms tumour gene *WT1* (essential for development of the bipotential gonad), the *AMH* gene, steroidogenic factor-1 (*SF1*), *DAX1*, *SRY* and *SOX* genes and a number of activating and inactivating mutations of the LH and FSH receptor genes (for reviews see [1, 2 and 10]). The clinical features of a number of genetic disorders of the reproductive system can be explained by understanding the process of fetal development (Table 13.1). For example, activating mutations of the LH receptor responsible for familial male precocious puberty (testotoxicosis) have no clinical correlates in females homozygous for the same mutation, as both LH and FSH are required for ovarian steroid production. Gonadotrophin deficiency itself, for example in Kallmann syndrome, idiopathic hypogonadotrophic hypogonadism [11] or caused by inactivating mutations of the β-subunits of LH and FSH [12,13], presents with developmental abnormalities. These include cryptorchidism, microphallus, delayed puberty, amenorrhoea and infertility, reflecting gonadotrophin-dependent processes.

**Table 13.1.** Genes involved in the development of the hypothalamo-pituitary-gonadal axis and clinical features associated with recognized mutations (data from [1, 2, 10 and 11]).

| Gene | Clinical features |
|---|---|
| *WT1* | WAGR syndrome,* Denys–Drash† syndrome |
| *SRY* | Complete gonadal dysgenesis, true hermaphroditism |
| *SOX9* | Campomelic dysplasia, XY sex reversal, gonadal/genital malformation |
| *AMH/AMH-R* | Persistent Müllerian duct syndrome |
| *Dax-1 (SF-1)* | Adrenal hypoplasia congenita-hypogonadal hypogonadism |
| *MTM-1* | Ambiguous genitalia, myotubular atrophy |
| *XH2* | XY gonadal dysgenesis, optic atrophy, mental retardation |
| Chromosome regions 9p, 10q, 18p (unidentified genes) | Complete or partial XY gonadal dysgenesis |
| LH-R inactivating | Male: varies – complete male pseudohermaphroditism – microphallus, cryptorchidism and hypospadias<br>Female: normal secondary sexual development, anovulatory amenorrhoea with cystic ovaries |
| LH-R activating | Male: familial male precocious puberty (testotoxicosis)<br>Female: clinically normal |
| FSH-R inactivating | Male: oligo/teratospermia<br>Female: hypergonadotrophic hypogonadism (resistant ovary syndrome) |
| FSH-R activating | Male: persistent spermatogenesis after hypophysectomy |
| *KAL* | X-linked Kallman syndrome |
| GnRH/GnRH-R | Hypogonadotrophic hypogonadism |
| Leptin/leptin-R | Obesity, hypogonadotrophic hypogonadism |

*Wilms tumour, aniridia, genitourinary anomalies, mental retardation.
†Nephrotic syndrome, Wilms tumour, gonadal dysgenesis.

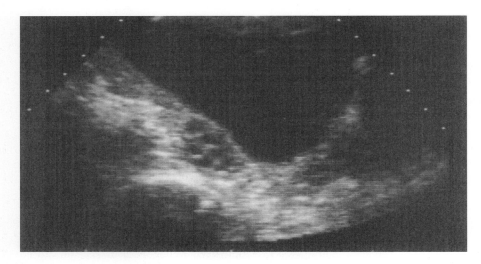

**Fig. 13.1.** Ultrasound scan showing a prepubertal ovary with a multifollicular appearance.

## Gonadal development in childhood and adolescence

During childhood, the reproductive system is quiescent but not inactive. In males, after a fall in testosterone concentrations at birth, there is a rise between the ages of 2 and 4 months associated with Leydig cell multiplication. After that, the testes remain relatively inactive associated with suppression of hypothalamo-pituitary-gonadal activity until the onset of puberty. Testicular size starts to increase at around 10 years of age, reflecting increased gonadotrophin secretion and growth of the seminiferous tubules, which form the bulk of the mature testis. Full testicular function depends primarily upon the actions of gonadotrophins and testosterone, but a wide range of humoral factors plays a part. These include other hormones and neuropeptides and locally produced peptides, growth factors and cytokines acting in an autocrine or paracrine fashion [14].

In females, removal of placental steroid negative feedback at birth results in the high levels of gonadotrophins seen in the first few months of postnatal life [15]. Levels decline by 1–3 years and remain low throughout childhood. However, detectable pulses of gonadotrophin secretion can be observed and mean serum concentration starts to rise by the age of 6, a change associated with an increase in the number of antral follicles and a subsequent rise in oestrogen concentrations [16].

By the age of 8 years, multifollicular ovaries can be observed by ultrasound scanning in all normal girls ([17]; see Fig. 13.1). Gametogenesis in the mature ovary occurs in granulosa cells, which lie within follicles in close proximity to the theca interna cells. LH receptors are localized on theca cells and develop on granulosa cells in response to FSH during the preovulatory phase of follicular growth. The two cell types are interdependent, such that androgens synthesized by theca cells diffuse into the granulosa layer, where they are metabolized to oestrogen by aromatase enzymes. FSH receptors are found exclusively on granulosa cells [18]. The effects of LH and FSH within the ovary are modulated by a number of hormones acting as co-gonadotrophins, including insulin ([19]; Fig. 13.2), growth hormone (GH) and insulin-

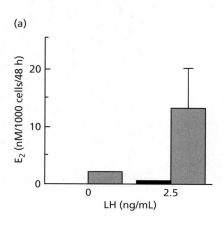

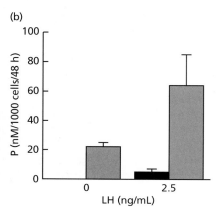

**Fig. 13.2.** Effect of FSH (5 ng/mL) with and without insulin (10 ng/mL) preincubation on LH-stimulated (a) oestradiol ($E_2$) and (b) progesterone (P) accumulation in granulosa cells from 4.5- to 8.5-mm follicles from a patient with normal ovaries. ■, FSH; ▨, insulin + FSH. From [19].

like growth factor I (IGF-I [20] ), and by a number of growth factors, peptide hormones and cytokines synthesized within the ovary itself [21,22].

The end of puberty in girls is marked by the menarche with establishment of regular ovulatory menses associated with adult ovarian morphology and characteristic cyclical changes in hypothalamo-pituitary-gonadal function.

## Menarche and the menstrual cycle

Over the last 150 years mean age at the menarche in European girls has declined from 16 to 13 years [23]. A number of factors influence the age at which menarche occurs, including genetic make-up, family size and birth order, exercise, chronic illness and socioeconomic status. Body weight is an important factor, demonstrated by the positive correlations that exist between birthweight and later menarche and between greater weight at 7 years and early menarche. These data support the theory that menarcheal age reflects fetal hypothalamic imprinting of patterns of gonadotrophin release that are modified by subsequent weight gain in childhood [24]. As mean age at the menopause remains unchanged, the net effect of earlier menarche is to prolong a woman's exposure to oestrogen with potential changes in risk of disease in later life. Early menarche appears to be a minor but significant risk factor for breast cancer but its

effects on other malignancies and osteoporosis remain to be fully established.

The establishment of a regular menstrual cycle represents the final stage of ovarian development and reflects maturity of the entire hypothalamo-pituitary-ovarian axis. The median length of the cycle is 28 days (range 25–31 days) and there is wide variation between women [25]. Irregular cycles are common at the two ends of reproductive life. Cycle length is often prolonged in the first 1–2 years after the menarche, and bleeding is erratic as a result of inadequate follicular development and the high prevalence of anovulatory cycles [26,27].

The menstrual cycle comprises a process of ovarian follicular maturation, ovulation of a dominant follicle and formation of a corpus luteum, with consequent hormonally mediated changes in the reproductive tract. It is traditionally divided into the follicular phase, during which follicular selection, maturation and ovulation occurs, and the luteal phase, which is characterized by high progesterone levels and endometrial differentiation (Fig. 13.3). Initiation of follicular growth occurs during the final days of the preceding cycle under the influence of rising FSH concentrations that follow the decline in oestradiol and progesterone levels. Follicular recruitment occurs during the first 4 days of the cycle, after which one follicle is selected to become dominant.

As oestradiol levels rise in the mid-follicular phase, FSH levels fall and maturation of the other follicles is suppressed.

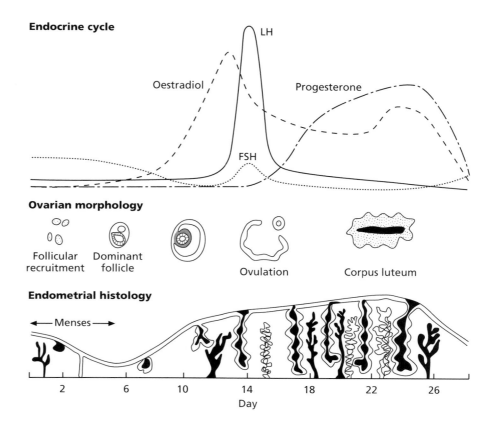

**Fig. 13.3.** The menstrual cycle. Hormonal, ovarian and endometrial histological changes during the menstrual cycle.

This process results in the ovulation of a single dominant follicle at days 13–15. The follicular phase is characterized by increasing oestrogen concentrations in proportion to follicular growth and the increasing number of granulosa cells. FSH induces aromatase activity and the development of LH receptors on granulosa cells. At the same time, LH stimulates theca interna cells to produce androgens that are aromatized to oestrogens in the granulosa. In the latter part of the follicular phase, LH contributes to the production of oestradiol and to the small amount of progesterone secreted by the preovulatory granulosa layer. As described above, locally produced peptides and growth factors modulate this process of gonadotrophin-induced steroidogenesis.

Follicular growth is associated with rising oestrogen concentrations, and just before ovulation there is a dramatic rise in oestrogen secretion that triggers the LH surge. In addition to inducing ovulation, the abrupt rise in LH stimulates the resumption of oocyte meiosis and initiates the process of luteinization of the granulosa layer. Granulosa lutein cells enlarge, become surrounded by cells of thecal origin and undergo vascularization to form the corpus luteum. The function of this is to secrete progesterone, allowing development of the oestrogen-primed endometrium before implantation of a fertilized ovum. In the absence of pregnancy and consequent hCG production by trophoblast cells of the early embryo, corpus luteum function declines at 9–11 days after ovulation when it starts to break down (luteolysis).

Ovulation and its associated endocrine changes are associated with changes in the endometrium characterized by cyclical angiogenesis. Endometrial stromal and epithelial cells possess steroid receptors and appear to mediate the production of a range of angiogenic factors that stimulate the growth of spiral arteries [28]. Endometrial glands start to develop in the follicular phase and after ovulation they become tortuous and dilated, producing intraluminal secretions by day 19. The stroma subsequently becomes oedematous and cells around the spiral arteries become enlarged and transformed into the predecidual layer. By the end of the luteal phase a well-developed sheet of decidual-like cells is established. In the absence of conception the decline in corpus luteum function means that the steroid support to the endometrial vascular supply is lost, resulting in cell death and shedding of the superficial endometrial layers during menstruation.

## Other endocrine and metabolic changes associated with puberty in girls

Hypothalamo-pituitary maturation in normal girls during puberty is associated with weight gain and changing body fat distribution. Fasting insulin levels rise at the onset of puberty, associated with peripheral insulin resistance [29] and increased concentrations of IGF-I. Insulin and IGF-I are important regulators of ovarian function. Insulin negatively regulates sex hormone-binding globulin (SHBG) concentra-

tions, altering free sex steroid levels and it also modulates the availability of IGF-binding protein 1 (IGFBP-1), which influences IGF-I activity. The features of hyperinsulinaemia, insulin resistance and elevated IGF-I levels characteristic of puberty are also found in women with the polycystic ovary syndrome (PCOS). Adolescent girls with irregular menstrual cycles appear to have many of the features of PCOS, and endocrinological evaluation shows a high proportion of them to have hyperandrogenaemia and polycystic ovaries, features that resolve with time in the majority (reviewed in [30] ). Conversely, undernutrition delays hypothalamo-pituitary maturation resulting in delayed puberty [31].

## Disorders of reproductive function presenting in childhood and adolescence

With the exception of genetic and intersex abnormalities, disorders of the reproductive system usually present in late childhood and adolescence with effects on normal pubertal and psychosexual development and, in the long term, on prospects for fertility.

Reproductive disorders in males present with the growth and developmental features of precocious or delayed puberty, whereas females commonly complain of abnormalities of the menstrual cycle. Menstruation that occurs before the youngest expected age (e.g. < 10 years in Western Europe and the USA) is an important sign and may indicate precocious ovarian function. Abnormal ovarian function in postpubertal females presents with irregular menstrual cycles, oligomenorrhoea or amenorrhoea.

Disorders of adrenal steroid hormone production also affect the reproductive system. Congenital adrenal hyperplasia (CAH) is an important cause of reproductive dysfunction presenting in children and adolescents of both sexes.

## Congenital adrenal hyperplasia

Over 90% of cases of congenital adrenal hyperplasia (CAH) are due to 21-hydroxylase deficiency (21-OHD). Other enzyme deficiencies described are 11β-hydroxylase, 3β-hydroxysteroid dehydrogenase (3β-HSD) and 17α-hydroxylase (17α-OHD). The spectrum of genetic, biochemical and clinical features of CAH in childhood are discussed in Chapter 21 but a number of issues are of particular importance in terms of the reproductive function of affected individuals.

Male infants with 21-OHD and 11β-OHD deficiencies have normal external genitalia at birth and develop progressive virilization, accelerated skeletal growth and, ultimately, short stature. Glucocorticoid replacement therapy can normalize growth velocity and the rate of physical development stature, but early puberty is the rule in these patients. Little is known about the fate of postpubertal males with 21-OHD; in theory they should be encouraged to continue therapy to avoid the development of testicular adrenal rests [32], although fertility appears to be less at risk than in women with 21-OHD [33]. Males with non-classic 21-OHD (NC21-OHD) are phenotypically normal but may have subfertility.

The situation is different for males with 3β-HSD and 17α-OHD who may be born with varying degrees of genital ambiguity, ranging from cryptorchidism and hypospadias to complete sex reversal (female genitalia). Such children not only require steroid replacement therapy but may also need gender assignment and surgery according to the degree of genital ambiguity. As with all children with inter-sex disorders, psychological support is essential and the long-term consequences to psychosexual well-being may be severe.

Female infants with classic 21-OHD and 11β-OHD may present at birth with genital ambiguity and often require surgery, including cliteroplasty and vaginal reconstruction followed by regular vaginal dilatation procedures. The fewer the surgical procedures the better is the outcome in terms of psychological adjustment, although long-term psychosexual effects are well recognized in terms of lack of sexual activity and low rates of marriage and childbearing compared with the normal population [34]. The fertility rate for women with classic 21-OHD is reduced, ranging from 0% in salt losers to around 60% full-term pregnancies in those with simple viril-izing disease [35]. Although it is possible to induce ovulation, even in salt-losers, other fertility problems include vaginal stricture, endometrial inadequacy, poor cervical mucus and poor oocyte quality. Improvements in surgical and medical management of these women show an increased rate of suc-cessful pregnancy [36]. Females with 3β-HSD deficiency have lesser degrees of masculinization. Those with 17α-OHD have varying degrees of failure to synthesize adrenal and gonadal hormones and may present in adolescence with primary amenorrhoea, hypergonadotrophic hypogonadism and absent axillary and pubic hair.

Females with NC21-OHD usually present in adolescence and early adulthood with hirsutism, acne, oligomenorrhoea and infertility, features that are clinically indistinguishable from PCOS. Androgen levels, including testosterone, andro-stenedione and dehydroepiandrosterone sulphate (DHEAS) are unhelpful in the differential diagnosis of the two conditions. The diagnosis of NC21-OHD depends upon demonstration of elevated basal and stimulated serum 17-hydroxyprogesterone concentrations (> 6 pmol/L and > 30 pmol/L 30 min after 250 µg of parenteral Synacthen respectively [37]). The majority of women with NC21-OHD develop polycystic ovaries, thought to be secondary to hyperandrogenaemia, although the exact mechanism for this remains uncertain. Glucocorticoid treatment may help to regulate menstrual cycles in women with NC21-OHD, but hirsutism usually responds better to the addition of anti-androgen therapy [38].

## Disorders of the reproductive system in male children and adolescents

### Cryptorchidism

The commonest disorder of the reproductive tract in male children is unilateral or bilateral undescended testes (UDT), a finding not associated with other congenital abnormalities in the majority of cases. The aetiology of UDT in the absence of identifiable endocrine or developmental pathology remains obscure, although the commonest cause is thought to be a defect in prenatal gonadotrophin or androgen secretion [5]. The incidence of UDT is rising [39] for reasons that are not clear, although the influence of environmental oestrogens or other toxins has been postulated.

The long-term effects of untreated UDT are well known in terms of subfertility and malignancy, both thought to be caused by temperature-induced degeneration and dysplasia within the UDT. Early surgical therapy is recommended to restore normal testicular function, and while there is debate about the exact optimal timing for orchidopexy there is gen-eral agreement that it should take place before 2 years of age to achieve the most favourable long-term results. Attempts to induce testicular descent by hormonal therapy with hCG or luteinizing hormone-releasing hormone (LHRH) have gener-ally proved ineffective [5].

### Precocious puberty

Precocious puberty is much less common in boys than in girls, and an underlying cause should always be sought and treated appropriately as described elsewhere (Chapter 12). The main long-term consequences of precocious puberty alone relate to short stature, as even treated children fail to attain their target height. This may have psychological impli-cations for some adult men.

### Hypogonadotrophic hypogonadism

Disorders of the hypothalamo-pituitary axis in prepubertal boys causing gonadotrophin-releasing hormone (GnRH) or gonadotrophin deficiency result in hypogonadotrophic hypogonadism (HH). The aetiology and clinical management of the underlying causes are discussed elsewhere (Chapter 12). In the long term, inadequate treatment of HH of what-ever cause in childhood and adolescence has profound effects on adult life. Delayed puberty, incomplete masculinization (poor secondary sexual characteristics), small testes and sub-fertility may all contribute to poor social and psychosexual adjustment. When coupled with other pituitary deficiencies, in particular GH deficiency leading to short stature and later features of the adult GH-deficiency syndrome, the prospects for normal socialization may be impaired, and there is evidence for low rates of marriage or stable sexual relationships in these patients [40]. Proper treatment of HH in adolescence is thus crucial for adult well-being.

Children with combined HH and GH deficiency should have induction of puberty after standard GH therapy, which should be continued in conjunction with testosterone replacement. After adequate induction of secondary sexual characteristics, testicular growth may be induced by a course of gonadotrophins, either using combination hCG/human menopausal gonadotrophin (hMG) or pulsatile GnRH therapy [41]. Recombinant FSH and HCG may replace the traditional therapies, and recombinant LH is likely to become available. Not only do gonadotrophins increase testicular volume, they also probably lead to improved spermatogenesis in the future. In patients with isolated HH there is no clear benefit of pulsatile GnRH over gonadotrophin therapy; both will induce testicular growth with subsequent fertility in half to one-third of subjects. Advances in the management of male infertility and the introduction of intracytoplasmic sperm injection (ICSI) with *in vitro* fertilization (IVF) have improved the outlook for fertility in men with subnormal sperm counts [42].

## Disorders of the reproductive system in female children and adolescents

Common disorders of the reproductive system in girls usually present with menstrual cycle irregularity. Oligomenorrhoea is defined as an intermenstrual interval of more than 6 weeks, whereas amenorrhoea indicates the absence of menses for more than 6 months. Amenorrhoea may be divided into primary and secondary groups. Patients complaining of primary amenorrhoea have never menstruated, whereas those with secondary amenorrhoea have lost previously existing menstrual function. In adolescent girls it is clearly essential to assess these symptoms in the context of pubertal development. It is also important to note that the distinction between primary and secondary amenorrhoea is largely artificial, so that many of the causes of secondary amenorrhoea may present in adolescence with primary amenorrhoea and, rarely, some girls with congenital lesions may menstruate [43].

## Primary amenorrhoea

Primary amenorrhoea is uncommon. The majority of cases are due to developmental abnormalities of the ovaries, genital tracts or external genitalia, with syndromes of gonadal dysgenesis accounting for about half of these. The causes of primary amenorrhoea are shown in Table 13.2. Many patients will have delayed puberty and it is important to identify those causes not directly related to the hypothalamo-pituitary-gonadal axis.

### Clinical assessment

The history should include detailed questions about the age of onset, synchrony and progression of pubertal development. Features that are of particular importance in identifying those girls with an underlying primary ovarian disorder, such as Turner syndrome, should be sought. These include coexistent growth failure, musculoskeletal abnormalities, cutaneous lesions, congenital heart disease, recurrent ear infections or deafness and structural renal anomalies. Examination should begin with height and weight and accurate assessment of pubertal stage. Particular attention should be paid to dysmorphic body features, ambiguous genitalia, inguinal herniae and palpable masses in the labia or a blind-ending vaginal canal.

The investigation of girls with primary amenorrhoea is largely dictated by the clinical findings. Measurement of basal gonadotrophin concentrations will distinguish primary from secondary ovarian failure. Ovarian ultrasound scanning is helpful to identify ovarian tissue and assess its morphology. The presence of multifollicular ovaries in a girl with delayed puberty suggests that the hypothalamo-pituitary-gonadal axis is functioning and puberty will eventually progress. Patients with PCOS occasionally present with

**Table 13.2.** Causes of primary amenorrhoea

| Ovarian disorders | |
| --- | --- |
| Gonadal dysgenesis | Turner syndrome, mixed gonadal dysgenesis, pure gonadal dysgenesis |
| Ovarian insensitivity | 17-Hydroxylase deficiency, 'ovarian resistance syndromes' |
| Gonadal irradiation | |
| Chemotherapy | |
| Polycystic ovary syndrome | |
| Genital tract disorders | Müllerian dysgenesis, disorders of genital differentiation |
| Hypothalamo-pituitary disease | Hypogonadotrophic hypogonadism, pituitary/hypothalamic tumours, radiotherapy/chemotherapy |
| Delayed puberty | Chronic illness, constituted delay, psychogenic |

primary amenorrhoea [44], and this also will be demonstrated on ultrasound scanning. Chromosome analysis should be performed if dysmorphic features are observed and in all cases of short stature and delayed puberty, as Turner mosaics may be phenotypically normal. The treatment of primary amenorrhoea is varied, being dictated by the clinical findings.

## Ovarian causes of primary amenorrhoea

### Syndromes of gonadal dysgenesis

The clinical presentation of patients with gonadal dysgenesis is variable, depending upon the underlying chromosomal abnormality. The complete absence of a second sex chromosome is associated with features of Turner syndrome ([45]; reviewed in [46]). Treatment of Turner syndrome involves the achievement of maximal height, induction of secondary sexual characteristics and the correction of somatic abnormalities where possible. The long-term psychosocial effects of Turner syndrome associated with short stature and with altered sense of femininity related to long-standing primary ovarian failure and infertility have been recognized. However, developments in the field of reproductive technology mean that fertility is now achievable in the context of IVF with ovum donation. Results using this technique in Turner women are good, with reported pregnancy rates of 20–25% [42].

The features associated with Turner syndrome may be modified by sex chromosome mosaicism or partial sex chromosome monosomy. In mosaic patients, the ratio of 45,XO to 45,XX primordial germ cells determines the degree of ovarian abnormality and the relationship between 45,XO and 45,XX cells in the periphery may be important in the development of somatic disorders. Patients with the most common chromatin-positive mosaicism, 45,XO/45,XX, are often of normal height, may menstruate and are occasionally fertile. More often, these patients have short stature and streak gonads but few other features of Turner syndrome. In other forms of gonadal dysgenesis the presentation and clinical management depend upon the degree of genital ambiguity and the need for reconstructive surgery, as discussed above.

### Ovarian resistance syndromes

In ovarian resistance syndromes the ovary is unable to respond to gonadotrophin stimulation and patients present with hypergonadotrophic hypogonadism, such as that seen in girls with 17α-hydroxylase deficiency. Primary ovarian failure, resulting from a variety of underlying causes, may present with primary amenorrhoea, but more commonly it develops later in life, causing secondary amenorrhoea. The long-term outlook for fertility is similar to that described for Turner girls.

### Gonadal irradiation and chemotherapy

The importance of gonadal irradiation and chemotherapy for malignant disease in childhood on reproductive function is becoming increasingly recognized and is discussed elsewhere (Chapter 19). When such therapy has been given early in childhood girls may present with primary amenorrhoea, although secondary amenorrhoea is a more common outcome.

### Polycystic ovary syndrome

PCOS usually presents with secondary amenorrhoea, although rarely young women with PCOS present with primary amenorrhoea [44].

### Other causes of primary amenorrhoea

A number of other mechanisms for primary amenorrhoea exist that are not directly caused by ovarian dysfunction, although primary amenorrhoea is the ultimate presenting feature. Thus developmental abnormalities of the genital tract (Müllerian dysgenesis) are relatively common, with congenital absence of the vagina being reported in 1 in 5000 live births [47]. The intersex disorders of genital differentiation are well recognized. Finally, any of the hypothalamo-pituitary disorders that generally present with secondary amenorrhoea may occur in childhood causing primary amenorrhoea, usually with features of delayed puberty and other anterior pituitary hormone deficiencies. Childhood chemotherapy or irradiation may also cause primary amenorrhoea of hypothalamic origin.

## Secondary amenorrhoea

The symptom of secondary amenorrhoea reflects a wide range of underlying pathology as shown in Table 13.3. The majority of these disorders occur in older women, although all of them may present in adolescent girls. As discussed above, the distinction between primary and secondary amenorrhoea is not absolute, so that occasionally patients with syndromes of gonadal dysgenesis present with secondary amenorrhoea, and those girls who have received treatment for malignant disease in childhood may present with either.

The relationship between nutrition and the reproductive system is under intensive investigation. The most common causes of secondary amenorrhoea in the adolescent population relate to body weight and it is important to recognize that both underweight and obese girls may present with disordered menstrual function.

### Clinical assessment of the patient with secondary amenorrhoea

A detailed menstrual history should be taken from all patients. A history of irregular cycles dating back to menarche is suggestive of PCOS and this may be associated with weight gain or obesity. The question of weight loss should be dealt with carefully and a detailed dietary history obtained as a patient with weight loss-related amenorrhoea might not necessarily be underweight at the time of presentation. The

**Table 13.3.** Causes of secondary amenorrhoea

| | |
|---|---|
| Primary ovarian failure | 'Resistant ovary syndrome'<br>Irradiation/chemotherapy<br>Gonadal dysgenesis<br>Postoperative |
| Secondary ovarian failure<br>  Hypothalamo-pituitary<br>  dysfunction | Hyperprolactinaemia<br>Hypothalamo-pituitary tumours<br>Sheehan syndrome<br>Empty sella syndrome<br>Irradiation/chemotherapy<br>Postoperative |
| Functional disorders | Weight loss/anorexia nervosa<br>Exercise<br>Psychogenic<br>Chronic illness |
| Polycystic ovary syndrome | |
| Genital tract disorders | |
| Functional ovarian tumours | |

amount of physical exercise should be reviewed. Symptoms of oestrogen deficiency may be present, and headaches and visual disturbance should be enquired after. Features suggestive of other endocrine disorders or known previous chemotherapy or radiotherapy should be established. A history of sexual activity or pelvic inflammatory disease is important and may not be proffered by younger patients unless specifically asked after.

The examination should begin with measurement of height and weight and the body mass index calculated [BMI = weight (kg)/height$^2$ (m$^2$); normal range 20–25 kg/m$^2$]. Signs of hyperandrogenism such as hirsutism, acne or virilization should be noted and the breasts examined for galactorrhoea. Features of other endocrine disorders may be present, and the visual fields should be assessed.

Investigations are initially aimed at establishing the site of the lesion. Thus basal FSH measurement will determine those patients with primary ovarian dysfunction. LH is also raised but this is non-specific as LH levels are also elevated in 60–70% of patients with PCOS. Serum prolactin and thyroid function should be measured although unsuspected thyroid disease is a rare cause of secondary amenorrhoea. The use of the GnRH test is of little or no value in the investigation of secondary amenorrhoea as it provides poor discrimination between patients with hypothalamic amenorrhoea and normal women [48]. Oestrogen activity may be inferred by the response to a progestagen challenge (e.g. vaginal bleeding after a course of medroxyprogesterone acetate, 5 mg daily by mouth for 5 days) or by demonstration of endometrial thickness of greater than 5 mm by ultrasound scanning. Direct measurement of serum oestradiol can be performed but the result may not reflect accurately the degree of oestrogenization. Pelvic ultrasound scanning, in skilled hands,

will distinguish between polycystic and multifollicular ovaries [17].

### Primary ovarian failure

The term primary ovarian failure (POF) is used to describe failure of ovarian function before the age of 40 years and is characterized by hypergonadotrophic hypogonadism. A number of underlying causes have been described, including the chromosomal and genetic abnormalities discussed above, galactosaemia, infections such as mumps, chemotherapy and radiotherapy treatment for malignant disease and autoimmunity [49]. Autoimmunity is an important cause of POF and may form part of the spectrum of multiple autoimmune endocrinopathy [50]. The syndrome usually presents in adult life with secondary amenorrhoea associated with symptoms of oestrogen deficiency such as hot flushes and dyspareunia. However, POF may present at any age [51] and should be considered in adolescent girls with secondary amenorrhoea in whom the diagnosis will be confirmed by the presence of elevated FSH concentrations. Treatment is with sex steroid replacement therapy and assisted reproduction with oocyte donation if and when desired.

## Body weight and ovarian function

The relationship between body weight and menstrual disorders has been recognized clinically for many years. The changes in body fat distribution, insulin, IGF-I and SHBG concentrations associated with maturation of the hypothalamo-pituitary-gonadal axis at puberty has been described. Recognition of the importance of insulin effects on the mature reproductive system (reviewed in [52]) and recent identification of leptin as an endocrine signal between adipose tissue and the hypothalamus [53] suggest at least some of the mechanisms whereby nutritional status may interact with gonadal function. The potential role of leptin as a mediator of the hypothalamo-pituitary dysfunction observed in starvation is supported by studies in mice in which the neuroendocrine changes associated with fasting were partially or fully normalized by leptin treatment [54]. Dramatic weight loss induced by leptin therapy in a girl shown to be leptin deficient has been described [55].

## Weight loss-related amenorrhoea

Weight loss-related amenorrhoea is the commonest cause of secondary amenorrhoea in young women, and in adolescent girls it may be associated with anorexia nervosa or other defined eating disorders. A similar clinical picture may be seen in girls with chronic illness. A BMI of less than 16 kg/m$^2$ is associated with severely impaired GnRH activity resulting in a prepubertal pattern of gonadotrophin secretion [54]. Less severe weight loss is also important, and in these patients the endocrine and ovarian morphological pattern exactly replicates that seen during normal puberty [17].

Treatment of weight loss-related amenorrhoea is weight gain; this requires the assistance of experienced dietitians. Patients who remain amenorrhoeic should be treated with hormone replacement therapy in the form of a low-dose combined oestrogen/progestagen preparation.

## Exercise-related amenorrhoea

This form of amenorrhoea, related to strenuous physical exercise, is also common in young women and the endocrine and ovarian changes are similar to those seen in girls with weight-related amenorrhoea. The treatment of choice is to reduce the exercise level, but young women such as athletes or ballet dancers may be unable or unwilling to do this. It is advisable to check oestrogen status, and replacement therapy should be offered to those who are oestrogen deficient [57].

Psychological factors may be important in patients with either weight loss-related or exercise-related amenorrhoea. Appropriate expert psychological and psychiatric support should be arranged and is mandatory in adolescent girls with anorexia nervosa.

## Polycystic ovary syndrome

The morphological appearance of polycystic ovaries can be observed in about one-quarter of asymptomatic adult women by ultrasound examination, making this the most common structural abnormality of the ovary [58]. Women with the classic syndrome of PCOS have disorders of menstrual function, hirsutism and obesity, reflecting hyperandrogenism and anovulation. Typically, these morphological and clinical abnormalities are associated with the biochemical features of raised testosterone and LH concentrations. However, there is a broad spectrum of presenting clinical features ranging from anovulatory women without hirsutism to those with regular menses and hirsutism. Elevated LH levels are not a universal finding [59].

Polycystic ovary syndrome appears to have a complex aetiology requiring both genetic and environmental triggers for its full expression. Extensive genetic studies have examined the potential role of a number of candidate genes in PCOS. These include genes coding for steroidogenic enzymes and those which affect the secretion and action of insulin and gonadotrophins. Studies in large numbers of families with PCOS suggest an oligogenic disorder in which a small number of key genes are involved and which interact with environmental, particularly nutritional, factors. Current evidence indicates that the P450 cholesterol side-chain cleavage gene (*CYP11a*, a rate-limiting stage in steroid biosynthesis), the insulin gene *VNTR* minisatellite region and the follistatin gene may all play a role in the aetiology of PCOS [60,61].

Patients with PCOS may present in adolescence, usually complaining of hirsutism and oligomenorrhoea or amenorrhoea. A clinical history of menstrual irregularity dating back to adolescence is common in women who present in later life and is regarded as a useful diagnostic symptom when differentiating between PCOS and other causes of hyperandrogenaemia. The first presentation in older girls and women may reflect the increasing adiposity required for full expression of the syndrome.

The association between obesity, hyperinsulinaemia, insulin resistance and PCOS is well recognized and is characterized by increased upper body fat mass, raised triglyceride and subnormal high-density lipoprotein (HDL)-cholesterol concentrations and relative glucose intolerance (reviewed in [62]). The relationship between hyperinsulinaemia and the hyperandrogenaemia and raised LH concentrations typical of PCOS is complex. Raised androgen levels reflect both alterations in intraovarian steroidogenesis [19–22,62] and suppression of SHBG concentrations, resulting in elevated free testosterone concentrations, the latter being reversible by weight reduction [63].

The mechanism whereby LH concentrations rise remains controversial, although it is likely, in part, to be secondary to altered steroid feedback from the ovary. Identification of leptin, which is produced by adipocytes, regulated by insulin and acts within the hypothalamus, suggests one potential regulatory pathway directly linked to weight gain [64].

Clinical management of PCOS in adolescence is aimed at regularization of the menstrual cycle and treatment of hirsutism. The first-line therapy in all obese girls should be weight reduction, which may be sufficient in itself to restore regular menstruation [63]. If oligomenorrhoea is present, induction of regular withdrawal bleeding is necessary because of the risk of endometrial hyperplasia and potential future neoplastic change. This may be achieved by cyclical progesterone therapy or, more usually in older adolescents, by a combined oral contraceptive preparation such as Dianette, containing oestrogen and the prostestogenic antiandrogen cyproterone acetate. Treatment of hirsutism depends upon its severity and the patient's perception of the degree of excess hair growth. Thus some girls may be content with the use of cosmetic measures such as depilatory creams, waxing or electrolysis, but in others the degree of psychological distress indicates a need for antiandrogen therapy. Successful treatment may be achieved with Dianette alone or in combination with high-dose cyproterone acetate or the 5α-reductase inhibitor finasteride [65]. Other antiandrogens are rarely indicated in adolescent girls. In all cases, patients should be warned that the response to treatment is slow and that improvement may not be seen for at least 6 months from commencement of therapy. In later life the successful treatment of infertility depends upon weight loss in obese subjects and may require antioestrogen therapy, gonadotrophin induction of ovulation or laparoscopic surgery [42].

The metabolic features of PCOS associated with insulin resistance suggest that they may have long-term health risks associated with type 2 diabetes and cardiovascular disease. As central obesity, glucose intolerance, high triglyceride and low HDL-cholesterol concentrations appear to be strong predictors of coronary heart disease in women, it seems sensible to introduce dietary and lifestyle advice to women with PCOS at an early age in an attempt to lower their future risk [66].

## Sex hormone replacement therapy

Many of the causes of reproductive dysfunction presenting in children and adolescents result in hypogonadism and require the institution of sex hormone replacement therapy. After the induction of puberty, long-term treatment is required for the avoidance of deficiency symptoms, maintenance of normal secondary sexual characteristics and preservation of psychosexual well-being.

The effects of oestrogen on skeletal bone mineral density have been widely reported in postmenopausal women, and studies in young women with oestrogen deficiency from a variety of causes suggest that early treatment is essential to maximize peak bone density [57]. Testosterone exerts similar protective effects on the skeleton in hypogonadal males (reviewed in [67]). Sex hormone replacement therapy should be combined with an adequate dietary calcium intake, including supplements where necessary.

Other benefits of hormone replacement therapy are less well described, largely due to a lack of prospective data on patients undergoing long-term treatment starting in adolescence. However, data from postmenopausal women suggest that oestrogen therapy reduces the mortality from cardiovascular disease and stroke [68], and it seems reasonable to assume that replacement therapy in young women will reduce any increased risk associated with oestrogen deficiency. The known adverse effects of testosterone therapy in men on HDL-cholesterol and plasma viscosity may be offset by reductions in blood pressure and serum triglycerides [67]. More recently, menopausal oestrogen therapy has been shown to have beneficial effects on the risk and age of onset of Alzheimer disease in women [69], and if these data are confirmed in prospective trials they may have major implications for oestrogen-deficient young women.

The risks of sex hormone replacement therapy in young people with hypogonadism are difficult to assess because of a lack of data for this patient group. The usual absolute contraindications to oestrogen replacement in postmenopausal women, such as genital tract malignancy and breast cancer, are unlikely to apply to the adolescent age group, although a strong family history of venous thrombosis may be important and indicate the need for a thrombophilia screen before the institution of long-term therapy. Although postmenopausal oestrogen therapy increases the risk ratio for breast cancer in long-term (over 10 years) postmenopausal users to about 1.3, the interactions between even longer treatment duration with age of onset of therapy and lack of pre-exposure of breast tissue to oestrogens are unknown. Similarly, there are few data on the incidence of prostate cancer in long-term testosterone users and the role of monitoring by serum prostate-specific antigen or ultrasonography is not established. Without evidence to the contrary, it seems likely that the risk–benefit analysis for young adults with hypogonadism is greatly in favour of sex hormone replacement, although careful follow-up for these patients should be undertaken.

## Summary

Normal development of the reproductive system involves a complex series of coordinated genetic, neurohormonal and nutritional inputs taking place over a number of years. Abnormalities presenting in childhood and adolescence have profound effects on pubertal development and on adult life. Early diagnosis and appropriate treatment, usually involving a multidisciplinary approach, are essential to achieve the best outcome in terms of psychosexual well-being and prospects for fertility in later life.

## References

1 Lim HN, Hawkins JR. Genetic control of gonadal differentiation. *Ballière's Clin Endocrinol Metab* 1998; 12: 1–16.
2 Rey R, Picard J-Y. Embryology and endocrinology of genital development. *Ballière's Clin Endocrinol Metab* 1998; 12: 17–33.

3 Lee MM, Donahoe PK. Müllerian inhibiting substance – a gonadal hormone with multiple functions. *Endocr Rev* 1993; 14: 152–64.

4 Huhtaniemi IL, Korenbrot CC, Jaffe RB. HCG binding and stimulation of testosterone biosynthesis in the human fetal testis. *J Clin Endocrinol Metab* 1977; 44: 963–7.

5 Hutson JM, Hasthorpe S, Heyns CF. Anatomical and functional aspects of testicular descent and cryptorchidism. *Endocr Rev* 1997; 18: 259–80.

6 Scorer CG. The descent of the testis. *Arch Dis Child* 1964; 39: 605–9.

7 Baker TG. A quantitative and cytological study of germ cells in human ovaries. *Proc R Soc London Biol* 1963; 158: 417–33.

8 Gougeon A. Regulation of ovarian follicular development in primates: facts and hypotheses. *Endocr Rev* 1996; 17: 121–55.

9 Huhtaniemi IL, Yamamoto M, Ranta T, Jalkanen J, Jaffe RB. Follicle-stimulating hormone receptors appear earlier in the primate fetal testis than in the ovary. *J Clin Endocrinol Metab* 1987; 65: 1210–14.

10 Misrahi M, Beau I, Meduri G *et al.* Gonadotrophin receptors and the control of gonadal steroidogenesis: physiology and pathology. *Balliere's Clin Endocrinol Metab* 1998; 12: 35–66.

11 Seminara SB, Hayes FJ, Crowley WF. Gonadotrophin-releasing hormone deficiency in the human (idiopathic hypogonadotrophic hypogonadism and Kallman's syndrome): pathophysiological and genetic considerations. *Endocr Rev* 1998; 19: 521–39.

12 Weiss J, Axelrod J, Whitcomb W *et al.* Hypogonadism caused by a single aminoacid substitution in the β-subunit of luteinising hormone. *N Engl J Med* 1992; 326: 179–83.

13 Matthews C, Chatterjee VK. Isolated deficiency of follicle stimulating hormone revisited. *N Engl J Med* 1997; 337: 642.

14 Gnessi L, Fabbri A, Spera G. Gonadal peptides as mediators of development and functional control of the testis: an integrated system with hormones and local environment. *Endocr Rev* 1997; 18: 541–609.

15 Winter JSD, Hughes IA, Reyes FI. Pituitary-gonadal steroid concentrations in man from birth to two years of age. *J Clin Endocrinol Metab* 1976; 42: 679–86.

16 Brook CGD, Jacobs HS, Stanhope R, Adams J, Hindmarsh P. Pulsatility of reproductive hormones: applications to the understanding of puberty and to the treatment of infertility. *Ballière's Clin Endocrinol Metab* 1987; 1: 23–41.

17 Adams J, Franks S, Polson D *et al.* Multifollicular ovaries: clinical and endocrine features and response to pulsatile gonadotrophin-releasing hormone. *Lancet* 1985; 2: 1375–9.

18 Leung PK, Steele GL. Intracellular signalling in the gonads. *Endocr Rev* 1992; 13: 476–98.

19 Franks S, Gilling-Smith C, Watson H, Willis D. Insulin action in the normal and polycystic ovary. *Endocr Metab Clin N Am* 1999; 28: 361–78.

20 Franks S. Growth hormone and ovarian function. *Ballière's Clin Endocrinol Metab* 1998; 12: 331–40.

21 Findlay JK. Growth factors in endocrinology – the ovary. *Ballière's Clin Endocrinol Metab* 1991; 5: 755–69.

22 Mason H, Franks S. Local control of ovarian steroidogenesis. *Ballière's Clin Obstet Gynaecol* 1997; 11: 261–79.

23 Baxter-Jones ADG, Helms P, Baines-Preece J, Preece M. Menarche in intensively trained gymnasts, swimmers and tennis players. *Ann Hum Biol* 1994; 21: 407–15.

24 Cooper C, Kuh D, Egger P, Wadsworth M, Barker D. Childhood growth and age at menarche. *Br J Obst Gynaecol* 1996; 103: 814–17.

25 Vollman RF. *The Menstrual Cycle.* Philadelphia: Saunders, 1977.

26 Apter D, Raisanen I, Ylostano P. Follicular growth in relation to serum hormonal patterns in adolescence compared with adult menstrual cycles. *Fertil Steril* 1987; 47: 82–8.

27 Fraser IS, Michie EA, Wide L. Pituitary gonadotrophin and ovarian function in adolescent dysfunctional uterine bleeding. *J Clin Endocrinol Metab* 1973; 37: 407–14.

28 Zhang L, Rees MCP, Bicknell R. The isolation and long term culture of normal human endometrial endothelium and stroma: expression of mRNAs for angiogenic polypeptides basally and on oestrogen and progesterone challenges. *J Cell Sci* 1995; 108: 323–31.

29 Amiel SA, Caprio S, Sherwin RS, Plewe G, Haymond MW, Tamborlane WV. Insulin resistance of puberty: a defect restricted to peripheral glucose metabolism. *J Clin Endocrinol Metab* 1991; 72: 277–82.

30 Porcu E, Venturoli S. Hirsutism and irregular menses in adolescence. In: Stanhope R, ed. *Adolescent Endocrinology.* Bristol: BioScientifica, 1998: 93–9.

31 Van der Spuy Z. Nutrition and reproduction. *Clin Obstet Gynecol N Am* 1985; 12: 579–604.

32 Willi U, Atares M, Prader A, Zachmann M. Testicular adrenal-like tissue (TALT) in congenital adrenal hyperplasia: detection by ultrasonography. *Pediatr Radiol* 1991; 21: 284–7.

33 Urban MD, Lee PA, Migeon CJ. Adult height and fertility in men with congenital virilizing adrenal hyperplasia. *N Engl J Med* 1978; 299: 10796–800.

34 Federman DD. Psychosexual adjustment in congenital adrenal hyperplasia. *N Engl J Med* 1987; 316: 209–11.

35 Mulaikal RM, Migeon CJ, Rock JA. Fertility rates in female patients with congenital hyperplasia due to 21-hydroxylase deficiency. *N Engl J Med* 1987; 326: 178–82.

36 Premawardhana LD, Hughes IA, Read GF, Scanlon MF. Longer term outcome in females with congenital adrenal hyperplasia (CAH): the Cardiff experience. *Clin Endocrinol* 1997; 46: 327–32.

37 Azziz R, Dewailly D, Owerbach D. Nonclassical adrenal hyperplasia: current concepts. *J Clin Endocrinol Metab* 1994; 78: 810–15.

38 Sprotzer P, Billaud L, Thalabard JC *et al.* Cyproterone acetate versus hydrocortisone treatment in late-onset adrenal hyperplasia. *J Clin Endocrinol Metab* 1990; 70: 642–6.

39 John Radcliffe Hospital Cryptorchidism Study Group. Cryptorchidism: an apparent substantial increase since 1960. *Br Med J* 1987; 293: 1401–4.

40 Dean HJ, McTaggart TL, Fisk DG, Friesen HG. The educational, vocational and marital status of growth hormone deficient adults treated with growth hormone during childhood. *Am J Dis Child* 1985; 139: 1105–10.

41 Quinton R, Bouloux PMG. Male hypogonadism, infertility and impotence. In: Ginsburg J, ed. *Drug Therapy in Reproductive Endocrinology.* London: Arnold, 1996: 242–58.

42 Davies MC. Management of infertility and the newer reproductive techniques: treatment opportunities and ethical implications. In: Stanhope R, ed. *Adolescent Endocrinology.* Bristol: BioScientifica, 1998: 59–67.

43 Franks S. Primary and secondary amenorrhoea. In: *Gynaecology Clinical Algorithms.* London: BMJ Publishing, 1989: 41–5.

44 Canales ES, Zarate A, Castelazo Ayala L. Primary amenorrhoea associated with polycystic ovaries. Endocrine, cytogenetic and therapeutic considerations. *Obstet Gynecol* 1971; 37: 205–10.

45 Turner HH. A syndrome of infantilism, congenital webbed neck and cubitus valgus. *Endocrinology* 1938; 23: 566–74.

46 Wood DF, Franks S. Hypogonadism in women. In: Grossman A, ed. *Clinical Endocrinology*, 2nd edn. Oxford: Blackwell Scientific Publications, 1998: 702–16.

47 Griffin JE, Edwards C, Madden JD, Harrod MJ, Wilson JD. Congenital absence of the vagina. The Mayer–Rokitansky–Kuster–Hauser syndrome. *Ann Intern Med* 1976; 85: 224–36.

48 Franks S. Diagnostic uses of LHRH. In: Shaw RW, Marshall JC, eds. *LHRH and its Analogues*. London: Wright, 1989: 80–91.

49 Anasti JN. Premature ovarian failure: an update. *Fertil Steril* 1998; 70: 1–15.

50 Hoek A, Schoemaker J, Drexhage HA. Premature ovarian failure and ovarian autoimmunity. *Endocr Rev* 1997; 18: 107–34.

51 Coulam CB. Premature gonadal failure. *Fertil Steril* 1982; 38: 645–55.

52 Dunaif A. Insulin resistance and polycystic ovary syndrome: mechanism and implications for pathogenesis. *Endocr Rev* 1997; 18: 774–800.

53 Zhang Y, Proenca R, Maffei M *et al*. Positional cloning of the mouse obese gene and its human homologue. *Nature* 1994; 372: 425–32.

54 Ahima RS, Prabakaran D, Mantzoros C *et al*. Role of leptin in the neuroendocrine response to fasting. *Nature* 1996; 382: 250–2.

55 Farooqi IS, Jebb SA, Langmack G *et al*. Effects of recombinant leptin therapy in a child with congenital leptin deficiency. *N Engl J Med* 1999; 341: 879–84.

56 Nillius SJ, Wide L. The pituitary responsiveness to acute and chronic administration of gonadotropin releasing hormone in acute and recovery stages of anorexia nervosa. In: Vigersky RA, eds. *Anorexia Nervosa*. New York: Raven Press, 1977: 225–411.

57 Davies MC, Hall ML, Jacobs HS. Bone mineral loss in young women with amenorrhoea. *Br Med J* 1990; 301: 790–3.

58 Polson DW, Adams J, Wadsworth J, Franks S. Polycystic ovaries – a common finding in normal women. *Lancet* 1988; 1: 870–2.

59 Franks S. The polycystic ovary syndrome. *New Engl J Med* 1995; 333: 853–61.

60 Franks S, Gharani N, Waterworth D *et al*. The genetic basis of polycystic ovary syndrome. *Hum Reprod* 1997; 12: 2641–8.

61 Urbanek M, Legro R, Driscoll D *et al*. Thirty seven candidate genes for polycystic ovary syndrome: strongest evidence for linkage is with follistatin. *Proc Natl Acad Sci USA* 1999; 96: 8573–8.

62 Holte J. Disturbances in insulin secretion and sensitivity in women with the polycystic ovary syndrome. *Ballière's Clin Endocrinol Metab* 1996; 10: 221–47.

63 Kiddy DS, Hamilton-Fairley D, Bush A *et al*. Improvement in endocrine and ovarian function during dietary treatment of obese women with polycystic ovary syndrome. *Clin Endocrinol* 1992; 36: 105–11.

64 Conway GS, Jacobs HS. Leptin: a hormone of reproduction. *Hum Reprod* 1997; 12: 633–5.

65 Venturoli S, Marescalchi O, Colombo FM *et al*. A prospective randomised trial comparing low dose flutamide, finasteride, ketoconazole and cyproterone acetate–estrogen regimens in the treatment of hirsutism. *J Clin Endocrinol Metab* 1999; 84: 1304–10.

66 McKeigue P. Cardiovascular disease and diabetes in women with polycystic ovary syndrome. *Ballière's Clin Endocrinol Metab* 1996; 10: 311–18.

67 Francis RM. The effects of testosterone on osteoporosis in men. *Clin Endocrinol* 1999; 50: 411–14.

68 Meade TW, Berra A. Hormone replacement therapy and cardiovascular disease. *Br Med Bull* 1992; 48: 276–308.

69 Tang MX, Jacobs D, Stern Y *et al*. Effect of oestrogen during menopause on risk and age of onset of Alzheimer's disease. *Lancet* 1996; 348: 429–32.

# 14 Disorders of water balance

## G. L. Robertson

## Introduction

The regulation of water balance in infants and children has not been studied extensively, but it is probably similar in principle to that in adults. Thus, the conceptual approach to disorders of water balance in paediatrics should be very similar if not identical to that in adults. In practice, however, the management of fluid and electrolyte disorders in infants and children presents special challenges owing to age-related differences in size, diet and development of the relevant renal, hormonal, cognitive, verbal and motor functions. These challenges are compounded by a paucity of normative data for thirst and antidiuretic function at various stages of growth and development. Therefore, although the principles described in this chapter will be drawn largely from studies in adults, the main qualitative and quantitative differences that are known to be present in infants and children will also be presented. The physiology and pathophysiology of water balance in premature infants encompasses an even wider range of special problems and will not be covered in this chapter.

## Body water: distribution, composition and turnover

Water is by far the largest constituent of the human body. In healthy infants at term, it constitutes 75–85% of body weight and is divided between the extracellular and intracellular compartments in a ratio of about 1.5:1 (Fig. 14.1). In the first 1–2 weeks after birth, total body water and weight decrease largely because of a diuresis of water and sodium chloride from the extracellular compartment. At the same time, the proportion of weight contributed by intracellular volume increases. Subsequently, as the infant begins to grow and gain body fat and muscle, the *proportion* of body weight contributed by intracellular water continues to increase while

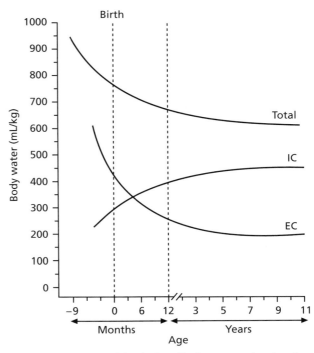

**Fig. 14.1.** The volume and distribution of body water as a function of age in infants and children [1]. IC, intracellular; EC, extracellular.

the *proportion* contributed by extracellular and total body water continues to decrease, eventually reaching near adult levels of about 40%, 20% and 60%, respectively, by early puberty.

The solute compositions of intracellular and extracellular fluid differ markedly, because most cell membranes possess an array of transport systems that actively accumulate or expel specific solutes [2]. Thus, sodium and chloride are the predominant solutes of plasma and interstitial fluid, whereas potassium, magnesium and various organic acids or phosphates are predominantly intracellular. Glucose, which requires an insulin-activated transport system to enter most somatic cells and is rapidly converted in those cells to glycogen or other metabolites, is present in significant amounts only in extracellular fluid. Bicarbonate is present in both compartments but is about three times more concentrated in extracellular fluid. Urea is unique among the major naturally occurring solutes in that it diffuses freely across most cell membranes and is therefore present in similar concentrations in all body fluids except the renal medulla, where it is concentrated to very high levels. The plasma concentration of sodium and its associated anions in infants and children are the same as in adults and, with the possible exception of the hours immediately after birth, there is no evidence that they change appreciably during growth and development.

Despite marked differences in the concentration of particular solutes in extracellular and intracellular fluid, the total solute concentration in these two compartments is always the same. This equilibrium is because most cell membranes are freely permeable to water [3]. Therefore, a change in the total concentration of solutes in one compartment creates an effective osmotic gradient that is rapidly eliminated by a net redistribution of water from or to the other compartment. The driving force for this rapid redistribution is the 'effective' osmotic pressure of the fluids on either side of the membrane. It is similar but not completely identical to the osmotic pressure as determined by freezing point or vapour pressure osmometry [4]. The latter is a physicochemical property determined by the total concentration of all of the solutes present, regardless of their ability to penetrate biological membranes. The 'effective' osmolality of a body fluid, on the other hand, is a biological property determined by the total concentration of only those solutes that do not equilibrate freely across the membranes of living cells. Thus, for example, sodium and chloride, which are actively excluded from the intracellular compartment, are osmotically effective whereas urea is not. Normally, the difference between the effective osmolality of body fluids and that determined by freezing point or vapour pressure osmometry is too small to be important, because more than 95% of the solute in plasma and extracellular fluid is due to sodium and its anions. However, in certain situations, such as chronic renal failure, effective osmolality may be considerably less than that determined by conventional osmometry, because the concentration of ineffective solutes such as urea is much higher than normal.

Because osmotic equilibrium is maintained by rapid shifts of water, any change in the concentration of an effective solute in one compartment changes the volume and osmolality of all compartments [5]. Thus, for example, a rise in the extracellular concentration of sodium and its anions induced by dehydration causes water to flow from the intracellular to the extracellular compartment. As a result, the water deficit distributes evenly throughout the body, causing a proportionally equal decrease in volume and increase in osmolality

**Table 14.1.** Basal rates of water excretion in healthy infants, children and adults ingesting diets typical for their age

| Route | At birth | 2 months | 30 months | Adults |
|---|---|---|---|---|
| Evaporation | 20–30 | 30–40 | 30–40 | 10–20 |
| Urine | 40–140 | 62–158 | 40–80 | 10–40 |
| Stool | 2–4 | 2–4 | 2–4 | 3–5 |
| Growth | – | 2–3 | 3–4 | – |
| Total | 62–174 | 96–205 | 75–128 | 23–65 |

Values are ranges in mL/kg/day.

in each of the compartments. Conversely, a fall in extracellular sodium and its anions induced by overhydration causes water to flow in the opposite direction, redistributing the excess to all compartments. However, if the total amount of electrolyte or other effective solute in one compartment changes (due, for example, to infusion of hypertonic saline or administration of a diuretic), the amount of water in the other compartments changes in the *opposite* direction [5]. In these acute situations, the cells as a whole behave essentially like perfect osmometers; that is, the observed changes in the volume and osmolality of extracellular fluid conform closely to theoretical expectations. However, deviations from this kind of ideal behaviour may occur when the disturbance in the salt and water balance is particularly severe and/or prolonged. Under these conditions, many cells appear to be able to counteract osmotically induced changes in volume by reversibly activating or deactivating intracellular solute [6,7]. In addition, these disturbances bring into play a variety of other homeostatic mechanisms that, by altering total body content of salt and/or water, gradually restore the balance to normal (see below). Because the plasma concentrations of sodium and its anions and other solutes are virtually the same in healthy infants, children and adults, their total and effective plasma osmolality are also the same.

Body water is also in a constant state of external flux because of obligatory evaporation, urination, eating and drinking (Table 14.1). The magnitude of the turnover varies widely from person to person or from time to time in the same person because the rate of intake and output are strongly affected by common variables such as diet, temperature, humidity and physical activity. In adults, for example, an increase in temperature and/or physical activity can cause as much as a 10- to 20-fold increase in the rate of evaporation from the skin and lungs [8]. In infants and children, this insensible loss is about twofold greater than in adults (Table 14.1) owing, presumably, to their greater ratio of surface area to weight. The rate of urine output also varies markedly depending on the level of urine concentration and the rate of solute excretion (Fig. 14.2). In healthy infants and young children, it is highly variable and usually much greater than in adults (Table 14.1). This variability and age-related difference

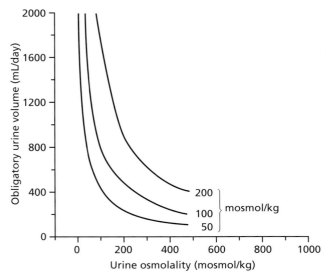

**Fig. 14.2.** Urinary flow as a function of urinary concentration at three different rates of solute excretion. Note that (1) changes in urine osmolality between 50 and 300 mosmol/kg have a much greater effect on urine flow than comparable changes between 300 and 600 mosmol/kg; and (2) changes in solute excretion rate have a much greater effect on urine flow when urine is dilute (osmolality < 300 mosmol/kg) than when it is concentrated (osmolality > 300 mosmol/kg).

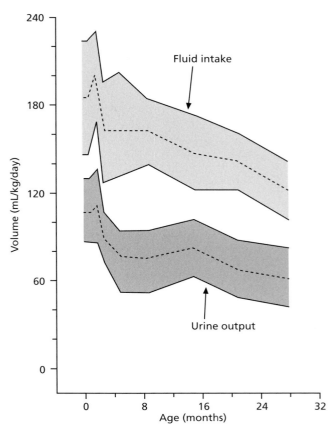

**Fig. 14.3.** Water intake and urine output as a function of age in healthy infants and children receiving *ad libitum* water and standard amounts of formula or baby food. Values are shown as the mean ± one standard deviation [9].

are most evident in the first few months after birth and gradually narrow over the next 2 years (Fig. 14.3). They probably result from several factors including an incompletely developed capacity to concentrate urine during the first months of life (Fig. 14.4) and the relatively large but variable amounts of water and/or solute contained in the different kinds of milk or formula customarily fed to infants (Table 14.2). As expected, the higher rates of insensible and urinary water loss in healthy infants and children are balanced by higher rates of total fluid intake (Fig. 14.3).

Despite the relatively high turnover of body water in healthy infants and children, plasma osmolality and its principal determinant, the concentration of sodium and its anions, are normally maintained within a remarkably narrow range somewhere between 275 and 295 mosmol/kg and between 135 and 145 mequiv/L respectively. This *osmotic* stability is achieved largely by the combined actions of the thirst mechanism and the antidiuretic hormone, arginine vasopressin (AVP), which continuously raise or lower total body water to keep it in balance with the concentration of sodium and its anions in the extracellular compartment. The *volume* of the extracellular and intracellular fluids is also kept relatively constant but this homeostatic function is subserved primarily by the mechanisms for regulating sodium excretion. This division of labour is useful to bear in mind when considering the physiology and pathophysiology of salt and water balance in humans.

## Physiology of water balance

### Antidiuretic function

#### Anatomy

The antidiuretic hormone, AVP, is produced by large neurosecretory neurones that form the posterior pituitary or neurohypophysis. These neurones originate primarily in cell bodies in the supraoptic nucleus of the hypothalamus and project into the sella turcica, where they terminate as bulbous enlargements on capillary networks that drain into the jugular vein via the sellar, cavernous and lateral venous sinuses (Fig. 14.5) [12]. A separate branch that arises in small cells of the paraventricular nucleus of the hypothalamus projects to the infundibulum and terminates on a capillary network that coalesces into the portal veins and perfuses the adenohypophysis before discharging into the systemic circulation. Smaller divisions of parvocellular neurones also project to many other areas of the brain, including the cerebral ventricles,

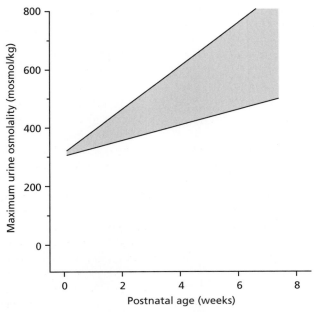

**Fig. 14.4.** Maximum urinary concentrating capacity as a function of age in 17 healthy infants. Shaded area indicates the range of the maximum urine osmolality values observed after administration of the vasopressin analogue DDAVP [10].

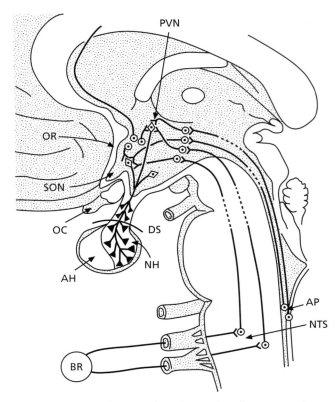

**Fig. 14.5.** Anatomy of the neurohypophysis and its afferent connections. Reproduced from [12]. PVN, paraventricular nucleus; OR, osmoreceptor; SON, supraoptic nucleus; OC, optic chiasm; DS, diaphragm sella; AN, adenohypophysis (anterior pituitary); NH, neurohypophysis (posterior pituitary); AP, area postrema; NTS, nucleus tractus solitarius; BR, baroreceptors.

where they appear to secrete directly into cerebrospinal fluid. The blood supply of the neurohypophysis comes from the superior and inferior hypophyseal arterial branches from the posterior communicating and intracavernous portion of the internal carotid. Microscopically, the neurohypophysis appears as a densely interwoven network of capillaries, pituicytes and large non-myelinated nerve fibres that contain many electron-dense, neurosecretory granules [13]. Magnocellular neurones displaying these features appear to be fully developed and functional at birth.

## Chemistry

AVP is a nonapeptide composed of a six-member disulphide ring and a three-member tail on which the carboxy-terminal

**Table 14.2.** Potential renal solute load (PRSL) of various milks and formulas

| Source | Nutrients | | | | | PRSL | |
|---|---|---|---|---|---|---|---|
| | Protein (g/L) | Na (mmol/L) | Cl (mmol/L) | K (mmol/L) | P (mmol/L) | (mosmol/L) | mosmol/100 kcal |
| Human milk | 10 | 7 | 11 | 13 | 5 | 93 | 14 |
| Formulas | | | | | | | |
|   Milk based | 15 | 8 | 12 | 18 | 11 | 135 | 20 |
|   Soy based | 20 | 10 | 16 | 21 | 16 | 177 | 26 |
| FDA limits | 30 | 17 | 28 | 34 | 27* | 277 | 41 |
| Cow's milk | 33 | 21 | 30 | 39 | 30 | 308 | 46 |
| Skimmed milk | 34 | 23 | 33 | 43 | 33 | 326 | 93 |

*Not established. PRSL consists of nitrogenous substances (urea, uric acid, creatine, and creatinine), sodium, potassium, chloride and phosphorous generated metabolically from nutrients assuming none used for growth or lost by the extrarenal route. Adapted from [11].

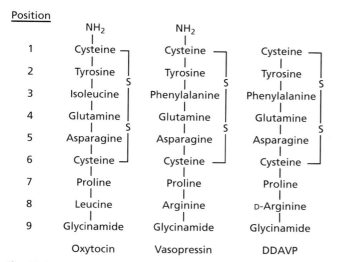

| Position | | | |
|---|---|---|---|
| 1 | Cysteine | Cysteine | Cysteine |
| 2 | Tyrosine | Tyrosine | Tyrosine |
| 3 | Isoleucine | Phenylalanine | Phenylalanine |
| 4 | Glutamine | Glutamine | Glutamine |
| 5 | Asparagine | Asparagine | Asparagine |
| 6 | Cysteine | Cysteine | Cysteine |
| 7 | Proline | Proline | Proline |
| 8 | Leucine | Arginine | D-Arginine |
| 9 | Glycinamide | Glycinamide | Glycinamide |
| | Oxytocin | Vasopressin | DDAVP |

**Fig. 14.6.** Primary structure of oxytocin, vasopressin and des-amino-D-arginine vasopressin (DDAVP). Reproduced from [12].

group is amidated (Fig. 14.6) [12]. It differs from oxytocin, another nonapeptide hormone produced by the neuro-hypophysis, only in the substitution of phenylalanine for isoleucine at position 3 and of arginine for leucine at position 8 in the tail of the molecule.

AVP is synthesized via a protein precursor that is composed of a signal peptide, the hormone moiety, a tripeptide linker, a binding protein known as neurophysin, a dipeptide linker and a glycosylated peptide known as copeptin (Fig. 14.7) [12]. The gene encoding the prohormone in humans is located on chromosome 20 [14]. It has three exons that code for (1) the signal peptide, AVP, a tripeptide linker and the variable, amino-terminal part of neurophysin; (2) the central, highly conserved portion of neurophysin; and (3) the variable, carboxy-terminal part of neurophysin, another linker and copeptin (Fig. 14.7) [15]. The gene for the oxytocin precursor is similar except that it lacks the part of the third exon that encodes the copeptin moiety in provasopressin. The

genes encoding AVP and oxytocin are located in close proximity on opposing strands of DNA [15,16] but are expressed exclusively in different neurones [17].

Like other peptide hormones destined for secretion, the protein precursor of AVP is translocated into the endoplasmic reticulum, where the signal peptide is removed by a peptidase and the prohormone folds and oligomerizes before transiting the Golgi apparatus into the neurosecretory granules. Binding of the N-terminus of the AVP moiety into a pocket formed by the N-terminal domain of the neurophysin moiety facilitates proper folding, intrachain disulphide bonding and oligomerization of neurophysin *in vitro* [18] and is thought to play an important role in production and trafficking of the hormones *in vivo*. As these granules move down the neurones towards the axon terminal, the prohormone is further cleaved by endopeptidases and exopeptidases, releasing AVP, its neurophysin and copeptin. The hormone is also amidated at its C-terminus by a mono-oxygenase and lyase [11], bound in insoluble complexes with neurophysin in neurosecretory granules and stored in the nerve terminals until they are released by a calcium-dependent exocytotic process similar to that described for other neurosecretory systems. Once in plasma, the AVP–neurophysin complex disassociates and the hormone circulates largely if not totally in a free form. In some unknown way, the secretion of AVP increases its synthesis, but this compensatory response develops gradually and may never completely offset the increased rate of release. Consequently, a chronic severe stimulus such as prolonged water deprivation may severely deplete the neurohypophyseal stores of vasopressin.

## Secretion

Of the many variables known to influence the release of vasopressin [12–19], the most important under physiological conditions is the effective osmotic pressure of body water. Specialized cells, known collectively as osmoreceptors, that

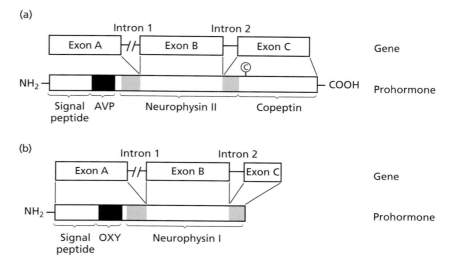

**Fig. 14.7.** Schematic structure of the preprohormones of vasopressin (a) and oxytocin (b) and the genes that encode them. Reproduced from [12].

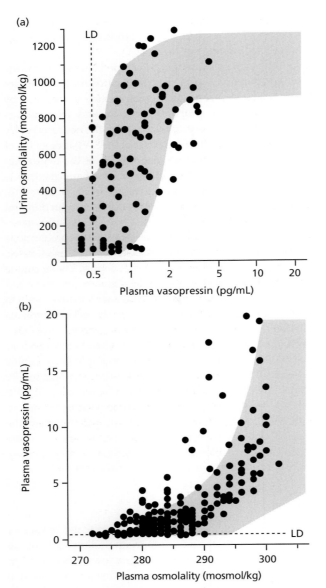

**Fig. 14.8.** Relationship of plasma vasopressin to urine (a) or plasma osmolality (b) in healthy infants and children. The values were obtained before and during a standard fluid deprivation test in 14 girls and eight boys, ages 0.4–6 years (unpublished). The shaded areas indicate the range of these relationships in healthy adults.

are located in the anterior hypothalamus near but separate from the supraoptic nucleus (Fig. 14.5) mediate this influence [20]. They also have a distinct blood supply from small, uncollateralized branches of the anterior cerebral and/or anterior communicating arteries [21].

The osmoregulatory mechanism operates like a discontinuous or 'set point' receptor (Fig. 14.8). Thus, at plasma osmolalities below a certain minimum or threshold level, plasma vasopressin is normally suppressed to low or undetectable concentrations. This suppression seems to require the action of inhibitory input (see the section 'Adipsic hypernatraemia'), suggesting that the osmoregulatory system is bimodal. It results in maximum urinary dilution and the development of a water diuresis that serves to prevent further expansion and dilution of body fluids. Above this threshold or 'set point', plasma vasopressin rises steeply in direct proportion to plasma osmolality. The slope of this relationship indicates that, on average, a rise in plasma osmolality of only 1% increases plasma vasopressin by approximately 1 pg/mL (1 pmol/L), an amount sufficient to significantly alter urinary concentration and flow (Fig. 14.8). This property does not differ appreciably between men and women, but can differ as much as 10-fold between healthy adults [22], apparently because of genetically determined differences in the rate of hormone secretion and/or clearance. The osmotic threshold for vasopressin secretion averages about 280 mosmol/kg in healthy adults but can also vary from 275 to 290 mosmol/kg [22]. These interindividual differences in the 'set' of the osmoregulatory system are also genetically determined but can also be altered by changes in blood volume and/or pressure.

The osmoregulatory mechanism is not equally sensitive to all plasma solutes. Sodium and its anions, which normally contribute more than 95% of the osmotic pressure of plasma, are the most potent solutes known in terms of their capacity to stimulate vasopressin release [23]. However, certain sugars, such as sucrose and mannitol, are also very effective when infused intravenously. In this respect therefore the control mechanism behaves like a true osmoreceptor. However, a rise in plasma osmolality due to urea or glucose causes little or no increase in plasma vasopressin unless insulin is deficient [24], in which case hyperglycaemia is weakly stimulatory. These differences in the response to various plasma solutes are independent of any recognized non-osmotic influence and are probably a property of the osmoregulatory mechanism *per se*.

The osmoregulation of vasopressin secretion in healthy infants and children has not been thoroughly studied. However, the osmoregulatory system appears well developed by late gestation in fetal sheep [25] and is fully functional in human infants and young children (Fig. 14.8). The only difference is that it appears to have a slightly greater gain or sensitivity and/or a lower threshold or 'set' than in adults.

Several non-osmotic variables also influence the secretion of vasopressin. One is a change in blood volume and/or pressure [12,19,26]. These haemodynamic influences are mediated primarily by neurogenic afferents that arise in pressure-sensitive receptors in the cardiac atria and large arteries. These travel via the vagal and glossopharyngeal nerves to the nucleus of the solitary tract where postsynaptic pathways ascend to the lateral parabrachial nucleus, the A1 region of the ventrolateral medulla, and the paraventricular and supraoptic nuclei. (Fig. 14.5) [12]. An acute reduction in blood pressure increases plasma vasopressin by an amount that is roughly proportional to the degree of hypotension

[12,19,26]. However, this stimulus–response relationship is exponential. Thus, small decreases of 5–10% usually have little effect whereas decreases of 20–30% increase plasma vasopressin to levels many times those required to produce maximum antidiuresis. The vasopressin response to changes in blood volume appears to be quantitatively and qualitatively similar to the response to blood pressure [12,19,26].

Changes in blood volume or pressure large enough to affect vasopressin secretion do not necessarily interfere with osmoregulation of the hormone. Instead, they appear simply to lower or raise the set of the osmoregulatory system, thereby increasing or decreasing the stimulatory effect of a given level of plasma osmolality [12,19,26]. Thus, the capacity to osmoregulate vasopressin is preserved and the hormone can still be fully suppressed if the effective osmotic pressure of body fluids falls below the new, lower set point. This interaction indicates that the osmoregulatory and baroregulatory systems, though different in location and function, ultimately converge and act on the same population of neurosecretory neurones [26].

The baroregulation of vasopressin secretion in infants and children has not been investigated. However, it too is probably fully developed and functional from birth, because the receptors and peripheral neural efferents that mediate the baroregulation of sympathetic activity and the renin–angiotensin system are functional and these efferents are similar if not identical to those that mediate vasopressin release.

Nausea is an extremely potent stimulus for vasopressin secretion in humans [12]. The pathways that mediate this effect have not been defined, but they probably involve the chemoreceptor trigger zone in the area postrema of the medulla (Fig. 14.5). It can be activated by a variety of drugs, including apomorphine, morphine, nicotine, alcohol, and conditions such as motion sickness. Its effect on vasopressin is instantaneous and extremely potent. Increases of 100–1000 times basal levels are not unusual, even when the nausea is transient and unaccompanied by vomiting or changes in blood pressure. Pretreatment with fluphenazine, haloperidol or promethazine in doses sufficient to prevent nausea completely abolishes the vasopressin response. This inhibition is specific for emetic stimuli, for it does not affect the vasopressin response to osmotic or haemodynamic stimuli. Water loading blunts but does not abolish the effect of nausea on vasopressin release, suggesting that osmotic and emetic influences interact in a manner similar to the interaction of osmotic and haemodynamic pathways.

The effect of nausea on vasopressin secretion in healthy infants and children has not been investigated. However, it is probably similar to that in adults because application of an emetic stimulus (ipecac) in children with a selective deficiency in osmoregulation elicits a marked rise in vasopressin that is quantitatively indistinguishable from that in adults (see 'Adipsic hypernatraemia').

Other non-osmotic stimuli for vasopressin release include acute hypoglycaemia, acute hypoxia and hypercapnia, as well as many drugs and hormones. Most of the drug effects are probably mediated via haemodynamic or emetic stimuli. The renin–angiotensin system has also been implicated in animals, but it is questionable whether it has any significant effect in humans. The secretion of vasopressin may also be autoregulated by a direct feedback effect of the hormone on the neurohypophysis. Non-specific stress caused by factors such as pain, emotion and physical exercise has long been thought to cause the release of vasopressin, but this effect is probably secondary to induction of another stimulus, such as the hypotension and/or nausea that usually accompanies stress-induced vasovagal reactions. In rats and adult humans, a variety of noxious stimuli capable of activating the pituitary–adrenal axis and sympathetic nervous system do not stimulate vasopressin secretion unless they also lower blood pressure or alter blood volume [12,19].

The effect of these other non-osmotic influences on vasopressin secretion in healthy infants and children has not been determined. However, like the osmotic and other non-osmotic influences, it is probably similar to that in adults.

## Distribution and clearance

The concentration of vasopressin in plasma is determined by the difference between its rates of production and removal from the vascular compartment. In healthy adults, vasopressin distributes rapidly into a space roughly equivalent in size to the extracellular compartment [12,19]. This initial, or 'mixing', phase has a half-life of 4–8 min and is virtually complete in 10–15 min. The rapid mixing phase is followed by a second, slower decline, which probably corresponds to the metabolic, or irreversible, phase of clearance. Studies with one immunoassay yielded mean values of 10–20 min by both steady-state and non-steady-state techniques [12,19]. Most metabolism probably occurs in the liver and kidney. The distribution and clearance of vasopressin in healthy infants and children has not been timed, but it is probably faster than in adults because cardiac output is also greater relative to their body weight and surface area.

Some vasopressin is excreted intact in the urine, but the amounts are quite small relative to the total metabolic clearance. In healthy, normally hydrated adults, the urinary clearance of vasopressin ranges from 0.1 to 0.6 mL per kilogram of body weight per minute under basal conditions and has never been found to exceed 2 mL per kilogram of body weight per minute, even in the presence of a solute diuresis [12,19]. The mechanisms involved in the excretion of vasopressin have not been defined with certainty, but the hormone is probably filtered at the glomerulus and variably reabsorbed at one or more sites along the tubule. The latter process may be linked in some way to the handling of sodium in the proximal nephron, because the urinary clearance of vasopressin varies as much as 20-fold in direct relation to solute clearance [12,19]. Consequently, measurements of vasopressin excretion do not provide a consistently reliable index of changes in plasma vasopressin and must be interpreted cautiously when glomerular filtration and/or solute clearance are inconstant or abnormal.

The urinary clearance of vasopressin in healthy infants and children has not been determined. However, it may be even lower than in adults, for the rate of glomerular filtration and sodium excretion are also much lower at birth and do not reach normal adult levels until 1–2 years of age [12].

## Biological actions

The most important if not the only significant action of vasopressin in humans is to conserve body water by reducing the rate of urine output. This antidiuretic effect is achieved by promoting the reabsorption of solute-free water in the distal and/or collecting tubules of the kidney [12]. In the absence of vasopressin, the luminal surfaces of the cells lining this portion of the nephron are largely impermeable to water and solutes. Hence, the relatively large volume of dilute tubular fluid issuing from the more proximal nephron passes unmodified as urine. In this condition, which is referred to as *water diuresis*, the urine is maximally dilute (osmolality less than 100 mosmol/kg) and the rate of urine flow approximates 0.1–0.2 mL/kg/min, depending on the rate of solute excretion. In the presence of vasopressin, water can penetrate the luminal surface of the principal cells in the distal and collecting tubules and passively back-diffuse down the osmotic gradient that normally exists between tubular fluid and the isotonic or hypertonic milieu of the renal cortex and medulla. Because water is reabsorbed without solute, the tubular fluid that remains to be excreted as urine is not only smaller in volume but also more concentrated. The magnitude of this antidiuretic effect varies as a direct function of the plasma vasopressin concentration (Fig. 14.8). The sensitivity of this relationship differs appreciably among healthy adults but, on average, an increase in plasma vasopressin of 0.5 pg/mL raises urine osmolality by 150–250 mosmol/kg. The effect of this change on the rate of urine flow varies as an inverse curvilinear function of urine osmolality and also depends on the solute load (Fig. 14.2). Thus, it is greatest during a water diuresis and smallest when the urine is already concentrated. The maximum antidiuresis is usually achieved at a plasma vasopressin concentration between 2 and 5 pg/mL. In adults excreting normal amounts of solute (10–20 mosmol/kg/day) this usually results in a maximum urine osmolality of approximately 1200 mosmol/kg and a minimum obligatory urine flow of about 10 mL/kg/day. If renal function is normal, urine flow can be reduced below this rate only by decreasing the solute load.

The cellular mechanism by which vasopressin increases the hydro-osmotic permeability of the distal nephron has now been elucidated [27]. It results from the insertion of water channels into the luminal surface of the principal cells that line the distal and collecting tubules. These water channels are formed by oligomers of a 29-kDa protein known as aquaporin 2. The gene that encodes aquaporin 2 in humans has been cloned and sequenced and localized to chromosome 12q13. It is expressed largely if not exclusively in the distal nephron. In the absence of vasopressin, the rate of production of aquaporin 2 decreases and most of it is stored in intracellular vesicles. In the presence of vasopressin, these vesicles move rapidly to the luminal surface and fuse with the membrane, thereby increasing the hydro-osmotic permeability of the cell. More prolonged stimulation by vasopressin also increases the production of aquaporin 2, which over the course of several hours further enhances urinary concentrating capacity.

The actions of vasopressin on aquaporin function and water permeability in the distal nephron are mediated by receptors on the serosal surface of principal cells in tubular epithelia [28]. These receptors have been designated V2 to distinguish them from those which mediate the putative extrarenal actions of vasopressin (see below). The gene encoding the V2 receptor has been cloned and sequenced and mapped to the distal long arm of the X chromosome. The receptor has a seven-transmembrane topography characteristic of G-protein-coupled receptors and uses cAMP (cyclic adenosine monophosphate) as a second messenger. Nonpeptides capable of competitively antagonizing the antidiuretic effect of vasopressin at V2 receptors have been developed and are undergoing testing for use in the treatment of patients with the syndrome of inappropriate antidiuresis (SIAD) and other disorders associated with excessive retention of free water (see 'Syndrome of inappropriate antidiuresis').

The effect of vasopressin on urine concentration in healthy infants and children has been studied more thoroughly than any other aspect of antidiuretic function. At birth, the capacity to dilute the urine is normal or even supranormal compared with adults, for osmolalities as low as 30–40 mosmol/kg can be achieved after a water load. However, the capacity to mount a maximum water diuresis is substantially reduced owing most probably to immaturity of the kidneys and the lower rate of glomerular filtration and sodium excretion [10]. Thus, newborns are unusually susceptible to water intoxication if given excessive amounts of fluid. On the other hand, they are unable to concentrate their urine much above 300 mosmol/kg (Fig. 14.4). The reason for this blunting of maximum concentrating capacity has not been determined but could be due to incomplete expression of V2 receptors, a deficiency of aquaporin 2 or decreased hypertonicity in the renal medulla due to a dietary lack of a urea-forming protein. Whatever the mechanism, the defect is not of much physiological consequence because it does not greatly impair the ability to conserve water (Fig. 14.2) and improves relatively quickly in the first few weeks after birth (Fig. 14.4). Thus, the relationship of urine osmolality to plasma vasopressin concentration in healthy infants and children differs only slightly from that in adults (Fig. 14.8).

Vasopressin may also inhibit water loss from skin and lungs. However, this extrarenal effect is easily overridden by other factors such as an increase in ambient temperature or physical activity, which, in adults, can raise insensible loss to more than 200 mL/kg/day [8]. Other extrarenal effects attributed to vasopressin include contraction or relaxation of smooth muscle in the gastrointestinal tract and arterioles, potentiation of ACTH (adrenocorticotrophic hormone) release, inhibition of pancreatic flow, stimulation of hepatic glycogenolysis, aggregation of platelets, and inhibition of stress-induced hyperthermia. These effects have been demonstrated only at supraphysiological concentrations of vasopressin and appear to be mediated by different receptors, designated $V1_A$ and $V1_B$, which are encoded by different genes [28], expressed in many tissues including arteries, liver and brain and coupled to phospholipase C instead of adenyl cyclase. It is not known if they play any significant role in human physiology or pathophysiology. Humans are resistant to the hypertensive effects of vasopressin and non-peptides that competitively antagonize the actions of vasopressin at $V1_A$ receptors do not reduce systemic arterial pressure in hypertensive or dehydrated adults.

## Thirst

Because the urinary and insensible loss of water cannot be reduced below a certain minimum level, some mechanism to ensure adequate replacement of these obligatory losses is essential to prevent dehydration. This indispensable role is fulfilled by the thirst mechanism [29]. When used in a physiological sense, *thirst* is defined as a conscious, inner sensation of a need or desire to drink. It may be accompanied by but is not synonymous with other sensations, such as dry mouth, that can result from anxiety, hyperpnoea or other variables unrelated to hydration status. Thirst also should be distinguished from other causes of drinking such as enjoyment of the flavour or stimulant effect of a beverage, hunger when nutrients can be ingested only in liquid form (e.g. in infants) or the currently fashionable beliefs in the therapeutic value of a high fluid intake. These incidental, non-dipsetic stimuli to drink often suffice to replace urinary and insensible losses for long periods. Sooner or later, however, the relatively fixed amounts of water that they provide fail to match accelerated losses caused by changes in diet, temperature or physical activity. When this occurs, the thirst mechanism comes into play to prevent dehydration.

## Dipsogenesis

As might be expected, thirst is stimulated by many of the same variables and afferent pathways that cause the release

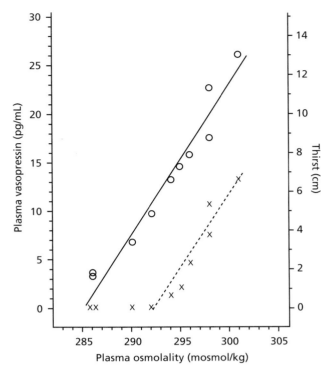

**Fig. 14.9.** The relationship of plasma vasopressin (O) and thirst (X) to plasma osmolality during hypertonic saline infusion in a healthy adult.

of vasopressin [29–32]. Of these, the most potent is a rise in effective plasma osmolality. It is mediated by osmoreceptors that also appear to be located in the anterior hypothalamus, near but not totally coincident with those that regulate vasopressin secretion [33]. Their functional properties differ only in that the osmotic threshold for thirst appears to be 'set' slightly higher than that for vasopressin release (Fig. 14.9). Normally, therefore, thirst begins when the effective osmotic pressure of plasma rises 1–2% above basal levels. Thereafter, it continues to increase in direct proportion to the level of hyperosmolality. This response is not dependent on a reduction in extracellular volume, as it is similar during the infusion of hypertonic saline and water deprivation. If potable water is freely available, the development of thirst stimulates an increase in intake [30], which serves to expand and dilute body fluids, thereby restoring plasma osmolality to normal. This mechanism is normally so effective that it prevents appreciable hypertonic dehydration even if urinary loss is markedly increased by a deficiency of vasopressin secretion or action (see 'Diabetes insipidus'). Basal water intake is also reduced by a fall in plasma osmolality of 1–2%, suggesting that there may also be an osmoregulated 'satiety' mechanism that helps to prevent overhydration when the capacity to mount a maximum water diuresis is impaired [32].

Hypovolaemia and/or hypotension are also dipsogenic. The degree of hypovolaemia and/or hypotension required to produce thirst in humans has not been defined but appears to be even greater than that needed to effect vasopressin release. The afferent pathways that mediate the haemodynamic influences on thirst have not been defined but are probably similar to those that mediate the baroregulation of vasopressin [34]. Haemodynamic stimuli also reset the osmotic threshold for thirst as they do for vasopressin.

The regulation of thirst in healthy infants and children has not been investigated. However, the osmoregulatory component at least is probably functional at birth because newborns with very high rates of urinary loss due to congenital nephrogenic diabetes insipidus exhibit a craving for water and will maintain relatively normal hydration if given sufficient amounts to drink. Their problem is that they have not yet developed the motor or verbal skills required to get the additional water themselves or make their needs clear to others. This handicap limits their ability to cope with disorders of water balance and necessitates special vigilance and skill on the part of parents and others responsible for their care.

## Disorders of water balance

### Deficiencies in vasopressin

#### Diabetes insipidus

Global deficiencies in vasopressin secretion or action result in diabetes insipidus (DI), a syndrome characterized by chronic excretion of abnormally large volumes of dilute urine. In adults and older children, the 24-h urine volume typically exceeds 50 mL/kg. In infants and young children, the upper limit of normal varies with age and ranges from more than 130 mL/kg at birth to 80 mL/kg at 2 years of age (Fig. 14.3). In all age groups, the osmolality of the 24-h urine collection is less than 300 mosmol/kg and the rate of fluid intake is increased commensurate with urine output. The signs and symptoms of DI are primarily urinary frequency, nocturia in adults and persistent enuresis or delayed toilet training in children. DI should be differentiated from other causes of urinary frequency. These include a reduced bladder capacity and diabetes mellitus or other forms of solute diuresis in which urine output is increased. These distinctions can usually be made quite easily by means of a voiding diary, tests for urinary glucose and estimates of 24-h urinary solute excretion. The last one, determined as the product of a 24-h urine volume and osmolality, is normally less than 20 mosmol/kg in adults but may be higher in infants and young children. DI can be subdivided into four basic types based on the cause of the antidiuretic defect.

*Pituitary diabetes insipidus*
The most common type of DI is caused by a primary deficiency of vasopressin secretion. It is referred to by a variety of names, including neurogenic, neurohypophyseal, pituitary, hypothalamic, central, cranial or vasopressin-responsive DI. It is almost always due to a deficiency of vasopressin-producing neurohypophyseal neurones caused by some genetic, developmental or acquired disorder (Table 14.3) [35–37]. Consequently, the hyperintense magnetic resonance signal usually emitted by the normal posterior pituitary is almost invariably absent [38,39]. In patients with some of the developmental or acquired forms of pituitary DI, magnetic resonance imaging (MRI) may also reveal other abnormalities such as a congenital malformation of the forebrain [40], a primary or metastatic tumour in the suprasellar region [41] or thickening of the pituitary stalk and/or basal meninges, which is commonly seen with histiocytosis and other granulomatous or chronic infectious diseases [42,43].

There are several forms of genetic or familial pituitary DI. The most common one is inherited in an autosomal dominant mode with virtually complete penetrance [44,45]. In these patients, the deficiency of vasopressin develops several months to several years after birth and usually increases in severity throughout childhood but is rarely if ever complete. The loss of vasopressin secretion appears to be due to selective, postnatal degeneration of the vasopressin-producing neurones, for autopsy studies show gliosis and a marked deficiency of magnicellular neurosecretory neurones in the supraoptic and, to a lesser extent, paraventricular nuclei of the hypothalamus. For unknown reasons, the DI remits spontaneously in some adults despite a continuing severe deficiency of vasopressin. Patients with the autosomal dominant form of familial pituitary DI invariably have a mutation in one allele of the gene that encodes the vasopressin–neurophysin II precursor (Fig. 14.10). The mutations differ widely in type and location and have been found in every area of the coding region except the part of the third exon that encodes the copeptin moiety. However, all of them are expected to alter one or more amino acids known or presumed to be crucial for removing the signal peptide and/or correctly folding the prohormone in the endoplasmic reticulum (ER). This pattern, as well as the clinical and autopsy evidence of progressive degeneration of vasopressin-producing neurones, suggests that the mutant alleles are cytotoxic because they direct the production of an abnormal precursor that cannot be folded and routed properly from the ER [44]. Expression studies *in vitro* support this hypothesis.

An autosomal recessive form of familial pituitary DI has also been reported recently [46]. In this family, three children of asymptomatic, consanguinous parents have pituitary DI. They were found to be homozygous for a single novel vasopressin–neurophysin II gene mutation that predicted the substitution of leucine for proline at position 7 in the vasopressin moiety. Their plasma appeared to contain high levels of immunoactive 7-leucine vasopressin, which bound poorly to V2 receptors *in vitro*. Presumably therefore their

**Table 14.3.** Causes of diabetes insipidus

*Pituitary*
Genetic
    Autosomal dominant (vasopressin–neurophysin gene)
    Autosomal recessive (vasopressin–neurophysin gene)
    Autosomal recessive – Wolfram syndrome – (chromosome 4p – *WFS 1* gene)
    X-linked recessive (chromosome Xq28)
Congenital malformations
    Midline craniofacial defects
    Holoprosencephaly
    Hypogensis of pituitary
Acquired
    Trauma – closed, penetrating
    Neoplasms – craniopharyngioma, dysgerminoma, meningioma, lymphoma, leukaemia
    Granulomas – neurosarcoid, histiocytosis, xanthoma disseminatum
    Infection – meningitis, encephalitis, toxoplasmosis
    Inflammatory – lymphocytic infundibuloneurohypophysitis
    Vascular – aneurysm (cavernous sinus)
    Hypoxic encephalopathy
    Idiopathic

*Nephrogenic*
Genetic
    X-linked recessive (vasopressin receptor-2 gene)
    Autosomal recessive (aquaporin 2 gene)
    Autosomal dominant (aquaporin 2 gene)
Acquired
    Drugs – lithium, demeclocycline, cisplatin, rifampin, foscarnet
    Metabolic – hypercalciuria, hypokalaemia
    Vascular – sickle cell disease and trait
    Granulomas – neurosarcoid
    Idiopathic

*Primary polydipsia*
Acquired
    Iatrogenic
    Psychogenic (schizophrenia, obsessive–compulsive disorder)
    Dipsogenic (abnormal thirst)
        Granulomas – neurosarcoid
        Infectious – tuberculous meningitis
        Head trauma – closed, penetrating
        Demyelinization – multiple sclerosis
        Drugs – lithium
        Idiopathic

DI is due to the production of a biologically inactive form of vasopressin rather than to the destruction of their neurophypophysis.

An X-linked, recessive form of familial pituitary DI has also been discovered recently [47]. In this kindred, obligate female carriers are completely unaffected, but males develop DI and a partial deficiency of vasopressin at or shortly after birth. These abnormalities can progress in severity with time and are associated with a very small or absent pituitary bright spot on MRI. Oxytocin production appears to be normal. The gene responsible for this form of familial pituitary DI has not been identified but has been traced to the Xq28 region.

The genes encoding the V2 receptor and vasopressin–neurophysin II are normal.

Other genetic defects can also cause pituitary DI as part of a constellation of other abnormalities. Wolfram syndrome, an autosomal recessive, neurodegenerative disorder that sometimes results in pituitary DI as well as diabetes mellitus, optic atrophy, deafness, and other abnormalities (DIDMOAD) [48] has now been linked to mutation of a novel chromosome 4p gene that encodes a putative transmembrane protein [49]. The mechanism by which this mutation causes the disease is unknown, but it appears to result in degeneration of vasopressin producing magnocellular neurones in the supraoptic

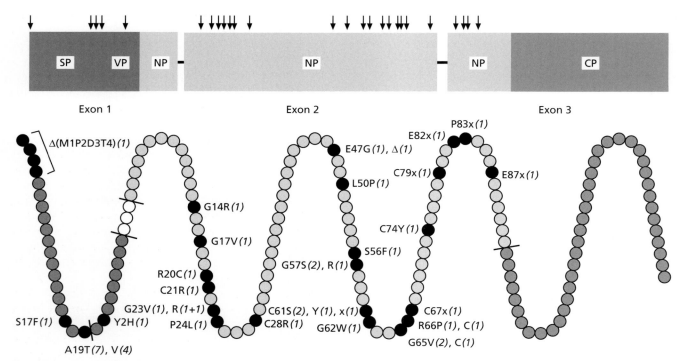

**Fig. 14.10.** Location and type of mutations in the vasopressin–neurophysin gene (top) and protein precursor in patients with the autosomal dominant form of familial pituitary diabetes insipidus. The amino acid changes predicted for the precursor are indicated by standard one-letter abbreviations placed before and after a number that refers to the position of the original residue in a particular part of the precursor. Deletions are indicated by 'Δ' and premature truncations by 'x'. The number in brackets after this code indicates the number of apparently unrelated families in which the mutation has been identified. Thus, the code A19T(7) at the bottom of the first bend in the precursor indicates that replacement of alanine (A) with threonine (T) at position 19 in the signal peptide has been found in seven families to date. Similarly, E47Δ(1) indicates the glutamic acid normally present at position 47 in neurophysin has been deleted in one family. Adapted from [12].

nucleus [50] and partial to severe deficiencies of vasopressin secretion in response to non-osmotic as well as osmotic stimuli [51]. Pituitary DI can also occur in familial congenital hypopituitarism, familial cerebellar ataxia, and congenital midline craniofacial defects associated with deletion of chromosome 7q. The genetic mechanisms involved are unknown.

Idiopathic forms of pituitary DI account for about half of all cases in adults. Many of them probably represent the 'burned-out' stage of infundibuloneurohypophysitis, a necrotizing inflammatory disorder of possible infectious or autoimmune aetiology [52]. Idiopathic pituitary DI appears to be less common in infants and young children, but it too may be due to neurohypophysitis [53,54] or an early stage of a germinoma [41] or histiocytosis [42,43].

It is important to note that the deficiency of vasopressin need not be complete for DI to occur [55]. It is necessary only that the level of plasma vasopressin required to concentrate the urine cannot be achieved at levels of plasma osmolality/ sodium below those that stimulate thirst and polydipsia. The extent to which secretory capacity must be reduced to produce this deficiency varies because of relatively large individual or situational differences in vasopressin metabolism, secretory reserve and the set of the osmoregulatory system.

However, studies of cell loss in the supraoptic nuclei after pituitary surgery [56], functional tests of vasopressin secretion in a large number of patients with diabetes insipidus of variable severity and aetiology [55] and theoretical considerations [57] all indicate that DI does not develop unless secretory capacity is reduced by more than 75%. Thus, there are probably many patients with lesser deficiencies of vasopressin who do not develop symptomatic DI unless metabolism of the hormone is increased or some inhibitory influence is imposed.

Recognition of the fact that many patients with pituitary DI retain a limited capacity to secrete vasopressin is the key to understanding many otherwise perplexing features of the disorder. For example, restricting water intake for only a few hours will often stimulate the remaining neurohypophyseal neurones to release enough hormone to concentrate the urine (Fig. 14.11) [55]. This response illustrates the relative nature of the vasopressin deficiency and shows that it is the compensatory increase in thirst and fluid intake that prevents these patients from using whatever residual secretory capacity they may have. Even when the vasopressin deficiency is so severe that fluid deprivation produces little or no increase in urine osmolality, a potent non-osmotic stimulus such as

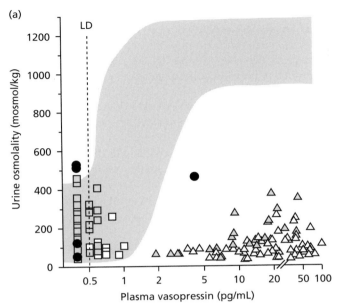

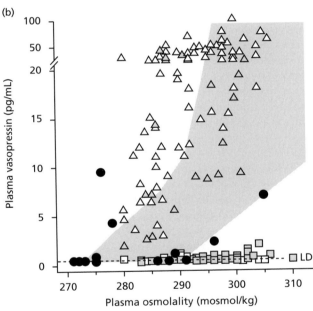

**Fig. 14.11.** Relationship of plasma vasopressin to urine (a) and plasma (b) osmolality before and during fluid deprivation/hypertonic saline infusion tests in infants and children with various types of diabetes insipidus (DI). The shaded areas represent the range of values in healthy infants and children. The values obtained in patients are shown by open and shaded squares (severe or partial pituitary DI, $n = 16$), open or shaded triangles (severe or partial nephrogenic DI, $n = 15$) and closed circles (primary polydipsia, $n = 2$).

Pituitary DI also alters the acute effect of vasopressin on urinary concentration. The most obvious change is a reduction in maximum concentrating capacity [55], which probably results from washout of the medullary concentration gradient and/or suppression of aquaporin 2 production. The severity of this defect is proportional to the severity of the basal polyuria and is independent of its cause [55]. Because of it, the level of urinary concentration produced initially by an acute increase in plasma vasopressin is usually subnormal. However, this blunting of maximum concentrating capacity is temporary and will repair within 24–48 h if the antidiuresis is sustained. Moreover, in patients with pituitary DI, the defect in maximum concentrating capacity is partly offset by enhanced sensitivity to the antidiuretic effect of very low levels of plasma vasopressin (Fig. 14.11). The cause of this apparent supersensitivity is unknown, but may be upward regulation of vasopressin receptors secondary to a chronic deficiency of the hormone.

Adults with pituitary DI are also reported to have decreased bone mineral density and serum osteocalcin that is not affected by treatment of the DI with DDAVP [58]. However, there is no evidence that they have an increased incidence of bone fractures or other symptoms of osteopenia. Pituitary DI *per se* is not associated with any obvious abnormalities in baroregulation, pituitary adrenal function, clotting or other physiological functions linked to V1 receptors. However, some of the diseases that cause DI can also damage one or more of these other systems. The osmoregulation of thirst is also normal in more than 90% of patients with pituitary DI but a few, most notably those with a history of head trauma, hypothalamo-pituitary surgery or a suprasellar malignancy, have either hypodipsia or hyperdipsia apparently due to associated damage to the osmoregulatory system. When present, these defects in thirst greatly complicate the management of DI (see below).

*Primary polydipsia*

DI can also result from a deficiency of vasopressin secretion that is secondary to excessive intake of water. This condition is usually referred to as primary polydipsia and can be subdivided into three types depending on the cause of the excessive fluid intake (Table 14.3). One type appears to be due to a primary defect in the osmoregulation of thirst and has been referred to as dipsogenic DI [59]. It may result from multifocal diseases involving the hypothalamus (e.g. neurosarcoid, tuberculous meningitis and multiple sclerosis) but is usually idiopathic. The exact location of the lesions responsible for the abnormal thirst has not been determined, but hyperdipsia can be produced experimentally in rats by lesioning the midbrain, septal nuclei and nucleus medianus. The second type of primary polydipsia is due to a more general cognitive defect associated with schizophrenia or other psychiatric disorders [60,61]. It is usually referred to as psychogenic polydipsia or compulsive water drinking. With rare exception,

nausea or a vasovagal reaction may release enough hormone to concentrate the urine. Consequently, when interpreting diagnostic or therapeutic procedures in these patients, it is necessary to be circumspect about the presence of drugs or associated diseases that can modify vasopressin secretion via non-osmotic mechanisms.

these patients do not complain of thirst and usually attribute their polydipsia to bizarre personal motives, such as a need to cleanse their system of poison. The third type of primary polydipsia is not associated with either increased thirst or overt mental illness but is prompted by the advice of physicians, nurses, folk practitioners or the lay media. It may be referred to as iatrogenic polydipsia. All three forms of primary polydipsia appear to be relatively uncommon in infants or young children and the psychogenic form occurs very rarely if at all.

The pathogenesis and pathophysiology of primary polydipsia is the opposite of the other forms of DI. Thus, excessive intake of water slightly reduces the effective osmotic pressure of body fluids, thereby inhibiting the secretion of vasopressin. This results in a water diuresis that compensates completely for the increased intake and stabilizes the osmolality of body fluids at a new, slightly lower level approximating the osmotic threshold for vasopressin secretion. The magnitude of the DI varies from patient to patient depending on the nature and/or intensity of the stimulus to drink. In those with dipsogenic DI, the osmotic threshold for thirst appears to be reset below that for vasopressin secretion [59]. Polydipsia reduces but does not completely relieve the desire to drink, as the resultant suppression of vasopressin produces a water diuresis that prevents the dilution of body water to the abnormally low level required to osmotically inhibit thirst. Thus, thirst, polydipsia and polyuria persist. In psychogenic polydipsia, the stimulus to drink is not driven by thirst. However, it may vary with the emotional state of the patient and, in adults, may exceed 20 L/day. Iatrogenic polydipsia is usually mild and rarely results in urine outputs of more than 5 L/day.

Primary polydipsia rarely results in water intoxication unless the capacity to dilute the urine and/or mount a maximum water diuresis is also impaired. In patients with the dipsogenic form, this impairment usually results from inappropriate administration of DDAVP but can also be caused by an increase in vasopressin secretion triggered by an acute non-osmotic stimulus such as nausea. In psychogenic polydipsia, water intoxication is much more frequent, occasionally fatal, and is usually due to inappropriate secretion of vasopressin that can take any of several forms, including downward resetting of the osmostat [61] (see 'Syndrome of inappropriate antidiuresis).

*Nephrogenic diabetes insipidus*

A primary defect in the antidiuretic action of vasopressin results in a syndrome commonly referred to as *nephrogenic diabetes insipidus*. It was first recognized as a familial disorder that was inherited in an X-linked recessive or semirecessive mode [62]. This form has now been linked to more than 150 different mutations of the gene on chromosome Xq28 that encodes the renal V2 receptor [63]. These mutations appear to impair V2 receptor function in a variety of ways including deficient

synthesis, misfolding and misrouting from the ER, increased degradation, decreased binding affinity for vasopressin and inefficient linkage to the second messenger. Recently, another form of familial nephrogenic DI, which is inherited in an autosomal recessive or autosomal dominant mode, has been discovered and linked to more than 15 different mutations in one or both alleles of the gene that encodes aquaporin 2 [64,65], the protein that forms the hydro-osmotic water channels activated by vasopressin in renal collecting tubules. In both forms of familial nephrogenic DI, the disease is present from birth. In the X-linked type, males who inherit the mutation are always affected and female carriers usually are not. Most of these mutations largely or completely abolish the antidiuretic effect of vasopressin, but a few affecting the V2 receptor result in partial resistance [66] that is characterized by a 10-fold or greater shift to the right in the dose–response curve (Fig. 14.11). As a result, many of them are able to concentrate their urine during a fluid deprivation test. Severe or partial nephrogenic DI can also be acquired as a result of other diseases or drugs (Table 14.3), the most notable of which is lithium. Drug-induced and other acquired forms of nephrogenic DI appear to be relatively uncommon in infants and children, who usually have one of the familial types.

The pathophysiology of nephrogenic DI is similar in most respects to pituitary DI. Thus, insensitivity to the antidiuretic effect of vasopressin also results in the excretion of increased volumes of dilute urine. This loss causes a decrease in body water and a slight rise in plasma osmolality, which, by stimulating the thirst mechanism, induces a compensatory increase in water intake. As a consequence, the osmolality of body fluid stabilizes at a new and higher level that approximates the osmotic threshold for thirst. Hypertonic dehydration does not occur unless fluid intake is somehow impaired. The only difference with pituitary DI is that plasma vasopressin is elevated under basal conditions as well as during a fluid deprivation test. For unknown reasons, this elevation is out of proportion to the relatively modest increase in plasma osmolality that is present (Fig. 14.11). The additional large increases in plasma vasopressin that occur during fluid deprivation may be sufficient to concentrate the urine in patients with partial resistance to the hormone (Fig. 14.11). Thus, their DI may temporarily cease if they become dehydrated as a result of fevers, vomiting, coma or other impediments to fluid intake. These disturbances are relatively common in infants and young children, and they may delay recognition of the DI in those with partial defects in vasopressin action or secretion. Unrecognized episodes of dehydration may also be responsible for the increased incidence of mental retardation in this disease. Children with untreated nephrogenic DI may also grow more slowly than normal, possibly because their thirst and polydipsia interferes with adequate intake of calories. Patients with mutations of the V2 receptor gene also lack the normal vasodepressor and coagulation factor response to DDAVP but these defects do not result in clinically appreciable defects in baroregulation or haemostasis.

*Differential diagnosis*

When DI is suspected, the diagnosis should be verified by determining the volume, osmolality and creatinine content of urine collected for 24 h under conditions of *ad libitum* fluid intake. If the patient is not toilet trained or has another condition that makes it difficult to accurately collect urine, the measurement of *ad libitum* fluid intake may be an acceptable substitute. In either case, the results should be interpreted from age-adjusted normal values (Fig. 14.3). Measuring the osmolality or specific gravity of a random urine sample is less reliable because it can give a false-negative result in a patient with partial pituitary or partial nephrogenic DI. Measurements of basal plasma osmolality or sodium under conditions of *ad libitum* fluid intake are rarely useful for diagnosing DI because they are usually within the normal range. However, they should be obtained as an elevated value serves to identify the occasional patient with associated hypodipsia who does not need and may be harmed by a fluid deprivation test.

If tests of the 24-h urine are normal, further evaluation for DI is not needed unless there is reason to suspect that it is being masked by a concomitant disease such as adrenal insufficiency or adipsic hypernatraemia (see 'Adipsic hypernatraemia' below). In that case, the tests of a 24-h urine collection should be repeated after the associated deficiency of cortisol or water is corrected.

If the 24-h urine collection confirms the presence of DI and the basal plasma osmolality and sodium are within normal limits, a fluid deprivation test should be performed. Because patients with a severe defect in the secretion or action of vasopressin can become significantly dehydrated in only a few hours, fluid deprivation should be performed during the day without prior restriction of eating or drinking and should be monitored closely, with hourly measurements of body weight, plasma osmolality or sodium, urine output and urine osmolality.

If fluid restriction does not result in concentration of the urine (osmolality > 300 mosmol/kg) before plasma osmolality and/or sodium reach 300 mosmol/kg and/or 146 mequiv/L, primary polydipsia, as well as partial defects in vasopressin secretion or action, are virtually excluded. The distinction between severe pituitary and severe nephrogenic DI usually can be made just by injecting 1–2 units of aqueous Pitressin or 1–2 μg of DDAVP and repeating the measurements of urine osmolality 1–2 h later. In this setting, a rise in urine osmolality of more than 50% is virtually diagnostic of severe pituitary (or gestational) DI, even though the maximum levels achieved may be markedly subnormal because of the temporary defect in renal concentrating capacity caused by the chronic polyuria *per se* [55]. Conversely, a rise in urine osmolality of less than 50% usually indicates severe

nephrogenic DI [55,67]. This criterion has a diagnostic accuracy of about 90%. However, it misdiagnoses about 10% of patients with severe pituitary DI because their secondary blunting of renal concentrating capacity is so severe that they cannot respond to DDAVP until sufficient time has elapsed to increase their renal medullary hypertonicity and aquaporin production. Because repair seems to begin within an hour or two of hormone treatment, the risk of misdiagnosis can be reduced by repeating the measurements of urine osmolality at 3–4 h and applying the same percentage criteria.

However, if fluid deprivation results in concentration of the urine, indirect criteria are unreliable for differentiating between primary polydipsia and a partial deficiency in vasopressin secretion or action [55,67]. The reason probably is that the secondary defect in renal concentrating capacity caused by the chronic polyuria starts to improve almost as soon as urinary concentration begins. Consequently, any further rise in urine osmolality that occurs after the administration of exogenous vasopressin or DDAVP can be due in whole or in part to continued improvement in the secondary defect rather than to correction of a primary deficiency in vasopressin secretion or action. The simplest and most effective way to avoid this problem is to directly measure vasopressin in aliquots of plasma and/or urine collected before and during the fluid deprivation test [55,67]. If the basal plasma vasopressin level is elevated (> 2 pg/mL), the patient probably has partial nephrogenic DI. However, if basal plasma vasopressin is suppressed (< 1 pg/mL), nephrogenic DI is unlikely and the hormonal response to osmotic stimulation can be used to differentiate between primary polydipsia and pituitary DI. To minimize diagnostic ambiguity, these vasopressin values should be analysed in relation to the concurrent plasma osmolality (Fig. 14.11) and at least one measurement should be made when the latter is above the normal range (> 295 mosmol/kg). This level of hypertonic dehydration is usually difficult to achieve by fluid restriction alone after urinary concentration begins. Therefore, it is usually necessary to give a supplemental infusion of hypertonic (3%) saline (0.1 mL/kg/min) to shorten the duration of the test. This infusion should be continued for 60–90 min or until plasma osmolality and/or sodium exceeds the upper limit of the normal range, at which point a final sample for measurement of vasopressin should be collected. With this approach, patients with partial pituitary DI can be differentiated easily from those with primary polydipsia or partial nephrogenic DI (Fig. 14.11). In most cases, the last two disorders can be distinguished by examining the relation of urine osmolality to the concurrent level of vasopressin before and during the fluid deprivation test (Fig. 14.1), although this interpretation may also be clouded by secondary defects in renal concentrating capacity.

As might be expected, most patients with pituitary DI also exhibit a subnormal rise in vasopressin secretion after haemodynamic, emetic and glucopenic stimuli. For

(a)

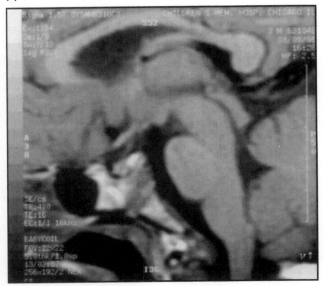

(b)

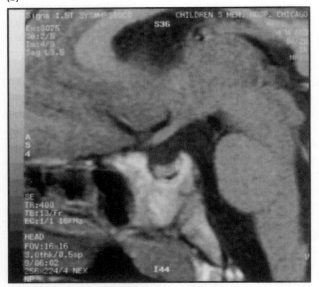

**Fig. 14.12.** Magnetic resonance image of the brain in pituitary DI. Both images are T₁ weighted and were obtained before infusion of gadolinium. (a) This is from a healthy 4-year-old boy and shows the hyperintense signal normally emitted by the posterior pituitary. (b) This is from a boy with the autosomal dominant form of familial pituitary DI and lacks the posterior pituitary bright spot.

diagnostic purposes, however, these non-osmotic tests of neurohypophyseal function do not appear to provide any particular advantage over dehydration/hypertonic saline infusion, and they are usually more stressful for the physician and the patient.

MRI of the brain is also useful in the differential diagnosis of DI [68]. In 80–90% of healthy children and adults, the posterior pituitary emits a hyperintense signal ('bright spot') on T₁ weighted, non-infused midsagittal images (Fig. 14.12). This bright spot is abnormally small or absent in most but possibly not all [69] patients with pituitary DI. This includes almost all patients with familial pituitary DI, even though their oxytocinergic neurones are apparently normal. In contrast, the pituitary bright spot is present in 80–90% of patients with primary polydipsia. Thus, MRI is very good for ruling out pituitary DI (if the bright spot is present) but is less reliable for ruling it in (if the bright spot is absent). When used as an aid in the differential diagnosis, MRI should always be performed with fat suppression techniques to avoid confusing fat in the marrow of the dorsum sella with the posterior pituitary bright spot. Fluid-filled cysts in the pars intermedia or posterior pituitary can also simulate the normal bright spot although they are usually rounder and less bean shaped. A false-positive result (absence of the bright spot) also may result if the images are more than 3 mm apart and none goes through or very near the midline of the brain.

The various types of DI can also be differentiated by their distinctive responses to a closely monitored therapeutic trial of DDAVP (see below) [67].

### Management

#### Pituitary diabetes insipidus

The treatment of choice for pituitary DI is a synthetic analogue of vasopressin known as DDAVP (desmopressin) (Fig. 14.6) [70]. The modifications in positions 1 and 8 of the molecule enhance its antidiuretic potency, eliminate its effects on V1 receptors, and increase significantly its resistance to metabolic degradation. Consequently, it has a much longer duration of action than the native molecule and can be given by parenteral, intranasal (i.n.) or oral routes. The most convenient mode of administration for chronic therapy is usually the nasal spray or tablet. The dose required to completely eliminate polyuria must be determined empirically but usually ranges from 10 to 20 μg i.n. or 100–400 μg by mouth every 8–12 h in older children and adults. The dose in infants and young children (< 3 years of age) is only slightly less owing, perhaps, to a relatively higher rate of metabolism of the drug. If administration by the intranasal or oral route is not possible or ineffective because of the age or condition of the child, DDAVP can also be given by injection (1–2 μg of DDAVP s.c. every 12–24 h).

The antidiuretic effect of parenteral, intranasal or oral DDAVP is usually evident within 60–120 min, although the maximum effect may not be achieved for 24–48 h owing to the transient blunting of the concentrating capacity caused by a chronic water diuresis. The antidiuresis is followed promptly by a 1–2% increase in body water and a similar small decrease in plasma osmolality and sodium, which immediately relieves the thirst and results in a commensurate reduction in *ad libitum* fluid intake. Consequently, the balance between water intake and output is quickly restored and plasma osmolality/sodium stabilize within the normal range.

In most adults and older children with pituitary DI, the DDAVP treatment can and should be continued indefinitely at doses that maintain the 24-h urine volume within the normal range. It is usually not necessary to allow periodic 'escape' from the antidiuretic effect because the thirst mechanism is normally so effective at down-regulating fluid intake to keep it in balance with output [30,32]. However, it is essential to educate these patients or their parents about the hazards of excessive fluid intake and the signs and symptoms of water intoxication. This should include an explanation of why fluid requirements vary from day to day and why they should be guided solely by thirst and not by any preset amount. They should also be equipped with a bracelet or wallet card indicating their diagnosis and treatment and instructed to have their plasma sodium checked periodically or any time that symptoms suggestive of water intoxication occur.

If DDAVP treatment results in hyponatraemia, it is not due to an excessive dose because the drug does not have a direct effect on plasma sodium and cannot reduce urine output below the level of water intake obligated by a standard diet. Rather, hyponatraemia is invariably due to excessive fluid intake that cannot be excreted because the level of antidiuresis produced by the drug cannot be reduced in response to the increase in hydration. The reason for the excessive fluid intake varies and usually can be determined from a careful interview. In most adults and older children, it can be traced to lack of understanding of and/or adherence to proscriptions against incidental, non-dipsetic drinking. This problem usually can be corrected by re-education or by limiting formula to the amounts required for nutrition and prohibiting the intake of juice, fizzy drinks and all other drinks except plain, unflavoured water. Sometimes, the excessive fluid intake is due to an exaggerated concern about the dangers of dehydration and can also be corrected by re-education. Occasionally, however, it is due to a defect in the osmotic suppression of thirst. If this appears to be present (i.e. if any degree of thirst persists despite the presence of hyponatraemia), the patient should be re-evaluated thoroughly to determine whether hyperdipsia is the sole cause of the DI or is associated with a primary deficiency in vasopressin secretion. This distinction is important because the approach to treatment of the two conditions should be different.

Erratic or decreased responses to intranasal or oral DDAVP usually result from poor absorption because of sinusitis, rhinitis or food. These problems can usually be alleviated by use of nasal decongestants or taking the tablets on an empty stomach. If not, it may be necessary to take DDAVP by injection or switch to another form of treatment. Resistance due to antibody production has not been observed with DDAVP.

The management of pituitary DI in infants, obtunded or postoperative patients differs slightly because their water intake may be determined partly or totally by factors other than thirst. The diet of infants and young children normally contains a relatively large amount of water obligating a commensurately higher urine output (Fig. 14.3). Therefore, their dose of DDAVP may need to be reduced to allow a mild or intermittent water diuresis. In addition, to prevent taste-induced drinking, the only non-dietary liquids allowed should be plain unflavoured water. In obtunded or postoperative patients, DDAVP should be infused or injected in doses sufficient to maintain urine output and osmolality within the age-adjusted normal range. Total fluid intake should be adjusted every 8 h to equal the sum of urine output plus an appropriate amount for insensible loss (4–12 mL/kg/day when body temperature is normal). If fluid intake cannot be restricted to the required level, the dose or frequency of DDAVP administration should be reduced sufficiently to allow periodic 'escape' in order to prevent water intoxication. The effectiveness of the regimen should be monitored by measuring plasma osmolality or sodium at least twice a day until fluid intake can be regulated solely by thirst or other measures of physiologic need.

In adults and adolescents, pituitary DI can also be treated with a variety of oral drugs, such as chlorpropamide, clofibrate, carbamazepine and chlorothiazide [70]. However, these treatments have more side-effects than DDAVP and they are probably best reserved for patients with unusual complications such as hyperdipsia or antibody-induced resistance to DDAVP.

The treatment of pituitary DI is usually lifelong, because recovery from a deficiency lasting more than a week is uncommon, even if the underlying cause is eliminated. In the few patients who appear to have a remission, it may not be due to a detectable improvement in vasopressin secretion [66]. It sometimes results from the development of a more serious problem, such as adrenal insufficiency, ectopic production of vasopressin by a malignancy or severe dehydration due to destruction of the thirst mechanism (see below). Therefore, tests to evaluate these possibilities should be undertaken in all patients who appear to have spontaneous remission of their DI.

The management of pituitary DI also requires a careful search for its cause (Table 14.3). At a minimum, this search should include radiographs of the chest and skull, visual field examination, and computerized tomography and/or MRI of the hypothalamo-pituitary area. If the initial MRI is unrevealing, it should be repeated every 6–12 months for several years because morphological evidence for an underlying cause such as dysgerminoma or histiocytosis may eventually emerge [41,71]. In some cases, a lumbar puncture may also be needed to identify a specific pathology, such as a dysgerminoma, which determines the choice of treatment. Because of the possible co-involvement of hypothalamic release factors, anterior pituitary function also should be evaluated even if there is no other evidence of intrasellar disease. In view of a recent report that adults with pituitary DI have osteopenia that is reversible with alendronate but not with DDAVP [58,72], bone densitometry may also be worthwhile.

*Primary polydipsia*

Iatrogenic and psychogenic polydipsia are rare in infants and children but they may occur in adolescents. The iatrogenic type should be addressed simply by education of the patient. The psychogenic type is refractory to the usual psychotropic drugs and other treatments. Management should be directed at preventing or recognizing and treating promptly the severe and occasionally fatal episodes of water intoxication to which these patients are prone. This includes the avoidance of smoking and all drugs and conditions capable of stimulating vasopressin secretion or otherwise impairing free water excretion. The abnormal thirst that causes dipsogenic DI also cannot be treated effectively at present. Fluid restriction reduces the polyuria, but it is usually difficult if not impossible to maintain because it almost invariably increases thirst. As would be expected, treatment with standard doses of DDAVP completely abolishes the polyuria in all forms of primary polydipsia. However, it is contraindicated in these patients because it has little or no effect on psychogenic polydipsia and only partially inhibits the thirst and polydipsia in patients with dipsogenic DI. Therefore, it invariably produces water intoxication [59]. This syndrome develops rapidly, usually within 24–48 h, and is characterized by varying levels of hyponatraemia as well as central nervous system symptoms and signs ranging from slight headache, dizziness and anorexia to nausea, vomiting, confusion, convulsions, coma and even death. Therefore, any time that DDAVP is used to diagnose or treat a patient in whom the dipsogenic or other forms of primary polydipsia cannot be excluded with certainty, the trial should be initiated in the hospital with close monitoring of fluid balance for the first 24–48 h. If hyponatraemia develops, the patient should be taken off treatment, started on complete fluid restriction and treated for acute SIAD (see below).

In most patients with dipsogenic DI, the nocturnal polyuria that is responsible for their nocturnal enuresis or nocturia can be treated safely with DDAVP. However, the drug must be given only at bedtime and the dose should be carefully titrated to ensure that its antidiuretic effect does not persist into the next day, when their polydipsia accelerates and water intoxication may develop. The patient should be warned against any other use of DDAVP, thiazide diuretics or other antidiuretic medications and should be informed of the potential hazards of nicotine and the many other drugs or illnesses that can stimulate release of endogenous vasopressin.

The management of dipsogenic DI should also include a search for the cause (Table 14.3) and possible associated defects in hypothalamic and anterior pituitary function. In addition to a history and a physical examination focused on other symptoms and signs, this search should include MRI of the brain and tests of baseline thyroid and adrenal function.

*Nephrogenic diabetes insipidus*

When caused by a metabolic disorder, such as hypercalcaemia or hypokalaemia, or a drug, such as amphotericin B, demeclocycline or lithium, nephrogenic DI can often be corrected if the cause is eliminated before secondary, irreversible renal damage occurs. However, if the DI has been present for more than 5 years or is genetic in origin, it can be reduced but not cured. In these patients, the polyuria, thirst and polydipsia can be decreased by 30–70% by reducing the urinary solute load (Fig. 14.2) and administering a thiazide diuretic [73], amiloride [74] and/or a prostaglandin synthetase inhibitor [75]. The thiazide diuretics work by inhibiting sodium reabsorption in the diluting segment of the nephron. The resultant reduction in body sodium causes a slight contraction of extracellular volume that stimulates increased reabsorption of glomerular filtrate in the proximal tubule, thereby decreasing delivery to the distal nephron. Thus, urinary volume as well as urinary dilution are reduced by a mechanism that does not require the action of vasopressin in the distal nephron but is critically dependent on net sodium excretion and contraction of the extracellular volume. The latter also produces secondary hyperaldosteronism, increased excretion of potassium and hydrogen ions and mild hypokalaemia necessitating increased intake of potassium. The mechanism by which amiloride reduces DI is probably similar to thiazides, except that it does not increase excretion of potassium or hydrogen. The prostaglandin inhibitors are thought to act by interfering with feedback inhibition of vasopressin action within the kidney. In adults and older children, decreasing the intake of protein and salt as much as possible can reduce urinary solute load. In infants and young children, more protein is required for growth but solute load can and should be minimized by feeding a formula (Table 14.2) or baby food with the lowest predicted renal solute load per calorie. DDAVP is ineffective in severe nephrogenic DI, but it can produce urine concentration in those with partial forms of the syndrome [66]. This treatment is impractical for long-term use, however, because the doses required are prohibitively expensive.

## Other deficiencies of vasopressin

### Enuresis and nocturia

Enuresis and nocturia are related syndromes characterized, respectively, by involuntary or voluntary excretion of urine during sleep [76]. Enuresis is normal in infants and children up to the age of 5 years. Thereafter, it declines in frequency reaching an incidence of about 1% from early adolescence until late middle age. Nocturia exhibits the reverse change, being very low until age 55, at which point it begins to increase progressively reaching an incidence of nearly 80% in elderly people. Occasionally, enuresis or nocturia is due to DI or another form of global polyuria. More often, however, it is due to a defect in bladder function or the production of abnormally large volumes of subnormally concentrated urine at night [76]. This nocturnal polyuria appears to be due to a nocturnal deficiency in the secretion or antidiuretic action of vasopressin. The cause of these selective nocturnal deficiencies is unknown, although a genetic defect may be involved in some children with enuresis [77].

The differential diagnosis of enuresis and nocturia in a child over 5 years of age includes DI, diabetes mellitus, a primary sleep disorder, defective bladder function and idiopathic nocturnal polyuria. If the patient is continent, these various causes can be distinguished most easily by having the patient keep a voiding diary in which the time and volume of each spontaneously voided urine is recorded. If this voiding diary reveals that the total urine output is normal and the proportion excreted from bedtime to the next morning is less than 25%, the enuresis or nocturia is probably due to a primary sleep disturbance or a urological defect that should be evaluated further by the appropriate specialists. However, if the voiding diary indicates that the total urine output is abnormally increased, the patient has global polyuria and should be evaluated further to determine whether it is due to uncontrolled diabetes mellitus or some form of diabetes insipidus (see above). However, if the voiding diary indicates that only the overnight urine volume is high (> 25% of the total in 8 h), the patient has nocturnal polyuria and will not benefit from further evaluation of antidiuretic function. In this situation, a trial of antidiuretic therapy is indicated.

The most effective treatment for enuresis or nocturia caused by nocturnal polyuria is a reduction in fluid intake after supper and/or administration of DDAVP at bedtime. The drug can be given by tablet, nasal insufflation or injection, but the dose required to eliminate the enuresis or nocturia is often twofold higher than in patients with pituitary or dipsogenic DI, possibly because nocturnal polyuria may also involve some resistance to the antidiuretic effect of the hormone. The only significant side-effect of DDAVP therapy for enuresis or nocturia is hyponatraemia [78]. This complication seems to be unusual and may be nearly eliminated by giving the drug as a single dose at bedtime and monitoring serum sodium from time to time. Treatment should be deferred in patients whose voiding diaries suggest primary polydipsia or another form of global polyuria until definitive investigations have been performed.

## Deficiency of thirst

### Hypernatraemia

A prolonged reduction in water intake has little or no clinical significance if it is matched by a commensurate reduction in water output. However, if the total amount of water obtained from food and beverage is less than the minimum obligatory output from the kidneys, lungs, skin and gastrointestinal tract, total body water decreases and the concentration of solute in body fluid increases. This change is evidenced by a proportionate rise in plasma osmolality and sodium. If the dehydration develops slowly, even moderate to severe elevations in plasma osmolality and sodium may be well tolerated and cause no obvious clinical abnormalities. The lack of effect may be partly due to adaptive increases in intracellular solute which serve to defend cell volume by counteracting the osmotically driven dehydration that would otherwise result [79]. However, if the hypertonic dehydration develops rapidly or is particularly severe, it usually results in overt clinical signs of hypovolaemia and damage to the brain and other organs (see below). The causes of inadequate fluid intake are numerous and can be divided between those with or without a primary defect in the thirst mechanism.

### Adipsic hypernatraemia

A global deficiency in thirst results in a syndrome characterized by chronic or recurrent episodes of severe hypertonic dehydration [30,79]. Besides hypernatraemia and mild to moderate signs of volume depletion (tachycardia, postural hypotension, azotaemia, hyperuricaemia, hypokalaemia, hyper-reninaemia and hyperaldosteronism), these patients report little or no thirst and usually refuse water when it is offered to them. They are often surprisingly alert and healthy appearing. However, they may also suffer a variety of complications, including chorea, confusion, coma, convulsions, paralysis, cerebral haemorrhage, rhabdomyolysis and acute renal failure [79,80]. They may also have hyperglycaemia and hyperlipidaemia that require insulin therapy until the dehydration is corrected.

The cause of deficient thirst is usually malformation or destruction of the osmoregulatory system by pathology involving the anterior hypothalamus [30,79,81]. These lesions can be induced by a variety of disorders (Table 14.4), including congenital malformations, tumours, granulomas, vascular occlusion, trauma, hydrocephalus, infections and idiopathic inflammation. In a few patients, no anatomic lesions have been identified. In all but one of the patients in whom the osmoregulation of vasopressin was evaluated, it has also been deficient presumably because the cells that mediate this control are located in much the same area of the anterior hypothalamus as the thirst osmoreceptors. This deficiency is usually selective because the neurohypophysis appears normal on the MRI and vasopressin secretion responds normally or even supranormally to haemodynamic, emetic or glucopenic stimuli (Fig. 14.13) [30,79,81]. Autopsy studies delineating the precise location and histological appearance of the lesions responsible for this syndrome have not been reported, but experiments in animals have shown that similar defects in thirst and/or vasopressin

**Table 14.4.** Causes of adipsic hypernatraemia

Genetic
   Autosomal recessive (Schinzel–Giedion syndrome)

Congenital malformations
   Septo-optic dysplasia
   Hypogenesis corpus callosum
   Microcephaly

Acquired
   Vascular
      Aneurysm or occlusion, anterior communicating artery
   Neoplasms
      Craniopharyngioma
      Germinoma
      Meningioma
      Glioma
   Granulomas
      Neurosarcoid
      Histiocytosis
   Trauma – closed and penetrating
   Other – hydrocephalus, cystic
   Idiopathic

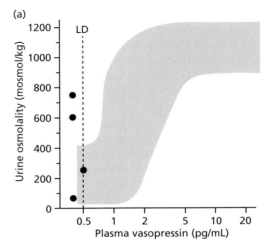

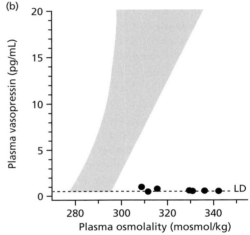

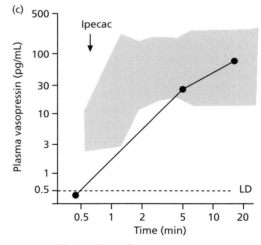

secretion can be produced by lesioning areas of the anterolateral hypothalamus near the supraoptic nuclei [20,33]. In a few patients with adipsic hypernatraemia, the neurohypophysis is also destroyed resulting in a global deficiency in vasopressin secretion [82].

The pathogenesis and pathophysiology of adipsic hypernatraemia are simple in principle. Because the thirst mechanism fails to stimulate the intake of enough water to replenish renal and extrarenal losses, total body water declines and becomes more concentrated, resulting in hypertonicity and hypernatraemia. The reduction in extracellular volume also decreases renal perfusion and increases plasma urea, plasma renin activity and aldosterone secretion. Consequently, sodium is maximally conserved and potassium is lost, aggravating the hypernatraemia and inducing hypokalaemia. The hypernatraemia and/or hypokalaemia, in turn, sometimes result in rhabdomyolysis and myoglobinuria, which in the presence of decreased renal perfusion may produce acute renal failure. The relationship between these changes and the severe carbohydrate intolerance and hyperlipidaemia that may also occur transiently during dehydration is unknown.

In hypodipsic patients, water output need not be increased for hypertonic dehydration to develop, because the amount of water in food is usually inadequate to replace even minimal obligatory urinary and insensible losses. Often, however, the development of dehydration is accelerated or exacerbated by an increase in urinary or insensible loss resulting from a deficiency in vasopressin or an increase in physical activity or ambient temperature. The deficiency of vasopressin that results from the loss of osmoreceptor stimulation

**Fig. 14.13.** The different effects of hypertonic and emetic stimuli on plasma vasopressin in a child with adipsic hypernatraemia. (a) and (b) The relationship of plasma vasopressin to urine and plasma osmolality, respectively, under dehydrated conditions. The shaded areas indicate the ranges of these relationships in healthy children. (c) The changes in plasma vasopressin that occurred after nausea and vomiting was induced by administration of ipecac. Note the log scale. The shaded area indicates the range of responses observed in healthy adults. Redrawn from [99]. LD, lower limit of detection of assay.

produces a constellation of clinical abnormalities different from that caused by a deficiency in the neurohypophysis itself. DI usually is not present when the patient presents with hypertonic dehydration because the deficiency in plasma vasopressin is not great enough to prevent concentration of the urine. However, during rehydration, plasma vasopressin and urine osmolality sometimes decrease to a level that results in DI, thereby interfering with complete correction of the dehydration. Originally, this pattern of premature urinary dilution during rehydration was attributed to upward resetting of the osmostat, an entity sometimes referred to as *essential hypernatraemia*. However, regression analysis of the relation between plasma osmolality and urine osmolality or plasma vasopressin has shown that this abnormality in antidiuretic function is usually if not always due to a reduction in the slope or sensitivity of the osmoregulatory system. In other patients with hypodipsic hypernatraemia, forced rehydration does not result in a water diuresis even if hyponatraemia develops. This paradoxical defect resembles that seen in the SIAD and appears to result from two different mechanisms. One is a continuous or fixed secretion of vasopressin due to a total loss of osmoregulatory function. In these patients, plasma vasopressin continues to circulate in small but biologically effective amounts, irrespective of increases or decreases in hydration. In the other type of dilutional defect, urine osmolality remains high even when plasma vasopressin is suppressed to low or undetectable levels. The cause of this abnormality is unknown but may involve supersensitivity of the kidney to the antidiuretic effect of low levels of plasma vasopressin.

Adipsic hypernatraemia should be differentiated from other causes of hypertonic dehydration caused by physical obstacles to drinking, such as prolonged immobilization, impaired consciousness or an environmental deficiency of potable water. It also should be distinguished from the hypernatraemia that occasionally results from excessive intake or retention of sodium due to errors in the preparation of infant formulas or excess production of aldosterone or other mineralocorticoids [79,83]. These distinctions can usually be made on the basis of the history, physical examination and routine laboratory determinations. If a patient with physical and laboratory signs of hypertonic dehydration (tachycardia, postural hypotension, haemoconcentration, azotaemia and hypokalaemia) is conscious and mobile, a lack of thirst or desire to drink is virtually diagnostic of adipsic hypernatraemia. If the patient is obtunded or otherwise unable to speak or drink, the diagnosis may be made by monitoring thirst and plasma vasopressin during rehydration or a subsequent infusion of hypertonic saline [30]. If hypernatraemia is associated with signs of extracellular volume expansion, it is probably due to an increase in total body sodium caused by excessive ingestion or retention. However, these forms of hypernatraemia are rapidly corrected by drinking unless the patient also has a deficiency in osmoti-

cally mediated thirst or some other impediment to water intake. The latter is the rule in infants and young children who have not yet developed the motor and verbal skills to obtain or ask for water. In this setting, the presence or absence of normal thirst can be determined in a conscious child by offering a bottle with water and observing the response.

The initial treatment of adipsic hypernatraemia should aim to replace the water deficiency and minimize further losses by treating DI or diabetes mellitus if either is present [79]. Hypokalaemia should also be treated particularly if it is associated with neuromuscular symptoms or hyperglycaemia. The dehydration should be corrected gradually over a 24- to 48-h period. Free water should be given orally if possible, but it also can be infused intravenously either as 0.45% saline or 2.5% dextrose (if hyperglycaemia is not present). The net increase in body water that must be achieved to correct the deficit can be estimated by the formula

$$\Delta H_2O = (P_{Na} - 140/140) \times (0.6\,BW),$$

where $\Delta H_2O$ is the water deficit in litres, $P_{Na}$ = the plasma sodium concentration in mequiv/L and BW is the body weight in kilograms. If the patient is less than 10 years of age, the value of 0.6 in the formula should be replaced with a higher value for total body water as indicated in Fig. 14.1. If hyperglycaemia is present, $P_{Na}$ should be corrected for dilution caused by a hydro-osmotic shift from intracellular to extracellular space. This correction can be made by increasing the measured serum sodium by 1 mequiv/L for every 36 mg/dL (2 mmol/L) that plasma glucose exceeds 90 mg/dL (5 mmol/L). The total amount of free water that needs to be given over a 24-h period to correct the hypernatraemia can be estimated from the formula

$$\text{total } H_2O = \Delta H_2O + U_{Vol} + IL,$$

where $U_{Vol}$ and IL are, respectively, the ongoing 24-h urine output and insensible water loss in litres. If the patient is afebrile and does not have DI or is receiving adequate amounts of DDAVP, the IL and $U_{Vol}$ should approximate the age-related values in Table 14.1. Fluid intake and urine output as well as plasma sodium, glucose and potassium should be monitored and the treatments adjusted as necessary to normalize values by 24–48 h.

The long-term management of patients with adipsic hypernatraemia should aim to prevent or minimize recurrences of hypertonic dehydration. The keystones of this management plan should be (1) to minimize urinary water losses by treating with DDAVP or chlorpropamide if DI is present (see above); and (2) to ensure that fluid intake is just sufficient to replace total water output. The latter objective can be quite challenging because both urinary and insensible loss can vary markedly from day to day, depending on unpredictable changes in DDAVP adsorption, dietary solute load, ambient temperature or physical activity. Moreover, too much water intake can be as dangerous as too little in these patients, because their ability to excrete excess water usually is impaired by either concomitant antidiuretic therapy or a loss of the normal ability to osmotically suppress endogenous vasopressin. Hence, they are also prone to retain water and develop hyponatraemia if their fluid intake is too high [82]. The best approach therefore is to teach the patient to drink according to a sliding scale based on daily changes in hydration as determined from changes in body weight [30,82]. The sliding scale can be made by assigning to each patient a target weight that corresponds to optimum hydration (e.g. a serum sodium of 140 mequiv/L) and a basal rate of water intake that approximates his or her rate of urine output and insensible loss under usual conditions of treatment, diet, temperature and activity (Table 14.1). The basal rate of water intake is increased or decreased each day by an amount equal to the difference between the actual weight and the assigned target weight. Checking serum sodium every week until the values stabilize and then checking it every month should monitor the effectiveness of this programme thereafter. In infants and children, the target weight needs to be recalibrated every 3–6 months to compensate for growth. Rigorous compliance with the regimen will usually succeed in maintaining the serum sodium concentration between 130 and 150 mequiv/L, which in most cases is sufficient to prevent frequent readmission for acute therapy. However, constant reinforcement of the regimen is usually necessary because compliance tends to decline when symptoms and signs of dehydration are absent for prolonged periods.

## Excess vasopressin

A sustained increase in the secretion or action of vasopressin results in the production of smaller volumes of more concentrated urine. If water intake is not reduced sufficiently to match the reduction in output, the excess water accumulates and dilutes body fluids, resulting in the development of hypotonic hyponatraemia. When it is mild or develops slowly, the hyponatraemia usually produces few or no symptoms and may go unrecognized for long periods of time. This tolerance may be because brain and many other cells appear to reversibly inactivate intracellular solute, thereby counteracting the osmotically driven swelling that would otherwise result from the fall in extracellular sodium concentration [7,79]. However, if the hyponatraemia develops rapidly (over 24–48 h) and/or is exceptionally severe (less than 120 mequiv/L), it usually results in symptoms and signs of water intoxication, which can range from mild headache or dizziness to anorexia, nausea, vomiting, confusion, coma, seizures and occasionally death. The causes of undiminished or increased water intake in the face of refractory antidiuresis are as varied as those in patients with primary polydipsia (see above). Infants and young children may be particularly susceptible to hyponatraemia because their nutritional needs obligate a relatively high rate of fluid intake. The causes of

the abnormal antidiuresis are also numerous and can be subdivided into primary and secondary disturbances in vasopressin secretion as well as vasopressin-independent types of impaired water excretion. Infants and children may be particularly susceptible to water intoxication because, in addition to the usual vasopressin-dependent and -independent forms of impaired water excretion, their glomerular filtration rate and distal delivery of filtrate is only about 25% of that in older children and adults [10].

### Syndrome of inappropriate antidiuresis

Osmotically inappropriate antidiuresis that cannot be accounted for by any recognized non-osmotic stimulus is generally attributed to a primary abnormality in the regulation of vasopressin secretion or action. The clinical syndrome that results from this abnormality is variously referred to as the syndrome of inappropriate antidiuresis (SIAD), euvolaemic hyponatraemia or type IIIA hyponatraemia. It was first described in two patients with bronchogenic carcinoma and has since been recognized in patients with several other types of tumours as well as many non-malignant diseases or drug treatments (Table 14.5) [84,85]. Most of these disorders and congenital midline malformations of brain can also cause SIAD in infants and children.

Plasma vasopressin is elevated or inadequately suppressed in most adults with SIAD [84]. In absolute terms, however, it is usually within the normal basal range, and can be recognized as 'inappropriate' only in relation to the concurrent hypotonic hyponatraemia. Except when the hormone is exogenous or made ectopically by a tumour [86], the cause of the inappropriately high plasma vasopressin is unknown. Presumably, the hormone is released from the neurohypophysis as a result of some abnormality in the gland or one of its regulatory afferents. Several different pathogenic mechanisms are probably responsible because measurements of plasma vasopressin during treatment with hypertonic saline infusion in adults have shown at least four distinct types of osmoregulatory dysfunction (Fig. 14.14) [84]. Type a is characterized by large and erratic fluctuations in plasma vasopressin that bear no relation whatever to the rise in plasma osmolality. It is found in about 25% of all patients with SIAD and appears to be due to a total loss of osmoreceptor control or intermittent stimulation by some unrecognized non-osmotic pathway. In the type b defect, plasma vasopressin remains fixed at an inappropriately high level until plasma osmolality rises into the normal range. At that point, plasma vasopressin begins to rise appropriately in close association with a further increase in plasma osmolality. This pattern also occurs in about 25% of all patients with SIAD. It could reflect a constant, non-suppressible 'leak' of vasopressin or selective loss of inhibitory input in the presence of an otherwise normal stimulatory component of a bimodal osmoregulatory system. The type c defect is the most common, occurring in at least 35% of all patients. It is characterized by increases

**Table 14.5.** Causes of syndrome of inappropriate antidiuresis (SIAD)

Congenital malformations
  Agenesis corpus callosum
  Other midline defects
Acquired
  Eutopic
    Neoplasms — carcinoma of lung
    Head trauma — closed, penetrating
    Infections
      Pneumonia, tuberculosis
      Abscess (lung or brain)
      Meningitis, encephalitis
    Vascular — cerebrovascular occlusions, haemorrhage
    Neurological
      Neuropathy
        Guillain–Barré syndrome
        Multiple sclerosis
        Amytrophic lateral sclerosis
      Hydrocephalus
      Psychosis
    Metabolic — acute porphyria
    Pulmonary — asthma, pneumothorax, positive pressure respiration
    Drugs — vincristine, cyclophosphamide, phenothiazines, tricyclic
        antidepressants monoamine oxidase inhibitors serotonin
        reuptake inhibitors
  Ectopic
    Drugs — vasopressin or DDAVP treatment
    Neoplasm — lung, duodenum, pancreas, thymus
    Mesothelioma, ganglioglioma

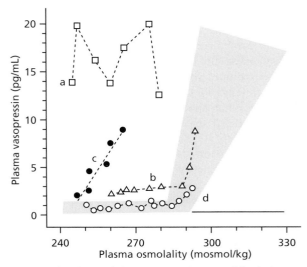

**Fig. 14.14.** The relation of plasma vasopressin to osmolality during hypertonic saline infusion in four adults (a–d) with the clinical syndrome of inappropriate antidiuresis [98].

in plasma vasopressin that correlate closely with acute increases in plasma osmolality and sodium produced by the saline infusion. Regression analysis of this relationship shows that the precision and sensitivity of the vasopressin response to osmolality are normal but the extrapolated threshold value is subnormal. Patients with this type of defect appear to have resetting of the osmostat and may exhibit clinical characteristics slightly different from those found in other forms of SIAD (see below). Type d is much less common than the other three osmoregulatory defects and may represent a basically different abnormality in antidiuretic function. In these unusual patients, vasopressin secretion appears to be stimulated and suppressed normally but urine osmolality remains fixed at a hypertonic level. The reason for this apparent dissociation between plasma vasopressin and urinary concentration has not been determined, but one recent study suggests that the antidiuretic effect is mediated via V2 receptors [87]. Plasma vasopressin in infants or children with SIAD has not been studied, but it is likely to exhibit the same abnormalities as in adults.

The pathophysiology of the fluid and electrolyte disturbance in SIAD is probably similar to that observed when healthy volunteers are treated with vasopressin [87]. In the latter, the administration of Pitressin or DDAVP in doses sufficient to maintain a fixed, maximum antidiuresis causes little or no decrease in plasma sodium unless fluid intake is maintained artificially at a level greater than total urinary and insensible output (about 30 mL/kg/day). Under these conditions, the excess water accumulates, expanding and diluting body fluids. When the expansion of body water exceeds 5–6%, the urinary excretion of sodium begins to increase. This natriuresis serves to ameliorate the extracellular volume expansion but also aggravates the hyponatraemia. The net result is that the hyponatraemia is due in roughly equal proportions to both a primary increase in body water and a secondary decrease in body sodium. If water intake is reduced to less than total urinary and insensible output, the entire series of events slowly reverses as body water decreases, sodium is retained and plasma osmolality and sodium return to their original levels even though vasopressin levels remain high [87]. These observations illustrate the critical importance of fluid intake in determining the effect of vasopressin on lowering serum sodium and increasing sodium excretion.

The abnormalities in adults with SIAD appear to be similar [79,84,88]. Total body water and the rate of sodium excretion are increased at least during the developmental phase. Plasma renin activity and aldosterone tend to be suppressed, whereas atrial natriuretic peptide is elevated, presumably because of the volume expansion. However, the patients differ from the experimental model in two important respects. One is that the excessive fluid intake in patients can be due either to inappropriate administration of fluids or to an associated abnormality in the osmoregulation of thirst. The other is that the antidiuretic defects in patients can vary enormously owing to the individual differences in the nature of their osmoregulatory defect (Fig. 14.14). The patients with downward resetting of the vasopressin osmostat (type c defect) are particularly noteworthy because they retain the capacity to maximally suppress their plasma vasopressin and develop a maximum water diuresis if their plasma osmolality and sodium decrease to the lower set point. Thus, unlike patients with other osmoregulatory defects, they are able to limit the severity of their hyponatraemia even if their fluid intake is very high.

The pathophysiology of SIAD in infants and children has not been studied extensively but is probably similar to that in adults. The only potential difference is the natriuretic response to volume expansion which may be attenuated due to a limited capacity to excrete a sodium load.

The major effects of hyponatraemia are in the central nervous system [79,84,88]. They include lethargy, dizziness, confusion, headache, anorexia, pathological reflexes, pseudobulbar palsy, coma, Cheyne–Stokes respiration and seizures. Postmortem studies in patients who died with hyponatraemia show cerebral oedema, herniation of the brain and, in a few cases, central myelinolysis. The severity of the neurological defects depends on several factors, including the degree of hyponatraemia, the rate of decline and the age of the patient. Unless the patient has epilepsy or another preexisting brain disease, seizures and coma usually do not occur until plasma sodium falls below 120 mequiv/L. If hyponatraemia is chronic or slow to develop, cerebral swelling and symptoms appear to be less severe, probably because brain cells are able to inactivate or excrete solute [88].

An SIAD-like syndrome, which can be referred to as hyponatraemia type IIIB, also occurs in some patients with secondary adrenal insufficiency [89]. The mechanism of the osmotically inappropriate secretion of vasopressin in these patients is uncertain but may be due to a direct effect of cortisol deficiency on the neurohypophysis. A deficiency of cortisol can also cause antidiuresis in patients with pituitary DI, suggesting that there may also be a vasopressin-independent effect on urine concentration. As in true SIAD, the development of hyponatraemia is dependent upon excessive water intake that, in some patients at least, may be due to an associated abnormality in thirst. Whatever the precise mechanism of the hyponatraemia, however, it is important to remember that patients with hyponatraemia because of an isolated glucocorticoid deficiency do not have hyperkalaemia or signs of hypovolaemia and can be reliably differentiated from patients with SIAD only by measuring plasma or urinary cortisol.

*Hypovolaemic hyponatraemia*
Osmotically inappropriate thirst and vasopressin secretion can also result from relatively large reductions in extracellular volume. This syndrome, which is also referred to as type II or hypovolaemic hyponatraemia, is often due to diuretic abuse in adults but can also result from a number of other salt- and water-depleting diseases, such as severe gastroenteritis, renal tubular acidosis, medullary cystic disease of the kidney and a deficiency of aldosterone, all of which also occur in infants and children.

The pathophysiology of hypovolaemic hyponatraemia is similar in principle to SIAD in that it results from impaired free-water excretion and a relatively high fluid intake. The major differences are that the increase in vasopressin is only partly responsible for the impaired water excretion, is secondary to a hypovolaemic stimulus and appears to be due largely if not totally to downward resetting of the osmostat [79]. Its antidiuretic effect is potentiated by decreased glomerular filtration and increased reabsorption of salt and water in the proximal nephron, both of which decrease delivery of filtrate to the distal nephron. Except in patients with mineralocorticoid deficiency, the increase in plasma renin activity that results from the hypovolaemia also stimulates aldosterone secretion, which further reduces the rate of sodium excretion and increases potassium excretion. Therefore, urinary sodium is usually low instead of high as in SIAD, and hypokalaemia may occur. Thirst and fluid intake are probably also increased as a result of downward resetting of the osmostat. The net effect is that total body water is decreased rather than expanded and most if not all of the decrease comes from the extracellular compartment. If anything, intracellular water is slightly expanded because of an osmotically driven redistribution from the extracellular to the intracellular space.

The cortisol and aldosterone deficiency caused by destruction of the adrenal cortex or some forms of congenital adrenal hyperplasia present a special case of hypovolaemic hyponatraemia. In these patients, urinary sodium excretion may be inappropriately high and hyperkalaemia rather than hypokalaemia is usually present. They can be distinguished from SIAD not only by the hyperkalaemia but also by hyperreninaemia and other signs of volume depletion.

*Hypervolaemic hyponatraemia*
Osmotically inappropriate thirst and vasopressin secretion can also result from a marked reduction in 'effective' blood volume. This syndrome, which is also referred to as hypervolaemic or type I hyponatraemia, usually occurs in patients with severe low-output congestive heart failure, advanced cirrhosis with ascites or nephrosis [90]. It is thought to be due to decreased cardiac output and/or a reduction in blood volume caused by a shift of salt and water from plasma to the interstitial space. This redistribution and the associated increase in sodium retention are responsible for the formation of oedema, which is the hallmark of this type of hyponatraemia.

The pathophysiology of hypervolaemic hyponatraemia also entails impaired water excretion in association with inadequate suppression of water intake. As in hypovolaemic hyponatraemia, the impaired water excretion is due to a combination of decreased distal delivery of filtrate and increased secretion of vasopressin, both of which are probably secondary to a hypovolaemic stimulus. When this impairment of water excretion is combined with inadequate suppression of water intake, hyponatraemia develops even though total body sodium is often increased by more than 25%. Thus, hypervolaemic hyponatraemia is distinguished from the other two types of hyponatraemia by the fact that total body sodium and water are markedly increased.

*Differential diagnosis*

The first step in evaluating a patient with hyponatraemia is to rule out hyperglycaemia as the cause. When plasma glucose or another solute such as mannitol is elevated, the effective osmotic pressure of the extracellular osmotic pressure is also increased and water enters quickly from the intracellular compartment until osmotic equilibrium is re-established. This influx of water dilutes the concentration of sodium in plasma and other extracellular compartments but does not completely reduce plasma osmolality to normal. Hence, this form of hyponatraemia is not associated with hypotonicity and can be easily recognized either by correcting the sodium level for the elevation in glucose (see treatment of adipsic hypernatraemia) or measuring the osmolality of heparinized plasma. Serum or ethylenediaminetetraacetic (edetic) acid (EDTA) plasma should not be used for osmolality measurements, as both are subject to significant artifacts caused by glucose or the anticoagulant itself.

Differentiating SIAD (type IIIA hyponatraemia) from the other forms of hypotonic hyponatraemia is a process of exclusion based largely on standard clinical assessment of the extracellular volume, thyroid function and adrenal function. Thus, patients with SIAD lack oedema and postural hypotension as well as any laboratory sign of or true or effective hypovolaemia. Their plasma urea, creatinine, urate and renin activity tend to be low and urinary sodium is high, at least in the developmental phase of the syndrome. Serum aldosterone may also be low and serum potassium is normal. Their thyroid function tests and morning plasma cortisol are also within normal limits, excluding the SIAD-like syndrome (hyponatraemia type IIIB) caused by hypothyroidism or hypoadrenalism. In contrast, the presence of oedema in a patient with severe heart failure, advanced cirrhosis or nephrosis is pathognomonic of hypervolaemic (type I) hyponatraemia. In these patients, urinary sodium is usually low (< 20 mequiv/day), and plasma renin activity, aldosterone, urea, creatinine and urate are often elevated because of a reduction in effective blood volume and glomerular filtration. Hypovolaemic (type II) hyponatraemia is characterized by signs and symptoms of volume depletion without oedema, and postural hypotension may be present. Thus, plasma urea, creatinine, urate and renin are usually increased. Urinary sodium is usually low unless the syndrome is caused by diuretic abuse,

primary renal sodium wasting or adrenal insufficiency in which case it may be high. Some degree of hypokalaemia is the rule, except in patients with aldosterone deficiency, in whom serum potassium is usually elevated. Measurements of plasma vasopressin are of no help in distinguishing between the various types of hypotonic hyponatraemia, as they are usually elevated to the same extent in all three types.

*Therapy*
*Syndrome of inappropriate antidiuresis*
The primary abnormality in vasopressin secretion can often be eliminated when the hormone is made ectopically, given exogenously or released from the neurohypophysis in response to certain non-essential drugs. If the inappropriate secretion of vasopressin is caused by chronic or recurrent nausea (as in patients receiving some forms of chemotherapy), it can also be eliminated by treatment with standard antiemetics. Most of the time, however, the abnormal vasopressin secretion cannot be corrected and must be allowed to run its course until spontaneous recovery occurs. Fortunately, this usually occurs within 2–3 weeks or as soon as the underlying cause is eliminated. Until such remission, the hyponatraemia can be stabilized or corrected by restricting water intake. To be effective, however, the *total* intake of water must be at least 30% less than the total of urinary and insensible output. This is particularly difficult in infants and young children because the water content of formula or baby food is relatively high. Moreover, even if the requisite level of fluid restriction is achieved, the rate of decrease in body water and rise in plasma sodium is usually no greater than about 1–2% a day. Therefore, additional measures are often needed, particularly if the hyponatraemia is symptomatic.

The hyponatraemia can also be corrected by intravenous infusion of hypertonic saline. Infusion of 3% saline at a rate of 0.05 mL/kg/min increases plasma osmolality and sodium by about 1% an hour. This approach is rational as well as effective, for it not only corrects the sodium deficiency but may also produce a mild solute diuresis that helps to reduce body water. Many physicians believe that hypertonic saline infusion is also safe [91], provided the plasma sodium is raised no more than 24 mequiv/L and no higher than 130–135 mequiv/L. However, others believe that raising plasma sodium more than 12 mequiv/L per day runs a serious risk of producing central pontine myelinolysis [92], a rare and often fatal neurological disorder characterized by quadriparesis, dysphagia, and dysarthria. Therefore, hypertonic saline should be used cautiously in patients with SIAD and only to the extent necessary to raise plasma sodium to asymptomatic levels. To guard against sudden rapid increases in plasma sodium caused by remission of the abnormal vasopressin secretion, changes in urine output as well as plasma sodium should be monitored at least every 2–4 h during the infusion. These caveats apply particularly to patients in whom the hyponatraemia has been present for more than 48 h because they usually have fewer symptoms and are more likely to have serious complications from too rapid correction of their hyponatraemia. The safety of hypertonic saline infusion for treatment of infants or young children with SIAD has not been systematically investigated and should be used with caution.

Body water can also be reduced by inhibiting the antidiuretic effects of vasopressin. Among the drugs currently available in the USA for this purpose, demeclocycline is probably the best [93]. At conventional doses of up to 1.2 g per day in adults, it causes a reversible form of nephrogenic DI in almost all patients with SIAD. This effect may require a week or more to manifest. Its mechanism of action has not been defined precisely but appears to involve a step distal to the generation of cAMP. Because of other catabolic as well as nephrotoxic effects, it may cause a rise in plasma urea, which is reversible when the drug is stopped. Demeclocycline can have serious or potentially lethal side-effects in patients with type I and type II hyponatraemia, and its efficacy and safety in treating infants and children with SIAD is unknown. Hence, its use should be monitored closely and restricted to patients with chronic SIAD that is not amenable to fluid restriction and is not associated with significant underlying cardiac, renal or hepatic disease. Lithium carbonate also causes a form of reversible nephrogenic DI but at conventional doses this effect is inconsistent and it is even more prone to produce undesirable side-effects. For these reasons, it is rarely used for treatment of SIAD or other forms of hyponatraemia.

Recently, potent non-peptide V2 receptor antagonists capable of blocking the antidiuretic effect of vasopressin have been developed and tested in humans [94]. Preliminary clinical trials in adults with SIAD or type I hyponatraemia indicate that these antagonists are both safe and effective in promoting a water diuresis and raising the plasma sodium in a dose-dependent manner [90,94]. They have not been tested in infants or children and are not yet available in the USA for routine use for treatment of SIAD or type I hyponatraemia in any age group.

Other measures that may be useful in the treatment of chronic SIAD include the administration of oral sodium chloride with or without frusemide [95]. This regimen works much like an osmotic diuretic in that it increases free-water excretion by increasing solute load. Much the same result can be obtained by giving urea by mouth, but the latter is unpalatable and may not be well accepted by patients. Florinef is also quite effective in the management of chronic SIAD. At doses ranging from 0.1 to 0.2 mg twice a day, it will usually maintain plasma sodium within the normal range. The mechanism is uncertain but may include some inhibition of fluid intake as well as increased retention of sodium. The principle side-effects are hypokalaemia, which can usually be avoided by dietary potassium supplements, and hypertension, which may require discontinuation of the treatment.

In patients with an SIAD-like disorder due to myxoedema or secondary adrenal insufficiency (hyponatraemia type IIIB), the abnormalities in salt and water balance can be corrected completely by treatment with thyroxine or cortisol. In a hypothyroid patient, thyroxine should not be started until a co-deficiency of cortisol has been excluded because the increase in metabolism caused by the treatment could provoke an adrenal crisis.

*Hypovolaemic (type II) hyponatraemia*
The fluid and electrolyte abnormalities in these patients can be corrected completely by correcting the cause of the hypovolaemia and/or restoring extracellular volume to normal. As their sodium deficit is relatively greater than their water deficit, the ideal combination is hypertonic, i.e. the ratio of sodium chloride to water should exceed 150 mequiv/L. However, this approach is necessary only if the hyponatraemia is severe and must be corrected quickly. In such a situation, an infusion of 3% saline at a rate of 0.1 mL/kg /min for 2 h will raise plasma sodium by almost 10 mequiv/L, an amount that is usually sufficient to eliminate the threat of serious neurological complications. In using this approach, it is again important not to raise the plasma sodium too far or too fast (see above). In most cases of hypovolaemic hyponatraemia, it is sufficient and probably preferable simply to give the salt and water by mouth or infuse isotonic saline with or without supplementary potassium. In addition, the cause of the sodium loss should be identified and, if possible, corrected. If the patient is hyperkalaemic or has other signs suggestive of primary adrenal dysfunction, blood for measurement of plasma cortisol, aldosterone and renin activity should be obtained immediately and parenteral cortisol should be administered pending completion of the assays. In no case should patients with this form of hypo-natraemia be treated by water restriction, demeclocycline, lithium, vasopressin antagonists or frusemide because these measures only aggravate the underlying hypovolaemia and may precipitate cardiovascular collapse.

*Hypervolaemic (type I) hyponatraemia*
As expected, the impaired water excretion and hyponatraemia in adults with congestive heart failure, nephrosis or advanced cirrhosis sometimes can be improved by increasing cardiac output [96] or shunting ascitic fluid into the vascular space [97]. Usually, however, the basic haemodynamic defect cannot be completely rectified, and other methods must be used to correct the oedema and hyponatraemia. As patients in this category have a greater increase in total body water than sodium, the most rational and effective therapy is to combine fluid restriction with the administration of an osmotic or loop diuretic [98]. Preliminary clinical experience with the non-peptide vasopressin antagonists indicates that,

when combined with fluid restriction, they are also quite effective and safe in promoting a water diuresis and correcting the hyponatraemia in patients with congestive heart failure or advanced cirrhosis [90]. However, they have not been tested in children and are not yet available for routine use. Patients with hypervolaemic hyponatraemia should never be treated with hypertonic saline or Florinef because they increase body sodium and worsen the oedema. Demeclocycline and lithium are also contraindicated because patients with hypervolaemic hyponatraemia are more likely to suffer severe side-effects.

# References

1 Friis-Hansen B. Water distribution in the newborn infant. *Acta Paediatr Scand* 1983; 305 (Suppl.): 7–11.

2 Hill LL. Body composition, normal electrolyte concentrations, and the maintenance of normal volume, tonicity, and acid–base metabolism. *Pediatr Clin N Am* 1990; 37(2): 241–56.

3 Leaf A, Chatillon JY, Wrong O, Tuttle EP Jr. The mechanism of the osmotic adjustment of body cells as determined in vivo by the volume of distribution of a large waterload. *J Clin Invest* 1954; 33: 1261–8.

4 Hendry EB. Osmolarity of human serum and of chemical solutions of biologic importance. *Clin Chem* 1961; 7: 156–64.

5 Darrow DC, Yanett H. Changes in distribution of body water accompanying increase and decrease in extracellular electrolytes. *J Clin Invest*, 1935; 14: 266–75.

6 Arieff AI, Guisado R, Lazarowitz VC. Pathophysiology of hyperosmolar states. In: Andreoli TE, Grantham JJ, Rector FC, eds. *Disturbances in Body Fluid Osmolality*. Bethesda: American Physiological Society 1977: 227–50.

7 Verbalis JG. Adaptation to acute and chronic hyponatremia: implications for symptomatology, diagnosis, and therapy. *Semin Nephrol* 1998; 18 (1): 3–19.

8 Adolph EF. *Physiology of Man in the Desert*. New York: Hofner, 1969.

9 Goellner MH, Ziegler EE, Fomon SJ. Urination during the first three years of life. *Nephron* 1981; 28: 174–8.

10 Aperia A, Zetterstrom R. Renal control of fluid homeostasis in the newborn infant. *Clin Perinatol* 1982; 9: 523–33.

11 Ziegler EE, Fomon SJ. Potential renal solute load of infant formulas. *J Nutr* 1989; 119 (Suppl. 12): 1785–8.

12 Robertson GL. The posterior pituitary. In: Frohman LA, Felig P. eds. *Endocrinology and Metabolism*. New York: McGraw-Hill, 2001.

13 Scharrer E, Scharrer B. Hormones produced by neurosecretory cells. *Recent Prog Horm Res* 1954; 10: 183–240.

14 Riddell DC, Mallonee R, Phillips JA, Parks JS, Sexton LA, Hamerton JL. Chromosomal assignment of human sequences encoding arginine vasopressin-neurophysin II and growth hormone releasing factor. *Somatic Cell Mol Genet* 1985; 11: 189–95.

15 Sausville E, Carney D, Battey J. The human vasopressin gene is linked to the oxytocin gene and is selectively expressed in a cultured lung cancer cell line. *J Biol Chem* 1985; 260: 10236–41.

16 Schmale H, Fehr S, Richter D. Vasopressin biosynthesis — from gene to peptide hormone. *Kidney Int* 1987; 32 (Suppl. 21): S8–13.

17 Mohr E, Bahnsen U, Kiessling C, Richter D. Expression of the vasopressin and oxytocin genes in rats occurs in mutually exclusive sets of hypothalamic neurons. *FEBS Lett* 1988; 242: 144–8.

18 Breslow E. The conformation and functional domains of neurophysins. In: Gross P, Richter D, Robertson GL, eds. *Vasopressin*. John Libbey Eurotext, 1993: 143–5.

19 Robertson GL. The regulation of vasopressin function in health and disease. *Recent Prog Horm Res* 1977; 33: 333–85.

20 Thrasher TN, Keil LC. Regulation of drinking and vasopressin secretion: Role of organum vasculosum laminae terminalis. *Am J Physiol* 1987; 253: R108–20 (*Regul Integrative Comp Physiol* 22).

21 Strong OS, Elwyn A. *Human Neuroanatomy*. Baltimore: Williams & Wilkins, 1948: 398.

22 Zerbe RL, Miller JZ, Robertson GL. The reproducibility and heritability of individual differences in osmoregulatory function in normal human subjects. *J Lab Clin Med* 1991; 117: 51–9.

23 Zerbe RL, Robertson GL. Osmoregulation of thirst and vasopressin secretion in human subjects: effect of various solutes. *Am J Physiol* 1983; 224: E607–14.

24 Vokes TP, Aycinena PR, Robertson GL. Effect of insulin on osmoregulation of vasopressin. *Am J Physiol* 1987; 252: E538–48 (*Endocrinol Metab* 15).

25 McDonald TJ, Li C, Nijland MJ, Caston-Balderrama A, Ross MG. Fos response of fetal sheep anterior circumventricular organs to osmotic challenge in late gestation. *Am J Physiol* 1998; 275 (2, Part 2): H609–14.

26 Robertson GL, Athar S, Shelton RL. Osmotic control of vasopressin function. In: Andreoli TE, Grantham JJ, Rector FC, eds. *Disturbances in Body Fluid Osmolality*. Bethesda: American Physiological Society, 1977: 125.

27 Knepper MA. Molecular physiology of urinary concentrating mechanism: regulation of aquaporin water channels by vasopressin. *Am J Physiol* 1997; 272 (*Renal Physiol* 41): F3–12.

28 Jard S. Vasopressin receptors. A historical survey. *Adv Exp Med Biol* 1998; 449: 1–13.

29 Ramsay DJ, Water. Distribution between compartments and its relationship to thirst. In: Ramsay DJ, Booth DA, eds. *Thirst – Physiological and Psychological Aspects*. London: Springer-Verlag, 1990: 23–52.

30 Robertson GL. Disorders of thirst in man. In: Ramsay DJ, Booth DA, eds. *Thirst – Physiological and Psychological Aspects*. London. Springer-Verlag, 1990: 453–75.

31 Rolls BJ. Physiological determinants of fluid intake in humans. In: Ramsay DJ, Booth DA, eds. *Thirst – Physiological and Psychological Aspects*. London: Springer-Verlag, 1990: 391–8.

32 Verbalis JG. Inhibitory controls of drinking: Satiation of thirst. In: Ramsay DJ, Booth DA, eds. *Thirst – Physiological and Psychological Aspects*. London: Springer-Verlag, 1990: 313–30.

33 McKinley MJ. Osmoreceptor for thirst. In: Ramsay DJ, Booth DA, eds. *Thirst – Physiological and Psychological Aspect*. London: Springer-Verlag, 1990: 77–91.

34 Thrasher TN. Volume receptors and the stimulation of water intake. In: Ramsay DJ, Booth DA, eds. *Thirst – Physiological and Psychological Aspects*. London: Springer-Verlag, 1990: 93–107.

35 Greger NG, Kirkland RT, Clayton GW, Kirkland JL. Central diabetes insipidus. 22 years' experience. *Am J Dis Child* 1986; 140 (6): 551–4.

36 Wang LC, Cohen ME, Duffner PK. Etiology of central diabetes insipidus in children. *Pediatr Neurol* 1994; 11: 273–7.

37  Robertson GL. Diabetes insipidus. *Endocrinol Metab Clin North Am* 1995; 24: 549–72.

38  Elster AD. Modern imaging of the pituitary. *Radiology* 1993; 187: 1–14.

39  Appignani B, Landy H, Barnes P. MR in idiopathic central diabetes insipidus of childhood. *Am J Neuroradiol* 1993; 14: 1407–10.

40  Masera N, Grant DB, Stanhope R, Preece MA. Diabetes insipidus with impaired osmotic regulation in septo-optic dysplasia and agenesis of the corpus callosum. *Arch Dis Child* 1994; 70 (1): 51–3.

41  Mootha SL, Barkovich AJ, Grumbach MM *et al.* Idiopathic hypothalamic diabetes insipidus, pituitary stalk thickening, and the occult intracranial germinoma in children and adolescents. *J Clin Endocrinol Metab* 1997; 82: 1362–7.

42  Carlson RA, Hattery RR, O'Connell EJ, Fontana RS. Pulmonary involvement by histiocytosis X in the pediatric age group. *Mayo Clin Proc* 1976; 51: 542–7.

43  Schmitt S, Wichmann W, Martin E, Zachmann M, Schoenle EJ. Pituitary stalk thickening with diabetes insipidus preceding typical manifestations of Langerhans cell histiocytosis in children. *Eur J Pediatr* 1993; 152: 399–401.

44  Hansen LK, Rittig S, Robertson GL. Genetic basis of familial neurohypophyseal diabetes insipidus. *Trends Endocrinol Metab* 1997; 8: 363–72.

45  Rutishauser J, Kopp P, Gaskill MB, Kotlar TJ, Robertson GL. A novel mutation (R97C) in the neurophysin moiety of prepro-vasopressin–neurophysin II associated with autosomal-dominant neurohypophyseal diabetes insipidus. *Mol Genet Metab* 1999; 67: 89–92.

46  Willcutts MD, Felner E, White PC. Autosomal recessive familial neurohypophyseal diabetes insipidus with continued secretion of mutant weakly active vasopressin. *Hum Mol Genet* 1999; 8: 1303–7.

47  Habiby RL, Robertson GL, Kaplowitz PB, Rittig S. A novel x-linked form of familial neurohypophyseal diabetes insipidus. *J Invest Med* 1996; 44: 341A.

48  Cremers CWRJ, Wijdeveld PGAB, Pinckers AJLG. Juvenile diabetes mellitus, optic atrophy, hearing loss, diabetes insipidus, atonia of the urinary tract and bladder, and other abnormalities (Wolfram syndrome). *Acta Paediatr Scand* 1977; 264: 1–16.

49  Inoue H, Tanizawa Y, Wasson J *et al.* A gene encoding a transmembrane protein is mutated in patients with diabetes mellitus and optic atrophy (Wolfram syndrome). *Nature Genet* 1998; 20: 143–8.

50  Gabreëls BATF, Swaab DF, de Kleijn DPV *et al.* The vasopressin precursor is not processed in the hypothalamus of wolfram syndrome patients with diabetes insipidus: evidence for the involvement of PC2 and 7B2. *J Clin Endocrinol Metab* 1998; 83: 4026–33.

51  Thompson CJ, Charlton J, Walford S *et al.* Vasopressin secretion in the DIDMOAD (Wolfram) syndrome. *Q J Med* 1989; 264: 333–45.

52  Imura H, Nakao K, Shimatsu A *et al.* Lymphocytic infundibulo-neurohypophysitis as a cause of central diabetes insipidus. *N Engl J Med* 1993; 329: 683–9.

53  Cemeroglu AP, Blaivas M, Muraszko KM, Robertson PL, Vazquez DM. Lymphocytic hypophysitis presenting with diabetes insipidus in a 14-year-old girl: case report and review of the literature. *Eur J Pediatr* 1997; 156: 684–8.

54  Maghnie M, Genovese E, Sommaruga MG *et al.* Evolution of childhood central diabetes insipidus into panhypopituitarism with a large hypothalamic mass: is 'lymphocytic infundibuloneuro-hypophysitis' in children a different entity? *Eur J Endocrinol* 1998; 139: 635–40.

55  Zerbe RL, Robertson GL. A comparison of plasma vasopressin measurements with a standard indirect test in the differential diagnosis of polyuria. *N Engl J Med* 1981; 305: 1539–46.

56  Maccubbin DA, Van Buren JM. A quantitative evaluation of hypothalamic degeneration and its relation to diabetes insipidus following interruption of the human hypophyseal stalk. *Brain* 1963; 46: 443–46.

57  Robertson GL. Osmoregulation of thirst and vasopressin secretion: Functional properties and their relationship to water balance. In: Schrier R, ed. *Vasopressin*. New York: Raven Press, 1985: 202–212.

58  Pivonello R, Colao A, Di Somma C *et al.* Impairment of bone status in patients with central diabetes. *J Clin Endocrinol Metab* 1998; 83: 2275–80.

59  Robertson GL. Dipsogenic diabetes insipidus: A newly recognized syndrome caused by a selective defect in the osmoregulation of thirst. *Trans Assoc Am Physicians C* 1987; 241–9.

60  Sleeper FH, Jellinek EM. A comparative physiologic, psychologic and psychiatric study of polyuric and nonpolyuric schizophrenic patients. *J Nerv Ment Dis* 1936; 83: 557–63.

61  Goldman MB, Luchins DJ, Robertson GL. Mechanisms of altered water metabolism in psychotic patients with polydipsia and hyponatremia. *N Engl J Med* 1988; 318: 397–403.

62  Forssman H. Two different mutations of X-chromosome causing diabetes insipidus. *Am J Hum Genet* 1955; 7: 21–7.

63  Bichet DG, Fujiwara TM. Diversity of nephrogenic diabetes insipidus mutations and importance of early recognition and treatment. *Clin Exp Nephrol* 1998; 2: 253–63.

64  Mulders SM, Bichet DG, Rijss JPL *et al.* An aquaporin-2 water channel mutant which causes autosomal dominant nephrogenic diabetes insipidus is retained in the golgi complex. *J Clin Invest* 1998; 102: 57–66.

65  Oksche A, Rosenthal W. The molecular basis of nephrogenic diabetes insipidus. *J Mol Med* 1998; 76: 326–37.

66  Robertson GL, McLeod JF, Zerbe RL, Baylis PH, Kovács L, Rittig S. Vasopressin function in heritable forms of diabetes insipidus. In: Gross P, Richter D, Robertson GL, eds. *Vasopressin*. Paris: John Libbey Eurotext, 1993: 493–503.

67  Robertson GL. Diabetes insipidus. *Endocrinol Metab Clin N Am* 1995; 24: 549–72.

68  Sato N, Ishizaka H, Yagi H, Matsumoto M, Endo K. Posterior lobe of the pituitary in diabetes insipidus: dynamic MR imaging. *Radiology* 1993; 186: 357–60.

69  Maghnie M, Genovese E, Bernasconi S, Binda S, Arico M. Persistent high MR signal of the posterior pituitary gland in central diabetes insipidus. *Am J Neuroradiol* 1997; 18: 1749–52.

70  Drincic AT, Robertson GL. Treatment of diabetes insipidus in adults. In: Meikle AW, eds. *Contemporary Endocrinology: Hormone Replacement Therapy*. Totowa, NJ: Humana Press, 1998; 21–38.

71  Catalina PF, Rodr'iguez Garc'ia M, de la Torre C, P'aramo C, Garc'ia-Mayor RV. Diabetes insipidus for five years preceding the diagnosis of hypothalamic Langerhans cell histicytosis. *J Endocrinol Invest* 1995; 18: 663–6.

72  Pivonello R, Faggiano A, DiSomma C *et al.* Effect of a short-term treatment with alendronate on bone density and bone markers in patients with central diabetes insipidus. *J Clin Endocrinol Metab* 1999; 84: 2349–52.

73 Earley LE, Orloff J. The mechanism of antidiuresis associated with administration of hydrochlorothiazide to patients with vasopressin resistant diabetes insipidus. *J Clin Invest* 1962; 41: 1988–97.

74 Alon U, Chan JCM. Hydrochlorothiazide-amiloride in the treatment of congenital nephrogenic diabetes insipidus. *Am J Nephrol* 1985; 5: 9–13.

75 Jakobsson B, Berg U. Effect of hydrochlorothiazide and indomethacin treatment on renal function in nephrogenic diabetes insipidus. *Acta Paediatr* 1994; 83: 522–5.

76 Nørgaard JP. Pathophysiology of nocturnal enuresis. *Scand J Urol Nephrol Suppl* 1991; 140: 1–35.

77 Eiberg H, Berendt I, Mohr J. Assignment of dominant inherited nocturnal enuresis (ENUR1) to chromosome 13q. *Nature Genet* 1995; 10: 354–6.

78 Bernstein SA, Williford SL. Intranasal desmopressin-associated hyponatremia: a case report and literature review. *J Fam Pract* 1997; 44(2): 203–8.

79 Kovacs L, Robertson GL. Disorders of water balance – hyponatremia and hypernatremia. *Bailliere's Clin Endocrinol Metab* 1992; 6(1): 107–27.

80 Han BK, Lee M, Yoon HK. Cranial ultrasound and CT findings in infants with hypernatremic dehydration. *Pediatr Radiol* 1997; 27: 739–42.

81 Papadimitriou A, Kipourou K, Manta C, Tapaki G, Philippidis P. Adipsic hypernatremia syndrome in infancy. *J Pediatr Endocrinol Metab* 1997; 10: 547–50.

82 Robertson GL. Abnormalities of thirst regulation. *Kidney Int* 1984; 25: 460–9.

83 Conley SB. Hypernatremia. *Pediatr Clin N Am* 1990; 37(2): 365–72.

84 Kovacs L, Robertson GL. Syndrome of inappropriate antidiuresis. *Endocrinol Metab Clin N Am* 1992; 21: 859–75.

85 Thiagarajan R, La Gamma E, Dey S, Blethen S, Wilson TA. Hyponatremia caused by a reset osmostat in a neonate with cleft lip and palate and panhypopituitarism. *J Pediatr* 1996; 128: 561–3.

86 George JM, Capen CC, Phillips AS. Biosynthesis of vasopressin in vitro and ultrastructure of a bronchogenic carcinoma. *J Clin Invest* 1972; 51: 141–8.

87 Leaf A, Bartter FC, Santos RF, Wrong O. Evidence in man that urinary electrolyte loss induced by pitressin is a function of water retention. *J Clin Invest* 1953; 32: 868–78.

88 Verbalis JG. Hyponatremia: epidemiology, pathophysiology, and therapy. *Curr Opin Nephrol Hypertens* 1993; 2: 636–52.

89 Oelkers W. Hyponatremia and inappropriate secretion of vasopressin (antidiuretic hormone) in patients with hypopituitarism. *N Engl J Med* 1989; 321: 492–6.

90 Schrier RW, Fassett RG, Ohara M, Martin PY. Vasopressin release, water channels, and vasopressin antagonism in cardiac failure, cirrhosis, and pregnancy. *Proc Assoc Am Physicians* 1998; 110: 407–11.

91 Ayus JC, Krothapalli RK, Arieff AI. Treatment of symptomatic hyponatremia and its relation to brain damage. *N Engl J Med* 1987; 317: 1190–5.

92 Sterns RH. The treatment of hyponatremia: First, do no harm, editorial. *Am J Med* 1990; 88: 557–60.

93 Cherrill DA, Stote RM, Birge JR, Singer I. Demeclocycline treatment in the syndrome of inappropriate antidiuretic hormone secretion. *Ann Intern Med* 1975; 83: 654–6.

94 Ohnishi A, Orita Y, Okahara R *et al*. Potent aquaretic agent – A novel nonpeptide selective vasopressin 2 antagonist (OPC-31260) in men. *J Clin Invest* 1993; 92: 2653–9.

95 Decaux G, Waterlot Y, Genette F, Mockel J. Treatment of the syndrome of inappropriate secretion of antidiuretic hormone with furosemide. *N Engl J Med* 1981; 304: 329–30.

96 Dzau VJ, Colucci WS, Williams GH, Curfman G, Meggs L, Hollenberg NK. Sustained effectiveness of converting enzyme inhibition in patients with severe congestive heart failure. *N Engl J Med* 1980; 302: 1373–9.

97 Yamahiro HW, Reynolds TB. Effects of ascitic fluid infusion on sodium excretion, blood volume and creatinine clearance in cirrhosis. *Gastroenterology* 1961; 40: 497.

98 Robertson GL. Thirst and vasopressin function in normal and disordered states of water balance. *J Lab Clin Med* 1983; 101(3): 351–71.

99 Schaff-Blass E, Robertson GL, Rosenfield RL. Chronic hypernatremia resulting from a congenital defect in osmoregulation of thirst and vasopressin. *J Pediatr* 1983; 102: 703–8.

# 15 Urogenital implications of endocrine disorders in children and adolescents

**D. T. Wilcox, Sarah Creighton, C. R. J. Woodhouse and P. D. E. Mouriquand**

## Introduction

The management of children born with ambiguous genitalia is complex. Gender assignment and the surgical correction of genital anomalies are urgent and crucial issues that must be coordinated from birth with complete consensus. The most difficult problem is that irreversible decisions are taken when significant limitations exist in our understanding of these malformations, their treatment and long-term outcomes. In addition, they are taken in a highly emotional context for the parents and when the patient cannot be consulted nor give informed consent.

A major pitfall is our limited understanding of sexuality. The external genitalia are the tip of an iceberg, yet the only part where the surgeon can act. To create the external appearance of a female does not necessarily mean that the child will accept the assignment and behave as a female. The surgical possibilities are limited and never completely satisfactory. Surgeons can create a 'vagina' that will allow penetration, but the extent to which it is sexually sensate or functional is uncertain. Creation of a penile organ [1] is more challenging as erectile tissue cannot be made. Operations to create a penis using other tissues have been performed for transsexual patients but have not been successful in children. Very few data have been published on the quality of sexual life after genital reconstruction in male or female patients.

## Male disorders

### Undescended testes

An undescended testis (UDT) is one that cannot be brought to the bottom of the scrotum without undue tension of the cord. It has an incidence at 3 months of 1.6%. The incidence at birth is 6.7%, with newborns weighing less than 2500 g having an incidence of cryptorchidism of 29%. The improvement between birth and 3 months is thought to be due to the post-natal androgen surge resulting in inguinoscrotal migration. Interestingly, the incidence of undescended testis appears to be increasing, although the reasons are unclear [2].

### Embryology

Testicular descent occurs in two steps and begins about the tenth week of gestation, shortly after sexual differentiation [3]. The two stages of descent, abdominal testicular descent and the migratory inguinoscrotal phase are separate and under different hormonal control. The transabdominal phase occurs between 10 and 15 weeks' gestation, when the testis moves from the urogenital ridge to the inguinal region. This occurs because the gubernaculum is attached to the caudal portion of the testis and to the inguinal region. The persistence and enlargement of the gubernaculum, which is responsible for this phase of descent, is under the control of anti-Müllerian hormone (AMH) [4,5]. In the second phase, between 28 and 35 weeks' gestation, the testis descends from the inguinal region to the scrotum under androgen control. The exact mechanism is unknown, but it is postulated that calcitonin gene-related peptide is released from the genitofemoral nerve causing gubernaculum migration [6]. The gubernaculum is canalized by the processus vaginalis and the testis travels through the processus into the scrotum.

There are three types of undescended testicle.

**1** True undescended: testes that have descended partially along the normal line of descent and then stopped, which can be further divided into palpable and impalpable.

**2** Ectopic: testes that have descended into an ectopic position in the superficial inguinal pouch, femoral region, perineal region, pubopenile or, rarely, the opposite scrotum [5].

**3** Retractile: testes that can be brought to the bottom of the scrotum, but are often pulled back into the inguinal canal because of cremester retraction [7] (Table 15.1).

Clinical examination of the testes is the most important pointer to management of boys with UDT. The child should be at ease, and the examination should be carried out in comfortable surroundings using warm hands. Inspection of the

**Table 15.1.** Classification of undescended testis

Impalpable
   Intra-abdominal
   Absent

Palpable
   True undescended
   Ectopic
   Retractile

scrotum will often reveal the location of the testis. If the scrotum is well developed, it suggests a retractile testis; if, however, the hemiscrotum is hypoplastic, it is likely that the testis is undescended. By retracting the suprapubic skin superiorly the scrotum and its contents become more visible. If the testis is still not seen, gentle palpation is required. It is important to start the examination lateral to the deep inguinal ring and then to move gently medially towards the scrotum along the line of the canal. This ensures that the testis which is mobile does not disappear unnoticed up the inguinal canal. Eighty per cent to 90% of testicles can be identified in this way [5]. Once the testicle is found, it should be manipulated as far as possible into the scrotum. If the testis has not been identified, the ectopic sites should be inspected. At the end of the examination, it should be possible to decide whether the testis is palpable; a palpable testis can be further classified into true undescended, ectopic or retractile.

Undescended testes have been imaged using a variety of modalities, including ultrasound, computerized tomography (CT), magnetic resonance imaging (MRI), arteriography and venography. It is now widely agreed that these techniques have a limited role in the diagnosis of UDT and are less accurate than an experienced examiner [8]. For bilateral impalpable testes, the differential diagnosis is between bilateral undescent or anorchia. They can be distinguished by a human chorionic gonadotrophin (hCG) test, the absence of a testosterone response indicating anorchia.

One investigative technique that is used is laparoscopy [9,10]. This accurately enables absent testes to be distinguished from the impalpable by the presence of blind-ending testicular vessels. If the testis is seen within the abdominal cavity, orchidopexy can be performed at the same time, either by laparoscopy or by an open surgical technique [11].

The indications for treatment are, first, the cosmetic and psychological benefits of having two testes in the scrotum. Second, as the undescended testis has an increased risk of malignancy, it enables easy palpation. Third, it places the testis in a lower temperature environment, which may improve the long-term chances of fertility.

Orchidopexy should be performed after 6 months of age as it is then unlikely that the testis will descend spontaneously [2]. Histological studies have shown a steady degeneration in germ cells from 12 months, worsening with age. Many surgeons now recommend orchidopexy before 2 years of age to minimize germ cell damage and improve chances of fertility but there are no long-term studies to prove this theoretical benefit [5,12,13].

There are two methods of bringing the undescended testis into the scrotum: hormonal and surgical. At present two types of hormone treatment are described, hCG and gonadotrophin-releasing hormone (GnRH). The rationale for these treatments is that both agents cause testosterone production, promoting testicular descent. Early studies reported good success with both hormonal therapies [14,15], but a double-blind randomized study showed a success rate of only 6–19% [16]. The poor success was probably because all retractile testes had been excluded, and, consequently, this study represents the true outcome of hormonal treatment of undescended testis. Some authors now suggest using hormonal therapy to distinguish retractile from undescended testes [13].

A surgical algorithm is outlined in Fig. 15.1. As 80–90% of testes are palpable, the majority can be brought down by a simple orchidopexy. For the few that are intra-abdominal, there is considerable controversy about the best approach. The options include:

**1** The Jones repair, in which the testicular vessels are mobilized in the retroperitoneum up to their origin [13,17].
**2** The two-stage Fowler–Stephens operation, where the testicular vessels are first divided and then using the vasal blood supply the testis is brought into the scrotum [11,18].
**3** Autotransplantation of the testis with a microvascular anastomosis with the inferior epigastric vessels [19]. In postpubertal men with unilateral maldescent, the quality of the testis seldom warrants orchidopexy. Orchidectomy, with or without prosthetic implantation, is preferred [13]. In bilateral cases, an attempt may be made to bring one testis down to preserve natural testosterone production and the other may be removed.

## Outcome

### Fertility

The evidence strongly suggests that the undescended testis is infertile if untreated. It is much less certain to what extent the normally descended partner of an undescended testis is fertile, or what the effect of orchidopexy is. It is difficult to discover whether any group of men defined by a condition in infancy grows up to be fertile. Retrospective questionnaires have a response rate of about 50–60%. The investigation of patients in fertility clinics picks out only those who are infertile from a pool of indeterminate size. In addition, there are the usual difficulties in defining fertility. Much of the literature in this field considers only the quality of semen, which is a poor guide to fertility.

With a few poorly documented exceptions, men with untreated bilateral UDT are infertile. All of 17 men

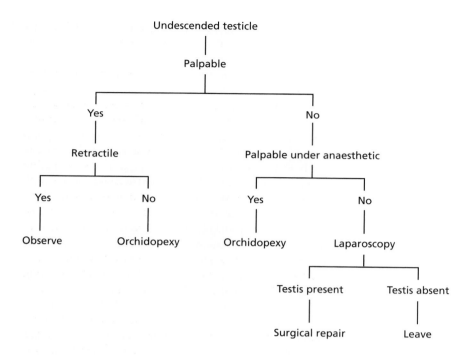

Undescended testicle

Palpable

Yes — No

Retractile — Palpable under anaesthetic

Yes — No    Yes — No

Observe — Orchidopexy    Orchidopexy — Laparoscopy

Testis present — Testis absent

Surgical repair — Leave

**Fig. 15.1.** Algorithm for the management of undescended testicle.

investigated by semen analysis or biopsy (admittedly in an infertility clinic) were sterile [20]. In a series of postpubertal men treated by orchidectomy for UDT, 36 of 52 testes had no germ cells on histology. Four per cent had carcinoma *in situ*. The higher the testis and the older the patient, the more severe were the histological changes. Twelve per cent of the patients presented with infertility (all having azoospermia), but the fertility of the other patients was not given [21].

In retrospective surveys, the incidence of infertility in men with treated bilateral maldescent is consistently higher than in those with unilateral maldescent [22]. There is a disproportionate number of men with bilateral UDT attending infertility clinics. In one large series, 6.25% of male attendees had a history of UDT, 60% of which were bilateral. In the men with bilateral maldescent, 80% were azoospermic [23]. Untreated unilateral UDT, on the other hand, is compatible with fertility, although there is still a disproportionate number of such men in infertility clinics who have abnormal sperm counts [20].

In a questionnaire survey of 363 men (from an original pool size that was not stated), a comparison was made with age-matched control subjects. It was found that the paternity rate in men with a permanent partner was the same in those with treated unilateral UDT as in the control subjects (73%). In the men with bilateral UDT, only 53% had children, and they appeared to have had more difficulty in the conception as shown by a longer 'trying time' [24].

Two studies have been performed on men with unilateral UDT of proven fertility who requested vasectomy. They were persuaded to have the vas of the normally descended testis tied first and the other side tied after an interval. Semen analysis between the operations was normal in only 1 of the 16 patients. This suggests that the undescended testis, even after orchidopexy, does not produce good sperm, at least when there is a normal testis in the scrotum [25,26]. It is compatible with the normal semen concentrations found in men with unilateral maldescent, regardless of the age of orchidopexy [27].

These observations are more in line with everyday experience than the rather gloomy view derived from a meta-analysis by Chilvers and Pike [28], who found that 43% of reported men with successfully treated UDT had azoospermia or oligozoospermia and that the same figure was found in untreated men.

Bilateral UDT are a more severe problem. Even with treatment, it is clear that there is a reduction in fertility. Aside from the disproportionate number of patients with this history in infertility clinics, up to 50% may have reduced sperm concentrations [27]. The observation that patients who were successfully treated by hCG injection rather than surgery is irrelevant as it may just be identifying a group of patients with retractile testes.

Experimentally, both children and rats with UDT have histological abnormalities on biopsy. In children, the numbers of germ cells and spermatogonia are reduced (or even absent) compared with normal [29]. It would appear that, before the first year of life, the biopsy appearances of unilateral UDT are similar to those of their normally descended pair. After 1 year of age, the histological fertility index deteriorates compared with both the descended pair and the expected for age [30].

In trans-scrotal rats, a mutant in which 85% have UDT, there is a good model for the condition in humans. Up to 14 days after birth, there is no difference in the histology of undescended and normal testes. Thereafter, the germ cells of the UDT deteriorate with an increase in Leydig cells. Early orchidopexy eliminates this deterioration [31].

When considering the effect of treatment, the age at which it is carried out is probably the most important factor. In the past, the surgery has been undertaken in mid- or late childhood, and it has been difficult to show any advantage for early surgery. In the series of Lee *et al.* [24] the distribution of patients with proven fertility could not be matched with the age at orchidopexy. However, that age ranged from 1 month to 15 years and only 21 of 184 patients were operated in the first 2 years of life.

In patients who were operated late (mean of 9.4 years), it has been suggested that semen quality can be improved by treatment with GnRH [32]. It remains to be seen whether this improvement will be maintained and translated into an improvement in paternity.

The present practice of paediatric surgeons is to perform orchidopexy in the first year or two of life. It will be some time before the results filter through to the adult population. However, with a cut-off age of 4 years for orchidopexy, it has been shown that no boy had severe impairment of testicular endocrine function or a sperm concentration below 25 million per millilitre [27]. This would be in line with the biopsy results and experimental findings.

It seems probable that men with unilateral UDT can have much the same fertility as normal men. Men with bilateral UDT, even with successful treatment, have a fertility rate of a half to two-thirds that of normal men.

## Testicular neoplasia

### Undescended testes

The majority of testicular neoplasms arise from the germ cells. It follows that gonads without germ cells cannot have such tumours, although they may develop one of the rare neoplasms arising from other cells. The most important group to consider is those who are born with UDT as these boys have an increased risk of germ cell neoplasia. The level of the risk is difficult to assess because of uncertainty about the true incidence of UDT and the variable (and rising) incidence of testis tumours in different countries. Furthermore, the original anatomical site probably affects the risk of the testis and whether the condition is unilateral or bilateral.

Sir Percival Pott apparently knew the increased risk in 1771 [12]. Three relatively early but much quoted studies gave a relative risk of 35–50 times normal [33–35]. However, more recent studies have given a much lower relative risk. Denmark has a particularly good cancer and population registry, and its data have a deserved reputation for accuracy.

Unfortunately, the incidence of germ cell neoplasia in Denmark is rising rapidly, so that the relative risk has constantly to be adjusted.

In a series of 509 boys with UDT treated between 1949 and 1960, the risk in boys with bilateral UDT was 9.3 times that of the age-matched population. Surprisingly, three of the four cases of neoplasia were seminomas occurring late in life, so that the risk was highest, on average, in the fourth decade of life [36]. There is a remarkable similarity in the relative risks in the majority of contemporary papers, but with wide confidence limits. The world mean relative risk for any UDT appears to be 5.4 with 95% confidence limits at 3.3 to 8.3 [28].

With a rising incidence of germ cell tumours, at least in Western Europe and the USA, it would be reasonable to expect the incidence in men with previous UDT to rise. It is therefore not surprising to find a newer study giving a relative risk of 7.5 for testicular cancer [37]. The most interesting feature of this study is that the relative risk of neoplasia in an UDT was greatly increased if the testis was biopsied (66.7 vs. 6.7). There was no clue in the operation notes of the orchidopexy to say why the biopsies had been carried out. The authors pointed out that there are two possible explanations: that biopsy does increase the risk of neoplasia, or that the surgeons have some means of identifying those patients who are at particular risk. All but one of the biopsies were normal. Whichever explanation is correct, it is worthy of further investigation.

It is possible that the infantile testis is vulnerable to even minor trauma. It has been shown that putting a suture through the testis to fix it in the scrotum at orchidopexy is the single most important prognostic factor for future infertility in boys with UDT. It is more significant even than the presence of bilateral maldescent [38]. The result of a biopsy of the testis at the time of orchidopexy does not alter the immediate management. It is not necessary to fix the testis in the scrotum with a suture. It is therefore better to avoid such trauma. Testicular biopsies should not be done at the time of orchidopexy, except as a part of a prospective study in which the prognostic information obtained would be of value.

The risk is higher when both testes are undescended. In the meta-analysis, the relative risk for those with bilateral UDT was 11.7 and for unilateral UDT 4.0 [28]. In the Danish study, the figures were 9.3 and 2.4 respectively. In unilateral cases, there is an increased risk of 1.7 for the normally descended testis [28]. Successful orchidopexy does not abolish the risk of neoplasia but does reduce it. Broadly speaking, the chance of later neoplasia in a boy born with unilateral UDT is one in 120 and with bilateral UDT is 1 in 44.

The higher the testis in the abdomen, the higher the risk. Smith [39] has quoted a figure of 1 in 20 but based on rather old data. Some intra-abdominal testes do not have germ cells and presumably do not develop tumours. On the other hand, in prune belly syndrome, where the testes are usually intra-abdominal, there have been three cases of neoplasia.

Carcinoma *in situ* of the testis is being found with increasing frequency in biopsies of UDT in the young. The higher the testis, the higher the incidence: 4 of 16 intra-abdominal testes, 3 of 44 inguinal testes and 1 of 30 normally descended testes in unilateral UDT in one series [40]. In a series of 300 Danish men (responders to a questionnaire to an original pool of 500), carcinoma *in situ* was found in five biopsies. In contrast, the same authors found no cases in the testes of 400 young men who died suddenly [41].

## Intersex

The other group of patients with an increased risk of testicular neoplasia is that with intersex. Management is frequently dictated by the possibility of malignancy. The majority are germ cell neoplasms, and so, again, some germ cells must be present in the gonad, even though primitive and small in number. The more dysplastic the germ cells, the higher the risk of neoplasia.

The highest risk is in poorly virilized 46,XY males with dysgenetic gonads. The babies are phenotypically female without genital ambiguity with normal internal female structures. With mixed gonadal dysgenesis, the genitalia are ambiguous and there is usually some fairly normal testicular tissue on one side. The gonads are either streaks or contain some testicular tissue and may be different on each side. The usual tumour is a gonadoblastoma. This is a mixed tumour of Sertoli cells and germ cells, with occasional Leydig cells. The gonadoblastoma never metastasizes and may even regress, but the germ cell portion becomes malignant in a third of cases. The endocrine cells may secrete active hormones, especially testosterone [42]. The tumours may occur, though rarely, *in utero* or in childhood [43], but the incidence rises rapidly after puberty and is highest at the usual age for germ cell tumours, the second and third decades.

In a series of 102 intersex patients at the Great Ormond Street Hospital for Children, 38 patients had gonadal dysgenesis, three of whom developed neoplasia at a median age of 2.5 years [44], but, in another series (of older patients), four of five cases occurred in the second decade [42]. Primary malignant dysgerminoma may occur occasionally in dysgenetic gonads. This is the name given to a seminoma arising in a gonad thought to be an ovary or of indeterminate type. In androgen insensitivity, especially in its complete form, seminomas occur. They are rare in childhood but commoner in the second and third decades. Three cases have been reported in siblings [45]. On testicular biopsy, abnormal cells can be seen that precede the development of carcinoma *in situ*. The finding of these cells in a male phenotype with 45,X/46,XY indicates a high risk of neoplasia developing and is an indication for gonadectomy [46].

True hermaphrodites, who account for about 10% of intersex patients, must, by definition, have both ovarian and testicular tissue. Most have a 46,XX karyotype but one-third have mosaic karyotypes. Testicular tissue develops in spite of the absence of a Y chromosome, usually in the form of an ovotestis. Those with a Y chromosome have a higher chance of having an identifiable testis and are at particular risk of having a germ cell neoplasm. A wide variety of tumours have been described, gonadoblastoma and seminoma/dysgerminoma being the commonest but teratoma, Brenner tumour and mucinous cystadenoma have also been reported [42]. In the ovarian gonad, a juvenile form of granulosa cell tumour occurs, 10% of which are malignant. They arise from ovarian mesenchyme and are oestrogen secreting. Characteristically, they recur many years after initial removal [47]. The management of the gonads in true hermaphroditism is dictated by the appropriateness of their type to the sex of rearing and by the risk of neoplasia. There is no increased risk of germ cell neoplasia in congenital adrenal hyperplasia (CAH), the commonest cause of intersex, but a scrotal mass may occur from gross hypertrophy of testicular adrenal rests [48].

## Hypospadias

Hypospadias is the result of hypoplasia of the ventral radius of the penis [49].

Embryologically, one can distinguish two types of hypospadias [50]: 25% involve the penile urethra, resulting from a failure of tubularization of the urethral plate (horizontal segment of the urogenital sinus) at the eleventh week of gestation. The remainder involve the glanular urethra, resulting from a failure occurring at 4 months of gestation.

The incidence of hypospadias seems to have doubled over the past 10 years in Western countries [51]. There is approximately 1 hypospadias for 300 male births. The exact cause of hypospadias is unknown, although endocrine and genetic factors are likely to be involved [52,53] and environmental factors may play a part.

Other research studies show that epidermal growth factors (EGFs) may be lacking on the ventral radius of the penis. In one study, the mean EGF value was low in skin adjacent to hypospadias defects compared with normal phallic skin, suggesting that inadequate expression of EGF may be related to the aetiology of hypospadias and to possible wound complications after surgery [54]. Some clinical and experimental studies are currently under way to introduce these missing factors after hypospadias surgery to improve the quality of healing [55].

Other studies in proximal hypospadias report enzymatic defects in the testosterone biosynthetic pathway [56]. Androgen receptor gene mutations seem rarely to be associated with isolated penile hypospadias [57–60]. Shima *et al.* [61] reported that the maximum testosterone response to human chorionic gonadotrophin stimulation was significantly decreased in boys with severe hypospadias in direct proportion to the degree of hypospadias. It does not seem that maternal serum human chorionic gonadotrophin during

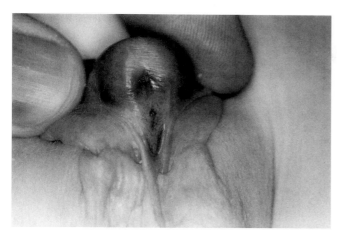

**Fig. 15.2.** Hypospadias showing the abnormal separation of the corpora spongiosum.

early pregnancy affects the formation of genitalia in boys [62]. Vascular defects could be involved in hypospadias as the frenular artery, which supplies the distal urethra, is constantly missing in boys with hypospadias.

Three associated anomalies are found in the hypospadiac penis: an ectopic opening of the urethral meatus, a ventral curvature of the penis (chordee) and a hooded foreskin with a marked excess of skin on the dorsal aspect of the penis and a lack of skin on the ventral. In fact, the chordee and the hooded foreskin are not constant, and one should be warned that a hypospadiac meatus may be found under a normally formed prepuce. Similarly, chordee may occur with a normally positioned meatus.

A careful examination of the ventral aspect of the penis shows that the corpus spongiosum, which normally surrounds the urethra, divides proximally to the ectopic urethral meatus into two pillars that extend laterally up to the glans cap (Fig. 15.2). The level of division of the corpus spongiosum is the best known criterion to define the severity of hypospadias. In fact, the position of the ectopic meatus is a poor indicator of severity since the urethra proximal to the meatus is often hypoplastic and also needs surgical reconstruction.

Penile chordee can be related to four different factors [63,64]. In 85% of cases it is related to the tethering of the shaft skin onto the underlying hypoplastic urethra and to the pillars of the divided spongiosum. In 10% of cases, the chordee is due to an abnormal tethering of the urethral plate onto the underlying corpora cavernosa and, in rare cases (5%), it is related also to asymmetrical development of the corpora cavernosa.

Hypospadias is usually isolated. Association with undescended testes has been reported in up to 10% of cases and should lead to endocrine and genetic investigation. Association with a utricular cavity sited at the back of the posterior urethra has been reported in 53% of cases of severe hypospadias and is another indication of possible hormonal impair-

ment. The utricular enlargement may be due to androgenic insufficiency during the critical period of organogenesis [65]. Scrotal transposition and micropenis can also be associated with hypospadias. Beyond the genitalia, hypospadias can be one aspect of a more complex syndrome, especially midline defects.

The inheritance of hypospadias is incompletely understood. It has been considered as an autosomal recessive condition but this has been questioned by Harris and Beaty [66], who suggest an autosomal dominant or co-dominant model. Whatever the mode of inheritance, the risk of hypospadias occurring in a brother or first-degree relative is 17–21% [67,68].

There are several classifications of hypospadias. In practice, one that can be used to decide surgical management is most useful [69] but there is no minor and major hypospadias. All cases are a surgical challenge, with many complications, even in the best hands.

In glanular hypospadias, the ectopic meatus lies on the glans. Although the abnormality may look quite minor, it can be associated with marked hypoplasia of the distal urethra and a glans tilt or chordee. This form is difficult to repair as expectations are high and the surgical techniques not entirely satisfactory. Hypospadias may be associated with a distal division of the corpus spongiosum associated with little or no chordee or with a proximal division of the corpus spongiosum associated with chordee. These abnormalities are often simpler to handle surgically, as techniques to correct the chordee and reconstruct a long length of urethra are well established.

The most challenging are patients who have already undergone several procedures that failed, leaving them with scarred tissues, abnormal meatus, strictures, urethral dehiscence, fistulae and, of course, bad cosmetic and psychological results.

## Surgical principles

Surgical techniques have been developing for more than 100 years but there is still no consensus and most paediatric urologists perform a single-stage hypospadias repair. However, some surgeons still recommend two-stage procedures [70].

In general, hypospadias surgery follows three main steps:
1 straightening the penis (i.e. correction of chordee);
2 reconstruction of the missing urethra (i.e. urethroplasty);
3 reconstruction of the tissues forming the ventral radius of the penis (i.e. glans, corpus spongiosum and skin).

## Correction of chordee

Degloving of the penile skin usually corrects the penile chordee related to the tethering of the ventral skin and to the two spongiosal pillars. If the chordee persists after degloving, freeing the urethral plate from the ventral surface of the corpora cavernosa from the glans cap down to the normal urethra surrounded by normal spongiosum allows a full straightening of the penis. In less than 5% of cases, the chordee still persists after these two manoeuvres and a dorsal plication of the corpora cavernosa is then needed [71].

## Urethroplasty

When the urethral plate (strip of urethral mucosa extending from the ectopic urethral meatus up the glans cap) [72] is fully dissected and the chordee fixed, the type of urethroplasty is decided. If the urethral plate is wide enough, it can be rolled to create a urethral tube (Thiersch–Duplay procedure) [73,74]. If the urethral plate is too narrow, a rectangle of tissue has to be isolated and applied to the urethral plate and stitched to its edges (onlay urethroplasty) [75–77]. This rectangle of tissue can either be from penile skin attached to the ventral edge of the ectopic urethral meatus (Mathieu flip-flap procedure) [78] or a pedicule of preputial mucosa (onlay island flap procedure) or a free graft of tissue, mainly buccal mucosa [79] (or, less frequently nowadays, bladder mucosa [80] or skin [81]). In rare cases, the urethral plate cannot be preserved, and a full substitution of the missing urethra has to be performed using a tube of pediculed preputial mucosa (Asopa–Duckett procedure) [82,83] or a tube of buccal mucosa.

Besides these standard procedures, other surgical techniques may be useful, such as the MAGPI (meatoplasty and glanuloplasty) reshaping of the glans for very distal hypospadias, although there is now less enthusiasm for this once popular [84] procedure. For the creation of a full length of urethra from urethral tissue alone, the plate may be split longitudinally and rolled into a tube (Snodgrass procedure [85]) or fully mobilized and then rolled (Koff procedure [86] and Turner–Warwick procedure). In total, more than 210 procedures have been described, which shows that none is completely satisfactory.

## The penile covering

Once the penis is straight and the urethra reconstructed, the next steps are the reconstruction of the new meatus (meatoplasty), the creation of a ventral glans (glanuloplasty) and a mucosal collar around it (Firlit procedure [87]), the reunion of the two spongiosal pillars over the neourethra (spongioplasty [88]) and the skin cover.

## Results

Both cosmetic and functional results have to be assessed after hypospadias surgery. A good result implies a slit-shaped meatus positioned at the top of the glans cap, a straight penis when erect, no redundant skin, regular suture lines, a straight and good urine stream with no spraying and no straining after one single operation.

The success rate by these criteria varies with the type of reconstruction and the experience of the surgeon. Hypospadias with a distal division of the corpus spongiosum can be corrected with a good result in over 90% of cases. When the division of the corpus spongiosum is proximal, a good result can be achieved in about 75–80% of cases. Buccal graft urethroplasties have good results (i.e. no further surgery) in only about 65% cases.

Success in glanular hypospadias is difficult to measure because parental expectations may not be achievable, even if there is a good technical result by surgical standards.

## Complications

The most common complication is an unsatisfactory cosmetic result with irregular suture lines, skin blobs and redundant ventral skin. When the ventral aspect of the glans is short and if there is no mucosal collar around the glans, the cosmetic result is disappointing (Fig. 15.3). The surgeon's and the patient's views on the cosmetic result are often very different [89].

Fistulae are the second most common complication and present with an abnormal stream or drops coming from the under-surface of the penis. Although late fistulation can occur, it is usually a complication of the first postoperative month. Fistulae may heal spontaneously when small and not associated with an urethral stricture but otherwise require surgical closure.

Strictures are less common nowadays as paediatric urologists tend to avoid circular anastomosis and prefer onlay urethroplasties. Meatal stenoses are usually simple to handle by performing a surgical meatal revision. Proximal stenoses are always severe and respond only transiently to urethral dilatation, which is an unacceptable manoeuvre in children. A repeat urethroplasty is often necessary to relieve the obstruction. Prolonged obstruction may cause abnormal bladder behaviour with high pressure voiding and eventually upper

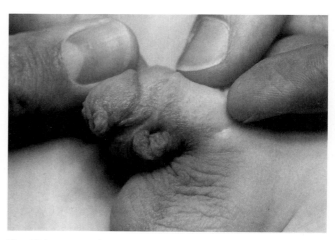

**Fig. 15.3.** Hypospadias: poor cosmetic result after multiple procedures.

urinary tract damage. It is therefore important to recognize urethral strictures and treat them promptly. Regular urine flow measurements are recommended after hypospadias surgery, especially if the child has to strain to empty his bladder.

Other complications such as urethral dehiscence, urethral prolapse, urethrocele, persistent chordee and urethral balanitis xerotica obliterans have also been reported.

Hypospadias surgery remains very challenging, with a significant complication rate even in the best hands. This surgery should be performed exclusively by surgeons experienced in the field. The complication rate may be reduced by the development of laser welding [90], which could replace sutures. The great progress that hypospadias surgeons expect is the introduction of preoperative hormonal or growth-factor stimulation. It is clear that the factors responsible for healing located on the ventral surface of the penis are deficient or insufficient. Pre-, peri- and postoperative therapy may considerably change the outcomes of this surgery [91–96].

The main problem in this type of surgery is to find a tissue to replace the missing urethra (neither skin nor buccal mucosa nor bladder mucosa are entirely satisfactory), and it is to be hoped that urothelial cell cultures will provide an easy to handle material for urethroplasty [97,98].

## Hypospadias: long-term outcomes

The techniques for the correction of hypospadias have changed considerably over the last 40 years. The operations on adults whose sexual function can be investigated are obsolete. There seems no doubt that the cosmetic results have improved, but the sexual results remain as controversial as ever. The greatest difficulty lies in the identification of a satisfactory control group to compare with the hypospadiac patient. Without control subjects it is impossible to know whether the myriad of sexual problems that have been identified are caused by the hypospadias.

### Success of the repair

Urologists are aware of the wide range of size and appearance of the penis. The growth of the penis with age has been documented (see the section 'Micropenis'), but its normal appearance has not. It has been established, however, that the meatus is not always at the tip of the penis. Thirteen per cent of apparently normal men have a hypospadiac meatus, and it is in the middle third of the glans in a further 32%. Most of these men thought they were normal, all voided normally and had sexual intercourse [99].

The cosmetic results are entirely observer dependent. Surgeons reviewing their own results have a somewhat rosy view of the outcome. For example, in a personal series of 220 men reviewed at a mean age of 18.4 years, the surgeon reported a good outcome with all patients having a straight erection and a normal, formed urinary stream. Unfortunately, 65% still had a degree of hypospadias that would, by current standards, require correction.

When there is an independent review, a more realistic outcome is seen. Summerlad [100] examined 60 patients operated by his predecessors with apparently successful repairs. He found that the meatus was rarely at the tip of the penis, and 22% had chordee even when flaccid. Almost none of the patients could void normally and 16 of 60 could not stand to void into a toilet bowl.

The patients themselves have an even gloomier view of the appearance. Up to 80% of adolescent patients are dissatisfied with their penile appearance, although only 38–44% sufficiently so to want further surgery [70,101]. There is also a difference in results depending on the attitude of the community to circumcision: in countries where childhood circumcision is routine, results are perceived to be better than in those where it is uncommon.

When there is a direct comparison between the opinions of the patient and the surgeon, there is almost no agreement. In a series where eight features of the penis were scored from 1 to 4 by patient and surgeon, the best outcome would have been a genital satisfaction score of 32 and the worst of 8. Surgeons gave a mean score of 29.1 and the patients gave a mean of 25.1, a difference that was statistically significant [89].

It is important to note, however, that three of the eight features were concerned with penile size, which cannot be altered by surgery. For the uncorrectable, size-related features, the patients gave a mean satisfaction score of 3.1 (out of four), whereas the surgeons gave a score of 3.9. For the features related to the surgical result the patient score was 3.2 and the surgeons' was 3.5. Much of the dissatisfaction seems to have been related to the circumcised appearance in a society where circumcision is unusual and is perceived to shorten the penis [89].

### Sexual function

Curiously, sexual function does not seem to be related to the success of the repair, although it is probably related to the degree of severity of the original hypospadias. All reported series record that most men have sexual intercourse, even though the quality and quantity may be difficult to decipher from the data. Figures for successful intercourse range from 77% to 90% [70,102,103]. Even in the most severely affected individuals intercourse still occurs. In a series of 19 patients born with ambiguous genitalia, subsequently determined to be caused by perineal hypospadias, it was reported that 63% had had intercourse. However, only four had a regular partner [104].

Two studies have shown that there was no difference in the number of sexual episodes or their perceived quality between hypospadiac subjects and control subjects (herniorrhaphy patients and circumcision patients respectively) [101,105]. This was despite the observation that the hypospadiac subjects had significantly more erectile problems such as curvature, shortness and pain than the controls [105].

When the components of male sexual function are analysed in more detail, differences from normal do appear. Chordee and other erectile deformities are more common than would be expected. In early series it seems that chordee was almost never corrected adequately in proximal hypospadias. Up to 60% of patients with penile and all patients with scrotal and perineal hypospadias had chordee in Kenawi's [103] series.

More recent series reporting on the current style of repair have much better results, especially with the use of artificial erections during surgery. Bracka [70] reported an 18% incidence of chordee in adult follow-up. Whatever else may be said about current techniques of hypospadias repair, it is usually possible to correct the chordee.

Ejaculation is a complex function. It begins with the formation of a bolus of semen in the prostatic urethra. The bolus is then expelled forcefully by the contraction of the prostatic urethral muscles against a closed bladder neck. Thus far, the hypospadiac male should be normal unless there is a major prostatic anomaly associated with intersexuality. The next stage is the expulsion of the semen by the bulbospongiosus muscle. In very proximal hypospadias, this muscle is likely to be absent. It is therefore not surprising to find that ejaculation is unsatisfactory in 63% of severe hypospadiac subjects, even though orgasm is normal in most [104]. Poor surgical results from the distal urethroplasty may cause a baggy urethra or even a diverticulum, further slowing the ejaculation. In more general reviews, authors state that ejaculation is normal although, by asking the right questions, Bracka [70] found that 33% had 'dribbling ejaculation' and 4% were dry.

Satisfaction with intercourse is particularly difficult to measure and series without control subjects are valueless. Most teenagers, exploring their sexuality, have anxieties that are unrelated to any penile abnormality, although a penis that is perceived to be abnormal may get the blame.

Where the result of surgery has been poor, with chordee and scars causing pain, it is reasonable to accept that intercourse will be unsatisfactory. Size may also be a cause of dissatisfaction, but even patients with micropenis can have normal intercourse. The hypospadiac penis is often said to be short. In part this may be because of the circumcised appearance, especially in countries where infant circumcision is unusual. However, where a formal measurement has been made, 20% of hypospadiac penises were below the 10th centile. The finding was most marked in the adolescents with four of seven being below the 10th centile [89].

In terms of episodes of sexual activity, number of partners, sexual problems and libido, there is no significant difference between hypospadiac subjects and control subjects (herniorrhaphy or circumcision patients) [89,105]. Similarly, there is little difference in the age of sexual debut compared either with control subjects or with established community norms.

There is conflict over the effect of the success of the repair. Bracka [70] made the interesting observation that those who were satisfied with the results of their repair had a sexual debut at a mean of 15.6 years of age, whereas those who were dissatisfied had a debut at 19 years. On the other hand, it has been reported that in a group of boys whose 'curative repair' was delayed beyond 12 years, 50% had their sexual debut before the definitive surgery [106]. It could be said that the experience of intercourse, acknowledged by the authors to be less satisfactory, drew attention to the shortcomings of the repair.

## Endocrine function

In uncomplicated cases of hypospadias it seems likely that the sex hormones are normal. In Bracka's [70] series, luteinizing hormone (LH), follicle-stimulating hormone (FSH) and testosterone were measured only in the first 100 patients because they were all normal. There do seem to be exceptions to this observation. In a series of 16 adults with mild hypospadias, the mean levels of LH and FSH were higher than in normal adults, but not outside the normal range. Testosterone concentrations were normal. Five patients who had grossly abnormal parameters distorted the means, but three of them were fertile [107]. Low levels of 5α-reductase have been reported [108].

## Fertility

It seems probable that boys with uncomplicated hypospadias are normally fertile. There have been no formal studies of a large cohort of hypospadiac patients. There is no excess of hypospadiac subjects in infertility clinics. In an apparently unselected group of 169 patients, 50% were found to have a sperm count below 50 million/mL and 25% below 20 million. More than half of those with the lowest sperm counts had associated anomalies such as UDT, which might have accounted for the poor result [70]. In a detailed study of 16 hypospadiac men, true oligo-astheno-teratozoospermia (OATS) was only found in the two patients with perineal hypospadias; low counts were seen in one of three with glanular and two of six with penile hypospadias, but other parameters were normal. With two minor exceptions of slightly elevated LH, all the patients had normal hormone profiles [109]. Perineal hypospadias is frequently associated with other genital anomalies and intersex, and it is not surprising to find a high incidence of azoospermia [110].

## Psychological consequences

There is much debate about the psychological consequences of hypospadias and nowhere is there a greater need for control patients in the analyses. The problem is the selection of the control subjects. In the studies quoted above, the control patients had had circumcision or a hernia repair [101,105]. In the very extensive psychological reviews undertaken by Berg *et al.* [111–113], the control patients had had appendicectomies. Faults can obviously be found with all of these control subjects, none having undergone the same scale of surgery as hypospadiac subjects. On the other hand, there is no other condition that could be compared with hypospadias in terms of diagnosis and surgical trauma.

From the uncontrolled series, it seems that about 20% of adults remembered their surgery as being traumatic [70,100]. A third of men avoided changing in public [100].

In the controlled studies, the main problems of hypospadiac subjects lie in sexual development discussed above. In Finland, where there is conscription, there is no difference in the success rate between members of the armed forces and in men who are cohabiting [105]. Similarly, there were no differences in IQ, general health or socioeconomic background in the Swedish men reviewed by Berg *et al.* In the Dutch study, there was no evidence that hypospadiac men had worse psychosocial adjustment than the age-matched control subjects [114].

It has been found in one study, however, that hypospadiac subjects are underachievers. Berg and Berg [112] found that they had lower ego strength and poor utilization of their mental resources. Their levels of hostility, general anxiety and castration were higher and they had lower self-esteem than the control appendicectomy patients. In childhood the boys had been shy, timid and isolated. As adults they showed neurotic (but not psychotic) disturbances and formed abnormal social and emotional relationships. They had less rewarding and less demanding jobs. Eventually, like the men in other studies, they did establish secure and long-lasting sexual partnerships. The outcome was not related to the original severity of the hypospadias [108,111–113].

These studies are open to some criticism, and the picture they paint is somewhat out of line with ordinary clinical observation. It appears that the authors anticipated psychological morbidity and set out to prove it. The majority of patients appear to have had a poor surgical result. Nonetheless, they are careful and detailed studies that cannot be dismissed out of hand. There is some corroborating evidence from similar (but less detailed) studies on severe hypospadiac subjects; however, many of the patients had ambiguous genitalia or even Reifenstein syndrome [104,110].

## Micropenis

There is a difficulty over the definition of micropenis. Strictly speaking, the term should be used only for patients with a recognizable endocrinopathy affecting all androgen-sensitive organs. For patients without a defined diagnosis, the better term is small penis, although this could include even the malformed penis [115]. As far as this section is concerned, the outcome is that of the small penis, rather than of the original diagnosis.

A growth curve has been drawn for the penis and, although it was based disproportionately on Caucasians, it has stood the test of time [116]. A micropenis is normally formed and more than 2.5 standard deviations (SD) below the mean stretched length for age. A micropenis at birth ranges from 1.75 to 2.7 cm, depending on the reference standards used [117,118].

## Penile enlargement

Early management is that of the underlying condition and the growth of the penis may be normal. Once the boy has passed puberty, further growth of the penis is unlikely. Furthermore, from the data available it would seem that where early androgen treatment has produced some penile growth, the position on the centile chart is not maintained. In other words, the penis is capable of only one growth spurt in response to androgens, and if that is used in childhood puberty will not have a further stimulating effect [119]. In rat experiments, early androgen treatment produces the shortest penis in adults, whereas treatment delayed until puberty or adolescence results in normal adult length [120].

Dihydrotestosterone cream has been used to stimulate penile growth. Both the penis and prostate show rapid growth. In a series of 22 children there was a mean increase in length of 53% in the first month and a further 18% in the second month of treatment. The series included four boys who had failed to respond to testosterone treatment [121]. Late treatment of a 12-year-old and a 17-year-old boy have been reported, but the responses were poor [122].

Surgical enlargement of the penis is limited by the inability to make erectile tissue. It is possible to gain length by releasing the corpora from the pubic bone by dividing the suspensory ligament, but the price is some loss of erectile stability. A new penis can be formed from skin flaps using the techniques developed for gender reassignment. Good technical results have been reported in boys with micropenis using both groin flaps and a microsurgical transfer of a forearm flap [123,124]. The microsurgical technique is claimed to allow return of sensation and even, with time, of erogenous sensation. No attempt was made to insert prostheses for erection, and there is no report on the sexual results (if any). Our opinion is that a small penis with natural erections is likely to allow better sexual function than a large but sexually insensate one.

## Sexuality

Sexuality with a small penis may be complex because of the underlying endocrinopathy. In those who do have androgens, either natural or medical, there is some conflict in the literature on the success of sexual function. Reilly and

Woodhouse [119] investigated 12 postpubertal patients with micropenis from a variety of causes using a semistructured questionnaire. Patients were included even if there was associated hypospadias, providing the penis conformed to the definition of micropenis. In spite of the very small penile shaft, even with erection, sexual function was claimed by the patients to be satisfactory. The views of their partners were not obtained.

The most surprising finding was the firmness with which they were established in the male role. None wanted gender reassignment and none cross-dressed. They regarded themselves as successful in sexual partnerships, which were stable and long-lasting. All were heterosexual, all had erections and orgasms and 11 of 12 ejaculated. Three-quarters had debut sexual intercourse at a mean age of 16.4 years (range 13.5–20 years). Vaginal penetration was usual, but there was an experimental attitude to positions and technique. Some men attributed the stability of their partnership to the extra care and trouble that had to be taken with intercourse. One had fathered a child [119].

It is difficult to be certain whether these data reflect reality as there is little supporting evidence in the literature. The patients reported by Money *et al.* [125] appear to have been less successful, but only three of nine complied with endocrine therapy, which may have altered androgen levels and thus libido. Five demonstrated normal male behaviour and six were heterosexual (one with sadistic tendencies). Three were homosexual and two had doubts about their male gender identity. Nonetheless, in strictly physical terms, they functioned well with normal erections [125].

Patients with perineal hypospadias, small penis and bilateral UDT may be in a similar situation. In a group of 18 adults thought to have ambiguous genitalia at birth, the sexual outcome was found to be poor. Eleven had 46,XY karyotype, six 45,X/46,XY and one 46,XX. Fifteen were satisfied with erections and orgasm, but only seven had ejaculated. Although 12 had had intercourse, in only six had it been within the previous 3 months [104].

It has been said that males with inadequate genitalia who are raised as males (especially those with cloacal exstrophy) grow up to be psychologically disturbed or even criminal. McClorie *et al.* [126] recommend that those whose stretched penile length is less than 2 cm after 1 month of treatment with testosterone should be reassigned as female. In his series of 25 cases of cloacal exstrophy, seven were raised as males. None of the three males reaching puberty had satisfactory sexual function, and two had spent long periods in psychiatric institutions or correctional establishments.

### Gender reassignment

Infants with intersex present one of the greatest challenges a paediatrician can face. In considering the sexual outcome in these and other men with gross genital anomalies, it is impor-tant to remember that there is no 'right answer'. Even with the most careful counselling and psychological care, 39% of children develop one or more general psychological disorders, regardless of the sex of rearing. Psychological intervention from birth reduces but does not abolish the problem [127].

Individuals must be helped to achieve that which is possible with the structures available. It is a mistake to amputate sexually sensitive organs without a definite medical reason. Furthermore, it is naïve to think that female sexuality is so simple that inadequate male genitalia can be 'cured' by gender reassignment: there is no evidence to show that the outcome of this policy is satisfactory. Indeed, evidence is emerging to suggest that the outcome is poor, and many individuals with ambiguous genitalia would prefer to keep that which they have, rather than have bits reconstructed to produce a copy of a specific sex [128].

It is difficult to know whether any society could cope with the idea of a child of undefined sex as Diamond [129] has suggested and as is vigorously championed by the Intersex Society of North America [130]. The entire structure of family, school and social life is built around the division into boys and girls. Failure to conform to such stereotypes would lack the support of parents [131] and might generate its own psychological morbidity. If surgical assignment of gender is to wait until the child has developed a gender identity, it follows that an undefined sex has to be accepted to some extent, at least in childhood. It would seem that such an arrangement is found in Papua New Guinea. There is a sizeable cohort of children with 5α-reductase deficiency that is recognized at birth; they are reared as a special group of males known as 'kwalatmala', but this policy is based on previous experience that the apparently female infant will 'become a man' at puberty rather than having a discrete third gender [132]. The same is true in the Dominican Republic.

Regardless of decisions made at birth, sympathetic support is required throughout childhood and adolescence [127]. Those who exhibit gender behaviour different from that assigned should not be regarded as abnormal, but adolescents who develop gender identity disorder (an artificial concept if the gender was undefined originally) should be fully supported in deciding to change assignment. It is particularly unhelpful to call sexual activity with individuals of the same sex 'homosexual behaviour' (as has been suggested in a review article) when the intersex individual is uncertain of a gender [133].

## Female

## Gonads

### Ovarian cysts

Cysts in the neonatal period were in the past considered rare but, with the advent of prenatal ultrasound, detection is much more frequent. The cysts are of germinal or Graafian origin and can be extremely mobile. Differential diagnosis includes urachal cysts, hydrocolpos and distal megaureter. The majority of these cysts resolve spontaneously during the neonatal period as, presumably, they are hormonally driven. As a general rule, cysts less than 5 cm in diameter that are asymptomatic can be managed conservatively with ultrasound follow-up. Larger cysts or those causing symptoms due to haemorrhage or infarction should be removed. Ovarian tissue should be conserved, although if torsion has already occurred it may prove to be impossible.

Functional ovarian cysts can occur at any time during female life. Follicular cysts are usually unilocular and lined with granulosa cells. Treatment is as described above with expectant management most appropriate for smaller asymptomatic cysts. Corpus luteum cysts occur after puberty. They can resolve spontaneously but are prone to rupture and bleeding and may present acutely. In McCune–Albright syndrome ovarian cysts may vary in size [134].

## Ovarian tumours

The commonest benign tumour in girls is a teratoma. They are small and can be bilateral in up to 15% of patients. Because of the small risk of malignant transformation they should be removed, the ovarian tissue being preserved if at all possible. Serous and mucinous cystadenomas are not common in children but can be found in older adolescents. They can be large and symptomatic and should be removed. Gonadoblastomas are rare and usually arise from dysgenetic gonads, often in a girl with an XY karyotype or Y-chromosome fragment. They are usually benign but can contain germ cells that subsequently become malignant. Thecomas are rare but can cause precocious puberty because of oestrogen secretion.

Malignant ovarian tumours in childhood are usually of germ cell origin. Treatment in a specialist centre is essential to achieve cure but also, if possible, to maintain fertility. Dysgerminoma is the commonest and treatment is initially operative. The tumour however, is very chemo- and radiosensitive and the prognosis is good. Endodermal sinus tumours are less common. They are extremely aggressive and treatment is surgical followed by aggressive chemotherapy.

## Genitalia

### Feminizing genitoplasty

Feminizing genitoplasty involves three procedures, a reduction in clitoral size, creation of a perineal vagina and formation of labia minora and majora. Feminizing genitoplasty may be necessary in a variety of endocrine and non-endocrine disorders, the most common being congenital adrenal hyperplasia. Regardless of the underlying cause, the surgical management remains similar.

Reduction of clitoral size may be necessary in some girls to normalize appearance and to aid development. This can be performed surgically by recessing the clitoris or by excision of clitoral corporal tissue. In less severe cases, it is possible to leave the clitoris, although enlarged, and wait for the patient's decision. Clitoral recession involves hiding the corporal bodies under the mons pubis or pubic rami, so reducing the external clitoral appearance. This can be used for minor cases of clitoromegaly, if required. For more severe cases, clitoral erection after recession is painful and results in a bulge below the mons. Consequently, clitoral recession is used rarely, except in minor cases, when observation might be more prudent.

Clitoral reduction is achieved by reducing corporal length either by plicating the corpora or, more commonly, by amputating the middle portion of the corpora and performing a corpora-corporal anastomosis. The glans of the clitoris is also reduced either by removing a midline wedge or by removing two lateral wedges of glanular tissue [135]. Before reducing the corpora, it is important to identify and dissect the neurovascular bundles supplying the glans so that sexual sensation is not diminished after surgery. When the clitoris has been reduced, a hood of shaft skin is used partially to cover the glans.

Labial reconstruction is performed using the available phallic shaft skin to create labia minora and the labioscrotal folds are used to create the labia majora [135,136].

### Vaginal reconstruction

Children born with ambiguous genitalia and vaginal anomalies range from girls with a short urogenital sinus and low confluence of the vagina and urethra to boys with severe undervirilization requiring a change of sex of rearing and no vagina. Operations to deal with these problems are varied. Broadly they can be divided into three: low vaginal repair, high vaginal repair and vaginal reconstruction. The type of repair used is dependent on the presence or absence of the vagina and the distance between the perineum and the confluence of the vagina and urogenital sinus. If the common channel is less than 3–4 cm, a low vaginal repair can be performed; greater than this and a high vaginal repair is necessary [137,138]. Endoscopy is therefore mandatory in all patients before surgical reconstruction [139].

#### *Low vaginal repair*
Low vaginal repairs are frequently combined with clitoral reduction procedures in patients with congenital adrenal hyperplasia. There are two commonly used techniques: posterior vaginal skin flap and, more recently, total urogenital mobilization.

A posterior vaginal skin flap is performed by creating an inverted U-shaped skin flap, with the apex situated over the future site of the vaginal orifice. Once the flap has been formed, the urogenital sinus is opened posteriorly until the vagina is identified. The apex of the skin flap is then rotated up to meet the posterior part of the vagina and sutured in place [140]. This technique creates a wide open vaginal orifice on the perineum, but half the vaginal circumference is made up of non-mucus-producing skin, which may produce both cosmetic and long-term functional complications.

Total urogenital mobilization, originally described for the urogenital repair of cloacal anomalies [137], has been adapted for the repair of the urogenital sinus associated with CAH [141,142]. In this technique, the whole of the urogenital sinus is mobilized from the perineum with no effort to separate the urethra from vagina. When the vaginal confluence has been mobilized, the common channel is excised and the individual urethral and vaginal orifices sutured [137]. This has the advantage that the vagina is created completely of vaginal tissue with no skin flap. There is the potential risk of stricture but, in Pena's [142] series of 43 girls, there have been no strictures.

### High vaginal repair

In a small number of girls, the vagina enters the urogenital sinus close to the urinary sphincter mechanism. Low vaginal techniques are inadequate in these patients. One method of repair involves a vaginal pull down and a variety of skin flaps to produce a skin-lined distal vagina [143]. There have been many modifications [136,144] of this method, which involve splitting the urogenital sinus posteriorly up to the vaginal orifice, suturing phallic shaft skin to the lateral sides of the opened urogenital sinus and tubularization to create the distal vagina [136].

Rarely, in very high lesions it is necessary to open the bladder to identify the vaginal entrance into the urogenital sinus [144]. Other methods of identifying and dissecting these very high lesions involve putting the patient prone and using the posterior approach first described by Pena and deVries [145] and subsequently modified [146]. All these methods are extremely challenging and require considerable surgical experience.

### Vaginal replacement

When the vagina is absent or very shortened, vaginal replacement is necessary. Vaginal agenesis is usually associated with an absent or poorly developed uterus. If a uterus is present but the vagina absent or imperforate, urgent problems with non-drainage of menstrual loss can arise. Presentation can be during childhood, particularly if part of a complex condition. Presentation in adolescence with primary amenorrhoea is also a common feature.

### Mayer–Rokitansky–Kuster–Hauser syndrome

This condition has an estimated incidence of 1:20 000 [147]. The commonest presentation is with primary amenorrhoea. The external genitalia and pubertal development are normal, but the vagina and uterus are absent. The diagnosis is made on ultrasound scan. Laparoscopy is rarely necessary. The uterus may exist as very rudimentary horns lying either side of the pelvic wall. Further investigations will reveal a normal female karyotype and normal ovaries in terms of site and function. The aetiology of this condition is as yet unknown, although familial cases have been described. Up to 40% of these women have urinary tract malformations, which may be minor or significant, and skeletal anomalies are present in up to 12%.

The psychological impact of this condition is enormous. The news that infertility is inevitable is deeply disturbing both to the patient and to her parents. Initial management should be geared towards exploring and trying to come to terms with the diagnosis. The vagina is often short, and further intervention is usually necessary before a normal sex life is possible. The use of vaginal dilators is the first line of management before surgical vaginal replacement is considered.

### Androgen insensitivity syndrome

The genetics and endocrinology of this condition are discussed in Chapter 6. The vagina is blind ending and usually shortened. The length of the vagina is variable; it may be just a skin dimple or may be several centimetres long. It is often possible to create a vagina by progressive dilatation, and this should always be tried before reconstructive surgery is considered.

## Treatment of vaginal agenesis

Vaginal dilators were first used in the treatment of vaginal agenesis in 1938. Frank described the use of graduated glass dilators as a non-surgical technique to produce an artificial vagina [148]. Since its description, it remains the technique of first choice. The repeated insertion of graduated dilators over a period of 2–3 months allows development of a vagina (Fig. 15.4). The technique is to apply gentle pressure and use the dilators regularly for 30 min three times a day. Once the vagina is capacious enough to allow intercourse, the dilators can be discontinued, as intercourse itself will stretch the vagina. The main key to success is the motivation of the patient, and success rates of 78% having 'normal sexual function' have been reported [149]. Methods to try to improve the technique such as a specially modified bicycle seat have been used with some success. Failure with dilators leads to surgical options.

## Surgical management

Williams vulvovaginoplasty was described in 1964 [150] but is rarely used nowadays. It involves using the labia majora to make a tubular horizontal vagina that is essentially external to the body. The surgery is simple and relatively non-invasive and may be most suitable where dissection to form a neovagina is impossible. Satisfactory results have been

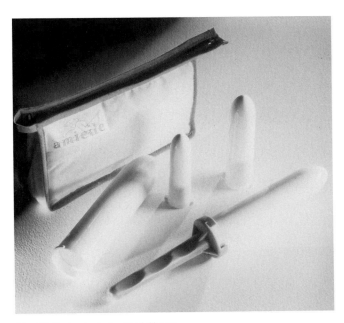

**Fig. 15.4.** Graduated vaginal dilators.

reported [151], but the vagina may still be short and the fact that it is external may mean there is not a real feeling of penetration during intercourse. It is possible that it allows for better clitoral stimulation, but there are few long-term follow-up data available.

The Vecchietti technique combines elements of surgery and vaginal dilatation. The technique relies on the principle of continuous pressure to form a vagina. An acrylic olive applies the pressure placed at the vaginal dimple. Threads from the olive are passed through the potential neovaginal space through the abdominal wall and connected to a traction device. The device is tightened over a period of 8–10 days. Recent modifications include performing the procedure laparoscopically, thus avoiding a laparotomy and prolonged hospital stay [152,153]. Reported success rates are high, although there are no long-term follow-up data available yet.

Split skin graft vaginoplasty is probably the most widely used technique [154,155]. An H-shaped incision is made over the vaginal dimple. Dissection is then performed between the bladder and rectum to form a neovagina. Morbidity is low, as the dissection is all extraperitoneal, although care must be taken with the angle of dissection to avoid damage to adjacent organs. A median raphe of tissue is encountered and must be divided. The next step is to line the cavity with a split skin graft. The cavity must then be kept open by a vaginal mould that is sutured into place. The mould is changed under general anaesthetic 1 week after the original surgery and then left in place for 6 weeks, except for cleaning.

Once the mould is removed, the patient must use vaginal dilators regularly. The duration of dilator use is not clear, but as stenosis is a major complication they should probably be used indefinitely unless replaced by regular intercourse. Complications include contraction of the graft and dyspareunia. The vagina may also be dry and require lubrication. The neovagina is at risk of premalignant and malignant change [156]. Good sexual function is reported in 80–90% of patients [149]. There are few long-term follow-up data available. Cali and Pratt [157] reported on 113 patients who were between 1 and 37 years old and had undergone McIndoe vaginoplasty. Of these, 90% were satisfied with sexual function, although 42% had some contracture of the vagina.

Other tissues such as amnion have also been used to line the neovagina [158]. Amnion can be obtained at elective caesarean section and avoids the disadvantage of scarring at the donor site. Good success rates have been reported in the short term [149,159], although dyspareunia is a problem. Amnion donation is, however, controversial and complicated to organize. Because of the risk of infection, the collected amnion should be frozen and stored. It is then cultured and, if sterile, can be used.

Peritoneum has been used to line a neovagina [160]. A space is created (as in the McIndoe procedure) and then an abdominal approach is used to free a cylinder of peritoneum and bring it down to line the neovagina. The top end of the vagina is then closed. Small series have produced good long-term results, although stenosis is again a problem necessitating the long-term use of vaginal dilators. Ward *et al.* [161] reported that 20 out of 21 women undergoing the procedure reported satisfactory coitus.

Different parts of the intestine in varying surgical modifications have been used as vaginal replacement. Baldwin [162] in 1904 used a loop of ileum. The complications surrounding the first few cases included death, and this led to the procedure being abandoned for nearly 60 years. Pratt [163], however, modified the operation and used sigmoid colon with success. The Ober–Meinreiken operation (also known as the Schubert–Schmidt procedure) used a loop of caecum to replace the vagina after exenteration for cancer, and this procedure has also been used in the treatment of intersex conditions. All bowel segment vaginoplasties require an abdominal and perineal approach, and a loop of bowel is brought down while retaining its blood supply. The distal end is sutured to the introitus, and the proximal end is closed. This type of surgery is indicated in patients who have extensive pelvic surgery and where dissection to form a neovagina by any other means is impossible. This would include major pelvic anomalies such as cloacal exstrophy as well as those who have failed with other simpler procedures.

The major advantage of this procedure is that contracture does not occur and dryness is not a problem. A good length of vagina can be achieved. The patients do, however, need to douche regularly as mucus discharge is a persistent and sometimes distressing problem. The vagina can prolapse outwards and can have an unsightly 'stoma-like' appearance. Adenocarcinoma of bowel segment vaginoplasties has also

**Table 15.2.** Commonest used techniques for vaginal replacement

| Method | Grade of surgery | Successful intercourse (%) [Ref. no.] | Number of patients and mean length of follow-up | Advantages | Disadvantages |
|---|---|---|---|---|---|
| Vaginal dilators | None | 46 [149] | 21 patients 7 months | No surgery | Contracture Dryness Requires motivation |
| Veccietti | Intermediate (laparoscopic) | 100 [153] | 6 patients 22 months | | Contracture Dryness |
| Williams | Minor | 100 [151] | 3 patients Follow-up not given | No contracture Non-invasive Good clitoral stimulation | Horizontal angle No feeling of penetration |
| McIndoe | Intermediate | 79 [157] | 71 patients 19 years | | Contracture Dryness Malignancy risk Donor site scarring |
| Davidov | Major | 98 [161] | 21 patients Follow-up not given | | Contracture |
| Amnion | Intermediate | 100 [159] | 15 patients 12 months | | Contracture ?Infection risk |
| Intestinal segment | Major | 80 | 10 patients 20.7 years | No contracture No dryness | May compromise bowel function Malignancy risk Mucus Stoma appearance and prolapse |

been reported [164]. Long-term good success in terms of sexual function have been reported in small studies [165,166].

## Sexual life after genital reconstruction

There are few data on long-term sexual function after reconstructive surgery of the genitalia. The evaluation of 'success rates' in vaginoplasty is difficult to standardize, and many papers do not specify their end points. Papers report 'normal' intercourse or 'normal' vaginal length without describing what they mean by 'normal'. In addition, most studies are small and follow-up periods short.

Clearly, the external appearance should be cosmetically acceptable, and full penetration without causing pain is essential. Other aspects such as orgasm and sensation are difficult to assess. It is impossible to separate physical difficulties from the psychological and psychosexual effects of the disease requiring genital surgery in the first place. Other associated problems may have a major impact on sexual response, and these include XY karyotype or infertility. If the uterus is present and functional, fertility will also be an aspect to consider when evaluating success. Comparison between

non-surgical use of vaginal dilators and different surgical methods is also imperative. Table 15.2 presents a comparison of the most frequently used methods of vaginal replacement with the success rates and complications.

It is clear that there are not enough follow-up data to counsel patients effectively about the choice of surgery. Some patients may prefer, on the basis of the above information, not to have surgery at all. Further long-term follow-up of psychological, sexual and gynaecological function following vaginal replacement is an essential next step in improving our management of this complex problem.

## Other congenital genital anomalies

### Buried penis

Buried penis is a congenital anomaly caused by a defect of the penile skin shaft associated with an abnormal tethering of the penis to the prepubic region, causing entrapment within the prepubic subcutaneous tissue of an otherwise normal penis. Various degrees of entrapment exist. This anomaly is often associated with a quite redundant prepubic fat pad and a tight foreskin, which further worsen the appearance of the genitalia. Although the incidence of this malformation has not been reported, it is not an unusual problem in paediatric urology practice (5–10 cases per year in a large centre).

In infants, the severe tightness of the foreskin can cause major urine flow obstruction with a huge foreskin pouch (preputial bladder), which fills up at each micturition and needs to be squeezed by the parents to empty. The worst thing to do is to circumcise these boys. Unfortunately it is not uncommon to see patients who underwent a circumcision with a consequent defect of shaft skin who end up with a major penile skin deficiency. No surgical procedure is entirely satisfactory and long-term outcomes are often disappointing. The principles are based on the transfer of preputial skin to the penile shaft and anchorage of the Buck's fascia at the base of the penis [167–171]. There is definitely a place for hormonal stimulation to allow penile growth. Parental pressure usually leads to surgery, although spontaneous improvement is likely to happen in many cases as buried penis is rare in the adult population [172].

## Congenital chordee without hypospadias

Congenital chordee without hypospadias is a much rarer condition than chordee associated with hypospadias. There is approximately one isolated chordee for 100 chordees associated with hypospadias [173]. We have already described in the section on hypospadias the possible causes of ventral chordee. The chordee can be lateral or dorsal (see the section 'Genitalia in bladder exstrophy, epispadias and cloacal exstrophy') associated or not with penile torsion. In these rare cases, the main cause is the asymmetrical development of the corpora cavernosa and asymmetrical distribution of the penile skin.

Surgery follows the same principles as described in the section 'Hypospadias' but often requires a corporeal plasty to rectify the curvature.

## Congenital absent penis (aphallia)

This is extremely rare. Sixty cases were reported in the literature in 1989 [174], 1 in 30 million births [175]. The more proximal the meatus, the higher is the incidence of other anomalies and the greater the number of neonatal deaths. Patients with postsphincteric urethral openings have a better prognosis than a presphincteric meatus (often associated with urointestinal communications). When these children survive, early feminization is recommended.

## Diphallia

Isolated diphallia is also extremely rare and may be associated with anomalies of the cloacal membrane [176]. Various degrees of duplication have been reported with associated anomalies, especially urethral duplication but also of the upper urinary and digestive tracts and of bones [177]. Each case must be treated individually in order to achieve the best functional and aesthetic result [178].

## Abnormal penile insertions (Robinow syndrome)

Features of the Robinow syndrome include a characteristic facies resembling that of a fetus, mesomelic brachymelia of the arms, bifid terminal phalanges of the hands and feet, vertebral and rib abnormalities, and hypoplastic external genitalia. The penile anomaly is due to abnormal insertion of the penile crura, resulting in a penis that appears shorter and more inferiorly placed between the legs [179].

## Scrotal transposition

The two hemiscrotums join above the penis like a saddle over a horse. Surgery is successful in repositioning each half of the scrotum under the penile shaft by rotating their upper attachments. This anomaly is often associated with urogenital anomalies (hypospadias, chordee, agenesis of one or both urinary tracts), gastrointestinal anomalies (predominantly imperforate anus) [180] and severe cardiovascular anomalies.

## Bifid scrotum

Bifid scrotums are quite common in cases of intersex and are often associated with other genital anomalies. It occurs if the genital swellings fail to fuse at the scrotal septum [181] and represents an aspect of the midline syndrome.

## Ectopic scrotum

Ectopic and accessory scrotums result from cleavage or abnormal migration of the genital swellings. They can be found anywhere on the perineum or inguinal canal area or even on the thigh. In most cases, the testis lies inside [182] as the gubernaculum joins the ectopic scrotum.

## Duplication anomalies

Duplication anomalies arise from failure at some point of the fusion of the paired Müllerian ducts. The true incidence of such anomalies is unknown. Many are entirely asymptomatic and found by chance. The incidence is higher in women with infertility and recurrent miscarriage. Uterine anomalies can be isolated but are also associated with an increased incidence of renal anomalies. Uterine anomalies, in particular duplication, are almost universal in girls with cloacal anomalies. Diethyl stilboestrol exposure also leads to an increased risk of Müllerian anomalies.

## Vaginal

Management of duplication anomalies depends on the type of anomaly and the symptoms. A longitudinal vaginal septum can cause painful intercourse. This condition is usually diagnosed on examination as it may be missed on ultrasound. Resection of the septum is straightforward and curative. Vaginal duplication is, however, often associated with a double uterus and cervix.

## Uterine

A double uterus is not usually an indication for surgery. Successful pregnancy is common. However, in some cases there may exist a bicornuate or septate uterus that may possess a non-communicating uterine horn. In this case when menstruation starts, the non-communicating horn will fill with blood and result in a haematometria. This causes severe dysmenorrhoea and is also associated with an increased incidence of endometriosis. A metroplasty is required.

## Transverse vaginal septum

This can be an isolated finding or in association with other anomalies as in McCusick–Kaufman syndrome which appears to be recessively inherited [183]. Presentation is with primary amenorrhoea and cyclical abdominal pain. It must be differentiated from an imperforate hymen, which has similar symptoms. An imperforate hymen is, however, easily diagnosed by a bluish bulge at the vagina, and simple surgical drainage is curative. With a transverse vaginal septum, the septum can be thick and treatment difficult. The approach to surgery depends on the position and thickness of the septum, which can be determined by ultrasound and magnetic resonance imaging if necessary (Fig. 15.5). If the septum is in the lower third of the vagina, blind dissection may be adequate to reach the haematometria and drain it. The septum is then excised and the upper and lower part of the vagina reanastomized. If the septum is high, a combined abdominal and vaginal approach is necessary. Occasionally, the septum is so large that either intestinal transposition or skin grafting is necessary to bridge the gap between the upper and the lower vagina. Fertility is possible in these patients as long as the cervix is normal and has been reported to be in the order of 40–50% [184]. Endometriosis may, however, be a significant problem and should be reduced by prompt diagnosis and treatment.

## Genitalia in bladder exstrophy, epispadias and cloacal exstrophy

Epispadias, bladder exstrophy and cloacal exstrophy are developmental abnormalities of increasing severity result-

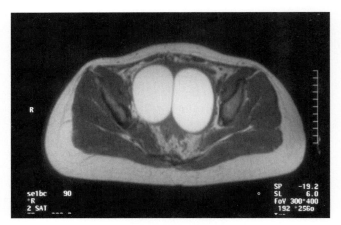

**Fig. 15.5.** MRI of a transverse vaginal septum.

ing from the interruption of the caudal delimitation of the embryo. The delimitation is the process allowing the three-dimensional rolling-up of the embryonic layers (ectoderm, mesoderm, entoderm), leading to the tubularization of the embryo (first 2 months of gestation) [185]. The consequence of this interruption is the partial or complete absence of cavitation and partitioning of the organs sitting in the pelvic cavity. The pelvic bony ring, the urethra, the bladder neck, the bladder and the bowels are open to the surface and not connected properly to the pelvic floor. Associated duplication of some internal pelvic organs is also common (bladder, vagina, uterus). The incidence of these malformations varies with the degree of severity: 1:117 000 births live births for epispadias (with a ratio of 5:1 male–female); 1:10 000 to 1:50 000 for bladder exstrophy (with a ratio of 5:1 to 6:1 male–female); 1:250 000 for cloacal exstrophy.

The genital problem in the boys is a short, broad penis worsened by the wide gap between the two pubic bones on the lower edge of which the corpora cavernosa normally attach. There is an associated dorsal penile chordee secondary to the malrotation of the corpora, which contributes to the difficulty of penetrative intercourse if not corrected. The testes are usually descended and the scrotum well formed, although stretched laterally by the distance between the two pubic bones. Testicular function is normal but ejaculation is often abnormal as a result of the absence of normally formed posterior urethra, absence of the bulbospongiosis and, possibly, as the consequence of some surgical procedures (Fig. 15.6a).

In females, the clitoris is split in two and the vagina opens very anteriorly. Pregnancy is possible (fertility is normal) but uterine prolapse is a severe complication of this abnormality and is due to the lack of pelvic muscle support (Fig. 15.6b).

Surgery of these complex malformations includes:
**1** closure of the bladder plate (associated with pelvic osteotomy) soon after birth;

(a)

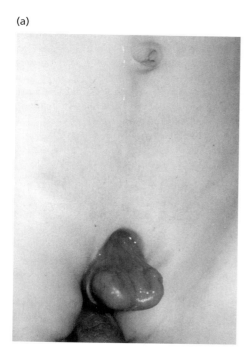

(b)

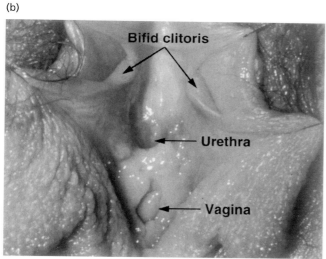

**Bifid clitoris**

**Urethra**

**Vagina**

**Fig. 15.6.** Epispadias in (a) a male and (b) a female patient.

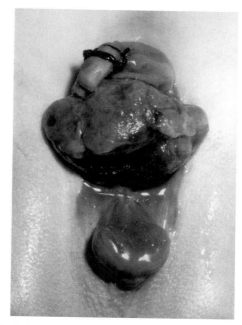

**Fig. 15.7.** Bladder exstrophy.

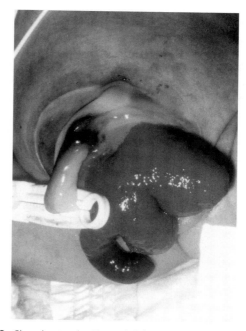

**Fig. 15.8.** Cloacal exstrophy. The anal cleft is at the bottom right of the picture. Above it and further to the right is half of the bladder, which is continuous with the exstrophied bowel (right of the umbilical clamp) with (below and darkened) the ileum prolapsed (like an intussusception) through the exstrophied bowel.

**2** reconstruction of the urethra between 18 months and 3 years of age;

**3** reconstruction of the bladder neck to achieve continence between 3 and 4 years of age.

The first two steps bring reasonably good results, but continence remains one of the most serious challenges in paediatric urology. Most 46,XY patients with bladder exstrophy (Fig. 15.7) are raised as males. Until now, most males with cloacal exstrophy have been raised as female, as the corporeal remnants are very poorly represented. Attempts to raise 46,XY cloacal exstrophies as males led to serious

psychological traumas (Fig. 15.8) [186]. However, evidence that they grow up as successful females is lacking and some paediatric urologists now are advocating maintaining them as males.

# References

1 Gilbert D, Winslow B, Gilbert D, Jordan D, Horton C. Transsexual surgery in the genetic female. *Clin Plast Surg* 1988; 15: 471.

2 Jackson MB, Chilvers C, Pike MC, Ansell P, Bull D for the John Radcliffe Hospital Cryptorchidism Study Group. Cryptorchidism: an apparent substantial increase since 1960. *Br Med J* 1986; 293: 1401–4.

3 Hutson J, Williams M, Fallat M, Attah A. Testicular descent: new insights into its hormonal control. In: Milligan S, ed. *Oxford Reviews of Reproductive Biology*. Oxford: Oxford University Press, 1990: 1–56.

4 Behringer R, Finegold M, Cate R. Müllerian inhibiting substance function during mammalian sexual development. *Cell* 1994; 79: 415.

5 Hutson J. Undescended testis, torsion and varicocele. In: O'Neil J, Rowe M, Grosfeld J, Fonkalsrud E, Coran A, eds. *Pediatric Surgery*, Vol. 2. St Louis: Mosby, 1998: 1087–109.

6 Hutson J. Normal and abnormal testicular descent. In: Stephens F, Smith E, Hutson J, eds. *Congenital Anomalies of Urinary and Genital Tracts*. Oxford: Isis Medical, 1996: 421–9.

7 Whitaker R. Undescended testis – the need for a standard classification. *Br J Urol* 1992; 70: 1–6.

8 Hrebinko R, Bellinger M. The limited role of imaging techniques in managing children with undescended testes. *J Urol* 1993; 150: 458.

9 Silber S, Cohen R. Laparoscopy for cryptorchidism. *J Urol* 1980; 124: 928.

10 Heiss K, Shandling B. Laparoscopy for the impalpable testes: experience with 53 testes. *J Pediatr Surg* 1992; 27: 175–9.

11 Bloom D. Two-step orchiopexy with pelviscopic clip ligation of the spermatic vessels. *J Urol* 1991; 145: 1030–3.

12 Hutson J. Undescended testis. In: Stringer M, Oldham K, Mouriquand P, Howard E, eds. *Paediatric Surgery and Urology: Long Term Outcomes*. London: W. B. Saunders, 1998: 603.

13 Rajfer J. Congenital anomalies of the testis and scrotum. In: Walsh P, Retik A, Darractott Vaughan E, Wein A, eds. *Campbell's Urology*, Vol. 2, 7th edn. Philadelphia: W. B. Saunders, 1998: 2172–92.

14 Job J, Canlorbe P, Garagorri J, Toublanc J. Hormonal therapy of cryptorchidism with human chorionic gonadotrophin. *Urol Clin N Am* 1982; 9: 405–12.

15 Hadziselimovic F. Treatment of cryptorchidism with GnRH. *Urol Clin N Am* 1982; 9: 413.

16 Rajfer J, Handelsman D, Swerdloff R *et al*. Hormonal therapy for cryptorchidism. A randomized double-blind study comparing human chorionic gonadotrophin and gonadotrophin releasing hormone. *N Engl J Med* 1986; 314: 466–70.

17 Jones P, Bagley F. An abdominal extraperitoneal approach for the difficult orchidopexy. *Br J Surg* 1979; 66: 14.

18 Ransley P, Vordermark J, Caldamone A, Bellinger M. Preliminary ligation of the gonadal vessels prior to orchidopexy for the intra-abdominal testis. A staged Fowler-Stephens procedure. *World J Urol* 1984; 2: 266.

19 Bianchi A. Management of the impalpable testis. *Pediatr Surg Int* 1990; 5: 48–53.

20 Scott L. Fertility in cryptorchidism. *Proc R Soc Med* 1962; 55: 1047.

21 Rogers E, Teahan S, Gallagher H *et al*. The role of orchiectomy in the management of postpubertal cryptorchidism. *J Urol* 1998; 159: 851.

22 Kumar D, Bremner D, Brown P. Fertility after orchiopexy for cryptorchidism: a new approach to assessment. *Br J Urol* 1989; 64: 516.

23 Plante P, Pontonnier F, Manst A. Cryptorchidie et sterilite. *J Urologie* 1982; 88: 147.

24 Lee P, O'Leary L, Songer N, Bellinger M, Laporte R. Paternity after cryptorchidism: lack of correlation with age at orchidopexy. *Br J Urol* 1995; 75: 704.

25 Eldrup J, Steven K. Influence of orchiopexy for cryptorchidism on subsequent fertility. *Br J Surg* 1980; 67: 269.

26 Alpert P, Klein R. Spermatogenesis in the unilateral cryptorchid testis after orchiopexy. *J Urol* 1983; 129: 301.

27 Taskinen S, Hovatta O, Wirkstrom S. Early treatment of cryptorchidism, semen quality and testicular endocrinology. *J Urol* 1996; 156: 82.

28 Chilvers C, Pike M. Epidemiology of undescended testis. In: Oliver R, Blandy J, Hope-Stone H, eds. *Urological and Genital Cancer*. Oxford: Blackwell Scientific Publications, 1989: 306.

29 Hadziselimovic F, Hecker E, Hergzoz B. The value of testicular biopsy in cryptorchidism. *Urol Res* 1984; 12: 171.

30 McAleer I, Packer M, Kaplan G, Scherz H, Krous H, Billamn G. Fertility index analysis in cryptorchidism. *J Urol* 1995; 153: 1255.

31 Zhou B, Hutson J, Hasthorpe S. Efficacy of orchidopexy on spermatogenesis in the immature mutant 'trans-scrotal' rat as a cryptorchid model by quantitative cytological analysis. *J Urol* 1998; 81: 290.

32 Hadziselimovic F, Hergzoz B. Treatment with luteinizing hormone releasing hormone analogue after successful orchiopexy markedly improves the chance of fertility later in life. *J Urol* 1997; 158: 1193.

33 Gilbert JB, Hamilton J. Studies in malignant testis tumours. III. Incidence and nature of tumours in ectopic testes. *Surg Gynecol Obstet* 1940; 76: 731.

34 Whitaker R. Management of the undescended testis. *Br J Hosp Med* 1970; 4: 25.

35 Campbell H. Incidence of malignant growth of the undescended testicle. *Arch Surg* 1942; 44: 353.

36 Giwercman A, Grindsted J, Hansen B, Jensen O, Skakkebaek N. Testicular cancer risk in boys with maldescended testis: a cohort study. *J Urol* 1987; 138: 1214.

37 Swerdlow A, Higgins C, Pike M. Risk of testicular cancer in a cohort of boys with cryptorchidism. *Br Med J* 1997; 314: 1507.

38 Coughlin M, Bellinger M, Laporte R, Lee P. Testicular suture: a significant risk factor for infertility among formerly cryptorchid men. *J Pediatr Surg* 1998; 33: 1790.

39 Smith R. Diagnosis and staging of testicular tumours. In: Skinner D, de Kernion J, eds. *Genitourinary Cancer*. Philadelphia: W. B. Saunders, 1978: 448.

40 Ford T, Parkinson M, Pryor J. The undescended testis in adult life. *Br J Urol* 1985; 57: 181.

41 Giwercman A, Muller J, Skakkebaek N. Carcinoma in situ of the undescended testis. *Semin Urol* 1988; 6: 110.

42 Savage M, Lowe D. Gonadal neoplasia and abnormal sexual differentiation. *Clin Endocrinol* 1990; 32: 519.

43 Manuel M, Katayama K, Jones H. The age of occurrence of gonadal tumours in intersex patients with a Y chromosome. *Am J Obset Gynecol* 1976; 124: 293.

44 Ramani P, Yeung C, Habeebu S. Testicular intratubular germ cell neoplasia in children and adolescents with intersex. *Am J Surg Pathol* 1993; 17: 1124.

45 O'Connell M, Ramsey H, Whang-Peng J, Wiernik P. Testicular feminisation syndrome in three siblings: emphasis on gonadal neoplasia. *Am J Med Sci* 1973; 265: 321.

46 Muller J, Skakkebaek N, Neilson O, Graem N. Cryptorchidism and testis cancer: atypical germ cells followed by carcinoma in situ in adult age. *Cancer* 1984; 54: 629.

47 Zaloudek C, Norris H. Granulosa cell tumours of the ovary in children: a clinical and pathologic review of 32 cases. *Am J Surg Pathol* 1982; 6: 503.

48 Cutfield R, Bateman J, Odell D. Infertility caused by bilateral testicular masses secondary to congenital adrenal hyperplasia (21-hydroxylase deficiency). *Fertil Steril* 1983; 40: 809.

49 Mouriquand P, Persad R, Sharma S. Hypospadias repair: current principles and procedures. *Br J Urol* 1995; 76 (Suppl. 3): 9–22.

50 Tuchmann-Duplessis H. *Embryologie – Organogenese*. Paris: Masson, 1970: 66–87.

51 Paulozzi L, Erickson J, Jackson R. Hypospadias trends in two US surveillance systems. *Pediatrics* 1997; 100: 831–4.

52 Albers N, Ulrichs C, Gluer S *et al*. Etiologic classification of severe hypospadias: Implications for prognosis and management. *J Pediatr* 1997; 131: 386–92.

53 Husmann D. Androgen receptor expression and penile growth during sexual maturation. *Dialogues Pediatr Urol* 1996; 19: 1–8.

54 El-Galley R, Smith E, Cohen C, Petros J, Woodard J, Galloway NTM. Epidermal growth factor and EGF receptor in hypospadias. *Br J Urol* 1997; 79: 116–19.

55 Atkinson J, Kosi M, Srikanth M, Takano K, Costin G. Growth hormone reverses impaired wound healing in protein-malnourished rats treated with corticosteroids. *J Pediatr Surg* 1992; 27: 1026–8.

56 Aaronson I, Carmak M, Key L. Defects of the testosterone biosynthetic pathway in boys with hypospadias. *J Urol* 1997; 157: 1884–8.

57 Sutherland R, Wiener J, Hicks J *et al*. Androgen receptors gene mutations are rarely associated with isolated penile hypospadias. *J Urol* 1996; 156: 828–31.

58 Gearhart J, Linhard H, Berkovitz G, Jeffs R, Brown T. Androgen receptor levels and 5 alpha reductase activities in preputial skin and chordee tissue of boys with isolated hypospadias. *J Urol* 1988; 140: 1243–6.

59 Bentvelsen F, Brinkmann A, Van der Linden J, Schroder F, Nijman J. Decreased immunoreactive androgen receptor levels are not the cause of isolated hypospadias. *Br J Urol* 1995; 76: 384–8.

60 Davits R, Van der Aker E, Scholtmeijer R, de Muinck Keizer Schramn S, Nijman R. Effect of parental testosterone therapy on penile development in boys with hypospadias. *Br J Urol* 1993; 71: 593–5.

61 Shima H, Ikoma F, Yabumoto H *et al*. Gonadotrophin and testosterone response in prepubertal boys with hypospadias. *J Urol* 1986; 135: 539–42.

62 Kiely E, Chapman R, Bajoria S, Hollyer J, Hurley R. Maternal serum human chorionic gonadotrophin during early pregnancy resulting in boys with hypospadias or cryptorchidism. *Br J Urol* 1995; 76: 389–92.

63 Mouriquand P. Controversies in Hypospadias Surgery. The urethral plate – Part 11. *Dial Ped Urol* 1996; 19 (8): 1–8.

64 Mouriquand P. Controversies in Hypospadias Surgery: Penile curvature – Part 1. *Dial Ped Urol* 1996; 19 (7): 1–8.

65 Shima H, Yabumotot H, Okamoto E, Orestano L, Ikoma F. Testicular function in patients with hypospadias associated with enlarged prostatic utricle. *Br J Urol* 1992; 69: 192–5.

66 Harris E, Beaty T. Segregation analysis of hypospadias: a re-analysis of published pedigree data. *Am J Med Gen* 1993; 45: 420.

67 Bauer S, Retik A, Colodny A. Genetic aspects of hypospadias. *Urol Clin N Am* 1981; 8: 559.

68 Stool C, Alembik Y, Roth M, Dott B. Genetic and environmental factors in hypospadias. *J Med Gen* 1990; 27: 559.

69 Mouriquand P. Hypospadias. In: Arwell JD (ed.) *Paediatric Surgery* London: Arnold, 1998: 603–16.

70 Bracka A. Hypospadias repair: the two-stage alternative. *Br J Urol* 1995; 76 (Suppl. 3): 31–41.

71 Baskin L, Duckett J, Ueoka K, Seibold J, Snyder H. Changing concepts of hypospadias curvature lead to more onlay island flap procedures. *J Urol* 1994; 151: 191–6.

72 Ransley P, Duffy P, Wollin M. Bladder exstrophy closure and epispadias repair. In: Dudley H, Carter D, Russel R, eds. *Operative Surgery*. London: Butterworth, 1988: 620–32.

73 Thiersh C. Uber die entstehungswise and operative behanldung der spispadie. *Arch Heitkunde* 1869; 10: 20–5.

74 Duplay S. De l'hypospade perineoscrotal et de son traitement chirurgical. *Arch Gen Med* 1874; 1: 613–57.

75 Elder J, Duckett J, Snyder H. Onlay island flap in the repair of mid and distal hypospadias without chordee. *J Urol* 1987; 138: 376–9.

76 Mollard P, Mouriquand P, Felfela T. Application of the onlay island flap urethroplasty to penile hypospadias with severe chordee. *Br J Urol* 1991; 68: 317–19.

77 Perovic S, Vukadinovic V. Onlay island flap urethroplasty for severe hypospadias: a variant of the technique. *J Urol* 1994; 151: 711–14.

78 Mathieu P. Traitement en un temps de l'hypospade balanique et juxuta-balanique. *J Chir* 1932; 39: 481–4.

79 Dessanti A, Rigamonti W, Merulla V, Faalchetti D, Caccia G. Autologous buccal mucosa graft for hypospadias repair: An initial report. *J Urol* 1992; 147: 1081–94.

80 Mollard P, Mouriquand P, Bringeon Bugmann P. Repair of hypospadias using a bladder mucosal graft in 76 cases. *J Urol* 1990; 142: 1548–50.

81 Mundy A. The long-term results of skin inlay urethroplasty. *Br J Urol* 1995; 75: 59–61.

82 Asopa H, Elhence E, Atria S, Bansal N. One stage correction of penile hypospadias using a foreskin tube. A preliminary report. *Int Surg* 1991; 55: 435.

83 Duckett J. The island flap technique for hypospadias repair. *Urol Clin N Am* 1981; 8: 503.

84 Duckett J. Magpi (meatoplasty and glanuloplasty): a procedure for subcoronal hypospadias. *Urol Clin North Am* 1981; 8: 513.

85 Snodgrass W. Tubularized, incised plate urethroplasty for distal hypospadias. *J Urol* 1994; 151: 464–5.

86 Koff S, Brinkman J, Ulrich J, Deighton D. Extensive mobilization of the urethral plate and urethra for repair of hypospadias: The modified Barcat technique. *J Urol* 1994; 151: 466–9.

87 Firlit C. The mucosal collar in hypospadias surgery. *J Urol* 1987; 137: 80–2.

88 Zaidi S, Hodapp J, Cuckow P, Mouriquand P. Spongioplasty in hypospadias repair. British Association of Urological Surgeons., 1997.

89 Mureau M, Slijper F, Koos Slob A, Verhulst F, Nijman R. Satisfaction with penile appearance after hypospadias surgery. *J Urol* 1996; 155: 703.

90 Miniberg D, Sosa R, Neidt G, Poe C. Laser welding of pedicle flap skin tubes. *J Urol* 1989; 142: 623–5.

91 Gearhart J, Jeffs R. The use of parenteral testosterone therapy in genital reconstructive surgery. *J Urol* 1987; 138: 1077–8.

92 Salcedo I, Serra M, Marrques A, Mendonca M, Seera L. Growth hormone solution applied directly to diabetic foot ulcers. Preliminary results. In: Saggese G, Stanhope R, eds. *Recent Advances on Growth and Growth Hormone Therapy.* Tel Aviv: Freund Publishing House, 1995: 203–16.

93 Scheuer S, Hanna M. Effect of nitroglycerin ointment on penile skin flap survival in hypospadias repair. *Urology* 1986; 27: 438–40.

94 Vinter-Jensen L, Juhl C, Dajanei E, Nielsen K, Djurrhus J. Chronic systemic treatment with epidermal growth factor induces smooth muscle hyperplasia and hypertrophy in the urinary tract of mature Goettingen minipigs. *Br J Urol* 1997; 79: 532–8.

95 Yi E, Shabalk A, Lacey D *et al.* Keratinocyte growth factor causes proliferation of urothelium in vivo. *J Urol* 1995; 154: 1566–70.

96 Wolfe J, Soble J, Ratliff T, Clayman R. Ureteral cell cultures II. Collagen production and response to pharmacologic agents. *J Urol* 1996; 156: 2067–72.

97 Baskin L, Macarak E, Duckett J, Snyder H, Howard P. Culture of urethral fibroblasts: Cell morphology, proliferation and extracellular matrix synthesis. *J Urol* 1993; 150: 1260–6.

98 Sabbagh W, Masters J, Duffy P, Herbage D, Brown R. In vitro assessment of a collagen sponge for engineering urothelial grafts. *Br J Urol* 1998; 82: 888–94.

99 Fichtner J, Filipas D, Mottrie A, Voges G, Hohenfellner R. Analysis of meatal location in 500 men: wide variation questions the need for meatal advancement in all pediatric hypospadias cases. *J Urol* 1995; 154: 833.

100 Summerlad B. A long term follow up of hypospadias patients. *Br J Plast Surg* 1975; 28: 324.

101 Mureau M, Slijper F, Nijman R, van der Meulen J, Verhulst F, Koos Slob A. Psychosexual adjustment of children and adolescents after different types of hypospadias. *J Urol* 1995; 154: 1902.

102 Johanson B, Avellan L. Hypospadias: a review of 299 cases operated 1957–1969. *Scand J Plastics Recon Surg* 1980; 14: 259.

103 Kenawi M. Sexual function in hypospadiacs. *Br J Urol* 1976; 47: 833.

104 Miller M, Grant D. Severe hypospadias with genital ambiguity: adult outcome after staged hypospadias repair. *Br J Urol* 1997; 80: 485.

105 Aho M, Tammela O, Somppi E, Tammela T. Sexual and social life of men operated for hypospadias and phimosis during childhood. *Eur J Urol* 2000; 37: 95–100.

106 Avellan L. Development of puberty, sexual debut and sexual function in hypospadias. *J Plast Recons Surg* 1976; 10: 29.

107 Gearhart J, Donohoue P, Brown T, Walsh P, Berkowitz D. Endocrine evaluation of adults with mild hypospadias. *J Urol* 1990; 144: 274.

108 Berg R, Berg G. Penile malformations, gender identity and sexual orientation. *Acta Psychiatr Scand* 1983; 68: 154.

109 Zubowska J, Jankowska J, Kula K, Owczarczk I, Garbowska-Gorska A. Clinical, hormonal and semiological data in adult men operated in childhood with hypospadias. *Endokrynologia Polska* 1979; 30: 565.

110 Eberle J, Uberreiter S, Radmyr C, Janetschek G, Marberger H, Bartsch G. Posterior hypospadias: long term follow up after reconstructive surgery in the male direction. *J Urol* 1993; 150: 1474.

111 Berg R, Berg G, Svensson J. Penile malformation and mental health. *Acta Psychiatr Scand* 1982; 66: 398.

112 Berg G, Berg R. Castration complex, evidence from men operated for hypospadias. *Acta Psychiatr Scand* 1983; 68: 143.

113 Berg G, Berg R, Edman G, Svensson J, Astrom G. Androgens and personality in normal men and men operated for hypospadias in childhood. *Acta Psychiatr Scand* 1983; 68: 167.

114 Mureau M, Slijper F, Van der Meulen J, Verhulst F, Slob A. Psychosexual adjustment of men who underwent hypospadias repair: a norm-related study. *J Urol* 1995; 154: 1351–5.

115 Allen T. The classification and the management of the micropenis: clinical classification. *Dialogues Pediatr Urol* 1989; 12: 3.

116 Schonfield W. Primary and secondary sexual characteristics. *Am J Dis Child* 1943; 65: 535.

117 Feldman K, Smith D. Fetal phallic growth and penile standards for new born male infants. *Pediatrics* 1975; 87: 395.

118 Flatau E, Josesfsberg Z, Reisner S, Bialik O, Laron Z. Penile size in the new born infant. *J Pediatr* 1975; 87: 663.

119 Reilly J, Woodhouse C. Small penis and the male sexual role. *J Urol* 1989; 142: 569.

120 Husmann D, Cain M. Microphallus: eventual size is dependent on the timing of androgen administration. *J Urol* 1994; 152: 734.

121 Choi S, Han S, de Kim D, Lignieres B. Transdermal dihydrotestosterone therapy and its effects on patients with microphallus. *J Urol* 1993; 150: 657.

122 Klugo R, Cerny J. Response of the micropenis to topical testosterone and gonadotrophins. *J Urol* 1978; 119: 667.

123 Gilbert D, Jordan G, Devine C, Winslow B, Schlossberg S. Phallic construction in prepubertal and adolescent boys. *J Urol* 1993; 149: 1521.

124 Perovic S. Phalloplasty in children and adolescents using the extended pedicle island groin flap. *J Urol* 1995; 154: 848.

125 Money J, Lehne G, Pirerre-Jerome F. Micropenis: gender, heterosexual coping strategy and behavioural health in nine pediatric cases followed into adulthood. *Comp Psychiatr* 1985; 26: 29.

126 McClorie G, Khoury A, Husmann D. Surgery for micropenis in childhood. *Dialogues Pediatr Urol* 1989; 12: 6.

127 Slijper F, Drop S, Molenaar J, de Muinck Keizer-Schrama M. Long term psychological evaluation of intersex children. *Arch Sex Behav* 1998; 27: 125.

128 Schober J. Feminising genitoplasty for intersex. In: Stringer M, Oldham K, Mouriquand P, Howard E, eds. *Paediatric Surgery and Urology: Long Term Outcome.* London: W. B. Saunders, 1999: 549.

129 Diamond M. Sex assignment considerations. *J Sexual Res* 1996; 22: 161.

130 Dreger A. Ethical issues in the medical treatment of intersexuality and 'ambiguous sex'. Hastings center report: 1998; 28: 24–55.

131 Glassberg K. Gender assignment and the pediatric urologist. *J Urol* 1999; 161: 1308.

132 Imperato-McGinley J, Miller M, Wilson J, Peterson R, Shackleton C. A cluster of male pseudohermaphrodites with 5 alpha reductase deficiency in Papua New Guinea. *Clin Endocrinol* 1991; 34: 293.

133 Aaronson I. Micropenis: medical and surgical implications. *J Urol* 1994; 152: 4.

134 Mauras N, Blizzard R. The McCune–Albright Syndrome. *Acta Endocrinol Scand* 1986; 279: 207–17.

135 Silver R, Gearhart J. Ambiguous Genitalia. In: Graham D, ed. *Glenn's Urologic Surgry,* 5th edn. Philadelphia: Lippincott-Raven Publishers, 1998: 859–70.

136 Passerini-Glazel G. A new one stage procedure for clitorovaginoplasty in severely masculinized female pseudohermaphrodites. *J Urol* 1989; 142: 565–8.

137 Pena A. Total urogenital mobilization – an easier way to repair cloacs. *J Pediatr Surg* 1997; 32 (2): 263–7.

138 Hendren W. Surgical approach to intersex problems. *Semin Pediatr Surg* 1998; 7: 8–18.

139 Hendren W. Surgical repair of the high vagina. *Dialogues Pediatr Urol* 1998; 21 (7): 1–8.

140 Hensle T, Kennedy W. Surgical management of intersexuality. In: Walsh PC, Retick A, Vaughan E, Wein A, eds. *Campbell's Urology,* Vol. 2. Philadelphia: W. B. Saunders, 1998: 2155–71.

141 Ludwikowski B, Oesh Hayward I, Gonzalez R. Total urogenital sinus mobilization: expanded applications. *Br J Urol Int* 1999; 83: 820–2.

142 Pena A. The transanorectal approach for the treatment of urogenital sinus. *Dialogues Pediatr Urol* 1998; 21 (7): 1–8.

143 Hendren W, Crawford F. Adrenogenital syndrome: The anatomy of the anomaly and its repair. *J Pediatr Surg* 1969; 4: 49–58.

144 Passerini-Glazel G. Vaginoplasty in severely virulized CAH females. *Dialogues Pediatr Urol* 1998; 21 (7): 1–8.

145 Pena A, deVries P. Posterior sagittal anorectoplasty: Important technical considerations and new applications. *J Pediatr Surg* 1982; 17: 796–811.

146 Rink R, Pope J, Kropp B *et al.* Reconstruction of the high urogenital sinus: early perineal prone approach without division of the rectum. *J Urol* 1997; 158: 1293–7.

147 Evans T, Poland M, Boving R. Vaginal malformations. *Am J Obstet Gynecol* 1981; 141: 910.

148 Frank R. The formation of an artificial vagina without operation. *Am J Obstet Gynecol* 1938; 35: 1053.

149 Rock J, Reeves L, Retto H, Baramki T, Zacur H, Jones H. Success following vaginal creation for mullerian agenesis. 1983; 39: 809–13.

150 Williams E. Congenital absence of the vagina: a simple operation for its relief. *Obstet Gynaecol Br Conmmonw* 1964; 71: 511.

151 Williams E. Uterovaginal agenesis. *Ann R Coll Surg Eng* 1976; 58: 226.

152 Gauwerky JFK, Wallwienger D, Bastert G. An endoscopically assisted technique for construction of a neovagina. *Arch Gynecol Obstet* 1992; 252: 59–63.

153 Veronikis D, McClure G, Nichols D. The Vecchietti operation for constructing a neonvagian: indications, instrumentations and techniques. *Obstet Gynecol* 1997; 90: 301–4.

154 Abbe R. A new method of creating a vagina in a case of congenital absence. *Med Rec* 1898; 54: 836–8.

155 McIndoe A, Bannister J. An operation for the cure of congenital absence of the vagina. *J Obstet Gynaecol Br Empire* 1938; 45: 490–4.

156 Hopkins M, Morley G. Squamous cell carcinoma of the neovagina. *Obstet Gynecol* 1987; 69: 525.

157 Cali R, Pratt J. Congenital absence of the vagina: long term results of vaginal reconstruction in 175 cases. *Am J Obstet Gynecol* 1968; 100: 752–63.

158 Morton K, Dewhurst C. Human amnion in the treatment of vaginal malformations. *Br J Obstet Gynaecol* 1986; 93: 50.

159 Ashworth M, Morton K, Dewhurst J, Lilford R, Bates R. Vaginoplasty using amnion. *Obstet Gynecol* 1986; 67: 443–6.

160 Davydov S. Modiferte kolpopsese aus peritonium der excavation rectouterin. *Gikekologiia Moskau* 1969; 45: 55–7.

161 Ward G, Panda S, Anwar K. Davydov's colpoclieses: vaginal construction using peritoneum. *Curr Obstet Gynaecol* 1998; 8: 224–6.

162 Baldwin J. The formation of an artificial vagina by intestinal transposition. *Ann Surg* 1904; 40: 398.

163 Pratt J. Sigmoidovaginostomy: a new method of obtaining satisfactory vaginal depth. *Am J Obstet Gynecol* 1961; 81: 535–45.

164 Ritchie R. Primary carcinoma of the vagina following a Baldwin reconstruction operation for congenital absence of the vagina. *Am J Obstet Gynecol* 1929; 18: 794.

165 Hendren W, Atala A. Use of bowel for vaginal reconstruction. *J Urol* 1994; 152: 752–7.

166 Martinez-Mora Isnard R, Castellvi A, Lopez-Ortez P. Neovagina in vaginal agenesis: surgical methods and long term results. *J Pediatr Surg* 1992; 27: 10–4.

167 Dwoskin J. Management of the 'concealed' penis. *Dialogues Pediatr Urol* 1993; 16: 1–8.

168 Boemers T, de Jong T. The surgical correction of buried penis. *J Urol* 1995; 154: 550–2.

169 Lim D, Barraza M, Stevens P. Correction of retractile concealed penis. *J Urol* 1995; 153: 1668–70.

170 Wollin M, Duffy P, Malone P, Ransley P. Buried penis: a novel approach. *Br J Urol* 1990; 65: 97–100.

171 Lipszyc E, Pfister C, Liard A, Mitrofanoff P. Surgical treatment of buried penis. *Eur J Pediatr Surg* 1997; 7: 292–5.

172 Donatucci C, Ritter E. Management of the buried penis in adults. *J Urol* 1998; 159: 420–4.

173 Hendren W, Caesar R. Chordee without hypospadias: experience of 33 cases. *J Urol* 1992; 147: 107–9.

174 Skoog S, Belman A. Aphallia: its classification and management. *J Urol* 1989; 141: 589–92.

175 Hendren W. The genetic male with absent penis and urethrorectal communication: experience with 5 patients. *J Urol* 1997; 157: 1469–74.

176 Najmaldin A, Gollow I, Stoodley N, Burge D. Diphallus and associated anomalies. *Pediatr Surg Int* 1989; 4: 360–2.

177 Zolfaghari A, Pourissa M, Hajialilou S, Amjadi M. True complete diphallia. *Scand J Urol Nephrol* 1995; 29: 233–5.

178 Dean J, Horton C. Diphallia and hindgut duplication. *Plast Reconst Surg* 1991; 87: 358–61.

179 Wilcox D, Quinn F, Ng C, Dicks-Mireaux C, Mouriquand P. Redefining the genital abnormality in the Robinow syndrome. *J Urol* 1997; 157: 2312–14.

180 Miller S. Transposition of the external genitalia associated with the syndrome of caudal regression. *J Urol* 1972; 108: 818.

181 Bloom D, Wan J, Key D. Disorders of the male external genitalia and inguinal canal. In: Kelalis King Belman, ed. *Clinical Pediatric Urology*, 3rd edn. Chicago: W. B. Saunders, 1992: 1024–5.

182 Lamma D, Kaplan G. Accessory and ectopic scrota. *Urology* 1977; 9: 149.

183 McKusick V, Weilbacher R, Gregg C. Recessive inheritance of a congenital malformation syndrome. *J Am Med Assoc* 1968; 204: 113.

184 Rock J, Zakur H, Dlugi A. Pregnancy success following surgical correction of an imperforate hymen and complete transverse vaginal septum. *Gynecology* 1982; 59: 448.

185 Mouriquand P. Congenital disorders of the bladder and urethra. In: Whitfield H, Hendry W, Kirby R, Duckett J, eds. *Textbook of Genitourinary Surgery*, 2nd edn. Oxford: Blackwell Scientific Publications, 1998: 205–21.

186 Husmann D, McClorie G, Churchill B. Phallic reconstruction in cloacal exstrophy. *J Urol* 1989; 142: 563–4.

# 16 Thyroid, parathyroid, adrenal and pancreas surgery

### R. C. G. Russell and T. R. Kurzawinski

## Introduction

Endocrine conditions requiring surgical intervention are uncommon in children and adolescent patients. Only a few centres and even fewer individual surgeons can draw on a wealth of experience, and a great divergence of opinions regarding management of these conditions exist. Contrasting views are enhanced further in that paediatric endocrine lesions often differ from their adult counterparts in histology, natural history and response to treatment [1]. Paediatric endocrine tumours are also less frequently malignant. Published literature lacks randomized trials assessing the value of different surgical interventions. Current treatments are therefore influenced by personal opinions and preferences based on individual experience. The quality of evidence in support of specific treatments is inadequate and should be improved by well-designed randomized studies. To this end, specialist centres dealing with sufficient numbers of cases and an increased collaboration between institutions on the national and the international levels must be encouraged. Institutions providing tertiary care will also be fundamental in accumulating significant endocrine, radiological, anaesthetic and pathology expertise and maintaining a high level of surgical skills.

The principle of management in paediatric surgical endocrinology is that the surgeon must work in conjunction with a paediatric endocrinologist who has the full support of a large adult endocrine unit and a well-equipped laboratory able to perform a whole array of measurements. Before an operation the exact diagnosis and possibility of associated syndromes and how these can affect the outcome should be fully discussed. The cornerstone of perioperative strategy in endocrinology is to control the effects of hormonal excess or deficiency, and new pharmaceutical agents have enabled physicians to do this with greater accuracy and precision. The strategy aiming to achieve this should be planned by the paediatric endocrinologist and the surgeon together. The role of an experienced anaesthetist able to monitor vital signs and biochemical parameters on a continuous basis, maintain patient stability during the operation and thus ensure smooth and rapid recovery cannot be underestimated.

The need for accurate imaging is fundamental and requires state-of-the-art ultrasound, a spiral computerized tomography (CT) scanner and magnetic resonance imaging (MRI). Recent advances in technology and imaging techniques have resulted in a significant improvement in the quality of images, providing the surgeon with an anatomical map on which he can design the operation. Localization of the lesion using appropriate imaging should be discussed with the relevant imaging specialists. Accurate preoperative staging usually dispenses with the need for the exploratory laparotomy.

Nuclear medicine is playing an increasing role in the management of endocrine problems. New radiopharmaceuticals and labelled antibodies are invaluable in providing additional information about the function of endocrine lesions and their accurate location, especially if aberrant. Recent progress in this field has made targeted radiotherapy (delivered to the site of the lesion) possible.

Close cooperation with a histopathologist and cytologist with a special interest in endocrine pathology is essential. The need for preoperative biopsy should be established and whether this would be helpful or merely contaminate the surgical field discussed. Image-guided core tissue biopsies or fine-needle cytology specimens can be reliably interpreted with the help of special stains and immunocytochemical markers to provide a pathological diagnosis. Reliable histology is important when deciding on the appropriate treatment and is useful in establishing the prognosis.

## The thyroid gland

### Benign thyroid disease

#### Multinodular goitre

The incidence and aetiology of multinodular goitre in children differs according to geographical background but worldwide it is caused most often by iodine deficiency. The thyroid can be diffusely enlarged initially but with time it becomes more nodular and autonomous, which can lead to subclinical and eventually overt hyperthyroidism. Serum thyroid-stimulating hormone (TSH), free thyroxine ($FT_4$) and free triiodothyronine ($FT_3$) should always be measured to assess thyroid function. In straightforward cases of multinodular goitre, imaging, such as thyroid scintigraphy or ultrasound, is not routinely indicated. When the patient presents with stridor or dyspnoea, CT scan or MRI should be performed to assess tracheal compression. CT scan and MRI are also 100% accurate in detecting retrosternal extension of the goitre. Aspiration cytology is indicated only if there is a strong clinical suspicion of thyroid malignancy [2].

Surgical treatment of young patients is indicated in the following situations [3]:

1 juvenile goitre of extraordinary size when sufficient regression is not expected;
2 tracheal or oesophageal compression;
3 retrosternal goitre;
4 conservative treatment is unsuccessful over a 2-year period;
5 autonomous adenoma;
6 thyroid cancer is suspected.

If hyperthyroidism develops in children with multinodular goitre, treatment with antithyroid drugs to achieve the euthyroid state followed by surgery is the treatment of choice. Thyroid surgery for neck discomfort or cosmesis is controversial.

Preoperative preparation consists of ascertaining that the patient is euthyroid and ensuring with the anaesthetist that the airway is satisfactory and will not present difficulty on intubation. A check of vocal cords is obligatory.

Bilateral subtotal thyroidectomy is the standard operation for multinodular goitre. If disease affects one lobe or isthmus only, lobectomy or isthmusectomy could be sufficient. Retrosternal goitres can be removed through a collar incision in the majority of patients and thoracotomy is rarely needed.

The results of surgery for multinodular goitre are good, with a rapid recovery after surgery. Most children leave hospital on the second or third postoperative day and return to full activity within 14 days. In the hands of an experienced surgeon the incidence of recurrent laryngeal damage and permanent hypoparathyroidism should be less than 5%. Voice change after surgery could be due to superior laryngeal nerve damage. Tracheomalacia and haemorrhage are the main causes of postoperative airway impairment.

The extent of surgery will determine the incidence of hypothyroidism and appropriate replacement therapy should be initiated if necessary. With adequate surgery the rate of goitre recurrence should be lower than 10%. The value of treatment with thyroxine to prevent recurrence of the multinodular goitre in the absence of hypothyroidism remains uncertain [2].

## Thyrotoxicosis

Thyrotoxicosis in children presents as a result of Graves disease or an autonomous nodule. The latter is extremely rare in childhood, but it is a definite indication for surgical treatment [4]. The main indications for surgery in Graves disease are failure of medical treatment to induce remission within a reasonable time scale and recurrence of thyrotoxicosis after successful therapy. Other indications include a large goitre and poor patient compliance.

Adequate control of thyrotoxicosis and its symptoms are essential and no patients with abnormal thyroid status should be submitted to surgical treatment. This is achieved with antithyroid drugs such as carbimazole or propylthiouracil but occasionally the addition of beta-blockers for symptomatic control is necessary. Thyroxine is sometimes given during treatment with antithyroid drugs if hypothyroidism develops. Some centres aim for this using the block replacement regimen [5].

Surgery for a solitary, hyperfunctioning autonomous nodule should be a thyroid lobectomy. For Graves disease, a near-total thyroidectomy is appropriate, leaving very small remnants, i.e. less than 3 g of tissue. The functional outcome after surgery is affected by the amount of remaining thyroid tissue and the accompanying lymphocytic thyroiditis. With more extensive resections 20–60% of patients become hypothyroid after the operation [6,7]. The more thyroid tissue that remains, the greater is the likelihood of recurrence of hyperthyroidism. In 558 operations for hyperthyroidism, thyrotoxicosis recurred in 12.7% [8]. To ensure prevention of recurrent hyperthyroidism, total thyroidectomy has been recommended, but this is not the general view [9]. A near-total thyroidectomy with immediate treatment with thyroxine replacement is the procedure of choice in the authors' institution.

## Thyroid carcinoma in children

Thyroid cancer is rare in childhood, but its incidence rises after the age of 5 and its overall incidence in children in England and Wales is 0.5 per million per year [10]. Its incidence worldwide has significantly decreased since 1970 as a result of the decline of radiotherapy for benign disease [11], but in Belarus it increased 62 times within 5 years of the Chernobyl nuclear accident, with a geographical distribution similar to $^{131}$I fallout [12–14]. About three-quarters of thyroid cancers in children are well-differentiated papillary and follicular tumours, but histological features of tumours in children aged less than 10 years are different from adult tumours [10]. Medullary thyroid cancers (MTCs), sporadic or more often associated with MEN2 (multiple endocrine neoplasia type 2) syndrome, are found in about 10% of children with thyroid malignancy [15]. Other malignancies such as lymphoma, sarcoma, teratoma and Hurtle cell tumour are very rare.

The commonest clinical presentation of a thyroid malignancy is a palpable, asymptomatic, solitary nodule in the neck [16]. The prevalence of thyroid nodularity in children is considerably less than in an adult population and has been estimated to be approximately 1.8% [17]. A solitary nodule in a child is much more alarming, since the incidence of malignancy in such a nodule is higher than in adults and varies from 18% to 46% [17,18].

A solitary thyroid nodule in a child should be assessed by a combination of clinical history (previous neck irradiation, family history) and examination (palpable nodule, lymphadenopathy). Solid nodules seen on ultrasound, which are 'cold' on scintigraphy, are highly indicative of malignancy. The diagnosis of cancer is established by fine-needle aspiration biopsy. Early diagnosis of medullary cancer can be made by measuring serum calcitonin levels, and screening children from families with MEN 2 syndrome is now possible because of the identification of the specific mutations of the *RET* proto-oncogene [12,19].

Surgery for differentiated thyroid cancer is the undisputed treatment of choice, but its extent and the need for postoperative adjuvant therapy is controversial. The fact that at the time of presentation 70–80% of children will have regional lymph nodes involved and 6–20% distant metastasis favours aggressive treatment [19]. Surgeons who see this as a decisive prognostic factor recommend total thyroidectomy, lymphadenectomy and adjuvant radioactive [131]I ablation therapy. This radical approach has been associated with lower recurrence rates but a higher rate of major complications, such as unilateral or bilateral recurrent laryngeal nerve injury and permanent hypoparathyroidism. Total thyroidectomy facilitates follow-up with serum thyroglobulin and total ablation with [131]I.

Some surgeons recommend more conservative surgery, e.g. thyroid lobectomy or subtotal thyroidectomy, and no postoperative treatment with radioactive iodine. The rationale is that differentiated carcinomas in young patients are less aggressive than in adults and their good prognosis is the result of yet unknown cellular and genetic factors rather than aggressive treatment. Less aggressive surgery should result in less morbidity. Treatment with thyroxine should be given to all patients regardless of the extent of surgery, as suppression of TSH levels improves the recurrence and survival rates [20]. The survival rates in children with well-differentiated carcinomas and median follow-up of 10–20 years is 90–100% [19].

Medullary carcinoma has a less favourable prognosis, and total thyroidectomy with resection of the involved lymph nodes is a universally accepted treatment. Postoperative follow-up by measuring serum calcitonin can detect early recurrence. Octeotride and metaiodobenzylguanidine (MIBG) scintigraphy can be useful in detecting metastatic medullary cancer. Treatment with therapeutic doses of radiation bound to octeotride or MIBG should be considered if adequate uptake is shown. It has been suggested that children with MEN2A syndrome should have a prophylactic total thyroidectomy performed before the age of 5–10 years, and children with MEN2B might benefit from it during the first year of life. This is, however, by no means universally accepted practice, for some of the patients have a minimally invasive variant of the tumour and nearly normal life expectancy without treatment [19,21].

## The parathyroid glands

Primary hyperthyroidism is very rare in children but can present in the neonatal period or later in childhood or adolescence [22].

### Neonatal hyperparathyroidism

Neonatal hyperparathyroidism is thought to be an autosomal recessive disease caused by mutation of the calcium-sensing receptor gene [23]. Only a few dozen cases have been reported in the world literature, but the true incidence of this condition is uncertain as many cases are misdiagnosed [24]. All reported cases have had chief-cell hyperplasia of all four glands. Symptoms such as muscle hypotonia and respiratory distress are caused by hypercalcaemia, which, if not diagnosed promptly, will lead to a life-threatening hypercalcaemic crisis.

Surgery appears to be the only therapy that offers a chance of a cure. Mortality associated with surgical treatment is nearly four times less than in medically managed patients [22]. Early attempts of a cure with subtotal parathyroidectomy failed, and total parathyroidectomy is the operation of choice. The resulting hypocalcaemia should be treated with permanent replacement therapy (calcium and vitamin D). Autotransplantation of fresh or cryopreserved parathyroid tissue has been traditionally recommended to maintain normal calcium levels after total parathyroidectomy [22,25], but transplantation of abnormal parathyroid tissue can cause recurrent hyperparathyroidism, which requires repeated excisions of transplanted tissue. This and the continuing improvement of replacement therapy might lead to a change of practice in the future.

### Primary hyperparathyroidism

Sporadic primary hyperparathyroidism is the commonest form of the disease in children and adolescents and is caused by a parathyroid adenoma (solitary more often than multiple) in the majority of cases [26]. The familial form of hyperparathyroidism, which could present alone or as a part of a multiple endocrine syndrome, is less common and most often due to parathyroid hyperplasia [27,28]. Hypercalcaemia resulting from parathyroid carcinoma is exceptionally rare, only five cases being reported [29].

Children with hyperparathyroidism are more often symptomatic than adults and commonly present with renal stones, bone disease, pancreatitis or vague, non-specific abdominal pain [30]. The incidence of symptoms correlates with high calcium concentrations and the size of the parathyroid adenomas [30]. Hypercalcaemic crisis is also a much more common presentation in younger patients than in adults [28]. Hyperparathyroidism in children tends to be diagnosed late because the diagnosis is often not considered. Diagnosis is confirmed by measuring serum levels of calcium, phosphate and parathyroid hormone. All young patients with hypercalcaemia as a result of hyperparathyroidism should be further investigated to determine whether the condition is familial [27].

Preoperative imaging of abnormal parathyroid glands has not been routinely performed in the past because careful exploration of all four parathyroids and excision of abnormal glands by an experienced surgeon ensured excellent results. However, ultrasound, MRI and sestamibi scan can be helpful in preoperative localization of the abnormal parathyroids if reoperation for persistent hypercalcaemia or unilateral exploration of the neck is planned.

Surgery is the best treatment for primary hyperparathyroidism and should be tailored according to the cause of the disease. All four glands (or more if accessory glands are present) should be visualized during neck exploration. In unequivocal cases of a single adenoma, it should be excised and biopsy of the remaining normal-looking glands should be avoided to prevent hypoparathyroidism postoperatively. Intraoperative parathyroid hormone (PTH) assay is a good way of assessing the completeness of the operation, but it is not widely used. If more than one gland looks abnormal, the pathology should be determined by intraoperative frozen section. Multiple adenomas should be excised and normal-looking glands marked. In the case of four-gland hyperplasia, total parathyroidectomy is recommended with long-term replacement therapy.

The results of surgery for primary hyperparathyroidism are excellent and recurrence of hypercalcaemia rare. In the hands of an experienced surgeon, a surgical cure rate of 95–99% should be achieved. Mortality is nil and morbidity (e.g. vocal cord palsy) minimal. Long-term follow-up is necessary.

## The adrenal gland

### Adrenal medulla

Tumours arising from the adrenal medulla include phaeochromocytoma, neuroblastoma and ganglioneuroma. The last two rarely have endocrine effects.

Phaeochromocytoma is a rare childhood tumour and accounts for 1% of hypertension in this age group [31].

Although 20% of all phaeochromocytomas are found in the paediatric population, they differ from the adult tumours in that more than 10% are bilateral and about half are at extra-adrenal sites, although 95% are within the abdomen [32,33]. Phaeochromocytomas can be sporadic or associated with familial syndromes, such as MEN2, von Hippel–Lindau or neurofibromatosis type 1, and this familial association is more common in children than in the adult population [34].

Hypertension, sweating, headache and visual blurring are the commonest symptoms of phaeochromocytoma [35]. Diagnosis is usually reached by confirming high concentrations of catecholamines and their metabolites in the urine, but occasionally serum catecholamine levels in response to suppression or provocative test are required. Preoperative localization of the tumour is essential. A CT scan or MRI of the abdomen should be performed, with particular emphasis on a sequence through the adrenal glands. MRI could be particularly useful for identifying unusual sites. Whole-body [131I]MIBG scan should be carried out to exclude thoracic or other extra-abdominal disease. Positron emission tomography (PET) scanning could be useful if tumours failed to concentrate MIBG [36]. Surgery should not proceed until the site of the disease has been accurately localized.

It is essential to have the effects of the catecholamine secretion completely controlled in the immediate preoperative period. As soon as the diagnosis has been made, the patient should be commenced on α-blocking agents, such as phenoxybenzamine. Beta-blockers, such as propranolol, are introduced to control the tachycardia and the cardiac dysrhythmias once the α-blockade is established. Even with α- and β-blockade, it is essential to dissuade the interventional radiologist from undertaking biopsy of the adrenal mass, as this can cause potentially fatal complications of acute hypertensive crisis or dysrhythmias. As a result of the ability to control the hypertension rapidly, prolonged preoperative preparation is unnecessary and conservative management of this condition is inappropriate as the tumours can be malignant. Patients with phaeochromocytoma tend to be hypovolaemic, experiencing an average 15% reduction of normal plasma volume, and careful fluid management before the operation is mandatory.

Children with phaeochromocytoma who have a high basal metabolic rate and high plasma concentrations of catecholamines are recognized as a poor anaesthetic risk. The anaesthetic must be approached with care to reduce the blood pressure in the immediate preoperative phase, during induction of anaesthesia and during mobilization of the tumour. Continuous electronic monitoring of arterial blood pressure and central venous pressure during the operation is essential. In an adequately blocked patient blood pressure during the operation should not fluctuate wildly, but surges of pressure can be controlled with phentolamine or with the vasodilator sodium nitroprusside. Great care is also required to maintain normal blood pressure after removal of the tumour, and this can usually be achieved with volume replacement. In hypotension unresponsive to volume replacement, infusion of catecholamines has limited effect owing to preoperative adrenergic blockade, and the administration of a vasopressor, such as angiotensin II, could be indicated. A urinary catheter is necessary to monitor urine output, which may well be poor initially because of the low plasma volume and high catecholamine concentrations.

Operation for phaeochromocytoma should be carefully planned with detailed knowledge of the radiological findings. Patients with unilateral sporadic adrenal tumours should undergo adrenalectomy, which was traditionally performed as an open procedure through either the transperitoneal or lumbar retroperitoneal approach. Recent advances in minimally invasive techniques and instrumentation have made laparoscopic removal of the adrenal glands possible [37,38]. In both open and laparoscopic surgery, careful dissection of the tumour and early ligation of the adrenal arteries feeding the tumour followed by ligation of the adrenal vein is required. Great care must be taken to ensure that the gland and the tumour within it are not ruptured. Excessive manipulation of the tumour should be avoided. Full exploration of the peritoneal cavity is unnecessary with accurate preoperative imaging.

The results of the surgical treatment for phaeochromocytoma in children are good. Reported mortality is between 0% and 3%, and perioperative morbidity can be prevented by adequate control of blood pressure [31,39]. Long-term results are influenced by the benign or malignant nature of the tumour. Most of the children remain normotensive and well but should be carefully followed up to detect recurrences or new phaeochromocytomas in the contralateral gland [34,35]. Comparison of laparoscopic and open adrenalectomy for phaeochromocytoma (historical controls) showed that the former is a safe technique with a low complication rate and frequency of intraoperative cardiovascular instabilities similar to the open procedure [37,38]. Postoperative hospital stay was significantly shorter and analgesia requirements less in the laparoscopic group [37].

Familial phaeochromocytomas are frequently bilateral but rarely malignant. Routine bilateral adrenalectomy is not indicated in these patients and good long-term results have been achieved by adrenal-sparing surgery [40,41]. Adrenal-preserving surgery can also be performed laparoscopically with good results [42].

## Adrenal cortex

Neoplasms of the adrenal cortex, although rare in childhood and adolescence, constitute the main indication for adrenalectomy in this age group. Patients with congenital adrenal hyperplasia resistant to medical therapy might be candidates for bilateral adrenalectomy to prevent the development of complications of androgen hypersecretion; however, only a

small number of operations for this indication have been reported [43,44].

Smaller adrenocortical tumours are usually benign and secrete one hormone, whereas larger lesions are more likely to be malignant and produce several hormones. In a series of 54 children with adrenocortical tumours, 94% secreted androgens, of which 36% were associated with glucocorticoids [45]. Abnormal hormone concentrations correlate well with clinical symptoms. Virilization is the commonest presentation, followed by Cushing syndrome and aldosteronism [46,47]. Abdominal examination may reveal a palpable mass [45,46]. The median time between the first symptoms and the diagnosis is about a year [46,47].

Preoperative evaluation should include CT scan or MRI of the abdomen to assess the site and size of the tumour and its relation to surrounding structures. Extra-adrenal sites are exceptionally rare. Biopsy of the tumour should be avoided to prevent tumour spillage, which will reduce chances of surgical cure. The endocrine effects of the tumour should be controlled and the patient presented to the surgeon in an optimal condition.

Smaller tumours can be removed laparoscopically but the majority of patients will require an open procedure. During the operation the tumour is removed with minimal trauma. Some of these tumours can be very large, particularly those associated with virilization. Such tumours require careful manipulation and handling so as not to breach the capsule. Enucleation of the tumour from the adrenal is inappropriate, and a complete adrenalectomy should be performed. Removal of the kidney without evidence of tumour involvement is contraindicated.

Postoperative care is required to maintain the electrolyte balance. Patients with Cushing syndrome may well require steroid supplementation in the immediate postoperative period to maintain blood pressure and well-being. Very careful follow-up of these patients is required, with slow withdrawal of steroid support to assess that the contralateral adrenal gland is functioning satisfactorily.

The malignant or benign nature of the adrenocortical tumours is undoubtedly the most important prognostic factor. Patients with small, functioning adenomas have an excellent prognosis. For smaller tumours, regardless of histology, the outcome can also be good. Of 20 children on the International Registry of Childhood Adrenocortical Tumours with tumours measuring less than 200 $cm^3$ or weighing less than 100 g after surgical removal, 18 were alive and with no evidence of recurrence at a median of 2.3 years [48]. Tumours larger than 200 $cm^3$ have a poor prognosis and patients with local invasion of the surrounding structures usually die [46,49]. Completeness of surgical resection is an independent prognostic factor. In a series of 54 children with adrenocortical tumours, of which half were less than 10 cm, the 5-year survival rate was 70% if the resection was microscopically complete, and only 7% if not [45]. Other factors such as age, delay of diagnosis or high levels of urinary androgens can be associated with an unfavourable outcome [46]. The role of adjuvant chemotherapy or chemotherapy for advanced or recurrent disease is uncertain [45,46].

## The pancreas

### Pancreatic neuroendocrine tumours

Pancreatic tumours originating from endocrine cells, both benign and malignant, are extremely rare in children. They can present in adolescence, which should prompt a search for MEN1. Diagnosis and treatment of these tumours is similar to those in an adult population. In case of insulinoma, pre- and intraoperative localization is of primary importance, and enucleation or formal pancreatic resection is usually curative. Malignant lesions confined to the pancreas (e.g. gastrinoma) should be treated by radical resection with lymphadenectomy. Patients with liver metastases from pancreatic endocrine tumours should be considered for liver resection, which could be curative. Percutaneous ablation of metastases with cryotherapy or a radiofrequency probe and angiographic embolization are helpful in controlling symptoms caused by an excess of hormones. To achieve this aim and to slow down the progression of disease, subcutaneous injections of the somatostatin analogue octeotride can be administered. Widespread metastatic disease can be treated with radioactive substances such as $^{125}I$ or yttrium attached to MIBG or octeotride [50,51].

### Neonatal hyperinsulinaemic hypoglycaemia

Neonatal hypoglycaemia can cause irreversible brain damage if not diagnosed and treated promptly. Hypoglycaemia can occur in normal neonates, especially if the first feeding is delayed for some hours, and is caused by developmental immaturity of liver mechanisms protecting against hypoglycaemia. However, the risk of hypoglycaemia in normal neonates decreases 12 h after birth, and after this time hyperinsulinism is the most common cause of neonatal hypoglycaemia.

Hyperinsulinism is characterized by hypoglycaemia and inappropriately elevated concentrations of insulin. *Transient hyperinsulinism* can be detected in infants of diabetic mothers or sick infants. *Persistent congenital hyperinsulinism* is the result of genetic mutations that cause focal or diffuse abnormalities of the β-cells of the pancreas. Maternal loss of chromosome 11p and inheritance of the paternal mutated gene *SUR1* cause the focal form of the disease, adenomatous hyperplasia. The diffuse form, characterized by overproduction of insulin by beta-cells, can be due to recessive mutations of *SUR1* and *KIR6.2* or dominant mutations of other genes. Hyperinsulinism due to the recessive mutations is more severe and cannot be controlled with diazoxide [52].

Surgical treatment is indicated for children who are unresponsive to medical therapy such as administration of diazoxide, glucagon, octeotride and dietary treatment and who require intravenous infusion of glucose at high doses to stabilize serum glucose.

The extent of pancreatic resection is the subject of controversy. Until recently, a 95% pancreatectomy was the preferred procedure for all patients who failed medical treatment. The earlier and more conservative approach of an 85% pancreatectomy, leaving much of the head of the pancreas *in situ*, proved less efficacious, with frequent recurrence of hypoglycaemia in up to 50% of cases. However, with the realization that the focal form of the disease could be responsible for as much as 40% of persistent hyperinsulinaemia, the opportunity has arisen to treat these patients with partial pancreatectomy. The success of the decision regarding the extent of pancreatectomy depends on the ability to distinguish between the focal and diffuse forms of the disease. This cannot be achieved clinically or biochemically, but can be done preoperatively by transhepatic selective catheterization of the pancreatic vein and blood sampling for insulin and C-peptide concentration. Further confirmation of the type of pathology responsible for hyperinsulinism can be obtained by intraoperative biopsy [53].

For diffuse hyperinsulinism 95% pancreatectomy is recommended. It is performed by mobilizing the body and tail of the pancreas from the left side across to the portal vein. In children there is a good plane of cleavage between the pancreas and splenic vessels and therefore a spleen-preserving pancreatectomy should be performed. The procedure is extended to the head of the gland and the uncinate process, which should be dissected cleanly from portal and superior mesenteric veins. The head of the pancreas is lifted from the C loop of the duodenum and away from the duodenal wall, leaving only a small amount of pancreas between the duodenum and the bile duct, which must be identified and carefully preserved. Partial pancreatectomy is recommended for patients with focal hyperinsulinism and the type of resection depends on the location of the focal adenomatous lesion.

Throughout surgery the blood glucose concentration is liable to fluctuate wildly. Thus, constant monitoring with a reliable glucose meter is essential, in combination with the ability to infuse either glucose during the mobilization or insulin after the excision of the gland. During the postoperative period, careful control of the blood glucose is essential, as it may rise or fall and require appropriate management.

Postoperative endocrine and exocrine pancreatic insufficiency can be caused by 95% pancreatectomy. The incidence of the diabetes increases with age and can be found in up to 50% of patients followed up for longer than 4 years, which is higher than previously thought [54]. Subclinical exocrine insufficiency, assessed by pancreatic function tests, exists in the majority of patients, but the proportion of patients reported to require enzyme supplements varies greatly from

10% to 60% [53,55]. Despite 95% pancreatectomy, hyperinsulinism and hypoglycaemia recur in 10–30% of patients, who require further medical treatment or more extensive, nearly total pancreatectomy [54]. Perioperative complications occur in 15% of patients undergoing 95% pancreatectomy, but this increases to 50% for near-total pancreatectomy. There should be no operative mortality. The results of partial pancreatectomy performed for focal disease are encouraging. None of the patients who had partial pancreatectomy for focal disease had recurrent hypoglycaemia, abnormal glucose tolerance or required further surgery [53].

## Conclusion

Paediatric endocrine surgery is a cooperative venture between paediatrician, surgeon, radiologist, pathologist and anaesthetist. The ideal environment for a paediatric endocrine unit providing all the necessary expertise is a large multispecialty hospital with an active adult endocrine unit. Expertise in adult endocrinology can be helpful, but the fact that many endocrine lesions in children behave differently should be recognized. Surgery requires an accurate endocrine diagnosis, localization of the disease, exact pathology either before or after the operation and careful monitoring throughout the procedure to counteract the endocrine effects of the disease process. With good teamwork results are excellent and the satisfaction from working with children is immense. Long-term monitoring is essential to ensure that recurrence of disease or hormonal deficiency does not occur, and that any replacement therapy needed is correctly administered.

## References

1 Gauderer MWL. Surgery for endocrinological diseases and malformations in childhood. In: Gauderer MWL, Angerpointner TA, eds. *Progress in Pediatric Surgery*, Vol. 26. Berlin: Springer Verlag, 1991: 1–2.

2 Hermus AR, Huysmans DA. Treatment of benign nodular thyroid disease. *N Engl J Med* 1998; 338: 1438–47.

3 Roher HD. *Endokrine Chirurgie*. Stuttgart: Thieme, 1987.

4 Singer PA, Cooper DS, Levy EG *et al.* Treatment guidelines for patients with hyperthyroidism and hypothyroidism. *J Am Med Assoc* 1995; 273: 808–12.

5 Raza J, Hindmarsh PC, Brook CGD. Thyrotoxicosis in children: thirty years' experience. *Acta Paediatr* 1999; 88: 937–41.

6 Farnell MB, van Heerden JA, McConahey WM, Carpenter HA, Wolff LH. Hypothyroidism after thyroidectomy for Graves' disease. *Am J Surg* 1981; 142: 535–9.

7 Buckingham BA, Costin G, Roe TF, Weitzman JJ, Kogut MD. Hyperthyroidism in children. *Am J Dis Child* 1981; 135: 112–17.

8 Muhlendahl KE, Helge H. Hyperthyreose im kindesalter. 2. Klinik und Therapie. *Padiatr Prax* 1978; 20: 601–16.

9 Perzik SL. The place of total thyroidectomy in the management of 909 patients with thyroid disease. *Am J Surg*; 1976; 132: 480–3.

10 Harach HR, Williams ED. Childhood thyroid cancer in England and Wales. *Br J Cancer* 1995; 72: 777–83.

11 Mehta MP, Goetowski PG, Kinsella TJ. Radiation induced thyroid neoplasms 1920 to 87: a vanishing problem? *Int J Radiat Oncol Biol Phys* 1989; 16: 1471–2.

12 Zimmerman D. Thyroid neoplasia in children. *Curr Opin Pediatr* 1997; 9: 413–18.

13 Bleuer JP, Averkin YI, Okeanov AE, Abelin T. The epidemiological situation of thyroid cancer in Belarus. *Stem Cells* 1997; 15 (Suppl. 2): 251–4.

14 Pacini F, Vorontsova T, Demidchik EP *et al.* Post-Chernobyl thyroid carcinoma in Belarus children and adolescents: comparison with naturally occuring thyroid carcinoma in Italy and France. *J Clin Endocrinol Metab* 1997; 82: 3563–9.

15 Bucksy P, Parlowsky T. Epidemiology and therapy of thyroid cancer in childhood and adolescence. *Exp Clin Endocrinol Diabetes* 1997; 105 (Suppl.): 70–3.

16 Hung W, Anderson KD, Chandra RS *et al.* Solitary thyroid nodules in 71 children and adolescents. *J Pediatr Surg* 1992; 27: 1407–9.

17 Raab SS, Silverman JF, Elsheikh TM, Thomas PA, Wakely PE. Pediatric thyroid nodules: disease demographics and clinical management as determined by fine needle aspiration biopsy. *Pediatrics* 1995; 95: 46–9.

18 McHenry C, Smith M, Lawrence AM, Jarosz H, Paloyan E. Nodular cancer disease in children and adolescence: a high incidence of carcinoma. *Am Surg* 1988; 54: 444–7.

19 La Quaglia MP, Telander RL. Differentiated and medullary thyroid cancer in childhood and adolescence. *Semin Pediatr Surg* 1997; 6: 42–9.

20 Mazzaferri EL, Jhiang SM. Long term impact on initial surgical and medical therapy on papillary and follicular thyroid cancer. *Am J Med* 1994; 97: 418–28.

21 Arts CH, Bax NM, Jansen M, Lips CJ, Vroom TM, van Vroonhoven TJ. Prophylactic total thyroidectomy in childhood for multiple endocrine neoplasia type 2A: preliminary results. *Ned Tijdschr Gemeeskd* 1999; 143: 98–104.

22 Ross AJ III. Parathyroid surgery in children. *Prog Pediatr Surg* 1991; 26: 48–59.

23 Cole DE, Janicic N, Salisbury SR, Hendy GN. Neonatal severe hyperparathyroidism, and familiar hypocalciuric hypercalcaemia: multiple different phenotypes associated with an inactivating Alu insertion mutation of the calcium-sensing receptor gene. *Am J Med Genet* 1997; 71: 251–2.

24 Blair JW, Carachi R. Neonatal primary hyperparathyroidism – a case report and review of the literature. *Eur J Pediatr Surg* 1991; 1 : 110–14.

25 Lutz P, Kane O, Pfersdorff A, Seiller F, Sauvage P, Levy JM. Neonatal primary hyperthyroidism: total parathyroidectomy with autotransplantation of cryopreserved parathyroid tissue. *Acta Paediatr Scand* 1986; 75: 179–82.

26 Loh KC, Duh QY, Shoback D, Gee L, Siperstein A, Clark OH. Clinical profile of primary hyperparathyroidism in adolescents and young adults. *Clin Endocrinol* 1998; 48: 435–43.

27 Levard G, Gaudelus J, Cessans C. Primary hyperparathyroidism in children. *Ann Chir* 1992; 46: 653–8.

28 Cronin CS, Reeve TS, Robinson B, Clifton-Bligh P, Guinea A, Delbridge L. Primary hyperparathyroidism in childhood and adolescence. *J Paediatr Child Health* 1996; 32: 397–9.

29 Meier DE, Snyder WH 3rd, Dickson BA, Margraf LR, Guzzetta PC Jr. Parathyroid carcinoma in a child. *J Pediatr Surg* 1999; 34: 606–8.

30 Harman CR, van Heerden JA, Farley DR, Grant CS, Thompson GB, Curlee K. Sporadic primary hyperparathyroidism in young patients: a separate disease entity? *Arch Surg* 1999; 134: 651–5.

31 Fonkalsrud EW. Pheochromocytoma in childhood. *Prog Pediatr Surg* 1991; 26: 103–11.

32 Revillon Y, Daher P, January D *et al*. Pheochromocytoma in children: 15 cases. *J Pediatr Surg* 1992; 27: 910–11.

33 Kaufman BH, Telander RL, van Heerden JA, Zimmerman D, Sheps SG, Dawson B. Phaeochromocytoma in the pediatric age group: current status. *J Pediatr Surg* 1983; 18: 879–84.

34 Caty MG, Coran AG, Geagen M, Thompson NW. Current diagnosis and treatment of pheochromocytoma in children. Experience with 22 consecutive tumours in 14 patients. *Arch Surg* 1990; 125: 978–81.

35 Ein SH, Pullerits J, Creighton R, Balfe JW. Pediatric pheochromocytoma. A 36 year review. *Pediatr Surg Int* 1997; 12: 595–8.

36 Shulkin BL, Thompson NW, Shapiro B, Francis IR, Sisson JC. Pheochromocytomas: imaging with 2-[fluorine-18]fluoro-2-deoxy-D-glucose PET. *Radiology* 1999; 212: 35–41.

37 Mobius E, Nies C, Rothmund M. Surgical treatment of pheochromocytomas: laparoscopic or conventional? *Surg Endosc* 1999; 13: 35–9.

38 Col V, de Canniere L, Collard E, Michel S, Donckier J. Laparoscopic adrenelectomy for phaeochromocytoma: endocrinological and surgical aspects of a new therapeutic approach. *Clin Endocrinol* 1999; 50: 121–5.

39 Telander RL, Zimmerman D, Kaufman BH, van Heerden JA. Pediatric endocrine surgery. *Surg Clin N Am* 1985; 65: 1551–87.

40 Neumann HPH, Bender BU, Reincke M, Eggstein S, Laubenberger J, Kirste G. Adrenal sparing surgery for phaeochromocytoma. *Br J Surg* 1999; 86: 94–7.

41 Albanese CT, Wiener ES. Routine total bilateral adrenelectomy is not warranted in childhood familial phaeochromocytoma. *J Pediatr Surg* 1993; 28: 1248–51.

42 Neumann HP, Reincke M, Bender BU, Elsner R, Janetschek G. Preserved adrenocortical function after laparoscopic bilateral adrenal sparing surgery for hereditary pheochromocytoma. *J Clin Endocrinol Metab* 1999; 84: 2608–10.

43 von Muhlendakl KE, Sippel WG. Adrenelectomy as a therapy in refractory adrenogenital syndrome. *Monatsschr Kinderheilkd* 1989; 137: 341–4.

44 Gunther DF, Bukowski TP, Ritzen EM, Wedell A, Van Wyk JJ. Prophylactic adrenelectomy of a three year old girl with congenital adrenal hyperplasia: pre and post operative studies. *J Clin Endocrinol Metab* 1997; 82: 3324–7.

45 Teinturier C, Pauchard MS, Brugieres L, Landais P, Chaussain JL, Bougneres PF. Clinical and prognostic aspects of adrenocortical neoplasms in childhood. *Med Pediatr Oncol* 1999; 32: 106–11.

46 Ribeiro RC, Sandrini Neto RS, Schell MJ, Lacerda L, Sambaio GA, Cat I. Adrenocortical carcinoma in children: a study of 40 cases. *J Clin Oncol* 1990; 8: 67–74.

47 Mayer SK, Oligny LL, Deal C, Yazbeck S, Gagne M, Blanchard H. Childhood adrenocortical tumours: case series and reevaluation of prognosis – a 24 year experience. *J Pediatr Surg* 1997; 32: 911–15.

48 Michalkiewicz EL, Sandrini R, Bugg MF *et al*. Clinical characteristics of small functioning adrenocortical tumours in children. *Med Pediatr Oncol* 1997; 28: 175–8.

49 Driver CP, Birch J, Gough DC, Bruce J. Adrenal cortical tumours in childhood. *Pediatr Hematol Oncol* 1998; 15: 527–32.

50 Vossen S, Goretzki PE, Goebel U, Willnow U. Therapeutic management of rare malignant pancreatic tumours in children. *World J Surg* 1998; 22: 879–82.

51 Jaksic T, Yaman M, Thorner P, Wesson DK, Filler RM, Shandling B. A 20-year review of paediatric pancreatic tumours. *J Pediatr Surg* 1992; 27: 1315–17.

52 Stanley CA, Baker L. The causes of neonatal hypoglycaemia. *N Engl J Med* 1999; 340: 1200–1.

53 Lonlay-Debeney P, Poggi-Travert F, Fournet JC *et al*. Clinical features of 52 neonates with hyperinsulinism. *N Engl J Med* 1999; 340: 1169–75.

54 Shilyansky J, Fisher S, Cutz E, Perlman K, Filler RM. Is 95% pancreatectomy the procedure of choice for treatment of persistent hyperinsulinaemic hypoglycaemia of the neonate? *J Pediatr Surg* 1997; 32: 342–6.

55 Cade A, Walters M, Puntis JW, Arthur RJ, Stringer MD. Pancreatic exocrine and endocrine function after pancreatectomy for persistent hyperinsulinaemic hypoglycaemia of infancy. *Arch Dis Child* 1998; 79: 435–9.

# 17 Brain tumours affecting growth and development

## E. R. Laws

## Introduction

The brain plays a central role in regulating growth and development. Beyond simple myelination and the development of neural connections is the role of the hypothalamus and other brain stem centres in regulating critical neurotransmitters and neurohormonal influences that provide for orderly growth and sexual maturation. The hypothalamus, under the control of the cerebral cortex and a variety of centres in the primitive portion of the developing brain, provides an internal clock for cerebral function that is presumed to include the timing of puberty. The pineal gland as a light-sensitive organ also plays a major role in natural rhythms, not only circadian but also those that may have influence on the state of alertness and certain psychological aspects of brain function.

## Developmental biology of the hypothalamus, pituitary and pineal

The hypothalamus, pituitary and pineal are all midline structures, and their development as composite organs with multiple connections is quite sophisticated. The embryogenesis of these three structures involves a series of sequential activations of genes related to the developing nervous system (homeobox genes), cellular differentiation of the pituitary, angiogenesis and neurotransmitter expression.

Markers have been developed for the location of cells involved in various aspects of growth and development and they can be traced both anatomically and physiologically. For most of these agents the physiology is well known, and the sequence of target organs affected by pituitary hormones under the control of releasing factors and inhibiting factors from the hypothalamus has been the subject of intense investigation. The overall tonic effects of pineal function are still to be elucidated.

## The histopathology and classification of tumours and other disorders affecting growth and development

### Hypothalamic lesions (Table 17.1)

The prototypical hypothalamic lesion that frequently is associated with precocious puberty is the hypothalamic hamartoma. Its presence in the midline, usually in the interpeduncular fossa, indicates that it has origins similar to

**Table 17.1.** Structural lesions producing hypothalamic dysfunction

Intrinsic hypothalamic lesions
  Hamartoma
  Glioma
  Langerhans cell histiocytosis
  Lipoma

Suprasellar lesions
  Craniopharyngioma
  Pituitary macroadenoma
  Dermoid/epidermoid tumour
  Rathke's cleft cyst
  Meningioma
  Arachnoid cyst
  Germinoma
  Aneurysm of the circle of Willis
  Sarcoid, tuberculosis
  Lymphocytic and granulocytic hypophysitis

Third ventricular lesions
  Glioma
  Ependymoma
  Colloid cyst
  Hydrocephalus
  Central neurocytoma

| Diagnosis | Number of cases | Percentage |
|---|---|---|
| Acromegaly (GH adenoma) | 468 | 18 |
| Prolactinoma | 861 | 33 |
| ACTH adenoma (Cushing disease and Nelson syndrome) | 433 | 16 |
| Non-functioning adenomas (gonadotrophic and null cell adenomas) | 855 | 32 |
| Miscellaneous adenomas | 28 | 1 |
| Total | 2645 | 100 |

**Table 17.2.** Incidence of various subtypes of pituitary adenoma (author's series)

the hypothalamus and the pituitary itself. Many hamartomas and gangliocytomas are hormonally active and can be stained for a variety of peptide-releasing and -inhibiting factors and for specific hormones as well [1,2].

Other lesions have a predilection for the hypothalamus and these include low-grade astrocytomas, Langerhans cell histiocytosis, dermoid and epidermoid tumours and inflammatory problems such as sarcoidosis. The hypothalamus can be indirectly affected by a number of lesions in the area, most commonly craniopharyngioma and germinoma, both of which tend to have their origins in the pituitary stalk and then extend to involve the hypothalamus.

## Pituitary stalk lesions

There are a few lesions that characteristically affect the pituitary stalk. These include granular cell tumours, choristomas [2], germinomas and occasionally pituitary tumours that primarily involve the stalk, as is sometimes seen in Cushing disease. As mentioned above, both craniopharyngiomas and germinomas may take origin from and appear primarily in the region of the pituitary stalk. The inflammatory condition, lymphocytic hypophysitis, often extends up to involve the infundibulum as well. These lesions have in common the production of diabetes insipidus.

## Anterior pituitary lesions

The most common anterior pituitary lesions are the benign pituitary adenomas, which can be categorized as either hyperfunctioning or non-functioning lesions [3,4]. They can occur from any of the five different types of anterior pituitary cells, and tumours involving combinations of these basic cell types are relatively common as well. The distribution of pituitary adenomas is seen in Table 17.2. In addition to pituitary tumours, there can be entirely intrasellar craniopharyngiomas, and the pituitary gland itself can be subject to the development of cysts and to inflammatory lesions such as lymphocytic hypophysitis, sarcoid and other granulomatous diseases.

## Pars intermedia lesions

The pars intermedia, which is located between the anterior and posterior lobes of the pituitary gland, can give rise to a number of lesions. The most common of these is the Rathke's cleft cyst, as this is the anatomic site of Rathke's cleft. One also can see small cysts, either liquid or colloid, in the same region, and some believe that a subcategory of adrenocorticotrophic hormone (ACTH)-secreting pituitary tumours associated with Cushing disease arises in the pars intermedia.

## Posterior pituitary lesions

Posterior pituitary tumours are rare. The most common is the pilocytic astrocytoma. One can also see hypothalamic hamartomas appearing in the posterior pituitary along with primary lesions called granular cell tumours or choristomas.

## Pineal lesions

A variety of different pathological entities can affect the pineal region [5]. The most common is the germinoma. A variety of other germ cell tumours, including embryonal cell carcinoma, choriocarcinoma and a variety of teratomas, benign and malignant, are also seen. The region may also be the site of benign and malignant primitive neuroectodermal tumours and meningiomas.

## Clinical presentation of intracranial lesions affecting growth and development

### Effects on growth and development

Pituitary tumours often affect growth and development [6,7]. Growth hormone (GH)-secreting tumours produce acromegaly in adults and, in children, lead to gigantism, usually an easily recognizable syndrome. The biochemistry of gigantism is similar to that of acromegaly with persistent elevation of serum GH concentrations, raised IGF-I (insulin-like growth factor I) levels and paradoxical GH responses to thyrotrophin-releasing hormone (TRH) and glucose loading. Care is needed in the tall pubertal patient as similar features can be recorded. The difference is the 24-h serum GH profile, which is persistently elevated in gigantism whereas the classic pulsatile pattern is observed in constitutional tall stature [8]. Other tumours such as hypothalamic hamartomas and some pineal tumours that result in precocious puberty may also have a secondary effect on growth, with an increase in sexual maturation, growth, bone age and bone density. Many non-functioning pituitary tumours and some prolactin-secreting pituitary tumours lead to a retardation of growth, as they diminish the pulsatile output of growth hormone from pressure effects [9,10]. This can also occur with craniopharyngiomas and is probably the major cause of short stature in children who have craniopharyngiomas [11]. Children with Cushing disease from a hypersecreting pituitary adenoma may develop short stature. Ultimately, this may arise from long-standing exposure to any adrenal androgen generated. In the short term, however, the more likely cause of the poor growth is the direct or indirect effect of the tumour on GH release coupled with the known inhibitory effect of corticotrophin-releasing hormone (CRH) on GH release [12]. The precise role of cortisol, which actually increases GH release in humans in the short-term, is not clear, although GH release is low in patients with Cushing disease [13].

## Effects on sexual maturation

Virtually any type of pituitary tumour and many hypothalamic lesions cause retardation in sexual maturation. The craniopharyngioma is the prototypical lesion producing the syndrome of dystrophic adiposity and sexual infantilism as described by Babinski and Fröhlich. These problems can also occur from hypothalamic disorders producing alterations of luteinizing hormone-releasing hormone (LHRH) and other hypothalamic hormones controlling pituitary function. Tumours that secrete excess levels of prolactin can themselves retard sexual development, particularly in the male. The syndrome of primary amenorrhoea can be produced by a whole spectrum of lesions, extending from pituitary tumours to craniopharyngiomas to histiocytosis to hydrocephalus with dilatation of the third ventricle [9]. As mentioned, both hypothalamic hamartomas and pineal tumours can produce precocious puberty. These syndromes can occur both in boys and girls and are quite dramatic when they appear. Unfortunately, they usually are irreversible, even when the offending lesion is successfully treated.

## Effects on vision and visual function

Tumours in the region of the sella and the suprasellar area can all produce difficulties with vision, primarily by compression of the optic nerves and optic chiasm. The most common lesions to do this are craniopharyngiomas and pituitary tumours with suprasellar extension. Other suprasellar lesions, such as epidermoid cysts, hypothalamic and optic gliomas and inflammatory lesions in the suprasellar region, can all produce visual compromise. The most common clinical finding of a suprasellar lesion is a bitemporal hemianopia, but if there is compression of either of the optic nerves or the optic tracts additional syndromes of visual loss can occur. Tumours in the region of the pineal gland produce their own set of characteristic visual problems. These include defective accommodation, difficulty in upward gaze, poor convergence and occasionally retractory nystagmus. Many patients have an afferent pupillary defect and some have disconjugate gaze.

## Effects on the circulation of cerebrospinal fluid and hydrocephalus

Any lesion in the pituitary area that grows towards the third ventricle can produce obstructive hydrocephalus by blocking one or both foramina of Monro. Hydrocephalus from this cause commonly accompanies cystic craniopharyngiomas in children but can occur with many other types of lesions as well. The sudden onset of obstructive hydrocephalus can be a medical emergency. When patients appear with symptoms and signs of increased intracranial pressure, the offending lesion must be dealt with directly or a cerebrospinal fluid (CSF) diversionary procedure such as a ventriculoperitoneal shunt must be carried out [14].

Tumours in the pineal region may also present with obstructive hydrocephalus, usually from obstruction of the aqueduct of Sylvius. Tumours in the pineal region can produce dorsal pressure on the midbrain, which is enough either to impair or occlude the flow of spinal fluid through the aqueduct. In this situation, progressive dilatation of the ventricular system can also occur and must be dealt with by removing the mass effect that compresses the aqueduct, by carrying out a CSF diversion, which can be done with a variety of shunt procedures or by performing a third ventriculostomy, which is another mechanism of bypassing posterior third ventricular obstruction [15,16].

## Increased intracranial pressure

There are two mechanisms for the production of increased intracranial pressure with tumours in the suprasellar or pineal region. These include mass effect from the size of a very large tumour taking up room within the closed compartment of the skull and the secondary effects of obstruction of CSF flow as noted above. Temporary alleviation of increased intracranial pressure can sometimes be accomplished with the use of steroid medications but most situations of increased intracranial pressure require surgical management, either with removal of the offending mass or the performance of a CSF diversionary procedure to relieve intracranial pressure.

## Other effects on brain and cerebral function

The impressive variety of different types of pathology that can occur in the suprasellar region includes lesions that can affect many important areas at the base of the skull. The effect on the visual system has been noted, but the hypothalamus itself can be directly affected, as can the mamillary bodies and septal region. This is a particular problem with the craniopharyngioma patient, in whom hypothalamic tumour extension or enthusiastic surgical tumour size reduction can lead to extensive damage to the hypothalamic nuclei [17]. Pressure or damage to the brain in these areas can produce varying degrees of difficulty with short-term memory and can even result in dementia. Tumours in the suprasellar region or the parasellar region may extend to involve the mesial aspect of the temporal lobe and thereby produce partial complex epilepsy.

## Diagnosis of tumours affecting growth and development

A variety of sophisticated endocrine tests are available for the characterization of patients with tumours that can alter growth, development or sexual maturation [18]. These include the pituitary hormones, which can be measured in their basal and activated states, and a number of peptide-releasing hormones and other factors that play important roles in the delicate balance that results in normal development.

Once an endocrine syndrome can be characterized clinically and by laboratory diagnosis, magnetic resonance imaging (MRI) provides highly sophisticated anatomic information allowing for the imaging analysis of the lesion and its affects on surrounding neural structures (Figs 17.1–17.5). Additional investigations may also include MRI with the rapid (5 s) acquisition of slices, which allows abnormalities of blood flow around tumours to be detected. This is particularly helpful where delineation of the lesion using conventional MRI has not aided the diagnosis. Consideration also needs to be given to petrosal sinus sampling, which can be helpful in differentiating pituitary from ectopic sources of ACTH production [19].

## Surgical management of brain tumours affecting growth and development

For tumours involving the sellar region the surgeon must determine whether a trans-sphenoidal route of access will be successful in dealing with the lesion or whether a craniotomy will be necessary. Basic principles involved in this determina-

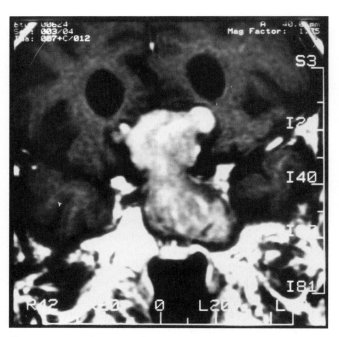

**Fig. 17.1.** Coronal MRI scan of a pituitary adenoma (null cell adenoma) with suprasellar extension and deformation of the hypothalamus.

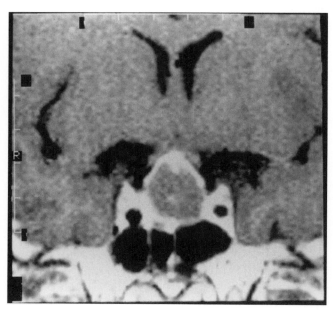

**Fig. 17.2.** Coronal MRI scan of an intrasellar craniopharyngioma with suprasellar extension and compression of the optic chiasm.

tion have to do primarily with the size of the sella. In patients with a large sella, in whom one expects a benign pituitary tumour, which is usually soft, the trans-sphenoidal approach is highly successful. Some craniopharyngiomas arise below the diaphragm of the sella and present as sellar and suprasellar masses with enlargement of the pituitary fossa. When this

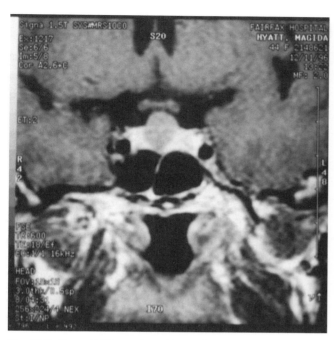

**Fig. 17.3.** Coronal MRI scan of a Rathke's cleft cyst.

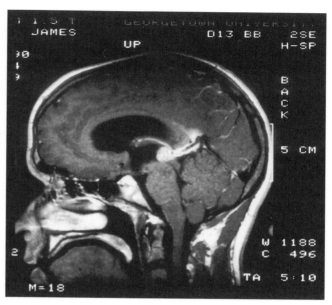

**Fig. 17.5.** Sagittal MRI scan of a pineal region germinoma. Note compression of the aqueduct of Sylvius and secondary hydrocephalus with dilatation of the lateral ventricle.

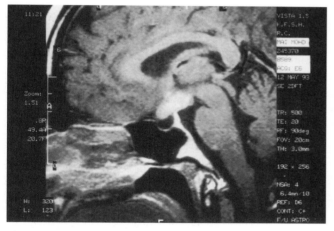

**Fig. 17.4.** Sagittal MRI scan of a hypothalamic glioma.

occurs, patients usually have hypopituitarism and a trans-sphenoidal approach may provide excellent management for the craniopharyngioma and allow the avoidance of the risks of a craniotomy [11,18,20].

When craniotomy is necessary for dealing with a suprasellar lesion, it is usually because the sella itself is small, compromising the amount of room necessary for effective surgical manipulation, or because the imaging studies suggest a different kind of pathology such as a meningioma, which would be unsuitably managed using trans-sphenoidal techniques.

There are a number of appropriate craniotomy approaches and these need to be tailored both to the anatomy and to the presumed pathology of the lesion to be considered. The most common craniotomy approach is a non-dominant subfrontal exposure of the sellar region. This can be done through a frontal craniotomy, a frontotemporal craniotomy, a bifrontal craniotomy or an extended pterional approach. Skull base approaches may occasionally be desirable and can provide expanded access. These include the fronto-orbital craniotomy and the transbasal approach. A transcranial trans-sphenoidal approach has been described and is occasionally useful, and one can approach craniopharyngiomas through the lamina terminalis, either with a subfrontal exposure or with an interhemispheric approach. Tumours that involve the third ventricle can be treated by using a transcallosal approach through a parasagittal craniotomy, and tumours of the pineal region can be approached posteriorly using either an infratentorial supracerebellar approach or a supratentorial transtentorial occipital approach, depending upon the nature and extension of the lesion.

Endoscopic techniques have been useful, both with intra-ventricular approaches and with trans-sphenoidal operations in the sellar region. The endoscope can also be effectively used in conjunction with the standard craniotomy when one requires visualization within the third ventricular region.

## Results of management of brain tumours affecting growth and development

Sophisticated surgical techniques can very often deal quite effectively with the tumours themselves and also with many of the secondary effects of the tumour [20]. In some cases impaired endocrine function can recover, particularly in patients harbouring pituitary adenomas where normal compressed pituitary gland may be preserved and may recover impaired function [21]. For most of the other syndromes, however, the difficulties in growth, development and sexual maturation persist, and therefore careful medical management with hormonal replacement therapy is necessary for these patients to achieve a normal and satisfactory quality of life. Fortunately, expertise and capabilities in this arena are improving as well, thus brightening the outlook for patients afflicted with these difficult lesions.

## References

1 Asa SL, Scheithauer BW, Bilbao JM *et al.* A case for hypothalamic acromegaly: a clinicopathological study of six patients with hypothalamic gangliocytomas producing growth hormone-releasing factor. *J Clin Endocrinol Me*tab 1984; 58: 796–803.

2 Scheithauer BW, Kovacs K, Randall RV, Horvath E, Okazaki H, Laws ER Jr. Hypothalamic neuronal hamartoma and adenohypophyseal neuronal choristoma: their association with growth hormone adenoma of the pituitary gland. *J Neuropathol Exp Neurol* 1983; 42: 648–63.

3 Thapar K, Kovacs K, Laws ER Jr. The classification and molecular biology of pituitary adenomas. *Adv Tech Standards Neurosurg* 1995; 22: 3–53.

4 Thapar K, Kovacs K, Laws ER Jr, Muller PJ. Pituitary adenomas: current concepts in classification, histopathology and molecular biology. *Endocrinologist* 1993; 3: 39–57.

5 Donat JF, Okazaki H, Gomez MR, Reagan TJ, Baker HL Jr, Laws ER Jr. Pineal tumours – a 53-year experience. *Arch Neurol* 1978; 35: 736–40.

6 Abboud CF, Laws ER Jr. Diagnosis of pituitary tumours. *Endocrinol Metab Clin N Am* 1988; 17: 241–80.

7 Kane LA, Leinung MC, Carpenter PC, Laws ER Jr, Zimmerman D. Pituitary adenomas in childhood and adolescence. *J Clin Endocrinol Metab* 1994; 79: 1135–40.

8 Hindmarsh PC, Stanhope R, Kendall BE, Brook CGD. Tall stature: a clinical, endocrinological and radiological study. *Clin Endocrinol* 1986; 25: 223–31.

9 Coulam CB, Laws ER Jr, Abboud CF, Randall RV. Primary amenorrhea and pituitary adenomas. *Fertil Steril* 1981; 35: 615–19.

10 Randall RV, Laws ER Jr, Abboud CF, Ebersold MJ, Kao PC, Scheithauer BW. Transsphenoidal microsurgical treatment of prolactin-producing pituitary adenomas: results in 100 patients. *Mayo Clinic Proc* 1983; 58: 108–21.

11 Laws ER Jr. Craniopharyngioma: diagnosis and treatment. *Endocrinologist* 1992; 2: 184–8.

12 Raza J, Massoud AF, Hindmarsh PC, Robinson ICAF, Brook CGD. Direct effects of corticotrophin releasing hormone on stimulated growth hormone secretion. *Clin Endocrinol* 1998; 48: 217–22.

13 Krieger DT. Rhythms in CRF, ACTH and corticosteroids. In: Kreiger DT, ed. *Endocrine Rhythms*. New York: Raven Press, 1979.

14 Abay EO, Laws ER Jr, Grado GL *et al.* Pineal tumours in children and adolescents – treatment by CSF shunting and radiotherapy. *J Neurosurg* 1981; 55: 889–95.

15 Marsh WR, Laws ER Jr. Shunting and irradiation of pineal tumours. *Clin Neurosurg* 1985; 32: 540–73.

16 Abboud CF, Laws ER Jr. Clinical endocrinological approach to hypothalamic- pituitary disease. *J Neurosurg* 1979; 51: 271–91.

17 DeVile CJ, Grant DB, Hayward RD, Stanhope R. Growth and endocrine sequelae of craniopharyngioma. *Arch Dis Child* 1996; 75: 108–14.

18 Laws ER Jr. Diagnosis and management of craniopharyngioma in children and adolescents. *Curr Opin Endocrinol Diabetes* 1996; 3: 110–14.

19 Oldfield EH, Doppman JL, Nieman LK *et al.* Petrosal sinus sampling with and without corticotropin-releasing hormone for the differential diagnosis of Cushing's syndrome. *N Engl J Med* 1991; 325: 897–905.

20 Laws ER Jr. Transsphenoidal microsurgery in the management of craniopharyngioma. *J Neurosurg* 1980; 52: 661–6.

21 Massoud AF, Powell M, Williams RA, Hindmarsh PC, Brook CGD. Transsphenoidal surgery for pituitary tumours. *Arch Dis Child* 1997; 76: 398–404.

# 18 Management of multiple endocrine neoplasia

## J. L. H. O'Riordan

## Introduction

Multiple endocrine neoplasia encompasses two syndromes, MEN1 and MEN2, that are distinct in the ways in which they affect the endocrine system. These differences relate not only to the clinical manifestations but also to the underlying genetic processes that lead to proliferation of the glands and hypersecretion of hormone.

MEN type 1 (previously referred to as multiple endocrine adenomatosis type 1 or MEA type 1) was first described by Erdheim in 1903, recording the finding at autopsy of four enlarged parathyroid glands in a patient who had acromegaly with a pituitary adenoma. The familial incidence of multiple endocrine tumours was described separately by Wermer and by Moldawer *et al.* in 1954. Thus, the eponyms Erdheim and Wermer syndromes were used for a while. It became clear that tumours of the parathyroid, pituitary and pancreas could occur in the same patient and that many members of a family could be affected. Later, when gastrinomas and prolactinomas could be recognized, it was appreciated that oversecretion in MEN1 affected not only parathyroid hormone (PTH), growth hormone (GH) and insulin but also involved hypersecretion of gastrin and prolactin in families or spontaneously.

Recognition of MEN2 was slower. Medullary carcinoma of the thyroid was recognized in the 1950s as a distinct form of thyroid tumour, often with deposition of amyloid. In 1961, before calcitonin had been discovered and had been found to be secreted by the parafollicular cells of the thyroid, Sipple described the association of phaeochromocytoma with carcinoma of the thyroid, so the condition is sometimes referred to as Sipple syndrome. It is now referred to as multiple endocrine neoplasia type 2 (MEN2) and subgroups of MEN2 have subsequently been recognized. In some of these, parathyroid tumours also occur, although different endocrine glands are generally involved in the two forms of MEN.

## Clinical features of MEN1

The clinical manifestations depend on which hormone is being oversecreted, be it PTH, prolactin, GH, insulin, gastrin or glucagon, so the clinical manifestations are variable [1]. Initially, it was thought that the features were reproducible within a family, so the different members would be affected similarly. This is not the case, and the phenotype therefore varies within a given kindred.

The most commonly affected gland is the parathyroid, which is involved in 95% of patients with MEN1. Hyperparathyroidism is often the first manifestation of the disease, either because it produces symptoms due, for example, to renal calculi or because biochemical screening is easier for this condition than for other glands. Hypercalcaemia is the critical feature. Measuring serum calcium is the simplest screening test and one that can be repeated over the years to see whether an individual is affected and the time at which hypercalcaemia developed. This can become apparent at widely different ages in different members of a family. In one it may be the cause of serious problems by the age of 20, whereas in others in the same family it may only become demonstrable in the fifth, sixth or seventh decades (Fig. 18.1). Thus a normal result with biochemical screening does not (in the context of either the parathyroid gland or for that matter any other test of glandular function) exclude the possibility that the disease would manifest later. In children, hyperparathyroidism can become symptomatic in this condition by 8 years of age, but it is quite unusual under the age of 15.

An important feature of the hyperparathyroidism in MEN1 is that multiple glands are affected, be they hyperplastic or adenomatous. It should be pointed out that the distinction between hyperplasia and adenoma of a gland or glands is generally not helpful as recognizing that an adenoma is present depends on finding a rim of normal tissue in a section, which is not a good criterion. Additional problems may arise as glands can be affected asynchronously, and a

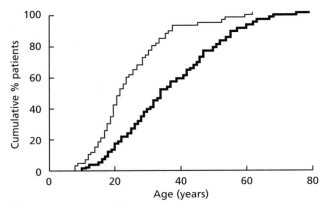

**Fig. 18.1.** Age-related onset of penetrance of MEN1. The ages and cumulative percentages of patients who had developed the first manifestation of MEN1 are shown for the symptomatic presenting group (n = 153) (bold line) and for the asymptomatic, biochemically detected group (n = 66) (thin line). Reproduced with permission [1].

gland that has seemed normal at initial surgery might be found to be enlarged at subsequent re-exploration of the neck, even if the patient has been normocalcaemic after the first operation, or even hypoparathyroid after the first operation, before hypercalcaemia recurs. Recurrence of hyperparathyroidism is frequent even when hypoparathyroidism has been produced initially. Another important feature of the condition is that males and females are affected equally, unlike the normal distribution in primary hyperparathyroidism in which the male–female ratio is 1:3.

Pancreatic tumours occur in about 40% of patients with MEN1. Of these, about two-thirds are gastrinomata, causing the Zollinger–Ellison syndrome, with severe peptic ulceration and sometimes diarrhoea. About a quarter of the patients have insulin-secreting tumours causing hypoglycaemic episodes, which may be the first manifestation of the presence of the syndrome. Glucagon-secreting tumours are rare in MEN. Even if the pancreatic tumour appears to be non-secreting, the presence of raised circulating pancreatic polypeptide is a useful tumour marker. Pancreatic tumours can also secrete GH-releasing hormone or parathyroid hormone-related peptide, although, again, this is uncommon.

The incidence of pituitary tumours in MEN1 has been reported variously as being between 10% and 30%. About two-thirds of these pituitary tumours secrete prolactin and perhaps a fifth of them secrete GH. Adrenocorticotrophic hormone (ACTH) overproduction is relatively less common (perhaps 5%), but in those in whom it does occur it is important because of the seriousness of Cushing disease. Carcinoid tumours are not common, occurring perhaps in a few per cent of patients with MEN1. They may arise in the stomach, bronchi or thymus and are serious because they can be malignant and metastasize and so be life-threatening, even though they do not produce the carcinoid syndrome. Other tumours

occurring uncommonly in MEN1 include phaeochromocytoma, teratoma of the testis and lipomata.

## Clinical features of MEN2

Three groups of MEN2 have been distinguished [2,3] on the basis of which tissues are affected. In familial medullary thyroid carcinoma (FMTC), there is involvement only of the C or parafollicular cells of the thyroid, so that, strictly speaking, this is not *multiple* endocrine neoplasia, but it has many features in common with other forms of MEN2 and so merits inclusion here. A few large families with this condition have been described and in these the tumours are of late onset and the mortality is low.

In MEN2A, apart from medullary carcinoma of the thyroid, there are phaeochromocytomata and parathyroid tumours. MEN2A is the most common form of MEN2, accounting for two-thirds of cases. Circulating calcitonin is a useful tumour marker and is generally raised by the age of 40 years in affected members of a family. In the population as a whole, the incidence of medullary carcinoma of the thyroid is probably only about 1 per million of population per year, and about a quarter of these are heritable. The tumours in MEN2A are malignant and have often metastasized from the thyroid locally to lymph glands, even when the primary tumour is only a centimetre in diameter. There may subsequently be distant metastases to lung or liver.

Measurement of circulating calcitonin, either in a basal state or after stimulation by administration of oral alcohol or an intravenous dose of pentagastrin, can indicate an abnormality at a stage at which there is no thyroid nodule but at which hyperplasia of the C cells may be found. Parathyroid lesions occur only in about 5–10% of affected individuals in a family, so that the penetrance is low. The parathyroid lesions may be adenomas or hyperplastic, and they cause hypercalcaemia that is sometimes symptomatic. Phaeochromocytoma occurs in about half of the affected members of a family with MEN2A. The tumours are usually benign (unless they are very large) and they cause hypertension that can be episodic and life-threatening as a result of over-release of adrenaline and noradrenaline.

As individuals in many families with MEN2A may have only medullary carcinoma of the thyroid, it is possible that some families classified as having familial medullary carcinoma of the thyroid really have MEN2A, in which only the medullary carcinoma of the thyroid has become apparent. Arbitrarily these families have been classified as having familial medullary thyroid carcinoma if there are at least four affected members none of whom has evidence of either phaeochromocytoma or hyperparathyroidism. In some families with otherwise typical MEN2A, there may be a skin lesion affecting the skin on the back between the scapulae; this is lichen amyloidosis. Another curious feature is the association in some cases with Hirschsprung disease. It should be noted also that familial phaeochromocytoma not associated with the other features of MEN2A can also occur, either with von Hippel–Lindau syndrome or with neurofibromatosis.

MEN2B is the least common form. Medullary carcinoma of the thyroid and phaeochromocytoma occur but hyperparathyroidism does not. The medullary carcinoma of the thyroid and the phaeochromocytoma present at about 20 years of age, in other words earlier than they do in MEN2A, and the tumours are more aggressive. A striking feature of this variant of the syndrome is the developmental abnormalities due to disorganized growth of peripheral nerve axons in the lips, mouth and conjunctivae. The facial appearance is characteristic with thick lips and nodules on the tongue and conjunctivae and there may be thickened corneal nerves. Abnormality of the nervous system in the intestine can also be shown on rectal biopsy. Hyperplasia of the intestinal autonomic nerve plexi causes abnormal intestinal motility in infancy and can lead to failure to thrive, with episodes of constipation and diarrhoea. The newborn infants may be 'floppy'. There may be skeletal abnormalities, such as pes cavus, slipped femoral epiphyses, pectus excavatum or bifid ribs. The child may have a Marfanoid appearance, but without lesions of the aorta, palate or lens. In men, impotence can occur because of neurological changes.

The C cells of the thyroid and the cells of the adrenal medulla are derived from neuroectoderm, as probably are the intestinal autonomic ganglia. The origin of the C cells was shown initially in studies of quail ultimobranchial bodies, the avian equivalent of C cells, which have a characteristic morphology. The parathyroid cells, however, are derived from endoderm of the third and fourth pharyngeal pouches, so their stem cells differ and expression of the mutant gene is not confined to a single lineage.

## The genetic basis of MEN1

The syndrome is inherited as an autosomal dominant condition. The gene, called *MEN1*, is at position 11q13, close to the centromere on chromosome 11. The coding part is approximately 9000 bases and the mRNA about 2800 basepairs, including a predicted protein containing 610 amino acids called menin. It has two nuclear localization signals near the carboxy terminus and is a nuclear protein. Human *MEN1* was first cloned by Chandrasekharappa *et al.* [4]. Shortly after that, the same gene was identified by The European Consortium [5]. In both cases, positional cloning techniques were used, and it was necessary to sequence a series of genes in the area. The murine homologue has also been cloned [6] and called *men1*; its structure is very similar. Critical to the identification of the gene in humans was finding mutations in families with MEN1, indicating that the correct gene had been sequenced.

Although the condition itself is inherited as an autosomal dominant, the mutation is recessive. This paradox is explained by Knudson's 'two-hit hypothesis'. In this extraordinary paper, Knudson [7] made sense out of seemingly confused data about the development of spontaneous and familial retinoblastomata. He reasoned that inheritance of an abnormal gene was the fundamental basis of the development of familial retinoblastoma but that this germline mutation was not sufficient on its own for tumorigenesis. There had to be a second mutation, this time a somatic mutation of the second copy (the normal copy) of the gene that the patient has before tumours develop.

The same is true for MEN1. Mutation of one parent's copy of the *MEN1* gene is the first hit. On its own, that cannot lead to tumour formation and there has to be a second hit, inactivating the normal copy of the gene that the other parent provides. That second hit is a somatic mutation. The earlier studies [8, 9] of the location of the *MEN1* locus on 11q13, which led ultimately to the gene being cloned 8 years later, also showed that loss of heterozygosity (LOH) occurred. In other words, when DNA from the patient's normal leucocytes and from the patient's tumour tissue were examined, it was found that some of the DNA present in the leucocytes was absent in the tumour. These deletions could be part of or even the whole of the long arm of chromosome 11. The effect of these deletions was to make it possible for the properties of the mutated gene, the first hit, to be expressed.

The mechanisms whereby the somatic mutations occur are not clear. It has been suggested that they may be attributable to the presence of sequences in the normal DNA that are subject to erroneous translation. This can be due to the presence of long tracts of either single nucleotides or shorter series of di- or even octonucleotides. These can be described in the 'replication–slippage model', with misalignment of the dinucleotide repeat in replication and subsequent excision of a single-stranded loop. On the basis of the finding of loss of heterozygosity, it was predicted that the *MEN1* gene would encode a tumour-suppressor protein. That menin is a nuclear protein was therefore to be expected.

It has been shown that menin interacts with JunD but not with other members of the Jun–Fos family members and the menin–JunD complex represses transcriptional activation mediated by JunD [10]. Mutations in menin disrupt menin interaction with JunD, suggesting that the tumour suppression function was dependent on direct binding to JunD and inhibition of JunD-activated transcription. Using deletion analysis, it has been shown that there are at least two independent nuclear localization signals in the carboxy-terminal quarter of the protein.

## Mutations causing MEN1

The germline mutation responsible for the development of

MEN1 has now been identified in over 100 families [10–12]. There has been great variation in the mutations, which include nonsense mutations, deletions, insertions, donor split-site mutations and missense mutations scattered throughout the coding region (Fig. 18.2). Only a small proportion of them occurred in more than one, apparently unrelated, family. It would seem likely that all these mutations result in loss of function.

While the germline mutation (the first hit) is consistent within a family, the second hit, the somatic mutation, is variable. It differs in tumours affecting separate tissues in one individual, for example in parathyroid or pancreas, and within a single tissue there may be differing forms of loss of heterozygosity. In different members of the same kindred, the second hit also varies with different degrees of loss of heterozygosity in the tumours examined. Those findings of course are in accord with the expectations of the Knudson hypothesis.

## The genetic basis of MEN2

By linkage analysis, the gene for MEN2 was shown to lie on chromosome 10q11.2. The clue as to the gene involved came from studies of a mutated mouse in which the *RET* proto-oncogene had been knocked out. *RET* is an acronym for *re*arranged in *t*ransfection assays using DNAs from human

lymphomas and gastric tumours. It was one of the candidate genes [2,3,13] for MEN2 as it was known to be in the relevant area. The phenotype of the mouse with the knockout of this gene included Hirschsprung disease, with which MEN2 is occasionally associated. Studies of the *RET* proto-oncogene in patients with MEN2 then showed that mutations were present.

RET is a glycoprotein member of the tyrosine kinase receptor family. It has an extracellular ligand-binding domain, a single transmembrane region and an intracellular tyrosine kinase domain. Binding to ligand causes dimerization of the extracellular domain and activation of the tyrosine kinase domain. Glial-derived neurotrophic factor (GDNF) has been shown to be a ligand for RET. It was known to be a trophic factor for dopaminergic neurones and, when the gene for GDNF was knocked out in mice, it was found that the phenotype included features of the RET knockout. Binding of GDNF to RET is indirect, occurring via a second protein, GDNF R-α, the receptor that is bound to the cell membrane lipid. This involvement of a second protein is unusual in tyrosine kinase receptors.

RET can exist in three different forms with between 1072 and 1114 amino acids. These distinct forms arise from alternative splicing of the gene, which consists of 55 kb with 21 exons. The protein has a signal sequence of 25 amino acids that is cleaved off when the peptide is secreted into the membrane. The extracellular domain is glycosylated and has

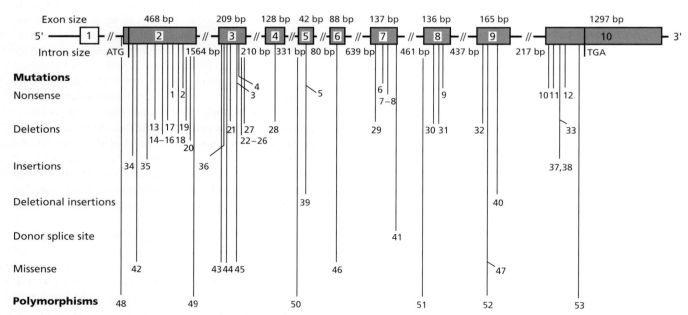

**Fig. 18.2.** schematic representation of the genomic organization of the *MEN1* gene. The human MEN1 gene consists of 10 exons that span more than 9 kb of genetic DNA and encodes a 610-amino-acid protein [4,5]. The 1.83-kb coding region is organized into nine exons (exons 2–10, hatched boxes) and eight introns [thicker horizontal line (not drawn to scale)]. The sizes of the exons (range 42–1 297 bp) and introns (range 80–1 564 bp) are shown, and the start (ATG) and the stop (TGA) sites in exons 2 and 10, respectively are indicated. Exon 1, the 5′ part of exon 2 and the 3′ part of exon 10 are untranslated (non-hatched boxes). The sites of the 47 mutations (12 nonsense mutations, 21 deletions, five insertions, two deletional insertions, one donor splice-site mutation and six missense mutations) and of six different polymorphisms are shown. Reproduced with permission [10].

a conserved cysteine-rich region near the membrane. Further out from the transmembrane domain is a region with homology to cadherin. Within the cell cytoplasm is the tyrosine kinase domain, with a short interkinase domain of 27 amino acids (Fig. 18.3).

In developmental studies in mice and rats, RET expression can be detected in neural crest-derived cells, which migrate from the hindbrain region into the posterior pharyngeal arches. From there, some give rise to the thyroid C cells and others to the vagal neural crest, which gives rise to intestinal autonomic nerves. RET is also expressed in trunk neural crest cells, including those that give rise to the chromaffin cells, which will form adrenal medulla. The endoderm of the pharyngeal pouches that gives rise to the parathyroid glands also expresses RET. Thus, the role of RET in the genesis of MEN2 is compatible with its expression at an early stage of

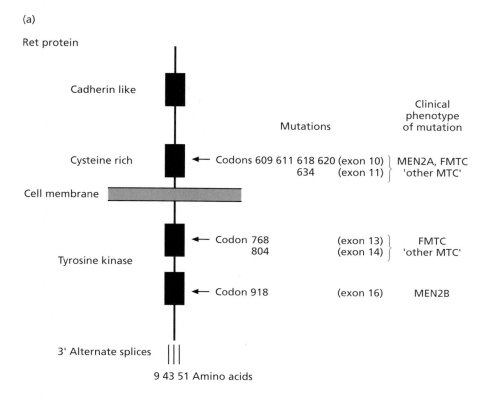

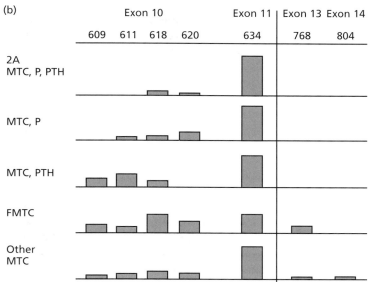

**Fig. 18.3.** (a) The main features of the protein encoded by the ret proto-oncogene, and the sites of the mutations in the different clinical varieties of MEN2. (b) Proportion of mutations in different codons of ret in different phenotypic subtypes of MEN2A, FMTC and other MTC families. Based on data from the International Ret Mutation Consortium. Reproduced with permission [2].

development. Its role in postnatal development cannot be assessed so easily, even in mice in which the gene has been knocked out, because they die at birth due to developmental failure.

The mutations causing MEN2 are all point mutations (Fig. 18.3) that result in tyrosine kinase being activated. In this respect, the situation, with gain of function, is quite different from that in MEN1, in which a variety of types of mutation occur (not just point mutations but deletions and splice-site mutations and so on) that all cause loss of function. The mutation in MEN2A and in FMTC usually lies in one of the five codons that encode the five cysteine residues in the cysteine-rich extracellular domain, and they result in amino acid substitutions. There is a correlation between the nature of the mutation and the resulting phenotype, although the patterns are not exclusive. In families with MEN2A, with medullary carcinoma of the thyroid plus phaeochromocytoma and hyperparathyroidism, the mutation is usually in codon 634. In contrast, when MEN2 occurs without a phaeochromocytoma, and also in isolated FMTC, codons 609, 611, 618 or 620 are usually involved. The mutation of codon 634 can result in any of the possible mutations allowed by the coding sequence, but the commonest results in the cysteine being replaced by tyrosine, which is the one most commonly associated with parathyroid disease. Mutations in the intracellular domain usually involve codon 804 in exon 14, and this seems to be associated with medullary thyroid carcinoma rather than phaeochromocytoma or parathyroid disease.

In MEN2B, the vast majority of families have a mutation of methionine with its replacement of threonine in codon 918 of exon 16 affecting the tyrosine kinase domain intracellularly. In two families with MEN2B, however, no mutation has been found in the coding region, so another alteration or another gene must be involved. In families with MEN2 associated with Hirschsprung disease, the mutations affect cysteine 618 or 620, so that the same mutation can give rise to different phenotypes in the same individual; the medullary carcinoma of the thyroid is the result of an activating mutation, whereas the Hirschsprung disease is the result of a loss of function.

## Identification of affected relatives

There are two ways in which affected individuals can be identified. The first relates to the use of standard clinical practice, and the second uses methods to exploit the advantages in molecular genetics.

### Clinical identification of affected relatives with MEN1

This involves recognizing the clinical effects of tumour development in particular glands, demonstrating hormone overproduction or showing that a tumour is present. Just as hyperparathyroidism is the most common initial manifestation of the disorder in the proband, so it is in other members of the kindred. Demonstrating the presence of hypercalcaemia is the simplest and most direct approach. However, it is often not present for a number of years, and its effects are generally delayed. However, if a pregnant woman is known to be affected by MEN1 and is hypercalcaemic, measurement of serum calcium in the neonate is essential as hypocalcaemia might be found as a consequence of suppression of the infant's parathyroid gland by maternal hypercalcaemia.

Development of hypercalcaemia can occur at very different ages in different members of the family, so it is reasonable to measure serum calcium periodically, starting from about the age of 10 and repeating every few years. In this way, excessive anxiety can be minimized and early diagnosis is achieved. If normocalcaemia is shown in an adult member of a kindred, further measurements are again reasonable, e.g. every 5 years.

Account has been taken of a number of facts when suggesting starting the tests at the age of about 10 years. One is that hyperparathyroidism is unusual before this age; another is that parathyroid surgery is much more difficult in children and best delayed until adult life. As MEN1 behaves as a pseudo-autosomal dominant, only half the members of a kindred will eventually manifest the disease, but prolonged screening will be necessary.

The other components of MEN are likely to produce symptoms, such as dyspepsia with the Zollinger–Ellison syndrome, hypoglycaemia in islet cell tumours, weight changes associated with ACTH overproduction or the effects of prolactin overproduction, such as galactorrhoea and infertility. It is reasonable to defer extensive investigation until clearly indicated, although some investigations can usefully be carried out in the presence of a well-established family history. These will include measurements of circulating prolactin to detect a prolactinoma and abdominal ultrasound looking for pancreatic tumours. Periodic clinical examination should be performed looking for some of the clinical manifestations, be they of hormone overproduction (such as in Cushing disease) or associated features such as lipomata.

### Clinical identification of affected relatives with MEN2

Clinical assessment will focus on looking for a thyroid nodule or for enlarged cervical lymph glands. If the family history is that of MEN2A, measurement of blood pressure is critical. However, unless there is hypertension or a history suggestive of episodic hypertension, more detailed investigations for phaeochromocytoma are unlikely to be helpful. With regard to the possibility of hyperparathyroidism, the comments made in relation to MEN1 apply.

The situation with MEN2B is rather different, as the thyroid tumours are more aggressive and develop at an earlier age. It is likely that affected children will develop the physical stigmata, such as the facial appearance. In terms of laboratory investigation, measurement of calcitonin has played a useful role, especially after stimulation with alcohol. If the basal calcitonin is grossly elevated for the particular method used, there is clear-cut support for the diagnosis. However, if it is borderline, it is of doubtful significance and stimulation tests may be useful.

## Genetic diagnosis of familial multiple endocrine neoplasia

As the genes causing MEN1 and MEN2 have been identified, it is now possible to tell by analysis of the relevant gene whether a member of a family is affected by the germline mutation. If the mutation in other members of that kindred has already been identified, it is relatively easy to use methods that focus on the relevant area of the gene using, for example, single-strand conformational polymorphism (SSCP) or enzyme digests specific to the region affected by the mutation. These approaches are valuable if the family mutation is known. It would be wise, however, to confirm that the postulated mutation is actually the correct one in a clearly affected member of the kindred before proceeding with the investigation of a patient whose phenotypic status needs to be established.

The situation is quite different if the mutation in the family is not known. This is particularly true in the case of familial MEN1, as the gene is large and the mutations that cause the clinical disorder can be spread all along the gene. In effect, the whole gene would have to be sequenced to identify a mutation causing MEN1 and, if a mutation were found, it would still have to be established that this was not a benign polymorphism.

In MEN2 the situation is different because the clinical disorder arises from mutation of only one of eight selected codons and one of these (namely 634) is the most commonly affected, and therefore the search can be very focused.

A number of critical questions have, however, to be considered. One is when a DNA test should be undertaken, if it is going to be done at all, and another is who should be screened. It is also important to consider the genetic counselling that is needed before and after the tests are done. In a survey [14] of interested healthcare professionals, 78% thought that, if the mutation in the family was known, DNA diagnosis should be performed before the age of 10 for MEN1, and 93% thought it appropriate in MEN2. The strongest case for doing this must be in MEN2B, as the medullary carcinomata in these patients are malignant and metastasize early, and a case can be made for total thyroidectomy at an early age.

In MEN1, when the development of the phenotype requires a second somatic mutation for a tumour to develop, no action is likely to follow unless there is other clinical evidence of tumour formation. That consensus can be questioned with regard to MEN1. It can be argued that a DNA test should be as late as possible so that a child is able to participate use-

fully with discussion, but it must be remembered that other concerns may make that difficult. It must also be realized that, by analogy with other conditions in which DNA diagnosis is possible, adverse reactions can follow when the mutation is found to be present but also when the mutation is found to be absent in the individual. This can certainly occur in more serious inherited disorders such as Huntington disease. It is perhaps less likely in MEN. Relief that further long-term follow-up is not needed in subjects without the mutation could be considerable: the reaction to the knowledge in patients with the mutation that long-term follow-up is certainly going to be necessary and that tumour development is likely will probably not be serious.

Genetic counselling is needed with an open discussion before a reasonable decision can be made, and it would be wise to consider who should be involved apart from the patient and his/her family. It is desirable for the individual to make his/her own decision, and advice will be needed from a well-informed source. This could be the endocrinologist, especially if the family has been known to the physician for a long time. It might also involve the family practitioner or a medical geneticist. Certainly, the decision needs to be made with great care and caution and should not be made after a single discussion. The availability of a precise genetic diagnosis adds to the strength of the clinical armamentarium, but it also adds to the challenge of good management of a patient and his/her family.

## Useful web sites

http://www3.ncbi.nlm.nih.gov/omim Search the data base by the OMIM no. (that is the reference number in Online Mendellian Inheritance In Man). For *MEN1* it is 131100, for *MEN2* it is 171400, and for the *RET* proto-oncogene it is 164761.

http://www.niddk.nih.gov/health/endo/pubs/FMEN1/FMEN1.htm This site gives information for professionals and for patients regarding MEN1.

http://endocrine.mdacc.tmc.edu/ This site gives information concerning laboratories in the USA and in the UK that can screen for *MEN2* mutations and educational information for patients.

## References

1 Trump D, Farren B, Wooding C *et al.* Clinical studies of multiple endocrine neoplasia type 1 (MEN1). *Q J Med* 1996; 89: 653–69 [published erratum appears in *Q J Med* 1996; 89: 957–8].

2 Ponder BAJ. Multiple endocrine neoplasia type 2. In: Vogelstein B, Kinzler KW, eds. *The Genetic Basis of Human Cancer.* New York: McGraw-Hill, 1998: 475–88.

3 Gagel RF, Cote GJ. Pathogenesis of medullary thyroid carcinoma. In: Fagin J, ed. *Thyroid Cancer.* Dordrecht: Kluwer, 1998; 85–103.

4 Chandrasekharappa SC, Guru SC, Manickam P *et al.* Positional cloning of the gene for multiple endocrine neoplasia-type 1. *Science* 1997; 276: 404–7.

5 Lemmens I, Van de Ven WJ, Kas K *et al.* The European Consortium on MEN1. Identification of the multiple endocrine neoplasia type 1 (MEN1) gene. *Hum Mol Genet* 1997; 6: 1177–83.

6 Bassett JH, Rashbass P, Harding B, Forbes SA, Pannett AA, Thakker RV. Studies of the murine homolog of the multiple endocrine neoplasia type 1 (MEN1) gene, men1. *J Bone Miner Res* 1999; 14: 3–10.

7 Knudson AG. Mutation and Cancer: statistical study of retinoblastoma. *Proc Natl Acad Sci USA* 1971; 68: 820–3.

8 Thakker RV, Bouloux P, Wooding C *et al.* Association of parathyroid tumors in multiple endocrine neoplasia type 1 with loss of alleles on chromosome 11. *N Engl J Med* 1989; 321: 218–24.

9 Friedman E, Sakaguchi K, Bale AE *et al.* Clonality of parathyroid tumors in familial multiple endocrine neoplasia type 1. *N Engl J Med* 321: 213–18 [published erratum appears in *N Engl J Med* 1989; 321: 1057].

10 Bassett JH, Forbes SA, Pannett AA *et al.* Characterization of mutations in patients with multiple endocrine neoplasia type 1. *Am J Hum Genet* 1998; 62 (2): 232–44.

11 Agarwal SK, Kester MB, Debelenko LV *et al.* Germline mutations of the MEN1 gene in familial multiple endocrine neoplasia type 1 and related states. *Hum Mol Genet* 1997; 6: 1169–75.

12 Giraud S, Zhang CX, Serova-Sinilnikova O *et al.* Germ-line mutation analysis in patients with multiple endocrine neoplasia type 1 and related disorders. *Am J Hum Genet* 1998; 63: 455–67.

13 Ponder BA, Smith D. The MEN II syndromes and the role of the ret proto-oncogene. *Adv Cancer Res* 1996; 70: 179–222.

14 Lips CJ. Clinical management of the multiple endocrine neoplasia syndromes: results of a computerized opinion poll at the Sixth International Workshop on Multiple Endocrine Neoplasia and von Hippel-Lindau disease. *J Intern Med* 1998; 243: 589–94.

# 19 The late endocrine consequences of curing childhood cancer

Helen A. Spoudeas

## Introduction

Improved therapeutic regimens and supportive care have increased survival rates of childhood cancer to 70% overall, and up to 95% in some leukaemias. This success has been tempered by the gradual evolution of long-term morbidity in more than 85% of survivors, particularly the youngest and most intensively treated, or where surgery has involved vital tissue (e.g. brain tumours). One in 1000 young adults is a survivor of childhood cancer, facing an uncertain future with significant cognitive, neuropsychological and endocrine impairment. Toxicity on other organ systems is receiving increasing attention.

Challenges for the future include preventing early death from late disease relapse or second primary tumours and also preventing chemotherapy-induced cardiotoxicity and endocrine-related disease, including hypopituitarism, obesity and their metabolic consequences. Improvements in quality of life must surely follow appropriate hormone replacement therapy, attempts to preserve fertility and neuropsychological rehabilitative strategies aimed at future employment, independence and successful peer relationships.

## The problems posed by a changing therapeutic baseline

Brain tumours and leukaemias/lymphomas account for more than 50% of childhood cancers. Both have, until recently, required whole-brain irradiation for a potential cure – in high doses (30–55 Gy) for brain tumours and lower doses (18–24 Gy) for leukaemia – this often being administered in combination with spinal irradiation as prophylaxis against neuraxial relapse and chemotherapy to eradicate micro-metastases. Even lower whole body doses (10–15 Gy) have formed part of the conditioning regimens for bone marrow transplantation in resistant disease. In ongoing attempts to minimize late neurotoxicity, cranial irradiation is being increasingly replaced by more aggressive chemotherapy, particularly for the youngest (< 3 years) and most vulnerable [1,2]. However, these drugs are not without neurotoxicity, particularly where the blood–brain barrier is disrupted [1], and new cancer treatments must be critically appraised longitudinally over many years.

The data on late organ toxicity comes from descriptive retrospective, cross-sectional studies in long-term survivors, and thus the aetiology is far from clear. Although irradiation is largely blamed, the few longitudinal studies before and after each treatment modality suggest that the tumour, or its surgery, also plays its part [3], but chemotherapy with irradiation is additively toxic [3–5]. Although long-term outcomes are important, particularly in endocrinology where final height and fertility are ultimate end points, retrospective studies relate to already outdated therapeutic regimens, and better surgical, supportive and rehabilitative opportunities affect recent outcomes.

Many brain tumour studies have included central (e.g. optic or suprasellar) tumours [6,7,8], which, by their proximity, mass effect or surgery, directly influence pituitary hormone secretion. When chemotherapy and radiotherapy have been administered in combination, it becomes difficult to site or differentiate the exact toxic effect of each therapeutic regimen, as multiple sites on the hypothalamo-pituitary target gland axes may be susceptible. Thus, it can be difficult to separate the gonadotoxic effect of alkylating agent chemotherapy from that of irradiation scatter from a spinal beam, or indeed to predict accurately the pubertal progress of a child who has received both cranial irradiation, with its potentially damaging effects on gonadotrophin secretion (either activation or depletion), together with other directly gonadotoxic radiation or chemotherapy.

Furthermore, endocrinopathies, skeletal irradiation, chemotherapy (which often includes potent glucocorticoids), malnutrition and prolonged ill-health all independently influence normal skeletal and sexual maturation processes and bone mineral accretion. This means there are many confounding factors when assessing, for example, the prevalence or aetiology of infertility or osteopenia in long-term survivors, particularly if the methods used are indirect rather than direct measures, such as DEXA (dual-energy X-ray absorptiometry) bone mineral density in a short population [9].

As physiological hormone secretion has been increasingly studied, it has become evident that the difficulties in accurately assessing damage to the endocrine system are compounded by the limitations of standard pharmacological stimulation tests, the mainstay of endocrine assessment [10]. These have been particularly noted before as well as after cranial radiation for leukaemia [11 and brain tumours [3] in the only studies that have prospectively assessed both measures of secretion. This observation has now been confirmed in cross-sectional studies [12,13].

## Principles of radiobiology

The radiosensitivity of a tissue is directly proportional to its mitotic activity and inversely proportional to its differentiation. Thus, highly active tissues such as skin and bone marrow are 'radiosensitive', whereas the specialized, mature and quiescent cells of the brain or bone are 'radioresistant', although the quiescent oocyte is a notable exception [14]. Nevertheless, if a quiescent cell is stimulated to divide, the radiation dose required to cause chromosome damage, mitotic delay and inhibition of DNA synthesis is similar in all tissues. Thus, all organ systems in the body will be damaged by irradiation, although the late effects on slowly or non-proliferating cell populations may emerge only with time. Other longer-term consequences include life-shortening, mutagenicity and carcinogenesis [15].

Radiation-induced mammalian cell death has two components. Radiosensitive tissues are susceptible to 'single-hit' non-reparable injury quantified by a high $\alpha$-coefficient. Slowly proliferating tissues, such as neural tissue, are more susceptible to 'multihit' injury, either the accumulation of sublethal injuries, the sum of which is lethal, and/or the progressive destruction of the cell's ability to repair itself, with resulting cell depletion, quantified by a high $\beta$-coefficient [16].

As $\beta$ is proportional to the square of the dose, fractionation effectively reduces 'multihit' mechanisms and enhances the therapeutic ratio between late effects and tumour control. Dose fractions larger than 2 Gy (not in general use in children) increase the injury relatively more to late- (neural) than to early-responding (tumour) tissues. Smaller fractions over the same treatment duration (hyperfractionation) may be further beneficial in reducing late toxicity, provided sufficient time (ideally > 6 h) is allowed between fractions for tissue repair. Although fractionation of the dose is generally considered beneficial, there is evidence to suggest the gonads are an exception to this rule [14,17].

With conventional external beam radiotherapy, late neuroendocrine toxicity depends on the volume of the brain irradi-ated, the fraction size, the interfraction interval, the age of the child, the total dose delivered and the time elapsed since injury. Irradiation scatter is greater for $^{60}$Co sources than for linear accelerators, which tend to have a more penetrating beam, but as the irradiation field for most childhood brain tumours (infratentorial) is so close to the pituitary margins (demarcated by the posterior clinoids), this is generally academic in terms of pituitary dose (at least 40–45 Gy). The highest estimated hypothalamo-pituitary doses (up to 70 Gy) occur after treatment for nasopharyngeal tumours, accounting for the high incidence of hypothalamo-pituitary deficits in these cases [18], whereas yttrium-90 implants and the newer stereotactic irradiation techniques, although more focused, have a very limited application in childhood malignancy.

## Chemotherapy, radiation and toxicity

A radiosensitizing effect of certain drugs is often postulated, but this would mean a change in cellular dose and survival characteristics ($\alpha$ and $\beta$) not often confirmed. Increased tumour or normal tissue responses to the concomitant administration of drugs and radiation usually represent additive effects. This may have significant implications in terms of long-term effects in late-responding tissues, as cumulative toxicity is not reduced by regeneration between the two modalities of treatment.

A few studies have now documented greater morbidity after such combinations than either regimen independently, not only on peripheral target glands, such as the thyroid [4], gonad [5] and skeleton [19], but also on central hormone secretion across a disrupted blood–brain barrier [3]. It is thus possible that the recent strategy of using chemotherapy to delay (but not omit) potentially curative (but neurotoxic) cranial irradiation in the youngest children with brain tumours [2] may cause additive injury evident only in the longer term.

## Consequences of cranial irradiation

### Panhypopituitarism

It has long been recognized that hypopituitarism may result after surgery or external radiotherapy directed at tumours lying within or close to the hypothalamo-pituitary axis, but there remained the possibility that this was due to compression effects from the underlying disease itself. However, reports of insidious hypopituitarism occurring in adults several years after irradiation for nasopharyngeal carcinoma, where estimated total doses to the hypothalamo-pituitary axis were often greatly in excess of 50 Gy [20], suggested a causative role for radiotherapy. This was supported by longitudinal studies in leukaemic children undergoing therapy [21] and in rhesus monkeys in which suppression of spontaneous and insulin-induced growth hormone (GH) release

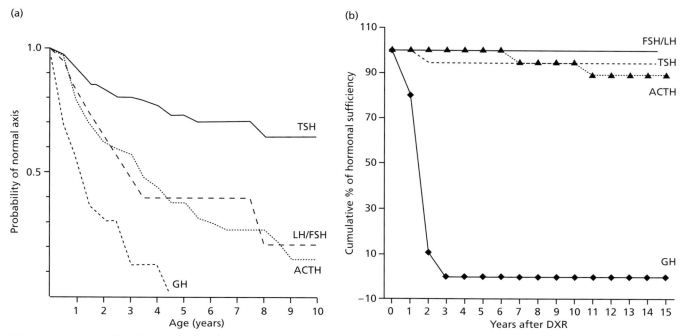

**Fig. 19.1.** (a) Ten-year life table analysis, in 37 of 165 adults with intrasellar or anatomically adjacent tumours, and normal postoperative hypothalamo-pituitary function, indicating the likelihood of an evolving endocrinopathy after 37.5–42.5 Gy pituitary irradiation in 15 fractions over 20–22 days (redrawn from [8]). GH is most sensitive, all adults are GH deficient within 5 years, whereas ACTH and gonadotrophins (LH and FSH) are increasingly affected over time (80% at 10 years). TSH is most resistant. (b) Ten-year probability of an evolving endocrinopathy occurring after a median estimated hypothalamo-pituitary irradiation dose (DXR) of at least 40 Gy in 1.8-Gy fractions, in 20 young adult survivors of resected posterior fossa brain tumours tested twice at the onset of growth failure and at completion of growth, who were otherwise asymptomatic (redrawn from [28]). GH deficiency was present in all patients tested at first assessment and was permanent. ACTH (10%) and TSH (5%) deficiencies were comparatively rare, and there was no case of gonadotrophin deficiency or hyperprolactinaemia over the duration of follow-up.

was observed within 1 year of 24 Gy and 40 Gy fractionated cranial irradiation doses [22].

Longitudinal provocation tests in adults with normal postoperative endocrinology subsequently irradiated for pituitary tumours purport to show the pure effect of local irradiation (20–45 Gy) on the evolving endocrinopathy, which is increasingly evident with time. This is both dose- and fractionation-dependent [23] and hierarchical in nature, GH being the most sensitive, then gonadotrophins and adrenocorticotrophic hormone (ACTH). Thyroid-stimulating hormone (TSH) is the most radioresistant [8] (Fig. 19.1a). However, only 20% (37/165) of the original cohort of patients were eligible for this analysis, the remainder having already experienced postoperative anterior pituitary deficiencies.

Slowly replicating neural cells may not at first demonstrate damage. Although toxicity has been attributed entirely to irradiation, delayed evidence of tumour- or surgery-induced neuronal injury may play a significant part. The vulnerability of GH secretion to cranial irradiation has been replicated in rats, but not the relative resistance of TSH, which was affected early, together with prolactin, perhaps reflecting their common developmental origin, whereas gonadotrophin and ACTH secretion were relatively preserved [24].

In children, anterior pituitary deficiencies were noted after irradiation doses > 50 Gy for orbital and middle ear tumours [25] and, more surprisingly, after lower whole-brain irradiation doses for cranial tumours (> 30 Gy) displaced from the pituitary or leukaemia neuraxial prophylaxis (24 Gy) [26]. However, the high prevalence of anterior pituitary deficiencies noted in the adult studies [8] has not been confirmed in childhood survivors of tumours distant from the central area (only 2–6%) [4–7,27,28], other than GH deficiency, despite similar pituitary doses and 10 years' follow-up. GH deficiency is the earliest and often only abnormality, and, in this situation, the deficit is permanent [28,29] (Fig. 19.1b).

The hypothalamo-pituitary axis of young children has been said to be more vulnerable to irradiation. Fewer adults [30] than children [31] treated with similar low-dose fractionated total body irradiation (TBI) develop subnormal GH responses to insulin-induced hypoglycaemia (insulin tolerance test) at the same short (2.4–2.8 years) follow-up time. Given their time and dose dependency, pituitary deficiencies are likely to be multiple, occurring frequently and rapidly in the youngest children receiving high-dose cranial irradiation for centrally placed tumours [18,25]. Compared with more distant tumours, they may be single, take longer to evolve

**Table 19.1.** Likely endocrine deficit according to cranial irradiation dose (brain tumours distant from pituitary area)

| Dose | Endocrinopathy |
|---|---|
| > 55–70 Gy | Hyperprolactinaemia, panhypopituitarism, adult GHD |
| 30–55 Gy | GH insufficiency, evolving endocrinopathy, pubertal GH insufficiency, early puberty, adult GHD |
| 18–24 Gy | GH neurosecretory disturbance, adult GHD, early puberty |
| 10–15 Gy | GH neurosecretory disturbance, adult GHD |

GHD, growth hormone deficiency.

or be qualitative rather than quantitative in nature soon after irradiation [3] or after lower doses used in leukaemia prophylaxis [11,32,33] and TBI [11,30,31], particularly if the fraction size is also reduced [26] (Table 19.1). This will result in a cohort of survivors emerging with an accruing potential for hormone replacement therapy when they are adults, because they had not previously been treated as children [33].

### Nature and site of the neuroendocrine defect

Whether postirradiation endocrinopathy be neural or vascular, hypothalamic or pituitary in origin, is still debated. The few studies on hypothalamic [34] and hypophyseal portal blood flow [35] do not suggest this is particularly compromised. The hypothalamus or its portal connections are deemed more radiosensitive than the pituitary, particularly after doses > 50 Gy [20], but diabetes insipidus, a typical hypothalamic disorder, which may pre-date the radiographic appearance of a suprasellar germinoma by as much as 20 years [36], has, as yet, not been reported after high-dose irradiation for non-central tumours [18].

Selective damage to hypothalamic control centres is suggested by discordant suppression of insulin-mediated and spontaneous GH release, with preservation of GH responses to other provocative agents acting through different central mechanisms, as seen in irradiated rhesus monkeys [22] and children with leukaemia [37] or brain tumours [3,12]. Pituitary hormone responses to their corresponding hypothalamic-releasing hormone stimuli may be delayed [8,20] or preserved [38,39] in the face of absent or attenuated responses to insulin-induced hypoglycaemia.

Elevations in prolactin have been deemed evidence of hypothalamic damage to inhibitory dopaminergic neurones [18,20] but vary in severity and permanence. They are more likely after high-dose radiotherapy for nasopharyngeal carcinoma or pituitary-related tumours, particularly those causing acromegaly; they are rare after treatment for extrasellar tumours in childhood [18]. The effects of previous pituitary surgery and residual tumour tissue, which may contain lactogenic as well as somatogenic activity, thus confuse the picture. We documented longitudinal *decreases* in basal and stimulated prolactin with *increases* in stimulated TSH within the normal range 6 and 12 months after craniospinal irradiation for posterior fossa tumours (median estimated pituitary dose 45 Gy), suggesting intact dopamine secretion (Fig. 19.2a,b). Nevertheless, we did note a decrease in both 24-h physiological TSH periodicity (Fig. 19.2c) and the normal, hypothalamically induced nocturnal TSH surge (Fig. 19.2d), suggestive of early postsurgical or irradiation-induced hypothalamic deficits in TRH and somatostatin (SS) release, which require further study [39].

Preserved GH responses to its hypothalamic-releasing hormone in the presence of suboptimal responses to other pharmacological tests [38,39] suggest a primary hypothalamic growth hormone-releasing hormone (GHRH) deficiency. However, given the tropic effects of GHRH [40], that the GHRH doses used were supraphysiological [41], that any response is highly dependent on endogenous SS tone [42] and that both GH secretion [3,13] and pituitary GHRH responses [35,38,39] decline with time in this situation, direct pituitary damage could also be a contributory factor. Somatotroph responses to physiological [41] GHRH doses are preserved 1 year after neurosurgery and radiation for non-central tumours [39], but these are suppressed in long-term survivors [35]. Despite pulsed infusions of alternating GHRH and/or SS clamp studies, pituitary damage has not been excluded, as normalization of GH output was not achieved and ultimately more prolonged GHRH priming may be necessary [35] (Fig. 19.3a,b).

The majority of late survivors of irradiation for non-central brain tumours retain much attenuated GH neuroregulatory responses to modulations of SS tone and GHRH [35,43], often with disordered pulsatility and an elevated baseline [3,35,39], suggestive of SS dysfunction as in animals after SS immuno-neutralization. After multiple pituitary insults, sensitive assays show that even greatly attenuated GH secretion is still pulsatile, albeit of slow frequency [44].

Prospective studies of GH secretory profiles in children undergoing cranial irradiation at low (10 Gy) [11] or high (30–50 Gy) [3] doses suggest that disturbances in GH pulse frequency are the earliest abnormality, coupled with discrepancies between good physiological and poor insulin-induced GH peaks, the latter provoking GH release by reducing SS tone. Physiological GH peak generation is additionally affected by the imposition of higher cranial irradiation doses. We have proposed that the disease itself and/or brain tumour surgery somehow disturb afferent or efferent hypothalamic connections determining the GH chemo-receptor response to hypoglycaemia, and that SS dysregulation is an early evolutionary abnormality resulting from insults other than just radiotherapy, eventually compounded by an evolving and irradiation-induced hypothalamic GHRH deficiency [3] and possible consequent pituitary dysfunction [35]. This occurs with increasing therapeutic intensity and

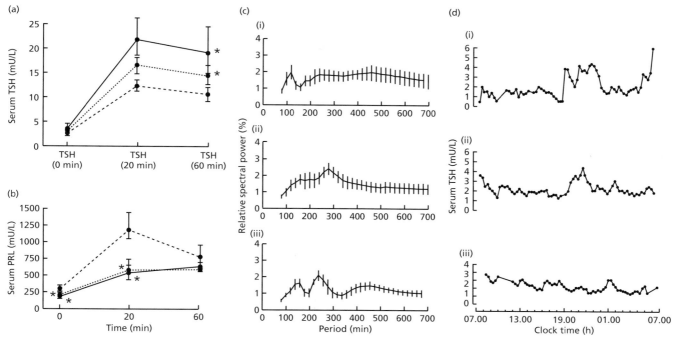

**Fig. 19.2.** Thyroid-stimulating hormone (TSH) (a) and prolactin (PRL) (b) release to their releasing-factor stimuli before (pre, – – –), 6 months (- - - - -) and 12 months (———) in seven prepubertal children with resected posterior fossa tumours tested longitudinally after craniospinal irradiation (without chemotherapy) (redrawn from [39]). Note the rise (within normal values) in basal and stimulated TSH levels and the fall in basal and stimulated PRL with time from irradiation. The asterisks indicate the significance of difference from preirradiation values. (a) The concentration of T$_4$ is pre 99 ± 8 nmol/L, 6 months 100 ± 8 nmol/L, 12 months 95 ± 5 nmol/L. (c) Periodicity (shown as relative spectral power) of TSH secretion before (i), 6 months (ii) and 12 months (iii) after craniospinal irradiation (without chemotherapy) in seven prepubertal children with resected posterior fossa tumours (redrawn from [39]). Note the slowing of the periodicity after radiotherapy. (d) Loss of TSH nocturnal surge in a representative, prepubertal individual followed longitudinally before (i) 6 months (ii) and 12 months (iii) after craniospinal irradiation for a posterior fossa tumour (redrawn from [39]). Group data in the seven individuals followed longitudinally confirmed that this was the result of an increase in 12-h daytime (nadir) secretion, without a corresponding increase in the nocturnal mean, peak secretion and is separate from recognized primary thyroid gland toxicity from the exit dose of the spinal irradiation beam [4].

time, and chemotherapy has an important additive central role [3] (Fig. 19.4a,b).

There are potential implications of differentiating between hypothalamic and pituitary disease. Intermittent pulsatile subcutaneous gonadotrophin-releasing hormone (GnRH) therapy can successfully induce puberty in both sexes, with resultant ovulatory cycles in girls and fertility in hypogonadotrophic females treated for pituitary tumours [45].

Continuous subcutaneous GHRH therapy, for periods up to 1 year, promotes growth in GH-deficient children with a presumed hypothalamic aetiology and also after irradiation therapy for brain tumours [46]. The response depends on the integrity of hypothalamic SS secretion and is generally less than that seen with GH alone. Were depot formulations of GHRH or the related orally active GH-releasing peptides to become widely available, they may prove a more physiological, cost-effective and user-friendly therapeutic option than GH therapy. Significant pituitary destruction would limit such therapeutic potential.

If it becomes possible to accurately site the damage, pre-irradiation endocrine strategies for protecting the area might

be attempted. However, such specific analogue or hormonal therapy to render the gonad 'quiescent', and hence more radioresistant, has been attempted with varied success in humans to date [47,48].

## Growth failure and growth hormone deficiency

GH deficiency is evidenced by retarded growth rate, disturbed physiological GH secretion (neurosecretory dysfunction) and/or attenuated peak GH responses to various pharmacological stimuli. It is the commonest pituitary deficit, affecting 60–100% of children receiving fractionated cranial doses of 30 Gy or more within 2–5 years, with resultant growth failure [6,7,27]. Although the effective radiobiological dose received by the hypothalamo-pituitary axis is the determining factor for the development and speed of onset of GH deficiency [23], no lowest 'safe' dose has been identified. Given that time is also an important determinant and that the somatotroph is a late-effects tissue, it is unlikely that such a phenomenon exists. The few prospective, longitudinal studies of physiological 24-h GH secretion before and after

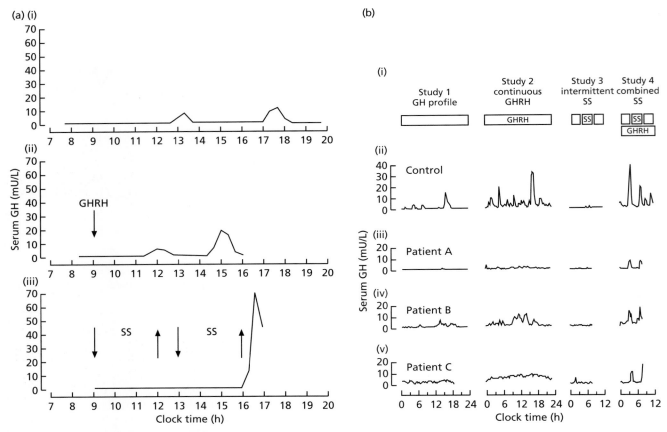

**Fig. 19.3.** (a) Attempts at improving the GH secretory pattern (i) of a prepubertal child just 1 year after 40 Gy of cranial irradiation for a temporoparietal tumour with continuous GHRH (ii) or pulsed somatostatin (iii) infusion on consecutive 12-h days. Both hypothalamic factors augment GH secretion but, in this case, early after irradiation, somatostatin withdrawal is relatively more potent, regularizing pulsatility (redrawn from [39]). (b). Study protocol (i). Typical GH profiles (over 12 h or 24 h) and responses to GHRH infusion, intermittent somatostatin (SS) withdrawal or a combination of both, in a control volunteer (ii) and for three adult survivors of childhood posterior fossa tumours with long-term postirradiation GH insufficiency (iii–v) (redrawn from [35]). Note that, in contrast to (a), GH secretion is grossly attenuated in long-term survivors of similar, non-central tumours. Continuous GHRH infusions, pulsed somatostatin infusion or a combination of both regularize secretion, but pituitary responses are not completely restored.

TBI (10 Gy) [11], cranial irradiation (24 Gy) for leukaemia [21,49] or non-central brain tumours (> 30 Gy) [3] suggest rather an evolving picture of neurosecretory disturbance with time and irradiation dose intensity, which is eventually severe and permanent [35,39].

Pulsatile GH neurosecretory abnormalities occur after cranial irradiation doses as low as 10 Gy delivered at a slow continuous rate in TBI [11] or after fractionated (2 Gy) doses of 18 Gy [32] and 24 Gy [50] for neuraxial prophylaxis for leukaemia, these being particularly evident in puberty. The lower dose of 18 Gy, now abandoned in the UK, seems no less damaging to growth [51], GH secretion [32] or cognition, although data interpretation may have been confounded by the studies being undertaken in series rather than in parallel. Other more favourable reports [49] assessed mean or peak GH secretion only, whereas much of the early postirradiation deficit may be confined to qualitative, subtle disturbances in periodicity and an inability adequately to

augment pubertal, if not prepubertal, GH secretion [32,50] (Fig. 19.5).

## The influence of chemotherapy and irradiation on growth

### Chemotherapy

Several groups have reported growth retardation during leukaemic chemotherapy and cranial irradiation, with moderate 'catch up' after cessation of maintenance therapy. However, percentages of children with significant height loss vary from 40% [52] to 70% [53] at 6-year follow-up, depending on the intensity of chemotherapy. Adjuvant chemotherapy aggravates the growth failure of children with brain tumours who have been given craniospinal irradiation [19].

A similarly poor short-term growth pattern has been described in children who received chemotherapy regimens alone without cranial irradiation [54,55] or TBI [56]. The

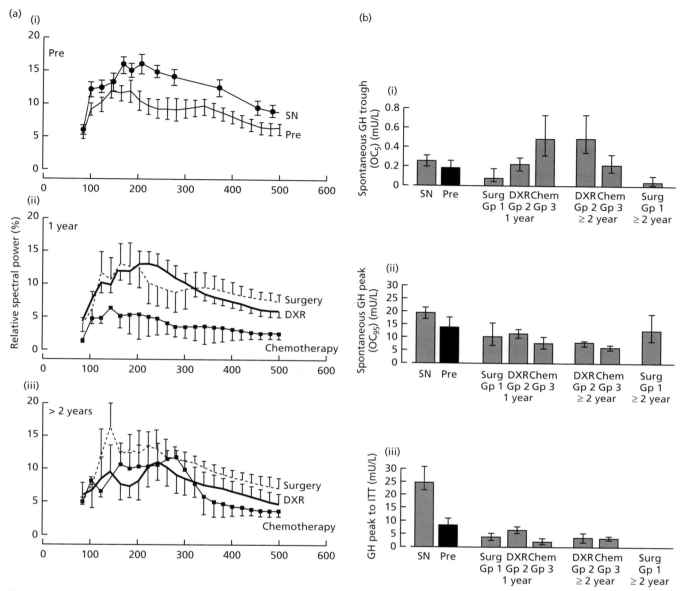

**Fig. 19.4.** (a) Periodicity (shown as relative Fourier transforms) of GH secretion in short-normal (SN) control subjects, and children with brain tumours before (pre) radiotherapy (i) and at 1 year (ii) and 2–5 years (iii) after neurosurgery alone (surgery), or with additional > 30 Gy cranial irradiation (DXR), and > 30 Gy DXR with adjuvant chemotherapy (chemotherapy) (redrawn from [3]). Note the diminution in oscillatory activity with time and intensity of therapy, suggesting compounding central hypothalamic disturbance by treatment modalities, evolving over time. (b) Relationship of spontaneous GH troughs ($OC_5$) (i) spontaneous GH peaks ($OC_{95}$) (ii) and stimulated peak GH responses to hypoglycaemia (ITT) (iii), with increasing therapeutic intensity and time in short-normal (SN) control subjects and children with brain tumours before (pre) radiotherapy and at 1 and 2–5 years after neurosurgery alone (Surg, Gp 1), or with additional > 30 Gy cranial irradiation (DXR, Gp 2), and > 30 Gy DXR with adjuvant chemotherapy (Chem, Gp 3) (redrawn from [3]). Note the wide variation in trough secretion across treated groups compared with control subjects, and the marked early discrepancy between spontaneous (preserved) and stimulated (attenuated) peaks, even in children treated with surgery only (Gp 1). This discrepancy becomes concordant with time and intensity of therapy as spontaneous GH secretion fails (redrawn from [3]).

lack of a difference between irradiated and non-irradiated groups in the first 6 months to 2 years after diagnosis suggests that irradiation does not play a major part in the initial decline in height SD scores. However, it does seem to be a significant factor in the continuous long-term deceleration,

as it was not so marked in the group given chemotherapy alone [54].

Studies *in vitro* [58] and in leukaemia subjects *in vivo* [55] have demonstrated that chemotherapeutic agents suppress osteoblast proliferation and enhance osteoclast activity.

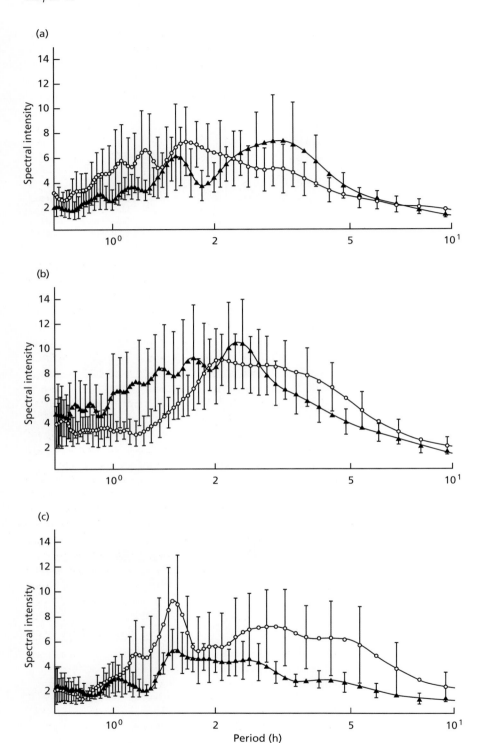

(a)

(b)

(c)

Period (h)

**Fig. 19.5.** Pooled estimate power spectra for GH secretion profiles of (a) prepubertal, (b) pubertal and (c) postpubertal normal (○) and cranially irradiated (18 Gy) (▲) children (redrawn from [32]). Note the spectral flattening of irradiated pubertal group in particular indicating random and chaotic GH pulsatility.

Glucocorticoids simultaneously administered may modify these actions [59] and also have their own negative effects on growth and bone mineralization. Leukaemia itself, associated sepsis or malnutrition cause a low bone turnover state, as evidenced by low markers of bone formation and degrada-

tion, and GH resistance. The former is aggravated by the initiation of chemotherapy, but disease control and thus weight gain follow. After glucocorticoid withdrawal, markers of bone and soft tissue turnover increase dramatically in concert with growth velocity, but this effect is reduced by high-dose

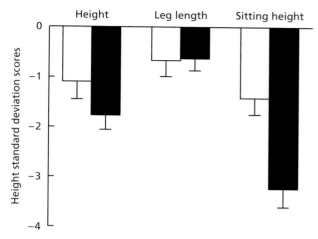

**Fig. 19.6.** Adult height without endocrine therapy of 33 patients irradiated in childhood for brain tumours (redrawn from [7]). All patients are short, but the greatest deficit is seen in the spine, even in those not receiving spinal irradiation. Although less severe, this suggests a subtle GH disturbance affecting pubertal (and hence) spinal growth. □, Cranial irradiation (*n* = 19); ■, craniospinal irradiation (*n* = 14).

i.v. (intravenous) methotrexate [55]. Our own prospective study in children before and after treatment for brain tumours is the first to also suggest that alkylating agents and antimetabolites cross the disrupted blood–brain barrier and are important additional factors contributing to irradiation effects on GH secretion centrally [3] (Fig. 19.4).

Not all leukaemia patients with growth failure have required investigation or therapy. Nevertheless, despite a temporary catch-up, possibly due to an attenuated pubertal spurt, 90% of 115 young (< 12 years) leukaemia subjects in continuous remission after 24 Gy of cranial irradiation suffer significant height deficits in adulthood of 1 or 2 standard deviations (SD) from pretreatment scores in 70% and 32% respectively. Spinal irradiation aggravated the problem [60].

Attenuated pubertal growth, seen only in children treated at a very young age (< 7 years) [54], accounts for the adult height deficit and accords with the pubertal neurosecretory abnormalities described in this situation [32,50] (Fig. 19.5). Although it has been suggested [61] that chemotherapy-induced vertebral lesions might explain the asymmetric body proportions (longer legs) of adult leukaemia survivors, particularly girls, treated with cranial (not spinal) irradiation alone, compromised pubertal, and hence spinal, growth could result from untreated pubertal GH deficiency. This is perhaps more likely given that similar disproportion is evident in a cohort of brain tumour survivors, even those not given spinal irradiation [7] (Fig. 19.6).

### Spinal irradiation
#### Hodgkin disease
Probert *et al.* [62] first described significant spinal growth impairment and resultant skeletal disproportion in children

with Hodgkin disease after 18 fractionated doses of 44 Gy to the midplane in both mantle and inverted 'y' fields. Estimated scattered vertebral doses to the remainder of the spine ranged from 40% to 100% despite shielding. The height deficit was worse in children irradiated under the age of 6 years and pubertally.

Spinal shortening also occurs after paravertebral nodal irradiation, particularly when doses exceed 35 Gy. Scoliosis or lordosis (possibly the result of asymmetric irradiation fields), aseptic/avascular necrosis of the femoral head or bilateral slipped femoral epiphyses have also been described. It is likely that steroid therapy is a major contributor to the latter problem.

#### Brain tumours
Children receiving craniospinal irradiation for brain tumours in doses of 27–35 Gy over 22–27 days have appreciably impaired spinal growth, and the younger the child at irradiation, the greater the subsequent skeletal disproportion [7,63]. The spine is not more vulnerable to such damage in puberty, but as spinal growth is a major component of the pubertal growth spurt, the deficit may only then become apparent, at a time when the potential for growth-promoting therapies is limited.

Thirty-three adult patients who were treated for brain tumours in childhood with a median hypothalamic radiation dose of 48 Gy (10–56 Gy), with or without a median spinal dose of 30 Gy (25–33 Gy) and who had achieved final height without endocrine intervention were all short compared with normal standards. The overall prevalence of GH deficiency in this study was 86%, but loss of sitting height was a major factor, causing further disproportionate shortening in the craniospinal group [7] (Fig. 19.6). The eventual height deficit after spinal irradiation has been estimated to be 9 cm when irradiation is given at 1 year, 7 cm at 5 years and 5.5 cm when given at 10 years [63], but it is likely to be greater with larger doses. Conversely, there is animal evidence that hyper-fractionation (1–1.25 Gy vs. 1.5–1.8 Gy to a total of 25 Gy in 8–9 days) decreases the deleterious effects on vertebral growth [64], but others have suggested that overall treatment duration must also be reduced [65].

#### Leukaemia
Almost 50% of those treated with craniospinal irradiation (24 Gy) for acute leukaemia demonstrated a height loss greater than 2 SD from pretreatment values compared with 32% of their peers receiving cranial irradiation (24 Gy) alone and intrathecal methotrexate. Furthermore, there was no period of catch-up growth observed in the craniospinal group, presumably because of the absence of a significant spinal growth spurt in puberty [60]. Chemotherapy and steroids adversely contributed to this growth failure by influencing physiological bone turnover, especially osteoblastic activity [55,58,59].

### Total body irradiation

Both single (7.5–10 Gy) and fractionated (12–15.75 Gy) TBI regimens cause multiple endocrinopathies that contribute to the documented high incidence of growth failure after this form of therapy [66,67]. It is progressive from the first year, with one-third of patients having heights less than 2 SD below the mean at 5 years [67]. Even after 7.5 Gy of total lymphoid irradiation (TLI) without cranial irradiation for aplastic anaemia, significant growth failure results [67], presumably the result of irradiation-induced skeletal damage to epiphyseal growth plates and bony matrix [62]. This probably explains in part the reported poor and disproportionate growth response to conventional doses of GH [68], the lack of correlation between peak GH secretion and height loss [69] or growth rate [56], and the accrual of further height deficits despite GH therapy in those followed to adult height [70]. There exist the additional adverse contributions of steroids and chemotherapy in the early phases [56] for significant graft-versus-host disease, and the subtle nature of GH neurosecretory disturbances after low cranial doses may also mean the expected therapeutic benefit is diminished accordingly.

Quoted figures for GH deficiency (to provocation) in those with growth failure increase with time and irradiation intensity, ranging from 42% for those transplanted in first remission to 87% in those given prior cranial irradiation, with corresponding height deficits of 1.7 SD after 4 years. This was not similarly observed after transplant conditioning regimens employing chemotherapy alone [66]. At present, patients should be warned that the pretreatment centile positions can be maintained only by GH therapy, and that further pubertal and adult height deficits are likely despite treatment (Fig. 19.7).

### Diagnosis and aetiology of growth hormone deficiency

The diagnosis of GH deficiency after lower cranial irradiation doses for leukaemia is complicated by discrepancies between subnormal growth velocities, peak GH responses to different provocative tests and 24-h measurements of pulsatile endogenous GH secretion [10,11,37]. In a prospective study of 23 leukaemic children undergoing continuous low-dose rate TBI (10 Gy), only subtle abnormalities in physiological GH frequency regulation were observed, but this relative normality contrasted with markedly suboptimal GH responses to insulin hypoglycaemia in the majority, often present before any irradiation [11]. Such discrepancies are not usually observed after the higher doses used in the treatment of brain tumours, except in the occasional report where children have been studied within 2 years of diagnosis [3] (Fig. 19.4b). This is presumably because of the greater speed and completeness with which GH deficiency develops.

Serum IGF-I (isulin-like growth factor I) and IGFBP-3 (IGF-binding protein 3) measurements give unreliable estimates of

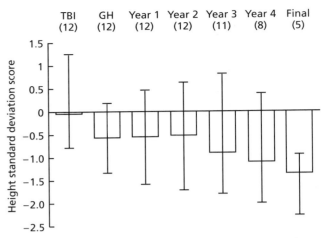

**Fig. 19.7.** Stature (expressed as height standard deviation scores SD) of 12 leukaemic children who were prepubertal at the time of TBI (TBI), followed longitudinally to adult height from the time of growth hormone replacement (GH) for confirmed GH deficiency. The numbers of subjects are shown in parentheses (redrawn from [70]). Note that institution of GH therapy initially maintains only the height position without 'catch-up growth', but GH subsequently fails to prevent an ongoing pubertal deficit to adult height.

GH secretion status in children, especially in those with brain tumours or leukaemia. Concentrations do not always reflect 24-h physiological GH secretion [13,39] or GH provocation tests [39,71], with IGFBP-3 being particularly poor in this regard. Suggested reasons include disruption of hypothalamic feedback controls [39], the disrupted peak and trough secretory pattern of GH [13], nutritional influences early in the disease [71], pubertal changes in hormone secretion and increased IGFBP-3 protease activity in malignancy. However, as the severity of GH deficiency evolves over time, the efficiency of the tests improves. In one study of long-term adult survivors (median 13 years since irradiation for posterior fossa tumours), serum IGF-I was 79% sensitive, 100% specific and 83% efficient at a cut-off of 217 µg/L; IGFBP-3 was 64% sensitive, 89% specific and 71% efficient at a cut-off of 2.42 mg/L compared with matched control subjects [13] (Fig. 19.8).

This lack of a gold standard for assessing GH secretory status probably accounts for the conflicting reports on the incidence and permanence of GH deficiency in leukaemia patients treated with lower cranial doses. Because of such discrepancies between tests, because of difficulties in standardizing a maximal stimulus for GH secretion and because the mechanisms by which the neuropeptides and insulin-induced hypoglycaemia stimulate GH release in man are as yet poorly understood, these data are not easy to interpret. However, such discrepancies may provide the clue to the aetiological factors implicated in the evolution of GH deficiency after irradiation.

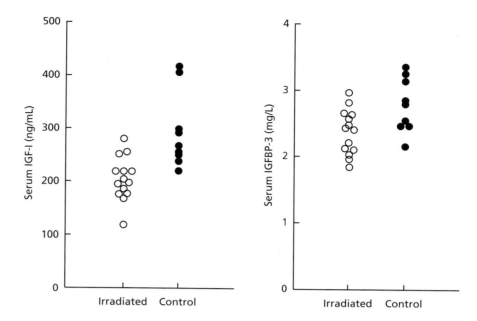

**Fig. 19.8.** Serum IGF-I and IGFBP-3 levels in long-term (13 years) adult survivors of cranial irradiation for posterior fossa tumours (○) and controls (●) (redrawn from [13]).

As hypothalamic dysregulation is dose- and time-dependent, it is not surprising that growth [51,60] and GH secretory abnormalities [32,50] may not be evident after lower doses of cranial irradiation (18 Gy and 24 Gy) in leukaemic children until puberty, when an amplitude-modulated increase in GH secretion is necessary to achieve a normal pubertal growth spurt. This evolving deficit also carries implications for those surviving into adult life, who are at significant risk of adult GH deficiency [33], with its attendant concerns on bone mineralization, body composition, lipid profile and quality of life.

## Precocious puberty

This is probably the second most common pituitary dysfunction after cranial irradiation, but its incidence is difficult to estimate because of possible compounding gonadal damage from chemotherapy [72,73] or scattered spinal beam irradiation [5] administered simultaneously. Gonadotrophin deficiency, which can prevent, disrupt or perturb pubertal development, is also possible [5], although it is more likely to be part of an evolving endocrinopathy after high-dose irradiation of pituitary or closely related tumours [8].

Precocious or early puberty may be a presenting feature of centrally placed tumours, but this tendency has also been detected after treatment for distant tumours, most commonly in girls [7,74]; it is directly related to the age at irradiation [74]. Despite potentially gonadotoxic chemotherapy and spinal irradiation in some, a tendency to early puberty was demonstrated in 39 children who were prepubertal at the time of cranial irradiation for brain tumours, more obviously girls, and this persisted even when those with central optic tract tumours were removed from the analysis [7] (Fig. 19.9).

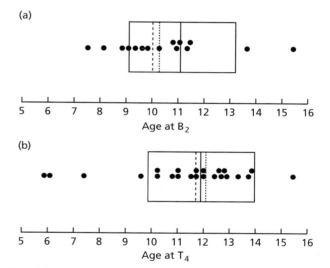

**Fig. 19.9.** Age at pubertal onset of 15 girls and 24 boys receiving 10–56 Gy of fractionated cranial irradiation for brain tumours distant from the hypothalamo-pituitary axis. The solid line boxes represent the mean ± 2 SD for normal children. The broken lines represent the study population medians with optic gliomas excluded (⋯⋯⋯) or included (– – –) (this study). (a) Breast stage 2; (b) testis volume 4 mL (redrawn from [7]).

Early puberty has been increasingly documented in children after lower cranial irradiation doses (24 or 18 Gy), particularly since the neuraxial prophylaxis for leukaemia has not included spinal irradiation [51,75]. It is possible that radiation damage to higher, as yet unidentified, inhibitory centres regulating the onset of puberty occurs at lower cranial doses and results in the premature activation of puberty, whereas higher radiation doses ablate hypothalamic GnRH or pituitary gonadotrophin release.

Reports that early puberty is more frequently observed in those treated at an early age (< 8 years) with 18 Gy compared with 24 Gy of cranial irradiation [51,75] lends support to this theory, and the absence of the phenomenon after the lower fractionated (12–15.75 Gy) or single fraction (7.5–10 Gy) cranial doses used in TBI is explained by the severe gonadotoxicity of such a regimen administered together with conditioning alkylating agent chemotherapy [76]. The observation that female leukaemia survivors treated with 18–20 Gy are also the group who experience the greatest risk of obesity [77] raises the interesting possibility that neuroregulatory changes in leptin secretion may be contributory to mediating the early puberty seen in this situation.

The importance of a premature puberty is twofold. First, it limits the time available for growth by leading to premature fusion of the epiphyses. Second, an early pubertal spurt due to sex steroids (or sustained growth at the expense of hyperinsulinism and obesity) may mask concomitant GH deficiency. The end result is an attenuated growth spurt, accelerated skeletal maturation and a compromised final adult height. If the radiotherapy fields have included the spine, further limitation of pubertal growth may occur. Attempts at delaying puberty with a GnRH analogue in combination with GH therapy increase short-term growth rate and predicted height but final height data are lacking, and such combinations have proved largely unsuccessful in idiopathic precocious puberty. It is likely that such unrecognized early puberty, delays in the initiation of GH therapy, suboptimal GH dosage schedules and skeletal damage have all contributed to the initial reports of a poor therapeutic response to GH in children after irradiation compared with children with idiopathic GH deficiency, which have now been refuted.

## Gonadal dysfunction (Tables 19.2 and 19.3)

The population of oocytes at birth is irreplaceable and declines exponentially by atresia with time [78] (Fig. 19.10). It can be reduced by radiation and cytotoxic injury, the latter possibly causing follicular maturation arrest. The apparently greater radiosensitivity of the ovary and the higher incidence of permanent menopause in women over the age of 40 (100% at 4 Gy) than in their younger peers (60% at 5–8 Gy) [17] is most readily explained by depletion in the initial pool of primordial follicles. Thus the size of the radiation dose required to cause permanent sterility is dependent on the age at irradiation or, more precisely, the number of oocytes that still remain [78]. The 50% lethal dose ($LD_{50}$) to the human oocyte is 4 Gy or less [79], and fractionation may be more deleterious [14,17]. Thus, despite absence of evidence of ovarian injury in childhood or early adulthood [80], subfertility and/or an early menopause are likely in many girls receiving direct or scattered ovarian irradiation or gonadotoxic chemotherapy.

**Table 19.2.** Gonadotoxic drugs

| Group | Proven gonadotoxicity | Dose likely to cause azoospermia (g/m²) |
|---|---|---|
| Alkylating agents | Cyclophosphamide | 19.0 |
| | Chlorambucil | 19.0 |
| | Melphalan | 1.4 |
| | Busulphan | |
| | Carmustine | |
| | Lomustine | |
| | Mechlorethamine | |
| | Procarbazine | 4.0 |
| | Cisplatin | 0.6 |
| | CCNU | 19.0 |
| | BCNU | 0.5 |
| Vinka alkaloids | Vinblastine | |
| Antimetabolites | Cytosine arabinoside | |

## Transplant preconditioning regimens

After single-fraction TLI or TBI, primary ovarian failure and secondary amenorrhoea affects all postmenarcheal women [81], and fractionation (12 Gy in 3 days) does not alleviate this [30]. Recovery of ovarian function has been reported in up to 10% of the youngest women [81], but only 4% have so far become parents [76]. In studies where conditioning regimens included cyclophosphamide, gonadal failure was 6–9 times more likely in those that received additional TBI [81]. However, those conditioned with combinations of high-dose busulphan/melphalan and cyclophosphamide (> 200 mg/kg) alone are also particularly compromised [76]. Concerns about adverse genetic effects on the offspring of those who have remained fertile have not been confirmed [82], but follow-up times are far too short and numbers are small.

By contrast to the ovary, the testicular germ cells are at all stages of development, the primitive spermatogonia being the most radiosensitive. For a short time after irradiation, the relatively radioresistant spermatocytes and spermatids mature to form spermatozoa, but azoospermia eventually results after fractionated testicular doses as low as 0.35 Gy. Complete recovery has been recorded within 9–18 months after single doses < 1 Gy, 2–3 years after 2–3 Gy and 5–12 years after 4–6 Gy, although fractionation prolongs this recovery [17].

Fertility is unlikely after direct testicular doses of 25–30 Gy given for testicular tumours or leukaemic relapse at any age [83,84], or after single (7.5–10 Gy) or fractionated (12–15 Gy) TBI [76]. All adult men are likely to be azoospermic after similar therapy, particularly after fractionated regimens [30], although there are occasional reports of recovery after many years [84]. Inhibin B, a product of both Sertoli and germ cells, correlates positively with testicular volume and sperm

**Table 19.3.** Best assessment of subfertility risk after current treatment for childhood cancer in UK by disease

| Risk of subfertility | | |
| --- | --- | --- |
| **Low** | **Medium** | **High** |
| 1. Acute lymphoblastic leukaemia | 1. Acute myeloid leukaemia | 1. Total body irradiation |
| 2. Wilms tumour | 2. Hepatoblastoma | 2. Localized radiotherapy: |
| 3. Soft tissue sarcoma: stage I | 3. Osteosarcoma | pelvic or testicular |
| 4. Germ cell tumours with | 4. Ewing's sarcoma | 3. Preconditioning chemotherapy |
| gonadal preservation and no RT | 5. Soft tissue sarcoma | for bone marrow transplant |
| 5. Brain tumour:* | 6. Neuroblastoma | 4. Hodgkin disease: |
| – Surgery only | 7. Hodgkin disease | alkylating agent-based therapy |
| – Cranial irradiation (< 24 Gy) | 'hybrid' therapy | 5. Soft tissue sarcoma: metastatic |
| | 8. Non-Hodgkin lymphoma | |
| | 9. Brain tumour: | |
| | – Craniospinal radiotherapy | |
| | – Cranial radiation* (> 24 Gy) | |
| | – Chemotherapy | |

Low risk , < 20%; high risk, > 80%; medium risk difficult to quantify.

Men more susceptible to subfertility after chemotherapy than women, but women may be at risk of premature menopause and males may continue to recover over time.

Insufficient evidence to be definitive, therefore best educated guide.

This table may be used as a guideline on which to base fertility counselling at onset of treatment.

*Infertility probably due to central hypothalamo-pituitary dysfunction rather than direct gonadal damage. Latter manifests by elevated gonadotrophins (FSH).

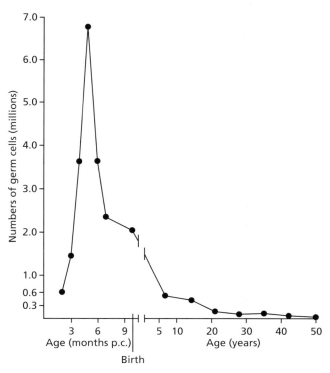

**Fig. 19.10.** The exponential decline of a fixed population of oocytes from the time of birth (redrawn from [78]). Months post coitum.

counts and negatively with follicle-stimulating hormone (FSH) and the presence of Sertoli cell only (SCO) tubules in testicular biopsies. It may prove an earlier and more sensitive marker than FSH for the detection of irradiation-induced subfertility [85].

The Leydig cell is more radioresistant than the germinal cell or the oocyte and has been said to tolerate doses up to 30 Gy in adults [17]. The effect is dose dependent, however, and partial Leydig cell dysfunction affects the majority treated for testicular tumours with fractionated doses of 30 Gy [84], whereas prepubertal boys treated for testicular leukaemic relapse (24 Gy in 12 fractions) are very likely to suffer profound and probably irreversible Leydig cell failure requiring sex steroids for the induction of puberty [83]. This is less common after reduced doses of 12 Gy [86], but pubertal delay and elevated gonadotrophins have been observed in 60% (27/45) of boys who were prepubertal at the time of TBI [66]. Although single doses of 7.5–10 Gy or fractionated doses of 12–15.75 Gy TBI may not prevent pubertal progression [66,86], sex steroid levels may be maintained only at the expense of an elevated gonadotrophin message.

### Craniospinal irradiation

The ovaries of young girls are not fixed. Their mobility makes them difficult to protect and particularly vulnerable to irradiation scatter from a spinal beam, estimated to be between 0.9 Gy and 2.5 Gy [73]. The scattered dose to the scrotum is less (0.4–1.2 Gy) [72]. The potentially gonadotoxic effect of such scatter is difficult to separate from that of alkylating agent or nitrogen mustard chemotherapy administered simultaneously. Some reports have attributed gonadal damage to spinal irradiation scatter [5], whereas others concluded that adjuvant chemotherapy was responsible [72,73].

Clayton *et al.* [72,73] have documented biochemical or clinical signs of gonadal damage in 20 of 29 boys and 18 of 21 girls irradiated for brain tumours with adjuvant alkylating agent, nitrosourea and procarbazine chemotherapy. Recovery was rare in boys treated prepubertally at a mean 4.5 years' follow-up but, excepting two children of each sex who developed gonadotrophin deficiency, neither sexual maturation nor the timing of menarche was prejudiced. Although the authors state that chemotherapy was undoubtedly the gonadotoxic agent, only four children of each sex had not received additional spinal irradiation.

In a series of 93 children treated for centrally displaced brain tumours, primary ovarian failure occurred in 43% overall but affected 64% of those given an additional 29–33 Gy of spinal irradiation with or without chemotherapy at a mean of 8.5 years. Chemotherapy had a significant gonadotoxic effect in the group given cranial irradiation alone, but the addition of spinal irradiation was the major gonadotoxic factor and was reflected in the lower incidence of boys (9%) similarly affected [5].

Craniospinal irradiation was also implicated as causing biochemical gonadal dysfunction in 49% of 97 leukaemic girls treated at an early age (4.8 years) and followed for 14 years. Only 9% of those given cranial irradiation alone suffered a similar fate, although both groups received identical chemotherapy. Gonadal dysfunction was directly dependent upon the spinal dose used (18 Gy vs. 24 Gy) and further compounded (93%) by additional abdominal (12 Gy) irradiation [87]. High gonadotrophins may not prevent menstruation [87] but may delay its onset. The longer-term implications upon fertility or early menopause have yet to be defined.

## Hodgkin disease

Both pelvic irradiation (30–45 Gy) and the alkylating agents used in the treatment of Hodgkin disease are gonadotoxic, and uterine integrity is also compromised by pelvic irradiation in the females [88]. Males are particularly susceptible to germ cell depletion and resultant azoospermia after six cycles of MOPP (mustine, vincristine, procarbazine and prednisolone) chemotherapy, with quoted figures up to 83% regardless of pubertal status and without additional irradiation [80]. Azoospermia persists for periods up to 10 years, with occasional reports of recovery and fatherhood after 11 years [80]. After platinum-based therapy for testicular germ cell tumours, temporary oligo/azoospermia is common, but recovery occurs earlier and is ongoing, with 50% being normospermic at 2 years and 80% at 5 years [89].

Oligospermia is the more usual problem after pelvic radiation, with doses of 20–45 Gy affecting about 50% of individuals, and recovery appears more likely than after chemotherapy (up to 88% within 26 months), particularly if gonadal shielding is used [80]. The total fractionated testicular dose from an inverted 'Y' with the best gonadal shielding has been estimated to be about 2 Gy [90].

Ovarian injury correlates with the volume and dose of irradiation and of chemotherapy, as well as the age of the patient at exposure. A satisfactory oophoropexy before inverted Y irradiation, with markers identifying both ovaries for lead shielding, reduces the estimated ovarian dose to 6–14% of the total pelvic dose (20–45 Gy) and increases the chances of fertility [80]. Sterility is more likely if the irradiation field is wider and oophoropexy inadequate and also more likely if modality therapy is combined or more than six cycles of MOPP chemotherapy are given. However, the majority of females (67–87%) achieve menarche at an average age and maintain normal menses [80]. Rates of subfertility or early menopause are unknown and, in the future, timed measurements of inhibin B and FSH early in the follicular phase of the menstrual cycle [91] may be helpful in assessing ovarian reserve in these patients.

## Gonadal protection strategies

By contrast to animal studies [92], the few human studies in patients with Hodgkin disease or testicular tumours do not support the concept that protection can be easily achieved by suppression of the pituitary–gonadal axis [48,93]. However, the timing of the intervention or its continuation beyond the completion of chemo/radiotherapy may be important [92]. It has been suggested that testosterone enhances recovery from documented azoo/oligospermia 6 months later if administered simultaneously with cyclophosphamide (total dose 120 mg/kg) during 8 months of therapy for nephrotic syndrome [47].

Recent developments in assisted reproductive technology (ART) have naturally focused attention on improving quality of life in cancer survivors by preserving fertility. Sperm banking before therapy has long been used in postpubertal adults, but this is increasingly being considered in younger and younger boys, raising concerns about valid consent (storage and use), as well as sperm maturity and quality. Spermatogenesis (even in the contralateral testis) may be impaired in patients with testicular cancer [94], Hodgkin disease [93] and other malignancies [95], semen quality being further compromised by long-term cryopreservation.

Techniques such as intracytoplasmic sperm injection (ICSI) have so improved efficiency that even survivors with the most severe forms of Sertoli cell only dysplasia may be able to parent their own genetic children, provided the 'single sperm' necessary can be identified and obtained by testicular extraction [96]. Adult studies harvesting stem cells before gonadotoxic therapy and reinjecting them into the seminiferous tubules after treatment to initiate spermatogenesis have already commenced [97], but *in vitro* maturation of immature spermatogonia remains elusive.

In postpubertal females it is now possible to cryopreserve oocytes (as well as embryos for those with established partners), but this is inefficient, requires a stimulated cycle and cannot help those who are prepubertal. Hence, alternative strategies are being explored. Pioneering experiments restoring temporary (2 years) fertility to 50% of castrate ewes by autotransplantation of cryopreserved ovarian cortical slices [98] has captured the imagination of many. However, given an individual's legally protected reproductive right, the quality (not quantity) of life issue, the absence of immediate therapeutic benefit, proven efficacy and risk–safety profiles, as well as the constantly changing chemotherapeutic (and hence gonadotoxic) baseline, it is questionable whether such experimentation is justified or ethical in children [99]. There must first be clarification of each nation's legal and moral position and, second, adequate counselling to ensure consent is truly informed, without pressure or bias.

## Thyroid dysfunction

Radiation damage to the thyroid gland includes hypothyroidism and thyroid tumours. In the majority of cases, the hypothyroidism is compensated by increased TSH concentration and thus not obviously manifest. It is dose and time dependent and has been documented after fractionated doses to the thyroid area in excess of 25 Gy [20]. Although some reports have suggested an increased incidence in the younger age group, this has not been confirmed by other studies [100].

After mantle irradiation doses of 36–44 Gy in 1.5- to 2-Gy fractions for Hodgkin disease in those under 16 years, prevalence rates, notably in the first 2 years, vary between 37% and 88% [100,101], with 25–53% being compensated and 0–58% overt. The use of a posterior spinal and laryngeal block at 30 Gy and 20 Gy, respectively, did not reduce the overall incidence of hypothyroidism (57%), but this was overt in fewer cases (5%) at a median follow-up of 65 months [102]. Transient hyperthyroidism has been reported after adjuvant MOPP chemotherapy [100], and one series documented primary thyroid dysfunction in 24 of 54 adults who did not receive radiotherapy [103].

Compensated, or, less commonly, frank hypothyroidism has been documented in 30–40% of children treated with craniospinal irradiation for brain tumours without chemotherapy, the majority occurring within 4 years. Adjuvant chemotherapy increases this risk [4,104]. A similar percentage develop thyroid dysfunction after TBI [66], usually compensated at first, progressing to overt hypothyroidism 5–10 years later. After 7.5–10 Gy of single-fraction TBI, 28% and

13% developed compensated and overt hypothyroidism respectively. After 12–15.75 Gy of fractionated TBI, these figures were decreased to 12% and 3%, respectively, although the latter group were followed for only half the number of years [66,105].

These figures have been proved to be overestimates, as one-third of those with compensated thyroid dysfunction recovered at a median of 60 months and there were no overt cases [106]. Although the same study documented a higher incidence of thyroid dysfunction after TLI for aplastic anaemia, these patients were followed for longer.

Although chemotherapy is additive to irradiation effects, it does not seem to play an important independent role in the pathogenesis of thyroid dysfunction, as it was not observed in a large series of 105 children transplanted for thalassaemia, and it was observed in only 1 of 50 transplanted for aplastic anaemia with conditioning chemotherapy but not TBI [105].

Elevations in TSH after spinal irradiation and TBI have been thought to reflect primary thyroid gland damage resulting from direct or scattered irradiation from the exit dose of the posterior spinal beam. Because of the recognized carcinogenic potential of megavoltage irradiation and prolonged TSH stimulation, annual thyroid palpation (with further ultrasound and needle biopsy evaluation of any nodules) and thyroid function tests ($fT_4$ and TSH) have always been advised, with institution of thyroxine replacement when TSH is elevated. However, increasing attention is being focused on the possibility of thyroid recovery now documented to occur after mantle irradiation [100], spinal irradiation used in brain tumours [104] and after TBI [106]. There remains the possibility that elevations in TSH may be a manifestation of higher irradiation damage to hypothalamic centres [39], although in the presence of a normal thyroid gland an increase in thyroxine levels should also follow.

## Adrenal function

Symptomatic ACTH deficiency after cranial irradiation for brain tumours not involving the hypothalamo-pituitary area has not been reported, but this may yet occur as survival is further prolonged. After estimated hypothalamo-pituitary doses of > 50 Gy to adults with brain tumours distant from that area, a recent report documented an 18–35% dose-related incidence of asymptomatic subnormal cortisol responses to metyrapone at 2–13 years' follow-up, although responses to corticotrophin-releasing factor were normal [18].

In our own series of 20 childhood survivors 10 years after cranial irradiation for posterior fossa tumours (estimated pituitary doses 40–45 Gy), all but two (who were asymptomatic and had normal low-dose ACTH responses) demonstrated normal (> 500 nmol/L) peak cortisol responses to hypoglycaemia with persistently suboptimal growth hormone responses [28] (Fig. 19.1b). As the childhood data contrast with the high incidence of ACTH insufficiency evolving after irradiation for pituitary/central tumours in adults after a similar interval and pituitary dose [8], this may be due to a late evolution of early surgical or tumour-related damage than simply to the purported irradiation therapy.

Clinical signs of cortisol deficiency may be non-specific, and the diagnosis may be missed by conventional dynamic tests such as insulin-induced hypoglycaemia [107]. Physiological ACTH and cortisol secretion profiles in children treated for leukaemia with 18-Gy or 24-Gy cranial prophylaxis 3.5–10 years previously showed no disruption in the amount or pattern of secretion compared with normal control subjects [108].

There has been little documentation in the medical literature of the possibility of hypoadrenalism after direct (TBI) or scattered (spinal) irradiation to the adrenals. This may be partly due to the lack of a suitable physiological test of intact adrenal function. Although most studies have documented normal cortisol responses to insulin-induced hypoglycaemia or 250 µg of ACTH (Synacthen), such tests may be pharmacological rather than physiological in their action and thus they may not detect subclinical damage [107,109]. A dose of 500 ng/1.73 m$^2$ Synacthen has been proposed as a physiological test of adrenal reserve [109] and was normal in all our 20 survivors of posterior fossa tumours [28]. The 24% incidence of subnormal adrenal 11-deoxycortisol responses to metyrapone after TBI in asymptomatic patients [66] suggests that subclinical adrenal damage is a possibility to consider with increasing time from therapy.

## Impaired bone mineralization

Any skeletal changes observed in cancer survivors may be as much due to nutritional as hormonal (GH and sex steroid) deficiencies. Skeletal irradiation [62], corticosteroids and antineoplastic agents [55,58,59] may additionally impair mineralization by direct actions on the growth plate or by indirectly inducing renal tubulopathies and mineral loss. Disease (e.g. leukaemia), prolonged bed rest and changes in vitamin D metabolism may all influence bone mineral density in children with malignancy. There is concern that a lower peak bone mass will eventually result in consequent osteoporosis in adult life.

Care needs to be taken in the interpretation of surrogate markers of bone mineral density (BMD), such as DEXA measurements at the lumbar spine (L1–L4). There are sex- and age-standardized reference charts for children, but they may be misleading in a short population (owing to GH deficiency and spinal irradiation), as they increase with body and vertebral size [9]. In adults, other femoral and distal radial sites may be used, but corrections should be made for size [9]. Volumetric densities, independent of bone size, measured with quantitative computerized tomography are the ideal [110].

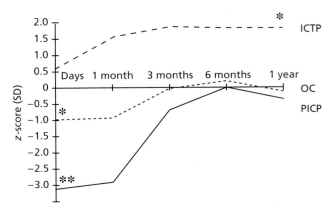

**Fig. 19.11.** Changes in serum markers of bone formation, type I collagen carboxy-terminal propeptide and osteocalcin (PICP and OC) and resorption type I collagen carboxy-terminal telopeptide (ICTP) (expressed as standard deviation scores, SDS) over time in newly diagnosed patients with malignancy, during chemotherapy. The asterisk indicates significant difference from normal standards (redrawn from [113]). Bone formation is suppressed at diagnosis and subsequently normalizes, but bone resorption continues, impairing development of peak bone mass.

Using such methodology, Gilsanz *et al.* [110] reported reduced lumbar spine volumetric bone density in 42 leukaemic survivors (mean age 12 years), 3–4 years after cessation of chemotherapy compared with control subjects, with a further difference between shorter irradiated (*n* = 29) and taller non-irradiated (*n* = 13) groups (z-scores –0.93 vs. 0.21). Nyssom *et al.* [111] documented a size-adjusted decrease in bone mass (lumbar spine DEXA, BMD) 10.7 years after diagnosis (aged 4 years) in 95 leukaemic survivors in first remission, who had never received skeletal irradiation. This occurred largely in those who were older (> 19 years), female and shorter at follow-up, and, by contrast to the other size-adjusted study of Gilsanz *et al.* [110] in a younger cohort, no effect of cranial irradiation was noted.

Two recent prospective longitudinal studies in children with newly diagnosed malignancies [112] or leukaemia [55] documented a negative bone turnover at diagnosis, with additional decreases in vitamin D metabolites in one [112] and GH resistance resulting from the disease in the other [55]. There is continuing increase in bone resorption and depletion of vitamin D metabolites at 12 months [112] and impaired accrual of cortical (femoral neck) but not trabecular (lumbar spine) bone. Thus, if peak bone mass is impaired, the aetiology is likely to be multifactorial, making intervention strategies harder to define (Fig. 19.11).

## Obesity

Excessive weight gain is a recognized complication of suprasellar (rather than intrasellar) tumours or their surgery/

radiotherapy. For some time, growth may be maintained in the face of GH deficiency, through increased IGF bioavailability modulated in turn by hyperinsulinaemia, which also drives the obesity [113]. The latter results from ventromedial hypothalamic lesions causing disinhibition of vagal tone at the pancreatic β-cell and can be normalized by truncal vagotomy [114].

The tendency to obesity observed in cranially irradiated youngsters without hypothalamic lesions is harder to explain [77,115] and just as difficult to treat. Whether the eventual insulin resistance is also primarily the result of increased vagal tone or secondary to hyperphagia involving central satiety centres is entirely unknown. Prior treatment with corticosteroids may be contributory, but cortisol secretion appears normal [108].

Obesity and insulin resistance now pose a significant medical challenge to prevent premature death from diabetes and cardiovascular disease in those who have already survived one life-threatening challenge. GH deficiency aggravates obesity, whereas GH therapy decreases fat mass and increases lean mass through direct actions on adipocytes, which are also the source of leptin, which decreases in parallel [116].

Both insulin and leptin levels are also suppressed by octreotide administration, which has been paradoxically successfully used to improve intractable insulin resistance in this situation [115]. Leptin signalling modulates energy balance via effects on hypothalamus and other tissues, maintaining adipose tissue mass within a finite (optimal) range. What role disturbances in leptin signalling might play in the evolution of obesity (or early puberty) after cranial irradiation remains to be elucidated, but adult GH replacement therapy may need to be considered in this situation, even in the absence of other significant endocrinopathies.

## Growth hormone therapy and tumour relapse

Concerns have been expressed that GH therapy is potentially mitogenic and may induce malignant transformation. However, the theoretical risk that GH may predispose to malignancy [117,118] remains scientifically unproven, at least when used in replacement doses [119]. GH treatment has not increased the relapse rate or occurrence of second primary malignancies [120], well documented in children irradiated for cancers and leukaemia, who have an estimated 7–20 times increased risk [15]. However, very large numbers of GH-treated individuals would need to be studied to achieve statistical certainty.

GH receptors are found on lymphocytes. If leukaemic transformation has taken place therefore GH could potentially accelerate this process. However, experiments in culture show that concentrations 10 times higher than those used therapeutically are needed [117]. However, the increase in

bleomycin-induced chromosomal fragility of lymphocytes from GH-treated children compared with control subjects and pretreatment values is of concern [118]. There are reports of leukaemia in 35 children treated with GH worldwide, but 19 of these had predisposing conditions.

In a large study of 6284 individuals treated with GH in the USA, relative risks (RR) for leukaemia were identified: three cases occurred in 59 736 patient–years of follow-up (RR 1.8, 95% CI 0.8–7.5), and this figure increased to six cases at 83 917 patient–years of follow-up (RR 2.6, 95% CI 1.2–5.2). Five of these six had previous cranial tumours, and all except one of these had previous irradiation [119].

It is also noteworthy that leukaemia has been reported in untreated patients with idiopathic GH deficiency [121]. Although lymphocyte subsets are normal in GH-deficient patients, consistent with the absence of clinical immunodeficiency, lymphocyte natural killer activity is reduced in some [122].

In the biggest postmarketing surveillance series in the USA and Canada, 29 000 children were treated with GH over 120 000 patient–years. Approximately 2800 of these patients start and stop GH each year. Taking all cases of leukaemia in North America, the risk ratio of GH-treated individuals developing leukaemia is 3.0 but, in children without a predisposing cause, this returns to 1.0, no different from the normal risk in childhood (L. L. Robison, personal communication).

Experiments with physiological doses of GH to improve the nitrogen wasting and cachexia of malignant disease in a rodent tumour-bearing model have shown beneficial effects on nutritional parameters without an increase in the rate of growth of the primary tumour compared with placebo-treated animals with a significant reduction in the number of pulmonary metastases [123]. Preliminary studies of GH therapy to improve cachexia in subjects with malignancy and AIDS are now being undertaken.

To achieve a maximal response to therapy, GH should be substituted early. However, most centres do not advocate introducing therapy within the first 1–2 years after treatment as this is the time of highest relapse rate. Most children treated for brain tumours will be deficient on pharmacological testing within that time. However, the diagnosis may be delayed or difficult in children treated with lower cranial irradiation doses for leukaemia because of the discrepancies previously described. Documentation of growth rates is of paramount importance, but supportive evidence from pharmacological or physiological tests is invariably required. There may be cases where further physiological assessment and even a GH therapeutic trial may prove necessary.

## Summary

There is now a wealth of evidence documenting that cranial irradiation results in hypothalamo-pituitary dysfunction if this area is included within the radiation field. Its incidence and time course, as well the number of anterior pituitary hormones affected, depends on the sensitivity of the hormone itself to such therapy, as well as the dose, fractionation and time elapsed since irradiation. The few prospective studies have also indicated that irradiation is not the only culprit; disease, surgery and chemotherapy play contributory roles at all levels of the hypothalamo-pituitary target gland axis. Where tumours have not involved the pituitary area, the GH axis is the most sensitive and the adrenal axis the most resistant to the effects of direct irradiation, although the incidence of the latter may be underestimated and may increase with time as survival is further prolonged. As endocrinopathies may evolve over many years, lifelong endocrine follow-up is necessary.

As the difficulties in interpreting growth rates in children with possible radiation-induced skeletal lesions and in evaluating the various pharmacological tests used in the diagnosis of GH deficiency are recognized, it seems increasingly important to define the aetiological factors implicated in the evolution of postirradiation GH deficiency. This becomes a real possibility as understanding of the factors underlying the neuroregulatory control of the GH axis increases. Such a strategy may not only help to identify the best biochemical test to perform in this situation but also the potentially most useful replacement therapy. Early detection and appropriate replacement therapy before clinical manifestations occur may carry important benefits in terms of normal pubertal and social development, growth, fertility and bone mineralization.

GH replacement therapy has been traditionally discontinued after the end of adolescence, but increasing reports of an important role for GH on atherogenic lipid profiles, body mass and bone density as well as general well-being suggest that such replacement therapy may need to be continued indefinitely in future years, particularly in those with multiple endocrinopathies or severe deficiency. Because of the potential hazards of indiscriminate replacement therapy and real concerns about GH mitogenicity, it becomes all the more important to define adequately normal ranges for pharmacological and physiological tests of GH release at all ages and to understand the factors implicated in their action.

Recognition of the causes and evolutionary changes leading to neuroendocrine sequelae can only assist oncologists and radiotherapists in effectively planning their treatment protocols to reduce morbidity as well as prolonging survival. This carries new challenges associated with addressing the causes of obesity and hyperinsulinaemia, defining the aetiology of premature puberty and attempts to preserve fertility, as well as directly improving psychosocial and neurorehabilitation.

## References

1 Mahoney DH Jr, Shuster JJ, Nitschke R *et al*. Acute neurotoxicity in children with B-precursor acute lymphoid leukaemia: an association with intermediate-dose intravenous methotrexate and intrathecal triple therapy – a pediatric oncology group study. *J Clin Oncol* 1998; 16: 1712–22.

2 Mulhern RK, Kepner JL, Thomas PR, Armstrong FD, Friedman HS, Kun LE. Neuropsychologic functioning of survivors of childhood medulloblastoma randomized to receive conventional or reduced-dose craniospinal irradiation; a pediatric oncology group study. *J Clin Oncol* 1998; 16: 1723–8.

3 Spoudeas HA, Hindmarsh PC, Matthews DRM, Brook CGD. Evolution of growth hormone (GH) neurosecretory disturbance after cranial irradiation for childhood brain tumours; a prospective study. *J Endocrinol* 1996; 150: 329–42.

4 Livesey EA, Brook CGD. Thyroid dysfunction after radiotherapy and chemotherapy of brain tumours. *Arch Dis Child* 1989; 64: 593–5.

5 Livesey EA, Brook CGD. Gonadal dysfunction after treatment of intracranial tumours. *Arch Dis Child* 1988; 63: 495–500.

6 Brauner R, Rappaport R, Prevot C *et al*. A prospective study of the development of growth hormone deficiency in children given cranial irradiation, and its relation to statural growth. *J Clin Endocrinol Metab* 1989; 68: 346–51.

7 Darendeliler F, Livesey EA, Hindmarsh PC, Brook CGD. Growth and growth hormone secretion in children following treatment of brain tumours with radiotherapy. *Acta Paediatr Scand* 1990; 79: 121–7.

8 Littley MD, Shalet SM, Beardwell CG, Ahmed SR, Applegate G, Sutton ML. Hypopituitarism following external radiotherapy for pituitary tumours in adults. *Q J Med* 1989; 70: 145–60.

9 Prentice A, Parsons TJ, Cole TJ. Uncritical use of bone mineral density in absorptiometry may lead to size-related artefacts in the identification of bone mineral determinants. *Am J Clin Nutr* 1994; 60: 837–42.

10 Spiliotis BE, August GP, Hung W, Sonis W, Mendelson W, Bercu BB. Growth hormone neurosecretory dysfunction: a treatable cause of short stature. *J Am Med Assoc* 1984; 251: 2223–30.

11 Ryalls M, Spoudeas HA, Hindmarsh PC *et al*. Short-term endocrine consequences of total body irradiation and bone marrow transplantation in children treated for leukaemia. *J Endocrinol* 1993; 136: 331–8.

12 Jorgensen EV, Schwartz ID, Hvizdala E *et al*. Neurotransmitter control of growth hormone secretion in children after cranial radiation therapy. *J Pediatr Endocrinol* 1993; 6: 131–42.

13 Achermann JC, Hindmarsh PC, Brook CGD. The relationship between the growth hormone and insulin-like growth factor axis in long-term survivors of childhood brain tumours. *Clin Endocrinol* 1998; 49: 639–45.

14 Coggle JE. The effect of radiation at the tissue level. In: *Biological Effects of Radiation*. London: Taylor & Francis, 1983: 89–109.

15 Hawkins MM, Draper GJ, Kingston JE. Incidence of second primary tumours among childhood cancer survivors. *Br J Cancer* 1987; 56: 339–47.

16 Withers HR. Biology of radiation oncology. In: Tobias JS, Thomas PRM, eds. *Current Radiation Oncology*, Vol. 1. London: Edward Arnold, 1994: 5–23.

17 Ash P. The influence of radiation on fertility in man. *Br J Radiol* 1980; 53: 271–8.

18 Constine LS, Woolf PD, Cann D *et al*. Hypothalamic-pituitary dysfunction after radiation for brain tumors. *N Engl J Med* 1993; 328: 87–94.

19 Olshan JS, Gubernick J, Packer RJ *et al.* The effects of adjuvant chemotherapy on growth in children with medulloblastoma. *Cancer* 1992; 70: 2013–17.

20 Samaan NA, Vieto R, Schultz PN *et al.* Hypothalamic, pituitary and thyroid dysfunction after radiotherapy to the head and neck. *Int J Radiat Oncol Biol Phys* 1982; 8: 1857–67.

21 Dacou-Voutetakis C, Xypolyta A, Haidas S, Constantinidis M, Papavasiliou C, Zannos-Mariolea L. Irradiation of the head. Immediate effect on growth hormone secretion in children. *J Clin Endocrinol Metab* 1977; 44: 791–4.

22 Chrousos GP, Poplack D, Brown T, O'Neill D, Schwade JG, Bercu BB. Effects of cranial radiation on hypothalamic-adeno-hypophyseal function: abnormal growth hormone secretory dynamics. *J Clin Endocrinol Metab* 1982; 54: 1135–9.

23 Littley MD, Shalet SM, Beardwell CG, Robinson EL, Sutton ML. Radiation-induced hypopituitarism is dose-dependent. *Clin Endocrinol* 1989; 31: 363–73.

24 Shalet SM, Fairhall KM, Sparks E, Hendry J, Robinson I. Radiosensitivity of hypothalamo-pituitary (HP) function in the rat is time and dose dependent (Abstract). *Horm Res* 1999; 51 (Suppl. 2): P103.

25 Richards GE, Wara WM, Grumbach MM, Kaplan SD, Sheline GE, Conte FA. Delayed onset of hypopituitarism: sequelae of therapeutic irradiation of central nervous system, eye, and middle ear tumours. *J Pediatr* 1976; 89: 553–9.

26 Shalet SM, Beardwell CG, Morris Jones PH, Pearson D. Growth hormone deficiency after treatment of acute leukaemia in children. *Arch Dis Child* 1976; 51: 489–93.

27 Clayton PE, Shalet SM. Dose dependency of time of onset of radiation-induced growth hormone deficiency. *J Pediatr* 1991; 118: 226–8.

28 Spoudeas HA, Charmandari E, Brook CGD. The effect of cranial irradiation for tumours distal to the pituitary on ACTH secretion (Abstract). *Horm Res* 2000; 53 (Suppl. 2): 549.

29 Clayton PE, Price DA, Shalet SM. Growth hormone state after completion of treatment with growth hormone. *Arch Dis Child* 1987; 62: 222–6.

30 Littley MD, Shalet SM, Morgenstern GR, Deakin DP. Endocrine and reproductive dysfunction following fractionated total body irradiation in adults. *Q J Med* 1991; 78: 2665–74.

31 Ogilvy-Stuart AL, Clark DJ, Wallace WHB *et al.* Endocrine deficit after fractionated total body irradiation. *Arch Dis Child* 1992; 67: 1107–10.

32 Crowne EC, Moore C, Wallace WHB *et al.* A novel variant of growth hormone (GH) insufficiency following low dose cranial irradiation. *Clin Endocrinol* 1992; 36: 59–68.

33 Brennan BMD, Rahim A, Mackie EM, Eden OB, Shalet SM. Growth hormone status in adults treated for acute lymphoblastic leukaemia in childhood. *Clin Endocrinol* 1998; 48: 777–83.

34 Chieng PU, Huang TS, Chang CC *et al.* Reduced hypothalamic blood flow after radiation treatment of nasopharyngeal cancer: SPECT studies in 34 patients. *Am J Nuclear Radiol* 1991; 12: 661–5.

35 Achermann J. *The Pathophysiology of Post-irradiation Growth Hormone Insufficiency.* MD Thesis, London University, 1997.

36 Charmandari E, Brook CGD. 20 years of experience in idiopathic central diabetes insipidus. *Lancet* 1999; 353: 2212–13.

37 Dickinson WP, Berry DH, Dickinson L *et al.* Differential effects of cranial irradiation on growth hormone responses to arginine and insulin infusion. *J Pediatr* 1978; 92: 754–7.

38 Lustig RH, Schriock EA, Kaplan SL, Grumbach MM. Effect of growth hormone-releasing factor on growth hormone release in children with radiation-induced growth hormone deficiency. *Pediatrics* 1985; 76: 274–9.

39 Spoudeas HA. *The Evolution of Growth Hormone Neurosecretory Disturbance During High Dose Cranial Irradiation and Chemotherapy for Childhood Brain Tumours.* MD Thesis, University of London, 1995.

40 Wells T, Flavell DM, Wells SE, Carmignac DF, Robinson ICAF. Effects of growth hormone secretagogues in the transgenic growth-retarded rat. *Endocrinology* 1997; 138: 580–7.

41 Spoudeas HA, Winrow AP, Hindmarsh PC, Brook CGD. Low dose growth hormone-releasing hormone tests: a dose response study. *Eur J Endocrinol* 1994; 131: 238–45.

42 Devesa J, Lima L, Lois N, Fraga C, Lechuga MJ, Arce V, Tresguerres JAF. Reasons for the variability in growth hormone (GH) responses to GHRH challenge: the endogenous hypothalamic-somatotroph rhythm (HSR). *Clin Endocrinol* 1989; 30: 367–77.

43 Ogilvy-Stuart AL, Wallace WHB, Shalet SM. Radiation and neuroregulatory control of growth hormone secretion. *Clin Endocrinol* 1994; 41: 163–8.

44 Toogood A, Nass RM, Pezzoli SS, O'Neill PA, Thorner MO, Shalet SM. Preservation of growth hormone pulsatility despite pituitary pathology, surgery, and irradiation. *J Clin Endocrinol Metab* 1997; 82: 2215–21.

45 Hall JE, Martin KA, Whitney HA, Landy H, Crowley WF Jr. Potential for fertility with replacement of hypothalamic gonadotropin-releasing hormone in long term female survivors of cranial tumours. *J Clin Endocrinol Metab* 1994; 79: 1166–72.

46 Ogilvy-Stuart AL, Stirling HF, Kelnar CJH, Savage MO, Dunger DB, Buckler JMH, Shalet SM. Treatment of radiation-induced growth hormone deficiency with growth hormone-releasing hormone. *Clin Endocrinol* 1997; 46: 571–8.

47 Masala A, Faedda R, Alagna S *et al.* Use of testosterone to prevent cyclophosphamide-induced azoospermia. *Ann Intern Med* 1997; 126: 292–5.

48 Howell SJ, Shalet SM. Pharmacological protection of the gonads. *Med Pediatr Oncol* 1999; 33: 41–5.

49 Marky I, Mellander L, Lannering B, Albertsson-Wikland K. A longitudinal study of growth and growth hormone secretion in children during treatment for acute lymphoblastic leukaemia. *Med Pediatr Oncol* 1991; 19: 258–64.

50 Moell C, Garwicz S, Westgren U, Wiebe T, Albertsson-Wikland K. Suppressed spontaneous secretion of growth hormone in girls after treatment for acute lymphoblastic leukaemia. *Arch Dis Child* 1989; 64: 252–8.

51 Uruena M, Stanhope R, Chessells JM, Leiper AD. Impaired pubertal growth in acute lymphoblastic leukaemia. *Arch Dis Child* 1991; 66: 1403–7.

52 Clayton PE, Shalet SM, Morris Jones PH, Price DA. Growth in children treated for acute lymphoblastic leukaemia. *Lancet* 1988; i: 460–2.

53 Kirk JA, Stevens MM, Raghupathy P *et al.* Growth failure and growth-hormone deficiency after treatment for acute lymphoblastic leukaemia. *Lancet* 1987; i: 190–3.

54 Hokken-Koelega ACS, Van Doorn JWD, Hahlen K, Stijnen T, De Muinck Keizer-Schrama SMPF, Drop SLS. Long-term effects of treatment for acute lymphoblastic leukaemia with and without

cranial irradiation on growth and puberty: a comparative study. *Pediatr Res* 1993; 33: 577–82.

55 Crofton PM, Ahmed SF, Wade JC *et al*. Effects of intensive chemotherapy on bone and collagen turnover and the growth hormone axis in children with acute lymphoblastic leukaemia. *J Clin Endocrinol Metab* 1998; 83: 3121–9.

56 Wingard JR, Plotnick LP, Freemer CS *et al*. Growth in children after bone marrow transplantation: busulfan plus cyclophosphamide versus cyclophosphamide plus total body irradiation. *Blood* 1992; 79: 1068–73.

57 Sklar C, Mertens A, Walter A *et al*. Final height after treatment for childhood acute lymphoblastic leukaemia: comparison of no cranial irradiation with 1800 and 2400 cGy cranial irradiation. *J Pediatr* 1993; 123: 59–64.

58 Robson H, Anderson E, Eden O, Isaksson O, Shalet S. Chemotherapeutic agents used in the treatment of childhood malignancies have direct effects on growth plate chondrocyte proliferation. *J Endocrinol* 1998; 157: 225–35.

59 Robson H, Anderson E, Eden O, Isaksson O, Shalet S. Glucocorticoid pre-treatment reduces the cytotoxic effects of a variety of DNA-damaging agents on rat tibial growth-plate chondrocytes in vitro. *Cancer Chemother Pharmacol* 1998; 42: 171–6.

60 Schriock EA, Schell MJ, Carter M, Hustu O, Ochs JJ. Abnormal growth patterns and adult short stature in 115 long-term survivors of childhood leukaemia. *J Clin Oncol* 1991; 9: 400–5.

61 Davies HA, Didcock E, Didi M, Ogilvy-Stuart A, Wales JKH, Shalet SM. Disproportionate short stature after cranial irradiation and combination chemotherapy for leukaemia. *Arch Dis Child* 1994; 70: 472–5.

62 Probert JS, Parker BR, Kaplan HS. Growth retardation in children after megavoltage irradiation of the spine. *Cancer* 1973; 32: 634–9.

63 Shalet SM, Gibson B, Swindell R, Pearson D. Effect of spinal irradiation on growth. *Arch Dis Child* 1987; 62: 461–4.

64 Hartsell WF, Hanson WR, Conterato DJ, Hendrickson FR. Hyperfractionation decreases the deleterious effects of conventional radiation fractionation on vertebral growth in animals. *Cancer* 1989; 63: 2452–5.

65 Wechsler-Jentzsch K, Huepfel H, Schmidt W, Wandl E, Kahn B. Failure of hyperfractionated radiotherapy to reduce bone growth arrest in rats. *Int J Radiat Oncol Biol Phys* 1992; 26: 427–31.

66 Sanders JE, Pritchard S, Mahoney P *et al*. Growth and development following marrow transplantation for leukaemia. *Blood* 1986; 68: 1129–35.

67 Bushouse S, Ramsay NKC, Pescovitz OH, Kim T, Robison LL. Growth in children following irradiation for bone marrow transplantation. *Am J Pediatr Hematol Oncol* 1989; 11: 134–40.

68 Papadimitriou A, Uruena M, Hamill G, Stanhope R, Leiper AD. Growth hormone treatment of growth failure secondary to total body irradiation and bone marrow transplantation. *Arch Dis Child* 1991; 66: 689–92.

69 Brauner R, Fontoura M, Zucker JM *et al*. Growth and growth hormone secretion after bone marrow transplantation. *Arch Dis Child* 1993; 68: 458–63.

70 Milikic V, Spoudeas HA, Achermann J, Bridges NA, Hindmarsh PC, Brook CGD. Growth after total body irradiation (TBI): response to growth hormone (GH) therapy (Abstract). *Horm Res* (Suppl.) 1995; 44: 217.

71 Nivot S, Benelli C, Clot JP *et al*. Nonparallel changes of growth hormone (GH) and insulin-like growth factor-1, insulin-like growth factor binding protein-3, and GH-binding protein, after craniospinal irradiation and chemotherapy. *J Clin Endocrinol Metab* 1994; 78: 597–601.

72 Clayton PE, Shalet SM, Price DA, Campbell RHA. Testicular damage after chemotherapy for childhood brain tumors. *J Pediatr* 1988; 112: 922–6.

73 Clayton PE, Shalet SM, Price DA, Morris-Jones PH. Ovarian function following chemotherapy for childhood brain tumours. *Med Pediatr Oncol* 1989; 17: 92–6.

74 Ogilvy-Stuart AL, Clayton PE, Shalet SM. Cranial irradiation and early puberty. *J Clin Endocrinol Metab* 1994; 78: 1282–6.

75 Mills JL, Fears TR, Robison LL, Nicholson HS, Sklar CA, Byrne J. Menarche in a cohort of 188, 1ong-term survivors of acute lymphoblastic leukaemia. *J Pediatr* 1997; 131: 598–602.

76 Sanders JE, Hawley J, Levy W. Pregnancies following high dose cyclophosphamide with or without high-dose busulphan or total body irradiation and bone marrow transplantation. *Blood* 1996; 87: 3045–52.

77 Odame I, Reilly JJ, Gibson BES, Donaldson MDC. Patterns of obesity in boys and girls after treatment of acute lymphoblastic leukaemia. *Arch Dis Child* 1994; 71: 147–9.

78 Baker TG. Radiosensitivity of mammalian oocytes with particular reference to the human female. *Am J Obstet Gynaecol* 1971; 110: 746–61.

79 Wallace WHB, Shalet SM, Hendry JH, Morris-Jones PH, Gattameneni HR. Ovarian failure following abdominal irradiation in childhood: the radiosensitivity of the human oocyte. *Br J Radiol* 1989; 62: 995–8.

80 Ortin TTS, Shostak CA, Donaldson SS. Gonadal status and reproductive function following treatment for Hodgkin's disease in childhood: the Stanford experience. *Int J Radiat Oncol Biol Phys* 1990; 19: 873–80.

81 Sanders JE, Buckner CD, Amos D, Levy W, Appelbaum FR, Doney K, Storb KM, Witherspoon RP, Thomas ED. Ovarian function following marrow transplantation for aplastic anemia or leukaemia. *J Clin Oncol* 1988; 6: 813–18.

82 Hawkins MM. Pregnancy outcome and offspring of childhood cancer. *Br Med J* 1994; 309: 1034.

83 Leiper AD, Grant DB, Chessells JM. Gonadal function after testicular radiation for acute lymphoblastic leukaemia. *Arch Dis Child* 1986; 61: 53–6.

84 Shalet SM, Tsatsoulis A, Whitehead E, Read G. Vulnerability of the human Leydig cell to radiation damage is dose-dependent. *J Endocrinol* 1989; 120: 161–5.

85 Foppiani L, Schlatt S, Simoni M, Weinbauer GF, Hacker-Klom U, Nieschlag E. Inhibin B is a more sensitive marker of spermatogenetic damage than FSH in the irradiated non-human primate model. *J Endocrinol* 1999; 162: 393–400.

86 Castillo LA, Craft AW, Kernhan J, Evans RGB, Aynsley-Green A. Gonadal function after 12-Gy testicular irradiation in childhood acute lymphoblastic leukaemia. *Med Pediatr Oncol* 1990; 18: 185–9.

87 Hamre MR, Robison LL, Nesbit ME *et al*. Effects of radiation on ovarian function in long term survivors of childhood leukaemia. A report from the children's cancer study group. *J Clin Oncol* 1987; 5: 1759–65.

88 Critchley HOD, Wallace WHB, Mamtola H, Higginson J, Shalet SM, Anderson DC. Ovarian failure after whole abdominal irra-

diation; the potential for pregnancy. *Br J Obstet Gynaecol* 1992; 99: 3392–4.

89 Lampe H, Horwich A, Norman A *et al.* Fertility after chemotherapy for testicular germ cell cancers. *J Clin Oncol* 1997; 15: 239–45.

90 Lushbaugh CC, Casarett GW. The effect of gonadal irradiation in clinical radiation therapy: a review. *Cancer* 1976; 37: 111–20.

91 Seifer DB, Scott RT, Bergh PA, Abrogast LK, Friedman CI, Mack CK, Danforth DR. Women with declining ovarian reserve may demonstrate a decrease in day 3 serum inhibin B before a rise in day 3 follicle-stimulating hormone. *Fertil Steril* 1999; 72: 63–5.

92 Meistrich ML, Kangasniemi M. Hormone treatment after irradiation stimulates recovery of rat spermatogenesis from surviving spermatogonia. *J Androl* 1997; 18: 80–7.

93 Chapman RM, Sutcliffe SB, Malpas JS. Male gonadal dysfunction in Hodgkin's disease. A prospective study. *J Am Med Assoc* 1981; 245: 1323–8.

94 Petersen PM, Skakkebaek N, Vistissen K, Rorth M, Giwercman A. Semen quality and reproductive hormones before orchiectomy in men with testicular cancer. *J Clin Oncol* 1999; 17: 941–7.

95 Padron OF, Sharma RK, Thomas AJ Jr, Agarwal A. Effects of cancer on spermatozoa quality after cryopreservation: a 12-year experience. *Fertil Steril* 1997; 67: 326–31.

96 Palermo GP, Schlegel PN, Scott Sills E *et al.* Births after intracytoplasmic injection of sperm obtained by testicular extraction from men with nonmosaic Klinefelter's syndrome. *N Engl J Med* 1998; 338: 588–90.

97 Radford JA, Shalet SM, Lieberman BA. Fertility after treatment for cancer: questions remain over ways of preserving ovarian and testicular tissue. *Br Med J* 1999; 319: 395–6.

98 Baird DT, Webb R, Campbell BK, Harkness LM, Gosden RG. Long-term ovarian function in sheep after ovariectomy and transplantation of autografts stored at –196C. *Endocrinology* 1999; 140: 462–71.

99 Spoudeas HA, Wallace WHB, Walker D. Is germ cell harvest and storage justified in minors treated for cancer? (letter). *Br Med J* 2000; 320: 316.

100 Devney RB, Sklar CA, Nesbit ME, Kim TH, Williamson JF, Robison LL, Ramsay NKC. Serial thyroid function measurements in children with Hodgkin disease. *J Pediatr* 1984; 105: 223–7.

101 Green EM, Brecher ML, Yakar D, Blumenson LE, Lindsay AN, Voorhess ML, MacGillivray M, Freeman AI. Thyroid function in pediatric patients after neck irradiation for Hodgkin disease. *Med Pediatr Oncol* 1980; 8: 127–36.

102 Mauch PM, Weinstein H, Botnick L, Belli J, Cassidy JR. An evaluation of long-term survival and treatment complications in children with Hodgkin's disease. *Cancer* 1983; 51: 925–32.

103 Sutcliffe SB, Chapman R, Wrigley PFM. Cyclical combination chemotherapy and thyroid function in patients with advanced Hodgkin's disease. *Med Pediatr Oncol* 1981; 9: 439–48.

104 Ogilvy-Stuart AL, Shalet SM, Gattameni HR. Thyroid function after treatment of brain tumors in children. *J Pediatr* 1991; 119: 733–7.

105 Sanders JE. The impact of marrow transplant preparative regimens on subsequent growth and development. *Semin Haematol* 1991; 28: 244–9.

106 Katsanis E, Shapiro RS, Robison LL *et al.* Thyroid dysfunction following bone marrow transplantation: long term follow–up of 80 pediatric patients. *Bone Marrow Transplant* 1990; 5: 335–40.

107 Tsatsoulis A, Shalet SM, Harrison J, Ratcliffe WA, Beardwell CG, Robinson EL. Adrenocorticotrophin (ACTH) deficiency undetected by standard dynamic tests of the hypothalamic-pituitary-adrenal axis. *Clin Endocrinol* 1988; 28: 225–32.

108 Crowne EC, Wallace WHB, Gibson S, Moore CM, White A, Shalet SM. Adrenocorticotrophin and cortisol secretion in children after low dose cranial irradiation. *Clin Endocrinol* 1993; 39: 297–305.

109 Crowley S, Hindmarsh PC, Holownia P, Honour JW, Brook CGD. The use of low doses of ACTH in the investigation of adrenal function in man. *J Endocr* 1991; 130: 475–9.

110 Gilsanz V, Carlson ME, Roe TF, Ortega JA. Osteoporosis after cranial irradiation for acute lymphoblastic leukaemia. *J Pediatr* 1990; 117: 238–44.

111 Nyssom K, Holm K, Michaelsen KF, Hertz H, Muller J, Molgaard C. Bone mass after treatment for acute lymophoblastic leukaemia in childhood. *J Clin Oncol* 1998; 16: 3752–60.

112 Arikowski P, Komulainen J, Riikonen P, Voutilainen R, Knip M, Kroger H. Alterations in bone turnover and impaired development of bone mineral density in newly diagnosed children with cancer: a 1-year prospective study. *J Clin Endocrinol Metab* 1999; 84: 3174–81.

113 Tiulpakov AN, Mazerkina AN, Brook CGD, Hindmarsh PC, Peterkova VA, Gorelyshev SK. Growth in children with craniopharyngioma following surgery. *Clin Endocrinol* 1998; 49: 733–8.

114 Smith DK, Sarfeh J, Howard L. Truncal vagotomy in hypothalamic obesity. *Lancet*, 1983; 1: 1330–1.

115 Lustig RH, Rose SR, Burghen GA *et al.* Hypothalamic obesity caused by cranial insult in children: altered glucose and insulin dynamics and reversal by a somatostatin agonist. *J Pediatr* 1999; 135: 162–8.

116 Randeva HS, Murray RD, Lewandowski K *et al.* Effects of growth hormone on components of the leptin system. *J Endocrinol* 2000; 164 (Suppl.): 135.

117 Zadik Z, Estrov Z, Karov Y, Hahn T, Barak Y. The effect of growth hormone and IGF-I on clonogenic growth of haematopoietic cells in leukaemic patients during active disease and during remission – a preliminary report. *J Pediatr Endocrinol* 1993; 6: 79–83.

118 Tedeschi B, Spadoni GL, Sanna ML *et al.* Increased chromosome fragility in lymphocytes of short normal children treated with recombinant human growth hormone. *Hum Genet* 1993; 91: 459–63.

119 Fradkin JE, Mills JL, Schonberger LB *et al.* Risk of leukaemia after treatment with pituitary growth hormone. *J Am Med Assoc* 1993; 270: 2829–32.

120 Swerdlow AJ, Reddinguis RE, Higgins CD *et al.* Growth hormone treatment of children with brain tumours and risk of tumour recurrence. *J Clin Endocrinol Metab* 2000; 85: 4444–9.

121 Redman GP, Shu S, Norris D. Leukaemia and growth hormone. *Lancet* 1988; i: 1335.

122 Kiess W, Doerr H, Butenandt O, Belohradsky BH. Lymphocyte subsets and natural-killer activity in growth hormone deficiency. *N Engl J Med* 1986; 314: 321.

123 Torosian MH, Donoway RB. Growth hormone inhibits tumor metastasis. *Cancer* 1991; 67: 2280–3.

# 20 The thyroid gland

**Rosalind S. Brown**

## Introduction

Thyroid dysfunction in infancy and childhood results in the metabolic abnormalities found in the adult and also affects growth and development. Because these thyroid hormone-dependent effects on tissue maturation are developmentally regulated and organ or tissue specific, the clinical consequences of thyroid dysfunction depend on the age of the infant or child.

Untreated hypothyroidism in the fetus or newborn infant results in permanent abnormalities in intellectual and/or neurological function, reflecting the crucial role of thyroid hormone on brain development. After the age of 3 years, when most thyroid hormone-dependent brain development is complete, hypothyroidism results in slow growth and delayed skeletal maturation, but there is usually no permanent influence on cognitive or neurological development.

## Thyroid hormonogenesis

The thyroid is composed of follicles that secrete thyroid hormone. They are composed of two types of cells that surround a central core of colloid. Thyroid hormone-secreting follicular cells, the major cellular constituent of the follicle, are interspersed with calcitonin-secreting parafollicular C cells, which are of neurogenic origin. A basal membrane surrounds the follicle and separates it from surrounding blood and lymph vessels as well as nerve terminals. The major constituent of the colloid is thyroglobulin (Tg), a very large iodinated, dimeric glycoprotein that functions as a thyroid hormone precursor and permits storage of iodine and of iodinated tyrosyl residues covalently bound within its protein structure.

The synthesis and secretion of thyroid hormone includes a complex series of events, each proceeding simultaneously in the same cell (Fig. 20.1) [1]. Dietary iodine ($I_2$) is converted to iodide in the gut and concentrated 20–40 times in the thyroid by an active transport mechanism involving the $Na^+/I^-$ symporter (NIS), located within the basal plasma membrane. At the same time, Tg, synthesized within the follicular cell, undergoes a number of post-translational steps to attain the proper tertiary and quaternary structure. These steps include glycosylation and folding, the latter with the aid of chaperone molecules. Tg is transported by exocytosis into the follicular lumen (colloid). Here, at the colloid apical cell membrane interface, Tg forms the backbone for a series of reactions that results in the oxidation of $I_2$ to an active intermediate and the iodination of tyrosyl residues ('organification') to form monoiodotyrosine (MIT) and di-iodotyrosine (DIT). Iodide oxidation and organification are both catalysed by thyroid peroxidase (TPO), a key membrane-bound, glycosylated haemoprotein enzyme. TPO also catalyses the coupling of iodotyrosines within the Tg molecule to form the thyroid hormones, triiodothyronine ($T_3$) and tetraiodothyronine or thyroxine ($T_4$). $T_3$ is formed by the coupling of one DIT and one MIT molecule; the coupling of two molecules of DIT results in $T_4$. Iodination also requires the generation of hydrogen peroxide.

Thyroid hormones stored in the colloid are released into the circulation by a series of steps that result initially in their incorporation into the apical surface of the follicular cell by a process known as endocytosis. The ingested colloid droplets fuse with apically streaming proteolytic enzyme-containing lysosomes to form phagolysosomes, wherein Tg hydrolysis occurs. The free MIT, DIT, $T_3$ and $T_4$ within the phagolysosomes are then released into the follicular cells. $T_3$ and $T_4$ released in this way diffuse from the thyroid follicular cell into the thyroid capillary blood. The released MIT and DIT are largely deiodinated by a deiodinase, the iodide re-entering the intracellular iodide pool to be reused for new hormone synthesis. Deiodination of $T_4$ to generate $T_3$ is a second source of $T_3$ within the thyroid.

Cloning of the genes for Tg, TPO and NIS in recent years has permitted a greater understanding of the events involved in thyroid hormonogenesis and their regulation at both a molecular and cell biological level. In addition, cloning of the

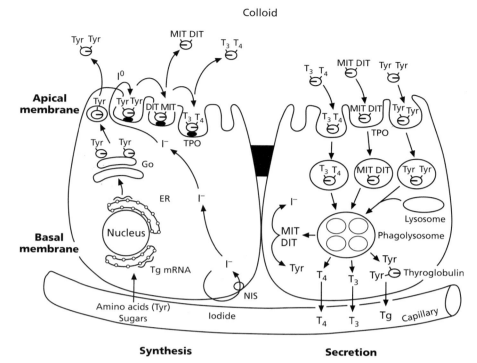

**Fig. 20.1.** Synthesis (left) and secretion (right) of thyroid hormones in thyroid follicular cells. Thyroglobulin (Tg) with its tyrosine (Tyr) residues is synthesized and transported to the apical membrane where it interacts with reactive iodine species to form iodotyrosines which couple to form triiodothyronine ($T_3$) and thyroxine ($T_4$). These products are stored in extracellular colloid. Secretion involves invagination and formation of intracellular colloid droplets that fuse with enzyme-laden lysosomes to form phagolysosomes in which Tg is hydrolysed to release iodotyrosines $T_3$ and $T_4$. The iodotyrosines are deiodinated and the iodide reused; $T_3$ and $T_4$ are released into the circulation. NIS, $Na^+/I^-$ symporter; Tyr, tyrosine; ⊖, Tg backbone; TPO, thyroid peroxidase; $I^-$, iodide; $I°$, iodide species; MIT, monoiodotyrosine; DIT, di-iodotyrosine; ER, endoplasmic reticulum; Go, Golgi apparatus. (Modified from Delange and Fisher [1]; see text for details.)

genes has elucidated the molecular basis of many of the inborn errors of thyroid hormonogenesis. Tg, TPO and NIS also serve as targets of immune attack in patients with autoimmune thyroid disease. In view of the location of TPO and Tg in the interior of the cell, these proteins are unlikely to be the primary trigger of immune attack but are accessible to the immune system after the cell has been injured.

## Regulation of thyroid function

### Thyrotrophin

The major regulator of thyroid function is thyrotrophin (thyroid-stimulating hormone, TSH), a glycoprotein hormone secreted by the pituitary gland. Like other pituitary glycoprotein hormones with which TSH shares structural homology, the TSH molecule is composed of the common α-subunit and a TSH-specific β-subunit. TSH stimulates both thyroid gland function and growth by binding to a specific receptor located on the basal plasma membrane [2]. The TSH receptor, which is a member of the subgroup 2, G-protein-coupled receptor superfamily, is composed of a large, extracellular domain, seven hydrophobic transmembrane-spanning regions and a short intracytoplasmic tail (Fig. 20.2). The N-terminal extracellular domain appears to be sufficient for binding the hormone; the cytoplasmic loops and C-terminal tail are important for signal transduction.

Through effects mediated primarily by the cyclic adeno-

sine monophosphate (cAMP) signal transduction pathway, TSH exhibits transcriptional control of the genes for Tg, TPO and NIS and stimulates an array of cellular events, including iodine uptake and organification, as well as thyroid hormone synthesis and secretion. TSH also stimulates follicular cell proliferation and growth. Although the effects of TSH are mediated primarily through the adenyl cyclase–protein kinase A signal transduction pathway, TSH at higher concentrations also stimulates the phosphoinositol–protein kinase C pathway.

In view of the pivotal importance of the TSH receptor in regulating thyroid function, it is not surprising that both germline and somatic mutations can lead to abnormalities of thyroid growth and function in patients (Fig. 20.2) [3]. In addition, unlike Tg and TPO, the TSH receptor is accessible to immune attack, as it is located not in the interior of the cell but at the basal plasma membrane adjacent to both the blood and lymphatic vessels. Thus, both stimulatory and blocking TSH receptor antibodies (Abs) may occur in patients and result in stimulation and/or inhibition of TSH-induced thyroid cell growth and function.

The secretion of TSH by the pituitary gland is under positive-feedback control by hypothalamic TSH-releasing hormone (TRH), a small tripeptide synthesized in the hypothalamus and transported to the pituitary by the portal vascular system. TSH secretion is under negative-feedback control by thyroid hormone, the latter acting at both the level of the hypothalamus and the pituitary gland. Dopamine, somatostatin and high doses of corticosteroids also inhibit

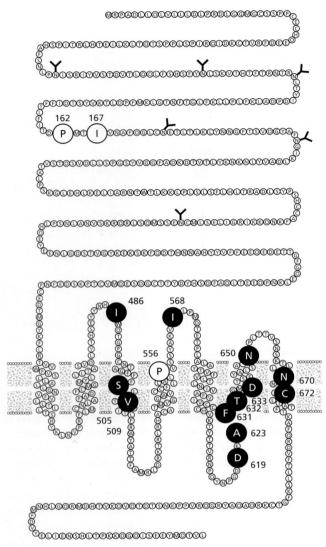

**Fig. 20.2.** Schematic representation of the human TSH receptor and the site of some disease-causing mutations. Like other members of the subgroup 2, G-protein-coupled receptor superfamily, the TSH receptor is composed of a large, extracellular domain, seven hydrophobic transmembrane-spanning regions and a short intracytoplasmic tail. The white symbols refer to loss-of-function mutations and the black symbols refer to gain-of-function mutations. Note the transmembrane location of the loss-of-function Pro556Leu mutation in the hyt/hyt mouse. (From Van Sande *et al.* [3], with permission.)

pituitary release of TSH. Decreasing environmental and/or body temperature increases TRH release.

## Iodide

Adequacy of dietary iodine is a critical regulator of thyroid gland function through adaptive mechanisms that respond to both its deficiency and its excess [1,4,5]. This is understandable because the major thyroid hormones $T_4$ and $T_3$ are 65% and 59% iodine by weight. The recommended daily consumption of iodine is 150 μg for adults, 90 μg for infants and children, 40 μg for premature infants and 200 μg for pregnant women [6].

In iodine deficiency, there is increased trapping of iodide as a result of TSH-independent and -dependent mechanisms. In addition, increased TSH secretion results in a stimulation of thyrocyte proliferation and hormonogenesis. However, because of the reduced iodine content, there is preferential synthesis and secretion of the less iodinated compounds (MIT and $T_3$) compared with DIT and $T_4$. Iodine deficiency also results in increased peripheral conversion of $T_4$ to $T_3$. The reverse is true in the presence of iodine excess.

Excess iodine inhibits a number of different steps in thyroid hormonogenesis, including organification of iodide and subsequent hormone synthesis (the Wolff–Chaikoff effect), Tg synthesis, hormone release and thyroid growth. Fortunately, under normal circumstances, the iodide-induced inhibition is transient and normal hormone synthesis resumes (adaptation to or escape from the Wolff–Chaikoff effect). The escape from the Wolff–Chaikoff effect appears to be due, at least in part, to a decrease in NIS mRNA and protein expression [5], with a resultant decreased iodide transport into the thyroid. This adaptation lowers the intrathyroidal iodine content below a critical inhibitory threshold, allowing organification of iodide to resume.

## Other

A wide variety of other extracellular stimulatory signals also have been shown to bind to thyroid membranes and affect thyroid function and/or growth *in vitro*, but their importance *in vivo* is not yet known [1]. These include adrenergic agents, growth factors and purinergic agents. It is of particular interest that thyroid cells contain thyroid hormone receptors, so that thyroid hormone itself could function as a regulator of thyroid function by a short loop-feedback mechanism. In addition, in patients with or without underlying autoimmune thyroid disease, cytokines, whether produced by infiltrating lymphocytes or by the thyroid follicular cells themselves, can directly modulate both thyroid function and growth.

## Thyroid hormone transport

$T_4$ and $T_3$ in the circulation are transported to their target cells in non-covalent linkage with carrier proteins [7]. These binding proteins produced in the liver include thyroxine-binding globulin (TBG), transthyretin and the secondary carrier protein albumin. TBG, although the least abundant, is the most important carrier protein for $T_4$; transthyretin is less important. Transthyretin does not bind $T_3$, and TBG is the major carrier protein, and albumin is a secondary carrier. In the euthyroid steady state, almost all circulating thyroid hormone

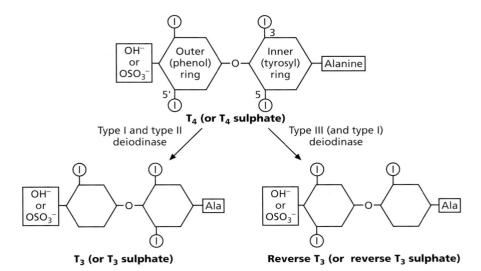

**Fig. 20.3.** Structure of the major thyroid hormones and the site of action of the monoiodothyronine deiodinase enzymes. The type I and type II deiodinases deiodinate the outer (phenol) ring, whereas the type III (and type I) deiodinases deiodinate the inner (tyrosyl) ring.

is bound to protein. This is especially true for $T_4$, 99.97% of which is bound, compared with 99.7% of $T_3$. Transport proteins function as an extrathyroidal storage pool of thyroid hormone that enable the release of free hormone on demand while at the same time protecting tissues from excessive hormone. However, they are not essential for normal thyroid function. Thus, the importance of thyroid hormone-binding proteins clinically lies in an appreciation of how abnormalities, whether secondary to genetic defects, drugs or illness may affect the assessment of thyroid function.

## Thyroid hormone metabolism

Thyroid hormone synthesized and secreted by the thyroid gland is both activated and inactivated by a series of monodeiodination steps in target tissues. Sulphation is an additional method of thyroid hormone metabolism of particular importance in the fetus [8,9]. In contrast to $T_4$, the sole source of which is the thyroid gland, only 20% of $T_3$ is derived by coupling of tyrosyl residues within the thyroid gland itself. The remainder is derived from conversion of $T_4$ to $T_3$ in peripheral tissues, primarily the liver, kidney, brain and pituitary gland.

$T_4$ and $T_3$ are thyronine molecules which consist of an inner (tyrosyl or $\alpha$) ring and outer (phenolic or $\beta$) ring (Fig. 20.3). Monodeiodination of the outer ring of $T_4$ results in $T_3$, which is three or four times more metabolically active than $T_4$ *in vivo*. Monodeiodination of the inner ring produces reverse $T_3$ ($rT_3$), a metabolically inactive metabolite (Fig. 20.3). Nearly all $rT_3$ (98%) is derived from peripheral conversion and only 2% from the thyroid gland. Progressive tissue monodeiodination results in a series of di-iodinated, monoiodinated and non-iodinated forms of thyronine, all of which are metabolically inactive.

Three selenoprotein iodothyronine monodeiodinase enzymes have been described [8,9]. Types I and II deiodinate the outer ring; there is one inner ring deiodinase (type III) (Fig. 20.3). Type I deiodinase is also capable of inner-ring monodeiodination, particularly of sulphated iodothyronines. These deiodinases are developmentally regulated and differ in both their tissue distribution and properties. The activity of the different deiodinases varies significantly between tissues. In the cerebral cortex, for example, > 50% of the intracellular $T_3$ is derived from the intracellular conversion of $T_4$ to $T_3$. In contrast, in liver, only 25% of the intracellular $T_3$ is generated from $T_4$, the remainder being derived from plasma. As a consequence of these variations in deiodinase activity, the relative amounts of $T_4$ and $T_3$ in the serum do not necessarily correspond to their intracellular proportions.

Type I deiodinase, responsible for most of the circulating $T_3$, is expressed predominantly in liver and kidney. In contrast, the highest concentration of type II deiodinase is in brain, pituitary, placenta and brown adipose tissue, whereas type III deiodinase is present predominantly in fetal tissues (liver, kidney) and placenta. Adaptive mechanisms in the activity of these deiodinases at a cellular level result in the preferential shunting of thyroid hormone to areas of need. For example, increased conversion of $T_4$ to $T_3$ by the fetal brain in the presence of hypothyroidism is a critical protective mechanism that accounts, in part, for the normal or near-normal cognitive outcome of babies with congenital hypothyroidism as long as postnatal therapy is early and adequate.

## Thyroid hormone action

Thyroid hormone has multiple effects in cells, including stimulation of thermogenesis, water and ion transport, acceleration of substrate turnover, and amino acid and lipid

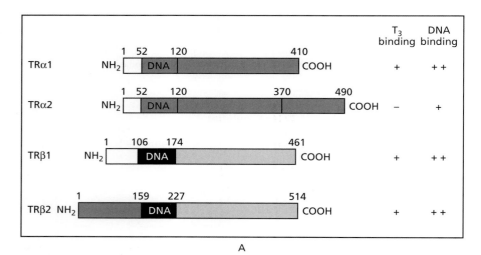

**Fig. 20.4.** The deduced amino acid structure and functional domains of the known thyroid hormone receptor (TR) subtypes (α and β) and isoforms (1 and 2). Note that, unlike the other TRs, Trα2 does not bind thyroid hormone. (From Brent [10] with permission.)

metabolism. Thyroid hormone also potentiates the action of catecholamines, an effect that is responsible for many of the clinical manifestations seen in patients with thyroid over-activity. Unique to infants and children is the stimulation of growth and development of various tissues, including the brain and skeleton.

Thyroid hormone initiates its action by binding to specific receptors located in the cell nucleus [10]. The binding of $T_3$ to the thyroid hormone receptor (TR) is 10 times higher than $T_4$. At least four TRs are known to exist, TRα1, TRα2, TRβ1 and TRβ2. The gene encoding the TRα subtype is located on chromosome 17, and the gene encoding the TRβ subtype is on chromosome 3; the respective isoforms (1 and 2) result from alternative splicing of the initial mRNA transcripts.

The TRs are composed of a carboxy-terminal portion, which is important for ligand binding and interactions between receptors, a DNA-binding domain with two loop structures known as 'zinc fingers' and an amino-terminal domain with no known function (Fig. 20.4); TRα2, unlike the other TRs, has a functional DNA-binding domain but does not bind $T_3$. TRs exist as monomers, homodimers or hetero-dimers with other nuclear proteins, such as the retinoid X receptors. The heterodimeric structure is the active form of the receptor. Forms of TR that bind DNA but do not bind hormone (such as Trα2 and certain TRβ mutants found in patients) may inhibit the binding of the other TRs to DNA ('dominant negative inhibition'). TRα1, TRβ1 and TRβ2 act to stimulate or suppress responsive genes. This activity requires the interaction of numerous co-activators and co-repressors. In the unliganded state TRs repress gene function.

Like the iodothyronine deiodinases, the various TRs are expressed differentially in tissues and are developmentally regulated. The highest concentration of TRβ1 mRNA is found in brain, liver, kidney and heart, whereas TRβ2 mRNA expression is restricted to pituitary and brain tissues. TRα1 and TRα2, on the other hand, are widely distributed among tissues.

## Ontogenesis of thyroid function and regulation in humans

The ontogeny of mature thyroid function is complex and involves an interaction between the thyroid gland and hypothalamo-pituitary development, as well as the matura-tion of mechanisms for thyroid hormone metabolism, thyroid hormone transport proteins and thyroid hormone action. In addition, the placenta plays a pivotal role not only by regulating the transport of essential factors such as iodine and hormones but by synthesizing and metabolizing hor-mones as well.

## Thyroid gland development

The thyroid gland is derived from the fusion of a medial outpouching from the floor of the primitive pharynx, the pre-cursor of the $T_4$-producing follicular cells, and bilateral evagi-nations of the fourth pharyngeal pouch, which give rise to the parafollicular or calcitonin (C)-secreting cells. Commitment towards a thyroid-specific phenotype as well as the growth and descent of the thyroid anlage into the neck results from the coordinate action of a number of novel, recently cloned transcription factors. These include the thyroid transcription factor (TTF)-1, TTF-2, and Pax8 [11,12]. TTF-1 is important for the development of both follicular cells and C cells, whereas Pax8 is involved only in thyroid follicular cell development. In addition, other homeodomain-containing or *Hox* genes (*Hoxa-3*, and the paralogous gene *Hoxb-3*) appear to regulate the expression of Pax8 and TTF-1 respectively [13]. It is of interest that each of these transcription factors also is expressed in a limited number of other cell types, suggesting that it is the specific combination of transcription factors, and possibly non-DNA-binding cofactors acting coordinately, that determine the specific phenotype of a cell.

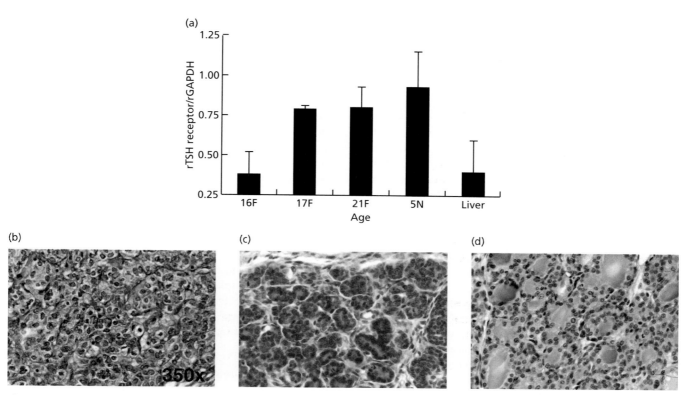

**Fig. 20.5.** Developmental regulation of thyrotrophin (TSH) receptor gene expression and its relation to thyroid morphology in the rat fetus (a). Before fetal day 17, the thyroid gland is difficult to recognize. On fetal day 17 (b), clusters of epithelial cells containing numerous mitoses and separated by a scanty stromal network are seen, coincident with up-regulation of TSH receptor gene expression. On fetal day 18 (c), clear evidence of follicular development is observed, which increases further on postnatal day 10 (d) (haematoxylin–eosin stain; 350× magnification). (Modified from Brown *et al.* [16] with permission.)

TTF-1, TTF-2 and Pax8 also regulate thyroid-specific gene expression [14]. Both TTF-1 and Pax8 stimulate expression of Tg and TPO mRNA; TTF-1 also regulates TSH receptor gene expression. In contrast, TTF-2, transiently expressed in the course of fetal thyroid gland development, has been postulated to repress thyroid-specific gene expression. Thus, TTF-2-null mutant mice develop one of two phenotypes. The thyroid gland either fails to develop or a sublingual thyroid gland is formed [15]. As predicted, the sublingual gland demonstrates evidence of thyroid differentiation, at least as indicated by Tg expression.

In the rat, at fetal day 15, despite early evidence of Tg, TPO and TSH receptor gene expression, the thyroid gland is difficult to distinguish from the surrounding structures and neither iodine organification, thyroid hormonogenesis nor evidence of a follicular structure is present. This suggests that TTF-1 and Pax8 are necessary but not sufficient for the expression of the fully differentiated thyroid phenotype. On fetal day 17, TSH receptor gene expression is significantly up-regulated, and this is accompanied by significant growth and by rapid development of both structural and functional characteristics (Fig. 20.5) [16].

At this time, expression of Tg and TPO mRNA is increased, thyroid follicles first appear on morphological examination,

TPO function can be demonstrated and there is evidence of thyroid hormonogenesis. These findings suggest that the TSH receptor plays an important role only at this later stage of development but is not involved earlier in gestation. In support of this hypothesis, hyt/hyt mice, which have a loss of function (Pro556-Leu) mutation in the transmembrane domain of the TSH receptor, have hypoplastic but normally located thyroid glands with a poorly developed follicular structure and severe hypothyroidism [17]. Similar findings are detected in babies born to mothers with potent TSH receptor-blocking Abs [18], as well as in babies with severe loss-of-function mutations of the TSH receptor [19].

Embryogenesis in man is largely complete by 10–12 weeks' gestation, equivalent to fetal day 15–17 in the rat [8,9]. At this stage, tiny follicle precursors are first seen, Tg can be detected in follicular spaces and evidence of iodine uptake and organification is first obtained. Low concentrations of $T_4$ and $T_3$ are detectable in fetal serum at 10–12 weeks (Fig. 20.5), although it is possible that a fraction of the thyroid hormone measurable at this early stage of the development is maternal in origin (Fig. 20.5).

Tg, first identified in the follicular spaces by 10–11 weeks, can be identified in the human fetal circulation at gestational age 27–28 weeks, but it is not known when Tg can first be detected in serum [8,9]. The secretion of a poorly iodinated thyroid hormone precursor and impaired clearance of this glycoprotein from the circulation by the immature liver results in a higher serum concentration of Tg in the premature fetus than at term.

Despite the fact that iodide uptake by the thyroid can be demonstrated at 10–11 weeks' gestation, the capacity of the fetal thyroid to reduce iodide trapping in response to excess iodide (the Wolff–Chaikoff effect) does not appear until 36–40 weeks' gestation (Fig. 20.5) [8,9]. Thus, premature infants are much more likely to develop hypothyroidism when exposed to excess iodine than are full-term babies.

## Maturation of the hypothalamo-pituitary-thyroid axis

TSH, first identified in the pituitary gland by 10–12 weeks, is detectable in fetal serum at levels of 3–4 mIU/L at gestational age 12 weeks and increases moderately over the last two trimesters to levels of 6–8 mU/L. This is accompanied by a parallel increase in fetal thyroid radioiodine uptake, and by a progressive increase in the serum concentrations of both total $T_4$ and free $T_4$ (Fig. 20.6) [8,9]. The serum concentration of TBG also increases during gestation as a consequence of placental oestrogen effects on the fetal liver. However, there is a progressive increase in the ratio of free $T_4$ to TSH concentration during the second half of gestation, suggesting changes in both the sensitivity of the pituitary thyrotroph to the negative-feedback effect of thyroid hormones and the thyroid follicular cell sensitivity to TSH.

Additional support for hypothalamo-pituitary maturation beginning early in the third trimester derives from the demonstration of an elevated serum TSH concentration in response to hypothyroxinaemia and a suppressed TSH in fetuses with hyperthyroidism due to maternal Graves disease at this stage of fetal development. A fetal TSH response to exogenously administered TRH has been demonstrated as early as 25 weeks' gestation. The fetal serum $T_3$ concentration remains low during gestation, a consequence of immaturity of the type I deiodinase.

Serum levels of TRH are higher in the fetal circulation than in maternal blood, the result both of extrahypothalamic TRH production (placenta and pancreas) and the decreased TRH-degrading activity in fetal serum [8]. The physiological significance of these increased levels of TRH in the fetal circulation is not known.

## Maturation of thyroid hormone metabolism

Activity of the type I deiodinase, a seleno-enzyme, is low throughout gestation. As a result, circulating $T_3$ concentrations in the fetus are low in the order of 50–60 ng/dL (~ 1 nmol/L) at birth. The concentrations of the specific substrates metabolized by this deiodinase, $rT_3$ and the sulphate conjugates of $T_4$, are markedly elevated in the fetal circulation and, to a considerable extent, in amniotic fluid [8,9]. The physiological rationale for the maintenance of reduced circulating $T_3$ concentrations throughout fetal life is unknown, but it has been suggested that its function may be to avoid tissue thermogenesis and potentiate the anabolic state of the rapidly growing fetus [8].

In contrast to type I deiodinase, types II and III deiodinases, highly expressed in brain and pituitary, are detectable by midgestation. As a consequence, fetal brain $T_3$ levels are 60–80% those of the adult by fetal age 20–26 weeks, despite the low levels of circulating $T_3$ [20]. In the presence of fetal hypothyroidism, type II deiodinase activity increases while type III (and type I) deiodinase decreases. These coordinated adjustments are of critical importance in preserving near-normal brain $T_3$ levels, providing that maternal $T_4$ levels are maintained at normal concentrations (see below).

## Maturation of thyroid hormone action

The ontogenesis of thyroid hormone-mediated responsiveness, like thyroid hormone metabolism, is tissue specific and developmentally regulated. For example, whereas thyroid

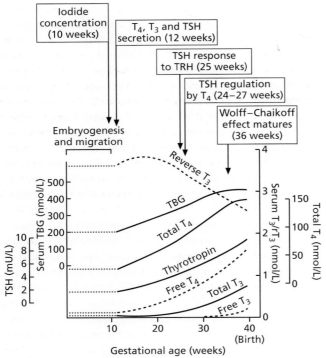

**Fig. 20.6.** Maturation of thyroid gland development and function during gestation. (From Brown and Larsen [9] with permission.)

hormone-mediated effects in the pituitary, brain and cartilage can be detected prenatally, thyroid hormone-dependent action in brown adipose tissue, liver, heart, skin, muscle and bone is apparent only postnatally. To what extent these differences are due to tissue-specific differences in the maturation of thyroid hormone transcriptional activity and action, as opposed to metabolism, is not known.

Tissue specificity of thyroid hormone action derives from multiple factors, including the predominant TR isoform expressed, the cofactor(s) involved and the type of receptor with which the TR partners. As a result, different genes are stimulated or inhibited in different tissues. For example, in brown adipose tissue, thyroid hormone action involves, in part, the stimulation of transcription of thermogenin, a unique protein that uncouples nucleotide phosphorylation and the storage of energy as ATP. This thyroid hormone-dependent action is particularly important in the perinatal period for the development of non-shivering thermogenesis.

In the brain, the action of thyroid hormone and its developmental regulation is more complex and less well understood [21]. At a functional level, thyroid hormone influences a diverse array of processes that lead to the establishment of neural circuits during a critical window of brain development. These processes include neurogenesis and neural cell migration (occurring predominantly between 5 weeks and 24 weeks), neuronal differentiation, dendritic and axonal growth, synaptogenesis, gliogenesis (late fetal to 6 months postpartum), myelination (second trimester to 24 months postpartum) and neurotransmitter enzyme synthesis. The absence of thyroid hormone appears to delay rather than eliminate the timing of critical morphological events or gene products, resulting in a disorganization of intercellular communication. However, the mechanism or mechanisms by which thyroid hormone mediates these effects remains unclear.

Consistent with a nuclear receptor-mediated mode of action, TRs are found in highest concentration in developing neurones and in multiple areas of the fetal brain, including the cerebrum, cerebellum, auditory and visual cortex. Thyroid hormone also stimulates a number of developmentally regulated genes, including neurogranin (a protein kinase substrate thought to be involved in long-term potentiation mechanisms), specific myelin genes and genes found in cerebellar Purkinje cells [21]. However, while these genes respond to $T_3$, it remains uncertain whether they represent a direct or indirect target of thyroid hormone action. There is evidence that the regulation of $T_3$ responsiveness might involve the altered timing of transcription suppressor factors as well as the appearance of enhancers.

Multiple lines of evidence suggest that it is the TRβ1 isoform that is the critical inducer of $T_3$-induced effects during central nervous system (CNS) development [9]. For example, the concentration of TRβ1 in the rat brain increases 40-fold between the time of birth and postnatal day 10 coincident

with the rise in serum $T_3$, and a high degree of saturation of TRs with $T_3$ has been demonstrated. In cerebellar Purkinje cells, where these changes in the β1 isoform have been especially well demonstrated, this increase in TRβ1 expression correlates well with specific effects of $T_3$-directed transcription of certain Purkinje cell genes. As the α1 and β2 mRNA isoforms are present before the increase in the β1 mRNA, it has been speculated that in the CNS $T_3$-induced induction of β1 TR may occur by its interaction with the α1 receptor.

Surprisingly, despite the multiple lines of evidence implicating TRβ in the mediation of $T_3$-induced effects during CNS development, apart from deafness, TRβ1 knockout mice do not exhibit any abnormalities in behavioural or brain neuroanatomical parameters nor in thyroid hormone-specific gene expression [22]. It is possible that the failure to demonstrate abnormalities in CNS development is due to redundancy in the system such that Trα1 (or even the retinoic acid receptor) compensates for the inactivated gene. Alternatively, more detailed studies might be required to demonstrate the CNS abnormality.

Another possibility is that the action of $T_4$ on the developing CNS involves, in part, a non-nuclear mechanism. For example, $T_4$-regulated actin polymerization appears to play an integral role in regulation of deiodinase activity through a non-nuclear mode of action; it has been proposed that the effect of $T_4$ on the actin cytoskeleton might be important in cellular migration, neurite outgrowth and dendritic spine formation [23]. It is of interest that the deafness found in the TRβ1 knockout mouse is a frequent finding in patients with severe endemic cretinism and in some patients with thyroid hormone resistance due to a deletion in the TRβ1 gene.

## The role of the placenta

The placenta plays an important role in fetal thyroid development and function by regulating the passage of certain maternal hormones, substrates and drugs and by serving as an important site of thyroid hormone metabolism [24]. Although the placenta also synthesizes some hormones that can affect the fetal thyroid (e.g. human chorionic gonadotrophin, TRH), these appear to have little influence on the fetus.

The important role of the placenta in regulating the passage of certain hormones and drugs is best demonstrated with the example of thyroid hormone. Under normal circumstances, the placenta has only limited permeability to thyroid hormone and the fetal hypothalamic-pituitary-thyroid system develops relatively independent of maternal influence. However, when the fetus is hypothyroid, there is an increased net flux of maternal thyroid hormone to the fetal compartment [25]. Thus, infants with the complete inability to synthesize $T_4$ because of an inherited absence of the TPO enzyme nonetheless have cord $T_4$ concentrations between 25% and 50% of normal [26]. Similar results are obtained in retrospective studies of cord serum in infants with sporadic congenital athyreosis.

This transplacental passage of maternal $T_4$ (coupled with the coordinate adjustments in brain deiodinase activity discussed above) plays a critical role in minimizing the adverse effects of fetal hypothyroidism. Not only may it help to explain the normal or near-normal cognitive outcome of hypothyroid fetuses as long as postnatal treatment is early and adequate, it may also provide a partial explanation for the relatively normal clinical appearance at birth of over 90% of infants with congenital hypothyroidism. By contrast, when both maternal and fetal hypothyroidism occur, whether this is due to severe iodine deficiency, potent TSH receptor blocking Abs, or maternal–fetal Pit1 deficiency, there is a significant impairment in neurointellectual development despite the initiation of early and adequate postnatal thyroid replacement [27–29]. Maternal hypothyroidism alone may be sufficient to result in mild cognitive and/or motor delay in the fetus [30–32], but this has not been a universal finding [33] and the long-term significance of the deficits found is not known.

The relative impermeability of the human placenta to thyroid hormone is due primarily to the presence of type III and, less so, to type II deiodinase, which serve to inactivate most of the thyroid hormone presented from the maternal or fetal circulation. The iodide released in this way can then be used for fetal thyroid hormone synthesis.

In contrast to thyroid hormone, the placenta is freely permeable to TRH and to iodide, the latter being essential for fetal thyroid hormone synthesis. The placenta is also permeable to certain drugs and to immunoglobulins of the IgG class. Thus, the administration to the mother of excess iodide, drugs (especially propylthiouracil or methimazole), the transplacental passage of TSH receptor Abs from mothers with severe Graves disease or primary myxoedema may have significant effects on fetal and neonatal thyroid function.

Maternal TSH does not cross the placenta. Similarly, Tg is undetectable in the serum of athyreotic infants, indicating the absence of any transplacental passage of this large protein.

## Thyroid function in the full-term and premature neonate, in the infant and during childhood

### The neonate

Marked changes occur in thyroid physiology at the time of birth in the full-term newborn (Fig. 20.7) [8,9]. One of the most dramatic is an abrupt rise in serum TSH that occurs within 30 min of delivery, reaching concentrations of 60–70 mU/L. This causes a marked stimulation of the thyroid, resulting in an approximate 50% increase in the serum $T_4$ and an increase of three- to fourfold in the concentration of serum $T_3$ within 24 h (Fig. 20.7). Studies in experimental animals suggest that the increase in TSH is a consequence of the relative hypothermia of the ambient extrauterine environment. The marked increase in $T_3$ is due not only to the increase in TSH but also to an increase in the type I deiodinase activity at

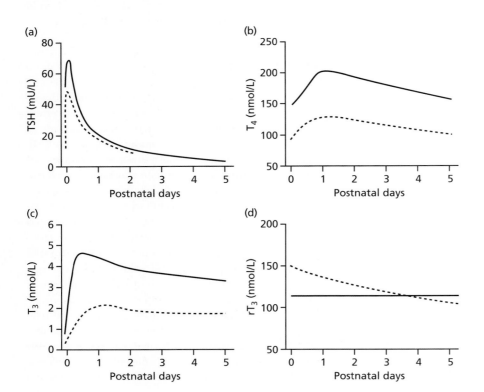

**Fig. 20.7.** Postnatal changes in the serum concentration of TSH (a), $T_4$ (b), $T_3$ (c) and $rT_3$ (d) in term babies (continuous line) compared with premature infants (broken line) in the first week of life. Note that the postnatal surge in TSH is followed by an increase in $T_4$ and $T_3$ concentrations in the first few days of life that subsequently decrease. Changes in premature infants are similar to those in term babies but are much less marked. -----, Premature; ———, term. (From Fisher and Klein [39], as modified by Brown and Larsen [9] with permission.)

the time of delivery. Not surprisingly, the elevated concentrations of the other substrates of type I deiodinase, reverse $T_3$ and $T_3$ sulphate, decrease relatively rapidly during the newborn period (Fig. 20.7). Increased activity of type II deiodinase leads to an increase in $T_3$ in brown adipose tissue at birth, which is required for optimal uncoupling protein synthesis and thermogenesis.

## The premature infant

Thyroid function in the premature infant reflects the relative immaturity of the hypothalamo-pituitary-thyroid axis found in infants of comparable gestational age *in utero*. Thus, in cord blood samples obtained by cordocentesis, there is a progressive increase in the TSH, TBG, $T_4$ and $T_3$ concentration in fetuses with increasing degrees of maturity (Fig. 20.8) [34]. After delivery, there is a surge in $T_4$ and TSH analogous to that observed in term infants, but the magnitude of the increase is less in premature neonates and there is a more dramatic fall in the $T_4$ concentration over the subsequent 1–2 weeks (Fig. 20.9). This decrease in the $T_4$ concentration is particularly significant in very low-birthweight infants (< 1.5 kg, approximately equivalent to < 30 weeks' gestation) in whom

the serum $T_4$ may occasionally be undetectable [35,36]. In most cases, the total $T_4$ is more affected than the free $T_4$, a consequence of abnormal protein binding and/or the decreased TBG in these babies with immature liver function. In addition to the aforementioned changes in $T_4$ and TSH concentrations, the serum $rT_3$ tends to stay higher and serum $T_3$ is reduced for longer in the premature newborn, reflecting the greater immaturity of the type I deiodinase system (Fig. 20.7).

The causes for the decrease in $T_4$ observed postnatally in premature infants are complex [36]. In addition to the clearance of maternal $T_4$ from the neonatal circulation, preterm babies have decreased thyroidal iodide stores. This is a particular problem in borderline iodine-deficient areas of the world. They are frequently sicker than their more mature counterparts, are less able to regulate iodide balance [37] and may be treated by drugs that affect neonatal thyroid function. In addition, as the capacity of the immature thyroid to adapt to exogenous iodide is reduced, there is an increased sensitivity to the thyroid-suppressive effects of excess iodide found in certain skin antiseptics and drugs to which these babies are frequently exposed (see below).

Despite the reduced total $T_4$ observed in some preterm babies, the TSH concentration is not significantly elevated

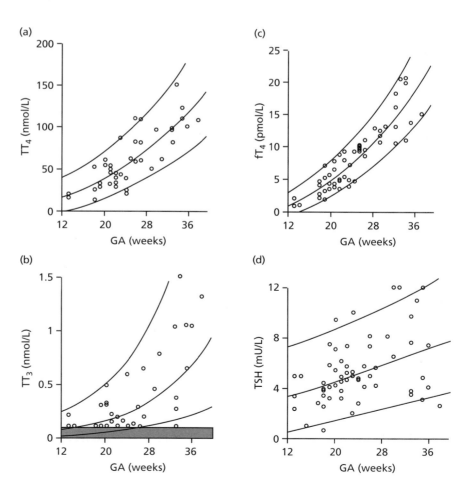

**Fig. 20.8.** Cord blood concentration of total $T_4$ ($TT_4$) (a), total $T_3$ ($TT_3$) (b), free $T_4$ ($fT_4$) (c) and TSH (d) in normal pregnancy. GA, gestationalage. (From Thorpe-Beeston *et al.* [*Thyroid* 2: 207–17] as modified by LaFranchi [36], with permission.)

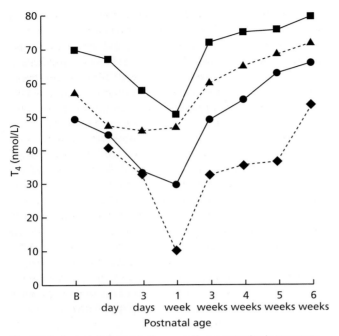

**Fig. 20.9.** Postnatal changes in the serum $T_4$ concentration in premature babies in the first 6 weeks of life. Note that in very premature infants no postnatal increase in the $T_4$ concentration in the first few days of life is observed. Instead, the $T_4$ concentration decreases with a nadir at 1 week of life. Values subsequently normalize by 3–6 weeks. ■, 30–31 weeks; ▲, 28–29 weeks; ●, 26–27 weeks; ◆, 23–25 weeks. (From Mercado *et al.* [35], with permission.)

in most of them. Transient elevations in TSH are seen in some, the finding of a TSH concentration > 40 mU/L being more frequent the greater the degree of prematurity. In one study, for example, the prevalence of a TSH concentration > 40 mU/L in very low-birthweight (< 1.5 kg) premature infants was eightfold higher and in low birthweight (1.5–2.5 kg) neonates twofold higher than the prevalence in term babies [38].

Although an elevated TSH concentration may reflect true primary hypothyroidism, the increase in TSH seen in preterm infants at several weeks of age may reflect the elevated TSH observed in adults recovering from severe illness. Such individuals may develop transient TSH elevations, which are associated with still reduced serum $T_4$ and $T_3$ concentrations. These have been interpreted as reflecting a 'reawakening' of the illness-induced suppression of the hypothalamo-pituitary axis. As the infant recovers from prematurity-associated illnesses, such as respiratory distress syndrome (RDS), a recovery of the illness-induced suppression of the hypothalamo-pituitary-thyroid axis would also occur.

## Infants and children

After the acute perturbations of the neonatal period there is a slow and progressive decrease in the concentrations of $T_4$,

free $T_4$, $T_3$ and TSH during infancy and childhood. The serum concentration of $rT_3$ remains unchanged or increases slightly. The most important aspect of thyroid physiology in the infant and child, however, is the markedly higher $T_4$ turnover in this age group relative to that in the adult. In infants, $T_4$ production rates are estimated to be in the order of 5–6 µg/kg/day, decreasing slowly over the first few years of life to about 2–3 µg/kg/day at ages 3–9 years [39]. This is to be contrasted with the production rate of $T_4$ in the adult, which is about 1.5 µg/kg/day. Serum Tg levels also fall over the first year of life, reaching concentrations typical of adults by about 6 months of age. The size of the thyroid gland increases slowly from approximately 1 g in the newborn by about 1 g per year until age 15, when it has achieved its adult size of about 15–20 g. The thyroid lobe is comparable to the terminal phalanx of the infant or child's thumb.

# Thyroid disease in infancy

## Congenital hypothyroidism

Congenital hypothyroidism (CH) is the commonest treatable cause of mental retardation. Worldwide, the most common cause of CH is iodine deficiency, a problem that continues to affect almost one billion people despite international efforts aimed at its eradication [1,6]. In areas where iodine deficiency is severe, CH is endemic ('endemic cretinism') and is characterized by mental retardation, short stature, deaf-mutism and neurological abnormalities. Both endemic cretinism and iodine deficiency have been the subject of several reviews [6,40,41].

### Screening for congenital hypothyroidism

In iodine-sufficient areas and in areas of borderline iodine deficiency, CH is usually sporadic and occurs in 1 in 3500–4000 infants. In order to achieve optimal neurological outcome, treatment must be initiated soon after birth, before affected infants are recognizable clinically. Neonatal screening programmes have therefore been introduced in most industrialized areas of the world. Elsewhere, such as Eastern Europe, South America, Asia, Oceania and Africa, neonatal screening programmes are under development.

By 1992, some 50 million infants had been screened for CH worldwide with 6000 cases detected annually [42]. Although there continues to be some disagreement whether minor neuro-intellectual sequelae remain in the most severely affected infants, accumulating evidence suggests that a normal outcome is possible as long as treatment is started sufficiently early and is adequate. Certainly, the main objective of screening, the eradication of mental retardation, has been achieved. In addition to the profound clinical benefit, it has been estimated that the cost–benefit ratio of neonatal screening programmes is approximately 10:1, a ratio that does not include the loss of tax income resulting from impaired intellectual capacity in the untreated but non-institutionalized person. Newborn screening also has permitted an elucidation of the prevalence of the various causes of CH, including a series of transient disorders found predominantly in premature infants. Of note is the fact that the incidence of CH has been found to be 4–5 times more common than phenylketonuria, for which screening programmes were developed first.

## Screening strategies for congenital hypothyroidism

Measurement of $T_4$ and/or TSH is performed on an eluate of dried whole blood collected on filter paper on days 1–4 of life. Two screening strategies for the detection of CH have evolved, a primary $T_4$/backup TSH method, favoured in North America, and a primary TSH/backup $T_4$ method, favoured in most parts of Europe and Japan. Whichever method is used, babies whose initial TSH is > 50 mU/L are most likely to have permanent CH, whereas a TSH between 20 and 49 mU/L is frequently a false positive or represents transient hypothyroidism. Transient CH is particularly common in premature infants in borderline iodine-deficient areas.

Each screening strategy has its advantages and disadvantages but the two approaches appear to be equivalent in the detection of babies with permanent forms of CH [44]. A primary $T_4$/backup TSH programme will detect primary, secondary or tertiary hypothyroidism (1 in 50 000 to 1 in 100 000 live births), babies with a low $T_4$ but delayed rise in the TSH concentration (7.5% of infants), TBG deficiency and hyperthyroxinaemia but may miss compensated hypothyroidism. A primary TSH strategy will detect frank and compensated hypothyroidism but will miss secondary or tertiary hypothyroidism, a delayed TSH rise, TBG deficiency and hyperthyroxinaemia. There are fewer false positives with a primary TSH strategy.

Both programmes will miss the rare infant whose $T_4$ level on initial screening is normal but who later develops low $T_4$ and elevated TSH concentrations (< 0.5% of infants, most commonly premature babies with transient hypothyroidism). In both strategies there is the very real possibility of human error failing to identify affected infants. This can occur because of poor communication, lack of receipt of specimens or the failure to test an infant who is transferred between hospitals during the neonatal period. Recently, with the development of more sensitive, non-radioisotopic TSH assays, Canada and some states in the USA have switched to a primary TSH programme.

Newborn screening was performed initially at between 3 and 4 days of life and the normal values derived reflected this postnatal age. The practice of early discharge from the hospital of otherwise healthy full-term infants has resulted in a greater proportion of babies being tested before this time. For example, it has been estimated that in North America 25% or more of newborns are discharged within 24 h of delivery and 40% in the second 24 h of life [43]. Because of the neonatal TSH surge and the dynamic changes in $T_4$ and $T_3$ concentrations that occur within the first few days of life, early discharge increases the number of false-positive results. In California, the ratio of false positive to confirmed CH has increased from 2.5:1 to approximately 5:1. Some programmes have responded by increasing their threshold value for TSH within the first day of life, but this increases the possibility of missing infants with a slowly rising TSH.

Another complicating factor is the increased survival of very premature infants. They greatly increase the cost of screening programmes because blood $T_4$ concentrations are lower and the incidence of transient hypothyroidism in them is much higher than in full-term babies. It has been estimated that very low-birthweight infants constitute only 0.8% of the population but increase the number of $T_4$ assays in a primary TSH programme by 9%. Very low-birthweight infants account for 8% of all TSH assays performed in a primary $T_4$ programme [44].

The paucity of appropriate standards for this high-risk group and inadequate data about whether these values should reflect the maternal contribution as found *in utero* at this age have constituted additional problems. Normal values according to gestational age (and/or birth weight) for cord blood $T_4$, free $T_4$, TSH and TBG [34], screening values for $T_4$ [38] and serum free $T_4$ and TSH in the first week of life [45], the last one using newer, more sensitive assay techniques, have been published.

## Thyroid dysgenesis

The causes of non-endemic CH and their relative frequencies are listed in Table 20.1. The most common cause (80–85% of cases) is thyroid dysgenesis, a sporadic disease. Thyroid dysgenesis may be due to the complete absence of thyroid tissue (agenesis) or it may be partial (hypoplasia); the latter often is accompanied by a failure to descend into the neck (ectopy). Females are affected twice as often as males and there are racial differences. Thyroid dysgenesis is less frequent among African Americans (1 in 32 000) and more common among Hispanics (1 in 2000) in the USA. Although a slightly higher incidence was originally reported in Western Europe (1 in 3300) and a slightly lower figure was reported in Japan (1 in 5700) than in North America (1 in 4500), these differences have decreased as screening protocols have been modified [44].

Genetic and environmental factors have both been implicated in the aetiology of thyroid dysgenesis but the cause is unknown in most cases. The occasional familial occurrence, the reported gender and ethnic differences, as well as the increased incidence in babies with Down syndrome [46], all

**Table 20.1.** Differential diagnosis of permanent congenital hypothyroidism

---

*Thyroid dysgenesis (1 in 4500)*
Aplasia
Hypoplasia with ectopy
Hypoplasia without ectopy

*Inborn errors of thyroid hormonogenesis (1 in 30 000)*
Decreased TSH responsiveness
    TSH receptor gene mutation
    G$_{sa}$ gene mutation
Failure to concentrate iodide
Abnormal organification of iodine
    Abnormal TPO enzyme
    Abnormal H$_2$O$_2$ generation
    Pendred syndrome

Defective Tg synthesis or transport
Abnormal iodotyrosine deiodinase

*Secondary and/or tertiary hypothyroidism (1 in 50 000–100 000)*
Hypothalamic abnormality
    Isolated TRH deficiency
    TRH resistance

    Associated with midline facial/brain dysmorphism
        Septo-optic hypoplasia
        Cleft lip, palate and/or absent corpus callosum ± septum pellucidum

    Pituitary abnormality
    Normal pituitary gland
        Abnormal TSH molecule
        POU1F1 deficiency
        PROP-1 deficiency

    Pituitary hypoplasia or aplasia
        Posterior pituitary ectopic
        Posterior pituitary eutopic
        (POU1F1 or PROP-1 deficiency)

*Thyroid hormone resistance (1 in 100 000)*

---

suggest that genetic factors might play a role in some cases. The transcription factors (TTF-1, TTF-2 and Pax8) would appear to be obvious candidate genes in the aetiology of thyroid dysgenesis in view of their important role in thyroid organogenesis and thyroid-specific gene expression. To date, however, abnormalities in these genes have been found in only a small proportion of affected patients.

A heterozygous deletion of the *TTF-1* gene has been described in a newborn infant with hypothyroidism, a normal-sized thyroid gland on scan, normal magnetic resonance imaging of the brain and respiratory failure [47]. These findings are of particular interest in view of the findings of abnormal thyroid, lung, pituitary and forebrain development in mice with a targeted disruption of the *TTF-1* gene [48]. No germline mutations in the *TTF-1* gene were found in a total of

76 CH patients studied by two different groups of investigators in Italy [49,50].

Abnormalities in Pax8 and TTF-2 appear to be similarly rare and germline mutations of the Pax8 gene were found in only 2 of 145 Italian patients with sporadic thyroid dysgenesis studied in one large series [51]. In one of these, the thyroid gland was hypoplastic and ectopic and in the other the thyroid gland was hypoplastic but located in a normal position in the neck. A missense mutation in the *TTF-2* gene has been reported recently in two siblings with the combination of thyroid agenesis, cleft palate, spiky hair and choanal atresia [52], abnormalities reminiscent of the findings in TTF-2 knockout mice that develop thyroid dysgenesis and cleft palate [15].

The rarity of abnormalities in the *TTF-1*, *TTF-2* and *Pax8* genes in patients with thyroid dysgenesis could be due to several reasons [53]. It is possible that, analogous to some mice with a targeted disruption in this gene, mutation of the *TTF-1* gene is not compatible with life. Alternatively, thyroid dysgenesis could be due to a somatic rather than a germline neomutation of one or other of these genes, which would not be identified by genetic analysis of peripheral lymphocytes. The aetiology of thyroid dysgenesis is probably multigenic (i.e. abnormalities in several genes might be necessary to produce the phenotype) and/or multifactorial (both genetic and environmental factors might be involved).

Maternal autoimmunity has been invoked as a potential cause of permanent CH but its role is controversial. There is no increased prevalence in the maternal circulation of TPO (formerly called microsomal) Abs, often used as a marker of autoimmunity [54]. Although both thyroid growth-blocking immunoglobulins and cytotoxic Abs have been reported in mothers of some babies with thyroid dysgenesis [55,56], evidence is lacking for an aetiological role. The original reports have not been confirmed [57].

### Inborn errors of thyroid hormonogenesis

Inborn errors of thyroid hormonogenesis are responsible for most of the remaining cases (10–15%) of CH. Defects include decreased TSH responsiveness, failure to concentrate iodide, defective organification of iodide due to an abnormality in the TPO enzyme or in the H$_2$O$_2$ generating system, defective Tg synthesis or transport, and abnormal iodotyrosine deiodinase activity (Table 20.1) [58,59].

The association of an organification defect with sensorineural deafness is known as Pendred syndrome. Unlike thyroid dysgenesis, the inborn errors of thyroid hormonogenesis usually have an autosomal recessive inheritance consistent with a single gene mutation. It is not surprising therefore that a molecular basis for many of these abnormalities has been identified, which include mutations in the genes for the TSH receptor, NIS, TPO and Tg. The gene for the iodotyrosine deiodinase enzyme has not been cloned. Pendred syndrome has been shown to be due to a defect in the pendrin gene on chromosome 7q22–31 [60]. Pendrin, a gene with sequence homology to several sulphate transporters, has been found to encode an apical iodide/chloride transporter [61].

All the inborn errors of thyroid hormonogenesis, except decreased TSH responsiveness, are associated with a normally placed ('eutopic') thyroid gland that may be increased in size at birth and this feature forms the basis for the clinical distinction from thyroid dysgenesis. In contrast, most babies with TSH resistance have a normal or hypoplastic eutopic gland that may in some cases mimic an abnormality of thyroid gland development [62,63]; in rare cases, no thyroid gland at all is discernible on thyroid imaging, a picture indistinguishable from thyroid agenesis [64]. Similar to the variability observed in thyroid gland size in this condition, the clinical findings in TSH resistance have varied from compensated to overt hypothyroidism depending on the severity of the functional defect. Some of the patients have a loss-of-function mutation of the TSH receptor, usually involving the extracellular domain [62–64]. Rarely, such a mutation involves the transmembrane domain, analogous to the hyt/hyt mouse (Fig. 20.2) [65]. In a few affected infants, a discrepancy between presumed 'athyreosis' on thyroid scintigraphy and the detection of either a 'normal' serum Tg concentration or glandular tissue on ultrasound examination has been noted, but this has not been a consistent finding.

The relative frequency of TSH receptor gene mutations as a cause of TSH resistance is not known. In one study, inactivating mutations of the TSH receptor gene were found in only 1 of 100 patients with CH, indicating that abnormalities in this gene are not a common cause of thyroid hypoplasia or aplasia [66]. A similar conclusion may be drawn from the failure to demonstrate linkage to the TSH receptor gene in 23 families in a majority of which there were two or more children affected by CH and in whom there was appreciable consanguinity of the parents [67]. Most familial cases of TSH resistance due to a loss of function mutation of the TSH receptor have an autosomal recessive form of inheritance.

TSH resistance may be due to an inactivating mutation of the stimulatory guanine nucleotide-binding protein ($Gs_\alpha$) gene [68]. This syndrome, known as pseudohypoparathyroidism type Ia or Albright's hereditary osteodystrophy, is characterized by a variable resistance to G-protein-coupled receptors, most commonly the parathyroid hormone receptor. Unlike loss-of-function mutations of the TSH receptor, Albright's hereditary osteodystrophy has an autosomal dominant inheritance with variable expression.

### Secondary and/or tertiary hypothyroidism

TSH deficiency due to a pituitary or hypothalamic abnormality accounts for < 5% of cases of CH detected by newborn screening (Table 20.1). TSH deficiency may be isolated or associated with other pituitary hormone deficiencies. Familial cases of both TSH and TRH deficiency have been described [58,59]. TRH resistance due to a mutation in the TRH receptor gene has been described in a child in whom secondary hypothyroidism was missed on newborn screening. In this patient, the diagnosis was suspected because of an absent TSH and prolactin response to TRH despite a normal pituitary gland on imaging [69].

TSH deficiency in association with other pituitary hormone deficiencies may be associated with abnormal midline facial and brain structures, particularly cleft lip and palate, and absent septum pellucidum and/or corpus callosum, and should be suspected in male infants with microphallus and prolonged hypoglycaemia [70]. Septo-optic dysplasia, has been shown to be due to a mutation in the *HESX-1* homeobox gene in some cases [71]. Non-dysmorphic causes of congenital hypopituitarism include pituitary hypoplasia, which is often associated with an ectopic posterior pituitary gland, and molecular defects in the genes for the transcription factors POU1F1 or PROP-1 [72,73]. POU1F1 (formerly called Pit1) is essential for the differentiation of thyrotrophs, lactotrophs and somatotrophs, and PROP-1, a homeodomain protein expressed briefly in the embryonic pituitary, is necessary for POU1F1 expression.

### Thyroid hormone resistance

Thyroid hormone resistance, although usually diagnosed later in life, may be identified in the newborn period by neonatal screening programmes that determine TSH. Affected babies are not usually symptomatic. Most cases result from a mutation in the TRβ gene and follow an autosomal dominant pattern of inheritance [74]. The incidence has been estimated to be 1 in 50 000.

### Transient congenital hypothyroidism

Estimates of the frequency of transient CH vary greatly depending on how this condition is defined (Table 20.2). A frequently quoted estimate is 10% of CH babies identified on newborn screening, or 1 in 40 000 neonates [8]. It is most common in premature infants, the frequency increasing with greater prematurity. Although iodine deficiency, iodine excess and drugs are common causes, in some cases the cause is unknown.

### Iodine deficiency and iodine excess

Transient hypothyroidism due to both iodine deficiency and iodine excess is more common in iodine-deficient areas [42]. In Belgium, for example, transient hypothyroidism was reported in 20% of premature infants, an eightfold higher prevalence than in North America. Administration of potassium iodide was successful in preventing the disorder.

**Table 20.2.** Differential diagnosis of transient congenital hypothyroidism

*Primary hypothyroidism*
  Prenatal or postnatal iodine deficiency or excess
  Maternal antithyroid medication
  Maternal TSH receptor blocking antibodies

*Secondary or tertiary hypothyroidism*
  Prenatal exposure to maternal hyperthyroidism
  Prematurity (particularly < 27 weeks' gestation)
  Drugs
    Steroids
    Dopamine

*Miscellaneous*
  Isolated TSH elevation
  Low $T_4$ with normal TSH
    Prematurity
    Illness
    Undernutrition
  Low-$T_3$ syndrome

Because newborn infants are so susceptible to the adverse effects of iodine deficiency, the serum TSH on newborn screening reflects the prevalence of iodine deficiency in a population [1]. Premature infants are particularly at risk not only because of decreased thyroidal iodine stores accumulated *in utero* but because of immaturity of the capacity for thyroid hormonogenesis, the hypothalamo-pituitary-thyroid axis and the ability to convert $T_4$ to $T_3$ [75]. Premature infants are in negative iodine balance for the first 1 or 2 weeks of postnatal life [37].

In addition to iodine deficiency, both the fetus and newborn infant are sensitive to the thyroid-suppressive effects of excess iodine, whether administered to the mother during pregnancy or directly to the baby [76]. This occurs because the fetus is unable to decrease thyroidal iodine uptake in response to an iodine load before 36 weeks' gestation. Other factors, including increased skin absorption and decreased renal clearance of iodine in premature infants, are also likely to play a role. Reported sources of iodine have included drugs (e.g. potassium iodide, amiodarone), radiocontrast agents (e.g. for intravenous pyelogram, oral cholecystogram, or amniofetography) and antiseptic solutions (e.g. povidone iodine) used for skin cleansing or vaginal douches. In contrast to Europe, iodine-induced transient hypothyroidism has not been documented frequently in North America [77].

### Maternal antithyroid medication

Transient neonatal hypothyroidism may develop in babies whose mothers are being treated with antithyroid medication [either propylthiouracil (PTU), methimazole (MMI), or carbimazole] for Graves disease. The fetus appears particularly sensitive to antithyroid drugs, even when the dose used in the mother is within recommended guidelines [78]. Babies with antithyroid drug-induced hypothyroidism characteristically develop a goitre that may be large enough to cause respiratory embarrassment. Both the hypothyroidism and goitre resolve spontaneously with clearance of the drug from the baby's circulation and replacement therapy is not usually required.

### Maternal thyrotrophin receptor antibodies

Maternal TSH receptor-blocking Abs, a population of Abs closely related to the TSH receptor-stimulating Abs in Graves disease, may be transmitted to the fetus in titres sufficient to cause transient CH. The incidence of this disorder has been estimated to be 1 in 180 000 [78]. TSH receptor-blocking Abs are most often found in mothers previously treated for Graves disease or who have the non-goitrous form of chronic lymphocytic thyroiditis ('primary myxoedema'). Occasionally, these mothers are not aware that they are hypothyroid and the diagnosis is made only after CH has been recognized in their infants. Unlike TSH receptor-stimulating Abs that mimic the action of TSH, TSH receptor-blocking Abs inhibit both the binding and the action of TSH. Because TSH-induced growth is blocked, these babies do not have a goitre. Similarly, inhibition of TSH-induced radioactive iodine uptake may result in a misdiagnosis of thyroid agenesis. The hypothyroidism usually resolves in 3 or 4 months.

Babies with TSH receptor-blocking Ab-induced hypothyroidism are difficult to distinguish at birth from babies with the more common thyroid dysgenesis, but they differ in a number of ways. They do not require lifelong therapy, and there is a high recurrence rate in subsequent offspring because of the tendency of the Abs to persist for many years in the maternal circulation. Unlike babies with thyroid dysgenesis in whom a normal cognitive outcome is found if postnatal therapy is early and adequate, babies with maternal-blocking Ab-induced hypothyroidism may have a permanent intellectual deficit if fetomaternal hypothyroidism was present *in utero* [29].

### Transient secondary and/or tertiary hypothyroidism

Babies born to mothers who were hyperthyroid during pregnancy occasionally develop transient hypothalamo-pituitary suppression. The hypothyroxinaemia is usually self-limited but may last for years and require replacement therapy [79]. In general, the titre of TSH receptor-stimulating Abs in these infants is lower than in those who develop transient neonatal hyperthyroidism. Other causes of transient secondary and tertiary hypothyroidism include prematurity (particularly < 27 weeks' gestation) and drugs used in neonatal intensive care units.

## Other abnormalities of thyroid function discovered on newborn screening

### Isolated hyperthyrotrophinaemia

Isolated hyperthyrotrophinaemia is most common in premature infants. Although some babies have 'compensated' hypothyroidism, the aetiology is not clear in others. In babies whose blood specimen is obtained within the first day or two of life because of early discharge, isolated hyperthyrotrophinaemia may be due to the postnatal cold-induced TSH surge. Maternal heterophile Abs that cross-react in the TSH radioimmunoassay have been implicated. Hyperthyrotrophinaemia of unknown aetiology has been reported in babies in Japan; the TSH normalized without treatment in the first year of life.

### Hypothyroxinaemia

Hypothyroxinaemia in the presence of a 'normal' TSH occurs most commonly in premature infants, in whom it is found in 50% of babies of less than 30 weeks' gestation [42]. Often the free $T_4$ is less affected than the total $T_4$. Because of this, and evidence that the hypothalamo-pituitary-thyroid axis begins to mature at midgestation, this hypothyroxinaemia in premature infants was thought to be normal. The recognition of an association between transient neonatal hypothyroxinaemia and subsequent problems in motor and cognitive development has led to a re-evaluation [36,81]. However, administration of L-$T_4$ to these premature infants with a low serum $T_4$ did not appear to affect subsequent performance.

The reasons for the hypothyroxinaemia of prematurity are complex. In addition to hypothalamo-pituitary immaturity, premature infants frequently have TBG deficiency due to both immature liver function and undernutrition: they may have 'sick euthyroid syndrome'.

Abnormalities in thyroid-binding proteins, particularly TBG and rarely transthyretin, may cause hypothyroxinaemia without associated hyperthyrotrophinaemia. The incidence of TBG deficiency is 1 in 5–12 000.

### Low $T_3$ syndrome

The $T_3$ concentration in premature infants is lower than in full-term infants because of immaturity of type 1 iodothyronine deiodinase. Premature infants are frequently undernourished and suffer from a variety of illnesses that aggravate the ability to convert $T_4$ to $T_3$. Serum $T_3$ values usually normalize within 2 months.

## Clinical manifestations

Clinical evidence of hypothyroidism is usually difficult to appreciate in the newborn period. Many of the classic features (large tongue, hoarse cry, facial puffiness, umbilical hernia, hypotonia, mottling, cold hands and feet and lethargy) are subtle and develop only with the passage of time. Figure 20.10 shows a baby with untreated CH diagnosed clinically compared with an infant in whom the diagnosis was made by newborn screening. Non-specific signs that suggest the diagnosis of CH include unconjugated hyperbilirubinaemia, gestation longer than 42 weeks, feeding difficulties, delayed passage of stools, hypothermia or respiratory distress in an infant weighing over 2.5 kg. A large anterior fontanelle and/or a posterior fontanelle > 0.5 cm is frequently present in affected infants but may not be appreciated.

(a)

(b)

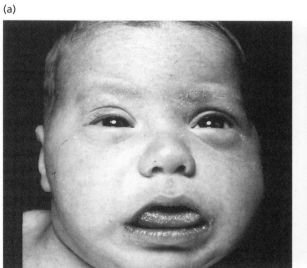
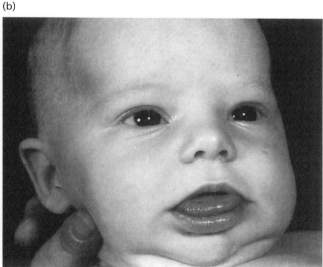

**Fig. 20.10.** Infant with severe, untreated congenital hypothyroidism diagnosed clinically before the advent of newborn screening (a), compared with an infant with congenital hypothyroidism identified through newborn screening (b). Note the striking difference in the severity of the clinical features.

In general, the extent of the clinical findings depends on the cause, severity and duration of the hypothyroidism. Babies in whom severe fetomaternal hypothyroidism was present *in utero* tend to be the most symptomatic at birth. Similarly, babies with athyreosis or a complete block in thyroid hormonogenesis tend to have more signs and symptoms at birth than infants with an ectopic thyroid, the most common cause of CH.

Babies with CH are of normal size at birth. However, if diagnosis is delayed, subsequent linear growth is impaired. The finding of palpable thyroid tissue suggests that the hypothyroidism is due to an abnormality in thyroid hormonogenesis or thyroid hormone action, or suggests that it will be transient.

## Laboratory evaluation

Infants detected by newborn screening should be evaluated without delay, preferably within 24 h. The diagnosis of CH is confirmed by the demonstration of a decreased concentration of $T_4$ and an elevated TSH ($> 20$ mU/L). Infants with permanent abnormalities of thyroid function have a serum TSH concentration $> 50$ mU/L. The serum $T_4$ concentration is much higher in full-term infants in the first 2 months of life (6.5–16.3 µg/dL, 84–210 nmol/L) than in adults for whom reference values are given in most laboratories. Normal values for thyroid function in the neonatal period have been published [82]. Measurement of $T_3$ is of little value in the diagnosis of CH.

A bone age X-ray is often performed to determine the duration and severity of the hypothyroidism *in utero*. A radionuclide scan (either $^{123}$I or [$^{99m}$Tc]pertechnetate) provides information about the location, size and trapping ability of the thyroid gland. Ectopic glands may be located anywhere along the pathway of thyroid descent from the foramen caecum to the anterior mediastinum. Thyroid imaging is helpful in verifying whether a permanent abnormality is present and aids in genetic counselling as thyroid dysgenesis is a sporadic condition whereas abnormalities in thyroid hormonogenesis are autosomal recessive. Scintigraphy with $^{123}$I, if available, is usually preferred because of the greater sensitivity and because $^{123}$I, unlike technetium, is organified. Imaging with $^{123}$I allows quantitative uptake measurements and tests for both iodine transport defects and abnormalities in thyroid oxidation. The lowest possible dose of $^{123}$I should be used. Pertechnetate is cheaper and more widely available. There is some disagreement whether a thyroid scan should be performed in all babies because of the unknown risk of radiation exposure, particularly in centres where $^{131}$I is used in large doses.

If there is no uptake on thyroid imaging, ultrasound should confirm the absence of thyroid tissue. Ultrasonography is also helpful to verify the presence of a eutopic thyroid gland if a transient abnormality is suspected or if a thyroid gland is palpable on clinical examination; the procedure is less sensitive than a radionuclide scan.

Apparent thyroid agenesis can be due to the presence of maternal TSH receptor-blocking Abs that completely inhibit TSH-induced thyroidal uptake of radioisotope, if present in a sufficiently high titre. Autoimmune thyroid disease in the mother or a history of a previously affected sibling should alert the physician to this diagnosis, but such information is not always known. A radioreceptor assay is appropriate for screening; bioassay can be carried out later if desired to demonstrate the biological action of the Abs.

In cases of TSH receptor Ab-induced CH, the blocking activity is extremely potent, half-maximal TSH binding inhibition being reported with as little as a 1:20 to 1:50 dilution of serum. A weak or borderline result should cause reconsideration of the diagnosis. TPO Abs, although frequently detectable in babies with blocking Ab-induced CH, are neither sensitive nor specific in predicting the presence of transient CH [79].

Other disorders that may mimic thyroid agenesis on thyroid scintigraphy include loss-of-function mutations of the TSH receptor, iodine excess or an iodide-concentrating abnormality. Potential clues to the diagnosis of a loss-of-function mutation of the TSH receptor include a normal Tg and/or evidence of a thyroid gland on ultrasound examination, despite the failure to visualize thyroid tissue on imaging studies. Verification of the diagnosis requires the demonstration of a genetic abnormality in the TSH receptor gene.

Measurement of urinary iodine is helpful if a diagnosis of iodine-induced hypothyroidism is suspected. An iodide-concentrating defect should be suspected in patients with a family history of CH, particularly if an enlarged thyroid gland is present. The detailed evaluation of infants suspected of having this and other abnormalities in thyroid hormonogenesis has been described elsewhere [59].

Serum Tg concentration, sometimes measured in the evaluation of babies with CH, reflects the amount of thyroid tissue present and the degree of stimulation. For example, Tg is undetectable in most patients with thyroid agenesis but Tg may be elevated in patients with abnormalities of thyroid hormonogenesis not involving Tg synthesis and secretion. It is intermediate in babies with an ectopic thyroid gland. Considerable overlap exists, which limits the value of Tg measurement in differential diagnosis. Measurement of Tg is most helpful when a defect in Tg synthesis or secretion is being considered. In the latter condition, the serum Tg concentration is low or undetectable despite the presence of an enlarged, eutopic thyroid gland.

In babies in whom hypothyroxinaemia unaccompanied by TSH elevation is found, a free $T_4$ should be measured, preferably by a direct dialysis method, and the TBG concentration should be evaluated as well. The finding of a low free $T_4$ in the presence of a normal TBG may suggest the diagnosis of secondary or tertiary hypothyroidism. In these cases, TRH testing will distinguish whether the abnormality is pituitary or hypothalamic. Pituitary function testing and brain imaging should also be performed in these infants.

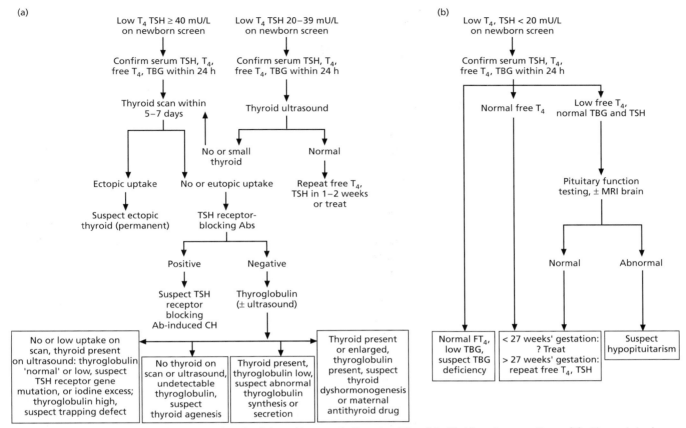

**Fig. 20.11.** Suggested approach to the investigation of an infant with congenital hypothyroidism. (Modified from Brown and Larsen [9] with permission.)

In premature, low-birthweight or sick babies in whom a low $T_4$ and 'normal' TSH are found, the free $T_4$ is frequently not as low as the total $T_4$. In these infants $T_4$ (and/or free $T_4$) and TSH should be measured every 2 weeks until the $T_4$ normalizes, because of the rare occurrence of delayed TSH rise. Similarly, any baby suspected of being hypothyroid clinically should have repeated thyroid function tests because of rare errors in the screening programme.

An approach to the investigation of infants with abnormal results on newborn thyroid screening is shown in Fig. 20.11(a,b).

## Therapy

Replacement therapy with L-$T_4$ should begin as soon as the diagnosis of CH is confirmed. Parents should be counselled regarding the causes of CH, the importance of compliance and the excellent prognosis in most babies if adequate therapy is initiated early. Educational materials should be provided. Treatment need not be delayed by imaging studies as long as they are before suppression of the serum TSH. An initial dosage of 10–15 µg/kg is recommended to normalize the $T_4$ as soon as possible [43,82].

Babies with compensated hypothyroidism may be started on a lower dose, whereas those with severe CH [e.g. $T_4 < 5$ µg/dL (64 nmol/L)], such as those with thyroid agenesis, should probably be started on a higher dose. Thyroxine tablets may be crushed and administered with juice or milk formula but care should be taken that all of the medicine has been swallowed. Thyroxine should not be given with substances that interfere with its absorption, such as iron, soya or fibre. Many babies will swallow the pills whole or chew the tablets with their gums before they have teeth. Liquid preparations are unstable and should not be used.

The aims of therapy are to normalize serum $T_4$ concentration as soon as possible, to avoid hyperthyroidism and to promote normal growth and development. Serum $T_4$ concentrations normalize in most infants within 1 week and the TSH within 1 month. Subsequent adjustments of doses are made according to the results of thyroid function tests and the clinical picture. Some infants develop supraphysiological serum $T_4$ values on this amount of thyroid replacement but the serum $T_3$ concentration usually remains normal, affected infants are not symptomatic and these short-term $T_4$ elevations are probably not associated with adverse effects on growth, skeletal maturation or cognitive development.

Normalization of the TSH concentration may sometimes be delayed because of relative pituitary resistance. In such cases, characterized by a normal or increased serum $T_4$ and an inappropriately high TSH level, the $T_4$ value is used to titrate the dose but non-compliance is the most common cause and should be excluded.

Current recommendations are to repeat $T_4$ and TSH at 2 and 4 weeks after initiation of treatment, every 1–2 months during the first year of life, every 2–3 months between 1 and 3 years of age and every 3–12 months thereafter until growth is complete [43]. In hypothyroid babies in whom an organic basis was not established at birth and in whom transient disease is suspected, a trial off replacement therapy can be initiated after 3 years of age, when most thyroid hormone-dependent brain maturation has occurred.

Whether or not premature infants with hypothyroxinaemia should be treated remains controversial [36,81]. Early retrospective investigations failed to document a difference in cognitive outcome in premature infants with hypothyroxinaemia compared with control subjects, but small numbers were studied. A relationship has been shown between severe hypothyroxinaemia and both developmental delay and disabling cerebral palsy in preterm infants < 32 weeks' gestation. Whether or not the poorer prognosis in these infants is causal or coincidental cannot be determined as the serum $T_4$ in premature infants reflects the severity of illness and risk of death. There are conflicting results on the effect of therapeutic intervention with $T_4$ or $T_3$ on neurocognitve outcome and mortality rate and respiratory function.

In the most thorough study to date, a placebo-controlled, double-blind trial of $T_4$ treatment, 8 µg/kg per day for 6 weeks, was carried out in 200 infants of less than 30 weeks' gestation [83]. Although overall no difference in cognitive outcome was found, there was an 18-point increase in the Bayley Mental Development Index score in the subgroup of $T_4$-treated infants < 27 weeks' gestation. Of some concern was the additional finding that treatment with $T_4$ was associated with a 10-point decrease in mental score ($P = 0.03$) in infants > 27 weeks' gestation. While further studies are needed, it would seem reasonable to treat any premature infant with a low $T_4$ and elevated TSH and to consider treatment of any infant < 27 weeks with a low $T_4$, whether or not the TSH is elevated. A dose of 8 µg/kg/day for these infants has been recommended. Whether or not to treat older premature infants with hypothyroxinaemia and what dosage to use remain uncertain [36,81]

## Prognosis

Numerous studies have been performed to evaluate the cognitive outcome of babies with CH detected on newborn screening [84]. In the initial reports, despite the eradication of severe mental retardation, the intellectual quotient (IQ) of affected infants was nonetheless 6–19 points lower than control babies. Though this IQ deficit was small, it was nonetheless significant as judged by a fourfold increase in the need for special education in affected children. In addition, sensorineural hearing loss, sustained attention problems and various neuropsychological variables were noted, although the frequency and severity of these abnormalities were much less than in the prescreening era. Those babies most likely to have permanent intellectual sequelae were infants with the most severe hypothyroidism *in utero* as determined by initial $T_4$ level [< 5 µg/dL (64 nmol/L)] and skeletal maturation at birth. These findings led to the widely held conclusion at the time that some cognitive deficits in the most severely affected babies might not be reversible by postnatal therapy.

In the initial programmes, an L-$T_4$ dosage of 5–8 µg/kg was used, and treatment was not initiated until 4–5 weeks of age. In contrast, accumulating data from a number of different studies have demonstrated that when a higher initial treatment dose is used (10–15 µg/kg) and treatment is initiated earlier (before 2 weeks) this development gap can be closed, irrespective of the severity of the CH at birth [84,85].

## Neonatal hyperthyroidism

### Transient neonatal hyperthyroidism

Unlike CH, which is usually permanent, neonatal hyperthyroidism is almost always transient. It results from the transplacental passage of maternal TSH receptor-stimulating Abs. Hyperthyroidism develops only in babies born to mothers with the most potent stimulatory activity in serum, 1% of mothers with Graves disease. The incidence at 1 50 000 newborns is approximately four times higher than that for transient neonatal hypothyroidism due to maternal TSH receptor-blocking Abs.

Some mothers have mixtures of stimulating and blocking Abs, the relative proportion of which may change over time. Not surprisingly, the clinical picture in the fetus and neonate of these mothers is complex, and depends not only on the relative proportion of each activity in the maternal circulation at any one time but on the rate of their clearance from the neonatal circulation after birth. Thus, one affected mother gave birth in turn to a normal infant, a baby with transient hyperthyroidism and one with transient hypothyroidism [86]. In another neonate, the onset of hyperthyroidism did not become apparent until 1–2 months postpartum, when the higher-affinity blocking Abs had been cleared from the neonatal circulation [87]. In the last case, multiple monoclonal TSH receptor-stimulating and -blocking Abs were cloned from peripheral lymphocytes in the mother's blood. Each monoclonal Ab recognized different antigenic determinants ('epitopes') on the receptor and had different functional properties [88]. Neonatal hyperthyroidism may occur in infants born to hypothyroid mothers, the maternal thyroid having been destroyed either by prior radioablation, surgery or destructive autoimmune processes so that potent thyroid-stimulating Abs present in the maternal circulation are silent in contrast to the neonate whose thyroid gland is normal.

### Clinical manifestations

Although maternal TSH receptor Ab-mediated hyperthyroidism may present *in utero*, the onset is usually towards the end of the first week of life. This is due both to the clearance of maternally administered antithyroid drugs from the infant's circulation and to the increased conversion of $T_4$ to $T_3$ after birth. The onset may be delayed if higher-affinity blocking Abs are present.

Fetal hyperthyroidism is suspected by fetal tachycardia (pulse greater than 160/min), especially if there is evidence of failure to thrive. Characteristic signs and symptoms include tachycardia, irritability, poor weight gain, and prominent eyes. Goitre may be related to maternal antithyroid drug treatment as well as to the neonatal Graves disease itself. Rarely, infants with neonatal Graves diseases present with thrombocytopenia, hepatosplenomegaly, jaundice and hypoprothrombinaemia, a picture that may be confused with congenital infections. Dysrhythmias and cardiac failure may develop and may cause death, particularly if treatment is delayed or inadequate. In addition to a 20% mortality rate in some older series, untreated fetal and neonatal hyperthyroidism is associated with premature closure of the cranial sutures (cranial synostosis), failure to thrive and developmental delay.

The half-life of TSH receptor Abs is 1–2 weeks. The duration of neonatal hyperthyroidism, a function of Ab potency and metabolic clearance rate, is usually 2–3 months but may be longer.

### Laboratory evaluation

Because of the importance of early diagnosis and treatment, fetuses and infants at risk for neonatal hyperthyroidism should undergo early clinical and biochemical assessment. A high index of suspicion is necessary in babies of women who have had thyroid ablation because a high titre of TSH receptor Abs would not be evident clinically. Similarly, women with persistently elevated TSH receptor Abs and with a high requirement for antithyroid medication are at an increased risk of having an affected child.

The diagnosis of hyperthyroidism is confirmed by the demonstration of an increased concentration of $T_4$, free $T_4$, $T_3$ and free $T_3$ accompanied by suppressed TSH. In the fetus, blood can be obtained by cordocentesis, and results should be compared with normal values during gestation. Fetal ultrasonography may help detect a goitre. Demonstration of a high titre of TSH receptor Abs in the baby or mother will confirm the aetiology of the hyperthyroidism and, in babies whose thyroid function testing is normal initially, indicate the degree to which the baby is at risk [89,90]. In general, babies likely to become hyperthyroid have the highest TSH receptor Ab titre, whereas if TSH receptor Abs are not detectable the baby is most unlikely to become hyperthyroid. In the latter case, it can be anticipated that the baby will be euthyroid, have transient hypothalamo-pituitary suppression or a transiently elevated TSH, depending on the relative contribution of maternal hyperthyroidism vs. the effects of maternal antithyroid medication. Therapy is rarely necessary, whether TSH receptor Abs are measured by radioreceptor assay or by bioassay. On the other hand, if TSH receptor Ab potency is intermediate, it is likely that the baby will be euthyroid, have a transiently elevated $T_4$ or transient hypothalamo-pituitary suppression.

The sensitivity of TSH receptor assays in different laboratories varies, so specific values recommended in the literature should be interpreted with caution, and, ideally, each laboratory should determine its own range. Close follow-up of all babies with abnormal thyroid function tests or detectable TSH receptor Abs is mandatory.

### Therapy

Treatment of the fetus is accomplished by maternal administration of antithyroid medication. The minimum dose of PTU or MMI necessary to normalize the fetal heart rate and render the mother euthyroid or slightly hyperthyroid is usually chosen. In the neonate, treatment is expectant. PTU (5–10 mg/kg/day) or MMI (0.5–1.0 mg/kg/day) can be used, initially in three divided doses. If the hyperthyroidism is severe, a strong iodine solution (Lugol's iodine, 1 drop every 8 h) is added to block the release of thyroid hormone immediately because the effect of PTU and MMI may be delayed for several days. Therapy with both PTU and iodine is adjusted subsequently, depending on the response. Propranolol (2 mg/kg/day in two or three divided doses) is added if sympathetic overstimulation is severe, particularly in the presence of pronounced tachycardia. If cardiac failure develops, treatment with digoxin should be initiated and propranolol should be discontinued.

Rarely, prednisone (2 mg/kg/day) is added for immediate inhibition of thyroid hormone secretion and decreased generation of $T_3$ from $T_4$ in peripheral tissues. Alternatively, sodium ipodate (0.5 g every 3 days), an iodine-containing radiocontrast material that inhibits both thyroid hormone secretion and the conversion of $T_4$ to $T_3$, has been used successfully as the sole treatment of neonatal hyperthyroidism [91]. Measurement of TSH receptor Abs in treated babies may be helpful in predicting when antithyroid medication can be safely discontinued. Lactating mothers on antithyroid medication can continue nursing as long as the dosage of PTU or MMI does not exceed 400 mg or 40 mg respectively. As the milk–serum ratio of PTU is one-tenth that of MMI, a consequence of pH differences and increased protein binding, PTU is preferable to MMI, although relatively low doses of MMI can be given to nursing mothers with no adverse effects on the baby [92]. At higher dosages of antithyroid medication, close supervision of the infant is advisable.

## Permanent neonatal hyperthyroidism

Rarely, neonatal hyperthyroidism is permanent and is due to a germline mutation in the TSH receptor resulting in its constitutive activation [93,94,95]. A gain-of-function mutation of the TSH receptor should be suspected if persistent neonatal hyperthyroidism occurs in the absence of detectable TSH receptor Abs in the maternal circulation. Most cases result from a mutation in exon 10 which encodes the transmembrane domain and intracytoplasmic tail (Fig. 20.2) [93,94]. Less frequently, a mutation encoding the extracellular domain has been described [95]. An autosomal dominant inheritance has been noted in many of these infants but other cases have been sporadic, arising from a *de novo* mutation. Early recognition is important because the thyroid function of affected infants is frequently difficult to manage medically. When diagnosis and therapy are delayed, irreversible sequelae, such as cranial synostosis and developmental delay may result. For this reason early, aggressive therapy with either thyroidectomy or even radioablation has been recommended.

# Thyroid disease in childhood and adolescence

## Hypothyroidism

### Chronic lymphocytic thyroiditis

The causes of hypothyroidism after the neonatal period are listed in Table 20.3. The most frequent is chronic lymphocytic thyroiditis (CLT), an autoimmune disease closely related to Graves disease [96]. Although lymphocyte and cytokine-mediated thyroid destruction predominates in CLT and Ab-mediated thyroid stimulation occurs in Graves disease, overlap may occur in some patients. Both goitrous (Hashimoto's thyroiditis) and non-goitrous (primary myxoedema) variants of thyroiditis have been distinguished. The disease has a striking predilection for females and a family history of autoimmune thyroid disease is found in 30–40% of patients. The most common age at presentation is adolescence but the disease may occur at any age, even infancy [97].

Patients with insulin-dependent diabetes mellitus, 20% of whom have positive thyroid Abs and 5% of whom have an elevated serum TSH level, have an increased prevalence of CLT, which may also occur as part of an autoimmune polyglandular syndrome (APS). In APS 1, also called APECED (autoimmune polyendocrinopathy, candidiasis, ectodermal dystrophy) syndrome, CLT is found in 10% of patients. APS 1 is associated with defective cell-mediated immunity and presents in childhood. It results from a mutation in the *AIRE* (autoimmune regulator) gene [98]. CLT and diabetes mellitus

**Table 20.3.** Differential diagnosis of juvenile hypothyroidism

*Primary hypothyroidism*
  Chronic lymphocytic thyroiditis
    Goitrous (Hashimoto's)
    Atrophic (primary myxoedema)
  Congenital abnormality
    Thyroid dysgenesis
    Inborn error of thyroid hormonogenesis
  Iodine deficiency (endemic goitre)
  Drugs or goitrogens
    Antithyroid drugs (PTU, MMI, carbimazole)
    Anticonvulsants
    Other (lithium, thionamides, aminosalicylic acid, aminoglutethimide)
    Goitrogens (cassava, water pollutants, cabbage, sweet potatoes, cauliflower, broccoli, soya beans)
  Miscellaneous
    Cistinosis
    Histiocytosis X
    Irradiation of the thyroid
      Radioactive iodine
      External irradiation of non-thyroid tumours
    Surgery

*Secondary or tertiary hypothyroidism*
  Congenital abnormality
  Acquired
    Hypothalamic or pituitary tumour (especially craniopharyngioma)
    Treatment of brain and other tumours
    Surgery
    Radiation

with or without adrenal insufficiency (APS 2, also referred to as Schmidt syndrome) tends to occur later in childhood or in the adult. In addition to these polyglandular syndromes, there is an increased incidence of CLT in patients with Down, Turner, Klinefelter and Noonan syndromes. CLT may be associated with chronic urticaria and with immune-complex glomerulonephritis [96].

Antibodies to Tg and TPO ('microsomal'), the thyroid Abs measured in routine clinical practice, are detectable in over 95% of patients with CLT. They are useful as markers of underlying autoimmune thyroid damage, TPO Abs being more sensitive and specific. TSH receptor Abs are also found in a small proportion of patients with CLT. When stimulatory TSH receptor Abs are present, they may give rise to a clinical picture of hyperthyroidism, the coexistence of CLT and Graves disease being known as hashitoxicosis. Blocking Abs, on the other hand, have been postulated to underlie both the hypothyroidism and the absence of goitre in some patients with primary myxoedema, but are detectable in only a minority of children [99]. In rare instances, the disappearance of blocking Abs has been associated with a normalization of thyroid function in previously hypothyroid patients [100].

Goitre, present in approximately two-thirds of children with CLT, results primarily from lymphocytic infiltration and, in some patients, from a compensatory increase in TSH. The role of Abs in goitrogenesis is controversial [101]. Contrary to previous beliefs, primary myxoedema probably arises as a result of independent immune mechanisms and does not represent the 'burned out' phase of CLT [99].

Children with CLT may be euthyroid or may have compensated or overt hypothyroidism. Rarely, they may experience an initial thyrotoxic phase due to the discharge of preformed $T_4$ and $T_3$ from the damaged gland. Alternatively, as indicated above, thyrotoxicosis may be due to concomitant thyroid stimulation by TSH receptor stimulatory Abs (Hashitoxicosis).

Long-term follow-up of children with CLT has suggested that, although most children who are hypothyroid initially remain hypothyroid, spontaneous recovery of thyroid function may occur, particularly in those with initial compensated hypothyroidism. On the other hand, some initially euthyroid patients will become hypothyroid over time [102]. Whether or not treatment is initiated, follow-up is necessary.

## Other causes of acquired hypothyroidism

### Thyroid dysgenesis and inborn errors of thyroid hormonogenesis

Occasionally, patients with thyroid dysgenesis escape detection by newborn screening and present later in childhood with non-goitrous hypothyroidism or with an enlarging mass at the base of the tongue or along the course of the thyroglossal duct. Similarly, children with inborn errors of thyroid hormonogenesis may be recognized later in childhood because of the detection of a goitre.

### Iodine and other micronutrient deficiency: natural goitrogens

Iodine deficiency continues to be a major public health problem. Endemic cretinism, the most serious consequence of iodine deficiency, occurs only in areas where the problem is most severe. Hypothyroidism in older infants, children and adults is seen in regions of moderate iodine deficiency. It develops when adaptive mechanisms fail, and may be exacerbated by the coincident ingestion of goitrogenic foods, such as cassava, soya beans, broccoli, cabbage, sweet potatoes and cauliflower, or by certain water pollutants. Iodine deficiency can be due to dietary restriction (for multiple food allergies) or the result of a fad [103]. Thiocyanate-containing foods (broccoli, sweet potatoes and cauliflower) block trapping and subsequent organification of iodine. Iodine deficiency also may be exacerbated by lack of selenium, a component of the selenocysteine thyroid hormone deiodinases.

### Drugs

A number of drugs used in children affect thyroid function, including antithyroid medication, some anticonvulsants, lithium, aminosalicylic acid and aminoglutethimide.

### Secondary or tertiary hypothyroidism

Secondary or tertiary hypothyroidism may be recognized later in childhood. They may develop as a result of acquired damage to the pituitary or hypothalamus by tumours (particularly craniopharyngioma), granulomatous disease, head irradiation, infection (meningitis), surgery or trauma. Other pituitary hormones are often affected, particularly growth hormone and gonadotrophins.

### Thyroid hormone resistance

Children with thyroid hormone resistance usually come to attention when thyroid function tests are performed because of poor growth, hyperactivity, a learning disability or other non-specific signs or symptoms. A small goitre may be present. The presentation is highly variable and some individuals may be completely asymptomatic, whereas others may have symptoms of both thyroid hormone deficiency and excess. In the past, some individuals have been classified as having selective pituitary resistance as distinct from generalized resistance to thyroid hormone because they appeared to have evidence of peripheral hypermetabolism in response to the elevated thyroid hormone levels. However, variable levels of expression of the mutant allele have not been demonstrated. Thus, it has been suggested that the variable clinical manifestations of this syndrome are a result of the genetic heterogeneity of the many cofactors that modulate thyroid hormone receptor (TR) expression [74].

Thyroid hormone resistance is most frequently caused by a point mutation in the hinge region or ligand-binding domain of the *TRβ* gene (Fig. 20.4). As a consequence, there is a dramatic reduction in $T_3$ binding. Less frequently, it results from impaired interaction with one of the cofactors involved in the mediation of thyroid hormone action [104]. Because these mutant TRs interfere with the function of the normal TRs, a dominant pattern of inheritance is seen. In contrast, in the single family with a deletion of all coding sequences of the *TRβ* gene, only homozygotes manifested resistance.

Rarely, thyroid hormone resistance may be found in patients with cystinosis.

### Miscellaneous causes of acquired hypothyroidism

The thyroid gland may be involved in generalized infiltrative (cystinosis), granulomatous (histiocytosis X) or infectious disease processes of sufficient severity to result in a disturbance in thyroid function. Hypothyroidism may be a long-term complication of mantle irradiation for Hodgkin disease or lymphoma. External irradiation of brain tumours in the posterior fossa of the brain may be associated with both primary and secondary hypothyroidism because of the inclusion of the neck in the radiation field.

## Clinical manifestations

The onset of hypothyroidism in childhood is insidious. Affected children are usually recognized either because of the detection of a goitre or because of poor growth, sometimes for several years before diagnosis. Because linear growth tends to be more affected than weight, affected children are relatively overweight for their height, although they rarely are significantly obese (Fig. 20.12). If the hypothyroidism is severe and long-standing, immature facies with an underdeveloped nasal bridge and immature body proportions (increased upper–lower body ratio) may be noted. Dental and skeletal maturation are delayed, the latter often significantly. Patients with secondary or tertiary hypothy-

roidism tend to be less symptomatic than those with primary disease.

The classic clinical manifestations of hypothyroidism can be elicited on careful evaluation; however, they are not often the presenting complaints. They include lethargy, cold intolerance, constipation, dry skin or hair texture and periorbital oedema. School performance is not usually affected, in contrast to the severe irreversible neurointellectual sequelae that occur in inadequately treated babies with CH.

Causes of hypothyroidism associated with a goitre (CLT, inborn errors of thyroid hormonogenesis, thyroid hormone resistance) should be distinguished from non-goitrous causes (primary myxoedema, thyroid dysgenesis, secondary or tertiary hypothyroidism). The typical thyroid gland in CLT is diffusely enlarged and has a rubbery consistency. Although the surface is classically described as 'pebbly' or bosselated, asymmetric enlargement occasionally occurs and must be distinguished from thyroid neoplasia. An enlarged pyramidal lobe superior to the isthmus can be found and may be confused with a thyroid nodule. A delayed relaxation time of the deep tendon reflexes may be seen in more severe cases.

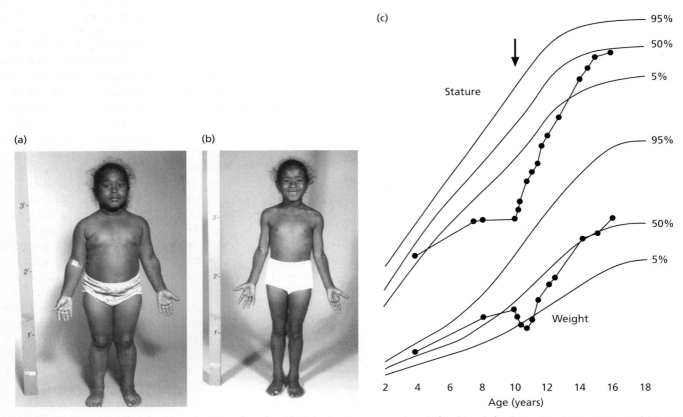

**Fig. 20.12.** Ten-year-old female with severe primary hypothyroidism due to primary myxoedema before (a) and after (b) treatment. Presenting complaint was poor growth. Note the dull facies, relative obesity and immature body proportions prior to treatment. At age 10 years she had not lost a deciduous tooth. After treatment was initiated (indicated by the arrow in c) she lost 6 teeth in 10 months and had striking catch-up growth. Bone age was 5 years at a chronological age of 10 years. TSH receptor-blocking antibodies were negative. (From Brown and Larsen [9], with permission.)

In patients with severe hypothyroidism of long-standing duration, the sella turcica may be enlarged due to thyrotrope hyperplasia. There is an increased incidence of slipped femoral capital epiphyses in hypothyroid children. The combination of severe hypothyroidism and muscular hypertrophy, which gives the child a 'Herculean' appearance, is known as the Kocher–Debre–Semelaign syndrome.

Puberty tends to be delayed in hypothyroid children, although sexual precocity has been described in long-standing severe hypothyroidism [105]. Females may menstruate but commonly have breast development with little sexual hair. Ovarian cysts may be demonstrated on ultrasonography due to follicle-stimulating hormone (FSH) secretion [106]. Galactorrhoea due to hyperprolactinaemia may occasionally occur. In boys, isolated testicular enlargement may be found.

## Laboratory evaluation

Measurement of TSH is the best initial screen for primary hypothyroidism. If the TSH is elevated, measurement of thyroxine will distinguish whether the child has compensated (normal free $T_4$) or overt (low free $T_4$) hypothyroidism.

Measurement of TSH is not helpful in secondary or tertiary hypothyroidism. Hypothyroidism in these cases is demonstrated by the presence of a low free $T_4$ with a low TSH. A hypothalamic cause vs. a pituitary origin of the hypothyroidism can be distinguished by TRH testing. Hypothalamic hypothyroidism is characterized by a delayed peak in TSH secretion (at 60–90 min in contrast to normal individuals in whom the peak is observed at 15–30 min). In hypopituitarism, there is little or no TSH response to TRH. Mild TSH elevation can be seen in individuals with hypothalamic hypothyroidism, a consequence of the secretion of a TSH molecule with impaired bioactivity but normal immunoreactivity. Thyroid hormone resistance is characterized by elevated levels of $T_4$ and $T_3$ and an inappropriately normal or elevated TSH concentration.

CLT is diagnosed by elevated titres of Tg and/or TPO Abs. Ancillary investigations (thyroid ultrasonography and/or thyroid scintigraphy) may be performed if thyroid Ab tests are negative or if a nodule is palpable, but these are rarely necessary. The typical picture of spotty uptake of radioactive iodine that is seen in adults is rare in children [107]. If thyroid Ab tests are negative and no goitre is present, ultrasonography and/or scan identify the presence and location of thyroid tissue and thereby distinguish primary myxoedema from thyroid dysgenesis. Inborn errors of thyroid hormonogenesis beyond a trapping defect are usually suspected by an increased radioiodine uptake and a large gland on scan.

## Therapy

In contrast to CH, rapid replacement is not essential in the older child. This is particularly true in children with long-standing, severe thyroid underactivity in whom rapid normalization may result in unwanted side-effects (deterioration in school performance, short attention span, hyperactivity, insomnia and behaviour difficulties) [108]. Replacement doses should be increased very slowly over several weeks to months. Severely hypothyroid children should also be observed closely for complaints of severe headache when therapy is initiated because of the rare development of pseudotumour cerebri [109]. In contrast, full replacement can be initiated at once without much risk of adverse consequences in children with mild hypothyroidism. Treatment of children with mild compensated hypothyroidism (normal $T_4$, TSH < 10–15 mU/L) is controversial. Some physicians treat all such patients, whereas others choose to reassess thyroid function in 3–6 months before initiating therapy because of the possibility that the thyroid abnormality will be transient.

The typical replacement dose of L-thyroxine in childhood is approximately 100 µg/m$^2$ or 4–6 µg/kg for children 1–5 years of age, 3–4 µg/kg for those ages 6–10 years and 2–3 µg/kg for those 11 years of age and older. In patients with a goitre, a somewhat higher L-thyroxine dosage is used to keep the TSH in the low-normal range (0.3–1.0 mU/L in an ultrasensitive assay) and thereby minimize its goitrogenic effect. Whether and how patients with thyroid hormone resistance should be treated is controversial [74].

After the child has received the recommended dosage for at least 8 weeks, free $T_4$ and TSH should be measured. Once a euthyroid state has been achieved, patients should be monitored every 6–12 months. Close attention is paid to interval growth and bone age as well as to the maintenance of a euthyroid state. Some children with severe, long-standing hypothyroidism at diagnosis may not achieve their adult height potential, even with optimal therapy, emphasizing the importance of early diagnosis and treatment [110]. Treatment is usually continued indefinitely.

## Asymptomatic goitre

Goitre occurs in 4–6% of schoolchildren in iodine-sufficient areas [111]. Like thyroid disease in general, there is a female preponderance, the female–male ratio being 2–3:1. Patients with goitre may be euthyroid, hypothyroid or hyperthyroid, euthyroid goitres being by far the most common. The most frequent cause of asymptomatic goitre is CLT.

## Colloid or simple (non-toxic) goitre

Colloid goitre is an important cause of euthyroid thyroid enlargement in childhood. Not infrequently there is a family history of goitre, CLT and Graves disease, leading to the suggestion that colloid goitre, too, might be an autoimmune disease. Thyroid growth immunoglobulins have been identified in a proportion of patients with simple goitre but their aetiological role is controversial [101]. It is important to distinguish patients with colloid goitre from CLT because of the risk of developing hypothyroidism in patients with CLT but not colloid goitre. Whereas many colloid goitres regress spontaneously, others undergo periods of growth and regression, resulting ultimately in large nodular thyroid glands later in life.

## Clinical manifestations and laboratory investigation

Evaluation of thyroid function by measurement of the serum TSH concentration is the initial approach to diagnosis. In euthyroid patients, the most common situation, CLT should be distinguished from colloid goitre. Clinical examination in both instances reveals a diffusely enlarged thyroid gland. Therefore, the distinction is dependent upon the presence of elevated titres of TPO and/or Tg Abs in CLT but not colloid goitre. All patients with negative thyroid Abs initially should have repeat examinations because some children with CLT will develop positive titres with time.

## Therapy

Thyroid suppression in children with a euthyroid goitre is controversial. There is no evidence of efficacy in CLT [111] and no long-term studies are available in children with colloid goitre. A therapeutic trial may be tried when the goitre is large. In some cases, surgery may be required for cosmesis.

## Painful thyroid

Painful thyroid enlargement is rare in paediatrics and suggests the probability of either acute (suppurative) or subacute thyroiditis. Occasionally, CLT may be associated with intermittent pain and be confused with the latter disorders. In acute thyroiditis, progression to abscess formation may occur rapidly so prompt recognition and antibiotic therapy is essential. Recurrent attacks and involvement of the left lobe suggest a pyriform sinus fistula between the oropharynx and the thyroid as the route of infection [112]. In the latter case, surgical extirpation of the sinus will prevent further attacks.

Subacute thyroiditis, unusual in childhood, is characterized by fever, general malaise, thyroid enlargement and tenderness [112]. Thyroid function tests may be normal or elevated, the result of the release of preformed $T_4$ and $T_3$ into the circulation. Unlike Graves disease, radioactive iodine uptake is low or absent. A low titre of TPO and Tg Abs may be found and the sedimentation rate is elevated. Characteristically the initial thyrotoxic phase persists for 1–4 weeks and is followed by a period of transient hypothyroidism as the thyroid gland recovers. Treatment is supportive and includes large doses of acetylsalicylic acid or other anti-inflammatory drugs. In severe cases corticosteroid medication may be helpful. Antithyroid medication is not indicated.

**Table 20.4.** Causes of thyrotoxicosis in childhood

Hyperthyroidism
    Diffuse toxic goitre (Graves disease)
    Nodular toxic goitre (Plummer disease)

TSH-induced hyperthyroidism
    TSH-producing pituitary tumour
    'Selective pituitary resistance' to thyroid hormone

Thyrotoxicosis without hyperthyroidism
    Chronic lymphocytic thyroiditis
    Subacute thyroiditis
    Thyroid hormone ingestion

## Hyperthyroidism

### Graves disease

The causes of hyperthyroidism in childhood and adolescence are indicated in Table 20.4. More than 95% of cases are due to Graves disease, an autoimmune disorder that, like CLT, occurs in a genetically predisposed population [96]. There is a strong female predisposition, the female–male ratio being 6–8:1. Graves disease is much less common in children than in adults, although it can occur at any age, especially in adolescence. Prepubertal children tend to have more severe disease, require longer medical therapy and achieve a lower rate of remission than pubertal children [113]. This appears to be particularly true in children who present at < 5 years of age [114]. Graves disease has been described in children with other autoimmune diseases, both endocrine and nonendocrine. These include diabetes mellitus, Addison disease, vitiligo, systemic lupus erythematosis, rheumatoid arthritis, myasthenia gravis, periodic paralysis, idiopathic thrombocytopenia purpura and pernicious anaemia. There is an increased risk of Graves disease in children with Down syndrome (trisomy 21).

Unlike CLT, in which thyrocyte damage is predominant, the major clinical manifestations of Graves disease are hyperthyroidism and goitre. Graves disease is caused by TSH receptor Abs that mimic the action of TSH. Binding of ligand results in stimulation of adenyl cyclase with subsequent thyroid hormonogenesis and growth. TSH receptor-blocking Abs inhibit TSH-induced stimulation of adenyl cyclase. Both stimulatory and blocking TSH receptor Abs bind to the extracellular domain of the receptor and appear to recognize linear epitopes as antigen in the context of a three-dimensional structure, but the specific epitope(s) with which they interact is different. Stimulatory Abs bind to the amino-terminal portion of the extracellular domain, whereas blocking Abs bind to the carboxy-terminal domain [115]. Studies using monoclonal TSH receptor Abs cloned from patients' peripheral lymphocytes and recombinant mutant TSH receptor have demonstrated that multiple TSH receptor Abs exist each with different specificities and functional activities [115]. In general, blocking Abs are more potent inhibitors of TSH binding than stimulatory ones.

The clinical assessment of TSH receptor Abs takes advantage of their ability to compete with radiolabelled TSH for binding to thyroid membranes (radioreceptor assay) or to stimulate (or inhibit) TSH-induced stimulation of adenyl cyclase (bioassay). Assays performed in different laboratories vary in sensitivity. A particular problem is that rat FRTL-5 cells, commonly used for bioassay of TSH receptor Abs, lose sensitivity with repeated passage. Technical improvements, including the development of reliable commercial radioreceptor assays and the availability of cultured cells transfected with human TSH receptor, have improved both the radioreceptor assay and the bioassay. TSH receptor Abs can be detected in 80–100% of patients with active Graves disease, whichever method is chosen for their detection (Fig. 20.13) [116]. Most children with Graves disease also have TPO and/or Tg Abs in their sera, but measurement of the latter is less sensitive and less specific than measurement of TSH receptor Abs [116].

### Rarer causes of hyperthyroidism

Hyperthyroidism may be caused by a functioning thyroid adenoma, by constitutive activation of the TSH receptor or may be seen as part of the McCune–Albright syndrome (Table 20.4). Hyperthyroidism may also be due to inappropriately elevated TSH secretion, the result of either a TSH-secreting pituitary adenoma or pituitary resistance to thyroid hormone (Table 20.4).

Miscellaneous causes of thyrotoxicosis without hyperthyroidism include the toxic phase of CLT, subacute thyroiditis and thyroid hormone ingestion (thyrotoxicosis factitia). Thyroxine may be abused by adolescents trying to lose weight or may be inadvertently eaten by toddlers. When the resultant thyrotoxicosis is severe, treatment with iopanoic acid may be effective [117].

### Clinical manifestations

All but a few children with Graves disease present with some degree of thyroid enlargement, and most have symptoms and signs of excessive thyroid activity, such as tremors, inability to fall asleep, weight loss despite an increased appetite, proximal muscle weakness, heat intolerance, headache and tachycardia. Often the onset is insidious. Shortened attention span and emotional lability may lead to severe behavioural and school difficulties. Some patients complain of polyuria and of nocturia, the result of an increased glomerular filtration rate. Acceleration in linear growth may occur, often accompanied by advancement in skeletal maturation (bone age). Adult height is not affected. In the adolescent child,

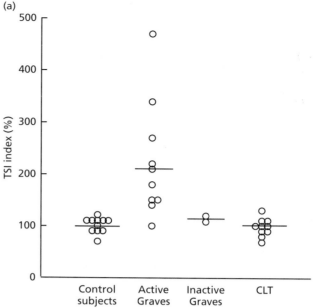

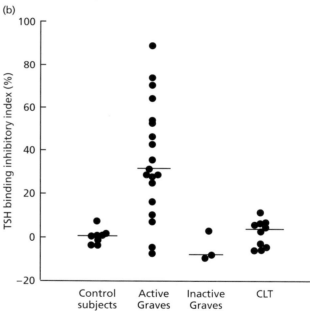

**Fig. 20.13.** TSH receptor antibodies in children and adolescents with Graves disease. Note that results are positive in a majority of patients whether a radioreceptor assay (○, a) or a bioassay (●, b) is used. (From Botero and Brown [116], with permission.)

puberty may be delayed. If menarche has occurred, secondary amenorrhoea is common. If sleep is disturbed, the patient may complain of fatigue.

Physical examination reveals a diffusely enlarged, soft or 'fleshy' thyroid gland, smooth skin and fine hair texture, excessive activity and a fine tremor of the tongue and fingers. A thyroid bruit may be audible. The finding of a thyroid nodule suggests the possibility of a toxic adenoma. The hands are often warm and moist. Tachycardia, a wide pulse pressure and a hyperactive precordium are common. *Café-au-lait* spots, particularly in association with precocious puberty, suggest a possible diagnosis of McCune–Albright syndrome, but if a goitre is absent thyrotoxicosis factitia should be considered. Severe ophthalmopathy is considerably less common in children than in adults, although a stare and mild proptosis are observed frequently.

## Laboratory evaluation

The clinical diagnosis of hyperthyroidism is confirmed by the finding of increased concentrations of circulating thyroid hormones. Suppressed TSH excludes rarer causes of thyrotoxicosis, such as TSH-induced hyperthyroidism and pituitary resistance to thyroid hormone in which the TSH is inappropriately 'normal' or slightly elevated. If these diseases are suspected, the free $\alpha$-subunit, which is elevated in patients with a pituitary TSH-secreting tumour, should be measured and a TRH test performed. Alternatively, elevated levels of $T_4$ in association with an inappropriately 'normal' levels of TSH may be due to an excess of thyroxine-binding globulins (either familial or acquired, for example as a result of oral contraceptive use) or the rarer binding-protein abnormalities (for example increased $T_4$ binding by a mutant albumin or familial dysalbuminaemic hyperthyroxinaemia). In the latter cases, free $T_4$ (and free $T_3$ measured by equilibrium dialysis) and serum TBG concentration will be normal.

If the diagnosis of Graves disease is unclear, TSH receptor Abs should be measured. The radioreceptor assay is appropriate for initial screening because it is sensitive and is technically relatively simple, rapid and reproducible. Bioassay, though of no advantage in screening, may be useful in the occasional Graves disease patient who is negative in the radioreceptor assay or in treated patients whose clinical picture is discordant with results in the radioreceptor assay [116]. Some individuals, initially negative in the radioreceptor assay, become positive several weeks later [116]. It has been hypothesized that TSH receptor Ab synthesis in these patients is restricted at first to lymphocytes residing within the thyroid gland itself, or, alternatively, that TSH receptor Abs escape detection because of binding by soluble TSH receptor circulating in serum. Measurement of TSH receptor Abs may be particularly useful in distinguishing the toxic phase of CLT and subacute thyroiditis (TSH receptor antibody negative) from patients with both CLT and Graves disease (Hashitoxicosis, TSH receptor antibody positive). As noted above, Tg and/or TPO Abs are often present but are less sensitive and specific than TSH receptor Abs in the diagnosis of Graves disease in childhood [116].

In contrast to adults, radioactive iodine uptake and scan are used to confirm the diagnosis of Graves disease only in atypical cases (for example, if measurement of TSH receptor Abs is negative and if the thyrotoxic phase of either CLT

or subacute thyroiditis or a functioning thyroid nodule is suspected).

## Therapy

The choice of which of the three therapeutic options (medical therapy, radioactive iodine or surgery) to use should be individualized and discussed with the patient and his/her family. Each approach has advantages and disadvantages [118]. Medical therapy with one of the thiouracil derivates (PTU or MMI) is used initially, although radioiodine is gaining increasing acceptance, particularly in non-compliant adolescents, in children who are mentally retarded, and in those about to leave home (for example, to go to college).

### Medical therapy

PTU, MMI and carbimazole (converted to MMI) exert their antithyroid effect by inhibiting the organification of iodine and the coupling of iodotyrosine residues on the Tg molecule to generate $T_3$ and $T_4$. MMI is preferred by many paediatric endocrinologists because, for an equivalent dose, it requires taking fewer tablets and has a longer half-life, an advantage in non-compliant adolescents. On the other hand, PTU but not MMI inhibits the conversion of $T_4$ to the more active isomer $T_3$, a potential advantage if the thyrotoxicosis is severe. The initial dose of PTU is 5 mg/kg/day given thrice daily and that of MMI is 0.5 mg/kg/day given daily or twice daily. Carbimazole is best given in a dose of 10–20 mg twice or thrice daily depending on the concentration of the free $T_4$.

In severe cases, a beta-adrenergic blocker (propranolol, 0.5–2.0 mg/kg/day given every 8 h) can be added to control cardiovascular overactivity until a euthyroid state is obtained.

The serum concentrations of $T_4$ and $T_3$ normalize in 4–6 weeks, but TSH concentration may not return to normal for several months. Therefore, measurement of TSH is useful as a guide to therapy only after it has normalized but not initially. Once the $T_4$ and $T_3$ have normalized, one can either decrease the dose of thioamide drug by 30% to 50% or, alternatively and better for the patient because there are fewer hospital attendances, wait until the TSH begins to rise and add a supplementary dose of L-thyroxine in a block-replacement regimen.

Approximately 50% of children will go into long-term remission within 4 years, with a continuing remission rate of 25% every 2 years for up to 6 years of treatment [119]. In patients treated with antithyroid drugs alone, a small drug requirement, small goitre, lack of eye signs and lower initial degree of hyperthyroxinaemia [$T_4 < 20\,\mu g/dL$ (250 nmol/L)] are favourable indicators that drug therapy can be tapered gradually and withdrawn. Body mass index (BMI) $< -0.5\%$ and older age (pubertal vs. prepubertal age) are associated with an increased likelihood of permanent remission

[113,114,120]. Persistence of TSH receptor Abs, on the other hand, indicates a high likelihood of relapse. Initial studies suggesting that combined therapy (i.e. antithyroid drug plus L-thyroxine) might be associated with an improved rate of remission [121] have not been confirmed [122].

Toxic drug reactions [erythematous rashes, urticaria, arthralgias, transient granulocytopenia (< 1500 granulocytes/mm$^3$) ] have been reported in 5–14% of children. Rarely, hepatitis, a lupus-like syndrome, thrombocytopenia and agranulocytosis (< 250 granulocytes/mm$^3$) may occur. Most reactions are mild and do not contraindicate continued use. In more severe cases, switching to the other thioamide is frequently effective. The risk of hepatitis and agranulocytosis appears greater within the first 3 months of therapy; there is some evidence that close monitoring of the white blood cell count during this initial time period may be useful in identifying agranulocytosis before the development of a fever and infection [123]. Many authors recommend also checking the white blood cell count and liver function tests before therapy, because Graves disease itself can be associated with abnormalities in these parameters. It is important to caution all patients to stop their medication immediately and consult their physician should they develop unexplained fever, sore throat, gingival sores or jaundice. Approximately 10% of children treated medically will develop long-term hypothyroidism later in life, a consequence of coincident cell and cytokine-mediated destruction and/or the development of TSH receptor-blocking Abs.

## Radioactive iodine

Definitive therapy with medical (radioactive iodine) or surgical thyroid ablation is usually reserved for patients who have failed drug therapy, developed a toxic drug reaction or are non-compliant but the nuisance of thyrotoxicosis should not be underestimated and long-continued antithyroid treatment should not lightly be continued indefinitely.

Radioactive iodine (RAI) is being favoured increasingly in some centres, even as the initial approach to therapy. The advantages are the relative ease of administration, the reduced need for medical follow-up and the lack of demonstrable long-term adverse effects [118,124]. Although a dose of 50–200 µCi of $^{131}$I per estimated gram of thyroid tissue has been used, the higher dose is recommended, particularly in younger children, in order to ablate the thyroid gland and thereby reduce the risk of future neoplasia. The size of the thyroid gland is estimated, based on the assumption that the normal gland is 0.5–1.0 g/year of age, maximum 15–20 g. The formula used is:

$$\frac{\text{Estimated thyroid weight in grams} \times 50\text{--}200\ \mu\text{Ci}^{131}\text{I}}{\text{Fractional}^{131}\text{I 24-h uptake}}$$

Radioactive iodine therapy should be used with caution in children under 10 years of age and particularly in those aged 5 years or less because of the increased susceptibility of the thyroid gland in the young to the proliferative effects of ionizing radiation. Almost all patients who developed papillary thyroid cancer after the Chernobyl disaster were less than 10 years at the time of the reactor malfunction [125,126]. Similarly, the risk of benign thyroid nodules after radioactive iodine therapy for Graves disease is greatest in the first decade of life. Pretreatment with antithyroid drugs before RAI therapy is not necessary, unless the hyperthyroidism is very severe.

Thyroid hormone concentrations may rise transiently 4–10 days after RAI administration owing to the release of preformed hormone from the damaged gland. Beta-blockers may be useful. Analgesics may be necessary for the discomfort of radiation thyroiditis. Other acute complications of RAI therapy (nausea, significant neck swelling) are rare. A therapeutic effect is usually seen within 6 weeks to 3 months.

Worsening of ophthalmopathy, described in adults after RAI, does not appear to be common in children, but if significant ophthalmopathy is present RAI therapy should be used with caution, and treatment with steroids for 6–8 weeks after RAI administration may be wise. In approximately 1000 children with Graves disease treated with RAI and followed for < 5 to > 20 years to date, there did not appear to be any increased rate of congenital anomalies in the offspring nor in the occurrence of thyroid cancer. However, the numbers of younger children treated with RAI and followed long-term are small.

## Surgery

Surgery is performed less frequently now than previously. Its major advantage is the immediate resolution of the hyperthyroidism. Near-total or subtotal thyroidectomy is performed, depending on whether the goal is to minimize the risk of recurrence or render the patient euthyroid. Surgery is appropriate for younger patients, those who have failed medical management, those who have a markedly enlarged thyroid, those who refuse radioactive iodine therapy and for the rare patient with eye disease in whom radioactive iodine therapy is contraindicated. Because of the potential complications of transient hypocalcaemia, recurrent laryngeal nerve paralysis, hypoparathyroidism and, rarely (as with all forms of surgery), death, this therapy should be performed only by an experienced thyroid surgeon. Occasionally unsightly keloid formation occurs at the site of the scar.

The child must be euthyroid before surgery to avoid thyroid storm. If medical management is inadequate for any reason, iodides (Lugol's solution, 5–10 drops t.i.d, or potassium iodide, 2–10 drops daily) are added for 7–14 days before surgery in order to decrease the vascularity of the gland.

After both medical and surgical thyroid ablation most patients become hypothyroid and require lifelong thyroid replacement therapy. On the other hand, if therapy is inadequate, hyperthyroidism may recur.

## Thyroid nodules

Thyroid nodules are uncommon in the first two decades of life in iodine-sufficient populations. Follicular adenomas and colloid cysts account for the majority of them, but they are more likely to be carcinomatous than are similar masses in adults. Causes of nodular enlargement also include CLT and embryological defects, such as intrathyroidal duct cysts or unilateral thyroid agenesis [127].

The most common form of cancer is papillary thyroid carcinoma, but other histological types found in the adult may occur also [127,128]. A high index of suspicion is necessary if the nodule is painless, of firm or hard consistency, if it is fixed to surrounding tissues, especially if it has undergone rapid growth, or if there is cervical adenopathy, hoarseness or dysphagia. Children exposed to high levels of radiation are at particularly high risk. Medullary thyroid carcinoma (MTC) should be considered if there is a family history of thyroid cancer or phaeochromocytoma and/or if the child has multiple mucosal neuromas and a marfanoid habitus, findings consistent with multiple endocrine neoplasia, types 2A and/or 2B.

Initial investigation includes evaluation of thyroid function and antithyroid Abs. A suppressed serum TSH concentration accompanied by an elevation in the circulating $T_4$ and/or $T_3$ suggests the possibility of a functioning nodule. Positive Abs, on the other hand, indicate the presence of underlying CLT. Thyroid scintiscan is often used to determine whether the nodule is 'cold', and ultrasound may provide information whether the nodule is solid or cystic. Unfortunately, although the finding of a functioning nodule, underlying CLT or a cystic component indicates that a malignancy is less likely, none of these findings completely excludes the possibility of thyroid carcinoma [129].

Fine-needle aspiration biopsy, popular in the investigation of thyroid carcinoma in adults, has been used increasingly in older children. Unfortunately, false-negative results have occurred occasionally with this technique, leading some to continue to favour immediate open excisional biopsy for all solitary, solid thyroid nodules or goitre-associated lymphadenopathy in childhood and adolescence. Despite an increased incidence of local spread and of pulmonary metastases at the time of diagnosis, the mortality rate is no greater in children than in adults [128,130].

Excision of the tumour or lobe is the appropriate treatment for benign tumours and cysts, whereas total thyroidectomy with preservation of the parathyroid glands and recurrent laryngeal nerves is the initial therapy for malignant thyroid tumours. The latter procedure is followed by radioablation if there is evidence of residual gland or tumour after surgery. After radioiodine therapy, the dose of thyroxine is adjusted to keep the serum TSH concentration suppressed (between 0.05 and 0.1 mU/L in sensitive assays). Measurement of serum Tg, a thyroid follicular cell-specific protein, is used to detect evidence of metastatic disease in differentiated forms of thyroid cancer, such as papillary or follicular cancer. This is best performed after a period (usually 6 weeks) of thyroxine withdrawal or after exogenous administration of recombinant TSH [131].

Measurement of circulating calcitonin is used as a tumour marker for MCT, a C-cell derived malignancy. Mutations of the *RET* proto-oncogene, detectable in nearly all familial forms of MTC, is of value in screening family members [132,133]. In families affected with multiple endocrine neoplasia type 2, screening of children as young as 5 years followed by total thyroidectomy has been successful in curing patients with microscopic MTC, an otherwise highly malignant neoplasm with a poor prognosis [133]. Some excellent reviews of childhood cancer and of medullary thyroid cancer have been published [127,132–134].

## References

1 Delange F, Fisher DA. The thyroid gland. In: Brook CGD, ed. *Clinical Paediatric Endocrinology*, 3rd edn. Oxford: Blackwell Science, 1995: 397–433.

2 Vassart G, Parmentier M, Libert F, Dumont J. Molecular genetics of the thyrotropin receptor. *Trends Endocrinol Metab* 1991; 2: 151–6.

3 Van Sande J, Parma J, Tonacchera M, Swillens S, Dumont J, Vassart G. Somatic and germline mutations of the TSH receptor gene in thyroid diseases. *J Clin Endocrinol Metab* 1995; 80: 2577–85.

4 Roti E, Colzani R, Braverman LE. Adverse effects of iodine on the thyroid. *Endocrinologist* 1997; 7: 245–54.

5 Eng PHK, Cordona GR, Fang S-L *et al*. Escape from the acute Wolff–Chaikoff effect is associated with a decrease in thyroid sodium/iodide symporter messenger ribonucleic acid and protein. *Endocrinology* 1999; 140: 3404–10.

6 Dunn JT. Iodine deficiency: consequences and prevention. *Thyroid Today* 1997; 20 (2): 1–9.

7 Robbins J. Thyroid hormone transport proteins and the physiology of hormone binding. In: Braverman LE, Utiger RD, eds. *Werner and Ingbar's the Thyroid*, 7th edn. Philadelphia: Lipincott Raven, 1995: 96–110.

8 Fisher DA. Disorders of the thyroid in the newborn and infant. In: Sperling MA, ed. *Pediatric Endocrinology*, Philadelphia: W. B. Saunders, 1996: 51–70.

9 Brown RS, Larsen PR. Thyroid gland development and disease in infancy and childhood. In: DeGroot L, Hennemann G, eds. *Thyroid Disease Manager*. http://www.thyroidmanager.org, 1999.

10 Brent GA. The molecular basis of thyroid hormone action. *N Engl J Med* 1994; 331: 847–53.

11 DiLauro R, Damante G, De Felice M *et al*. Molecular events in the differentiation of the thyroid gland. *J Endocrinol Invest* 1995; 18: 117–19.

12 Zannini M, Avantaggiato V, Biffali E *et al*. TTF-2, a new forkhead protein, shows a temporal expression in the developing thyroid which is consistent with a role in controlling the onset of differentiation. *EMBO J* 1997; 11: 3185–97.

13 Manley NR, Capecchi MR. The role of Hoxa-3 in mouse thymus and thyroid development. *Development* 1995; 121: 1989–2003.

14 Damante G, Di Lauro R. Thyroid-specific gene expression. *Biochim Biophys Acta* 1994; 1218: 255–66.

15 De Felice M, Ocitt C, Biffali E *et al.* A mouse model for hereditary thyroid dysgenesis and cleft palate. *Nature Genet* 1998; 19: 395–8.

16 Brown RS, Shalhoub V, DeVito W, Joris I, Lian J, Stein G. Developmental regulation of thyrotropin receptor gene expression in the fetal and neonatal rat thyroid: relation to thyroid morphology and to thyroid-specific gene expression. *Endocrinology* 2000; 141: 340–5.

17 Stein SA, Shanklin DR, Krulich L, Roth MG, Chubb CM, Adams PM. Evaluation and characterization of the hyt/hyt hypothyroid mouse: II. Abnormalities of TSH and the thyroid gland. *Neuroendocrinology* 1987; 49: 509–19.

18 Brown RS, Bellisario RL, Botero D *et al.* Incidence of transient congenital hypothyroidism due to maternal thyrotropin receptor-blocking antibodies in over one million babies. *J Clin Endocrinol Metab* 1996; 81: 1147–51.

19 Abramowicz MJ, Duprez L, Parma J, Vassart G, Heinrichs C. Familial congenital hypothyroidism due to inactivating mutation of the thyrotropin receptor causing profound hypoplasia of the thyroid gland. *J Clin Invest* 1997; 99: 3018–24.

20 Costa A, Arisio R, Benedetto C, Bertino E *et al.* Thyroid hormones in tissues from human embryos and fetuses. *J Endocrinol Invest* 1991; 14: 559–68.

21 Oppenheimer JH, Schwartz HL. Molecular basis of thyroid hormone-dependent brain development. *Endocr Rev* 1997; 18: 462–75.

22 Forrest D, Vennstrom B. Review. Functions of thyroid hormone receptors in mice. *Thyroid* 2000; 10: 41–52.

23 Farwell AP, Tranter P, Leonard JL. Thyroxine-dependent regulation of integrin–laminin interactions in astrocytes. *Endocrinology* 1995; 136: 3909–15.

24 Roti E, Gnudi A, Braverman LE. The placental transport, synthesis and metabolism of hormones and drugs which affect thyroid function. *Endocr Rev* 1983; 4: 131–49.

25 Calvo R, Obregon MJ, Ruiz de Ona C, Escobar del Rey F *et al.* Congenital hypothyroidism as studied in rats: crucial role of maternal thyroxine (T4) but not of 3,5,31 triiodothyronine (T3) in the protection of the fetal brain. *J Clin Invest* 1990; 86: 889–99.

26 Vulsma T, Gons MH, DeVijlder JMM. Maternal fetal transfer of thyroxine in congenital hypothyroidism due to a total organification defect of thyroid dysgenesis. *N Engl J Med* 1989; 321: 13–16.

27 Xue-Yi C, Zin-Min J, Zhi-hong Dou *et al.* Timing of vulnerability of the brain to iodine deficiency in endemic cretinism. *N Engl J Med* 1994; 331: 1739–44.

28 DeZegher F, Pernasetti F, Vanhole C *et al.* The prenatal role of thyroid hormone evidenced by fetomaternal Pit-1 deficiency. *J Clin Endocrinol Metab* 1995; 80: 3127–30.

29 Matsuura N, Konishi J and the transient hypothyroidism study group in Japan. *Endocrinol Japan* 1990; 37: 369–79.

30 Man EB, Brown JF, Serunian SA. Maternal hypothyroxinemia: psychoneurological deficits of progeny. *Ann Clin Lab Series* 1991; 21: 227–78.

31 Haddow JE, Palomaki GE, Allan WC *et al.* Maternal thyroid deficiency during pregnancy and subsequent neuropsychological development of the child. *N Engl J Med* 1999; 341: 549–55.

32 Pop VJ, Kuijpens JL, van Boar AL *et al.* Low maternal free thyroxine concentrations during early pregnancy are associated with impaired psychomotor development in infancy. *Clin Endocrinol* 1999; 50: 149–55.

33 Liu H, Momotani N, Noh JY, Ishikawa N, Takebe K, Ito K. Maternal hypothyroidism during early pregnancy and intellectual development of the progeny. *Arch Intern Med* 1994; 154: 785–7.

34 Thorpe-Beeston JG, Nicolaides KH, Felton CG, Butler J, McGregor AM. Maturation of the secretion of thyroid hormone and thyroid-stimulating hormone in the fetus. *N Engl J Med* 1991; 324: 532–6.

35 Mercado M, Yu VYH, Symonowicz W *et al. Early Human Dev* 1988; 16: 131–41.

36 LaFranchi S. Thyroid function in the preterm infant. *Thyroid* 1999; 9: 71–8.

37 Ares S, Escobar-Morreale HF, Quero J *et al.* Neonatal hypothyroxinemia: effects of iodine intake and premature birth. *J Clin Endocrinol Metab* 1997; 82: 1704–12.

38 Frank JE, Faix JE, Hermos R *et al.* Thyroid function in very low birth weight infants: effects in neonatal hypothyroidism screening. *J Pediatr* 1996; 128: 548–54.

39 Fisher DA, Klein AH. Thyroid development and disorders of thyroid function in the newborn. *N Engl J Med* 1981; 304: 702–12.

40 Boyages SC. Clinical review 49: Iodine deficiency disorders. *J Clin Endocrinol Metab* 1993; 77: 587–91.

41 Boyages SC, Halpern JP. Endemic cretinism: towards a unifying hypothesis. *Thyroid* 1993; 3: 59–69.

42 Delange F. Neonatal screening for congenital hypothyroidism: results and perspectives. *Horm Res* 1997; 48: 51–61.

43 LaFranchi SH, Dussault JH, Fisher DA *et al.* American Academy of Pediatrics and American Thyroid Association. Newborn screening for congenital hypothyroidism: recommended guidelines. *Pediatrics* 1993; 91: 1203–9.

44 Klein RZ, Mitchel ML. Hypothyroidism in infants and children. In: Braverman LE, Utiger RD, eds. *Werner and Ingbar's the Thyroid*, 7th edn. Philadelphia: Lipincott Raven, 1995: 984–8.

45 Adams LM, Emery JR, Clark SJ *et al.* Reference ranges for newer thyroid function tests in premature infants. *J Pediatr* 1995; 126: 122–7.

46 Fort P, Lifshitz F, Bellisario R *et al.* Abnormalities of thyroid function in infants with Down syndrome. *J Pediatr* 1984; 104: 545–9.

47 DeVriendt K, VanHole C, Matthijs G *et al.* Deletion of thyroid transcription factor-1 gene in an infant with neonatal thyroid dysfunction and respiratory failure. *N Engl J Med* 1998; 338: 1317–18.

48 Kimura S, Hara Y, Pineau T *et al.* The T/epb null mouse: thyroid-specific enhancer-binding protein is essential for the organogenesis of the thyroid, lung, ventral forebrain, and pituitary. *Genes Dev* 1996; 10: 60–9.

49 Perna MG, Civitareale D, De Filippis V *et al.* Absence of mutations in the gene encoding thyroid transcription factor-1 (TTF-1) in patients with thyroid dysgenesis. *Thyroid* 1997; 7: 377–81.

50 Lapi P, Macchia PE, Chiovato L *et al.* Mutations in the gene encoding thyroid transcription factor-1 (TTF-1) are not a frequent cause of congenital hypothyroidism (CH) with thyroid dysgenesis. *Thyroid* 1997; 7: 383–7.

51 Macchia PE, Lapi P, Krude H *et al.* Pax8 mutations associated with congenital hypothyroidism caused by thyroid dysgenesis. *Nature Genet* 1998; 19: 83–6.

52 Clifton-Blighe RJ, Wentworth JM, Heinz P *et al.* Mutation of the gene encoding human TTF-2 associated with thyroid agenesis, cleft palate and choanal atresia. *Nature Genet* 1998; 19: 399–401.

53 Abramowicz MJ, Vassart G, Refetoff S. Probing the cause of thyroid dysgenesis. *Thyroid* 1997; 7: 325–6.

54 Dussault JH, Letarte J, Guyda H *et al.* Lack of influence of thyroid antibodies on thyroid function in the newborn infant and on a mass screening programme for congenital hypothyroidism. *J Pediatr* 1980; 96: 385–9.

55 Van der Gaag RD, Drexhage HA, Dussault JH. Role of maternal immunoglobulins blocking TSH-induced thyroid growth in sporadic forms of congenital hypothyroidism. *Lancet* 1985; 1: 246–50.

56 Bogner U, Gruters A, Sigle B *et al.* Cytotoxic antibodies in congenital hypothyroidism. *J Clin Endocrinol Metab* 1989; 68: 671–5.

57 Brown RS, Keating P, Mitchell E. Maternal thyroid-blocking immunoglobulins in congenital hypothyroidism. *J Clin Endocrinol Metab* 1990; 70: 1341–6.

58 Medeiros-Neto G. Clinical and molecular advances in inherited disorders of the thyroid system. *Thyroid Today* 1996; 19 (3): 1–13.

59 Gruters A, Finke R, Krude H, Meinhold H. Etiological grouping of permanent congenital hypothyroidism with a thyroid gland in situ. *Horm Res* 1994; 41: 3–9.

60 Kopp P. Pendred's syndrome: identification of the genetic defect a century after its recognition. *Thyroid* 1999; 9: 65–9.

61 Royau IE, Suzuki K, Mori A *et al.* Pendrin, the protein encoded by the Pendred Syndrome gene (PDS), is an apical porter of iodide in the thyroid and is regulated by thyroglobulin in FRTL-5 cells. *Endocrinology* 2000; 141: 839–45.

62 Sunthornthepvarakul T, Gottschalk ME, Hayashi Y *et al.* Brief report: resistance to thyrotropin caused by mutations in the thyrotropin-receptor gene. *N Engl J Med* 1995; 332: 155–60.

63 Biebermann H, Schoneberg T, Krude H *et al.* Mutations of the human thyrotropin receptor gene causing thyroid hypoplasia and persistent congenital hypothyroidism. *J Clin Endocrinol Metab* 1997; 82: 3471–80.

64 Gagne N, Parma J, Deal C *et al.* Apparent congenital athyreosis contrasting with normal plasma thyroglobulin levels and associated with inactivating mutations in the thyrotropin receptor gene: are athyreosis and ectopic thyroid distinct entities? *J Clin Endocrinol Metab* 1998; 83: 1771–5.

65 Stein SA, Oates EL, Hall CR *et al.* Identification of a point mutation in the thyrotropin receptor of the hyt/hyt hypothyroid mouse. *Mol Endocrinol* 1994; 8: 129–38.

66 Krude H, Biebermann H, Gopel W *et al.* The gene for the thyrotropin receptor (TSHR) as a candidate gene for congenital hypothyroidism with thyroid dysgenesis. *Exp Clin Endocrinol Diabetes* 1996; 104 (Suppl.): 117–20.

67 Ahlbom BE, Yaqoob M, Larsson A *et al.* Genetic and linkage analysis of familial congenital hypothyroidism: exclusion of linkage to the TSH receptor gene. *Hum Genet* 1997; 99: 186–90.

68 Levine MA, Jap T-S, Hung W. Infantile hypothyroidism in two sibs: an unusual presentation of pseudohypoparathyroidism type 1a. *J Pediatr* 1985; 107: 919–22.

69 Collu R, Tang J, Castagne J *et al.* A novel mechanism for isolated central hypothyroidism: inactivating mutations in the thyrotropin-releasing hormone receptor gene. *J Clin Endocrinol Metab* 1997; 82: 1561–5.

70 Brown RS, Bhatia V, Hayes E. An apparent cluster of congenital hypopituitarism in central Massachusetts: magnetic resonance imaging and hormonal studies. *J Clin Endocrinol Metab* 1991; 72: 12–18.

71 Dattani MT, Martinez-Barbera JP, Thomas PQ *et al.* HESX1: a novel homeobox gene implicated in septo-optic dysplasia. *Horm Res* 1998; 50 (Suppl.): 8.

72 Parks JS, Adess ME, Brown MR. Genes regulating hypothalamic and pituitary development. *Acta Paed Suppl* 1997; 423: 28–32.

73 Rosenbloom AL, Almonte AS, Brown MR *et al.* Clinical and biochemical phenotype of familial anterior hypopituitarism from mutation of the PROP1 gene. *J Clin Endocrinol Metab* 1999; 84: 50–7.

74 Weiss RE, Refetoff S. Treatment of resistance to thyroid hormone – Primum non nocere (editorial). *J Clin Endocrinol Metab* 1999; 84: 401–4.

75 Fisher DA. Editorial: The hypothyroxinemia of prematurity. *J Clin Endocrinol Metab* 1997; 82: 1701–3.

76 l'Allemand D, Gruters A, Beyer P *et al.* Iodine in contrast agents and skin disinfectants is the major cause for hypothyroidism in premature infants during intensive care. *Horm Res* 1987; 28: 42–9.

77 Brown RS, Bloomfield S, Bednarek FJ *et al.* Routine skin cleansing with povidone-iodine is not a common cause of transient neonatal hypothyroidism in North America: a prospective, controlled study. *Thyroid* 1997; 7: 395–400.

78 Cheron RG, Kaplan MM, Larsen PR *et al.* Neonatal thyroid function after propylthiouracil therapy for maternal Graves' disease. *N Engl J Med* 1981; 304: 525–8.

79 Brown RS, Bellisario RL, Botero D *et al.* Incidence of transient congenital hypothyroidism due to maternal thyrotropin receptor-blocking antibodies in over one million babies. *J Clin Endocrinol Metab* 1996; 81: 1147–51.

80 Mandel SH, Hanna CE, LaFranchi SH. Diminished thyroid-stimulating hormone secretion associated with neonatal thyrotoxicosis. *J Pediatr* 1986; 109: 662–5.

81 Fisher DA. The hypothyroxinemia of prematurity (editorial). *J Clin Endocrinol Metab* 1997; 82: 1701–3.

82 Fisher DA. Clinical review 19: management of congenital hypothyroidism. *J Clin Endocrinol Metab* 1991; 72: 523–9.

83 van Wassenaer AG, Kok JH, de Vijlder JJM *et al.* Effects of thyroxine supplementation on neurologic development in infants born at less than 30 weeks' gestation. *N Engl J Med* 1997; 336: 21–6.

84 Van Vliet G. Neonatal hypothyroidism. *Treatment Outcome Thyroid* 1999; 9: 79–84.

85 New England Congenital Hypothyroidism Collaborative. Effects of neonatal screening for hypothyroidism: Prevention of mental retardation by treatment before clinical manifestations. *Lancet* 1981; 2: 1095–8.

86 Fort P, Lifshitz F, Pugliese M *et al.* Neonatal thyroid disease: differential expression in three successive offspring. *J Clin Endocrinol Metab* 1988; 66: 645–7.

87 Zakarija M, McKenzie JM. Immunoglobulin G inhibitor of thyroid-stimulating antibody is a cause of delay in the onset of neonatal Graves' disease. *J Clin Invest* 1983; 72: 1352–6.

88 Kohn LD, Suzuki K, Hoffman WH *et al.* Characterization of monoclonal thyroid-stimulating and thyrotropin binding-inhibiting autoantibodies from a Hashimoto's patient whose children had intrauterine and neonatal thyroid disease. *J Clin Endocrinol Metab* 1997; 82: 3998–4009.

89 Matsuura N, Konishi J, Fujeda K *et al.* TSH-receptor antibodies in mothers with Graves' disease and outcome in their offspring. *Lancet* 1988; 2: 14–17.

90 Tamaki H, Amino N, Aozasa M *et al.* Universal predictive criteria for neonatal overt thyrotoxicosis requiring treatment. *Am J Perinatol* 1988; 5: 152–8.

91 Karpman BA, Rapoport B, Filetti S *et al.* Treatment of neonatal hyperthyroidism due to Graves' disease with sodium ipodate. *J Clin Endocrinol Metab* 1987; 64: 119–23.

92 Azizi F. Effect of methimazole treatment of maternal thyrotoxicosis on thyroid function in breast-feeding infants. *J Pediatr* 1996; 128: 855–8.

93 de Roux N, Polak M, Couet J *et al.* A neomutation of the thyroid-stimulating hormone receptor in a severe neonatal hyperthyroidism. *J Clin Endocrinol Metab* 1996; 81: 2023–6.

94 Holzapfel H-P, Wonerow P, von Petrykowski W *et al.* Sporadic congenital hyperthyroidism due to a spontaneous germline mutation in the thyrotropin receptor gene. *J Clin Endocrinol Metab* 1997; 82: 3879–84.

95 Grüters A, Schoneberg T, Biebermann H *et al.* Severe congenital hyperthyroidism caused by a germ-line neo mutation in the extracellular portion of the thyrotropin receptor. *J Clin Endocrinol Metab* 1998; 83: 1431–6.

96 Brown RS. Thyroid disease in infancy, childhood, and adolescence. In: Braverman LE, ed. *Contemporary Endocrinology.* Totowa, NJ: Humana Press, 1997: 81–102.

97 Foley TP, Abbassi V, Copeland KC, Draznin MB. Brief report: Hypothyroidism caused by chronic autoimmune thyroiditis in very young infants. *N Engl J Med* 1994; 330: 466–8.

98 Scott HS, Heino M, Peterson P *et al.* Common mutations in autoimmune polyendocrinopathy-candidiasis-ectodermal dystrophy patients of different origins. *Mol Endocrinol* 1998; 12: 1112–19.

99 Matsuura N, Konishi J, Yuri K *et al.* Comparison of atrophic and goitrous auto-immune thyroiditis in children: clinical, laboratory and TSH-receptor antibody studies. *Eur J Pediatr* 1990; 149: 529–33.

100 Takasu N, Yamada T, Takasu K *et al.* Disappearance of thyrotropin-blocking antibodies and spontaneous recovery from hypothyroidism in autoimmune thyroiditis. *New Engl J Med* 1992; 326: 513–18.

101 Brown RS. Immunoglobulins affecting thyroid growth: a continuing controversy. *J Clin Endocrinol Metab* 1995; 80: 1506–8.

102 Maenpaa J, Raatikka M, Rasanen J *et al.* Natural course of juvenile autoimmune thyroiditis. *J Pediatr* 1985; 107: 898–904.

103 Pacaud D, Van Vliet G, Delvin E *et al.* A third world endocrine disease in a 6-year old North American boy. *J Clin Endocrinol Metab* 1995; 80: 2574–6.

104 Weiss RE, Hayashi Y, Nagaya T *et al.* Dominant inheritance of resistance to thyroid hormone not linked to defects in the thyroid hormone receptor a or b genes may be due to a defective cofactor. *J Clin Endocrinol Metab* 1996; 81: 4196–203.

105 Van Wyk J, Grumbach M. Syndrome of precocious menstruation and galactorrhea in juvenile hypothyroidism: an example of hormonal overlap in pituitary feedback. *J Pediatr* 1960; 57: 416–35.

106 Anasti JN, Flack MR, Froehlich J *et al.* A potential novel mechanism for precocious puberty in juvenile hypothyroidism. *J Clin Endocrinol Metab* 1995; 80: 276–9.

107 Alos N, Huot C, Lambert R *et al.* Thyroid scintigraphy in children and adolescents with Hashimoto disease. *J Pediatr* 1995; 127: 951–3.

108 Rovet JF, Daneman D, Bailey JD. Psychologic and psychoeducational consequences of thyroxine therapy for juvenile acquired hypothyroidism. *J Pediatr* 1993; 122: 543–9.

109 Van Dop C, Conte FA, Koch TK *et al.* Pseudotumor cerebri associated with initiation of levothyroxine therapy for juvenile hypothyroidism. *N Engl J Med* 1983; 308: 1076–80.

110 Rivkees SA, Bode HH, Crawford JD. Long-term growth in juvenile acquired hypothyroidism: the failure to achieve normal adult stature. *N Engl J Med* 1988; 318: 599–602.

111 Rother KI, Zimmerman D, Schwenk WF. Effect of thyroid hormone treatment on thyromegaly in children and adolescents with Hashimoto disease. *J Clin Endocrinol Metab* 1994; 124: 599–601.

112 Brown RS. Thyroiditis. In: Rakel, ed. *Conn's Current Therapy.* Philadelphia: W. B. Saunders, 1987: 535–6.

113 Shulman DI, Muhar I, Jorgensen EV *et al.* Autoimmune hyperthyroidism in prepubertal children and adolescents: comparison of clinical and biochemical features at diagnosis and responses to medical therapy. *Thyroid* 1997; 7: 755–60.

114 Segni M, Leonardi E, Mazzoncini B, Pucarelli I, Pasquino AM. Special features of Graves' disease in early childhood. *Thyroid* 1999; 9: 871–7.

115 Tahara K, Ban T, Minegishi T *et al.* Immunoglobulin from Graves' disease patients interact with different sites on TSH receptor/LH-CG chimeras than either TSH or immunoglobulins from idiopathic myxoedema. *Biochem Biophys Res Commun* 1991; 179: 70–7.

116 Botero D, Brown RS. Bioassay of thyrotropin receptor antibodies with Chinese hamster ovary cells transfected with recombinant human thyrotropin receptor: clinical utility in children and adolescents with Graves' disease. *J Pediatr* 1998; 132: 612–18.

117 Brown RS, Cohen JH III, Braverman LE. Successful treatment of massive acute thyroid hormone poisoning with iopanoic acid. *J Pediatr* 1998; 132: 903–5.

118 Rivkees SA, Sklar C, Freemark M. Clinical review 99: the management of Graves' disease in children, with special emphasis on radioiodine treatment. *J Clin Endocrinol Metab* 1998; 83: 3767–76.

119 Collen RJ, Landaw EM, Kaplan SA *et al.* Remission rates of children and adolescents with thyrotoxicosis treated with antithyroid drugs. *Pediatrics* 1980; 65: 550–5.

120 Glaser NS, Styne DM. Predictors of early remission of hyperthyroidism in children. *J Clin Endocrinol Metab* 1997; 82: 1719–32.

121 Hashizume K, Ichikawa K, Sakurai A *et al.* Administration of thyroxine in treated Graves' disease. Effects on the level of antibodies to thyroid-stimulating hormone receptors and on the risk of recurrence of hyperthyroidism. *N Engl J Med* 1991; 324: 947–53.

122 McIver B, Rae P, Beckett G *et al.* Lack of effect of thyroxine in patients with Graves' hyperthyroidism who are treated with an antithyroid drug. *N Engl J Med* 1996; 334: 220–4.

123 Tajiri J, Joguchi S, Murakami T *et al.* Antithyroid drug-induced agranulocytosis: the usefulness of routine white blood cell count monitoring. *Arch Intern Med* 1990; 150: 621–4.

124 Levy WJ, Schumacher OP, Gupta M. Treatment of childhood Graves' disease. *Cleveland Clin J Med* 1988; 55: 373–82.

125 Nikiforov Y, Gnepp DR, Fagin JA. Thyroid lesions in children and adolescents after the Chernobyl disaster: implications for

the study of radiation tumorigenesis. *J Clin Endocrinol Metab* 1996; 81: 9–14.

126 Pacini F, Vorontsova T, Demidchik EP *et al.* Post-Chernobyl thyroid carcinoma in Belarus children and adolescents: Comparison with naturally occurring thyroid carcinoma in Italy and France. *J Clin Endocrinol Metab* 1997; 82: 3563–9.

127 Hung W. Nodular thyroid disease and thyroid carcinoma. *Pediatr Ann* 1992; 21: 50–7.

128 Schlumberger M, De Vathaire F, Travagli JP *et al.* Differentiated thyroid carcinoma in childhood: long term follow-up of 72 patients. *J Clin Endocrinol Metab* 1987; 65: 1088–94.

129 Flannery TK, Kirkland JL, Copeland KC, Bertuch AA, Karaviti LP, Brandt ML. Papillary thyroid cancer: a pediatric perspective. *Pediatrics* 1996; 98: 464–6.

130 Zimmerman D, Hay ID, Gough IR *et al.* Papillary thyroid carcinoma in children and adults: Long-term follow-up of 1039 patients conservatively treated at one institution during three decades. *Surgery* 1988; 104: 1157–66.

131 Ladenson PW, Braverman LE, Mazzaferri EL *et al.* Comparison of administration of recombinant human thyrotropin with withdrawal of thyroid hormone for radioactive iodine scanning in patients with thyroid carcinoma. *N Engl J Med* 1997; 337: 888–96.

132 Wohllk N, Cote GJ, Evans DB, Goepfert H, Ordonez NG, Gagel RF. Application of genetic screening information to the management of medullary thyroid carcinoma and multiple endocrine neoplasia type 2. *Endocrinol Metab Clin N Am* 1996; 25 (1): 1–25.

133 Lairmore TC, Frisella MM, Wells SA Jr. Genetic Testing and early thyroidectomy for inherited medullary thyroid carcinoma. *Ann Med* 1996; 28: 401–6.

134 Zimmerman D. Thyroid neoplasia in children. *Curr Opin Pediatr* 1997; 9: 413–18.

# 21 The adrenal cortex and its disorders

Walter L. Miller

## Embryology, anatomy and history

The adrenal cortex produces three categories of steroid hormones. *Mineralocorticoids*, principally aldosterone, regulate renal retention of sodium, which influences electrolyte balance, intravascular volume and blood pressure. *Glucocorticoids*, principally cortisol, are named for their carbohydrate-mobilizing activity but influence a wide variety of bodily functions. *Adrenal androgens* modulate the mid-childhood growth spurt and regulate some secondary sexual characteristics in women; their overproduction may result in virilism.

### Embryology

The cells of the adrenal cortex are mesodermal, in contrast to the ectodermal adrenal medulla. Between the fifth and sixth week of fetal development, the 'gonadal ridge' develops near the rostral end of the mesonephros. These cells give rise to the steroidogenic cells of the gonads and the adrenal cortex. The adrenal and gonadal cells separate, with the adrenal cells migrating retroperitoneally and the gonadal cells migrating caudally. Between the seventh and eight week, the adrenal cells are invaded by sympathetic neural cells that give rise to the adrenal medulla. By the end of the eight week, the adrenal has become encapsulated and is clearly associated with the upper pole of the kidney, which at this time is much smaller than the adrenal.

The fetal adrenal cortex consists of an outer 'definitive' zone, the principal site of glucocorticoid and mineralocorticoid synthesis and a much larger 'fetal' zone that makes androgenic precursors for the placental synthesis of oestriol. The fetal adrenal gland is huge in proportion to other structures. At birth, the adrenals weigh 8–9 g, roughly twice the size of adult adrenals, and represent 0.5% of total body weight, compared with 0.0175% in the adult.

## Anatomy

The adrenals derive their name from their anatomical location, located on top of the upper pole of each kidney. Unlike most other organs, the arteries and veins serving the adrenal do not run in parallel. Arterial blood is provided by several small arteries arising from the renal and phrenic arteries, the aorta and, sometimes, the ovarian and left spermatic arteries. The veins are more conventional, with the left adrenal vein draining into the left renal vein and the right adrenal vein draining directly into the vena cava. Arterial blood enters the sinusoidal circulation of the cortex and drains towards the medulla, so that medullary chromaffin cells are bathed in very high concentrations of steroid hormones.

The adrenal cortex consists of three histologically recognizable zones: the *glomerulosa* is immediately below the capsule, the *fasciculata* is in the middle and the *reticularis* lies next to the medulla, constituting 15%, 75% and 10%, respectively, of the adrenal cortex in the older child and adult. The zones appear to be distinct functionally as well as histologically but considerable overlap exists, and immunocytochemical data show that the zones physically interdigitate. After birth, the large fetal zone begins to involute and disappears by 1 year of age. The definitive zone simultaneously enlarges, but two of the adult zones, the glomerulosa and the fasciculata, are not fully differentiated until about 3 years of age and the reticularis may not be fully differentiated until about 15 years of age.

## History

The adrenal glands were first described in 1563 by the Italian anatomist Bartolomeo Eustaccio, better known for the eustacian tube of the ear [1]. Medical interest in them as something other than an anatomical curiosity began in the mid-nineteenth century with Addison's classic description of adrenal insufficiency and Brown-Sequard's experimental creation of similar disorders in animals subjected to adrenalectomy. The signs and symptoms of glucocorticoid excess

**Table 21.1.** Physical characteristics of human genes encoding steroidogenic enzymes

| Enzyme | Number of genes | Gene size (kb) | Chromosomal location | Exons (*n*) | mRNA size (kb) |
|---|---|---|---|---|---|
| P450scc | 1 | > 20 | 15q23–q24 | 9 | 2.0 |
| P450c11 | 2 | 9.5 | 8q21–22 | 9 | 4.2 |
| P450c17 | 1 | 6.6 | 10q24.3 | 8 | 1.9 |
| P450c21 | 2 | 3.4 | 6p21.1 | 10 | 2.0 |
| P450aro | 1 | > 52 | 15q21.2 | 10 | 3.5, 2.9 |
| 3β-HSD-I and -II | 2 | 8 | 1p13 | 4 | 1.7 |
| 11β-HSD-I | 1 | 7 | 1 | 6 | 1.6 |
| 11β-HSD-II | 1 | 6.2 | 16p22 | 5 | 1.6 |
| 17β-HSD-I | 2 | 3.3 | 17q21 | 6 | 1.4, 2.4 |
| 17β-HSD-II | 1 | > 40 | 16q24 | 5 | 1.5 |
| 17β-HSD-III | 1 | > 60 | 9q22 | 11 | 1.4 |
| Adrenodoxin | 1 | > 30 | 11q22 | 5 | 1.0, 1.4, 1.7 |
| Adrenodoxin reductase | 1 | 11 | 17q24–q25 | 12 | 2.0 |
| P450 reductase | 1 | < 22 | 7p15→q35 | ? | 2.5 |
| 5α-Reductase – type 1 | 1 | > 35 | 5p15 | 5 | 2.4 |
| 5α-Reductase – type 2 | 1 | > 35 | 2p23 | 5 | 2.4 |

due to adrenal tumours were well known by 1932, when Cushing described the pituitary tumours that cause what is now known as Cushing syndrome [2]. Effects of adrenalectomy on salt and water metabolism were reported in 1927, and by the late 1930s Selye [3] had proposed the terms 'glucocorticoid' and 'mineralocorticoid' to distinguish the two broad categories of actions of adrenal extracts.

Numerous adrenal steroids were painstakingly isolated and their structures determined during the 1930s in the laboratories of Reichstein [4] and Kendall [5], leading to their sharing the 1950 Nobel Prize in medicine. Many of these steroids were synthesized chemically, providing pure material for experimental purposes. The observation in 1949 that glucocorticoids ameliorated the symptoms of rheumatoid arthritis [6] greatly stimulated interest in synthesizing new pharmacologically active analogues of naturally occurring steroids. The structures of the various adrenal steroids suggested precursor–product relationships, leading in 1950 to the first treatment of congenital adrenal hyperplasia with cortisone by both Wilkins [7] and Bartter [8]. This opened a vigorous era of clinical investigation of the pathways of steroidogenesis in a variety of inherited adrenal and gonadal disorders. The association of cytochrome P450 with 21-hydroxylation was made in 1965 [9], and some of the steroidogenic enzymes were then isolated in the 1970s. It was not until the genes for most of these enzymes were cloned in the 1980s that it became clear which proteins participated in which steroidal transformations [10]. The identification of these genes (Table 21.1) then led to an understanding of the genetic lesions causing heritable disorders of steroidogenesis. At the same time, studies of steroid hormone action led to the discovery of steroid hormone receptors in the 1960s, but it was not until they were cloned that their biology was understood [11].

## Steroid hormone synthesis

### Early steps: cholesterol uptake, storage and transport

The adrenal gland can synthesize cholesterol *de novo* from acetate but most of its cholesterol comes from plasma low-density lipoproteins (LDL) derived from dietary cholesterol [12]. Adequate concentrations of LDL will suppress 3-hydroxy-3-methylglutaryl coenzyme A (HMGCoA) reductase, the rate-limiting enzyme in cholesterol synthesis. Adrenocorticotrophic hormone (ACTH), which stimulates adrenal steroidogenesis, also stimulates the activity of HMGCoA reductase, LDL receptors and uptake of LDL-cholesterol. LDL-cholesterol esters are taken up by receptor-mediated endocytosis, and are then stored directly or converted to free cholesterol and used for steroid hormone synthesis [13]. Storage of cholesterol esters in lipid droplets is controlled by the action of two opposing enzymes, cholesterol esterase (cholesterol ester hydrolase) and cholesterol ester synthetase. ACTH stimulates the esterase and inhibits the synthetase, thus increasing the availability of free cholesterol for steroid hormone synthesis [14].

### Steroidogenic enzymes

#### Cytochrome P450

Most steroidogenic enzymes are members of the cytochrome P450 group of oxidases. Cytochrome P450 is a generic term for a large number of oxidative enzymes, all of which have about 500 amino acids and contain a single haem group [15].

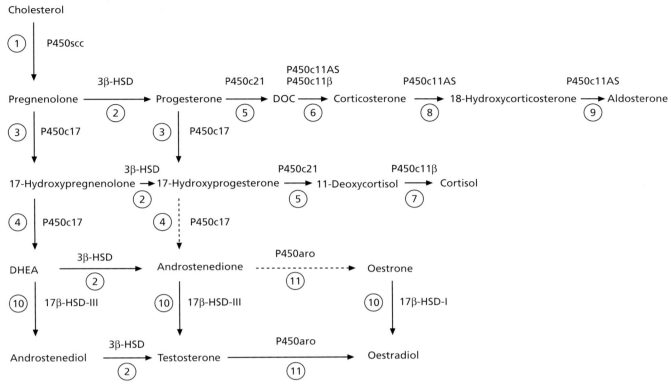

**Fig. 21.1.** Principal pathways of human adrenal steroid hormone synthesis. Other quantitatively and physiologically minor steroids are also produced. The names of the enzymes are shown by each reaction and the traditional names of the enzymatic activities correspond to the circled numbers. Reaction 1, mitochondrial cytochrome P450scc mediates 20α-hydroxylation, 22-hydroxylation and cleavage of the C20–22 carbon bond. Reaction 2, 3β-HSD mediates 3β-hydroxysteroid dehydrogenase and isomerase activities, converting $\Delta^5$ steroids to $\Delta^4$ steroids. Reaction 3, P450c17 catalyses the 17α-hydroxylation of pregnenolone to 17-hydroxy-pregnenolone and of progesterone to 17-OH-progesterone. Reaction 4, the 17,20-lyase activity of P450c17 converts 17-OH-pregnenolone to DHEA; only insignificant amounts of 17-hydroxy-progesterone are converted to $\Delta^4$ androstenedione by human P450c17, although this reaction occurs in other species. Reaction 5, P450c21 catalyses the 21-hydroxylation of progesterone to DOC and of 17-OH-progesterone to 11-deoxycortisol. Reaction 6, DOC is converted to corticosterone by the 11-hydroxylase activity of P450c11AS in the zona glomerulosa and by P450c11β in the zona fasciculata. Reaction 7, 11-deoxycortisol undergoes 11β-hydroxylation by P450c11β to produce cortisol in the zona fasciculata. Reactions 8 and 9, the 18-hydroxylase and 18-oxidase activities of P450c11AS convert corticosterone to 18-OH-corticosterone and aldosterone, respectively, in the zona glomerulosa. Reactions 10 and 11 are found principally in the testes and ovaries. Reaction 10, 17β-HSD-III converts DHEA to androstenediol and androstenedione to testosterone, while 17β-HSD-I converts oestrone to oestradiol. Reaction 11, testosterone may be converted to oestradiol and androstenedione may be converted to oestrone by P450aro.

They are termed P450 (pigment 450) because all absorb light at 450 nm in their reduced states [16]. It is sometimes stated that certain steroidogenic enzymes are P450-dependent enzymes. This is a misnomer, as it implies a generic P450 cofactor to a substrate-specific enzyme; the P450 *is* the enzyme binding the steroidal substrate and catalysing the steroidal conversion on an active site associated with the haem group. Most cytochrome P450 enzymes are found in the endoplasmic reticulum of the liver, where they metabolize countless endogenous and exogenous toxins, drugs, xenobiotics and environmental pollutants. Despite this huge variety of substrates, there are probably fewer than 200 types of cytochrome P450 [15,17,18]. Thus, most, if not all, P450 enzymes can metabolize multiple substrates, catalysing a broad array of oxidations. This theme recurs with each adrenal P450 enzyme.

Five distinct P450 enzymes are involved in adrenal steroido-genesis (Fig. 21.1). P450scc, found in adrenal mitochondria, is the cholesterol side chain cleavage enzyme catalysing the series of reactions formerly termed 20,22-desmolase. Two distinct isozymes of P450c11, P450c11β and P450c11AS, also found in mitochondria, catalyse 11β-hydroxylase, 18-hydroxy-lase and 18-methyl oxidase activities. P450c17, found in the endoplasmic reticulum, catalyses both 17α-hydroxylase and 17,20-lyase activities, and P450c21 catalyses the 21-hydroxy-lation of both glucocorticoids and mineralocorticoids. In the gonads (and elsewhere) P450aro in the endoplasmic reticu-lum catalyses aromatization of androgens to oestrogens.

### Hydroxysteroid dehydrogenases

In addition to the cytochrome P450 enzymes, a second class of enzymes termed hydroxysteroid dehydrogenases (HSDs) is also involved in steroidogenesis [19]. These enzymes have molecular masses of about 35–45 kDa, do not have haem groups and require NAD$^+$ or NADP$^+$ as cofactors. Whereas most steroidogenic reactions catalysed by P450 enzymes are due to the action of a single form of P450, each of the reactions catalysed by HSDs can be catalysed by at least two, often very different, isozymes. Members of this family include the 3α- and 3β-hydroxysteroid dehydrogenases, the two 11β-hydroxysteroid dehydrogenases and a series of 17β-hydroxysteroid dehydrogenases; the 5α-reductases are unrelated to this family.

## P450scc

Conversion of cholesterol to pregnenolone in mitochondria is the first, rate-limiting and hormonally regulated step in the synthesis of all steroid hormones. This involves three distinct chemical reactions, 20α-hydroxylation, 22-hydroxylation and cleavage of the cholesterol side chain to yield pregnenolone and isocaproic acid. Early studies showed that 20-hydroxycholesterol, 22-hydroxycholesterol and 20,22-hydroxycholesterol could all be isolated from adrenals in significant quantities, suggesting that three separate and distinct enzymes were involved. However, protein purification studies and *in vitro* reconstitution of enzymatic activity show that a single protein, termed P450scc (where scc refers to the *s*ide *c*hain *c*leavage of cholesterol) encoded by a single gene on chromosome 15 [20], catalyses all the steps between cholesterol and pregnenolone [21–23]. These three reactions occur on a single active site [24] that is in contact with the hydrophobic bilayer membrane [16]. Deletion of the gene for P450scc in the rabbit eliminates all steroidogenesis [25], indicating that all steroidogenesis is initiated by this one enzyme.

### Transport of electrons to P450scc: adrenodoxin reductase and adrenodoxin

P450scc functions as the terminal oxidase in a mitochondrial electron transport system. Electrons from NADPH (reduced form of nicotinamide adenine dinucleotide phosphate) are accepted by a flavoprotein, termed adrenodoxin reductase, that is loosely associated with the inner mitochondrial membrane [26]. Adrenodoxin reductase transfers the electrons to an iron–sulphur protein termed adrenodoxin, which is found in the mitochondrial matrix [27] or loosely adherent to the inner mitochondrial membrane [28]. Adrenodoxin then transfers the electrons to P450scc (Fig. 21.2). Adrenodoxin reductase and adrenodoxin serve as generic electron transport proteins for all mitochondrial P450s and not just for those involved in steroidogenesis; hence, these proteins are also termed ferredoxin oxidoreductase and ferredoxin. Adrenodoxin forms a 1:1 complex with adrenodoxin reductase, then dissociates, then subsequently reforms an analogous 1:1 complex with P450scc or P450c11, thus functioning as an

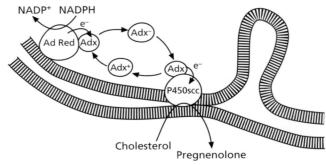

**Fig. 21.2.** Electron transport to mitochondrial forms of cytochrome P450. Adrenodoxin reductase (Ad Red), a flavoprotein loosely bound to the inner mitochondrial membrane, accepts electrons (e$^-$) from NADPH, converting it to NADP$^+$. These electrons are passed to adrenodoxin (Adx), an iron–sulphur protein in solution in the mitochondrial matrix that functions as a freely diffusible electron shuttle mechanism. Electrons from charged adrenodoxin (Adx$^-$) are accepted by any available cytochrome P450 such as P450c11 or P450scc shown here. The uncharged adrenodoxin (Adx$^+$) may then be again bound to adrenodoxin reductase to receive another pair of electrons. For P450scc, three pairs of electrons must be transported to the P450 to convert cholesterol to pregnenolone. The flow of cholesterol into the mitochondria is facilitated by StAR, which is not shown in this diagram.

indiscriminate diffusible electron shuttle mechanism [29–31]. Adrenodoxin reductase is a membrane-bound mitochondrial flavoprotein that receives electrons from NADPH [26]. The single human adrenodoxin reductase gene [32,33] and the single functional adrenodoxin gene [34] are expressed in all human tissues [35,36], indicating that there are generic mitochondrial electron transfer proteins whose roles are not limited to steroidogenesis.

### Cholesterol transport into mitochondria

The chronic regulation of steroidogenesis by ACTH is at the level of gene transcription [37,38], but the acute regulation, where cortisol is released within minutes of a stimulus, is at the level of cholesterol access to P450scc. When either steroidogenic cells or intact rats are treated with inhibitors of protein synthesis, such as cycloheximide, the acute steroidogenic response is eliminated, suggesting that a short-lived, cycloheximide-sensitive protein acts at the level of the mitochondrion [23] as the specific trigger to the acute steroidogenic response [39,40]. Several candidate factors were proposed for this acute trigger, including the so-called steroidogenesis activator peptide (SAP), SCP-2, the peripheral benzodiazepine receptor complex (PBR) and its endogenous ligand, endozepine (also termed diazepam-binding inhibitor, DBI) (for review see [41]). The role of the PBR/endozepine system remains uncertain; substantial data indicate that this system participates in the slow, chronic delivery of cholesterol to the inner mitochondrial membrane (for review see [42]) but it is clear that the 'acute trigger' of steroidogenesis is the steroidogenic acute regulatory protein (StAR) [41].

StAR was first identified as short-lived 30- and 37-kDa phosphoproteins that were rapidly synthesized when steroidogenic cells were stimulated with trophic hormones [43–45]. Mouse StAR was then cloned from Leydig MA-10 cells in 1994 and could induce steroidogenesis when transfected back into these cells [46]. The central role of StAR was definitively proven by showing that it promoted steroidogenesis in non-steroidogenic COS-1 cells co-transfected with StAR and the cholesterol side chain cleavage enzyme system and by finding that mutations of StAR caused congenital lipoid adrenal hyperplasia [47]. Thus StAR is the acute trigger that is required for the rapid flux of cholesterol from the outer to the inner mitochondrial membrane, which is needed for the acute response of aldosterone to angiotensia II, of cortisol to ACTH and of sex steroids to an LH pulse.

Some steroidogenesis is independent of StAR; when non-steroidogenic cells are transfected with StAR and the P450scc system, they convert cholesterol to pregnenolone at about 14% of the StAR-induced rate [47,48]. Furthermore, some steroidogenic tissues, including the placenta and the brain, utilize mitochondrial P450scc to initiate steroidogenesis [49,50] but do not express StAR [51]. The mechanism of StAR-independent steroidogenesis is unknown. It is possible that it occurs spontaneously, without any triggering protein, or that some other protein may exert StAR-like activity to promote cholesterol flux without StAR's rapid kinetics. The mechanism of StAR's action is unknown, but it is clear that StAR acts on the outer mitochondrial membrane and does not need to enter the mitochondria to be active, as deletion of up to 62 N-terminal residues confines StAR to the cytoplasm without reducing activity [52,53]. StAR appears to undergo structural changes while interacting with the outer mitochondrial membrane [54].

## 3β-Hydroxysteroid dehydrogenase/$\Delta^5 \rightarrow \Delta^4$ isomerase

Once pregnenolone is produced from cholesterol, it may undergo 17α-hydroxylation by P450c17 to yield 17-hydroxypregnenolone or it may be converted to progesterone, the first biologically important steroid in the pathway. A single 42-kDa microsomal enzyme, 3β-hydroxysteroid dehydrogenase (3β-HSD) catalyses both the conversion of the hydroxyl group to a keto group on carbon 3 and the isomerization of the double bond from the B ring ($\Delta^5$ steroids) to the A ring ($\Delta^4$ steroids) [55–57]. Thus a single enzyme converts pregnenolone to progesterone, 17α-hydroxypregnenolone to 17α-hydroxyprogesterone, dehydroepiandrosterone (DHEA) to androstenedione and androstenediol to testosterone. As is typical of hydroxysteroid dehydrogenases, there are two isozymes of 3β-HSD, encoded by separate genes. The enzyme catalysing 3β-HSD activity in the adrenals and gonads is the type II enzyme [58,59]; the type I enzyme, encoded by a closely linked gene with identical intron/exon organization, catalyses 3β-HSD activity in placenta, breast and 'extraglandular' tissues enzyme [58,60].

## P450c17

Both pregnenolone and progesterone may undergo 17α-hydroxylation, to 17α-hydroxypregnenolone and 17α-hydroxyprogesterone (17-OHP) respectively. 17α-Hydroxyprogesterone may also undergo cleavage of the C17,20 carbon bond to yield dehydroepiandrosterone (DHEA); however, very little 17-OHP is converted to androstenedione because the human P450c17 enzyme catalyses this reaction at only 3% of the rate for conversion of 17α-hydroxypregnenolone to DHEA [61,62]. These reactions are all mediated by P450c17. This P450 is bound to smooth endoplasmic reticulum, where it accepts electrons from a P450 oxidoreductase. As P450c17 has both 17α-hydroxylase activity and C-17,20-lyase activity, it is the key branch point in steroid hormone synthesis. If neither activity of P450c17 is present, pregnenolone is converted to mineralocorticoids; if 17α-hydroxylase activity is present but 17,20-lyase activity is not, pregnenolone is converted to cortisol; if both activities are present, pregnenolone is converted to sex steroids (Fig. 21.1).

17α-Hydroxylase and 17,20 were once thought to be separate enzymes. The adrenals of prepubertal children synthesize ample cortisol but virtually no sex steroids (i.e. they have 17α-hydroxylase activity but not 17,20-lyase activity), until adrenarche initiates production of adrenal androgens (i.e. turns on 17,20-lyase activity) [63]. Furthermore, patients have been described lacking 17,20-lyase activity but retaining normal 17α-hydroxylase activity [64]. However, purification of pig testicular microsomal P450c17 to homogeneity and *in vitro* reconstitution of enzymatic activity show that both 17α-hydroxylase and 17,20-lyase activities reside in a single protein [65,66], and cells transformed with a vector expressing P450c17 cDNA acquire both 17α-hydroxylase and 17,20-lyase activities [67,68]. P450c17 is encoded by a single gene on chromosome 10q24.3 [69,70] that is structurally related to the genes for P450c21 (21-hydroxylase) [71].

Thus, the distinction between 17α-hydroxylase and 17,20-lyase is functional and not genetic or structural. The factors involved in determining whether a steroid molecule will remain on the single active site of P450c17 and undergo 17,20 bond cleavage after 17α-hydroxylation remains unknown. P450c17 prefers $\Delta^5$ substrates, especially for 17,20 bond cleavage, consistent with the large amounts of DHEA secreted by both the fetal and adult adrenal. Furthermore, the 17α-hydroxylase reaction occurs more readily than the 17,20-lyase reaction. An additional important factor is the abundance of electron donors for P450c17.

## Electron transport to P450c17: P450 oxidoreductase and cytochrome b₅

P450c17 (and P450c21) receive electrons from a membrane-bound flavoprotein, termed P450 oxidoreductase, which is a

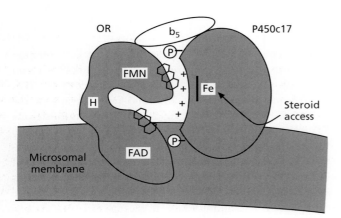

**Fig. 21.3.** Electron transport to microsomal forms of cytochrome P450. This figure shows the interactions of P450c17 with its redox partners; the interactions of other P450 proteins may be simpler, as most microsomal P450 proteins are not phosphorylated and do not interact with cytochrome $b_5$. The FAD moiety of P450 oxidoreductase (OR) picks up electrons from NADPH (not shown) and transfers them to its FMN (flavin mononucleotide) moiety. The FAD and FMN groups are in distinct protein domains connected by a flexible protein hinge (H). The FMN domain approaches the redox partner binding site of the P450, shown as a concave region. The active site containing the steroid lies on the side of the plane of the haem ring (Fe) opposite from the redox partner binding site. Cytochrome $b_5$ allosterically facilitates the interaction between OR and P450c17 to favour 17,20-lyase activity. Phosphoserine residues (P) also promote 17,20-lyase activity.

different protein from the mitochondrial flavoprotein, adrenodoxin reductase. P450 oxidoreductase receives two electrons from NADPH and transfers them one at a time to the P450 [72,73]. The first electron is transferred rapidly but transfer of the second is slow [74]. Electron transfer for the lyase reaction is promoted by the action of cytochrome $b_5$ as an allosteric factor rather than as an alternative electron donor [62]. 17,20-Lyase activity also requires the phosphorylation of serine residues on P450c17 by a cyclic adenosine monophosphate (cAMP)-dependent protein kinase [75] (Fig. 21.3). Because the adrenal endoplasmic reticulum contains many more molecules of P450c17 and of P450c21 than of P450 oxidoreductase, the P450s compete with one another for the reducing equivalents provided by the reductase.

The availability of electrons appears to determine whether P450c17 performs only 17α-hydroxylation or also performs 17,20 bond cleavage, as increasing the ratio of P450 oxidoreductase or cytochrome $b_5$ to P450c17 *in vitro* or *in vivo* increases the ratio of 17,20-lyase activity to 17α-hydroxylase activity. Competition between P450c17 and P450c21 for available 17-hydroxyprogesterone does not appear to be important in determining whether 17-OHP undergoes 21-hydroxylation or 17,20 bond cleavage [76]. However, increasing the ratio of P450 oxidoreductase to P450c17 increases 17,20-lyase activity (the testis contains three to four times more P450 oxidoreductase activity than does the adrenal).

Thus, the regulation of 17,20-lyase activity, and consequently of DHEA production, depends on factors that facilitate the flow of electrons to P450c17. These are high concentrations of P450 oxidoreductase, the presence of cytochrome $b_5$ and serine phosphorylation of P450c17 [77].

## P450c21

After the synthesis of progesterone and 17-hydroxyprogesterone, these steroids are hydroxylated at the 21 position to yield deoxycorticosterone (DOC) and 11-deoxycortisol respectively (Fig. 21.1). The nature of the 21-hydroxylating step has been of great clinical interest because disordered 21-hydroxylation causes more than 90% of all cases of congenital adrenal hyperplasia. The clinical symptoms associated with this common genetic disease are complex and devastating. Decreased cortisol and aldosterone synthesis often lead to sodium loss, potassium retention and hypotension, which will lead to cardiovascular collapse and death within the month after birth if not treated appropriately. Decreased synthesis of cortisol *in utero* leads to overproduction of ACTH and consequent overstimulation of adrenal steroid synthesis; as the 21-hydroxylase step is impaired, 17-OHP accumulates because P450c17 converts only miniscule amounts of 17-OHP to androstenedione. However, 17-hydroxypregnenolone also accumulates and is converted to DHEA and subsequently to androstenedione and testosterone, resulting in severe prenatal virilization of female fetuses [78–80].

Congenital adrenal hyperplasia (CAH) has been extensively studied clinically. Variations in the manifestations of the disease, and especially the number of patients without apparent defects in mineralocorticoid activity, suggested that there were two separate 21-hydroxylating enzymes that were differentially expressed in the zones of the adrenal specifically synthesizing aldosterone or cortisol. However, characterization of the P450c21 protein [81] and gene cloning show that there is only one 21-hydroxylase encoded by a single functional gene on chromosome 6p21 [82–84]. As this gene lies in the middle of the major histocompatibility locus, disorders of adrenal 21-hydroxylation are closely linked to specific human leucocyte antigen (HLA) types [85].

Adrenal 21-hydroxylation is mediated by P450c21 found in smooth endoplasmic reticulum. P450c21 uses the same P450 oxidoreductase used by P450c17 to transport electrons from NADPH. 21-Hydroxylase activity has also been described in a broad range of adult and fetal extra-adrenal tissues [86]. However, extra-adrenal 21-hydroxylation is not mediated by the P450c21 enzyme found in the adrenal [87]; the nature of the enzyme(s) responsible for extra-adrenal 21-hydroxylation is unknown. As a result, patients having absent adrenal 21-hydroxylase activity may still have appreciable concentrations of 21-hydroxylated steroids in their plasma.

## P450c11β and P450c11AS

Two closely related enzymes, P450c11β and P450c11AS, catalyse the final steps in the synthesis of both glucocorticoids and mineralocorticoids [88,89]. These two isozymes have 93% amino acid sequence identity [90] and are encoded by tandemly duplicated genes on chromosome 8q21–22 [91]. Like P450scc, the two forms of P450c11 are found on the inner mitochondrial membrane and use adrenodoxin and adrenodoxin reductase to receive electrons from NADPH [92]. By far the more abundant of the two isozymes is P450c11β, which is the classic 11β-hydroxylase that converts 11-deoxycortisol to cortisol and 11-deoxycorticosterone to corticosterone. The less abundant isozyme, P450c11AS, is found only in the zona glomerulosa, where it has 11β-hydroxylase, 18-hydroxylase and 18-methyl oxidase (aldosterone synthase) activities; thus P450c11AS is able to catalyse all the reactions needed to convert DOC to aldosterone [93,94].

P450c11β, which is principally involved in synthesis of cortisol, is encoded by a gene (*CYP11B1*) primarily induced by ACTH via cAMP and suppressed by glucocorticoids such as dexamethasone. The existence of two distinct functional genes is confirmed by the identification of mutations in each that cause distinct genetic disorders of steroidogenesis. Thus patients with disorders in P450c11β have classic-11β-hydroxylase deficiency but can still produce aldosterone [95], whereas patients with disorders in P450c11AS have rare forms of aldosterone deficiency (so-called corticosterone methyl oxidase deficiency) while retaining the ability to produce cortisol [96–98].

## 17β-Hydroxysteroid dehydrogenase

Androstenedione is converted to testosterone, DHEA to androstenediol and oestrone to oestradiol by a series of short-chain dehydrogenases called 17β-hydroxysteroid dehydrogenases (17β-HSDs), sometimes also termed 17-oxidoreductase or 17-ketosteroid reductase [99,100]. The terminology for this enzyme varies, as this is the only readily reversible step in steroidogenesis; hence, different names are used for a single enzyme, depending on the direction of the reaction being studied. This is the most complex and confusing step in steroidogenesis because there are several different 17β-HSDs: some are preferential oxidases whereas others are preferential reductases, they differ in their substrate preference and sites of expression, there is inconsistent nomenclature, especially with the rodent enzymes, and some proteins termed 17β-HSD actually have very little 17β-HSD activity and are principally involved in other reactions [19].

Type I 17β-HSD (17β-HSD-I), also known as oestrogenic 17β-HSD, is a cytosolic protein first isolated and cloned from the placenta, where it produces oestriol, and is expressed in ovarian granulosa cells, where it produces oestradiol [56,101–103]. 17β-HSD-I uses NADPH as its cofactor to catalyse its

reductase activity. The three-dimensional structure of human 17β-HSD-I has been determined by X-ray crystallography [104,105]. No genetic deficiency syndrome for 17β-HSD-I has been described.

17β-HSD-II is a microsomal oxidase that uses NAD$^+$ to inactivate oestradiol to oestrone and testosterone to $\Delta^4$ androstenedione. 17β-HSD-II is found in the placenta, liver, small intestine, prostate, secretory endometrium and ovary. In contrast to 17β-HSD-I, which is found in placental synctiotrophoblast cells, 17β-HSD-II is expressed in endothelial cells of placental intravillous vessels, consistent with its apparent role in defending the fetal circulation from transplacental passage of maternal oestradiol or testosterone [106]. No deficiency state for 17β-HSD-II has been reported.

17β-HSD-III, the androgenic form of 17β-HSD, is a microsomal enzyme that is apparently expressed only in the testis [107]. This is the enzyme that is disordered in the classic syndrome of male pseudohermaphroditism, which is often termed 17-ketosteroid reductase deficiency [107,108].

An enzyme termed 17β-HSD-IV was initially identified as an NAD$^+$-dependent oxidase with activities similar to 17β-HSD-II [109], but this peroxisomal protein is primarily an enoyl-CoA hydratase and 3-hydroxyacyl-CoA dehydrogenase [110,111]. 17β-HSD-V, originally cloned as a 3α-hydroxysteroid dehydrogenase [112], catalyses the reduction of $\Delta^4$ androstenedione to testosterone [113], but its precise role is unclear and no deficiency state has been described.

## Steroid sulphotransferase and sulphatase

Steroid sulphates may be synthesized directly from cholesterol sulphate or may be formed by sulphation of steroids by cytosolic sulphotransferases. Steroid sulphates may also be hydrolysed to the native steroid by steroid sulphatase. Deletions in the steroid sulphatase gene on chromosome Xp22.3 cause X-linked ichthyosis [114,115]. In the fetal adrenal and placenta, diminished or absent sulphatase deficiency reduces the pool of free DHEA available for placental conversion to oestrogen, resulting in low concentrations of oestriol in the maternal blood and urine. The accumulation of steroid sulphates in the stratum corneum of the skin causes the ichthyosis. Steroid sulphatase is also expressed in the fetal rodent brain, possibly converting peripheral DHEAS to active DHEA [116,117].

## Aromatase: P450aro

Oestrogens are produced by the aromatization of androgens, including adrenal androgens, by a complex series of reactions catalysed by a single microsomal aromatase, P450aro [118,119]. This typical cytochrome P450 is encoded by a single, large gene on chromosome 15q21.1. This gene uses several different promoter sequences, transcriptional start sites and alternatively chosen first exons to encode aromatase mRNA in different tissues under different hormonal regulation. Aromatase expression in the extraglandular tissues, especially adipose tissue, can covert adrenal androgens to oestrogens. Aromatase in the epiphyses of growing bone can convert testosterone to oestradiol, accelerating epiphyseal maturation and terminating growth [119]. Although it has traditionally been thought that aromatase activity is needed for embryonic and fetal development, infants and adults with genetic disorders in this enzyme have been described recently, showing that fetoplacental oestrogen is not needed for normal fetal development [120,121].

## 5α-Reductase

Testosterone is converted to the more potent androgen dihydrotestosterone by 5α-reductase, an enzyme found in testosterone's target tissues. There are two distinct forms of 5α-reductase. The type I enzyme, found in the scalp and other peripheral tissues, is encoded by a gene on chromosome 5; the type II enzyme, the predominant form found in male reproductive tissues, is encoded by a structurally related gene on chromosome 2p23 [122]. The syndrome of 5α-reductase deficiency, a disorder of male sexual differentiation, is due to a wide variety of mutations in the gene encoding the type II enzyme [123]. The type 1 and 2 genes show an unusual pattern of developmental regulation of expression. The type 1 gene is not expressed in the fetus; it is expressed briefly in the skin of the newborn and then remains unexpressed until its activity and protein are again found after puberty. The type 2 gene is expressed in fetal genital skin, in the normal prostate and in prostatic hyperplasia and adenocarcinoma. Thus, the type I enzyme may be responsible for the pubertal virilization seen in patients with classic 5α-reductase deficiency and the type II enzyme may be involved in male pattern baldness [122].

## 11β-Hydroxysteroid dehydrogenase

Although certain steroids are categorized as glucocorticoids or mineralocorticoids, cloning and expression of the 'mineralocorticoid' (glucocorticoid type II) receptor shows that it has equal affinity for both aldosterone and cortisol [124]. However, cortisol does not act as a mineralocorticoid *in vivo*, even though cortisol concentrations can exceed aldosterone concentrations by 100- to 1000-fold. In mineralocorticoid-responsive tissues, such as the kidney, cortisol is enzymatically converted to cortisone, a metabolically inactive steroid [125]. The interconversion of cortisol and cortisone is mediated by two isozymes of 11β-hydroxysteroid dehydrogenase (11β-HSD), each of which has both oxidase and reductase activity, depending on the cofactor available [126].

The type I enzyme (11β-HSD-I) is expressed mainly in glucocorticoid-responsive tissues, such as the liver, testis, lung and proximal convoluted tubule. 11β-HSD-I can catalyse both the oxidation of cortisol to cortisone using $NADP^+$ as its cofactor ($K_m$ 1.6 μM), or the reduction of cortisone to cortisol using NADPH as its cofactor ($K_m$ 0.14 μM); the reaction catalysed depends on which cofactor is available, but the enzyme can only function with high (micromolar) concentrations of steroid [127,128]. 11β-HSD-II catalyses only the oxidation of cortisol to cortisone using NADH and can function with low (nanomolar) concentrations of steroid ($K_m$ 10–100 nM) [129,130]. 11β-HSD-II is expressed in mineralocorticoid-responsive tissues and thus serves to 'defend' the mineralocorticoid receptor by inactivating cortisol to cortisone, so that only 'true' mineralocorticoids, such as aldosterone or deoxycorticosterone, can exert a mineralocorticoid effect. Thus, 11β-HSD-II prevents cortisol from overwhelming renal mineralocorticoid receptors [125], and in the placenta and other fetal tissues 11β-HSD-II [131,132] also inactivates cortisol. The placenta also has abundant $NADP^+$, favouring the oxidative action of 11β-HSD-I, so that in placenta both enzymes protect the fetus from high maternal concentrations of cortisol [126].

## Fetal adrenal steroidogenesis

Adrenocortical steroidogenesis begins early in embryonic life, probably around week 6 of gestation. Fetuses affected with genetic lesions in adrenal steroidogenesis can produce adrenal androgen sufficient to virilize a female fetus to a nearly male appearance, and this masculinization of the genitalia is complete by the twelfth week of gestation [79,133]. The definitive zone of the fetal adrenal produces steroid hormones according to the pathways in Fig. 21.1. By contrast, the large fetal zone of the adrenal is relatively deficient in 3β-HSD-II activity because it contains very little mRNA for this enzyme [134]. The fetal adrenal has relatively abundant 17,20-lyase activity of P450c17; low 3β-HSD and high 17,20-lyase activity account for the huge amount of DHEA and its sulphate (DHEAS) produced by the fetal adrenal for conversion to oestrogens by the placenta.

The fetal adrenal has considerable sulphotransferase activity but little steroid sulphatase activity, also favouring conversion of DHEA to DHEAS. The resulting DHEAS cannot be a substrate for adrenal 3β-HSD-II; instead, it is secreted, 16α-hydroxylated in the fetal liver and then acted on by placental 3β-HSD-I, 17β-HSD-I and P450aro to produce oestriol; the substrates can also bypass the liver to yield oestrone and oestradiol. Placental oestrogens inhibit adrenal 3β-HSD activity, providing a feedback system to promote production of DHEAS [135]. Fetal adrenal steroids account for 50% of the oestrone and oestradiol and 90% of the oestriol in the maternal circulation.

Although the fetoplacental unit produces huge amounts of DHEA, DHEAS and oestriol, as well as other steroids, they do not appear to serve an essential role. Successful pregnancy is wholly dependent on placental synthesis of progesterone, which suppresses uterine contractility and prevents spontaneous abortion, but fetuses with genetic disorders of adrenal and gonadal steroidogenesis develop normally, reach term gestation and undergo normal delivery.

Mineralocorticoid production is required postnatally, oestrogens are not required and androgens are needed only for male sexual differentiation [136]. It is not clear if human fetal development requires glucocorticoids, but, if so, the small amount of maternal cortisol that escapes placental inactivation suffices [136–138].

The regulation of steroidogenesis and growth of the fetal adrenal are not fully understood, but both are related to ACTH. ACTH effectively stimulates steroidogenesis by fetal adrenal cells *in vitro* [139,140], and excess ACTH is clearly involved in the adrenal growth and overproduction of androgens in fetuses affected with congenital adrenal hyperplasia. Prenatal treatment of such fetuses by orally administering dexamethasone to the mother at 6–10 weeks' gestation can significantly reduce fetal adrenal androgen production and thus reduce the virilization of female fetuses.

The hypothalamo-pituitary-adrenal axis functions very early in fetal life [141], but anencephalic fetuses, which lack pituitary ACTH, have adrenals that contain a fairly normal complement of steroidogenic enzymes and retain their capacity for steroidogenesis. Thus, it appears that fetal adrenal steroidogenesis is regulated by both ACTH-dependent and ACTH-independent mechanisms.

## Regulation of steroidogenesis

### The hypothalamo-pituitary-adrenal axis

The principal steroidal product of the human adrenal is cortisol, which is mainly secreted in response to ACTH (corticotrophin) produced in the pituitary; secretion of ACTH is stimulated mainly by corticotrophin-releasing factor (CRH) from the hypothalamus. Hypothalamic CRH is a 41-amino-acid peptide synthesized mainly by neurones in the paraventricular nucleus. These same hypothalamic neurones also produce arginine vasopressin (AVP, also known as antidiuretic hor-

mone or ADH) [142]. Both CRH and AVP are proteolytically derived from larger precursors with the AVP precursor containing the sequence for neurophysin, which is the AVP-binding protein. CRH and AVP travel through axons to the median eminence, which releases them into the pituitary portal circulation, although most AVP axons terminate in the posterior pituitary [143]. Both CRH and AVP stimulate the synthesis and release of ACTH, but they appear to do so by different mechanisms. CRH functions principally by receptors linked to the protein kinase A pathway, stimulating production of intracellular cAMP, whereas AVP appears to function via protein kinase C and intracellular $Ca^{2+}$ [144]. It is fairly clear that CRH is the more important physiological stimulator of ACTH release, although maximal doses of AVP can elicit a maximal ACTH response. When given together, CRH and AVP act synergistically, as would be expected from their independent mechanisms of action.

### ACTH and POMC

Pituitary ACTH is a 39-amino-acid peptide derived from pro-opiomelanocortin (POMC), a 241-amino-acid protein. POMC undergoes a series of proteolytic cleavages, yielding several biologically active peptides [145,146] (Fig. 21.4). The N-terminal glycopeptide (POMC 1–75) can stimulate steroidogenesis and may function as an adrenal mitogen [147]. POMC 112–150 is ACTH 1–39; POMC 112–126 and POMC 191–207 constitute α- and β-MSH (melanocyte-stimulating hormone) respectively. POMC 210–241 is β-endorphin. POMC is produced in small amounts by the brain, testis and placenta, but this extrapituitary POMC does not contribute significantly to circulating ACTH. Malignant tumours will commonly produce 'ectopic ACTH' in adults and rarely in children; this ACTH derives from ectopic biosynthesis of the same POMC precursor [145]. Only the first 20–24 amino acids of ACTH are needed for its full biological activity, and synthetic ACTH 1–24 is widely used in diagnostic tests of adrenal function. The shorter forms of ACTH have a shorter half-life than does native ACTH 1–39. POMC gene transcription is stimulated by CRH and is inhibited by glucocorticoids [148].

**Fig. 21.4.** Structure of human prepro-opiomelanocortin. The numbers refer to amino acid positions, with no. 1 assigned to the first amino acid of POMC after the 26-amino-acid signal peptide. The α-, β- and γ-MSH regions, which characterize the three 'constant' regions, are indicated by *diagonal lines*; the 'variable' regions are *solid*. The amino acid numbers shown refer to the N-terminal amino acid of each cleavage site; because these amino acids are removed, the numbers do not correspond exactly with the amino acid numbers of the peptides as used in the test. CLIP, corticotrophin-like intermediate lobe peptide.

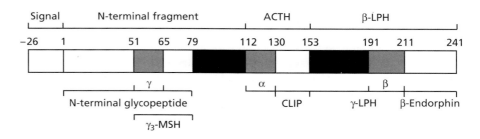

## Actions of ACTH

ACTH stimulates steroidogenesis by interacting with receptors that stimulate the production of cAMP, which elicits acute and long-term effects. ACTH, acting via cAMP, stimulates the biosynthesis of LDL receptors and the uptake of LDL, which provides most of the cholesterol used for steroidogenesis [12]. ACTH via cAMP also stimulates transcription of the gene for HMGCoA reductase, the rate-limiting step in cholesterol biosynthesis, but adrenal biosynthesis of cholesterol is quantitatively much less important than the uptake of LDL-cholesterol [13].

Cholesterol is stored in steroidogenic tissues as cholesterol esters in lipid droplets. ACTH stimulates the activity of cholesterol esterase while inhibiting cholesterol ester synthetase, thus increasing the intracellular pool of free cholesterol, the substrate for P450scc [14,149]. The esterase is similar to gastric and lingual lipases [150]. Finally, ACTH facilitates transport of cholesterol into mitochondria, by stimulating the synthesis and phosphorylation of StAR, thus increasing the flow of free cholesterol into the mitochondria. All of these actions occur within minutes and constitute the acute effect of ACTH on steroidogenesis. The adrenal contains relatively modest amounts of steroid hormones; thus, release of preformed cortisol does not contribute significantly to the acute response to ACTH, which occurs by the rapid provision of large supplies of cholesterol to mitochondrial P450scc [41,151].

Long-term chronic effects of ACTH are mediated directly at the level of the steroidogenic enzymes. ACTH via cAMP stimulates the accumulation of the steroidogenic enzymes and their mRNAs by stimulating the transcription of their genes [38]. Thus, ACTH increases both the uptake of the cholesterol substrate and its conversion to steroidal products. The stimulation of this steroidogenesis occurs at each step in the pathway, not only at the rate-limiting step, P450scc.

The role of ACTH and other peptides derived from POMC in stimulating growth of the adult adrenal remain uncertain [152,153]. However, in the fetal adrenal, ACTH stimulates the local production of insulin-like growth factor II [140,154], basic fibroblast growth factor [155] and epidermal growth factor [156]. These, and possibly other factors, work together to mediate ACTH-induced growth of the fetal adrenal [157].

## Diurnal rhythms of ACTH and cortisol

Plasma concentrations of ACTH and cortisol are high in the morning and low in the evening. Peak ACTH levels are usually seen at 04.00–06.00 h and peak cortisol levels follow at about 08.00 h. Both ACTH and cortisol are released episodically in pulses every 30–120 min throughout the day, but the frequency and amplitude is greater in the morning. The basis of this diurnal rhythm is complex and poorly understood. The hypothalamic content of CRH itself shows a diurnal rhythm, with peak content at about 04.00 h. At least four factors appear to play a role in the rhythm of ACTH and cortisol. These interdependent factors include intrinsic rhythmicity of synthesis and secretion of CRH by the hypothalamus, light–dark cycles, feeding and inherent rhythmicity in the adrenal, possibly mediated by adrenal innervation [158].

Dietary rhythms may play as large a role as light–dark cycles [159,160], since animal experiments show that altering the time of feeding can overcome the ACTH/cortisol periodicity established by a light–dark cycle. In normal human subjects, cortisol is released before lunch and supper but not at these times in persons eating continuously during the day. Thus, glucocorticoids, which increase blood glucose, appear to be released at times of fasting and are inhibited by feeding [161,162].

As all parents know, infants do not have a diurnal rhythm of sleep or feeding. They acquire such behavioural rhythms in response to the environment long before they acquire a rhythm of ACTH and cortisol. The diurnal rhythms begin to be established at 6–12 months but are often not well established until after 3 years of age [163]. Once the rhythm is well established in the older child or adult, it is changed only with difficulty. When people move time zones, their ACTH/cortisol rhythms generally take 15–20 days to adjust.

Physical stress (major surgery, severe trauma, blood loss, high fever or serious illness) increases the secretion of both ACTH and cortisol, but minor surgery and minor illnesses (upper respiratory infections) have little effect [164,165]. Infection, fever and pyrogens can stimulate the release of interleukin 1 (IL-1) and IL-6, which stimulate secretion of CRH, and also IL-2 and tumour necrosis factor (TNF), which stimulate release of ACTH, providing further stimulus to cortisol secretion during inflammation [166]. Most psychoactive drugs, such as anticonvulsants, neurotransmitters and antidepressants, do not affect the diurnal rhythm of ACTH and cortisol, although cyproheptidine (a serotonin antagonist) suppresses ACTH release.

## Adrenal: glucocorticoid feedback

The hypothalamo-pituitary-adrenal axis is a classic example of an endocrine feedback system. ACTH increases production of cortisol and cortisol decreases production of CRH and ACTH [148,167]. Like the acute and chronic phases of the action of ACTH on the adrenal, there are acute and chronic phases of the feedback inhibition of ACTH (and presumably CRH) [167]. The acute phase, which occurs within minutes, inhibits release of ACTH (and CRH) from secretory granules. With prolonged exposure, glucocorticoids inhibit ACTH synthesis by directly inhibiting the transcription of the gene for POMC. Some evidence also suggests that glucocorticoids can inhibit steroidogenesis at the level of the adrenal fasciculata cell itself, but this appears to be a physiologically minor component of the regulation of cortisol secretion.

## Mineralocorticoid secretion: the renin–angiotensin system

Renin is a serine protease enzyme synthesized primarily by the juxtaglomerular cells of the kidney. It is also produced in a variety of other tissues, including the glomerulosa cells of the adrenal cortex [168]. The role of adrenally produced renin is not well established; it appears to maintain basal levels of P450c11AS, but it is not known whether angiotensin II is involved in this action [169]. Renin is synthesized as a precursor (406 amino acids) that is cleaved to pro-renin (386 amino acids) and finally to the 340-amino-acid protein found in plasma [170]. Decreased blood pressure, upright posture, sodium depletion, vasodilatory drugs, kallikrein, opiates and β-adrenergic stimulation all promote release of renin. Renin enzymatically attacks angiotensinogen, the renin substrate, in the circulation.

Angiotensinogen is a highly glycosolated protein and therefore has a highly variable molecular weight, from 50 000 to 100 000 Da. Renin proteolytically releases the amino-terminal 10 amino acids of angiotensinogen, referred to as angiotensin I. This decapeptide is biologically inactive until converting enzyme, an enzyme found primarily in the lungs and blood vessels, cleaves off its two carboxy-terminal amino acids, to produce an octapeptide termed angiotensin II. Converting enzyme can be inhibited by captopril and related agents useful in the diagnosis and treatment of hyper-reninaemic hypertension.

Angiotensin II has two principal actions, both of which increase blood pressure. It directly stimulates arteriolar vasoconstriction within a few seconds and it stimulates synthesis and secretion of aldosterone within minutes [171]. Increased plasma potassium is a powerful and direct stimulator of aldosterone synthesis and release [172,173].

Aldosterone, secreted by the glomerulosa cells of the adrenal cortex, has the greatest mineralocorticoid activity of all naturally occurring steroids. It causes renal sodium retention and potassium loss, with a consequent increase in intravascular volume and blood pressure. Angiotensin II functions through receptors that stimulate production of phosphatidylinositol, mobilize intracellular and extracellular $Ca^{2+}$ and activate protein kinase C [174]. These intracellular second messengers then stimulate transcription of the P450scc gene by means independent of those used by ACTH and cAMP [175]. Potassium ions increase uptake of $Ca^{2+}$, with consequent hydrolysis of phosphoinositides to increase phosphotidylinositol. Thus, angiotensin II and potassium work at different levels of the same intracellular second-messenger pathway, but these differ fundamentally from the action of ACTH.

Although the renin–angiotensin system is clearly the major regulator of mineralocorticoid secretion, ACTH, and possibly other POMC-derived peptides such as $\gamma_3$-MSH, can also promote secretion of aldosterone when used in high concentrations in animal systems [176,177]. The relevance of physiological concentrations in human beings has not been established. Ammonium ions, hyponatraemia, dopamine antagonists and some other agents can also stimulate secretion of aldosterone; atrial natriuretic factor is a potent physiological inhibitor of aldosterone secretion [178].

## Adrenal androgen secretion and the regulation of adrenarche

DHEA, DHEAS and androstenedione, which are almost exclusively secreted by the adrenal zona reticularis, are generally referred to as adrenal androgens because they can be converted peripherally to testosterone. These steroids have little if any capacity to bind to and activate androgen receptors and are hence only androgen precursors, not true androgens. The fetal adrenal secretes large amounts of DHEA and DHEAS, and these steroids are abundant in the newborn; their concentrations fall rapidly as the fetal zone of the adrenal involutes after birth.

After the first year of life, the adrenals of young children secrete small amounts of DHEA, DHEAS and androstenedione until the onset of adrenarche, usually around age 7–8, preceding the onset of puberty by about 2 years. Adrenarche is independent of puberty, the gonads or gonadotrophins, and the mechanism by which its onset is triggered remains unknown [63]. The secretion of DHEA and DHEAS continues to increase during and after puberty and reaches maximal values in young adulthood, after which there is a slow, gradual decrease in the secretion of these steroids in elderly people ('adrenopause') (Fig. 21.5) [179]. Despite the increases in the adrenal secretion of DHEA and DHEAS during adrenarche, circulating concentrations of ACTH and cortisol do not change with age. Thus ACTH plays a permissive role in adrenarche but does not trigger it. Searches for hypothetical polypeptide hormones that might specifically stimulate the zona reticularis have been unsuccessful [180,181].

Recent studies of adrenarche have focused on the roles of 3β-HSD and P450c17. The abundance of 3β-HSD protein in the zona reticularis appears to decrease with the onset of adrenarche [182–184], and the adrenal expression of cytochrome $b_5$, which fosters the 17,20-lyase activity of P450c17, is confined almost exclusively to the zona reticularis [185,186]. Both of these factors would strongly favour the production of DHEA [187]. Exaggerated adrenarche has been found in association with insulin resistance, and girls with this condition appear to be at a much higher risk of developing the polycystic ovarian syndrome as adults [188–190]. Recent evidence suggests that infants born small for gestational age may be at increased risk for this syndrome [191]. Evidence is accumulating to suggest that replacement of DHEA after adrenopause may improve memory and a sense of well-being in elderly people [192].

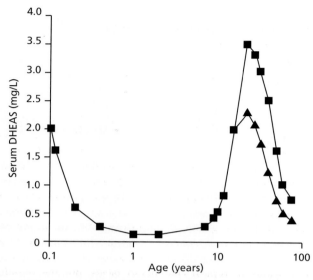

**Fig. 21.5.** Concentrations of DHEAS as a function of age. Note that the *x*-axis is on a log scale. ■, Males; ▲, females.

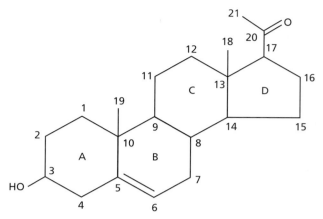

**Fig. 21.6.** Structure of pregnenolone. The carbon atoms are indicated by numbers and the rings are designated by letters according to standard convention. Pregnenolone is derived from cholesterol, which has a six-carbon side chain attached to carbon 21. Pregnenolone is a '$\Delta^5$ compound', having a double bond between carbons 5 and 6; the action of 3β-hydroxysteroid dehydrogenase/isomerase moves this double bond from the B ring to carbon numbers 4 and 5 in the A ring, forming $\Delta^4$ compounds. All of the major biologically active steroid hormones are $\Delta^4$ compounds.

## Plasma steroids and their disposal

### Structure and nomenclature

All steroid hormones are derivatives of pregnenolone (Fig. 21.6). Pregnenolone and its derivatives that contain 21 carbon atoms are often termed $C_{21}$ steroids. Each carbon atom is numbered, indicating the location at which the various steroidogenic reactions occur (e.g. 21-hydroxylation, 11-hydroxylation). The 17,20-lyase activity of P450c17 cleaves the bond between carbon atoms 17 and 20, yielding $C_{19}$ steroids, which include all the androgens. P450aro converts $C_{19}$ androgens to $C_{18}$ oestrogens. With the exception of oestrogens, all steroid hormones have a single unsaturated carbon–carbon double bond. Steroids having this double bond between carbon atoms 4 and 5, including all the principal biologically active steroids, are termed $\Delta^4$ steroids; their precursors, having a double bond between carbon atoms 5 and 6, are termed $\Delta^5$ steroids. The two isozymes of 3β-HSD convert $\Delta^5$ to $\Delta^4$ steroids.

A rigorous, logically systematic and unambiguous chemical terminology has been formulated to describe accurately the structure of all the steroid hormones and all their conceivable derivatives. However, this terminology is unbelievably cumbersome (e.g. cortisol is 11β,17α,21-trihydroxy-pregn-4-ene-3,20-dione, and dexamethasone is 9α-fluoro-11β,17α,21-trihydroxyprena-1,4-diene-3,20-dione). Therefore, we use only the standard trivial names.

Before the structures of the steroid hormones were determined in the 1930s, Reichstein, Kendall and others identified them as spots on paper chromatograms and designated them A, B, C, etc. Unfortunately, some persist in using this out-moded terminology more than 60 years later, so that corticosterone is sometimes termed 'compound B', cortisol 'compound F', and 11-deoxycortisol 'compound S.' This archaic terminology obfuscates the precursor–product relationships of the steroids, confuses students and should not be used.

### Circulating steroids

Although over 50 different steroids have been isolated from adrenocortical tissue, the main pathways of adrenal steroidogenesis include only a dozen or so steroids of which only a few are secreted in sizable quantities. The adult secretion of DHEA and cortisol are each about 20 mg/24 h and the secretion of corticosterone, a weak glucocorticoid, is about 2 mg/24 h [193]. Although glucocorticoids, such as cortisol, and mineralocorticoids, such as aldosterone, are both needed for life and hence are of 'equivalent' physiological importance, diagrams such as Fig. 21.1 fail to indicate that these steroids are not secreted in molar equivalents. The adult secretion rate of aldosterone is only about 0.1 mg/24 h. This 100- to 1000-fold molar difference in the secretory rates of cortisol and aldosterone must be borne in mind when considering the effects of steroid-binding proteins in plasma and when conceptualizing the physiological manifestations of incomplete defects in steroidogenesis due to single amino acid changes causing the partial loss of activity of a steroidogenic enzyme.

Most circulating steroids are bound to plasma proteins, including corticosteroid-binding globulin (CBG, also termed transcortin), albumin and $\alpha_1$-acid glycoprotein [194,195]. CBG has a very high affinity for cortisol but a relatively low binding capacity; albumin has a low affinity and high capacity; $\alpha_1$-acid glycoprotein is intermediate for both variables. The result is that about 90% of circulating cortisol is bound to CBG and a little more is bound to other proteins. These steroid-binding proteins are not transport proteins, as the biologically important steroids are water soluble in physiologically effective concentrations, and absence of CBG does not cause a detectable physiological disorder. However, these plasma proteins do act as a reservoir for steroids. This ensures that all peripheral tissues will be bathed in approximately equal concentrations of cortisol, which greatly diminishes the physiological effect of the great diurnal variation in cortisol secretion.

Synthetic glucocorticoids do not bind significantly to CBG and bind poorly to albumin, partially accounting for their increased potencies, which are also associated with increased receptor-binding affinities. Aldosterone is not bound well by any plasma protein; hence, changes in plasma protein concentration do not affect plasma aldosterone concentrations but greatly influence plasma cortisol concentrations. Oestradiol and testosterone bind strongly to a different plasma protein termed sex steroid-binding globulin and also bind weakly to albumin.

Because steroids are hormones it is often thought that the concentration of 'free' (i.e. unbound) circulating steroids determines biological activity. However, the target tissues for many steroid hormones contain enzymes that modify those steroids. Thus many actions of testosterone are actually due to dihydrotestosterone produced by local $5\alpha$-reductase; cortisol will have differential actions on various tissues due to the presence or absence of $11\beta$-HSD, which inactivates cortisol to cortisone. Similar peripheral metabolism occurs via 'extraglandular' 21-hydroxylase, P450aro, $3\beta$-HSD and $17\beta$-HSD. Thus circulating steroids are both classic hormones and precursors to locally acting autocrine or paracrine factors.

## Steroid catabolism

Only about 1% of circulating plasma cortisol and aldosterone are excreted unchanged in the urine; the remainder is metabolized by the liver. A large number of hepatic metabolites of each steroid is produced, most containing additional hydroxyl groups and linked to a sulphate or glucuronide moiety, rendering them more soluble and readily excretable by the kidney. A great deal is known about the various urinary metabolites of the circulating steroids because their measurement in pooled 24-h urine samples has been an important means of studying adrenal steroids. Although the measurement of urinary steroid metabolites by modern mass spectrometric techniques remains an important research tool [196–198], the development of separation techniques and of specific and highly sensitive radioimmunassays for each of the steroids in plasma has greatly reduced the need to measure their excreted metabolites in clinical practice.

## Clinical and laboratory evaluation of adrenal function

### Clinical evaluation

Primary adrenal deficiency or hypersecretion are generally evident before performing laboratory tests. Patients with chronic adrenal insufficiency have weakness, fatigue, anorexia, weight loss, hypotension and hyperpigmentation. Patients with acute adrenal insufficiency have hypotension, shock, weakness, apathy, confusion, anorexia, nausea, vomiting, dehydration, abdominal or flank pain, hyperthermia and hypoglycaemia.

Early signs of glucocorticoid excess include increased appetite, weight gain and growth arrest without a concomitant delay in bone age. Chronic glucocorticoid excess in children results in typical cushingoid facies, but the buffalo hump and centripetal distribution of body fat characteristic of Cushing disease in adults are seen only in long-standing undiagnosed disease.

Mineralocorticoid excess is characterized by hypertension, but patients receiving very low sodium diets (e.g. the newborn) are not hypertensive, as mineralocorticoids increase blood pressure primarily by retaining sodium and thus increasing intravascular volume.

Deficient adrenal androgen secretion will compromise the acquisition of virilizing secondary sexual characteristics (pubic and axillary hair, comedones, axillary odour) in female adolescents. Moderate hypersecretion of adrenal androgens is characterized by mild signs of virilization, whereas substantial hypersecretion of adrenal androgens is characterized by accelerated growth with a disproportionate increase in bone age, increased muscle mass, acne, hirsutism, deepening of the voice and more profound degrees of virilism. A key feature of any physical examination of a virilized male is careful examination and measurement of the testes. Bilaterally enlarged testes suggest true (central) precocious puberty; unilateral testicular enlargement suggests testicular tumour; prepubertal testes in a virilized male indicate an extratesticular source of androgen, such as the adrenal.

Imaging studies are of limited use in adrenocortical disease. Computerized tomography (CT) will rarely detect pituitary tumours secreting ACTH and magnetic resonance imaging (MRI) will detect less than half of them, even with gadolinium enhancement. The small size, odd shape and location near other structures also compromise the use of imaging techniques for the adrenals. Patients with Cushing disease or congenital adrenal hyperplasia have modestly enlarged adrenals, but these are often not detectable by imaging with any useful degree of certainty. The gross enlargement of the adrenals in congenital lipoid adrenal hyperplasia, their hypoplasia in adrenal hypoplasia congenita or in the hereditary ACTH unresponsiveness syndrome can be imaged as can many malignant tumours, but most adrenal adenomas are too small to be detected. Thus imaging studies may establish the presence of pituitary or adrenal tumours but never exclude them.

## Laboratory evaluation

### Steroid measurements

Plasma cortisol is measured by a variety of techniques including radioimmunoassay, immunoradiometric assay and high-performance liquid chromatography (HPLC). Other procedures, such as fluorimetric assays and competitive protein-binding assays, are useful research tools but are not in general clinical use. It is of considerable importance to know what procedure one's laboratory is using and precisely what it is measuring, because laboratories may have different normal values and most central hospital and commercial

laboratories are designed primarily to serve adult, rather than paediatric, patients. Tables 21.2 and 21.3 summarize the normal plasma concentrations for a variety of steroids.

All immunoassays have some degree of cross-reactivity with other steroids, and most cortisol immunoassays detect cortisol and cortisone, which are readily distinguished by HPLC. As the newborn's plasma contains mainly cortisone rather than cortisol during the first few days of life, comparison of newborn data obtained by HPLC to published standards obtained by immunoassays may incorrectly suggest adrenal insufficiency.

With the notable exception of DHEAS, most adrenal steroids exhibit a diurnal variation based on the diurnal rhythm of ACTH. Because the stress of illness or hospitalization can increase adrenal steroid secretion and because diurnal rhythms may not be well established in children under 3 years of age, it is best to obtain two or more samples for the measurement of any steroid [199,200].

**Table 21.2.** Mean sex steroid concentration in infants and children

| | PROG | 17-OHP | DHEA | DHEAS | $\Delta^4$ A | E$_1$ | E$_2$ | T M | T F | DHT M | DHT F |
|---|---|---|---|---|---|---|---|---|---|---|---|
| Cord blood | 1100 | 62 | 21 | 6400 | 3.0 | 52 | 30 | 1.0 | 0.9 | 0.2 | 0.2 |
| Premature babies | 11 | 8.1 | 28 | 11 000 | 7.0 | | | 4.2 | 0.4 | 1.0 | 0.1 |
| Term newborns | | 1.1 | 20 | 4400 | 5.2 | | | 6.9 | 1.4 | 0.9 | 0.3 |
| Infants | 1.0 | 1.0 | 3.8 | 820 | 0.7 | <0.1 | <0.1 | 6.6 | <0.4 | 1.4 | <0.1 |
| Children | | | | | | | | | | | |
|   1–6 years | | | 1.0 | 270 | 0.9 | <0.1 | <0.1 | 0.2 | | 0.1 | |
|   6–8 years | | | 3.1 | 540 | 0.9 | <0.1 | <0.1 | 0.2 | | 0.1 | |
|   8–10 years | | | 5.6 | 1400 | 0.9 | <0.1 | <0.1 | 0.2 | | 0.1 | |
| Males | | | | | | | | | | | |
|   Pubertal stage I | 0.6 | 1.3 | 5.6 | 950 | 0.9 | 0.0 | 0.0 | 0.2 | | <0.1 | |
|   Pubertal stage II | 0.6 | 1.6 | 10 | 2600 | 1.6 | 0.1 | 0.0 | 1.4 | | 0.3 | |
|   Pubertal stage III | 0.8 | 2.0 | 14 | 3300 | 2.4 | 0.1 | 0.1 | 6.6 | | 0.7 | |
|   Pubertal stage IV | 1.1 | 2.6 | 14 | 5400 | 2.8 | 0.1 | 0.1 | 13 | | 1.2 | |
|   Pubertal stage V | 1.3 | 3.3 | 17 | 6300 | 3.5 | 0.1 | 0.1 | 19 | | 1.6 | |
|   Adult | 1.1 | 3.3 | 16 | 7300 | 4.0 | 0.1 | 0.1 | 22 | | 1.7 | |
| Females | | | | | | | | | | | |
|   Pubertal stage I | 0.6 | 1.0 | 5.6 | 1100 | 0.9 | 0.1 | 0.0 | 0.2 | | 0.1 | |
|   Pubertal stage II | 1.0 | 1.6 | 11 | 1900 | 2.3 | 0.1 | 0.1 | 0.7 | | 0.3 | |
|   Pubertal stage III | 1.3 | 2.3 | 14 | 2500 | 4.2 | 0.1 | 0.1 | 0.9 | | 0.3 | |
|   Pubertal stage IV | 9.2 | 2.9 | 15 | 3300 | 4.5 | 0.1 | 0.2 | 0.9 | | 0.3 | |
|   Pubertal stage V | 5.1 | 3.6 | 19 | 4100 | 6.0 | 0.2 | 0.4 | 1.0 | | 0.3 | |
| Adult | | | | | | | | | | | |
|   Follicular | 1.0 | 1.5 | 16 | 4100 | 5.8 | 0.2 | 0.2 | 1.0 | | 0.3 | |
|   Luteal | 24 | 5.4 | 16 | 4100 | 5.8 | 0.4 | 0.5 | 1.0 | | 0.3 | |

PROG, progesterone; 17-OHP, 17-hydroxyprogesterone; DHEA, dehydroepiandrosterone; DHEAS, DHEA sulphate; $\Delta^4$ A, androstenedione; E$_1$, oestrone; E$_2$, oestradiol; T, testosterone; DHT, dihydrotestosterone; M, male; F, female.
All values are in nmol/L.
Data adapted from Endocrine Sciences, Tarzana, CA.

**Table 21.3.** Mean glucocorticoid and mineralocorticoid concentrations

| | Cortisol | DOC | Corticosterone | 18-OH-corticosterone | Aldosterone | Plasma renin activity |
|---|---|---|---|---|---|---|
| Cord blood | 360 | 5.5 | 19 | | 2.4 | 50 |
| Premature babies | 180 | | | 5.5 | 2.8 | 222 |
| Newborns | 140 | | 6.6 | 9.7 | 2.6 | 58 |
| Infants | 250 | 0.6 | 16 | 2.2 | 0.8 | 33 |
| Children (08.00 h) | | | | | | |
|   1–2 years | 110–550 | | | 1.8 | 0.8 | 15 |
|   2–10 years | as adults | 0.3 | | 1.2 | 0.3→0.8* | 8.3 |
|   10–15 years | as adults | | | 0.7 | 0.1→0.6* | 3.3 |
| Adults (08.00 h) | 280–550 | 0.2 | 12 | 0.6 | 0.2→0.4* | 2.8→4.0* |
| Adults (16.00 h) | 140–280 | | 3.8 | | | |

DOC, deoxycorticosterone.

All values in nmol/L except plasma renin activity (μg/L/s).

*Two values separated by an arrow indicate those in supine and upright posture.

## Plasma renin

Renin is not generally measured directly but is assayed by its enzymatic activity. Plasma renin activity (PRA) is simply an immunoassay of the amount of angiotensin I generated per milliliter of serum per hour at 37°C. In normal serum, the concentration of both renin and angiotensinogen (the renin substrate) are limiting. Therefore, another test, plasma renin content (PRC), measures the amount of angiotensin I generated in 1 h at 37°C in the presence of excess concentrations of angiotensinogen. Immunoassays for renin itself are being developed but are not yet available clinically.

Plasma renin activity is sensitive to dietary sodium intake, posture, diuretic therapy, activity and sex steroids. Because PRA values can vary widely, it is best to measure renin twice, once in the morning after overnight supine posture and then again after maintenance of upright posture for 4 h [201]. A simultaneous 24-h urine for total sodium excretion is generally needed to interpret PRA results. Decreased dietary and urinary sodium, decreased intravascular volume, diuretics and oestrogens will increase PRA. Sodium loading, hyperaldosteronaemia and increased intravascular volume decrease PRA.

The greatest use of renin measurements is in the evaluation of hypertension and in the management of CAH. However, several additional situations require assessment of the renin–angiotensin system. Children with simple virilizing adrenal hyperplasia who do not have clinical evidence of urinary salt wasting (hyponatraemia, hyperkalaemia, acidosis, hypotension, shock) may nevertheless have increased PRA, especially when dietary sodium is restricted. This was an early clinical sign that this form of 21-hydroxylase deficiency (21-OHD) was simply a milder form of the more common, severe, salt-wasting form. Treatment of simple virilizing 21-OHD with sufficient mineralocorticoid to suppress PRA into the normal range will reduce the child's requirement for glucocorticoids, thus maximizing final adult height. Children with CAH need to have their mineralocorticoid replacement therapy monitored routinely by measuring PRA. Measurement of angiotensin II is also possible in some research laboratories, but most antibodies to angiotensin II strongly cross-react with angiotensin I. Thus, PRA remains the most useful way of evaluating the renin–angiotensin–aldosterone system.

## Urinary steroid excretion

The measurement of 24-h urinary excretion of steroid metabolites is one of the oldest procedures for assessing adrenal function and is still useful. Examination of the total 24-h excretion of steroids eliminates the fluctuations seen in serum samples as a function of time of day, episodic bursts of ACTH and steroid secretion and transient stress (such as a visit to the clinic or difficult venepuncture). Collection of a complete 24-h urinary sample can be difficult in the infant or small child. Two consecutive 24-h collections should be obtained. Because of the diurnal and episodic nature of steroid secretion, one should never obtain 8- or 12-h collections and attempt to infer the 24-h excretory rate from such partial collections.

Urinary 17-hydroxycorticosteroids, assayed by the colorimetric Porter–Silber reaction, measures 17,21-dihydroxy-20-ketosteroids by the generation of a coloured compound after treatment with phenylhydrazine [202]. The reaction is highly specific for the major urinary metabolites of cortisol and cortisone. It will also measure metabolites of 11-deoxycortisol.

Measurement of 17-hydroxycorticosteroids is being replaced by measurement of urinary free cortisol, thus avoiding the non-specificity and drug interference problems inherent in 17-hydroxycorticosteroids. In adults, the test is highly reliable in the diagnosis of Cushing syndrome. Free cortisol is extracted from the urine and measured by immunoassay or HPLC, providing the advantage of specificity; furthermore, unlike 17-hydroxycorticosteroids, urinary free cortisol is not increased in exogenous obesity [203]. The upper limit of normal for urinary free cortisol excretion for children is 80 μg/m$^2$/day and that for 17-hydroxycorticosteroids is 5 mg/m$^2$/day [204]. Some clinical experience indicates that urinary 17-hydroxycorticosteroids may be more reliable for the diagnosis of Cushing disease in children, possibly due to greater experience with 17-hydroxycorticosteroids [205].

Urinary 17-ketosteroids, assayed by the Zimmerman reaction, measure 17-ketosteroids by the generation of a coloured compound after treatment with *meta*-dinitrobenzine and acid [206]. The reaction principally measures metabolites of DHEA and DHEAS and thus correlates with adrenal androgen production. Androstenedione will contribute significant 17-ketosteroids and, if an alkali extraction is not used, oestrone will also contribute. The principal androgens, testosterone and dihydrotestosterone, have hydroxyl rather than keto groups on carbon 17; hence, their metabolic products are not measured as 17-ketosteroids. A wide variety of drugs, including penicillin, nalidixic acid, spironolactone and phenothiazines, as well as non-specific urinary chromagens, can spuriously increase values of 17-ketosteroids. Measurement of urinary 17-ketosteroids remains a useful, inexpensive screening test, and some clinicians prefer to follow 17-ketosteroids to monitor therapy of CAH, but measurements of plasma steroids have now replaced the use of urinary 17-ketosteroids in most centres.

Urinary 17-ketogenic steroids are occasionally confused with urinary 17-ketosteroids because of the similarity of the names; however, 17-ketogenic steroids are used to measure urinary metabolites of glucocorticoids, not sex steroids. Although some laboratories continue to perform measurements of 17-ketogenic steroids, this obsolete assay no longer has a place in modern paediatric practice.

## Plasma ACTH and other POMC peptides

Accurate immunoassay of plasma ACTH is available in most centres, but its measurement remains more difficult and variable than the assays for most other pituitary hormones [207]. Samples must be drawn into a plastic syringe containing heparin or ethylenediamine tetraacetic acid (EDTA) and transported quickly in plastic tubes on ice, as ACTH adheres to glass and is quickly inactivated. Elevated plasma ACTH concentrations can be informative but most assays cannot detect low or low-normal values, and such values can be spurious if the samples are handled badly. In adults and older children with well-established diurnal rhythms of ACTH, normal 08.00 h values rarely exceed 50 pg/mL, whereas 20.00 h values are usually undetectable. Patients with Cushing disease often have normal morning values but consistently elevated afternoon and evening ones can suggest the diagnosis. Patients with the ectopic ACTH syndrome have values from 100 to 1000 pg/mL.

The carboxy portion of POMC [β-lipotrophic hormone (β-LPH), POMC 153–241] is released from POMC in equimolar amounts with ACTH. β-LPH has a longer circulating plasma half-life than ACTH, is more stable in the laboratory and is easier than ACTH to assay [208]. Such assays may be a useful adjunct to ACTH assays but routine measurement of β-LPH is not available.

## Secretory rates

The secretory rates of cortisol and aldosterone (or other steroids) can be measured by administering a small dose of tritiated cortisol or aldosterone and measuring the specific activity of one or more known metabolites in a 24-h urine collection. This procedure permitted measurement of certain steroids, such as aldosterone, before specific immunoassays became available. The procedures have provided much information about the normal rate of production of various steroids. On the basis of this procedure, most authorities have agreed that children and adults secrete about 12 mg of cortisol per square metre of body surface area per day. However, more recent studies indicate a rate of 6–9 mg/m$^2$ in children and adults [209,210]. Such differences are of considerable importance in estimating 'physiological replacement' doses of glucocorticoids.

## Dexamethasone suppression test

Administration of small doses of dexamethasone, a potent synthetic glucocorticoid, will suppress secretion of pituitary ACTH and of adrenal cortisol. Originally described by Liddle [211] in 1960, the dexamethasone suppression test remains the most useful procedure for distinguishing whether glucocorticoid excess is due primarily to pituitary disease or adrenal disease. As dexamethasone also suppresses adrenal androgen secretion, this test is useful for distinguishing between adrenal and gonadal sources of sex steroids. A dexamethasone suppression test requires the measurement of basal values and those obtained in response to both low- and high-dose dexamethasone. Variations of the test are common, notably the single 1.0-mg dose in adults [212] or 0.3 mg/m$^2$ in children [213]. This is a useful outpatient screening procedure for distinguishing Cushing syndrome from exogenous obesity. It can be useful for the same purpose in adolescents and older children but is otherwise of limited utility in paediatrics. An overnight high-dose dexamethasone suppression test is probably more reliable than the standard 2-day, high-dose test in differentiating adults with Cushing disease from those with the ectopic ACTH syndrome. However, the utility of this test in paediatric patients has not been established.

**Table 21.4.** Responses of adrenal steroids to a 60-min ACTH test

|  | Infants | | Prepubertal | | Pubertal | |
| --- | --- | --- | --- | --- | --- | --- |
|  | Basal | Stimulated | Basal | Stimulated | Basal | Stimulated |
| 17-OH-pregnenolone | 6.8 |  | 1.7 | 9.6 | 3.6 | 24 |
| 17-OHP | 0.8 | 5.8 | 1.5 | 5.8 | 1.8 | 4.8 |
| DHEA | 1.4 |  | 2.4 | 4.3 | 9.0 | 19 |
| 11-Deoxycortisol | 2.3 |  | 1.8 | 5.8 | 1.7 | 4.9 |
| Cortisol | 280 | 830 | 360 | 830 | 280 | 690 |
| DOC | 0.6 | 2.4 | 0.2 | 1.7 | 0.2 | 1.7 |
| Progesterone | 1.1 | 3.2 | 1.1 | 4.0 | 1.9 | 4.8 |

All values are mean values in nmol/L.
Data adapted from Endocrine Sciences, Tarzana, CA.

## Stimulation tests

Direct stimulation of the adrenal with ACTH is a rapid, safe and easy way to evaluate adrenocortical function. The original ACTH test consisted of a 4- to 6-h infusion of 0.5 units/kg of ACTH (1–39) to stimulate adrenal cortisol secretion maximally. It diagnoses primary adrenal insufficiency (Addison disease). In secondary adrenal insufficiency, some steroidogenic capacity is present and some cortisol is produced in response to the ACTH.

This ACTH test has been replaced in clinical practice by the 60-min test, when a single bolus of ACTH (1–24) is administered intravenously and cortisol values are measured at 0 and 60 min [214]. Normal responses are shown in Table 21.4 [215]. Synthetic ACTH (1–24) (cosyntropin) is preferred as it has a more rapid action and shorter half-life than ACTH (1–39). The usual dose is 0.1 mg in newborns, 0.15 mg in children up to 2 years of age and 0.25 mg for children over the age of 2 years and adults. All of these doses are pharmacological.

A very low-dose (1 μg) test may be useful in assessing adrenal recovery from glucocorticoid suppression [216]. Newer data show that maximal steroidal responses can be achieved after only 30 min, but the best available standards are for a 60-min test.

One of the widest uses of intravenous ACTH tests in paediatrics is in diagnosing congenital adrenal hyperplasia (CAH). Stimulating the adrenal with ACTH increases steroidogenesis, resulting in accumulation of steroids proximal to the disordered enzyme. For example, inspection of Fig. 21.1 shows that impaired activity of P450c21 (21-hydroxylase) should lead to the accumulation of progesterone and 17-hydroxyprogesterone (17-OHP). However, progesterone does not accumulate in appreciable quantities, because it, too, is converted to 17-OHP. Measuring the response of 17-OHP to a 60-min or 6-h challenge with ACTH is the single most powerful and reliable means of diagnosing 21-OHD. Comparing the patient's basal to ACTH-stimulated values of 17-OHP against those from large numbers of well-studied patients usually

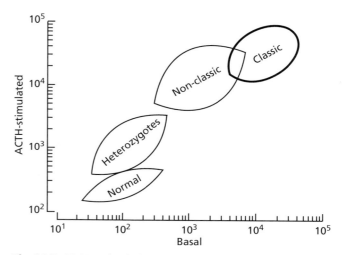

**Fig. 21.7.** 17-OHP values before and after stimulation with ACTH in normal subjects, patients with CAH and heterozygotes.

permits the discrimination of normal persons, heterozygotes, patients with non-classic CAH and patients with classic CAH, although there inevitably is some overlap between groups [217] (Fig. 21.7). Measurement of testosterone or $\Delta^4$ androstenedione in response to ACTH can distinguish normal persons from patients with classic CAH, but heterozygotes and patients with cryptic CAH have values overlapping both normal and classic CAH (Fig. 21.7).

Longer ACTH tests of up to 3 days have also been used to evaluate adrenal function, but it is important to remember that ACTH has both acute and chronic effects. Thus, short tests measure only the acute effects of ACTH, the maximal stimulation of pre-existing steroidogenic machinery. A 3-day test will examine the more chronic effects of ACTH to stimulate increased capacity for steroidogenesis by increasing the synthesis of steroidogenic machinery. Few situations exist where a 3-day intramuscular ACTH test is indicated, although it is useful in diagnosing the rare syndrome of hereditary unresponsiveness to ACTH [218].

Insulin-induced hypoglycaemia is another commonly used test. The hypoglycaemia stimulates the release of counter-regulatory hormones (ACTH and cortisol, growth hormone, epinephrine and glucagon) that have actions to increase plasma glucose concentrations. Most patients experience hunger, irritability, diaphoresis and tachycardia; when these are followed by drowsiness or sleep, blood sugar levels are probably below acceptable limits. If this occurs, a blood sample should be obtained and 2 mL/kg of 25% glucose given intravenously, to a maximum of 100 mL [219].

### Metyrapone test

Metyrapone blocks the action of P450c11β and, to a much lesser extent, P450scc. It is thus a chemical means of inducing a transient deficiency of 11-hydroxylase activity, which results in decreased cortisol secretion and subsequent increase in ACTH secretion. Metyrapone testing is done to assess the capacity of the pituitary to produce ACTH in response to a physiological stimulus. This test is useful in evaluating the hypothalamo-pituitary axis in the presence of central nervous system lesions after neurosurgery or long-term suppression by glucocorticoid therapy [220]. Patients with a previous history of hypothalamic, pituitary or adrenal disease or those who have been withdrawn from glucocorticoid therapy should be re-evaluated with a metyrapone test or with an insulin tolerance test. A normal response indicates recovery of the hypothalamo-pituitary-adrenal axis and predicts that the patient will respond normally to the stress of surgery.

Metyrapone is generally given orally as 300 mg/m² every 4 h for a total of six doses (24 h). Unlike many other drugs, it is appropriate to continue to increase the dose in older or overweight patients, but the total dose should not exceed 3.0 g [221]. Blood should be obtained for cortisol, 11-deoxycortisol and ACTH before and after the test, and a 24-h urine collection should be obtained before and during the test for 17-hydroxycorticosteroids. In a normal response to metyrapone, cortisol decreases, ACTH increases and 11-deoxycortisol (the substrate for P450c11β) increases greatly, to about 5 μg/dL. Metabolites of 11-deoxycortisol result in a doubling in urinary 17-hydroxycorticosteroids excretion. Adults and older children can be tested with the administration of a single oral dose of 30 mg/kg at midnight, given with food to reduce the gastrointestinal irritation [221]. Blood samples are drawn at 08.00 h the mornings before and after administering the drug.

### CRH testing

CRH is now generally available as a test of pituitary ACTH reserve [222]. It remains experimental in adults and little experience has been gained from children. Early data suggest that it may be useful for distinguishing hypothalamic from pituitary causes of ACTH deficiency and may also be a useful

adjunct in establishing the diagnosis of Cushing disease [223].

## Genetic lesions in steroidogenesis

Autosomal recessive disorders disrupt each of the steps in the pathway shown in Fig. 21.1. Most result in diminished synthesis of cortisol. In response to adrenal insufficiency, the pituitary synthesizes increased amounts of POMC and ACTH, which promotes increased steroidogenesis; ACTH and possibly other peptides derived from the amino-terminal end of POMC also stimulate adrenal hypertrophy and hyperplasia. Thus the term congenital adrenal hyperplasia (CAH) refers to a group of diseases traditionally grouped together on the basis of the most prominent finding at autopsy.

In theory, CAH is easy to understand. A genetic lesion in one of the steroidogenic enzymes interferes with normal steroidogenesis. The signs and symptoms of the disease derive from deficiency of the steroidal end product and the effects of accumulated steroidal precursors proximal to the blocked step. Thus, reference to the pathways in Fig. 21.1 and a knowledge of the biological effects of each steroid should permit one to deduce the manifestations of the disease.

In practice, CAH can be confusing, both clinically and scientifically. The key clinical, laboratory and therapeutic features of each form are summarized in Table 21.5. Because each steroidogenic enzyme has multiple activities and many extra-adrenal tissues contain enzymes that have similar activities, the complete elimination of a specific adrenal enzyme may not result in the complete elimination of its steroidal products from the circulation. In the past, disorders of steroidogenic enzymes had to be studied by examining their steroid metabolites in serum and urine, an indirect approach that led to numerous misconceptions about the steroidogenic processes. The cloning of the genes for the steroidogenic enzymes has now permitted the direct study of these diseases, altering traditional views substantially.

## Congenital lipoid adrenal hyperplasia

Lipoid CAH, the most severe genetic disorder of steroid hormone synthesis, is characterized by the absence of significant concentrations of all steroids, high basal ACTH and plasma renin activity. Steroid responses to long-term treatment with high doses of ACTH or hCG (human chorionic gonadotrophin) are absent. The adrenals are grossly enlarged with cholesterol and cholesterol esters [224–227]. These findings indicate a lesion in the first step in steroidogenesis, the conversion of cholesterol to pregnenolone, and have led to other names for lipoid CAH, including 20,22-desmolase deficiency and P450scc deficiency because other errors in steroidogenesis were in steroidogenic enzymes [227–232]. However, the P450scc gene is normal in these patients [232],

**Table 21.5.** Clinical and laboratory findings in the congenital adrenal hyperplasias

| Enzyme deficiency | Presentation | Laboratory findings | Therapeutic measures |
|---|---|---|---|
| Lipoid CAH (StAR) | Salt-wasting crisis<br>Male pseudohermaphroditism | Low/absent levels of all steroid hormones<br>Decreased/absent response to ACTH<br>Decreased/absent response to hCG in male pseudohermaphroditism<br>↑ ACTH and PRA | Glucocorticoid and mineralocorticoid replacement<br>Oestrogen replacement at age ≥ 12 years<br>Gonadectomy of male pseudohermaphrodite and salt supplementation |
| 3β-HSD | Salt-wasting crisis<br>Male and female pseudohermaphroditism | ↑Δ$^5$ steroids before and after ACTH<br>↑Δ$^5$/Δ$^4$ serum steroids<br>Suppression of elevated adrenal steroids after glucocorticoid administration<br>↑ ACTH and PRA | Glucocorticoid and mineralocorticoid replacement<br>Salt supplementation<br>Surgical correction of genitalia<br>Sex hormone replacement as necessary |
| P450c21 | *Classic form:*<br>Salt-wasting crisis<br>Female pseudohermaphroditism<br>Pre- and postnatal virilization<br>*Non-classic form:*<br>Premature adrenarche, menstrual irregularity, hirsutism, acne, infertility | ↑ 17-OHP before and after ACTH<br>↑ Serum androgens and urine 17-ketosteroids<br>Suppression of elevated adrenal steroids after glucocorticoid treatment<br>↑ ACTH and PRA | Glucocorticoid and mineralocorticoid replacement<br>Salt supplementation<br>Surgical repair of female pseudo-hermaphroditism |
| P450c11β | Female pseudohermaphroditism<br>Postnatal virilization in males and females | ↑ 11-deoxycortisol and DOC before and after ACTH<br>↑ Serum androgens and urine 17-ketosteroids<br>Suppression of elevated steroids after glucocorticoid administration<br>↑ ACTH and ↓ PRA<br>Hypokalaemia | Glucocorticoid administration<br>Surgical repair of female pseudohermaphroditism |
| P450c11AS | Failure to thrive<br>Weakness<br>Salt loss | Hyponatraemia, hyperkalaemia<br>↑ Corticosterone<br>↓ Aldosterone and ↑ PRA | Mineralocorticoid replacement<br>Salt supplementation |
| P450c17 | Male pseudohermaphroditism<br>Sexual infantilism<br>Hypertension | ↑ DOC, 18-OHDOC, corticosterone, 18-hydroxycorticosterone<br>Low 17α-hydroxylated steroids and poor response to ACTH<br>Poor response to hCG in male pseudohermaphroditism<br>Suppression of elevated adrenal steroids after glucocorticoid administration<br>↑ ACTH and ↓ PRA<br>Hypokalaemia | Glucocorticoid administration<br>Surgical correction of genitalia and sex steroid replacement in male pseudohermaphroditism consonant with sex of rearing<br>Oestrogen replacement in female at ≥ 12 years<br>Testosterone replacement if reared as male (rare) |

as are the mRNAs for adrenodoxin reductase and adrenodoxin [232]. The normal P450scc system plus the accumulation of cholesterol esters in the affected adrenal suggested that the lesion lay in a factor involved in cholesterol transport to the mitochondria. After initial unsuccessful searches for this factor [232,233], the steroidogenic regulatory protein (StAR) was cloned in 1994 [46] and was quickly identified as the disordered step in lipoid CAH [47,234]. Thus lipoid CAH is the only disorder in steroid hormone biosynthesis that is not caused by a disrupted steroidogenic enzyme.

Lipoid CAH provided a gene knockout of nature, elucidating the complex physiology of the StAR protein [235]. Trans-fection of non-steroidogenic cells with the P450scc system with and without StAR showed that StAR promotes steroidogenesis by increasing the movement of cholesterol into mitochondria but that, in the absence of StAR, steroidogenesis proceeds at about 14% of the StAR-induced level [47,48,151,234]. This observation led to the two-hit model of lipoid CAH [48]. The first hit is the loss of StAR itself, leading to a loss of most but not all steroidogenesis, with a compensatory rise in ACTH and LH. These hormones increase cellular cAMP, which increases biosynthesis of LDL receptors, their uptake of LDL-cholesterol and *de novo* synthesis of cholesterol. In the absence of StAR, this increased intracellular cholesterol accumulates as in a storage disease causing the second hit, which is the mitochondrial and cellular damage caused by the accumulated cholesterol, cholesterol esters and their auto-oxidation products [48].

The two-hit model explains the unusual clinical findings in lipoid CAH. In the fetal testis, which is steroidogenically very active under the tropic stimulation of hCG [236], the Leydig cells are destroyed early in fetal life, eliminating testosterone biosynthesis. An affected 46,XY fetus does not undergo normal virilization and is born with female external genitalia and a blind vaginal pouch. The Sertoli cells remain undamaged and continue to produce Müllerian inhibitory hormone, so that the phenotypically female 46,XY fetus has no cervix, uterus or fallopian tubes. The steroidogenically active fetal zone of the adrenal is similarly affected, eliminating most fetal adrenal DHEA biosynthesis and the fetoplacental production of oestriol; midgestation maternal and fetal oestriol levels are thus very low [237].

The definitive zone of the fetal adrenal, which differentiates into the zonae glomerulosa and fasciculata, normally produces very little aldosterone, and, as fetal salt and water metabolism are maintained by the placenta, stimulation of the glomerulosa by angiotensin II generally does not begin until birth. Consistent with this, many newborns with lipoid CAH do not have a salt-wasting crisis until after several weeks of life, when chronic stimulation then leads to cellular damage [48]. However, patients with lipoid CAH born in dry climates tend to develop a salt-wasting crisis very early, presumably reflecting chronic compensated hypovolaemia in the mother with secondary stimulation of the fetal renin–angiotensin system, so that damage to the glomerulosa begins before birth [48].

The two-hit model also explains the spontaneous feminization of affected 46,XX females who are treated in infancy and reach adolescence. The fetal ovary makes no steroids and contains no steroidogenic enzymes [236]; consequently the ovary remains undamaged until it is first stimulated by gonadotrophins at the time of puberty, when it produces some oestrogen by StAR-independent steroidogenesis. Continued stimulation results in cholesterol accumulation and cellular damage, so that biosynthesis of progesterone in the latter part of the cycle is impaired. Because gonadotrophin stimulation recruits individual follicles and does not promote steroidogenesis in the whole ovary, most follicles remain undamaged and available for future cycles. Cyclicity is determined by the hypothalamo-pituitary axis and remains normal. With each new cycle, a new follicle is recruited and more oestradiol is produced by StAR-independent steroidogenesis. Although net ovarian steroidogenesis is impaired, enough oestrogen is produced (especially in the absence of androgens) to induce breast development, general feminization, monthly oestrogen withdrawal and cyclic vaginal bleeding [48,238]. However progesterone synthesis in the latter half of the cycle is disturbed by the accumulating choles-

terol esters so that the cycles are anovulatory. Measurements of oestradiol, progesterone and gonadotrophins throughout the cycle in affected adult females with lipoid CAH confirms this model [239]. Similarly, examination of StAR-knockout mice confirms the two-hit model [240]. Thus, examination of patients with lipoid CAH has elucidated the physiology of the StAR protein in each steroidogenic tissue.

Genetic analysis of patients with lipoid CAH has revealed numerous mutations in the StAR gene [48,241]. These data reveal two distinct genetic clusters. As first reported in 1985 [227], lipoid CAH is common in Japan and about 65–70% of affected Japanese alleles and virtually all affected Korean alleles carry the mutation Q258X [47,48,241,242]. The carrier frequency for this mutation appears to be about 1 in 300 [48,242], so that one in every 250 000–300 000 newborns in these countries is affected, giving a total of about 500 patients in Japan and Korea. A second genetic cluster is found among Palestinian Arabs, most of whom carry the mutation R182L [48].

Many other mutations have been found throughout the gene but all amino acid replacement (missense) mutations are found in the carboxy-terminal 40% of the protein, suggesting that this is the biologically important domain [48,235]. Spectroscopic analysis of these mutant proteins indicates that they have lost activity because they are substantially misfolded [243]. Deletion of only 10 carboxy-terminal residues reduces StAR activity by half [52], and deletion of 28 carboxy-terminal residues by the common Q258X mutation eliminates all activity. By contrast, deletion of the first 62 amino-terminal residues has no effect on StAR activity, even though this deletes the entire mitochondrial leader sequence and forces StAR to remain in the cytoplasmic compartment [52]. Physical studies and partial proteolysis indicate that residues 63–193 of StAR (i.e. the domain that lacks most of the crucial residues identified by missense mutations) are protease resistant; this constitutes a 'pause–transfer' sequence, which permits the bioactive loosely folded carboxy-terminal molten globule domain to have increased interaction with the outer mitochondrial membrane [54].

Treatment of lipoid CAH is straightforward if the diagnosis is made. Physiological replacement with glucocorticoids, mineralocorticoids and salt will permit survival to adulthood [226,227]. The differential diagnosis includes 3β-HSD deficiency and adrenal hypoplasia congenita (AHC). The glucocorticoid requirement is less than in the virilizing adrenal hyperplasias, because it is not necessary to suppress excess adrenal androgen production. Growth in these patients should be normal [227]. Genetic males have female external genitalia and should undergo orchiectomy and be raised as females [48,226,227].

## 3β-Hydroxysteroid dehydrogenase deficiency

3β-HSD deficiency is a rare cause of glucocorticoid and mineralocorticoid deficiency that is fatal if not diagnosed early [244]. In its classic form, genetic females have cliteromegaly and mild virilization because the fetal adrenal overproduces large amounts of DHEA, a small portion of which is converted to testosterone by extra-adrenal 3β-HSD type I. Genetic males also synthesize some androgens by peripheral conversion of adrenal and testicular DHEA, but the concentrations are insufficient for complete male genital development so that these males have a small phallus and severe hypospadias.

There are two functional human genes for 3β-HSD: the type I gene is expressed in the placenta and peripheral tissues [58,60] and the type II in the adrenals and gonads [245,246]. Genetic and endocrine studies of 3β-HSD deficiency show that both the gonads and the adrenals are affected as a result of a single mutated 3β-HSD-II gene that is expressed in both tissues. However, considerable hepatic 3β-HSD activity persists in the face of complete absence of adrenal and gonadal activity due to the enzyme encoded by the 3β-HSD-I gene, thus complicating the diagnosis of 3β-HSD deficiency. Genetic studies have identified numerous mutations causing 3β-HSD deficiency, all in the type II gene [247–251]. Mutations have never been found in 3β-HSD-I, presumably because this would prevent placental biosynthesis of progesterone, resulting in a spontaneous first-trimester abortion.

The presence of peripheral 3β-HSD activity complicates the hormonal diagnosis of this disease. Affected infants should have low concentrations of 17-OHP, yet some newborns with 3β-HSD deficiency have very high concentrations of serum 17-OHP, approaching those seen in patients with classic 21-OHD [252]. These are due to extra-adrenal 3β-HSD-I. The adrenal of a patient with 3β-HSD-II deficiency will secrete very large amounts of the principal $\Delta^5$ compounds, pregnenolone, 17-hydroxypregnenolone and DHEA. Some of the secreted 17-hydroxypregnenolone is converted to 17-OHP by 3β-HSD-I. This 17-OHP is not effectively picked up by the adrenal for subsequent conversion to cortisol because the circulating concentrations are below the $K_m$ of P450c17. The ratio of the $\Delta^5$ to the $\Delta^4$ compounds remains high, consistent with the adrenal and gonadal deficiency of 3β-HSD [252]. Thus, the principal diagnostic test in 3β-HSD deficiency is intravenous administration of ACTH with measurement of the three $\Delta^5$ compounds and their corresponding $\Delta^4$ compounds.

Mild or 'partial' defects of adrenal 3β-HSD activity have been reported on the basis of ratios of $\Delta^5$ steroids to $\Delta^4$ steroids after an ACTH test that exceed 2 or 3 SD (standard deviations) above the mean. The patients are typically young girls with premature adrenarche or young women with a history of premature adrenarche and complaints of hirsutism, virilism and oligomenorrhoea [253–255]. However, the 3β-HSD-II genes are normal in these patients, and even patients with mild 3β-HSD-II mutations have ratios of $\Delta^5$ to $\Delta^4$ steroids that exceed 8 SD above the mean [250,256–258]. The basis of

the mildly elevated ratios of $\Delta^5$ to $\Delta^4$ steroids in these hirsute individuals with normal 3β-HSD genes is unknown. In adult women, the hirsutism can be ameliorated and regular menses restored by suppressing ACTH with 0.25 mg of dexamethasone given orally each day but such treatment is contraindicated in girls who have not yet reached final height.

## 17α-Hydroxylase/17,20-lyase deficiency

P450c17 is the single enzyme that has both 17α-hydroxylase and 17,20-lyase activities. Deficient 17α-hydroxylase activity and deficient 17,20-lyase activity have been described as separate genetic diseases, but it is now clear that they represent different clinical manifestations of different lesions in the same gene. P450c17 deficiency is fairly rare, although over 120 cases have been reported on clinical grounds [259]. Deficient 17α-hydroxylase activity results in decreased cortisol synthesis, overproduction of ACTH and stimulation of the steps proximal to P450c17. The patients may have mild symptoms of glucocorticoid deficiency but this is not life-threatening as the lack of P450c17 results in the overproduction of corticosterone, which also has glucocorticoid activity. This is similar to the situation in rodents, whose adrenals lack P450c17 [260] and consequently produce corticosterone as their glucocorticoid. Affected patients overproduce DOC in the zona fasciculata, which causes sodium retention, hypertension and hypokalaemia and also suppresses plasma renin activity and aldosterone secretion from the zona glomerulosa. When P450c17 deficiency is treated with glucocorticoids, DOC secretion is suppressed and plasma renin activity and aldosterone concentrations rise to normal [261].

The absence of 17α-hydroxylase and 17,20-lyase activities in complete P450c17 deficiency prevents the synthesis of adrenal and gonadal sex steroids. As a result, affected females are phenotypically normal but fail to undergo adrenarche and puberty [262], and genetic males have absent or incomplete development of the external genitalia [263]. The classic presentation is a teenage female with sexual infantilism and hypertension. The diagnosis is made by finding low or absent 17-hydroxylated $C_{21}$ and $C_{19}$ plasma steroids and low urinary 17-hydroxycorticosteroids and 17-KS, which respond poorly to stimulation with ACTH. Serum levels of DOC, corticosterone and 18-hydroxy-corticosterone are elevated, show hyper-responsiveness to ACTH and are suppressible with glucocorticoids.

The single gene for P450c17 has been cloned [71] and localized to chromosome 10q24.3 [69,70]. The molecular basis of 17α-hydroxylase deficiency has been determined in several patients by cloning and sequencing of the mutated gene, identifying at least 26 distinct mutations [77], which include 12 mutations that cause frameshifts or premature translational termination: as expected, none of these mutants has any detectable 17α-hydroxylase or 17,20-lyase activity. Eleven missense and in-frame mutations have been found, most of which also eliminate all activity, whereas others, such as P342T, reduce both activities by 80%.

Selective deficiency of the 17,20-lyase activity P450c17 has been reported in about a dozen cases [259], which initially led to the incorrect conclusion that 17α-hydroxylase and 17,20-lyase are separate enzymes. One of the original patients had two wholly inactivating mutations [264], which led to a corrected diagnosis of the patient as having complete 17α-hydroxylase deficiency [265]. Thus, because both the 17α-hydroxylase and 17,20-lyase activities of P450c17 are catalysed by the same active site, it was not clear that a syndrome of isolated 17,20-lyase deficiency could exist until two patients with genital ambiguity, normal excretion of 17-hydroxycorticosteroids and markedly reduced production of $C_{19}$ steroids were studied [266]. One was homozygous for the P450c17 mutation R347H and the other homozygous for R358Q. Both mutations changed the distribution of surface charges in the redox partner binding site of P450c17 [266]. When expressed in transfected cells, both mutants retained nearly normal 17α-hydroxylase activity but had no detectable 17,20-lyase activity [266,267]. Enzymatic competition experiments proved that the mutations did not affect the substrate binding site [267]. When an excess of both P450 oxidoreductase and cytochrome $b_5$ was provided, some 17,20-lyase activity was restored, demonstrating that the loss in lyase activity was caused by impaired electron transfer [267]. A third patient with similar findings has been reported with the mutation F417C, but the enzymology of that mutation has not been studied in detail [268].

A detailed computer-graphic model of P450c17 has been built and tested by numerous computational, enzymatic and mutagenesis approaches, which show that the model is an excellent representation of the human enzyme [269]. This model accurately predicts the effects of all known mutations, including those with partial retention of both activities and those causing selective 17,20-lyase deficiency. The model identifies both Arg-347 and Arg-358 and several other arginine and lysine residues in the redox partner binding site; mutations of these residues all cause varying degrees of selective loss of 17,20-lyase activity [266,267,269,270]. Another example of the critical nature of redox partner interactions comes from the sole reported case of cytochrome $b_5$ deficiency; this patient was a male pseudohermaphrodite but was not evaluated hormonally [271]. The central role of electron transfer in 17,20-lyase activity is now well established.

## 21-Hydroxylase deficiency

21-OHD is due to mutations in the gene encoding adrenal P450c21, is one of the most common inborn errors of metabolism and accounts for about 95% of CAH. Because of success in diagnosis and treatment in infancy, many patients with severe forms of 21-OHD have reached adulthood, so management issues in CAH concern all age groups. Detailed

reviews of the complex physiology and molecular genetics of this disorder have appeared [78–80,272–274].

### Pathophysiology

For patients with a complete absence of P450c21, the clinical manifestations can be deduced from Fig. 21.1. Inability to convert progesterone to DOC results in aldosterone deficiency causing severe hyponatraemia ($Na^+$ often below 110 mmol/L), hyperkalemia ($K^+$ often above 10 mmol/L) and acidosis (pH often below 7.1) with concomitant hypotension, shock, cardiovascular collapse and death. As the control of fluids and electrolytes in the fetus can be maintained by the placenta and the mother's kidneys, the salt-losing crisis develops only after birth, usually during the second week of life.

The inability to convert 17-OHP to 11-deoxycortisol results in cortisol deficiency, which impairs postnatal carbohydrate metabolism and exacerbates cardiovascular collapse because a permissive action of cortisol is required for full pressor action of catecholamines. Although the role of cortisol in fetal physiology is not well established [136], cortisol deficiency is also manifested prenatally. Low fetal cortisol stimulates ACTH secretion, which stimulates adrenal hyperplasia and transcription of the genes for all the steroidogenic enzymes, especially for P450scc, the rate-limiting enzyme in steroidogenesis. This increased transcription increases enzyme production and activity, with consequent accumulation of non-21-hydroxylated steroids, especially 17-OHP. As the pathways in Fig. 21.1 indicate, these steroids are converted to testosterone.

In the male fetus, the testes produce large amounts of mRNA, for the steroidogenic enzymes and concentrations of testosterone are high in early to midgestation [236]. This testosterone differentiates external male genitalia from the pluripotential embryonic precursor structures. In the male fetus with 21-OHD, the additional testosterone produced in the adrenals has little if any demonstrable phenotypic effect. In a female fetus, the ovaries lack steroidogenic enzyme mRNAs and are quiescent [236]; no sex steroids or other factors are needed for differentiation of the female external genitalia [275]. The testosterone inappropriately produced by the adrenals of the affected female fetus causes varying degrees of virilization of the external genitalia. This can range from mild cliteromegaly, with or without posterior fusion of the labioscrotal folds, to complete labioscrotal fusion that includes a urethra traversing the enlarged clitoris (Fig. 21.8). These infants have normal ovaries, fallopian tubes and a uterus, but have ambiguous external genitalia or may be sufficiently virilized so that they appear to be male, resulting in errors of sex assignment at birth.

The diagnosis of 21-OHD is suggested by genital ambiguity in females, a salt-losing episode in either sex or rapid growth and virilization in males. Plasma 17-OHP is markedly elevated and hyper-responsive to stimulation with ACTH

(a)

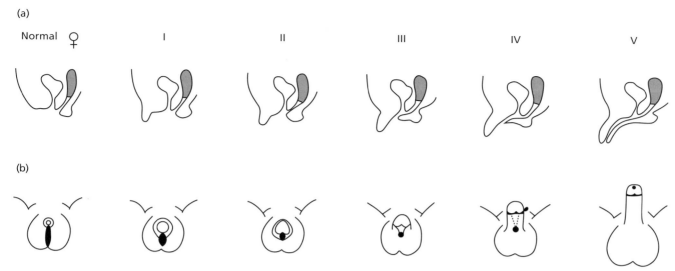

(b)

**Fig. 21.8.** Virilization of the external genitalia. A continuous spectrum is shown from normal female to normal male in both saggital section (a) and perineal views (b), using the staging system of Prader. Disorders of external genitalia can occur either by the virilization of a normal female, as in congenital adrenal hyperplasia, or because of an error in testosterone synthesis in the male. In females with congenital adrenal hyperplasia due to 21-OHD, the degree of virilization correlates poorly with the presence or absence of clinical signs of salt loss.

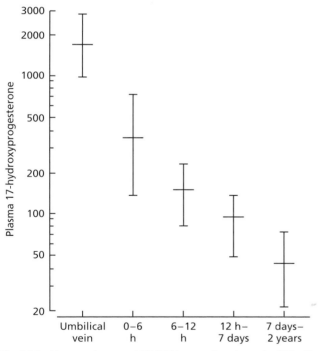

**Fig. 21.9.** Means and ranges of 17-OHP in normal newborns (ng/100 mL). Note that values can be very high and quite variable for the first 24 h of life.

(Fig. 21.7). Measurement of 11-deoxycortisol, 17-OHP, DHEA and androstenedione is important to distinguish from other forms of CAH and because adrenal or testicular tumours can also produce 17-OHP [276]. High newborn 17-OHP values that rise further after ACTH can also be seen in 3β-HSD and P450c11 deficiencies [252]. 17-OHP is normally high in cord blood but falls to normal newborn levels after 12–24 h (Fig. 21.9) so that assessment of 17-OHP should not be made in the first 24 h of life. Premature infants and term infants under severe stress (e.g. with cardiac or pulmonary disease) may have persistently elevated 17-OHP concentrations with normal 21-hydroxylase.

## Clinical forms of 21-OHD

There is a broad spectrum of clinical manifestations of 21-OHD, depending on the mutations of the P450c21 alleles. The different forms are not different diseases but rather a spectrum of manifestations, ranging from severe salt wasting to clinically unapparent forms that may be normal variants. Thus, the disease forms described are mainly for clinical convenience.

### Salt-wasting 21-OHD

Salt wasting is due to a complete deficiency of P450c21 activity, effectively eliminating both glucocorticoid and mineralocorticoid synthesis. Females are frequently diagnosed at birth because of masculinization of the external genitalia. After appropriate resuscitation of the cardiovascular collapse, acidosis and electrolyte disorders, the mineralocorticoids and glucocorticoids can be replaced orally and the ambiguous genitalia corrected with a series of plastic surgical procedures. The steroidal replacement management is difficult because of the rapidly changing needs of a growing infant or child. Drug doses must be adjusted frequently and there is considerable individual variability in what constitutes physiological replacement. As underdosage of glucocorticoids can be life-threatening, especially during illness, most paediatricians have tended to err 'on the safe side', so the children have received inappropriately large doses. It is not possible to compensate for growth lost during the first 2 years of life, when it is fastest, so these children almost always end up short. Female survivors may have sexual dysfunction, marry with a low frequency and have decreased fertility [277–281]. Males are not generally diagnosed at birth and they either come to medical attention during the salt-losing crisis that follows 5–15 days later or they die, invariably having been diagnosed incorrectly.

### Simple virilizing 21-OHD

Virilized females with elevated concentrations of 17-OHP but who do not suffer a salt-losing crisis have long been recognized as having the 'simple virilizing' form of CAH. The existence of this clinical variant first led to the incorrect belief that there were distinct 21-hydroxylases in the zona glomerulosa and in the zona fasciculata. Males often escape diagnosis until age 3–7 years, when they develop pubic, axillary and facial hair and phallic growth. The testes remain of prepubertal size in CAH, whereas gonadotrophic stimulation in true precocious puberty results in pubertal-sized testes. These children grow rapidly and are tall for age when diagnosed, but their bone age advances at a disproportionately rapid rate so that adult height is compromised.

Untreated or poorly treated children may fail to undergo normal puberty, and boys may have small testes and azoospermia because of the feedback effects of the adrenally produced testosterone. When treatment is begun at several years of age, suppression of adrenal testosterone secretion may remove tonic inhibition of the hypothalamus, occasionally resulting in true central precocious puberty requiring treatment with a gonadotrophin-releasing hormone (GnRH) agonist. High concentrations of ACTH in some poorly treated boys may stimulate enlargement of adrenal rests in the testes. These enlarged testes are usually nodular, unlike the homogeneously enlarged testes in central precocious puberty. Because the adrenal normally produces 100–1000 times as much cortisol as aldosterone, mild defects (amino acid replacement mutations) in P450c21 are less likely to affect mineralocorticoid than cortisol secretion. Thus, patients with simple virilizing CAH simply have a less severe disorder of P450c21. This is reflected physiologically by the increased plasma renin activity seen in these patients after moderate salt restriction.

### Non-classic 21-OHD

Many people have very mild forms of 21-OHD. These may be evidenced by mild to moderate hirsutism, virilism, menstrual irregularities and decreased fertility in adult women (so-called late-onset CAH) [282–284], or there may be no phenotypic manifestations at all, other than an increased response of plasma 17-OHP to an intraveneous ACTH test (so-called cryptic CAH) [285]. Despite the minimal manifestations of

this disorder, these individuals have hormonal evidence of a mild impairment in mineralocorticoid secretion, as predicted from the existence of a single adrenal 21-hydroxylase [286].

There has been considerable debate about how to classify patients principally because each diagnostic category represents a picture in a spectrum of disease due to a spectrum of genetic lesions in the P450c21 gene. Furthermore, because many different mutant P450c21 alleles are common in the general population, most patients are compound heterozygotes, carrying a different mutation in the alleles inherited from each parent. Finally, many factors other than the specific mutations found in P450c21 influence the clinical phenotype, including the presence of extra-adrenal 21-hydroxylases (other than P450c21), undiagnosed P450c21 promoter mutations and variations in androgen sensitivity. Discordances between genotype and phenotype are to be expected.

### Incidence of 21-OHD

Perinatal screening for elevated concentrations of serum 17-OHP in several countries yielded an incidence of 1 in 14 000 for 'classic' CAH (i.e. salt-wasting and simple virilizing CAH) and 1 in 60 for heterozygous carriers [287]. This calculation has now been confirmed through the screening of 1.9 million newborns in Texas [288]. The overall incidence was 1 in 16 000 and, because of the large numbers involved, an ethnic breakdown was possible showing an incidence of 1 in 15 600 Caucasians, 1 in 14 500 Hispanics (primarily Mexican Americans of indigenous American ancestry) and 1 in 42 300 African Americans [288]. Because about 20% of the African American gene pool is of European descent, the calculated incidence in individuals of wholly African ancestry is about 1 in 250 000.

Non-classic 21-OHD is much more common, but the data vary: 1 in 27 for Ashkenazi Jews, 1 in 53 for Hispanics, 1 in 63 for Yugoslavs, 1 in 333 for Italians and 1 in 1000 for other whites have been reported [289–291]. This indicates that one-third of Ashkenazi Jews, one-quarter of Hispanics, one-fifth of Yugoslavs, one-ninth of Italians and one-fourteenth of other Caucasians are heterozygous carriers. However, carrier rates of 1.2% [283] to 6% [292,293] for Caucasian populations that were not subdivided further have been recorded. These differences reflect the small populations examined and the errors that arise when hormonal data are used to distinguish individuals with non-classic CAH from heterozygous carriers of classic CAH. This error can be ameliorated by careful measurement of 17-OHP before and after stimulation with ACTH (Fig. 21.7) [79].

In homozygotes for both classic and non-classic CAH, serum concentrations of 21-deoxycortisol rise in response to ACTH but ACTH-induced 21-deoxycortisol remains normal in heterozygotes for both classic and non-classic CAH [294]. However, these studies have classified individuals by hormonal phenotype without examining the P450c21 genes directly to establish these incidences. Therefore, the diagnosis

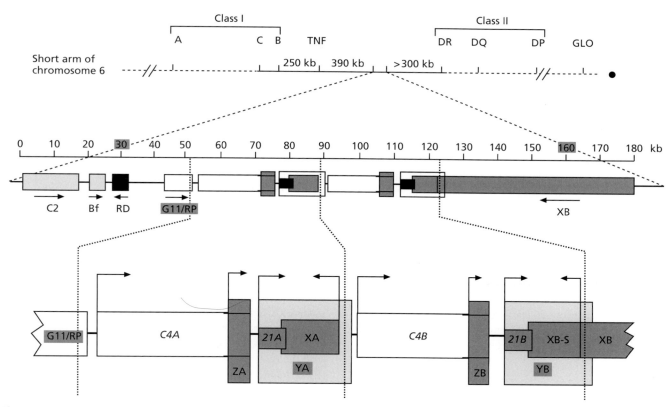

**Fig. 21.10.** Genetic map of the HLA locus containing the genes for P450c21. The top line shows the p21.1 region of chromosome 6, with the telomere to the left and the centromere to the right. Most HLA genes are found in the class I and class II regions; the class III region containing the P450c21 genes lies between these two. The second line shows the scale (in kilobases) for the diagram immediately below, showing (from left to right) the genes for complement factor C2, properedin factor Bf and the RD and G11/RP genes of unknown function; arrows indicate transcriptional orientation. The bottom line shows the 21-hydroxylase locus on an expanded scale, including the C4A and C4B genes for the fourth component of complement, the inactive *CYP21A* gene (21A) and the active *CYP21B* gene (21B) that encodes P450c21. XA, YA and YB are adrenal-specific transcripts that lack open reading frames. The *XB* gene encodes the extracellular matrix protein tenascin-X; *XB-S* encodes a truncated adrenal-specific form of the tenascin-X protein whose function is unknown. ZA and ZB are adrenal-specific transcripts that arise within the *C4* genes and have open reading frames, but it is not known if they are translated into protein; however, the promoter elements of these transcripts are essential components of the CYP21A and CYP21B promoters. The arrows indicate transcriptional orientation. The vertical dotted lines designate the boundaries of the genetic duplication event that led to the presence of A and B regions.

of non-classic CAH requires family studies, as the hormonal data (17-OHP responses to ACTH) in these individuals may be indistinguishable from those for unaffected heterozygous carriers of the more severe forms. The high incidence, lack of mortality and lack of decreased fertility in most individuals with non-classic CAH indicate that this is probably a variant of normal and not a disease in the classic sense. Nevertheless, patients may seek help for virilism and menstrual disorders.

## Genetics of the 21-hydroxylase locus

### 21-Hydroxylase genes

There are two 21-hydroxylase loci, a functional gene formally termed *CYP21A2* and a non-functional pseudogene formally termed *CYP21A1P* [295]. These genes, P450c21B (functional gene) and P450c21A (pseudogene), are duplicated in tandem with the *C4A* and *C4B* genes encoding the fourth component of serum complement [296,297] (Fig. 21.10). Although the

P450c21A locus is transcribed into two alternately spliced, adrenal-specific mRNAs, neither of them encodes a protein [298]: only the P450c21B gene encodes adrenal 21-hydroxylase. The P450c21 genes consist of 10 exons, are about 3.4 kb long and differ in only 87 or 88 of these bases [82–84]. This high degree of sequence similarity indicates that these two genes are evolving in tandem through intergenic exchange of DNA. The P450c21 genes of mice [299] and cattle [300,301] are also duplicated and linked to leucocyte antigen loci, but only the P450c21B gene functions in human beings, only the P450c21A gene functions in mice [302,303] and both genes function in cattle [304]. Sequencing of the gene duplication boundaries shows that the human locus, duplicated after mammalian speciation [305], is consistent with data that indicate that other mammals have single P450c21 gene copies [306].

### HLA linkage

The 21-hydroxylase genes lie within the class III region of the human major histocompatibility complex (MHC) (Fig. 21.10). The P450c21 locus lies about 600 kb from HLA-B and about 400 kb from HLA-DR. HLA typing has been widely used for prenatal diagnosis and to identify heterozygous family members. Statistical associations (linkage disequilibrium) are well established between CAH and certain specific HLA types. Salt-losing CAH is associated with HLA-B60 and HLA-40 in some populations [307] and the rare HLA type Bw47 is very strongly associated with salt-losing CAH [308,309]. HLA-Bw51 is often associated with simple virilizing CAH in some populations [310], and 30–50% of haplotypes for non-classic CAH carry HLA-B14 [311]. HLA-B14 is often associated with a duplication of the *C4B* gene [312,313]. By contrast, all HLA-B alleles can be found linked to CAH. HLA-identical individuals in a single family may have different clinical features of 21-OHD despite HLA identity [314–317], possibly representing extra-adrenal 21-hydroxylation, *de novo* mutations or multiple genetic crossover events. In one family with clinically non-concordant HLA-identical siblings, the Southern blotting pattern of P450c21 genes digested with *Eco*RI showed a within-generation genetic rearrangement not detectable by other means [316].

### C4 *genes*

The tandemly duplicated *C4A* and *C4B* loci produce proteins that can be distinguished functionally and immunologically; the C4B protein has substantially more haemolytic activity, despite greater that 99% sequence identity with C4A [318,319]. The *C4A* gene is always 22 kb long but there are long (22 kb) and short (16 kb) forms of *C4B* because of a variation in one intron [320,321]. The 3′ ends of the *C4* genes are only 2466 bp upstream from the transcriptional start sites of the P450c21 genes. Promoter sequences needed for the transcription of the human P450c21B gene lie within intron 35 of the *C4B* gene [322] and also initiate the transcription of the 'Z transcripts', which have an open reading frame but whose translational status is unclear [323].

### *Other genes in the 21-hydroxylase locus*

In addition to the P450c21 and C4 genes, there are numerous other genes within 100 kb of the P450c21 gene (Fig. 21.10). The genes for complement factor C2 and properdin factor Bf lie 80–100 kb 5′ to the P450c21 gene and have the same transcriptional orientation (i.e. lie on the same strand of DNA). Lying just 3′ of the Bf gene is the RD gene, so called because it encodes a protein with a long stretch of alternating arginine (R) and aspartic acid (D) residues [324]. This gene lies on the opposite strand of DNA from the complement and P450c21 genes and is expressed in all tissues but its function is unknown [325]. Thirteen other putative genes have been identified lying between the gene for TNF and C4A, but no functions have been ascribed to them [326].

A pair of genes, XA and XB, is duplicated with the C4 and P450c21 genes. These lie on the strand of DNA opposite from

the C4 and P450c21 genes and overlap the 3′ end of P450c21. The last exon of XA and XB lies within the 3′ untranslated region of exon 10 in P450c21A and P450c21B respectively [327]. Although the human XA locus was truncated during the duplication of the ancestral C4-P450c21-X genetic unit, the XA gene is abundantly transcribed in the adult and fetal adrenal [305]. By contrast, the XB gene encodes a large extracellular matrix protein (tenascin X) that is expressed in a wide variety of adult and fetal tissues, especially connective tissue [328,329]. The XB gene spans about 65 kb of DNA and includes 43 exons encoding a 12-kb mRNA [328,330]. The XB gene also encodes a short truncated form of tenascin X having unknown function and arising from an intragenic promoter [331].

Identification of a patient with a 'contiguous gene syndrome' comprising a deletion of both the P450c21B and XB genes demonstrated that deficiency of tenascin X results in Ehlers–Danlos syndrome (EDS) [332]. EDS can also be caused by mutations in collagen genes and genes for collagen-modifying enzymes. Studies in cattle indicate that tenascin X is associated with and stabilizes collagen fibrils [333], thus explaining the related phenotype of mutations in tenascin X and collagen-associated genes. Although the various transcripts from the XA and XB genes are complementary to the mRNA for P450c21 and the other transcripts that arise from the P450c21 promoters [298], these RNAs do not form RNA/RNA duplexes *in vivo* [334] and hence do not regulate P450c21.

### P450c21 gene lesions causing 21-OHD

21-OHD can be caused by P450c21B gene deletions, gene conversions and apparent point mutations. Most of the point mutations in the P450c21B gene are actually small gene conversion events [78,80,335], so that gene conversions account for about 85% of the lesions in 21-OHD. The P450c21 genes are autosomal, hence each person has two alleles, one contributed by each parent. Most patients with 21-OHD are compound heterozygotes, having different lesions on their two alleles. Because gene deletions and large conversions eliminate all P450c21B gene transcription, these lesions will cause salt-losing 21-OHD in the homozygous state. Some microconversions, such as those creating premature translational termination, are also associated with salt-losing CAH. Milder forms (simple virilizing and non-classic 21-OHD) are associated with amino acid replacements in the P450c21 protein caused by gene microconversion events. Patients with these forms of CAH are usually compound heterozygotes bearing a severely disordered allele and a mildly disordered allele so that the clinical manifestations are based on the nature of the mildly disordered allele.

### *Mapping of P450c21 genes in normal subjects and in 21-OHD*

Although the P450c21B and P450c21A loci differ by only 87 or 88 nucleotides, they can be distinguished by restriction endonuclease digestion and Southern blotting. The P450c21A locus is characterized by 3.2- and 2.4-kb *Taq*I fragments and 12-kb *Bgl*II fragments, whereas the functional P450c21B gene is characterized by 3.7- and 2.5-kb *Taq*I fragments and 11-kb *Bgl*II fragments. Two unusual and related features of the 21-hydroxylase locus complicate its analysis. First, the gene deletions in this locus are most unusual in that they extend 30 kb from one of several points in the middle of P450c21A to the precisely homologous point in P450c21B. Thus, the 15% of alleles that carry deletions do not yield a typical Southern blotting pattern with a band that is a different size from that of the normal, unless one uses very rare cutting enzymes and analyses the resulting large DNA fragments by pulsed-field gel electrophoresis. The second unusual feature of this locus is that gene conversions are extremely common [336,337].

### Gene conversions

If a segment of gene A replaces the corresponding segment of the related gene B, the structure of recipient gene B is said to be 'converted' to that of donor gene A. The hallmark of gene conversion is that the number of closely related genes remains constant, but their diversity decreases. Two types of gene conversions commonly cause 21-OHD, large gene conversions that can be mistaken for gene deletions and small microconversions that resemble point mutations. When a large gene conversion causes 21-OHD, the *Taq*I digestion pattern of the P450c21B gene is converted to that of the P450c21A. This conversion changes the 5' end of the P450c21B sequence to the 5' end of P450c21A.

The relative frequency of large gene conversions compared with gene deletions in 21-OHD was controversial, principally because initial studies used relatively small groups of patients from single locations or ethnic groups. A study of 68 French patients showed that 12.5% of the mutant alleles had large gene conversions, 12.5% had gene deletions and 75% had microconversions [313]. A compilation of the world literature on the genetics of 21-OHD found that 19% of mutant alleles had gene deletions, 8% large gene conversions, 67% microconversions and 6% uncharacterized lesions [80] (Fig. 21.11). Such statistics must be viewed with caution because there is considerable ascertainment bias in favour of the more severely affected patients [313] and because some studies excluded mildly affected patients. Thus, the above statistics are weighted in favour of gene deletions and large conversions, which can only yield a phenotype of salt-wasting 21-OHD.

### Point mutations (microconversions) causing 21-OHD

About 75% of mutated P450c21 genes appear to be structurally intact by Southern blotting and thus appear to carry point mutations [313,336]. Many mutant P450c21B genes causing 21-OHD have been cloned and sequenced (Table 21.6), revealing that a relatively small number of mutations cause the condition, virtually all of which are also found in

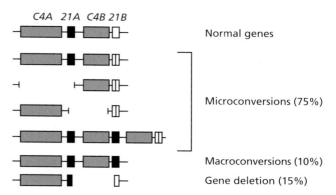

**Fig. 21.11.** Classes of genetic rearrangements causing 21-OHD. Deletions or duplications of the *C4A* and *C4B* genes can occur with or without associated lesions in the P450c21B gene. Note that all 'point mutations' in P450c21B are actually 'microconversion'. Many authors combine the 'gene deletion' and 'macroconversion' groups because these are difficult to distinguish by Southern blotting as both result in a loss of the P450c21B gene, but the genotypes are clearly distinct, as shown.

**Table 21.6.** Microconversions of the P450c21B gene that cause 21-hydroxylase deficiency

| Mutation | Location | Associated phenotypes | Activity |
|---|---|---|---|
| Pro-30→Leu | Exon 1 | NC/SV | 30–60% |
| A→G | Intron 2 | SV/SW | Minimal |
| 8-bp deletion | Exon 3 | SW | 0 |
| Ile-172→Asn | Exon 4 | SV | 3–7% |
| Ile-236→Asp | | | |
| Val-237→Glu | Exon 6 | SW | 0 |
| Met-239→Lys | | | |
| Val-281→Leu | Exon 7 | NC | 18±9% |
| Gly-292→Ser | Exon 7 | SW | |
| T insertion at 306 | Exon 7 | SW | 0 |
| Gly-318→Stop | Exon 8 | SW | 0 |
| Arg-339→His | Exon 8 | NC | 20–50% |
| Arg-356→Trp | Exon 8 | SV/SW | 2% |
| Pro-453→Ser | Exon 10 | NC | 20–50% |
| GG→C at 484 | Exon 10 | SW | 0 |

the P450c21A pseudogene. These observations indicate that most CAH alleles bearing apparent point mutations actually carry microconversions [78,80,335].

### Effects of known point mutations on 21-hydroxylase activity

There are three changes in the P450c21A pseudogene that render its product non-functional. Each results in an altered reading frame and/or premature stop codon, hence eliminating all activity; all of these, the C→T transition at codon 318, the 8-bp deletion in exon 3 and the T insertion in exon 7, have been found in P450c21B alleles that cause severe salt-losing 21-OHD. Three closely clustered base changes alter the normal amino acid sequence Ile–Val–Glu–Met at codons 236–239 in exon 6 to Asn–Glu–Glu–Lys in both P450c21A and in a small number of genes causing severe salt-losing 21-OHD. There is no assayable 21-hydroxylase activity when this sequence is expressed *in vitro*.

The most common lesion in classic 21-OHD is an A→G change in the second intron, 13 bases upstream from the normal 3′ splice acceptor site of this intron, a microconversion found in over 25% of severely affected alleles. This intronic mutation causes abnormal splicing of the mRNA precursor, destroying activity. However, a small portion of this mRNA may be spliced normally in some patients so that the phenotypic presentation is variable; most such patients are salt losers, but some are not salt-losing. This intron 2 microconversion is often associated with the Ser/Thr polymorphism at codon 268; this is a true polymorphism as S268T does not alter enzymatic activity [338]. The microconversion R356W, which is found in about 10% of severely affected alleles [339], eliminates all detectable activity [340], apparently because it changes a residue in the binding site for P450 oxidoreductase [269]. This mutation may retain slight activity and has been found in simple virilizing cases. Other, extremely rare mutations have been described in single individuals [341–343].

### Missense mutations causing simple virilizing 21-OHD

The microconversion I172N is the most common cause of simple virilizing 21-OHD [340,344,345]. Ile-172 is conserved in the other known mammalian P450c21 genes and may contribute to the hydrophobic interactions needed to maintain the correct conformation of the enzyme. When Ile-172 was changed to Asn, Leu, Gln or His and the constructed mutants were expressed in mammalian cells, the mutant constructions yielded only 3–7% of the 21-hydroxylase activity of normal P450c21 [340,346]. The intron 2 microconversion is occasionally seen in simple virilizing cases. The microconversion P30L is generally associated with non-classic 21-OHD but is found in some patients with the simple virilizing form.

### Missense mutations causing non-classic 21-OHD

The most common mutation causing non-classic 21-OHD is V281L. This microconversion is seen in all patients with the non-classic form linked to HLA-B14 and HLA-DR1 but is also found in patients with other HLA types. This mutation does not alter the affinity of the enzyme for substrate but drastically reduces its $V_{max}$ [347]. The microconversion P30L is found in about 15–20% of non-classic alleles. In addition, the mutations R339H and P453S have been associated with the non-classic form [348,349]. Initial surveys of the mutations in P450c21A failed to reveal these mutations, suggesting that they are bona fide point mutations rather than gene microconversions. Examination of large numbers of P450c21A pseudogenes shows that at least the P453S mutation is polymorphic in about 20% of P450c21A pseudogenes, and hence also represents a microconversion event.

### Structure–function inferences from P450c21 mutations

Each P450c21 missense mutation appears to occur in a functional domain of P450c21. By analogy with the membrane-anchoring domain of hepatic P450IIB, amino acids 167–178 of P450c21, including the crucial Ile-172 residue, appear to constitute a similar domain [340]. By analogy with the computationally inferred structure of the closely related enzyme P450c17 [269], Arg-356 may be part of the redox partner binding site, Val-281 appears to participate in coordinating the haem moiety, and Cys-428 is the crucial cystine residue in the haem binding site found in all cytochrome P450 enzymes. All these mutations can arise by gene microconversions. The N-terminal region of P450c21, including Pro-30, appears to be required for membrane insertion and enzyme stability [350]. Finding most mutations in the amino-terminal portion of P450c21 is consistent with finding most gene conversion and gene deletion events occurring in exons 1–8 of the P450c21B gene. Changes in exons 9 and 10 are very rare, possibly as a result of evolutionary pressure to retain the 3′ untranslated and 3′ flanking DNA of the P450c21B gene, as this DNA also contains the 3′ end of the XB gene [327,328].

### Prenatal diagnosis and treatment of 21-OHD

The prenatal diagnosis and therapy of 21-OHD are being actively pursued but prenatal therapy remains experimental and controversial [273,351–354]. The fetal adrenal is active in steroidogenesis from early in gestation, so a diagnosis can be made by amniocentesis and measurement of amniotic fluid 17-OHP [355–357]. Concentrations of $\Delta^4$ androstenedione are also elevated in the amniotic fluid of fetuses with 21-OHD, providing a potentially useful adjunctive assay [358]. However, amniotic fluid concentrations of 17-OHP and $\Delta^4$ androstenedione are reliable only for identifying fetuses affected with severe salt-losing 21-OHD, because these steroids may not be elevated above the broad range of normal in the non-salt-losing or non-classic forms [359,360].

If a fetus is known to be at risk because the parents are known heterozygotes, 21-OHD can be diagnosed by HLA typing of fetal amniocytes or by analysis of fetal amniocyte DNA. If the fetus has the same HLA type as the previously affected child, the fetus will be affected; a fetus that shares one parent's HLA type with the index case will be a heterozygous carrier and a fetus having both haplotypes differing from the index case will be unaffected. HLA typing of cultured amniocytes requires previous linkage analysis of the affected child and parents. Only HLA-A and HLA-B can be reliably determined in cultured amniocytes, although some HLA-B alleles are expressed weakly in amniocytes. There is a relatively high incidence of HLA-B homozygosity among 21-OHD patients. HLA-B loci are frequently identical between parents and patients, some HLA-B antigens may cross-react and amniocytes may not express HLA-DR antigens, further limiting the usefulness of HLA typing.

Experimental prenatal treatment requires early and accurate prenatal diagnosis. Female fetuses affected with 21-OHD begin to become virilized at about 6–8 weeks' gestation at the same time that a normal male fetal testis produces large amounts of testosterone, causing fusion of the labioscrotal folds, enlargement of the genital tubercle into a phallus and the formation of the phallic urethra [275]. The adrenals of affected female fetuses can produce concentrations of testosterone that may approach those in a normal male, resulting in varying degrees of masculinization of the external genitalia. If fetal adrenal steroidogenesis is suppressed in an affected fetus, the virilization can theoretically be reduced or eliminated. Several studies have reported the successful application of this approach by administering dexamethasone to the mother as soon as pregnancy is diagnosed [361–365]. This can be done only when the parents are known to be heterozygotes by having already had an affected child. However, even in such pregnancies, only one in four fetuses will have CAH. Furthermore, as no prenatal treatment is needed for male fetuses affected with CAH, only one in eight pregnancies of heterozygous parents would harbour an affected female fetus that might potentially benefit from prenatal treatment and seven would have been treated unnecessarily.

The efficacy, safety and desirability of such prenatal treatment remain highly controversial [80,141,273,351–354,357,364–367]. It is not known precisely when the fetal hypothalamus begins to produce CRH, when the fetal pituitary begins to produce ACTH, whether all fetal ACTH production is regulated by CRH, nor whether these hormones are suppressible by dexamethasone in the early fetus. Although there is considerable evidence that pharmacological doses of glucocorticoids do not harm pregnant women, no such data exist for the fetus. Pregnant women with diseases such as nephrotic syndrome and systemic lupus erythematosus are generally treated with prednisone, which does not reach the fetus because it is inactivated by placental 11β-HSD. Treatment of a fetus requires the use of fluorinated steroids that escape metabolism by these enzymes, and few data are available about the long-term use of such agents throughout gestation. The available preliminary studies indicate that the response of the fetal genital anatomy to treatment is generally good if the treatment is started very early (before week 6); thereafter, the virilization is reduced but may not be eliminated, so that at least one reconstructive surgical procedure may still be needed in the infant [141,356–368].

Successful treatment requires dexamethasone doses of 20 μg/kg of maternal body weight. For a 70-kg woman, this is 1.4 mg, which is equivalent to that in the low-dose dexamethasone suppression test and at least three times physiological replacement. The fetus normally develops in the presence of very low cortisol concentrations (100 nmol/L, 3.6 μg/dL)

[138], which are only about 20% of the corresponding maternal level. Thus the doses used in prenatal treatment appear to achieve effective concentrations of active glucocorticoid that may be 10–15 times physiological for the fetus. Treatment of pregnant rats with 20 μg/kg dexamethasone predisposes the fetuses to hypertension in adulthood [369], and some studies indicate that even moderately elevated concentrations of glucocorticoids can be neurotoxic [370–374]. Thus prenatal treatment of CAH remains an experimental and controversial therapy that should be done only in research centres. Follow-up studies of very long duration are needed to evaluate its effects fully, especially on the seven fetuses treated unnecessarily.

### Diagnosis

The key diagnostic manoeuvre in all forms of 21-OHD is the measurement of the 17-OHP response to intravenous synthetic ACTH. Individual patient responses must be compared with age- and sex-matched data from normal children [215] (Table 21.4 and Fig. 21.7). Other ancillary tests are listed in Table 21.5.

Plasma renin activity and its response to salt restriction constitute an especially useful test. Most patients with simple virilizing 21-OHD have high plasma renin activity, which increases further on sodium restriction, confirming that these patients are partially mineralocorticoid deficient and can maintain a normal serum sodium only by hyperstimulation of the zona glomerulosa. Mineralocorticoid therapy in these patients returns plasma volume to normal and eliminates the hypovolemic drive to ACTH secretion. Thus, mineralocorticoid therapy often permits the use of lower doses of glucocorticoids in patients with simple virilizing CAH, optimizing growth in children and diminishing unwanted weight gain in adults.

Long-term management is difficult and requires clinical and laboratory evaluation. Growth should be measured at 3- to 4-month intervals, along with an annual assessment of bone age. Each visit should be accompanied by measurement of urinary 17-KS and serum $\Delta^4$ androstenedione, DHEA, DHEA sulphate and testosterone. Measurement of 3α-androstenediol glucuronide may also be useful. In general, plasma 17-OHP is not a useful indicator of therapeutic efficacy because of its great diurnal variation and hyper-responsiveness to stress (e.g. clinic visits).

### Treatment

Although Wilkins *et al.* [7] and Bartter *et al.* [8] first demonstrated effective treatment of 21-OHD with cortisone in 1950, the management of this disorder remains difficult. Overtreatment with glucocorticoids causes delayed growth, even when the degree of overtreatment is insufficient to produce signs and symptoms of Cushing syndrome. Undertreatment results in continued overproduction of adrenal androgens, which hastens epiphiseal maturation and closure, again

**Table 21.7.** Potency of various therapeutic steroids (set relative to the potency of cortisol)

| Steroid | Anti-inflammatory glucocorticoid effect | Growth-retarding glucocorticoid effect | Salt-retaining mineralocorticoid effect | Plasma half-life (min) | Biological half-life (h) |
|---|---|---|---|---|---|
| Cortisol (hydrocortisone) | 1.0 | 1.0 | 1.0 | 80–120 | 8 |
| Cortisone acetate (oral) | 0.8 | 0.8 | 0.8 | 80–120 | 8 |
| Cortisone acetate (i.m.) | 0.8 | 1.3 | 0.8 | | 18 |
| Prednisone | 3.5–4 | 5 | 0.8 | 200 | 16–36 |
| Prednisolone | 4 | | 0.8 | 120–300 | 16–36 |
| Methyl prednisolone | 5 | 7.5 | 0.5 | | |
| Betamethasone | 25–30 | | 0 | 130–330 | |
| Triamcinolone | 5 | | 0 | | |
| Dexamethasone | 30 | 80 | 0 | 150–300 | 36–54 |
| 9α-Fluorocortisone | 15 | | 200 | | |
| DOC acetate | 0 | | 20 | | |
| Aldosterone | 0.3 | | 200–1000 | | |

resulting in compromised growth and other manifestations of androgen excess.

Doses of glucocorticoids should be based on the expected normal cortisol secretory rate. Widely cited classic studies have reported that the secretory rate of cortisol is $12.5 \pm 3$ mg/m$^2$/day [375–377] and have led most authorities to recommend doses of 10–20 mg of hydrocortisone (cortisol) per m$^2$ per day. However, the cortisol secretory rate is actually substantially lower, at $6–7 \pm 2$ mg/m$^2$/day [209,210]. Newly diagnosed patients, especially newborns, do require substantially higher initial dosages to suppress their hyperactive CRH/ACTH/adrenal access.

The glucocorticoid used is important. Most tables of glucocorticoid dose equivalencies are based on their equivalence in anti-inflammatory assays. However, the growth-suppressant equivalences of various glucocorticoids do not parallel their anti-inflammatory equivalencies [378]. Thus, long-acting synthetic steroids such as dexamethasone have a disproportionately greater growth-suppressant effect and must be avoided when treating growing children and adolescents (Table 21.7). Most authorities favour the use of oral hydrocortisone or cortisone acetate in three divided daily doses in growing children. However, adults and older teenagers who already have fused their epiphyses may be managed very effectively with prednisone or dexamethasone.

Only one oral mineralocorticoid preparation, fludrocortisone (9α-fluorocortisol), is generally available. It must be given as crushed tablets, not as a suspension, which delivers the medication unreliably. When the oral route is not available in severely ill patients, mineralocorticoid replacement is achieved through intravenous hydrocortisone plus sodium chloride. Hydrocortisone (20 mg) has a mineralocorticoid effect of about 100 µg of 9α-fluorocortisol (Table 21.7). Mineralocorticoids are unique in pharmacology in that their doses are not based on body mass or surface area. In fact, newborns are

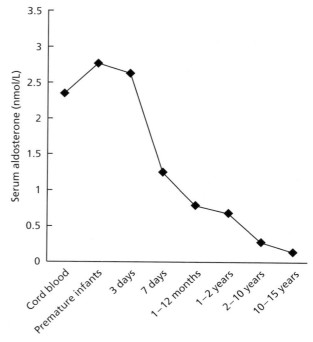

**Fig. 21.12.** Concentrations of aldosterone as a function of age.

quite insensitive to mineralocorticoids, as reflected by their high serum aldosterone concentrations (Fig. 21.12), and require larger doses than do adults (100–200 µg/day). In older children, the replacement dose of 9α-fluorocortisol is 50–150 µg daily. A mineralocorticoid is useless unless adequate sodium is presented to the renal tubules. Thus, additional salt supplementation, usually 1–2 g of NaCl per day in the newborn, is also needed. Patients with severe salt-losing CAH can sometimes discontinue mineralocorticoid replacement and salt supplementation as adults. They certainly need lower doses, possibly because they become more sensitive to the mineralocorticoid action of hydrocortisone via a developmental decrease in renal 11β-HSD activity, which normally inactivates cortisol to cortisone.

## Lesions in isozymes of P450c11: 11β-hydroxylase deficiency, corticosterone methyl oxidase deficiency and glucocorticoid-suppressible hypertension

There are two distinct forms of 11-hydroxylase. P450c11β mediates the 11β-hydroxylation of 11-deoxycortisol to cortisol and that of DOC to corticosterone in the zonae fasciculata and reticularis. P450c11AS, aldosterone synthase, is found only in the zona glomerulosa and mediates 11β-hydroxylation, 18-hydroxylation and 18-oxidation; thus, it is the sole enzyme required to convert DOC to aldosterone. Deficient P450c11β activity is a rare cause of CAH in persons of European ancestry but accounts for about 15% of cases in both Moslem and Jewish Middle Eastern populations [379]. Severe deficiency of P450c11β decreases the secretion of cortisol, causing CAH and virilization of affected females. However, because one of the steroids that accumulates in P450c11β deficiency, DOC, is a mineralocorticoid, these patients can retain sodium.

Although DOC is less potent than aldosterone, it is secreted at high levels in 11β-hydroxylase deficiency, so that salt is retained and the serum sodium remains normal. Overproduction of DOC frequently leads to hypertension; as a result, 11β-hydroxylase deficiency is often termed 'the hypertensive form of CAH'. However, newborns often manifest mild, transient salt loss [379,380], presumably as a result of the normal newborn resistance to mineralocorticoids (Fig. 21.12); this may lead to incorrect diagnosis and treatment. Thus, there may be a poor correlation between DOC concentrations, serum potassium and blood pressure or between the degree of virilization in affected females and the electrolyte and cardiovascular manifestations [79]. The diagnosis is established by demonstrating elevated basal concentrations of DOC and 11-deoxycortisol which hyperrespond to ACTH; a normal or suppressed plasma renin activity is also a hallmark of this disease [381].

The genetic lesions causing 11β-hydroxylase deficiency are in the *CYP11B1* gene that encodes P450c11β. In a study of Sephardic Jews of Moroccan ancestry, 11 of 12 affected alleles bore the mutation R448H [95] but at least two frameshifts, four premature stop codons and five amino acid replacement mutations have also been described in other populations [88]. A milder, non-classic form of 11β-hydroxylase deficiency, analogous to non-classic 21-OHD has been reported in otherwise asymptomatic women with hirsutism, virilism and menstrual irregularities [379,382]. However, true non-classic 11β-hydroxylase deficiency is rare; only two of five hyperandrogenaemic women who had 11-deoxycortisol

values more than three times higher than the 95th percentile in response to stimulation with ACTH had mutations of P450c11β, all of which retained 15–37% of normal activity [383]. Repeated ACTH testing in two of the three women who lacked mutations showed much lower (but still elevated) 11-deoxycortisol values. Thus, just as in the case of non-classic 3β-HSD deficiency, an abnormal steroid response to ACTH is not sufficient to diagnose a genetic lesion.

P450c11AS, the isozyme of P450c11β that is 93% identical in its amino acid sequence, is expressed exclusively in the zona glomerulosa, where it catalyses 11β-hydroxylase, 18-hydroxylase and 18-methyl oxidase activities. Both P450c11AS and P450c11β are expressed in the human and both can convert DOC to corticosterone, but the conversion of corticosterone to 18-hydroxycorticosterone and subsequently to aldosterone is performed exclusively by P450c11AS. Disorders of P450c11AS cause the so-called corticosterone methyl oxidase (CMO) deficiencies, wherein aldosterone biosynthesis is impaired while the zona fasciculata and reticularis continue to produce corticosterone and DOC. The absence of aldosterone biosynthesis will generally result in a salt-wasting crisis in infancy, at which time the normal secretory rate of DOC is insufficient to meet the newborn's mineralocorticoid requirements (similarly to the newborn with P450c11β deficiency).

These infants typically present with hyponatraemia, hyperkalaemia and metabolic acidosis, but the salt-wasting syndrome is typically less severe than in patients with 21-OHD or lipoid CAH because of the persistent secretion of DOC. The patients may recover spontaneously and grow to adulthood without therapy. This probably reflects the increasing sensitivity to mineralocorticoid action with advancing age in childhood, as reflected by the usual age-related decrease in serum aldosterone (Fig. 21.12). Consistent with this, plasma renin activity is markedly elevated in affected children but may be normal in affected adults [384].

CMOI deficiency results from a complete loss of P450c11AS activity so that no 18-hydroxylase or 18 methyl oxidase activity persists, eliminating the biosynthesis of 18OH-corticosterone and aldosterone while preserving the biosynthesis of corticosterone by P450c11β. Thus the diagnosis for CMOI deficiency is usually based on an increased ratio of corticosterone to 18OH-corticosterone [97]. Only three cases of CMOI deficiency have been fully characterized genetically, including a frameshift mutation [385], a premature stop codon [386] and the missense mutation R384P [387].

CMOII deficiency results from amino acid replacement mutations in P450c11AS that selectively delete the 18-methyl oxidase activity while preserving the 18-hydroxylase activity. The diagnosis of CMOII deficiency requires an increased 18OH-corticosterone and very low aldosterone concentration. CMOII deficiency is common in Sephardic Jews of Iranian origin, where all affected individuals appear to be homozygous for two different mutations, R181W and V385A [96]. Family members who were homozygous for only one of these mutations were clinically unaffected; both mutations are required to cause disease.

The distinction between CMOI and CMOII is not always clear. One patient with the clinical history and hormonal phenotype of CMOII had two mutations on each parental allele [98]. The mother's allele carried R181W and a deletion/frameshift mutation that deleted all activity; the father's allele carried T318M and V386A. Thr-318 is predicted to be the universally conserved Thr residue in all P450 enzymes that participates in cleavage of the dioxygen bond of $O_2$ to create the iron–oxy intermediate required for P450 catalysis. When the T318M/V386A double mutant was recreated *in vitro* there was no detectable activity [98]. These data would have predicted the CMOI phenotype instead of the patient's CMOII phenotype.

Another patient was homozygous for the missense mutations E198A and V386A. When re-created *in vitro* the double mutant enzyme behaved similarly to the mutant enzyme found in the Iranian Jewish CMOII patients, but the patient's clinical phenotype was CMOI [388]. This patient also carried R173K, which is a normally occurring polymorphism that has no affect on the enzyme's $K_m$ or $V_{max}$ [389]. Thus the distinction between CMOI and CMOII is not precise and these disorders should be regarded as different degrees of severity on a clinical spectrum, just as the various forms of 21-OHD.

Rats have four *CYP11B* genes encoding three P450c11 enzymes but there are only two *CYP11B* genes in the human genome, encoding P450c11β and P450c11AS [390]. This genetic anatomy is reminiscent of the P450c21A and P450c21B genes. Although gene conversion can cause CMOII deficiency [391], gene conversion appears to be much rarer than in the P450c21 locus. This may be due to the higher recombinational frequency in the HLA region carrying the P450c21 genes, or it may be related to the abundant antisense transcripts produced in the P450c21 locus [298,334].

Although gene conversion events in the P450c11 locus are rare, an unusual gene duplication causes glucocorticoid-suppressible hyperaldosteronism [392–394]. This homologous recombination event creates a third P450c11 gene, which fuses the 5′ flanking DNA of the P450c11β gene onto the gene for P450c11AS. In two such patients the genetic crossover occurred in intron 2 and in intron 3 or exon 4 in two other patients [393]. All these hybrid genes produce a hybrid P450c11 that retains aldosterone synthase activity; however, as the hybrid gene has P450c11β regulatory regions, its transcription is induced by ACTH and cAMP, as is the normal P450c11β gene. Thus, these patients make P450c11AS in response to physiology that should stimulate P450c11β. The excess P450c11AS causes hyperaldosteronism and hypertension, which is then suppressible by glucocorticoid suppression of ACTH, which normally suppresses P450c11β.

It is conceivable that localized microconversions, similar to those that cause most cases of 21-OHD, could insert sequences crucial for aldosterone synthase activity into the

**Table 21.8.** Causes of adrenal insufficiency

Primary adrenal insufficiency
 Autoimmune adrenalitis
 Autoimmune polyglandular syndromes (types I and II)
 Tuberculosis, fungal infections
 Sepsis
 AIDS
 Congenital adrenal hyperplasia
 Adrenal haemorrhage or infarction
 Congenital adrenal hypoplasia
 Adrenoleucodystrophy
 Primary xanthomatosis
 Unresponsiveness to ACTH

Secondary adrenal insufficiency
 Withdrawal from glucocorticoid therapy
 Hypopituitarism
 Hypothalamic tumours
 Irradiation of the CNS

P450c11β gene. Expression of chimeric proteins produced *in vitro* identified the residues Ser-288 and Val-320 as important for this activity [395]. Similarly, activating mutations that increase the aldosterone synthase activity of P450c11AS have been created *in vitro* [396]. However, examination of large numbers of patients with low-renin hypertension has failed to show mutations in this gene system, other than the gene conversions that cause glucocorticoid suppressible hypertension [389–398].

## Adrenal insufficiency

Besides CAH, many other conditions cause adrenal insufficiency, including ACTH deficiency and primary adrenal disorders. Primary adrenal insufficiency is commonly termed Addison disease, a vague term that encompasses many disorders (Table 21.8). Up to World War II, most patients with 'Addison disease' had tuberculosis of the adrenal but over 80% of contemporary adult patients have autoimmune adrenalitis, and the term *Addison disease* is now widely used to indicate an autoimmune or idiopathic cause.

## Chronic primary adrenal insufficiency

### Autoimmune adrenalitis

Autoimmune adrenalitis is most commonly seen in 25- to 45-year-old adults, about 70% of whom are women. The incidence in adults is about 1 in 25 000. The incidence in children is unknown but much less. Boys constitute about 75% of patients [399]. Chronic adrenal insufficiency is suggested by poor weight gain or weight loss, weakness, fatigue, anorexia,

**Table 21.9.** Signs and symptoms of adrenal insufficiency

Features shared by acute and chronic insufficiency
  Anorexia
  Apathy and confusion
  Dehydration
  Fatigue
  Hyperkalaemia
  Hypoglycaemia
  Hyponatraemia
  Hypovolaemia and tachycardia
  Nausea and vomiting
  Postural hypotension
  Salt craving
  Weakness

Features of acute insufficiency (adrenal crisis)
  Abdominal pain
  Fever

Features of chronic insufficiency (Addison disease)
  Decreased pubic and axillary hair
  Diarrhoea
  Hyperpigmentation
  Low-voltage electrocardiogram
  Small heart on X-ray
  Weight loss

hypotension, hyponatraemia, hypochloraemia, hyperkalaemia, frequent illnesses, nausea and vague gastrointestinal complaints (Table 21.9), reflecting chronic deficiency of both glucocorticoids and mineralocorticoids. Early in the course of autoimmune adrenalitis one may see signs of glucocorticoid deficiency (weakness, fatigue, weight loss, hypoglycaemia, anorexia) without signs of mineralocorticoid deficiency [hyponatraemia, hyperkalaemia, acidosis, tachycardia, hypotension, low voltage on electrocardiogram (ECG), small heart on chest X-ray] or evidence of mineralocorticoid deficiency without glucocorticoid deficiency. Thus, an initial clinical presentation that spares one category of adrenal steroids does not mean it will be spared in the long run. The symptoms listed in Table 21.9 can be seen in chronic adrenal insufficiency that is either primary or secondary.

In primary chronic adrenal insufficiency, the low concentrations of plasma cortisol stimulate the hypersecretion of ACTH and other POMC peptides, including the various forms of melanocyte-stimulating hormone (MSH), which is characterized by hyperpigmentation of the skin and mucous membranes. Such hyperpigmentation is most prominent in skin exposed to sun and in extensor surfaces such as knees, elbows and knuckles. The diagnosis is suggested by the signs and symptoms, verified by a low morning cortisol level with a high ACTH and confirmed by a minimal response of cortisol to a 60-min intravenous ACTH test. Associated findings may include the appearance of a small heart on chest

X-ray, anaemia, azotaemia, eosinophilia, lymphocytosis and hypoglycaemia. Treatment consists of physiological glucocorticoid and mineralocorticoid replacement therapy.

The diagnosis of an autoimmune cause is based on finding circulating antiadrenal antibodies. In many cases the adrenal antigens are the steroidogenic P450 enzymes, especially P450c21 [400,401]. It is not clear how these enzymes reach immune cells to elicit an antibody response, or whether there are clinical correlations with the spectrum of which enzymes become the antigens giving rise to a cytoxic immune response. Autopsy studies show lymphocytic infiltration of the adrenal cortex.

Autoimmune dysfunction of other endocrine tissues is frequently associated with autoimmune adrenalitis [402]. Approximately half of adult patients with lymphocytic adrenalitis also have disease of another endocrine system and high titres of antibodies specific to the affected tissues. The term *Schmidt syndrome* refers to the relatively common association of thyroiditis and/or diabetes mellitus with autoimmune adrenal insufficiency [403]. This disease triad, which is seen mainly in adults, is sometimes termed *type 2 autoimmune polyglandular syndrome* and is linked to HLA-DR3 and HLA-DR4 [404]. In older children and adults, primary ovarian failure (but not primary testicular failure) is seen in about one-quarter of patients with primary lymphocytic autoimmune adrenalitis.

Hypoparathyroidism, pernicious anaemia and chronic mucocutaneous candidiasis are often seen without adrenalitis in girls [402], but when adrenalitis is also present boys and girls are affected equally. This associated group of disorders is more common in children than adults and is sometimes termed *type 1 autoimmune polyglandular syndrome*. It may also include atrophic gastritis, hypergonadotrophic hypogonadism, chronic active hepatitis, alopecia or vitiligo. Unlike type 2 autoimmune polyglandular syndrome, a specific HLA association has not been found.

## Metabolic causes

Metabolic disorders cause chronic primary adrenal insufficiency, including adrenoleukodystrophy (Schilder disease), primary xanthomatosis (Wolman disease), cholesterol ester storage disease, hereditary unresponsiveness to ACTH and adrenal hypoplasia congenita.

*Adrenoleukodystrophy* is caused by mutations in a gene on chromosome Xq28a termed ALDP, but the mechanism by which these mutations cause the disease is unclear [405,406]. This X-linked disorder is seen almost exclusively in males, although a rare severe infantile autosomal recessive form also occurs. The disease is characterized by high ratios of $C_{26}$ to $C_{22}$ very-long-chain fatty acids in plasma and tissues, permitting diagnosis of carriers and affected fetuses as well as individual patients [407]. Symptoms commonly develop in mid-childhood, but a variant of the disorder, adrenomyeloneuropathy, presents in early adulthood [408]. Both adrenoleukodystrophy and adrenomyeloneuropathy are caused by mutations in the gene for ALDP. The same mutation causes both forms of the disease, so it is likely that other genetic loci are also involved [409].

Earliest findings are associated with the central nervous system leukodystrophy and include behavioural changes, poor school performance, dysarthria and poor memory, progressing to severe dementia. Symptoms of adrenal insufficiency usually appear after symptoms of white-matter disease but adrenal insufficiency may be the initial finding in some children [410]. By contrast, adrenomyeloneuropathy begins with adrenal insufficiency in childhood and adolescence and signs of neurological disease follow 10–15 years later. Dietary therapy with so-called Lorenzo's oil has not been effective [409].

*Wolman disease* and cholesterol ester storage disease appear to be two allelic variants in the secreted form of lysozomal acid lipase (cholesterol esterase) that mobilizes cholesterol esters from adrenal lipid droplets [411]. The gene for this enzyme on chromosome 10q has been cloned, and the mutations in it causing one case of Wolman disease have been identified [412]. Because insufficient free cholesterol is available to P450scc, there is adrenal insufficiency. The disease is less severe than congenital lipoid adrenal hyperplasia with respect to steroidogenesis and patients may survive for several months after birth. However, the disease affects all cells, not just steroidogenic cells, as all cells must store and utilize cholesterol; hence, the disorder is relentless and fatal.

Vomiting, steatorrhoea, failure to thrive, hepatosplenomegaly and adrenal calcification are the usual presenting findings. The diagnosis is established by bone marrow aspiration yielding foam cells containing large lysosomal vacuoles engorged with cholesterol esters and is confirmed by finding absent cholesterol esterase activity in fibroblasts, leucocytes or marrow cells. Cholesterol ester storage disease appears to be a milder defect in the same enzyme, generally presenting in childhood or adolescence among the 10 reported cases.

*Hereditary unresponsiveness to ACTH* (familial glucocorticoid deficiency) can present as an acute adrenal crisis precipitated by an intercurrent illness in an infant or with the signs and symptoms of chronic adrenal insufficiency in childhood [218]. Unlike patients with autoimmune adrenalitis or other forms of destruction of adrenal tissue, patients with hereditary unresponsiveness to ACTH continue to produce mineralocorticoids normally because production of aldosterone by the adrenal zona glomerulosa is regulated principally by the renin–angiotensin system. Thus, the presenting picture consists of failure to thrive, lethargy, pallor, hyperpigmentation, delayed milestones and hypoglycaemia (often associated with seizures), but serum electrolytes are normal and dehydration is seen only as part of the precipitating intercurrent illness. The disorder is transmitted as an autosomal recessive trait. Some but not all affected patients have mutations of the gene encoding the ACTH receptor on chromosome 18p11, indicating the heterogeneous nature of the defect [413].

*Triple A (Allgrove) syndrome* is a rare disorder consisting of ACTH-resistant *a*drenal (glucocorticoid) deficiency, *a*chalasia of the cardia and *a*lacrima [414]. The disorder appears to be autosomal dominant and resembles ACTH resistance, but mutations in the ACTH receptor have been excluded [218]. Many patients also have progressive neurological symptoms, including intellectual impairment, sensorineural deafness, peripheral neuropathies and autonomic dysfunction [218,415].

*Adrenal hypoplasia congenita* (AHC, congenital adrenal hypoplasia) is generally caused by mutations of the *DAX-1* gene on chromosome Xp21 [416]. This gene encodes a nuclear transcription factor that participates at various steps in the differentiation of adrenal and gonadal tissues, as well as in gonadotrophin expression, so that successfully treated children may not enter puberty [417]. In this disorder, the definitive zone of the fetal adrenal does not develop and the fetal zone is vacuolated and cytomegalic. Poor function of the fetal zone results in low maternal oestriol concentrations during pregnancy but parturition is normal. Neonatal glucocorticoid and mineralocorticoid deficiencies manifest with a typical salt-wasting crisis and respond well to replacement therapy. Deletions of the *DAX-1* gene may also encompass adjacent genes, causing glycerol kinase deficiency, Duchenne muscular dystrophy and mental retardation [416,417]. Genetic 46,XY males with adrenal hypoplasia have normal male external genitalia, but in 46,XX females the distinction between adrenal hypoplasia congenita and congenital lipoid adrenal hyperplasia cannot be made hormonally and requires imaging of the adrenals, which are small in adrenal hypoplasia and large in lipoid CAH.

### Other causes

Chronic adrenal insufficiency may be due to causes other than these. Adrenal hypoplasia, haemorrhage and infections, all discussed below as causes of acute primary adrenal insufficiency, may spare some adrenal tissue, leaving severely compromised, rather than totally absent, adrenal function. The result, as with autoimmune adrenalitis, is a chronic disorder with insidious onset of the broad range of non-specific findings described above. Tuberculosis, fungal infections and amyloidosis may cause a similar clinical picture.

## Acute primary adrenal insufficiency

Acute adrenal crisis occurs most commonly in the child with undiagnosed chronic adrenal insufficiency who is subjected to an additional stress such as major illness, trauma or surgery. The major presenting symptoms and signs include abdominal pain, fever, hypoglycaemia with seizures, weakness, apathy, nausea, vomiting, anorexia, hyponatraemia, hypochloraemia, acidaemia, hyperkalaemia, hypotension, shock, cardiovascular collapse and death. Treatment consists of fluid and electrolyte resuscitation, ample doses of glucocorticoids, chronic glucocorticoid and mineralocorticoid replacement and treatment of the precipitating illness.

*Massive adrenal haemorrhage* with shock due to blood loss can occur in large infants who have had a traumatic delivery [418]. A flank mass is usually palpable and can be distinguished from renal vein thrombosis by microscopic rather than gross haematuria. The diagnosis is confirmed by computerized tomography or ultrasonography [419]. Massive adrenal haemorrhage is more commonly associated with meningococcaemia (Waterhouse–Fridrichsen syndrome). Meningitis is often, but not always, present. The characteristic petechial rash of meningococcaemia can progress rapidly to large ecchymoses; the blood pressure drops and respirations become laboured, frequently leading rapidly to coma and death. Immediate intervention with intravenous fluids, antibiotics and glucocorticoids is not always successful. A similar adrenal crisis may also occur rarely with septicaemia from *Streptococcus*, *Pneumococcus* or diphtheria.

## Secondary adrenal insufficiency

Chronic adrenal insufficiency may result from insufficient tropic stimulation of the adrenal and tissue insensitivity to adrenal steroids. Insufficient tropic stimulation of the adrenal can be due to idiopathic hypopituitarism, central nervous system tumours that damage the cells producing CRH and/or POMC or chronic suppression of these cells by long-term glucocorticoid therapy.

*Idiopathic hypopituitarism* (multiple anterior pituitary hormone deficiency) is a hypothalamic rather than a pituitary disorder. The deficient secretion of growth hormone, gonadotrophins, thyroid-stimulating hormone and ACTH is due to insufficient stimulation of the pituitary by the corresponding hypothalamic hormones. Isolated growth hormone deficiency, a common disorder, and isolated ACTH deficiency, a rare disorder, are variants of this theme. In hypopituitarism from most causes, growth hormone secretion is generally lost first, followed in order by gonadotrophins, TSH and ACTH. Combined deficiency of growth hormone and ACTH will strongly predispose the patient to hypoglycaemia, as both hormones act to raise plasma glucose. Patients with ACTH deficiency, either with or without deficiency of other anterior pituitary hormones, have a relatively mild form of adrenal insufficiency. Mineralocorticoid secretion is normal, whereas cortisol secretion is reduced but not absent. However, adrenal reserve is severely compromised by the chronic understimulation of biosynthesis of the steroidogenic enzymes.

Because some cortisol synthesis continues, the diagnosis may not be apparent unless a CRH or metyrapone test of pituitary ACTH production capacity and an intravenous ACTH test of adrenal reserve are performed. This can be especially true when TSH deficiency is a component of hypopituitarism. The hypothyroidism resulting from TSH deficiency will result in slowed metabolism of the small amount of cortisol produced and therefore protects the patient from the symptoms of adrenal insufficiency. Treatment of the hypothyroidism with thyroxine will accelerate metabolism of the small amounts of cortisol, thus unmasking adrenal insufficiency due to ACTH deficiency and, on occasion, can precipitate an acute adrenal crisis. Careful evaluation of the pituitary–adrenal axis is required in hypopituitarism with secondary hypothyroidism. Many clinicians will choose to 'cover' a patient with small doses of glucocorticoids (one-quarter to one-half of physiological replacement) during initial treatment of such secondary hypothyroidism.

*Hypothalamic tumours,* such as craniopharyngioma [420], are associated with ACTH deficiency in about 25% of patients, perhaps more in tumours such as germinoma and astrocytoma [421]. Adrenal insufficiency is rarely the presenting complaint but may contribute to the clinical picture. After surgery and radiotherapy, the great majority of these patients have ACTH deficiency as part of their pituitary damage and all patients should receive glucocorticoid coverage during treatment, irrespective of the status of the hypothalamo-pituitary-adrenal axis at the time the tumour is identified. Cortisol is required for the kidney to excrete free water. Treatment of secondary adrenal insufficiency in some central nervous system tumours can unmask a previously unapparent deficiency of antidiuretic hormone (ADH) and thus precipitate diabetes insipidus.

*Long-term glucocorticoid therapy* can suppress POMC gene transcription and the synthesis and storage of ACTH. Furthermore, long-term therapy apparently decreases the synthesis and storage of CRH and diminishes the abundance of receptors for CRH in the pituitary. Therefore, recovery of the hypothalamo-pituitary axis from long-term glucocorticoid therapy entails recovery of multiple components in a sequential cascade and often requires considerable time. Patients successfully withdrawn from glucocorticoid therapy or successfully treated for Cushing disease may exhibit a fairly rapid normalization of plasma cortisol values while continuing to have diminished adrenal reserve for over 6 months.

Glucocorticoid therapy of pregnant women can suppress the fetal adrenal. Treatment of pregnant women with cortisone or prednisone will result in minimal suppression of the fetal adrenal, because placental 11β-HSD converts the biologically active form of these steroids, cortisol and prednisolone, back to their biologically inactive parent compounds. Thus, when radiolabelled cortisol or prednisolone is administered to a pregnant woman, the equilibrium concentrations in maternal plasma are 10 times higher than those in cord plasma. However, dexamethasone is a poor substrate for 11β-HSD, so that administration of low doses to a pregnant woman can affect fetal adrenal steroidogenesis.

**Table 21.10.** Aetiology of Cushing syndrome in infancy

| | Males | Females |
|---|---|---|
| Adrenal tumours (n = 48) | | |
| Carcinoma | 5 | 20 |
| Adenoma | 4 | 16 |
| Not defined | 2 | 1 |
| Ectopic ACTH syndrome | 1 | 1 |
| Nodular adrenal hyperplasia | 1 | 4 |
| Undefined adrenal hyperplasia | 2 | 2 |
| ACTH-producing tumour | 1 | 0 |
| Total | 16 | 44 |

Data from Miller *et al.* [424].

## Adrenal excess

### Cushing syndrome

The term *Cushing syndrome* describes any form of glucocorticoid excess. *Cushing disease* designates hypercortisolism due to pituitary overproduction of ACTH. The related disorder caused by ACTH of non-pituitary origin is termed the *ectopic ACTH syndrome*. Other causes of Cushing syndrome include adrenal adenoma, adrenal carcinoma and multinodular adrenal hyperplasia. All these are distinct from *iatrogenic Cushing syndrome,* which is the clinical constellation resulting from administration of supraphysiological quantities of ACTH or glucocorticoids.

Although generally described in great detail and illustrated with striking photographs in endocrine texts, Cushing disease is rare in adults [422] but 25% of patients referred to large centres are children, so it is clear that the disorder is more common in children than previously recognized. Many patients first seen as adults actually experienced the onset of symptoms in childhood or adolescence. Harvey Cushing's original patient was a young woman of only 23 years whose history and clinical features indicated long-standing disease [2]. In adults and children over 7 years of age, the most common cause of Cushing syndrome is Cushing disease [423]. In infants and children under 7 years, adrenal tumours predominate. Among 60 infants under 1 year of age with Cushing syndrome, 48 had adrenal tumours [424] (Table 21.10).

### Clinical findings

The physical features of Cushing syndrome are familiar. Central obesity, 'moon facies', hirsutism and facial flushing are seen in over 80% of adults. Striae, hypertension, muscular weakness, back pain, buffalo hump fat distribution, psychological disturbances, acne and easy bruising are also very commonly described (35–80%). These are the signs of advanced

**Table 21.11.** Findings in 39 children with Cushing disease

| Sign/symptom | Number of patients | % |
|---|---|---|
| Weight gain | 36/39 | 92 |
| Growth failure | 31/37 | 84 |
| Ostopenia | 14/19 | 74 |
| Fatigue | 26/39 | 67 |
| Hypertension | 22/35 | 63 |
| Delayed or arrested puberty | 21/35 | 60 |
| Plethora | 18/39 | 46 |
| Acne | 18/39 | 46 |
| Hirsutism | 18/39 | 46 |
| Compulsive behaviour | 17/39 | 44 |
| Striae | 14/39 | 36 |
| Bruising | 11/39 | 28 |
| Buffalo hump | 11/39 | 28 |
| Headache | 10/39 | 26 |
| Delayed bone age | 2/23 | 13 |
| Nocturia | 3/39 | 8 |

Data from Devoe *et al.* [425].

Cushing disease. When annual photographs of such patients are available, it is often apparent that the features can take 5 years or longer to develop. Thus, the classic cushingoid appearance will usually not be the initial picture seen in the child with Cushing syndrome.

The earliest, most reliable indicators of hypercortisolism in children are weight gain and growth arrest [425] (Table 21.11); any overweight child who stops growing should be evaluated for Cushing syndrome. The obesity of Cushing disease in children is initially generalized rather than centripetal and a buffalo hump is evidence of long-standing disease. Psychological disturbances, especially compulsive overachieving behaviour, are seen in about 40% of children and adolescents with Cushing disease [425] and are distinctly different from the emotional lability and depression typically seen in adults [426]. An underappreciated aspect is the substantial degree of bone loss and undermineralization in these patients [425,427]. It is likely that Cushing disease is generally regarded as a disease of young adults because the diagnosis was missed, rather than absent, during adolescence. Rarely, Cushing syndrome caused by adrenal carcinoma and the ectopic ACTH syndrome can produce a rapid fulminant course.

### Cushing disease

The recent development of transsphenoidal surgical approaches to the pituitary has led to pituitary exploration in large numbers of patients with Cushing disease. Among adults, over 90% of such patients have identifiable pituitary microadenomas [426,428], which are generally 2–10 mm in diameter, are not encapsulated, have ill-defined boundaries and are frequently detectable with a contrast-enhanced pituitary MRI. They are often identifiable only by minor differences in their appearance and texture from surrounding tissue, so the frequency of surgical cure is correlated with the technical skill of the surgeon. Although histological techniques may not distinguish the tumour from normal tissue, molecular biological techniques confirm increased synthesis of POMC in these tissues [429]. Among children and adolescents, about 80–85% of those with Cushing disease have surgically identifiable microadenomas [205,430]. Although removal of the tumour usually appears curative, 20% of such 'cured' patients suffer relapse and manifest Cushing disease again within about 5 years, so that the net cure rate is 70–75% [425,431]. Transsphenoidal surgery offers the best initial approach for rapid and complete cure of most patients, thus maximizing final height, which is typically reduced by 1.5–2.0 SD by the long-term hypercortisolism [425,432].

The high cure rate of transsphenoidal microadenomectomy in Cushing disease indicates that the majority of patients have primary disease of the pituitary itself, rather than secondary hyperpituitarism resulting from hyperstimulation of the pituitary by CRH or other agents. Careful follow-up studies of these patients confirm this [425,430,431]. In most postoperative patients, the circadian rhythms of ACTH and cortisol return to normal, ACTH and cortisol respond appropriately to hypoglycaemia, cortisol is easily suppressed by low doses of dexamethasone and the other hypothalamo-pituitary systems return to normal.

Some patients with Cushing disease have no identifiable microadenoma and some 'cured' patients relapse. This suggests that this smaller population of patients may have a primary hypothalamic disorder. Effective treatment of Cushing disease with cyproheptidine, a serotonin antagonist, has been reported in adults, further suggesting a hypothalamic disturbance. Thus, present clinical investigation suggests that Cushing disease is usually caused by a primary pituitary adenoma but that sometimes it is caused by hypothalamic dysfunction. Microsurgery can be curative in the former but not the latter. Unfortunately, no diagnostic manoeuvre is available to distinguish the two possibilities, so transsphenoidal exploration remains the preferred initial therapeutic approach to the patient with Cushing disease.

Other therapeutic approaches include hypophysectomy, pituitary irradiation, cyproheptidine, adrenalectomy and drugs that inhibit adrenal function. All have significant disadvantages, especially in children. Hypophysectomy eliminates pituitary secretion of growth hormone, TSH and gonadotrophins, causing growth failure, hypothyroidism and failure to progress in puberty.

Pituitary irradiation has been touted to avoid many of these problems, but the deficiency of various pituitary hormones may be obscured by delayed onset, and the delayed onset in elimination of the hypersecretion of ACTH will further compromise the final adult height of the child with Cushing disease. Furthermore, large doses of radiation increase the risk of cerebral arteritis, leukoencephalopathy, leukaemia, glial neoplasms, bone tumours involving the skull and congenital defects in subsequent offspring.

Cyproheptidine has met with virtually no success in paediatric Cushing disease, in part due to the unacceptable side-effects (weight gain, irritability, hallucinations) often seen with the doses needed.

Adrenalectomy is the preferred approach when two transsphenoidal procedures fail. In addition to the obvious effects of eliminating normal production of glucocorticoids and mineralocorticoids, removal of the adrenal eliminates the physiological feedback inhibition of the pituitary. In some adults, this results in the development of pituitary macroadenomas, producing very large quantities of ACTH. These can expand and impinge on the optic nerves and can produce sufficient POMC to yield enough MSH to produce profound darkening of the skin (Nelson syndrome), but this is rarely seen in children. There is little paediatric experience with ketoconazole and other drugs that inhibit steroidogenesis, but these may provide a useful form of therapy for selected patients. Metyrapone is not useful for long-term therapy. *Ortho, para*-DDD (mitotane), an adrenolytic agent, may be used to effect a chemical adrenalectomy, but its side-effects of nausea, anorexia and vomiting are severe.

## Other causes of Cushing syndrome

*The ectopic ACTH syndrome* is commonly seen in adults with oat cell carcinoma of the lung, carcinoid tumours, pancreatic islet cell carcinoma and thymoma. Ectopically produced POMC and ACTH are derived from the same gene that produces pituitary POMC [145], but it is not sensitive to glucocorticoid feedback in the malignant cells. This phenomenon permits distinction between pituitary and ectopic ACTH by suppressibility of the former by high doses of dexamethasone. Although the ectopic ACTH syndrome is rare in children, it has been described in infants younger than 1 year of age. Associated tumours have included neuroblastoma, phaeochromocytoma and islet cell carcinoma of the pancreas [433]. The ectopic ACTH syndrome is typically associated with ACTH concentrations 10–100 times higher than those seen in Cushing disease.

Adults and children with this disorder may show little or no clinical evidence of hypercortisolism, probably due to the typically rapid onset of the disease and to the general catabolism associated with malignancy. Unlike patients with Cushing disease, patients frequently have hypokalaemic alkalosis, presumably because the extremely high levels of ACTH stimulate the production of DOC by the adrenal fasciculata and may also stimulate the adrenal glomerulosa in the absence of hyper-reninaemia [433].

*Adrenal tumours*, especially adrenal carcinomas, are the more typical cause of Cushing syndrome in infants and small children [434] (Table 21.10). They occur with much greater

**Table 21.12.** Diagnostic values in various causes of Cushing syndrome

| Test | | Normal values | Adrenal carcinoma | Nodular adrenal adenoma | Adrenal hyperplasia | Cushing disease | Ectopic ACTH syndrome |
|---|---|---|---|---|---|---|---|
| Plasma cortisol | AM | >14 | ↑ | ↑ | ↑ | ± | ↑↑ |
| concentration | PM | <8 | ↑ | ↑ | ↑ | ↑ | ↑↑ |
| Plasma ACTH | AM | <100 | ↓ | ↓ | ↓ | ↑ | ↑↑ |
| concentration | PM | <50 | ↓ | ↓ | ↓ | ↑ | ↑↑ |
| Low-dose dex | Cortisol | <3 | No Δ | No Δ | No Δ | * | No Δ |
| suppression | ACTH | <30 | No Δ | No Δ | No Δ | * | No Δ |
| | 17-OHCS | <2 | No Δ | No Δ | No Δ | * | No Δ |
| High-dose dex | Cortisol | ↓↓ | No Δ | No Δ | † | ↓ | No Δ |
| suppression | ACTH | ↓↓ | No Δ | No Δ | † | ↓ | No Δ |
| | 17-OHCS | ↓↓ | No Δ | No Δ | † | ↓ | No Δ |
| IV ACTH test | Cortisol | >20 | No Δ | ±↑ | ±↑ | ↑ | No Δ |
| Metyrapone test | Cortisol | ↓ | ±↓ | No Δ | ±↓ | ↓ | ±↓ |
| | 11-Deoxycortisol | ↑ | ±↑ | No Δ | ±↑ | ↑ | ±↑ |
| | ACTH | ↑ | No Δ | No Δ | ±↑ | ↑ | No Δ |
| | 17-OHCS | ↑ | No Δ | No Δ | ± | ↑ | No Δ |
| 24-h urinary excretion | 17-OHCS | | ↑↑ | ↑ | ↑ | ↑ | ↑ |
| (basal) | 17-ketosteroids | | ↑↑ | ±↑ | ↑ | ↑ | ↑ |
| Plasma concentration | DHEA or DHEAS | | ↑↑ | ↓ | ±↑ | ↑ | ↑ |

Dex, dexamethasone. Cortisol concentration in mg/dL. ACTH concentration in pg/mL. 17-OHCS in mg/24 h.
*Incomplete response, i.e. ±.
†Usually no Δ.

frequency in girls for unknown reasons [435]. Adrenal adenomas almost always secrete cortisol with minimal secretion of mineralocorticoids or sex steroids. By contrast, adrenal carcinomas tend to secrete both cortisol and androgens [436]. Congenital bodily asymmetry (hemihypertrophy) may be associated with adrenal adenoma or carcinoma, with or without association with the Beckwith–Wiedemann syndrome. CT and MRI are useful in the diagnosis of adrenal tumours. The treatment is surgical, although the prognosis for adrenal carcinoma is generally poor. A few patients have done well with adjunctive therapy with *ortho, para*-DDD. Size is the best guide to differentiating adenoma (< 10 cm) from carcinoma.

*ACTH-independent multinodular adrenal hyperplasia* is a rare entity characterized by the secretion of both cortisol and adrenal androgens [437]. It is seen in infants, children and young adults, with females affected more frequently. Familial instances have been seen [438] and many of these have an autosomal dominant disorder (Carney syndrome), consisting of pigmented lentigines and blue naevi on the face, lips and conjuctivae and a variety of tumours including schwannomas, Sertoli cell tumours and atrial myxomas. This disorder, linked to loci on chromosome 2, accounts for up to 80% of patients who have *bilateral* micronodular adrenal hyperplasia [439,440]. Because the hypercortisolism is resistant to suppression with high doses of dexamethasone and because both glucocorticoids and sex steroids are produced, this entity was difficult to distinguish from the ectopic ACTH syndrome before plasma ACTH assays became available. Adrenalectomy is usually indicated, although some successes have been reported with subtotal resections. A form of multinodular adrenal hyperplasia is occasionally seen in the McCune–Albright syndrome, suggesting that this form of adrenal hyperfunction may be associated with a G-protein defect.

### Differential diagnosis

The suspicion of Cushing syndrome in children is usually raised by weight gain, growth arrest, mood change and change in facial appearance (plethora, acne, hirsutism). The diagnosis may be subtle and difficult when it is sought early in the natural history of the disease. Absolute elevations of concentrations of plasma ACTH and cortisol are often absent. Rather than finding morning concentrations of cortisol > 20 µg/dL or of ACTH > 50 pg/mL, it is more typical to find mild, often equivocal elevations in the afternoon and evening values. This loss of diurnal rhythm, evidenced by continued secretion of ACTH and cortisol throughout the afternoon, evening and night-time, is usually the earliest reliable laboratory index of Cushing disease. Values for ACTH and cortisol are typically extremely high in the ectopic ACTH syndrome, whereas cortisol is elevated but ACTH suppressed in adrenal tumours and in multinodular adrenal hyperplasia (Table 21.12).

The performance of low- and high-dose dexamethasone suppression tests can be useful. Two days of baseline (control) data should be obtained. Low-dose dexamethasone (20 μg/kg/day) should be given, divided into equal doses given every 6 h for 2 days followed by high-dose dexamethasone (80 μg/kg/day) given in the same fashion. Values at 08.00 h and 20.00 h for ACTH and cortisol and 24-h urine collections for 17-OHS, 17-ketosteroids, free cortisol and creatinine (to monitor the completeness of the collection) should be obtained on each of the 6 days of the test. Because of variations due to episodic secretion of ACTH, 08.00 h and 20.00 h blood values should be drawn in triplicate: on the hour and 15 and 30 min after. In patients with exogenous obesity or other non-Cushing disorders, cortisol, ACTH and urinary steroids will be suppressed readily by low-dose dexamethasone. Plasma cortisol should be less than 5 μg/100 mL, ACTH less than 20 pg/mL and 24-h urinary 17-OHS less than 1 mg/g of creatinine. Patients with adrenal adenoma, adrenal carcinoma or the ectopic ACTH syndrome will have values relatively insensitive to both low- and high-dose dexamethasone, although some patients with multinodular adrenal hyperplasia may respond to high-dose suppression. Patients with Cushing disease classically respond with a suppression of ACTH, cortisol and urinary steroids during the high-dose treatment, but not during the low-dose treatment. However, some children, especially those early in the course of their illness, may exhibit partial suppression in response to low-dose dexamethasone. Thus, if the low dose that is given exceeds 20 μg/kg/day or if the assays used are insufficiently sensitive to distinguish partial from complete suppression, false-negative tests may result. In general, the diagnosis of Cushing disease is considerably more difficult to establish in children than in adults.

## Virilizing and feminizing adrenal tumours

Most virilizing adrenal tumours are carcinomas producing a mixed array of androgens and glucocorticoids. Virilizing and feminizing adrenal adenomas are rare. Virilizing tumours in boys have a presentation similar to that of simple virilizing CAH [441] with phallic enlargement, erections, pubic and axillary hair, increased muscle mass, deepening of the voice, acne and scrotal thinning; testicular size will be prepubertal. Elevated concentrations of testosterone in young boys alter behaviour, with increased irritability, rambunctiousness, hyperactivity and rough play without evidence of libido. Diagnosis is based on hyperandrogenaemia that is insuppressible by glucocorticoids. The treatment is surgical; all such tumours should be handled as if they are malignant, with care exerted not to cut the capsule and seed cells onto the peritoneum. The pathological distinction between adrenal adenoma and carcinoma is difficult.

Feminizing adrenal tumours are extremely rare. P450aro, the enzyme aromatizing androgenic precursors to oestrogens, is not normally found in the adrenals but is found in peripheral tissues such as fat. It is not known whether most feminizing adrenal tumours exhibit ectopic adrenal production of this enzyme, whether some other enzyme mediates aromatization in the tumour or whether these are truly androgen-producing, virilizing tumours occurring in a setting where there is unusually effective peripheral aromatization of adrenal androgens. Feminizing adrenal (or extra-adrenal) tumours can be distinguished from true (central) precocious puberty in girls by the absence of increased circulating concentrations of gonadotrophins and by a prepubertal response of luteinizing hormone to an intravenous challenge of GnRH. In boys, such tumours will cause gynaecomastia, which will resemble the benign gynaecomastia that often accompanies puberty. However, as with virilizing adrenal tumours, testicular size and the gonadotrophin response to GnRH testing will be prepubertal. The diagnosis of a feminizing tumour in a pubertal boy can be extremely difficult but is usually suggested by an arrest in pubertal progression and can be proved by the persistence of circulating plasma oestrogens after administration of testosterone.

## Conn syndrome

Conn syndrome, characterized by hypertension, polyuria, hypokalaemic alkalosis and low plasma renin activity due to an aldosterone-producing adrenal adenoma, is well described in adults but is exquisitely rare in children. The diagnostic task is to differentiate primary aldosteronism from physiological secondary hyperaldosteronism occurring in response to another physiological disturbance. Any loss of sodium, retention of potassium or decrease in blood volume will result in hyper-reninaemic secondary hyperaldosteronism. Renal tubular acidosis, treatment with diuretics, salt-wasting nephritis or hypovolaemia due to nephrosis, ascites or blood loss are typical settings for physiological secondary hyperaldosteronism. Primary aldosteronism is characterized by hypertension and hypokalaemic alkalosis. The cause is a small adrenal adenoma, usually confined to one adrenal. Both adrenals need to be explored surgically because adrenal vein catheterization is not possible in children and is difficult in adults.

## Glucocorticoid therapy and withdrawal

Since their introduction into clinical medicine in the early 1950s, glucocorticoids have been used to treat virtually every known disease [442]. At present their rational use falls into two broad categories, replacement in adrenal insufficiency and pharmacotherapeutic use. The latter category is largely related to the anti-inflammatory properties of glucocorticoids, but also includes their actions to lyse leukaemic leucocytes, lower plasma calcium concentrations and reduce increased intracranial pressure. Virtually all of these actions are mediated through glucocorticoid receptors, which are found in most cells. Because there appears to be only one major type of glucocorticoid receptor, all glucocorticoids affect all tissues containing such receptors. Thus, with the exception of the distinction between glucocorticoids and mineralocorticoids, tissue-specific, disease-specific or response-specific analogues of naturally occurring glucocorticoids cannot be produced. The only differences among the various glucocorticoid preparations are their ratio of glucocorticoid to mineralocorticoid activity, their capacity to bind to various binding proteins, their molar potency and their biological half-life. Dexamethasone is commonly used in reducing increased intracranial pressure and brain oedema. Neurosurgical experience indicates that the optimal doses are 10–100 times those that would thoroughly saturate all available receptors, suggesting that this action of dexamethasone may not be mediated through the glucocorticoid receptor.

Glucocorticoids are so termed because of their major actions to increase plasma concentrations of glucose. This occurs by their induction of the transcription of the genes encoding the enzymes of the Embden–Myerhoff glycolytic pathway and other hepatic enzymes that divert amino acids, such as alanine, to the production of glucose. Thus, the co-ordinated action to increase the transcription of these genes can result in increased plasma concentrations of glucose, obesity and muscle wasting. The other features of Cushing syndrome are similarly attributable to the increased transcriptional activity of specific glucocorticoid-sensitive genes.

## Replacement therapy

Glucocorticoid replacement therapy is complicated by undesirable side-effects, with even minor degrees of overtreatment or undertreatment. Overtreatment can cause the signs and symptoms of Cushing syndrome and even minimal overtreatment can impair growth. Undertreatment will cause the signs and symptoms of adrenal insufficiency (Table 21.9) only if the extent of undertreatment (dose and duration) is considerable. However, undertreatment may impair the individual's capacity to respond to stress.

To optimize paediatric glucocorticoid replacement therapy, physicians have gauged their therapy to resemble the endogenous secretory rate of cortisol. Most authorities recommend treatment equivalent to a secretory rate of 12.5 mg of cortisol per metre squared of body surface area per day, 9.5–15.5 mg/m$^2$/day. The time-honoured value of 12.5 mg/m$^2$ may be too high, and appropriate replacement may be as low as 6 mg/m$^2$ in younger children and 9 mg/m$^2$ in older children and adolescents [209,210].

The management of the delicate balance between over- and undertreatment is confounded by considerable variation in the normal cortisol secretory rate among different children of the same size and the probability that most conventional guidelines err on the side of overtreatment. Additional factors must, however, be considered in tailoring a specific child's glucocorticoid replacement regimen.

The specific form of adrenal insufficiency influences therapy. When treating autoimmune adrenalitis or any other form of Addison disease, it is prudent to err slightly on the side of undertreatment. This will eliminate the possibility of glucocorticoid-induced iatrogenic growth retardation and permit the pituitary to continue to produce normal to slightly elevated concentrations of ACTH. This ACTH will continue to stimulate the remaining functional adrenal steroidogenic machinery and provide a convenient means of monitoring the effects of therapy. By contrast, when treating CAH, the adrenal should be suppressed more completely, as any adrenal steroidogenesis will result in the production of unwanted androgens, with their consequent virilization and rate of advancement of bony maturation that is more rapid than the rate of advancement of height.

The presence or absence of associated mineralocorticoid deficiency is important. Children with mild degrees of mineralocorticoid insufficiency, such as those with simple virilizing CAH, may continue to have mildly elevated ACTH values, suggesting insufficient glucocorticoid replacement in association with elevated PRA. In some children, the ACTH is elevated in response to chronic, compromised hypovolaemia, attempting to stimulate the adrenal to produce more mineralocorticoid. In these children, who do not manifest overt signs and symptoms of mineralocorticoid insufficiency, treatment with mineralocorticoid replacement may permit one to decrease the amount of glucocorticoid replacement needed to suppress plasma ACTH and urinary 17-ketosteroids. This reduction in glucocorticoid therapy reduces the likelihood that adult height will be compromised.

The specific formulation of glucocorticoid is of great importance. Potent, long-acting glucocorticoids, such as dexamethasone or prednisone, are preferred in the treatment of adults but are rarely appropriate for children. Small, incremental dose changes are more easily carried out with weaker glucocorticoids. It is easy to change from 25 to 30 mg of hydrocortisone but virtually impossible to change from an equivalent 0.5–0.6 mg of dexamethasone. The efficacy of attempting to mimic the physiological diurnal variation in steroid hormone secretion remains controversial. As ACTH and cortisol concentrations are high in the morning and low in the evening, it is intellectually and logically appealing to attempt to duplicate this circadian rhythm in replacement therapy. However, the results do not clearly indicate that better growth is achieved by giving relatively larger doses in the morning and lower doses at night.

This probably reflects the fact that ACTH and cortisol secretion are episodic throughout the day and that this well-established circadian variation is not smooth. The pattern of high in the morning and low in the evening is only an averaged result. Furthermore, the adrenal releases cortisol episodically throughout the day in response to various physiological demands (hypoglycaemia, exercise, stress, etc.); thus, under normal circumstances the plasma concentrations are high when the clearance and disposal rates are also high. A planned programme of replacement therapy cannot possibly anticipate these day-to-day variations.

Finally, dosage equivalents among various glucocorticoids can be misleading (Table 21.7) because most preparations of glucocorticoids are intended for pharmacotherapeutic use rather than replacement therapy and because the most common indication for pharmacological doses of glucocorticoids is for their anti-inflammatory properties.

All of these variables explain why there is little unanimity in recommendations for designing a glucocorticoid replacement regimen. An understanding of them will permit appropriate monitoring of the patient and encourage the physician to vary the treatment according to the responses and needs of the individual child.

## Commonly used glucocorticoid preparations

Numerous chemical derivatives and variants of the naturally occurring steroids are commercially available in a huge array of dosage, forms, vehicles and concentrations, all carrying confusing and uninformative brand names. Choosing the appropriate product can be simplified by considering only the most widely used steroids listed in Table 21.7. There are four relevant considerations.

First, the glucocorticoid potency of the various drugs is generally calculated and described according to the anti-inflammatory potency. The pharmaceutical industry has chosen this standard for convenience and because the majority of their sales are to physicians using pharmacological doses of these steroids to achieve anti-inflammatory effects.

Second, the growth-suppressant effect of a glucocorticoid preparation may be significantly different from its anti-inflammatory effect. This is due to differences in half-life, metabolism and protein binding and receptor affinity (potency), but it is not due to receptor specificity as all known receptor-mediated effects of glucocorticoids are mediated through a single type of receptor.

Third, the mineralocorticoid activity of various glucocorticoid preparations varies widely. Both glucocorticoid and mineralocorticoid hormones can bind to both glucocorticoid (type I) and mineralocorticoid (type II) receptors, and most authorities now regard these as two different types of glucocorticoid receptors and find that there is no true specific mineralocorticoid receptor. Mineralocorticoid activity is intimately related to the activity 11β-HSD, which metabolizes glucocorticoids but not mineralocorticoids to a form that cannot bind the receptor. Thus, the relative mineralocorticoid potency of various steroids is determined by both their affinity for the type II receptor and their resistance to the activity of 11β-HSD. An understanding that some commonly used glucocorticoids, such as cortisol, cortisone, predniso-

lone and prednisone, have significant mineralocorticoid activity is especially important when large doses are used as stress doses in a patient on replacement therapy. Stress doses of the glucocorticoid preparation may provide sufficient mineralocorticoid activity to meet physiological needs, so mineralocorticoid supplementation is not needed.

Fourth, the plasma half-life and biological half-life of the various preparations may be discordant and vary widely. This is mainly related to binding to plasma proteins, hepatic metabolism and hepatic activation. For example, cortisone and prednisone are biologically inactive (and even have mild steroid antagonist actions) until they are metabolized by hepatic 11β-HSD-I to their active forms, cortisol and prednisolone. Thus, the relative glucocorticoid potency of these preparations will also be affected by hepatic function. Cortisone and prednisone are cleared more rapidly in patients receiving drugs such as phenobarbital or phenytoin, which induce hepatic enzymes, and are cleared more slowly in patients with liver failure.

In addition to these chemical considerations, the route of administration is critical. Glucocorticoids are available for oral, intramuscular, intravenous, intrathecal, intra-articular, inhalant and topical use on skin, mucous membranes and conjunctivae. Each preparation is designed to deliver the maximal concentration of steroid to the desired tissue while delivering less steroid systemically. All the preparations are absorbed to varying extents, so that the widely used inhalant preparations used to treat asthma can, in sufficient doses, cause growth retardation and other signs of Cushing syndrome.

In general, and in contradistinction to many other drugs, orally administered steroids are absorbed rapidly but incompletely, whereas intramuscularly administered steroids are absorbed slowly but completely. Thus, if the secretory rate of cortisol is $8 \text{ mg/m}^2$ of body surface area, the intramuscular or intravenous replacement dose of cortisol (hydrocortisone) would be $8 \text{ mg/m}^2$. However, because only about one-half of an oral dose is absorbed intact, the oral equivalent would be about 15–20 mg of hydrocortisone. The efficiency of absorption of glucocorticoids can vary considerably depending on diet, gastric acidity, bowel transit time and other individual factors. Thus the dosage equivalents listed in Table 21.7 are only general approximations. The equivalencies shown are estimated biological equivalencies with a broad range of variability and are not physical chemical equivalents.

ACTH can also be used for glucocorticoid therapy by its action to stimulate endogenous adrenal steroidogenesis. Although intravenous and intramuscular ACTH are useful in diagnostic tests, the use of ACTH as a therapeutic agent is no longer favoured, principally because it will stimulate synthesis of mineralocorticoids and adrenal androgens as well as glucocorticoids. Furthermore, the need to administer ACTH parenterally further diminishes its usefulness.

Intramuscular ACTH (1–39) in a gel form is the treatment of choice for infantile spasms, and possibly also for other forms of epilepsy in infants resistant to conventional anticonvulsants. Whether this action is mediated by ACTH itself, by other peptides in the biological preparation, by ACTH-induced adrenal steroids or by ACTH-responsive synthesis of novel 'neurosteroids' [443] in the brain has not been determined. When pharmacological doses of ACTH are used therapeutically, as in infantile spasms, the patient should be given a low-sodium diet to ameliorate steroid hypertension.

Although greatly elevated concentrations of ACTH, as in the ectopic ACTH syndrome, cause pituitary suppression, treatment with daily injections of ACTH results in less hypothalamo-pituitary suppression than treatment with equivalent doses of oral glucocorticoids, presumably because the effect on the adrenal is transient. Adrenal suppression obviously does not occur in ACTH therapy. Because the effects of ACTH on adrenal steroidogenesis are highly variable, it is even more difficult to determine dosage equivalencies for ACTH and oral steroid preparations than it is among the various steroids. A very rough guide from studies in adults is that 40 units of ACTH (1–39) gel is approximately equivalent to 100 mg of cortisol.

## Pharmacological steroid therapy

Pharmacological doses of glucocorticoids are used in an endless variety of clinical situations. The choice of glucocorticoid preparation to be used is guided by pharmacological parameters (described above and in Table 21.7) and by custom (e.g. the use of betamethasone rather than dexamethasone to induce fetal lung maturation in impending premature deliveries).

Pharmacological doses of glucocorticoids administered for more than 1 or 2 weeks will cause signs and symptoms of iatrogenic Cushing syndrome. These are similar to the glucocorticoid-induced findings in Cushing disease but may be more severe because of the high doses involved (Table 21.13). Iatrogenic Cushing syndrome is not associated with adrenal androgen effects and mineralocorticoid effects are rare.

**Table 21.13.** Complications of high-dose glucocorticoid therapy

| Short-term therapy | Long-term therapy |
| --- | --- |
| Gastritis | Gastric ulcers |
| Growth arrest | Short stature |
| ↑ Appetite | Weight gain |
| Hypercalciuria | Osteoporosis, fractures |
| Glycosuria | Slipped epiphyses |
| Immune suppression | Ischaemic bone necrosis |
| Masked symptoms of infection, especially fever and inflammation | Poor wound healing |
| Toxic psychoses | Catabolism |
| | Cataracts |
| | Bruising (capillary fragility) |
| | Adrenal/pituitary suppression |
| | Toxic psychosis |

Alternate-day therapy can decrease the toxicity of pharmacological glucocorticoid therapy, especially suppression of the hypothalamo-pituitary-adrenal axis and growth. The basic premise of alternate-day therapy is that the disease state can be suppressed with intermittent therapy, while there is significant recovery of the hypothalamo-pituitary-adrenal axis during the off-day. Alternate-day therapy requires the use of a short-acting glucocorticoid administered once in the morning of each therapeutic day to ensure that the 'off' day is truly 'off'. Long-acting glucocorticoids, such as dexamethasone, should not be used for alternate-day therapy; results are best with oral prednisone or methyl prednisolone.

## Withdrawal of glucocorticoid therapy

Withdrawal of glucocorticoid therapy can lead to symptoms of glucocorticoid insufficiency. When glucocorticoid therapy has been used for only 1 week or 10 days, therapy can be discontinued abruptly, even if high doses have been used [444]. Although only one or two doses of glucocorticoid are needed to suppress the hypothalamo-pituitary-adrenal axis, this axis recovers very rapidly from short-term suppression. When therapy has persisted for 2 weeks or longer, recovery of hypothalamo-pituitary-adrenal function is slower and tapered doses of glucocorticoids are indicated. Acute discontinuation of therapy in such patients will lead to symptoms of glucocorticoid insufficiency, the so-called steroid withdrawal syndrome. This symptom complex does not include salt loss, as adrenal glomerulosa function regulated principally by the renin–angiotensin system remains normal. However, blood pressure can fall abruptly, as glucocorticoids are required for the action of catecholamines in maintaining vascular tone.

The most prominent symptoms of the steroid withdrawal syndrome include malaise, anorexia, headache, lethargy, nausea and fever. In reducing pharmacological doses of glucocorticoids, it might appear logical to reduce the dosage precipitously to physiological replacement doses. This is rarely successful and occasionally disastrous. Even when given physiological replacement, patients who have been receiving pharmacological doses of glucocorticoids experience steroid withdrawal.

Although the mechanism is not known, it is most likely that long-term pharmacological glucocorticoid therapy inhibits transcription of the gene(s) for glucocorticoid receptors, thus reducing the number of receptors per cell. If this is so, physiological concentrations of glucocorticoids will elicit subphysiological cellular responses, resulting in the steroid withdrawal syndrome. Thus, it is necessary to taper gradually from the outset. The duration of glucocorticoid therapy is a critical consideration in designing a glucocorticoid withdrawal programme. Therapy for a couple of months will completely suppress the hypothalamo-pituitary-adrenal axis but will not cause adrenal atrophy. Therapy of years' duration may result in almost total atrophy of the adrenal fasciculata/reticularis, which may require a withdrawal regimen that takes months.

Procedures for tapering steroids are empirical. Their success is determined by the length and mode of therapy and by individual patient responses. Patients who have been on alternate-day therapy can be withdrawn more easily than those receiving daily therapy, especially daily therapy with a long-acting glucocorticoid such as dexamethasone. In patients on long-standing therapy, a 25% reduction in the previous level of therapy is generally recommended weekly. When withdrawal is done with steroids other than cortisone or cortisol, measurement of morning cortisol values can be a useful adjunct. Morning cortisol values of 10 μg/dL or more indicate that the dose can be reduced safely.

Even after the successful discontinuation of therapy, the hypothalamo-pituitary-adrenal axis is not wholly normal and may be incapable of responding to severe stress for 6–12 months after successful withdrawal from long-term, high-dose glucocorticoid therapy. Evaluation of the hypothalamus and pituitary by a CRH or metyrapone test and evaluation of adrenal responsiveness to pituitary stimulation with an intravenous ACTH test should be done at the conclusion of a withdrawal programme and 6 months thereafter. The results of these tests will indicate if there is a need for steroid cover in acute surgical stress or illness.

## Stress doses of glucocorticoids

The cortisol secretory rate increases significantly during physiological stress such as trauma, surgery, or severe illness. Patients receiving glucocorticoid replacement therapy or those recently withdrawn from pharmacological therapy need cover with stress doses. The indications for this cover and the appropriate dose are controversial and difficult to establish; most practitioners prefer to err on the safe side of steroid overdosage. This is a good tactic in the short term but can have a significant effect on growth over a period of years.

It is generally said that doses 3–10 times physiological replacement are needed for the stress of surgery. The stress accompanying a surgical procedure can vary greatly. Modern techniques of anaesthesiology, better anaesthetic, analgesic and muscle-relaxing drugs and increased awareness of the particular needs of children in managing intraoperative fluids and electrolytes have greatly reduced the stress of surgery. In the past, a significant portion of such stress had to do with pain and hypovolaemia, but these should be minimized in contemporary practice. Similarly, part of the stress of acute illness is fever and fluid loss, factors now familiar to all paediatricians. Although it remains appropriate and necessary to give about three times physiological requirements during such periods of stress, it is probably not necessary to give much higher doses. Similarly, it is not necessary

to triple a child's physiological replacement regimen during simple colds, upper respiratory infection, otitis media or after immunizations.

The preparation of the hypoadrenal patient on replacement therapy for surgery is simple if planned in advance. Although stress doses of steroids can be administered intravenously by the anaesthetist during surgery, this may be suboptimal. Doses administered as an intravenous bolus are short acting and may not provide cover throughout the procedure. The transition from ward to theatre to recovery room usually involves a transition among three or more teams of personnel, increasing the risk for error. Because intramuscularly administered cortisone acetate has a biological half-life of about 18 h, we recommend intramuscular administration of twice the day's physiological requirement at 18 h before surgery and again at 8 h before surgery. This provides the patient with a body reservoir of glucocorticoid throughout the surgical and immediate postoperative period. Regular therapy at two to three times physiological requirements can then be reinstituted on the day after the surgical procedure.

## Mineralocorticoid replacement

Replacement therapy with mineralocorticoids is indicated in salt-losing CAH and in syndromes of adrenal insufficiency that affect the zona glomerulosa. Only one mineralocorticoid, 9α-fluorocortisol (Fluorinef) is currently available. There is no parenteral mineralocorticoid preparation, so hydrocortisone plus salt must be used.

Mineralocorticoid doses used are essentially the same irrespective of the size or age of the patient. Newborns are quite insensitive to mineralocorticoids and may require larger doses than adults. The replacement dose of 9α-fluorocortisol is usually 50–100 μg daily; sodium must be available to the nephrons for mineralocorticoids to promote reabsorption of sodium.

Cortisol has significant mineralocorticoid activity and when given in stress doses provides adequate mineralocorticoid activity so that mineralocorticoid replacement can be interrupted. Because 9α-fluorocortisol can be administered only orally and because this may not be possible in the postoperative period, the appropriate drug for glucocorticoid replacement is cortisol or cortisone, which have mineralocorticoid activity, rather than a synthetic steroid such as prednisone or dexamethasone, which have little mineralocorticoid activity.

## References

1 Gaunt R. History of the adrenal cortex. In: Greep RO, Astwood EB, eds. *Handbook of Physiology: Endocrinology*. Washington, DC: American Physiological Society, 1975: 1–12.

2 Cushing H. The basophil adenomas of the pituitary body and their clinical manifestations. *Bull Johns Hopkins Hosp* 1932; 50: 137–95.

3 Selye H. The general adaptation syndrome and the diseases of adaptation. *J Clin Endocrinol* 1946; 6: 117–230.

4 Steiger M, Reichstein T. Desoxy-cortico-steron (21-oxyprogesterone) aus Δ 5–3-xoy-atio-cholensaure. *Helv Chim Acta* 1937; 20: 1164.

5 Kendall EC, Mason HL, McKenzie BF, Myers CS, Koelsche GA. Isolation in crystalline form of the hormone essential to life from the supranetal cortex: Its chemical nature and physiologic properties. *Trans Assoc Am Physicians* 1934; 49: 147.

6 Hench PS, Kendall EC, Slocumb CH, Polley HF. The effect of a hormone of the adrenal cortex (17-hydroxy-11-dehydrocorticosterone compound E) and of pituitary adrenocorticotropic hormone on rheumatoid arthritis. *Proc Staff Meet Mayo Clin* 1949; 24: 181–97.

7 Wilkins L, Lewis RA, Klein R, Rosenberg E. The suppression of androgen secretion by cortisone in a case of congenital adrenal hyperplasia. *Bull Johns Hopkins Hosp* 1950; 86: 249–52.

8 Bartter FC, Forbes AO, Leaf A. Congenital adrenal hyperplasia associated with the adrenogenital syndrome: An attempt to correct its disordered hormonal pattern. *J Clin Invest* 1950; 29: 797.

9 Cooper DY, Levin S, Narasimhulu S, Rosenthal O, Estabrook RW. Photochemical action spectrum of the terminal oxidase of mixed function oxidase systems. *Science* 1965; 145: 400–2.

10 Miller WL. Molecular biology of steroid hormone synthesis. *Endocr Rev* 1988; 9: 295–318.

11 Evans RM. The steroid and thyroid hormone receptor superfamily. *Science* 1988; 240: 889–95.

12 Gwynne JT, Strauss JF III. The role of lipoproteins in steroidogenesis and cholesterol metabolism in steroidogenic glands. *Endocr Rev* 1982; 3: 299–329.

13 Brown MS, Kovanen PT, Goldstein JL. Receptor-mediated uptake of lipoprotein-cholesterol and its utilization for steroid synthesis in the adrenal cortex. *Rec Prog Horm Res* 1979; 35: 215–57.

14 Strauss JF III, Miller WL. Molecular basis of ovarian steroid synthesis. In: Hillier SG, ed. *Ovarian Endocrinology.* Oxford: Blackwell Scientific Publications, 1991: 25–72.

15 Gonzalez FJ. The molecular biology of cytochrome P450s. *Pharmacol Rev* 1989; 40: 243–88.

16 Hall PF. Cytochromes P450 and the regulation of steroid syntheses. *Steroids* 1986; 48: 131–96.

17 Black SD, Coon MJ. P-450 cytochromes. Structure and function. *Adv Enzymol Relat Areas Mol Biol* 1987; 60: 35–87.

18 Nebert DW, Gonzalez FJ. P-450 genes. Structure, evolution and regulation. *Annu Rev Biochem* 1987; 56: 945–93.

19 Penning TM. Molecular endocrinology of hydroxysteroid dehydrogenases. *Endocr Rev* 1997; 18: 281–305.

20 Chung B, Matteson KJ, Voutilainen R, Mohandas TK, Miller WL. Human cholesterol side-chain cleavage enzyme, P450scc: cDNA cloning, assignment of the gene to chromosome 15 and expression in the placenta. *Proc Natl Acad Sci USA* 1986; 83: 8962–6.

21 Shikita M, Hall PF. Cytochrome P-450 from bovine adrenocortical mitochondria: An enzyme for the side chain cleavage of cholesterol. I. Purification and properties. *J Biol Chem* 1973; 248: 5596–604.

22 Shikita M, Hall PF. Cytochrome P-450 from bovine adrenocortical mitochondria: An enzyme for the side chain cleavage of cholesterol. II. Subunit structure. *J Biol Chem* 1973; 248: 5605–10.

23 Simpson ER. Cholesterol side-chain cleavage, cytochrome P450 and the control of steroidogenesis. *Mol Cell Endocrinol* 1979; 13: 213–27.

24 Lambeth JD, Pember SO. Cytochrome P-450scc–adrenodoxin complex: Reduction properties of the substrate-associated cytochrome and relation of the reduction states of haem and iron-sulfur centers to association of the proteins. *J Biol Chem* 1983; 258: 5596–602.

25 Yang X, Iwamoto K, Wang M, Artwohl J, Mason JI, Pang S. Inherited congenital adrenal hyperplasia in the rabbit is caused by a deletion in the gene encoding cytochrome P450 cholesterol side-chain cleavage enzyme. *Endocrinology* 1993; 132: 1977–82.

26 Kimura T, Suzuki K. Components of the electron transport system in adrenal steroid hydroxylase. *J Biol Chem* 1967; 242: 485–91.

27 Gnanaiah W, Omdahl JL. Isolation and characterization of pig kidney mitochondrial ferredoxin: NADP+ oxidoreductase. *J Biol Chem* 1986; 261: 12649–54.

28 Hanukoglu I, Suh BS, Himmelhoch S, Amsterdam A. Induction and mitochondrial localization of cytochrome P450scc system enzymes in normal and transformed ovarian granulosa cells. *J Cell Biol* 1990; 111: 1373–81.

29 Lambeth JD, Seybert D, Kamin H. Ionic effects on adrenal steroidogenic electron transport: The role of adrenodoxin as an electron shuttle. *J Biol Chem* 1979; 254: 7255–64.

30 Hanukoglu I, Spitsberg V, Bumpus JA, Dus KM, Jefcoate CR. Adrenal mitochondrial cytochrome P450scc: Cholesterol and adrenodoxin interactions at equilibrium and during turnover. *J Biol Chem* 1981; 256: 4321–8.

31 Coghlan VM, Vickery LE. Expression of human ferredoxin and assembly of the [2Fe–2S] center in *Escherichia coli. Proc Natl Acad Sci USA* 1989; 86: 835–9.

32 Solish SB, Picado-Leonard J, Morel Y *et al.* Human adrenodoxin reductase: Two mRNAs encoded by a single gene of chromosome 17cen→q25 are expressed in steroidogenic tissues. *Proc Natl Acad Sci USA* 1988; 71: 7104–8.

33 Lin D, Shi Y, Miller WL. Cloning and sequence of the human adrenodoxin reductase gene. *Proc Natl Acad Sci USA* 1990; 87: 8516–20.

34 Chang C-Y, Wu D-A, Lai C-C, Miller WL, Chung B. Cloning and structure of the human adrenodoxin gene. *DNA* 1988; 7: 609–15.

35 Picado-Leonard J, Voutilainen R, Kao L, Chung B, Strauss JF III, Miller WL. Human adrenodoxin: Cloning of three cDNAs and cycloheximide enhancement in JEG-3 cells. *J Biol Chem* 1988; 263: 3240–4.

36 Brentano ST, Black SM, Lin D, Miller WL. cAMP post-transcriptionally diminishes the abundance of adrenodoxin reductase mRNA. *Proc Natl Acad Sci USA* 1992; 89: 4099–103.

37 Moore CCD, Miller WL. The role of transcriptional regulation in steroid hormone biosynthesis. *J Steroid Biochem Mol Biol* 1991; 40: 517–25.

38 Hum DW, Miller WL. Transcriptional regulation of human genes for steroidogenic enzymes. *Clin Chem* 1993; 39: 333–40.

39 Ferguson JJ. Protein synthesis and adrenocorticotropin responsiveness. *J Biol Chem* 1963; 238: 2754–9.

40 Garren LD, Ney RL, Davis WW. Studies on the role of protein synthesis in the regulation of corticosterone production by ACTH *in vivo. Proc Natl Acad Sci USA* 1965; 53: 1443–50.

41 Stocco DM, Clark BJ. Regulation of the acute production of steroids in steroidogenic cells. *Endocr Rev* 1996; 17: 221–44.

42 Papadopoulos V. Peripheral-type benzodiazepine/diazepam binding inhibitor receptor: Biological role in steroidogenic cell function. *Endocr Rev* 1993; 14: 222–40.

43 Pon LA, Hartigan JA, Orme-Johnson NR. Acute ACTH regulation of adrenal corticosteroid biosynthesis: rapid accumulation of a phosphoprotein. *J Biol Chem* 1986; 261: 13309–16.

44 Epstein LF, Orme-Johnson NR. Regulation of steroid hormone biosynthesis: identification of precursors of a phosphoprotein targeted to the mitochondrion in stimulated rat adrenal cortex cells. *J Biol Chem* 1991; 266: 19739–45.

45 Stocco DM, Sodeman TC. The 30 kDa mitochondrial protein induced by hormone stimulation in MA-10 mouse Leydig tumour cells are processed from larger precursors. *J Biol Chem* 1991; 266: 19731–8.

46 Clark BJ, Wells J, King SR, Stocco DM. The purification, cloning and expression of a novel luteinizing hormone-induced mitochondrial protein in MA-10 mouse Leydig tumour cells. Characterization of the steroidogenic acute regulatory protein (StAR). *J Biol Chem* 1994; 269: 28314–22.

47 Lin D, Sugawara T, Strauss JF III, Clark BJ, Stocco DM, Saenger P, Rogol A, Miller WL. Role of steroidogenic acute regulatory protein in adrenal and gonadal steroidogenesis. *Science* 1995; 267: 1828–31.

48 Bose HS, Sugawara T, Strauss JF III, Miller WL. The pathophysiology and genetics of congenital lipoid adrenal hyperplasia. *N Engl J Med* 1996; 335: 1870–8.

49 Moore CCD, Hum DW, Miller WL. Identification of positive and negative placental-specific basal elements, a transcriptional repressor and a cAMP response element in the human gene for P450scc. *Mol Endocrinol* 1992; 6: 2045–58.

50 Mellon SH, Deschepper CF. Neurosteroid biosynthesis: Genes for adrenal steroidogenic enzymes are expressed in the brain. *Brain Res* 1993; 629: 283–92.

51 Sugawara T, Holt JA, Driscoll D *et al.* Human steroidogenic acute regulatory protein (StAR): Functional activity in COS-1 cells, tissue-specific expression and mapping of the structural gene to 8p11.2 and an expressed pseudogene to chromosome 13. *Proc Natl Acad Sci USA* 1995; 92: 4778–82.

52 Arakane F, Sugawara T, Nishino H *et al.* Steroidogenic acute regulatory protein (StAR) retains activity in the absence of its mitochondrial targeting sequence: Implications for the mechanism of StAR action. *Proc Natl Acad Sci USA* 1996; 93: 13731–6.

53 Arakane F, Kallen CB, Watari H *et al.* The mechanism of action of steroidogenic acute regulatory protein (StAR): StAR acts on the outside of mitochondria to stimulate steroidogenesis. *J Biol Chem* 1998; 273: 16339–45.

54 Bose HS, Whittal RM, Baldwin MA, Miller WL. The active form of the steroidogenic acute regulatory protein, StAR, appears to be a molten globule. *Proc Natl Acad Sci USA* 1999; 96: 7250–5.

55 Thomas JL, Myers RP, Strickler RC. Human placental 3β-hydroxy-5-ene-steroid dehydrogenase and steroid 5→4-ene-isomerase: purification from mitochondria and kinetic profiles, biophysical characterization of the purified mitochondrial and microsomal enzymes. *Steroid Biochem* 1989; 33: 209–17.

56 Luu-The V, Lechance Y, Labrie C *et al.* Full length cDNA structure and deduced amino acid sequence of human 3β-hydroxy-5-ene steroid dehydrogenase. *Mol Endocrinol* 1989; 3: 1310–12.

57 Lorence MC, Murry BA, Trant JM, Mason JI. Human 3β-hydroxysteroid dehydrogenase/$\Delta^5 \rightarrow \Delta^4$ isomerase from placenta: Expression in nonsteroidogenic cells of a protein that catalyzes the dehydrogenation/isomerization of $C_{21}$ and $C_{19}$ steroids. *Endocrinology* 1990; 126: 2493–8.

58 Lachance Y, Luu-The V, Labrie C *et al.* Characterization of human 3β-hydroxysteroid dehydrogenase/$\Delta^5$-$\Delta^4$-isomerase gene and its expression in mammalian cells. *J Biol Chem* 1990; 265: 20469–75.

59 Rhéaume E, Lachance Y, Zhao HL *et al.* Structure and expression of a new complementary DNA encoding the almost exclusive 3β-hydroxysteroid dehydrogenase/$\Delta^5$-$\Delta^4$-isomerase in human adrenals and gonads. *Mol Endocrinol* 1991; 5: 1147–57.

60 Lorence MC, Corbin CJ, Kamimura N, Mahendroo MS, Mason JI. Structural analysis of the gene encoding human 3β-hydroxysteroid dehydrogenase/$\Delta^5 \rightarrow \Delta^4$ isomerase. *Mol Endocrinol* 1990; 4: 1850–5.

61 Lin D, Black SM, Nagahama Y, Miller WL. Steroid 17α-hydroxylase and 17,20 lyase activities of P450c17: Contributions of serine[106] and P450 reductase. *Endocrinology* 1993; 132: 2498–506.

62 Auchus RJ, Lee TC, Miller WL. Cytochrome $b_5$ augments the 17,20 lyase activity of human P450c17 without direct electron transfer. *J Biol Chem* 1998; 273: 3158–65.

63 Sklar CA, Kaplan SL, Grumbach MM. Evidence for dissociation between adrenarche and gonadarche: Studies in patients with idiopathic precocious puberty, gonadal dysgenesis, isolated gonadotropin deficiency and constitutionally delayed growth and adolescence. *J Clin Endocrinol Metab* 1980; 51: 548–56.

64 Zachmann M, Vollmin JA, Hamilton W, Prader A. Steroid 17,20 desmolase deficiency: a new cause of male pseudohermaphroditism. *Clin Endocrinol* 1972; 1: 369–85.

65 Nakajin S, Hall PF. Microsomal cytochrome P450 from neonatal pig testis. Purification and properties of a $C_{21}$ steroid side-chain cleavage system (17α-hydroxylase-$C_{17,20}$ lyase). *J Biol Chem* 1981; 256: 3871–6.

66 Nakajin S, Shinoda M, Haniu M, Shively JE, Hall PF. $C_{21}$ steroid side-chain cleavage enzyme from porcine adrenal microsomes. Purification and characterization of the 17α-hydroxylase/$C_{17,20}$ lyase cytochrome P450. *J Biol Chem* 1984; 259: 3971–6.

67 Zuber MX, Simpson ER, Waterman MR. Expression of bovine 17α-hydroxylase cytochrome P450 cDNA in non-steroidogenic (COS-1) cells. *Science* 1986; 234: 1258–61.

68 Lin D, Harikrishna JA, Moore CCD, Jones KL, Miller WL. Missense mutation Ser[106]→Pro causes 17α-hydroxylase deficiency. *J Biol Chem* 1991; 266: 15992–8.

69 Matteson KJ, Picado-Leonard J, Chung B, Mohandas TK, Miller WL. Assignment of the gene for adrenal P450c17 (17α-hydroxylase/17,20 lyase) to human chromosome 10. *J Clin Endocrinol Metab* 1986; 63: 789–91.

70 Fan YS, Sasi R, Lee C, Winter JSD, Waterman MR, Lin CC. Localization of the human CYP17 gene (cytochrome P450, 17α) to 10q24.3 by fluorescence *in situ* hybridization and simultaneous chromosome banding. *Genomics* 1992; 14: 1110–11.

71 Picado-Leonard J, Miller WL. Cloning and sequence of the human gene encoding P450c17 (steroid 17α-hydroxylase/17,20 lyase): Similarity to the gene for P450c21. *DNA* 1987; 6: 439–48.

72 Yamano S, Aoyama T, McBride OW, Hardwick JP, Gelboin HV, Gonzalez FJ. Human NADPH-P450 oxidoreductase: Complementary DNA cloning, sequence, vaccinia virus-mediated

expression and localization of the CYPOR gene to chromosome 7. *Mol Pharmacol* 1989; 35: 83–8.

73 Wang M, Roberts DL, Paschke R, Shea TM, Masters BSS, Kim JJP. Three-dimensional structure of NADPH-cytochrome P450 reductase: Prototype for FMN- and FAD-containing enzymes. *Proc Natl Acad Sci USA* 1997; 94: 8411–16.

74 Oprian DD, Coon MJ. Oxidation-redcution states of FMN and FAD in NADPH-cytochrome P450 reductase during reduction by NADPH. *J Biol Chem* 1982; 257: 8935–44.

75 Zhang L, Rodriguez H, Ohno S, Miller WL. Serine phosphorylation of human P450c17 increases 17,20 lyase activity: implications for adrenarche and for the polycystic ovary syndrome. *Proc Natl Acad Sci USA* 1995; 92: 10619–23.

76 Yanagibashi K, Hall PF. Role of electron transport in the regulation of the lyase activity of C-21 side-chain cleavage P450 from porcine adrenal and testicular microsomes. *J Biol Chem* 1986; 261: 8429–33.

77 Miller WL, Auchus RJ. Biochemistry and genetics of human PW50c17. In: Hughes IA, Clark AJL, eds. *Andrenal Disease in Childhood*. Basel: Karger, 2000; 63–92.

78 Miller WL, Morel Y. Molecular genetics of 21-hydroxylase deficiency. *Annu Rev Genet* 1989; 23: 371–93.

79 New MI, White P, Pang S, Dupont B, Speiser PW. The adrenal hyperplasias. In: Scriver CR, Beaudet A, Sly S, Valle D, eds. *The Metabolic Basis of Inherited Disease*. New York: McGraw-Hill, 1989: 1881–917.

80 Morel Y, Miller WL. Clinical and molecular genetics of congenital adrenal hyperplasia due to 21-hydroxylase deficiency. *Adv Hum Genet* 1991; 20: 1–68.

81 Kominami S, Ochi H, Kobayashi Y, Takemori S. Studies on the steroid hydroxylation system in adrenal cortex microsomes: purification and characterization of cytochrome P450 specific for steroid 21 hydroxylation. *J Biol Chem* 1980; 255: 3386–94.

82 Higashi Y, Yoshioka H, Yamane M, Gotoh O, Fujii-Kuriyama Y. Complete nucleotide sequence of two steroid 21-hydroxylase genes tandemly arranged in human chromosome: a pseudogene and genuine gene. *Proc Natl Acad Sci USA* 1986; 83: 2841–5.

83 White PC, New MI, Dupont B. Structure of the human steroid 21-hydroxylase genes. *Proc Natl Acad Sci USA* 1986; 83: 5111–15.

84 Rodrigues NR, Dunham I, Yu CY, Carroll MC, Porter RR, Campbell RD. Molecular characterization of the HLA-linked steroid 21-hydroxylase B gene from an individual with congenital adrenal hyperplasia. *EMBO J* 1987; 6: 1653–61.

85 Dupont B, Oberfield SE, Smithwick ER, Lee TD, Levine LS. Close genetic linkage between HLA and congenital adrenal hyperplasia (21-hydroxylase deficiency). *Lancet* 1977; ii: 1309–12.

86 Casey ML, MacDonald PC. Extra-adrenal formation of a mineralocorticoid: Deoxycorticosterone and deoxycorticosterone sulphate biosynthesis and metabolism. *Endocr Rev* 1982; 3: 396–403.

87 Mellon SH, Miller WL. Extra-adrenal steroid 21-hydroxylation is not mediated by P450c21. *J Clin Invest* 1989; 84: 1497–502.

88 White PC, Curnow KM, Pascoe L. Disorders of steroid 11β-hydroxylase isozymes. *Endocr Rev* 1994; 15: 421–38.

89 Fardella CE, Miller WL. Molecular biology of mineralocorticoid metabolism. *Ann Rev Nutrition* 1996; 16: 443–70.

90 Mornet E, Dupont J, Vitek A, White PC. Characterization of two genes encoding human steroid 11β-hydroxylase (P45011β). *J Biol Chem* 1989; 264: 20961–7.

91 Wagner MJ, Ge Y, Siciliano M, Wells DE. A hybrid cell mapping panel for regional localization of probes to human chromosome 8. *Genomics* 1991; 10: 114–25.

92 Chua SC, Szabo P, Vitek A, Grzeschik K-H, John M, White PC. Cloning of cDNA encoding steroid 11β-hydroxylase, P450c11. *Proc Natl Acad Sci USA* 1987; 84: 7193–7.

93 Curnow KM, Tusie-Luna M, Pascoe L *et al.* The product of the CYP11B2 gene is required for aldosterone biosynthesis in the human adrenal cortex. *Mol Endocrinol* 1991; 5: 1513–22.

94 Kawamoto T, Mitsuuchi Y, Toda K *et al.* Role of steroid 11β-hydroxylase and 18-hydroxylase in the biosynthesis of glucocorticoids and mineralocorticoids in humans. *Proc Natl Acad Sci USA* 1992; 89: 1458–62.

95 White PC, Dupont J, New MI, Lieberman E, Hochberg Z, Rösler A. A mutation in CYP11B1 (Arg 448→His) associated with steroid 11β-hydroxylase deficiency in Jews of Moroccan origin. *J Clin Invest* 1991; 87: 1664–7.

96 Pascoe L, Curnow K, Slutsker L, Rösler A, White PC. Mutations in the human CYP11B2 (aldosterone synthase) gene causing corticosterone methlyoxidase II deficiency. *Proc Natl Acad Sci USA* 1992; 89: 4996–5000.

97 Ulick S, Wang JZ, Morton H. The biochemical phenotypes of two inborn errors in the biosynthesis of aldosterone. *J Clin Endocrinol Metab* 1992; 74: 1415–20.

98 Zhang G, Rodriguez H, Fardella CE, Harris DA, Miller WL. Mutation T318M in P450c11AS causes corticosterone methyl oxidase II deficiency. *Am J Hum Genet* 1995; 57: 1037–43.

99 Labrie F, Luu-The V, Lin SX, Labrie C, Simard J, Breton R, Bélanger A. The key role of 17β-hydroxysteroid dehydrogenases in sex steroid biology. *Steroids* 1997; 62: 148–58.

100 Moghrabi Nandersson S. 17β-Hydroxysteroid dehydrogenases: physiological roles in health and disease. *Trends Endocrinol Metab* 1998; 9: 265–70.

101 Peltoketo H, Isomaa V, Mäenlavsta O, Vihko R. Complete amino acid sequence of human placental 17β-hydroxysteroid dehydrogenase deduced from cDNA. *FEBS Lett* 1988; 239: 73–7.

102 Gast MJ, Sims HF, Murdock GL, Gast PM, Strauss AW. Isolation and sequencing of a complementary deoxyribonucleic acid clone encoding human placental 17β-estradiol dehydrogenase: identification of the putative cofactor binding site. *Am J Obstet Gynecol* 1989; 161: 1726–31.

103 Tremblay Y, Ringler GE, Morel Y *et al.* Regulation of the gene for estrogenic 17-ketosteroid reductase lying on chromosome 17cen→q25. *J Biol Chem* 1989; 264: 20458–62.

104 Ghosh D, Pleuteu VZ, Zhu DW *et al.* Structure of human estrogenic 17β-hydroxysteroid dehydrogenase at 2.2 Å resolution. *Structure* 1995; 3: 503–13.

105 Sawicki MW, Erman M, Puranen T, Vihko P, Ghosh D. Structure of the ternary complex of human 17β-hydroxysteroid dehydrogenase type 1 with 3-hydroxyestra-1,3,5,7-tetraen-17-one (equilin) and NADP+. *Proc Natl Acad Sci USA* 1999; 96: 840–5.

106 Takeyama J, Sasano H, Suzuki T, Iinuma K, Nagura Handersson S. 17β-Hydroxysteroid dehydrogenase types 1 and 2 in human placenta: an immunohistochemical study with correlation to placental development. *J Clin Endocrinol Metab* 1998; 83: 3710–15.

107 Geissler WM, Davis DL, Wu L *et al.* Male pseudohermaphroditism caused by mutations of testicular 17β-hydroxysteroid dehydrogenase 3. *Nature Genet* 1994; 7: 34–9.

108 Andersson S, Geissler WM, Wu L *et al.* Molecular genetics and pathophysiology of 17β-hydroxysteroid dehydrogenase 3 deficiency. *J Clin Endocrinol Metab* 1996; 81: 130–6.

109 Adamski J, Normand T, Leenders F *et al.* Molecular cloning of a novel widely expressed human 80 kDa 17β-hydroxysteroid dehydrogenase IV. *Biochem J* 1995; 311: 437–43.

110 Leenders F, Tesdorpf JG, Markus M, Engel T, Seedorf U, Adamski J. Porcine 80-kDa protein reveals intrinsic 17β-hydroxysteroid dehydrogenase, fatty acyl-CoA-hydratase/dehydrogenase and sterol transfer activities. *J Biol Chem* 1996; 271: 5438–42.

111 van Grunsven EG, van Berkel E, Ijlst L *et al.* Peroxisomal D-hydroxyacyl-CoA dehydrogenase deficiency: Resolution of the enzyme defect and its molecular basis in bifunctional protein deficiency. *Proc Natl Acad Sci USA* 1998; 95: 2128–33.

112 Lin HK, Jez JM, Schlegel BP, Peehl DM, Pachter JA, Penning TM. Expression and characterization of recombinant type 2 3α-hydroxysteroid dehydrogenase (HSD) from human prostate: demonstration of bifunctional 3α/17β-HSD activity and cellular distribution. *Mol Endocrinol* 1997; 11: 1971–84.

113 Dufort I, Rheault P, Huang XF, Soucy P, Luu-The V. Characteristics of a highly labile human type 5 17β-hydroxysteroid dehydrogenase. *Endocrinology* 1999; 140: 568–74.

114 Yen PH, Allen E, Marsh B, Mohandas T, Shapiro LJ. Cloning and expression of steroid sulphatase cDNA and the frequent occurrence of deletions: Implications for X-Y interchange. *Cell* 1987; 49: 443–54.

115 Ballabio A, Shapiro LJ. Steroid sulphatase deficiency and X-linked icthiosis. In: Schriver CR, Beaudet AL, Sly WS, Valle D, eds. *The Metabolic and Molecular Basis of Inherited Disease.* New York: Mc-Graw-Hill, 1995: 2999–3022.

116 Compagnone NA, Salido E, Shapiro LJ, Mellon SH. Expression of steroid sulphatase during embryogenesis. *Endocrinology* 1997; 138: 4768–73.

117 Compagnone NA, Mellon SH. Dehydroepiandrosterone. A potential signalling molecule for neocortical organization during development. *Proc Natl Acad Sci USA* 1998; 95: 4678–83.

118 Simpson ER, Mahendroo MS, Means GD *et al.* Aromatase cytochrome P450, the enzyme responsible for estrogen biosynthesis. *Endocr Rev* 1994; 15: 342–55.

119 Grumbach MM, Auchus RJ. Estrogen: consequences and implications of human mutations in synthesis and action. *J Clin Endocrinol Metab* 1999; 84: 4677–94.

120 Ito Y, Fisher CR, Conte FA, Grumbach MM, Simpson ER. Molecular basis of aromatase deficiency in an adult female with sexual infantilism and polycystic ovaries. *Proc Natl Acad Sci USA* 1993; 90: 11673–7.

121 Conte FA, Grumbach MM, Ito Y, Fisher CR, Simpson ER. A syndrome of female pseudohermaphrodism, hypergonadotropic hypogonadism and multicystic ovaries associated with missense mutations in the gene encoding aromatase (P450arom). *J Clin Endocrinol Metab* 1994; 78: 1287–92.

122 Thigpen AE, Silver RI, Guileyardo JM, Casey ML, McConnell JD, Russell DW. Tissue distribution and ontogeny of steroid 5α-reductase isozyme expression. *J Clin Invest* 1993; 92: 903–10.

123 Wilson JD. The role of androgens in male gender role behaviour. *Endocr Rev* 1999; 20: 726–37.

124 Arriza JL, Weinberger C, Cerelli G, Glaser TM, Handelin BL, Housman DE, Evans RM. Cloning of human mineralocorticoid receptor DNA. Structural and functional kinship with the glucocorticoid receptor. *Science* 1987; 237: 268–75.

125 Funder JW, Pearce PT, Smith R, Smith I. Mineralocorticoid action: Target tissue specificity is enzyme, not receptor, mediated. *Science* 1988; 242: 583–5.

126 White PC, Mune T, Agarwal AK. 11β-Hydroxysteroid dehydrogenase and the syndrome of apparent mineralocorticoid excess. *Endocr Rev* 1997; 18: 135–56.

127 Agarwal AK, Tusie-Luna M-T, Monder C, White PC. Expression of 11β-hydroxysteroid dehydrogenase using recombinant vaccinia virus. *Mol Endocrinol* 1990; 4: 1827–32.

128 Moore CCD, Mellon SH, Murai J, Siiteri PK, Miller WL. Structure and function of the hepatic form of 11β-hydroxysteroid dehydrogenase in the squirrel monkey, an animal model of glucocorticoid resistance. *Endocrinology* 1993; 133: 368–75.

129 Brown RW, Chapman KE, Edwards CRW, Seckl JR. Human placental 11β-hydroxysteroid dehydrogenase: evidence for and partial purification of a distinct NAD⁺-dependent isoform. *Endocrinology* 1993; 132: 2614–21.

130 Rusvai E, Náray-Fejes-Tóth A. A new isoform of 11β-hydroxysteroid dehydrogenase in aldosterone target cells. *J Biol Chem* 1993; 268: 10717–20.

131 Krozowski Z, MaGuire JA, Stein-Oakley AN, Dowling J, Smith R, Eandrews RK. Immunohistochemical localization of the 11β-hydroxysteroid dehydrogenase type II enzyme in human kidney and placenta. *J Clin Endocrinol Metab* 1995; 80: 2203–9.

132 Hirasawa G, Sasono H, Suzuki T *et al.* 11β-Hydroxysteroid dehydrogenase type 2 and mineralocorticoid receptor in human fetal development. *J Clin Endocrinol Metab* 1999; 84: 1453–8.

133 Miller WL, Levine LS. Molecular and clinical advances in congenital adrenal hyperplasia. *J Pediatr* 1987; 111: 1–17.

134 Voutilainen R, Ilvesmaki V, Miettinen PJ. Low expression of 3β-hydroxy-5-ene steroid dehydrogenase gene in human fetal adrenals *in vivo*; adrenocorticotropin and protein kinase C-dependent regulation in adrenocortical cultures. *J Clin Endocrinol Metab* 1991; 72: 761–7.

135 Fujieda K, Faiman C, Feyes FI, Winter JSD. The control of steroidogenesis by human fetal adrenal cells in tissue culture: IV. The effects of exposure to placental steroids. *J Clin Endocrinol Metab* 1982; 54: 89–94.

136 Miller WL. Steroid hormone biosynthesis and actions in the materno-feto-placental unit. *Clin Perinatol* 1998; 25: 799–817.

137 Pasqualini JR, Nguyen BL, Uhrich F, Wiqvist N, Diczfalvay E. Cortisol and cortisone metabolism in the human fetoplacental unit at midgestation. *J Steroid Biochem* 1970; 1: 209–19.

138 Kari MA, Raivio KO, Stenman U-H, Voutilainen R. Serum cortisol, dehydroepiandrosterone sulphate and sterol-binding globulins in preterm neonates: Effects of gestational age and dexamethasone therapy. *Pediatr Res* 1996; 40: 319–24.

139 DiBlasio AM, Voutilainen R, Jaffe RB, Miller WL. Hormonal regulation of mRNAs for P450scc (cholesterol side-chain cleavage enzyme) and P450c17 (17α-hydroxylase/17,20 lyase) in cultured human fetal adrenal cells. *J Clin Endocrinol Metab* 1987; 65: 170–5.

140 Voutilainen R, Miller WL. Coordinate tropic hormone regulation of mRNAs for insulin-like growth factor II and the cholesterol side-chain cleavage enzyme, P450scc, in human steroidogenic tissues. *Proc Natl Acad Sci USA* 1987; 84: 1590–4.

141 New MI, Wilson RC. Steroid disorders in children: congenital adrenal hyperplasia and apparent mineralocorticoid excess. *Proc Natl Acad Sci USA* 1999; 96: 12790–7.

142 Sawchenko PE, Swanson LW, Vale WW. Co-expression of corticotropin-releasing factor and vasopressin immunoreactivity in parvocellular neurosecretory neurons of the adrenalectomized rat. *Proc Natl Acad Sci USA* 1984; 81: 1883–7.

143 Whitnall MH, Mezey E, Gainer H. Co-localization of corticotropin-releasing factor and vasopressin in median eminence neurosecretory vesicles. *Nature* 1985; 317: 248–50.

144 Aguilera G, Harwood JP, Wilson JX, Morell J, Brown JH, Catt KJ. Mechanisms of action of corticotropin-releasing factor and other regulators of corticotropin release in rat pituitary cells. *J Biol Chem* 1983; 258: 8039–45.

145 Miller WL, Johnson LK, Baxter JD, Robert JL. Processing of the precursor to corticotropin and β-lipotropin in man. *Proc Natl Acad Sci USA* 1980; 77: 5211–15.

146 Whitfeld PL, Seeburg PH, Shine J. The human pro-opiomelanocortin gene: Organization, sequence and interspersion with repetitive DNA. *DNA* 1982; 1: 133–43.

147 Lowry PJ, Silas L, McLean C, Linton EA, Estivariz FE. Pro-gamma-melanocyte-stimulating hormone cleavage in adrenal gland undergoing compensatory growth. *Nature* 1983; 306: 70–3.

148 Lundblad JR, Roberts JL. Regulation of proopiomelanocortin gene expression in pituitary. *Endocr Rev* 1988; 9: 135–58.

149 Jefcoate CR, McNamara BC, DiBartolomeis MS. Control of steroid synthesis in adrenal fasciculata. *Endocr Res* 1986; 12: 315–50.

150 Anderson RA, Sando GN. Cloning and expression of cDNA encoding human lysosomal acid lypase/cholesterol ester hyrolase. *J Biol Chem* 1991; 266: 22479–84.

151 Miller WL, Strauss JF III. Molecular pathology and mechanism of action of the steroidogenic acute regulatory protein, StAR. *J Steroid Biochem Mol Biol* 1999; 69: 131–41.

152 Dallman MF. Control of adrenocortical growth in vivo. *Endocr Rev* 1985; 10: 213–42.

153 Townsend S, Dallman MF, Miller WL. Rat insulin-like growth factors-I and -II mRNAs are unchanged during compensatory adrenal growth but decrease during ACTH-induced adrenal growth. *J Biol Chem* 1990; 265: 22117–22.

154 Voutilainen R, Miller WL. Developmental and hormonal regulation of mRNAs for insulin-like growth factor and steroidogenic enzymes in human fetal adrenals and gonads. *DNA* 1988; 7: 9–15.

155 Mesiano S, Mellon SH, Gospodarowicz D, Di Blasio AM, Jaffe RB. Basic fibroblast growth factor expression is regulated by corticotropin in the human fetal adrenal: a model for adrenal growth regulation. *Proc Natl Acad Sci USA* 1991; 88: 5428–32.

156 Mesiano S, Mellon SH, Jaffe RB. Mitogenic action, regulation and localization of insulin-like growth factors in the human fetal adrenal gland. *J Clin Endocrinol Metab* 1993; 76: 968–76.

157 Mesiano S, Jaffe RB. Role of growth factors in the developmental regulation of the human fetal adrenal cortex. *Steroids* 1997; 62: 62–72.

158 Moore-Ede MC, Czeisler CA, Richardson GS. Circadian timekeeping in health and disease. Part 1. Basic properties of circadian pacemakers. *N Engl J Med* 1983; 309: 469–76.

159 Follenius M, Brandenberger G, Hietter B. Diurnal cortisol peaks and their relationships to meals. *J Clin Endocrinol Metab* 1982; 55: 757–61.

160 Goldman J, Wajchenberg BL, Liberman B, Nery M, Achando S, Germek OA. Contrast analysis for the evaluation of the circadian rhythms of plasma cortisol androstenedione and testosterone in normal men and the possible influence of meals. *J Clin Endocrinol Metab* 1985; 60: 164–7.

161 Quigley ME, Yen SS. A mid-day surge in cortisol levels. *J Clin Endocrinol Metab* 1979; 49: 945–7.

162 Wallace WH, Crowne EC, Shalet SM, Moore C, Gibson S, Littley MD, White A. Episodic ACTH and cortisol secretion in normal children. *Clin Endocrinol* 1991; 34: 215–21.

163 Onishi S, Miyazawa G, Nishimura Y *et al.* Postnatal development of circadian rhythm in serum cortisol levels in children. *Pediatrics* 1983; 72: 399–404.

164 Dempsher DP, Gann DS. Increased cortisol secretion after small hemorrhage is not attributable to changes in adrenocorticotropin. *Endocrinology* 1983; 113: 86–93.

165 Udelsman R, Norton JA, Jelenich SE *et al.* Responses of the hypothalamic-pituitary-adrenal and renin-angiotensin axes and the sympathetic system during controlled surgical and anesthetic stress. *J Clin Endocrinol Metab* 1987; 64: 986–94.

166 Chrousos GP. The hypothalamic-pituitary-adrenal axis and immune-mediated inflammation. *N Engl J Med* 1995; 332: 1351–62.

167 Keller-Wood ME, Dallman MF. Corticosteroid inhibition of ACTH secretion. *Endocr Rev* 1984; 5: 1–24.

168 Deschepper CF, Mellon SH, Cumin F, Baxter JD, Ganong WF. Analysis by immunocytochemistry and in situ hybridization of renin and its mRNA in kidney, testis, adrenal and pituitary of the rat. *Proc Natl Acad Sci USA* 1986; 83: 7552–6.

169 Sander M, Ganten D, Mellon SH. Role of adrenal renin in the regulation of adrenal steroidogenesis by ACTH. *Proc Natl Acad Sci USA* 1994; 91: 148–52.

170 Hardman JA, Hort YJ, Catanzaro DF, Tellam JT, Baxter JD, Morris BJ, Shine J. Primary structure of the human renin gene. *DNA* 1984; 3: 457–68.

171 Kramer RE, Gallant S, Brownie AC. Actions of angiotensin II on aldosterone biosynthesis in the rat adrenal cortex. *J Biol Chem* 1980; 255: 3442–7.

172 McKenna TJ, Island DP, Nicholson WE, Liddle GW. The effects of potassium on early and late steps in aldosterone biosynthesis in cells of the zona glomerulosa. *Endocrinology* 1978; 105: 1411–16.

173 Farese RV, Larson RE, Sabir MA, Gomez-Sanchez CE. Effects of angiotensin II, K⁺, adrenocorticotropin, serotonin, adenosine 3′,5′-monophosphate, A23187and EGTA on aldosterone synthesis and phospholipid metabolism in the rat adrenal zona glomerulosa. *Endocrinology* 1983; 113: 1377–86.

174 Barrett PQ, Bollag WB, Isales CM, McCarthy RT, Rasmussen H. The role of calcium in angiotensin II-mediated aldosterone secretion. *Endocr Rev* 1989; 10: 496–518.

175 Moore CCD, Brentano ST, Miller WL. Human P450scc gene transcription is induced by cyclic AMP and repressed by 12-*O*-tetradecanolyphorbol-13-acetate and A23187 by independent *cis*-elements. *Mol Cell Biol* 1990; 10: 6013–23.

176 Gullner HG, Gill JR Jr. Beta endorphin selectively stimulates aldosterone secretion in hypophysectomized, nephrectomized dogs. *J Clin Invest* 1983; 71: 124–8.

177 Yamakado M, Franco-Saenz R, Mulrow PJ. Effect of sodium deficiency on beta-melanocyte-stimulating hormone stimula-

tion of aldosterone in isolated rat adrenal cells. *Endocrinology* 1983; 113: 2168–72.

178 Atarashi K, Mulrow PJ, Franco-Saenz R. Effect of atrial peptides on aldosterone production. *J Clin Invest* 1985; 76: 1807–11.

179 Orentreich N, Brind JL, Rizer RL, Vogelman JH. Age changes and sex differences in serum dehydroepiandrosterone sulphate concentrations throughout adulthood. *J Clin Endocrinol Metab* 1984; 59: 551–5.

180 Mellon SH, Shively JE, Miller WL. Human proopiomelanocortin (79–96), a proposed androgen stimulatory hormone, does not affect steroidogenesis in cultured human fetal adrenal cells. *J Clin Endocrinol Metab* 1991; 72: 19–22.

181 Penhoat A, Sanchez P, Jaillard C, Langlois D, Begeot M, Saez JM. Human proopiomelanocortin (79–96), a proposed cortical androgen stimulating hormone, does not affect steroidogenesis in cultured human adult adrenal cells. *J Clin Endocrinol Metab* 1991; 72: 23–6.

182 Endoh A, Kristiansen SB, Casson PR, Buster JE, Hornsby PJ. The zona reticularis is the site of biosynthesis of dehydroepiandrosterone and dehydroepiandrosterone sulphate in the adult human adrenal cortex resulting from its low expression of 3β-hydroxysteroid dehydrogenase. *J Clin Endocrinol Metab* 1996; 81: 3558–65.

183 Gell JS, Carr BR, Sasano H, Atkins B, Margraf L, Mason JI, Rainey WE. Adrenarche results from development of a 3β-hydroxysteroid dehydrogenase-deficient adrenal reticularis. *J Clin Endocrinol Metab* 1998; 83: 3695–701.

184 Dardis A, Saraco N, Rivarola MA, Belgorosky A. Decrease in the expression of the 3β-hydroxysteroid dehydrogenase gene in human adrenal tissue during prepuberty and early puberty: Implications for the mechanism of adrenarche. *Pediatr Res* 1999; 45: 384–8.

185 Yanase T, Sasano H, Yubisui T, Sakai Y, Takayanagi R, Nawata H. Immunohistochemical study of cytochrome $b_5$ in human adrenal gland and in adrenocortical adenomas from patients with Cushing's syndrome. *Endocr J* 1998; 45: 89–95.

186 Mapes S, Corbin C, Tarantal A, Conley A. The primate adrenal zona reticularis is defined by expression of cytochrome $b_5$, 17α-hydroxylase/17,20-lyase cytochrome, P450 (P450c17): and NADPH-cytochrome P450 reductase (reductase) but not 3β-hydroxysteroid dehydrogenase/Δ5–4 isomerase (3β-HSD). *J Clin Endocrinol Metab* 1999; 84: 3382–5.

187 Miller WL. The molecular basis of adrenarche – an hypothesis. *Acta Pediatr* 1999; 88 (Suppl. 433): 60–6.

188 Ibañez L, Potau N, Virdis R *et al.* Postpubertal outcome in girls diagnosed of premature pubarche during childhood: Increased frequency of functional ovarian hyperandrogenism. *J Clin Endocrinol Metab* 1993; 76: 1599–603.

189 Oppenheimer E, Linder B, DiMartino-Nardi J. Decreased insulin sensitivity in prepubertal girls with premature adrenarche and acanthosis nigricans. *J Clin Endocrinol Metab* 1995; 80: 614–18.

190 Ibañez L, Potau N, Zampolli MNP, Virdis R, Vicens-Calvet E, Carrascosa A. Hyperinsulinemia in postpubertal girls with a history of premature pubarche and functional ovarian hyperandrogenism. *J Clin Endocrinol Metab* 1996; 81: 1237–43.

191 Ibanez L, Potau N, Marcos MV, de Zegher F. Exaggerated adrenarche and hyperinsulinism in adolescent girls born small for gestational age. *J Clin Endocrinol Metab* 1999; 84: 4739–41.

192 Arlt W, Callies F, van Vlijmen JC *et al.* Dehydroepiandrosterone replacement in women with adrenal insufficiency. *N Engl J Med* 1999; 341: 1013–20.

193 Zumoff B, Fukushima DK, Hellman L. Intercomparison of four methods for measuring cortisol production. *J Clin Endocrinol Metab* 1974; 38: 169–75.

194 Hammond GL. Molecular properties of corticosteroid binding globulin and the sex-steroid binding proteins. *Endocr Rev* 1990; 11: 65–79.

195 Rosner W. The functions of corticosteroid-binding globulin and sex hormone-binding globulin: recent advances. *Endocr Rev* 1990; 11: 80–91.

196 Shackleton CH, Gustafsson JA, Mitchell FL. Steroids in newborns and infants. The changing pattern of urinary steroid excretion during infancy. *Acta Endocrinol* 1973; 74: 157–67.

197 Stewart PM, Corrie JET, Shackleton CHL, Edwards CRW. Syndrome of apparent mineralocorticoid excess. A defect in the cortisol–cortisone shuttle. *J Clin Invest* 1988; 82: 340–9.

198 Fu GK, Lin D, Zhang MYH *et al.* Cloning of human 25-hydroxy vitamin D-1α-hydroxylase and mutations causing vitamin D-dependant rickets type I. *Mol Endocrinol* 1997; 11: 1961–70.

199 Weitzman ED, Fukushima D, Nogeire C, Roffwarg H, Gallagher TF, Hellman L. Twenty-four hour pattern of the episodic secretion of cortisol in normal subjects. *J Clin Endocrinol Metab* 1971; 33: 14–22.

200 Veldhuis JD, Iranmanesh A, Johnson ML, Lizarralde G. Amplitude but not frequency, modulation of adrenocorticotropin secretory bursts gives rise to the nyctohaemral rhythm of the corticotropic axis in man. *J Clin Endocrinol Metab* 1990; 71: 452–63.

201 Laragh JH, Sealey J, Brunner HR. The control of aldosterone secretion in normal and hypertensives man abnormal renin aldosterone patterns in low renin hypertension. *Am J Med* 1972; 53: 649–63.

202 Porter CC, Silber RH. A quantitative color reaction for cortisone and related 17,21-dihydroxy-ketosteroids. *J Biol Chem* 1950; 185: 201–7.

203 Murphy BE. Clinical evaluation of urinary cortisol determinations by competitive protein-binding radioassay. *J Clin Endocrinol Metab* 1968; 28: 343–8.

204 Franks RC. Urinary 17-hydroxycorticosteroid and cortisol excretion in childhood. *J Clin Endocrinol Metab* 1973; 36: 702–5.

205 Styne DM, Grumbach MM, Kaplan SL, Wilson CB, Conte FA. Treatment of Cushing's disease in childhood and adolescence by transcriptional microadenomectomy. *New England J Med* 1984; 310: 889–94.

206 Appleby JI, Gibson G, Normyberski JK, Stubbs RD. Indirect analysis of corticosteroids: The determination of 17-hydroxycorticosteroids. *Biochem J* 1955; 60: 453–60.

207 Raff H, Findling JW. A new immunoradiometric assay for corticotropin evaluated in normal subjects and patients with Cushing's syndrome. *Clin Chem* 1989; 35: 596–600.

208 Gibson S, Crosby SR, White A. Discrimination between beta-endorphin and beta-lipotrophin in human plasma using two-site immunoradiometric assays. *Clin Endocrinol* 1993; 39: 445–53.

209 Linder BL, Esteban NV, Yergey AL, Winterer JC, Loriaux DL, Cassorla F. Cortisol production rate in childhood and adolescence. *J Pediatr* 1990; 117: 892–6.

210 Kerrigan JR, Veldhuis JD, Leyo SA, Iranmanes HA, Rogol AD. Estimation of daily cortisol production and clearance rates in normal pubertal males by deconvolution analysis. *J Clin Endocrinol Metab* 1993; 76: 1505–10.

211 Liddle GW. Tests of pituitary-adrenal suppressibility in the diagnosis of Cushing's syndrome. *J Clin Endocrinol Metab* 1960; 20: 1539–60.

212 Tyrrell JB, Findling JW, Aron DC, Fitzgerald PA, Forsham PH. An overnight high-dose dexamethasone suppression test for rapid differential diagnosis of Cushing's syndrome. *Ann Intern Med* 1986; 104: 180–6.

213 Hindmarsh PC, Brook CG. Single dose dexamethasone suppression test in children: dose relationship to body size. *Clin Endocrinol* 1985; 23: 67–70.

214 Dickstein G, Shechner C, Nicholson WE *et al.* Adrenocorticotropin stimulation test: effects of basal cortisol level, time of day and suggested new sensitive low dose test. *J Clin Endocrinol Metab* 1991; 72: 773–8.

215 Lashansky G, Saenger P, Fishman K *et al.* Normative data for adrenal steroidogenesis in a healthy pediatric population: Age and sex-related changes after ACTH stimulation. *J Clin Endocrinol Metab* 1991; 73: 674–86.

216 Crowley S, Hindmarsh PC, Holownia P, Honour JW, Brook CG. The use of low doses of ACTH in the investigation of adrenal function in man. *J Endocrinol* 1991; 130: 475–9.

217 New MI, Lorenzen F, Lerner AJ *et al.* Genotyping steroid 21-hydroxylase deficiency: Hormonal reference data. *J Clin Endocrinol Metab* 1983; 57: 320–6.

218 Clark AJ, Weber A. Adrenocorticotropin insensitivity syndromes. *Endocr Rev* 1998; 19: 828–43.

219 Shah A, Stanhope R, Matthew D. Hazards of pharmacological tests of growth hormone secretion in childhood. *Br Med J* 1992; 304: 173–4.

220 Avgerinos PC, Yanovski JA, Oldfield EH, Nieman LK, Cutler GB Jr. The metyrapone and dexamethasone suppression tests for the differential diagnosis of the adrenocorticotropin-dependent Cushing syndrome: a comparison. *Ann Intern Med* 1994; 121: 318–27.

221 Spiger M, Jubiz W, Meikle AW, West CD, Tylor FH. Single-dose metyrapone test: review of a four-year experience. *Arch Intern Med* 1975; 135: 698–700.

222 Chrousos GP, Schuermeyer TH, Doppman J, Oldfield EH, Schulte HM, Gold PW, Loriaux DL. NIH conference. Clinical applications of corticotropin-releasing factor. *Ann Intern Med* 1985; 102: 344–58.

223 Riddick L, Chrousos GP, Jeffries S, Pang S. Comparison of adrenocorticotropin and adrenal steroid responses to corticotropin-releasing hormone versus metyrapone testing in patients with hypopituitarism. *Pediatr Res* 1994; 36: 215–20.

224 Sandison AT. A form of lipoidosis of the adrenal cortex in an infant. *Arch Dis Child* 1955; 30: 538–41.

225 Prader A, Siebenmann RE. Nebenniereninsuffizienz bie kongenitaler Lipoidhyperplasie der Nebennieren. *Helv Paed Acta* 1957; 12: 569–95.

226 Kirkland RT, Kirkland JL, Johnson CM, Horning MG, Librik L, Clayton GW. Congenital lipoid adrenal hyperplasia in an eight-year-old phenotypic female. *J Clin Endocrinol Metab* 1973; 36: 488–96.

227 Hauffa BP, Miller WL, Grumbach MM, Conte FA, Kaplan SL. Congenital adrenal hyperplasia due to deficient cholesterol side-chain cleavage activity (20,22 desmolase) in a patient treated for 18 years. *Clin Endocrinol* 1985; 23: 481–93.

228 Camacho AM, Kowarski A, Migeon CJ, Brough A. Congenital adrenal hyperplasia due to a deficiency of one of the enzymes involved in the biosynthesis of pregnenolone. *J Clin Endocrinol Metab* 1968; 28: 153–61.

229 Degenhart HJ, Visser KHA, Boon H, O'Doherty NJD. Evidence for deficiency of 20α cholesterol hydroxylase activity in adrenal tissue of a patient with lipoid adrenal hyperplasia. *Acta Endocrinol* 1972; 71: 512–18.

230 Koizumi S, Kyoya S, Miyawaki T *et al.* Cholesterol side-chain cleavage enzyme activity and cytochrome P450 content in adrenal mitochondria of a patient with congenital lipoid adrenal hyperplasia (Prader disease). *Clin Chim Acta* 1977; 77: 301–6.

231 Matteson KJ, Chung B, Urdea MS, Miller WL. Study of cholesterol side chain cleavage (20,22 desmolase) deficiency causing congenital lipoid adrenal hyperplasia using bovine-sequence P450scc oligodeoxyribonucleotide probes. *Endocrinology* 1986; 118: 1296–1305.

232 Lin D, Gitelman SE, Saenger P, Miller WL. Normal genes for the cholesterol side chain cleavage enzyme, P450scc, in congenital lipoid adrenal hyperplasia. *J Clin Invest* 1991; 88: 1955–62.

233 Lin D, Chang YJ, Strauss JF III, Miller WL. The human peripheral benzodiazepine receptor gene. Cloning and characterization of alternative splicing in normal tissues and in a patient with congenital lipoid adrenal hyperplasia. *Genomics* 1993; 18: 643–50.

234 Tee MK, Lin D, Sugawara T *et al.* T→A transversion 11 bp from a splice acceptor site in the gene for steroidogenic acute regulatory protein causes congenital lipoid adrenal hyperplasia. *Hum Mol Genet* 1995; 4: 2299–305.

235 Miller WL. Congenital lipoid adrenal hyperplasia: the human gene knockout of the steroidogenic acute regulatory protein. *J Mol Endocrinol* 1997; 17: 227–40.

236 Voutilainen R, Miller WL. Developmental expression of genes for the steroidogenic enzymes P450scc (20,22 desmolase), P450c17 (17α-hydroxylase/17,20 lyase) and P450c21 (21-hydroxylase) in the human fetus. *J Clin Endocrinol Metab* 1986; 63: 1145–50.

237 Saenger P, Klonari Z, Black SM *et al.* Prenatal diagnosis of congenital lipoid adrenal hyperplasia. *J Clin Endocrinol Metab* 1995; 80: 200–5.

238 Bose HS, Pescovitz OH, Miller WL. Spontaneous feminization in a 46,XX female patient with congenital lipoid adrenal hyperplasia caused by a homozygous frame-shift mutation in the steroidogenic acute regulatory protein. *J Clin Endocrinol Metab* 1997; 82: 1511–15.

239 Fujieda K, Tajima T, Nakae J *et al.* Spontaneous puberty in 46,XX subjects with congenital lipoid adrenal hypreplasia. *J Clin Invest* 1997; 99: 1265–71.

240 Caron K, Soo S-C, Wetsel W, Stocco D, Clark B, Parker K. Targeted disruption of the mouse gene encoding steroidogenic acute regulatory protein provides insights into congenital lipoid adrenal hyperplasia. *Proc Natl Acad Sci USA* 1997; 94: 11540–5.

241 Nakae J, Tajima T, Sugawara T *et al.* Analysis of the steroidogenic acute regulatory protein (StAR) gene in Japanese patients with congenital lipoid adrenal hyperplasia. *Hum Mol Genet* 1997; 6: 571–6.

242 Yoo H, Kim G. Molecular and clinical characterization of Korean patients with congenital lipoid adrenal hyperplasia. *J Pediatr Endocrinol Metab* 1998; 11: 707–11.

243 Bose HS, Baldwin MA, Miller WL. Incorrect folding of steroidogenic acute regulatory protein (StAR) in congenital lipoid adrenal hyperplasia. *Biochemistry* 1998; 37: 9768–75.

244 Bongiovanni AM, Kellenbenz G. The adrenogenital syndrome with deficiency of 3β-hydroxysteroid dehydrogenase. *J Clin Invest* 1962; 41: 2086–92.

245 Lachance Y, Luu-The V, Verreault H, Dumont M, Leblanc G, Labrie F. Characterization and expression of human type II 3β hydroxysteroid dehydrogenase/Δ5–Δ4 isomerase (3β-HSD) gene, the almost exclusive 3β-HSD species expressed in the adrenals and gonads. *DNA Cell Biol* 1991; 10: 701–11.

246 Rheaume E, Lachance Y, Zhao H *et al.* Structure and expression of a new cDNA encoding the major 3β-hydroxysteroid dehydrogenase/Δ5–Δ4 isomerase. *Mol Endocrinol* 1991; 5: 1147–57.

247 Rheaume E, Simard J, Morel Y *et al.* Congenital adrenal hyperplasia due to point mutations in the type II 3β-hydroxysteroid dehydrogenase gene. *Nature Genet* 1992; 1: 239–45.

248 Chang YT, Kappy MS, Iwamoto K, Wang X, Pang S. Mutations in the type II 3β-hydroxysteroid dehydrogenase gene in a patient with classic salt-wasting 3β-HSD deficiency congential adrenal hyperplasia. *Pediatr Res* 1993; 34: 698–700.

249 Simard J, Rhéaume E, Sanchez R *et al.* Molecular basis of congenital adrenal hyperplasia due to 3β-hydroxysteroid dehydrogenase deficiency. *Mol Endocrinol* 1993; 7: 716–28.

250 Morel Y, Mébarke F, Rhéaume E, Sanchez R, Forest MG, Simard J. Structure–function relationships of 3β-hydroxysteroid dehydrogenase: Contribution made by the molecular genetics of 3β-hydroxysteroid dehydrogenase deficiency. *Steroids* 1997; 62: 176–84.

251 Moisan AM, Ricketts ML, Tardy V *et al.* New insight into the molecular basis of 3β-hydroxysteroid dehydrogenase deficiency: identification of eight mutations in the HSD3B2 gene eleven patients from seven new families and comparison of the functional properties of twenty-five mutant enzymes. *J Clin Endocrinol Metab* 1999; 84: 4410–25.

252 Cara JF, Moshang T Jr, Bongiovanni AM, Marx BS. Elevated 17-hydroxy-progesterone and testosterone in a newborn with 3β-hydroxysteroid dehydrogenase deficiency. *N Engl J Med* 1985; 313: 618–21.

253 Rosenfield RL, Rich BH, Wolfsdorf JI *et al.* Pubertal presentation of congenital Δ5–3β hydroxysteroid dehydrogenase deficiency. *J Clin Endocrinol Metab* 1980; 51: 345–53.

254 Pang S, Levine LS, Stoner E *et al.* Nonsalt-losing congenital adrenal hyperplasia due to 3β-hydroxysteroid dehydrogenase deficiency with normal glomerulosa function. *J Clin Endocrinol Metab* 1983; 56: 808–18.

255 Pang SY, Lerner AJ, Stoner E, Levine LS, Oberfield SE, Engel I, New MI. Late-onset adrenal steroid 3β-hydroxysteroid dehydrogenase deficiency. I. A cause of hirsutism in pubertal and postpubertal women. *J Clin Endocrinol Metab* 1985; 60: 428–39.

256 Chang YT, Zhang L, Alkaddour HS *et al.* Absence of molecular defect in the Type II 3β-hydroxysteroid dehydrogenase (3β-HSD) gene in premature pubarche children and hirsute female patients with moderately decreased adrenal 3β-HSD activity. *Pediatr Res* 1995; 37: 820–4.

257 Sakkal-Alkaddour H, Zhang L, Yang X *et al.* Studies of 3β-hydroxysteroid dehydrogenase genes in infants and children manifesting premature pubarche and increased adrenocorticotropin-stimulated Δ5-steroid levels. *J Clin Endocrinol Metab* 1996; 81: 3961–5.

258 Pang S. The molecular and clinical spectrum of 3β-hydroxysteroid dehydrogenase deficiency disorder. *Trends Endocrinol Metab* 1998; 9: 82–6.

259 Yanase T, Simpson ER, Waterman MR. 17α-hydroxylase/17,20 lyase deficiency: From clinical investigation to molecular definition. *Endocr Rev* 1991; 12: 91–108.

260 Voutilainen R, Tapanainen J, Chung B, Matteson KJ, Miller WL. Hormonal regulation of P450scc (20,22-desmolase) and P450c17 (17α-hydroxylase/17,20-lyase) in cultured human granulosa cells. *J Clin Endocrinol Metab* 1986; 63: 202–7.

261 Scaroni C, Opocher G, Mantero F. Renin-angiotensin-aldosterone system: a long-term follow-up study in 17α–hydroxylase deficiency syndrome. *Hypertension (Clin Exp Theory Pract)* 1986; A8: 773–80.

262 Biglieri EG, Herron MA, Brust N. 17α-Hydroxylation deficiency in man. *J Clin Invest* 1966; 15: 1945–54.

263 New MI, Suvannakul L. Male pseudohermaphroditism due to 17α-hydroxylase deficiency. *J Clin Invest* 1970; 49: 1930–41.

264 Yanase T, Waterman MR, Zachmann M, Winter JSD, Simpson ER, Kagimoto M. Molecular basis of apparent isolated 17,20-lyase deficiency: Compound heterozygous mutations in the C-terminal region (Arg(496)→Cys, Gln(461)→Stop) actually cause combined 17α-hydroxylase/17,20-lyase deficiency. *Biochim Biophys Acta* 1992; 1139: 275–9.

265 Zachmann M, Kenpken B, Manella B, Navarro E. Conversion from pure 17,20 desmolase to combined 17,20-desmolase/17α-hydroxylase deficiency with age. *Acta Endocrinol* 1992; 127: 97–9.

266 Geller DH, Auchus RJ, Mendonça BB, Miller WL. The genetic and functional basis of isolated 17,20 lyase deficiency. *Nature Genet* 1997; 17: 201–5.

267 Geller DH, Auchus RJ, Miller WL. P450c17 mutations R347H and R358Q selectively disrupt 17,20-lyase activity by disrupting interactions with P450 oxidoreductase and cytochrome b5. *Mol Endocrinol* 1999; 13: 167–75.

268 Biason-Lauber A, Leiberman E, Zachmann M. A single amino acid substitution in the putative redox partner-binding site of P450c17 as cause of isolated 17,20 lyase deficiency. *J Clin Endocrinol Metab* 1997; 82: 3807–12.

269 Auchus RJ, Miller WL. Molecular modeling of human P450c17 (17α-hydroxylase/17,20-lyase): Insights into reaction mechanisms and effects of mutations. *Mol Endocrinol* 1999; 13: 1169–82.

270 Lee-Robichaud P, Akhtar ME, Akhtar M. Control of androgen biosynthesis in the human through the interaction of Arg[347] and Arg[358] of CYP17 with cytochrome b5. *Biochem J* 1998; 332: 293–6.

271 Giordano SJ, Kaftory A, Steggles AW. A splicing mutation in the cytochrome b5 gene from a patient with congenital methemoglobinemia and pseudohermaphrodism. *Hum Genet* 1994; 93: 568–70.

272 Miller WL. The congenital adrenal hyperplasias. *Endocrinol Metab Clin N Am* 1991; 20: 721–49.

273 Miller WL. Genetics, diagnosis and management of 21-hydroxylase deficiency. *J Clin Endocrinol Metab* 1994; 78: 241–6.

274 White PC. Genetic diseases of steroid metabolism. *Vitam Horm* 1994; 49: 131–95.

275 Grumbach MM, Conte FA. Disorders of sex differentiation. In: Wilson JD, Foster DW, Kronenberg HM, eds. *William's Textbook of Endocrinology*, 9th edn. Philadelphia, PA: W. B. Saunders, 1998: 1303–425.

276 Solish SB, Goldsmith MA, Voutilainen R, Miller WL. Molecular characterization of a Leydig cell tumour presenting as congenital adrenal hyperplasia. *J Clin Endocrinol Metab* 1989; 69: 1148–52.

277 Dittmann RW, Kappes ME, Kappes MH. Sexual behaviour in adolescent and adult females with congenital adrenal hyperplasia. *Psychoneurodorinology* 1992; 17: 153–70.

278 Mulaikal RM, Migeon CJ, Rock JA. Fertility rates in female patients with congenital adrenal hyperplasia due to 21-hydroxylase deficiency. *N Engl J Med* 1987; 316: 178–82.

279 Kuhnle U, Bollinger M, Schwarz HP, Knorr D. Partnership and sexuality in adult female patients with congenital adrenal hyperplasia. First results of a cross-sectional quality-of-life evaluation. *J Steroid Biochem Mol Biol* 1993; 45: 123–6.

280 Meyer-Bahlburg HFL, Gruen RS, New MI *et al.* Gender change from female to male in classical congenital adrenal hyperplasia. *Horm Behav* 1996; 30: 319–32.

281 Zucker KJ, Bradley SJ, Oliver G, Blake J, Fleming S, Hood J. Psychosexual development of women with congenital adrenal hyperplasia. *Horm Behav* 1996; 30: 300–18.

282 Migeon CJ, Rosenwask Z, Lee PA, Urban MD, Bias WB. The attenuated form of congenital adrenal hyperplasia as an allelic form of 21-hydroxylase deficiency. *J Clin Endocrinol Metab* 1980; 51: 647–9.

283 Chrousos GP, Loriaux DL, Mann DL, Cutler GB. Late-onset 21-hydroxylase deficiency mimicking idiopathic hirsutism or polycystic ovarian disease: An allelic variant of congenital virilizing adrenal hyperplasia with a milder enzymatic defect. *Ann Intern Med* 1982; 96: 143–8.

284 Kohn B, Levine LS, Pollack MS *et al.* Late-onset steroid 21-hydroxylase deficiency: a variant of classical congenital adrenal hyperplasia. *J Clin Endocrinol Metab* 1982; 51: 817–27.

285 Levine LS, Dupont B, Lorenzen F *et al.* Genetic and hormonal characterization of the cryptic 21-hydroxylase deficiency. *J Clin Endocrinol Metab* 1981; 53: 1193–8.

286 Fiet J, Gueux B, Gourmelen M *et al.* Comparison of basal and adrenocorticotropin-stimulated plasma 21-desoxycortisol and 17-hydroprogesterone values as biological markers of late-onset adrenal hyperplasia. *J Clin Endocrinol Metab* 1988; 66: 659–67.

287 Pang S, Wallace MA, Hofman L *et al.* Worldwide experience in newborn screening for classical congenital adrenal hyperplasia due to 21-hydroxylase deficiency. *Pediatrics* 1988; 81: 866–74.

288 Therrell BLJ, Berenbaum SA, Manter-Kapanke V *et al.* Results of screening 1.9 million Texas newborns for 21-hydroxylase-deficient congenital adrenal hyperplasia. *Pediatrics* 1998; 101: 583–90.

289 Speiser PW, Dupont B, Rubinstein P, Piazza A, Kastelan A, New MI. High frequency of nonclassical steroid 21-hydroxylase deficiency. *Am J Hum Genet* 1985; 37: 650–67.

290 Sherman SL, Aston CE, Morton NE, Speiser PW, New MI. A segregation and linkage study of classical and nonclassical 21-hydroxylase deficiency. *Am J Hum Genet* 1988; 42: 830–8.

291 Dumic M, Brkljacic L, Speiser PW *et al.* An update on the frequency of nonclassic deficiency of adrenal 21-hydroxylase in the Yugoslav population. *Acta Endocrinol* 1990; 122: 703–10.

292 Chetkowski RJ, DeFazio J, Shamonki I, Judd HL, Chang RJ. The incidence of the late-onset congenital adrenal hyperplasia due to 21-hydroxylase deficiency among hirsute women. *J Clin Endocrinol Metab* 1984; 58: 595–8.

293 Kuttenn F, Couillin P, Girard F *et al.* Late-onset adrenal hyperplasia in hirsutism. *N Engl J Med* 1985; 313: 222–31.

294 Gourmelen M, Gueux B, Pham-Huu-Trung MT, Fiet J, Raux-Demany MC, Girard F. Detection of heterozygous carriers for 21-hydroxylase deficiency by plasma 21-deoxycortisol measurement. *Acta Endocrinol* 1987; 116: 507–12.

295 Nebert DW, Nelson DR, Coon MJ *et al.* The P450 superfamily: Update on new sequences, gene mapping and recommended nomenclature. *DNA Cell Biol* 1991; 10: 1–14.

296 Carroll MC, Campbell RD, Porter RR. Mapping of steroid 21-hydroxylase genes to complement component C4 genes in HLA, the major histocompatibility locus in man. *Proc Natl Acad Sci USA* 1985; 82: 521–5.

297 White PC, Grossberger D, Onufer BJ *et al.* Two genes encoding steroid 21-hydroxylase are located near the genes encoding the fourth component of complement in man. *Proc Natl Acad Sci USA* 1985; 82: 1089–93.

298 Bristow J, Gitelman SE, Tee MK, Staels B, Miller WL. Abundant adrenal-specific transcription of the human P450c21A 'pseudogene'. *J Biol Chem* 1993; 268: 12919–24.

299 Amor M, Tosi M, Duponchel C, Steinmetz M, Meo T. Liver cDNA probes disclose two cytochrome P450 genes duplicated in tandem with the complement C4 loci of the mouse H-2S region. *Proc Natl Acad Sci USA* 1985; 82: 4453–7.

300 Chung B, Matteson KJ, Miller WL. Cloning and characterization of the bovine gene for steroid 21-hydroxylase (P450c21). *DNA* 1985; 4: 211–19.

301 Skow LE, Womack JE, Petresh JM, Miller WL. Synteny mapping of the genes for steroid 21-hydroxylase, alpha-A-crystalline class I bovine leukocyte antigen (BoLA) in cattle. *DNA* 1988; 7: 143–9.

302 Parker KL, Chaplin DD, Wong M, Seidman JG, Smith JA, Schimmer BP. Expression of murine 21-hydroxylase in mouse adrenal glands and in transfected Y1 adrenocortical tumour cells. *Proc Natl Acad Sci USA* 1985; 82: 7860–4.

303 Chaplin DD, Galbraith LJ, Seidman JG, White PC, Parker KL. Nucleotide sequence analysis of murine 21-hydroxylase genes: mutations affecting gene expression. *Proc Natl Acad Sci USA* 1986; 83: 9601–5.

304 John ME, Okamura T, Dee A *et al.* Bovine steroid 21-hydroxylase: Regulation of biosynthesis. *Biochemistry* 1986; 25: 2846–53.

305 Gitelman SE, Bristow J, Miller WL. Mechanism and consequences of the duplication of the human C4/P450c21/Gene X locus. *Mol Cell Biol* 1992; 12: 2124–34.

306 Geffrotin C, Chardon P, DeAndres-Cara DR, Feil R, Renard C, Vaiman M. The swine steroid 21-hydroxylase gene (CYP21): Cloning and mapping within the swine leukocyte antigen locus. *Anim Genet* 1990; 21: 1–13.

307 Partanen J, Koskimies S, Sipila I, Lipsanen V. Major histocompatibility-complex gene markers and restriction fragment analysis of steroid 21-hydroxylase (CYP21) and complement C4 genes in classical adrenal hyperplasia patients in a single population. *Am J Hum Genet* 1989; 44: 660–70.

308 Dupont B, Pollack MS, Levine LS, O'Neill GJ, Hawkins BR, New MI. Congenital adrenal hyperplasia: Joint report from the eight international histocompatibility workshop. In: Terasaki PI, ed. *Histocompatibility Testing 1980*. Berlin: Springer Verlag, 1981: 693–706.

309 Fleischnick E, Awdeh ZL, Raum D *et al*. Extended MHC haplotypes in 21-hydroxylase deficiency congenital adrenal hyperplasia: Shared genotypes in unrelated patients. *Lancet* 1983; i: 152–6.

310 Holler W, Scholz S, Knorr D, Bidlingmaier F, Keller E, Ekkehard DA. Genetic differences in the salt-wasting, simple virilizing and nonclassical types of congenital adrenal hyperplasia. *J Clin Endocrinol Metab* 1985; 60: 757–63.

311 Pollack MS, Levine LS, O'Neill GL. HLA linkage and B14, DR1, BfS haplotype association with the genes for late onset and cryptic 21-hydroxylase deficiency. *Am J Hum Genet* 1981; 33: 540–50.

312 Speiser PW, New MI, White P. Molecular genetic analysis of nonclassical steroid 21-hydroxylase deficiency associated with HLA-B14DR1. *N Engl J Med* 1988; 319: 19–23.

313 Morel Y, Andre J, Uring-Lambert B, Hauptman G *et al*. Rearrangements and point mutations of P450c21 genes are distinguished by five restriction endonuclease haplotypes identified by a new probing strategy in 57 families with congenital adrenal hyperplasia. *J Clin Invest* 1989; 83: 527–36.

314 Rosenbloom NR, Smith DW. Varying expression for salt-losing in related patients with congenital adrenal hyperplasia. *Pediatrics* 1966; 38: 215–19.

315 Stoner E, DiMartina J, Kuhnle U, Levine LS, Oberfield SE, New M. Is salt-wasting in congenital adrenal hyperplasia genetic? *Clin Endocrinol* 1986; 24: 9–20.

316 Morel Y, David M, Forest MG *et al*. Gene conversions and rearrangements cause discordance between inheritance of forms of 21-hydroxylase deficiency and HLA types. *J Clin Endocrinol Metab* 1989; 68: 592–9.

317 Sinnott PJ, Dyer PA, Price DA, Harris R, Strachan T. 21-hydroxylase deficiency families with HLA identical affected and unaffected sibs. *J Med Genet* 1989; 26: 10–17.

318 Isenman DE, Young JR. The molecular basis for the difference in immune hemolysis activity of the Chido and Rodgers isotypes of human complement component C4. *J Immunol* 1984; 132: 3019–27.

319 Law SKA, Dodds AW, Porter RR. A comparison of the properties of two classes, C4A and C4B, of the human complement component C4. *EMBO J* 1984; 3: 1819–23.

320 Carroll MC, Campbell RD, Bentley DR, Porter RR. A molecular map of the human major histocompatibility class III region lining complement genes C4, C2 and factor B. *Nature* 1984; 307: 237–41.

321 Yu CY, Belt KT, Giles CM, Campbell RD, Porter RR. Structural basis of the polymorphism of the human complement components C4A and C4B: gene size, reactivity and antigenicity. *EMBO J* 1986; 5: 2873–81.

322 Wijesuriya S, Zhang G, Dardis A, Miller WL. Transcriptional regulatory elements of the human gene for cytochrome P450c21 (steroid 21-hydroxylase) lie within intron 35 of the linked C4B gene. *J Biol Chem* 1999; 274: 38097–106.

323 Tee MK, Babalola GO, Aza-Blanc P, Speek M, Gitelman SE, Miller WL. A promoter within intron 35 of the human C4A gene initiates adrenal-specific transcription of a 1kb RNA. Location of a cryptic CYP21 promoter element? *Hum Mol Genet* 1995; 4: 2109–16.

324 Lévi-Strauss M, Carroll MC, Steinmetz M, Meo T. A previously undetected MHC gene with an unusual periodic structure. *Science* 1988; 240: 201–4.

325 Speiser PW, White PC. Structure of the human RD gene: a highly conserved gene in the class III region of the major histocompatibility. *DNA* 1989; 8: 745–51.

326 Sargent CA, Dunham I, Campbell RC. Identification of multiple HTF-island associated genes in the major histocompatibility complex class III region. *EMBO J* 1989; 8: 2305–12.

327 Morel Y, Bristow J, Gitelman SE, Miller WL. Transcript encoded on the opposite strand of the human steroid 21-hydroxylase/complement component/C4 gene locus. *Proc Natl Acad Sci USA* 1989; 86: 6582–6.

328 Bristow J, Tee MK, Gitelman SE, Mellon SH, Miller WL, Tenascin X. A novel extracellular matrix protein encoded by the human XB gene overlapping P450c21B. *J Cell Biol* 1993; 122: 265–78.

329 Burch GH, Bedolli MA, McDonough S, Rosenthal SM, Bristow J. Embryonic expression of tenascin-X suggests a role in limb, muscle and heart development. *Dev Dynamics* 1995; 203: 491–504.

330 Speek M, Barry F, Miller WL. Alternate promoters and alternate splicing of human tenascin-X, a gene with 5' and 3' ends buried in other genes. *Hum Mol Genet* 1996; 5: 1749–58.

331 Tee MK, Thomson AA, Bristow J, Miller WL. Sequences promoting the transcription of the human XA gene overlapping P450c21A correctly predict the presence of a novel, adrenal-specific, truncated form of Tenascin-X. *Genomics* 1995; 28: 171–8.

332 Burch GH, Gong Y, Liu W *et al*. Tenascin-X deficiency is associated with Ehlers–Danlos syndrome. *Nature Genet* 1997; 17: 104–8.

333 Elefteriou F, Exposito J, Garrone R, Lethias C. Characterization of the bovine Tenascin-X. *J Biol Chem* 1997; 272: 22866–74.

334 Speek M, Miller WL. Hybridization of complementary mRNAs for (P450c21 steroid 21-hydroxylase) and Tenascin-X is prevented by sequence-specific binding of nuclear proteins. *Mol Endocrinol* 1995; 9: 1655–65.

335 White PC, Tusie-Luna MT, New MI, Speiser PW. Mutations in steroid 21-hydroxylase (CYP21). *Hum Mutat* 1994; 3: 373–8.

336 Matteson KJ, Phillips JA III, Miller WL *et al*. P450XXI (steroid 21-hydroxylase) gene deletions are not found in family studies of congenital adrenal hyperplasia. *Proc Natl Acad Sci USA* 1987; 84: 5858–62.

337 Miller WL. Gene conversions, deletions and polymorphisms in congenital adrenal hyperplasia. *Am J Hum Genet* 1988; 42: 4–7.

338 Donohoue PA, Neto RS, Collins MM, Migeon CJ. Exon 7 Nco I restriction site within CYP21B (steroid 21-hydroxylase) is a normal polymorphism. *Mol Endocrinol* 1990; 4: 1354–62.

339 Higashi Y, Hiromasa T, Tanae A *et al*. Effects of individual mutations in the P-450 ($C_{21}$) pseudogene on P-450 ($C_{21}$) activity and their distribution in patient genomes of congenital steroid 21-hydroxylase deficiency. *J Biochem* 1991; 109: 638–44.

340 Chiou SH, Hu MC, Chung B-C. A missense mutation of Ile$^{172}$→Asn or Arg$^{356}$→Trp causes steroid 21-hydroxylase deficiency. *J Biol Chem* 1990; 256: 3549–52.

341 Wedell A, Ritzen E, Haglund-Stengler B, Luthman H. Steroid 21-hydroxylase deficiency: Three additional mutated alleles and establishment of phenotype–genotype relationships of common mutations. *Proc Natl Acad Sci USA* 1992; 89: 7232–6.

342 Wedell A, Luthman H. Steroid 21-hydroxylase (P450c21): a new allele and spread of mutations through the pseudogene. *Hum Mol Genet* 1993; 91: 236–40.

343 Wedell A, Luthman H. Steroid 21-hydroxylase deficiency: Two additional mutations in salt-wasting disease and rapid screening of disease-causing mutations. *Hum Mol Genet* 1993; 2: 499–504.

344 Amor M, Parker KL, Globerman H, New MI, White PC. Mutation in the *CYP21B* gene (Ile-172-Asn) causes steroid 21-hydroxylase deficiency. *Proc Natl Acad Sci USA* 1988; 85: 1600–4.

345 Urabe K, Kimura A, Harada F, Iwanage T, Sasazuki T. Gene conversion in steroid 21-hydroxylase genes. *Am J Hum Genet* 1990; 46: 1178–86.

346 Hu MC, Chung B-C. Expression of human 21-hydroxylase (P450c21) in bacterial and mammalian cell – A system to characterize normal and mutant enzymes. *Mol Endocrinol* 1990; 4: 893–8.

347 Wu DA, Chung B. Mutations of P450c21 (steroid 21-hydroxylase) at Cys$^{428}$, Val$^{281}$, or Ser$^{268}$ result in complete, partial, or no loss of enzymatic activity. *J Clin Invest* 1991; 88: 519–23.

348 Helmburg A, Tusie-Luna M, Tabarelli M, Kofler R, White PC. R339H and P453S: CYP21 mutations associated with nonclassic steroid 21-hydroxylase deficiency that are not apparent gene conversion. *Mol Endocrinol* 1992; 6: 1318–22.

349 Owerbach D, Sherman L, Ballard AL, Azziz R. Pro453 to Ser mutation in CYP21 is associated with non-classic steroid 21-hydroxylase deficiency. *Mol Endocrinol* 1992; 6: 1211–15.

350 Hsu L, Hu M, Cheng H, Lu J, Chung B. The N-terminal hydrophobic domain of P450c21 is required for membrane insertion and enzyme stability. *J Biol Chem* 1993; 268: 14682.

351 Seckl JR, Miller WL. How safe is long-term prenatal glucocorticoid treatment? *J Am Med Assoc* 1997; 277: 1077–9.

352 Miller WL. Prenatal treatment of congenital adrenal hyperplasia – A promising experimental therapy of unproven safety. *Trends Endocrinol Metab* 1998; 9: 290–3.

353 Ritzen EM. Prenatal treatment of congenital adrenal hyperplasia: a commentary. *Trends Endocrinol Metab* 1998; 9: 293–5.

354 Miller WL. Dexamethasone treatment of congenital adrenal hyperplasia – an experimental therapy of unproven safety. *J Urol* 1999; 162: 537–40.

355 Forest MG, Bétuel H, Couillin P, Boué A. Prenatal diagnosis of congenital adrenal hyperplasia (CAH) due to 21-hydroxylase deficiency by steroid analysis in the amniotic fluid of mid-pregnancy: comparison with HLA typing in 17 pregnancies at risk for CAH. *Prenatal Diagnosis* 1981; 1: 197–207.

356 Forest MG, Bétuel H, David M. Prenatal treatment in congenital adrenal hyperplasia due to 21-hydroxylase deficiency: update 88 of the French multicentric study. *Endocr Res* 1989; 15: 277–301.

357 Pang SY, Clark A. Newborn screening, prenatal diagnosis and prenatal treatment of congenital adrenal hyperplasia due to 21-hydroxylase deficiency. *Trends Endocrinol Metab* 1990; 1: 300–7.

358 Pang S, Levine LS, Cederqvist LL *et al.* Amniotic fluid concentrations of $\Delta^5$ and $\Delta^4$ steroids in fetuses with congenital adrenal hyperplasia due to 21-hydroxylase deficiency and in anencephalic fetuses. *J Clin Endocrinol Metab* 1980; 51: 223–9.

359 Pang S, Pollack MS, Loo M *et al.* Pitfalls of prenatal diagnosis of 21-hydroxylase deficiency congenital adrenal hyperplasia. *J Clin Endocrinol Metab* 1985; 61: 89–97.

360 Hughes IA, Dyas J, Riad-Fahmy D, Laurence KM. Prenatal diagnosis of congenital adrenal hyperplasia: reliability of amniotic fluid steroid analysis. *J Med Genet* 1987; 24: 344–7.

361 Forest MG, David M, Morel Y. Prenatal diagnosis and treatment of 21-hydroxylase deficiency. *J Steroid Biochem Mol Biol* 1993; 45: 75–82.

362 Speiser PW, New MI. Prenatal diagnosis and management of congenital adrenal hyperplasia. *Clin Perinatol* 1994; 21: 631–45.

363 Mercado AB, Wilson RC, Cheng KC, Wei JQ, New MI. Prenatal treatment and diagnosis of congenital adrenal hyperlasia owing to 21-hydroxylase deficiency. *J Clin Endocrinol Metab* 1995; 80: 2014–20.

364 Forest MG, Morel Y, David M. Prenatal treatment of congenital adrenal hyperplasia. *Trends Endocrinol Metab* 1998; 9: 284–9.

365 Lajic S, Wedell A, Bui T-H, Ritzen E, Holst M. Long-term somatic follow-up of prenatally treated children with congenital adrenal hyperplasia. *J Clin Endocrinol Metab* 1998; 83: 3872–80.

366 Migeon C. Comments about the need for prenatal treatment of congenital adrenal hyperplasia due to 21-hydroxylase deficiency. *J Clin Endocrinol Metab* 1990; 70: 836.

367 Pang S, Pollack MS, Marshall RN, Immken LD. Prenatal treatment of congenital adrenal hyperplasia due to 21-hydroxylase deficiency. *N Engl J Med* 1990; 322: 111–15.

368 Speiser PW, Laforgia N, Kato K *et al.* First trimester prenatal treatment and molecular genetic diagnosis of congenital adrenal hyperplasia (21-hydroxylase deficiency). *J Clin Endocrinol Metab* 1990; 70: 838–48.

369 Benediktsson R, Lindsay R, Noble J, Seckl JR, Edwards CRW. Glucocorticoid exposure *in utero*: a new model for adult hypertension. *Lancet* 1993; 341: 339–41.

370 Wolkowitz OM. Prospective controlled studies of the behavioural and biological effects of exogenous corticosteroids. *Psychoneuroendocrinology* 1994; 19: 233–55.

371 Trautman PD, Meyer-Bahlburg HFL, Postelnek J, New MI. Effects of early prenatal dexamethasone on the cognitive and behavioural development of young children: Results of a pilot study. *Psychoneuroendocrinology* 1995; 20: 439–49.

372 Seeman TE, McEwen BS, Singer BH, Albert MS, Rowe JW. Increase in urinary cortisol excretion and memory declines: MacArthur studies on successful aging. *J Clin Endocrinol Metab* 1997; 82: 2458–65.

373 Kalmijn S, Launer LJ, Stolk RP *et al.* A prospective study on cortisol, dehydroepiandrosterone sulphate and cognitive function in the elderly. *J Clin Endocrinol Metab* 1998; 83: 3487–92.

374 Laue L, Cutler GJ. 21-Hydroxylase deficiency: Overview of treatment. *Endocrinologist* 1992; 2: 291.

375 Kenny FM, Preeyasombat C, Migeon CJ. Cortisol production rate; II. Normal infants, children and adults. *Pediatrics* 1966; 37: 34–42.

376 Kenny F, Taylor F, Richards C. Reference standards for cortisol production and 17-hydroxy corticosteroid excretion during growth: Variation in the pattern of excretion of radiolabeled cortisol metabolites. *Metabolism* 1970; 19: 280–90.

377 Peterson KE. The production of cortisol and corticosterone in children. *Acta Paediatr Scand Suppl* 1980; 281: 2–38.

378 Styne DM, Richards GE, Bell JJ *et al.* Growth patterns in congenital adrenal hyperplasia – correlation of glucocorticoid therapy with stature. In: Lee P, Plotnick L, Kowarski A, Migeon C, eds. *Congenital Adrenal Hyperplasia*. Baltimore: University Park Press, 1977: 247–61.

379 Zachmann M, Tassinari D, Prader A. Clinical and biochemical variability in congenital adrenal hyperplasia due to 11β-hydroxylase deficiency. *J Clin Endocrinol Metab* 1983; 56: 222–9.

380 Holcombe JH, Keenan BS, Nichols BL, Kirkland RT, Clayton GW. Neonatal salt loss in the hypertensive form of congenital adrenal hyperplasia. *Pediatrics* 1980; 65: 777–81.

381 Sonino N, Levine LS, Vecsci P, New MI. Parallelism of 11- and 18-hydroxylation demonstrated by urinary free hormones in man. *J Clin Endocrinol Metab* 1980; 51: 557–60.

382 Azziz R, Boots LR, Parker CR Jr, Bradley E Jr, Zacur HA. 11β-hydroxylase deficiency in hyperandrogenism. *Fertil Steril* 1991; 55: 733–41.

383 Joehrer K, Geley S, Stasser-Wozak E *et al.* CYP11B1 mutations causing non-classic adrenal hyperplasia due to 11β-hydroxylase deficiency. *Hum Mol Genet* 1997; 6: 1829–34.

384 Rösler A. The natural history of salt-wasting disorders of adrenal and renal origin. *J Clin Endocrinol Metab* 1984; 59: 689–700.

385 Mitsuuchi Y, Kawamoto T, Miyahara K *et al.* Congenitally defective aldosterone biosynthesis in the humans: Inactivation of the P-450c18 gene (CYP11B2) due to nucleotide deletion in CMO I deficient patients. *Biochem Biophys Res Commun* 1993; 190: 864–9.

386 Peter M, Fawaz L, Drop S, Visser H, Sippell W. Hereditary defect in biosynthesis of aldosterone: aldosterone synthase deficiency 1964–97. *J Clin Endocrinol Metab* 1997; 82: 3525–8.

387 Geley S, Jöhrer K, Peter M *et al.* Amino acid substitution R384P in aldosterone synthase causes corticosterone methyloxidase type I deficiency. *J Clin Endocrinol Metab* 1995; 80: 424–9.

388 Portrat-Doyen S, Tourniaire J, Richard O *et al.* Isolated aldosterone synthase deficiency caused by simultaneous E198D and V386A mutations in the CYP11B2 gene. *J Clin Endocrinol Metab* 1998; 83: 4156–61.

389 Fardella CE, Rodriguez H, Montero J *et al.* Genetic variation in P450c11AS in Chilean patients with low renin hypertension. *J Clin Endocrinol Metab* 1996; 81: 4347–51.

390 Zhang G, Miller WL. The human genome contains only two CYP11B (P450c11) genes. *J Clin Endocrinol Metab* 1996; 81: 3254–6.

391 Fardella CE, Hum DW, Rodriguez H *et al.* Gene conversion in the CYP11B2 gene encoding aldosterone synthase (P450c11AS) is associated with, but does not cause, the syndrome of corticosterone methyl oxidase II deficiency. *J Clin Endocrinol Metab* 1996; 81: 321–6.

392 Lifton R, Dluhy RG, Powers M *et al.* A chimaeric 11β-hydroxylase/aldosterone synthase gene causes glucocorticoid-remediable aldosteronism and human hypertension. *Nature* 1992; 335: 262–5.

393 Pascoe L, Curnow K, Slutsker L *et al.* Glucocorticoid-suppressible hyperaldosteronism results from hybrid genes created by unequal crossover between CYP11B1 and CYP11B2. *Proc Natl Acad Sci USA* 1992; 89: 8327–31.

394 Dluhy RG, Lifton RP. Glucocorticoid-remediable aldosteronism. *J Clin Endocrinol Metab* 1999; 84: 4341–4.

395 Curnow KM, Mulatero P, Emeric-Blanchouin N, Aupetit-Faisant B, Corvol P, Pascoe L. The amino acid substitutions Ser288Gly and Val320Ala convert the cortisol producing enzyme, CYP11B1, into an aldosterone producing enzyme. *Nature Struct Biol* 1997; 4: 32–5.

396 Fardella CE, Rodriguez H, Hum DW, Mellon SH, Miller WL. Artificial mutations in P450c11AS (aldosterone synthase) can increase enzymatic activity: a model for low-renin hypertension? *J Clin Endocrinol Metab* 1995; 80: 1040–3.

397 Mulatero P, Curnow KM, Aupetit-Faisant B *et al.* Recombinant CYP11B genes encode enzymes that can catalyze conversion of 11-deoxycortisol to cortisol, 18-hydroxycortisoland 18-oxocortisol. *J Clin Endocrinol Metab* 1998; 83: 3996–4001.

398 Takeda Y, Furukawa K, Inaba S, Miyamori I, Mabuchi H. Genetic analysis of aldosterone synthase in patients with idiopathic hyperaldosteronism. *J Clin Endocrinol Metab* 1999; 84: 1633–7.

399 Spinner MW, Blizzard RM, Childs B. Clinical and genetic heterogeneity in idiopathic Addison's disease and hypoparathyroidism. *J Clin Endocrinol Metab* 1968; 28: 795–804.

400 Uibo R, Aavik E, Peterson P *et al.* Autoantibodies to cytochrome P450 enzymes P450scc, P450c17 and P450c21 in autoimmune polyglandular disease types I and II and in isolated Addison's disease. *J Clin Endocrinol Metab* 1994; 78: 323–8.

401 Colls J, Betterle C, Volpato M, Prentice L, Smith BR, Furmaniak J. Immunoprecipitation assay for autoantibodies to steroid 21-hydroxylase in autoimmune adrenal diseases. *Clin Chem* 1995; 41: 375–80.

402 Ahonen P, Myllarniemi S, Sipila I, Perheentupa J. Clinical variation of autoimmune polyendocrinopathy-candidiasis- ectodermal dystrophy (APECED) in a series of 68 patients. *N Engl J Med* 1990; 322: 1829–36.

403 Neufeld M, Maclaren NK, Blizzard RM. Two types of autoimmune Addison's disease associated with different polyglandular autoimmune (PGA) syndromes. *Medicine* 1981; 60: 355–62.

404 Maclaren NK, Riley WJ. Inherited susceptibility to autoimmune Addison's disease is linked to human leukocyte antigens-DR3 and/or DR4, except when associated with type I autoimmune polyglandular syndrome. *J Clin Endocrinol Metab* 1986; 62: 455–9.

405 Ligtenberg MJ, Kemp S, Sarde CO *et al.* Spectrum of mutations in the gene encoding the adrenoleukodystrophy protein. *Am J Hum Genet* 1995; 56: 44–50.

406 Watkins PA, Gould SJ, Smith MA *et al.* Altered expression of ALDP in X-linked adrenoleukodystrophy. *Am J Hum Genet* 1995; 57: 292–301.

407 Watkins PA, Naidu S, Moser HW. Adrenoleukodystrophy: biochemical procedures in diagnosis, prevention and treatment. *J Inherit Metab Dis* 1987; 10: 46–53.

408 Moser HW, MoSeries AE, Singh I, O'Neill BP. Adrenoleukodystrophy: survey of 303 cases: biochemistry, diagnosis and therapy. *Ann Neurol* 1984; 16: 628–41.

409 Moser HW. Adrenoleukodystrophy. *Curr Opin Neurol* 1995; 8: 221–6.

410 Sadeghi-Nejad A, Senior B. Adrenomyeloneuropathy presenting as Addison's disease in childhood. *N Engl J Med* 1990; 322: 13–16.

411 Schmitz G, Assman G. Acid lipase deficiency: Wolman's disease and cholesteryl ester storage disease. In: Scirer C, Beaudet A, Sly W, Valle D, eds. *The Metabolic Basis of Inherited Disease*. New York: McGraw-Hill, 1989: 1623–44.

412 Anderson RA, Byrum RS, Coates PM, Sando GN. Mutations at the lysosomal acid cholesteryl ester hydrolase gene locus in Wolman disease. *Proc Natl Acad Sci USA* 1994; 91: 2718–22.

413 Weber A, Clark AJ. Mutations of the ACTH receptor gene are only one cause of familial glucocorticoid deficiency. *Hum Mol Genet* 1994; 3: 585–8.

414 Allgrove J, Clayden GS, Grant DB, Macaulay JC. Familial glucocorticoid deficiency with achalasia of the cardia and deficient tear production. *Lancet* 1978; 1: 1284–6.

415 Grant DB, Barnes ND, Dumic M *et al.* Neurological and adrenal dysfunction in the adrenal insufficiency/alacrima/achalasia (3A) syndrome. *Arch Dis Child* 1993; 68: 779–82.

416 Zanaria E, Muscatelli F, Bardoni B *et al.* An unusual member of the nuclear hormone receptor superfamily responsible for X-linked adrenal hypoplasia congenita. *Nature* 1994; 372: 635–41.

417 Burris TP, Guo W, McCabe ER. The gene responsible for adrenal hypoplasia congenita, DAX-1, encodes a nuclear hormone receptor that defines a new class within the superfamily. *Recent Prog Horm Res* 1996; 51: 241–59.

418 Black J, Williams DI. Natural history of adrenal haemorrhage in the newborn. *Arch Dis Child* 1973; 48: 183–90.

419 Dahlberg PJ, Goellner MH, Pehling GB. Adrenal insufficiency secondary to adrenal hemorrhage. Two case reports and a review of cases confirmed by computed tomography. *Arch Intern Med* 1990; 150: 905–9.

420 Thomsett MJ, Conte FA, Kaplan SL, Grumbach MM. Endocrine and neurologic outcome in childhood craniopharyngioma: Review of effect of treatment in 42 patients. *J Pediatr* 1980; 97: 728–35.

421 Sklar CA, Grumbach MM, Kaplan SL, Conte FA. Hormonal and metabolic abnormalities associated with central nervous system germinoma in children and adolescents and the effect of therapy: report of 10 patients. *J Clin Endocrinol Metab* 1981; 52: 9–16.

422 Carpenter PC. Diagnostic evaluation of Cushing's syndrome. *Endocrinol Metab Clin North Am* 1988; 17: 445–72.

423 McArthur RG, Cloutier MD, Hayles AB, Sprague RG. Cushing's disease in children. Findings in 13 cases. *Mayo Clin Proc* 1972; 47: 318–26.

424 Miller WL, Townsend JJ, Grumbach MM, Kaplan SL. An infant with Cushing's disease due to an adrenocorticotropin-producing pituitary adenoma. *J Clin Endocrinol Metab* 1979; 48: 1017–25.

425 Devoe DJ, Miller WL, Conte FA *et al.* Long-term outcome of children and adolescents following transsphenoidal surgery for Cushing Disease. *J Clin Endocrinol Metab* 1997; 82: 3196–202.

426 Tyrrell JB, Brooks RM, Fitzgerald PA, Cofoid PB, Forsham PH, Wilson CB. Cushing's disease. Selective trans-sphenoidal resection of pituitary microadenomas. *N Engl J Med* 1978; 298: 753–8.

427 Hermus AR, Smals AG, Swinkels LM *et al.* Bone mineral density and bone turnover before and after surgical cure of Cushing's syndrome. *J Clin Endocrinol Metab* 1995; 80: 2859–65.

428 Boggan JE, Tyrrell JB, Wilson CB. Transsphenoidal microsurgical management of Cushing's disease. Report of 100 cases. *J Neurosurg* 1983; 59: 195–200.

429 Miller WL, Johnson LK. Synthesis and glycosylation of proopiomelanocortin in a Cushing tumour. *J Clin Endocrinol Metab* 1982; 55: 441–6.

430 Magiakou MA, Mastorakos G, Oldfield EH *et al.* Cushing's syndrome in children and adolescents. Presentation, diagnosis and therapy. *N Engl J Med* 1994; 331: 629–36.

431 Leinung MC, Kane LA, Scheithauer BW, Carpenter PC, Laws ER Jr, Zimmerman D. Long term follow-up of transsphenoidal surgery for the treatment of Cushing's disease in childhood. *J Clin Endocrinol Metab* 1995; 80: 2475–9.

432 Magiakou MA, Mastorakos G, Chrousos GP. Final stature in patients with endogenous Cushing's syndrome. *J Clin Endocrinol Metab* 1994; 79: 1082–5.

433 Styne DM, Isaac R, Miller WL *et al.* Endocrine, histological and biochemical studies of adrenocorticotropin-producing islet cell carcinoma of the pancreas in childhood with characterization of proopiomelanocortin. *J Clin Endocrinol Metab* 1983; 57: 723–31.

434 Loridan L, Senior B. Cushing's syndrome in infancy. *J Pediatr* 1969; 75: 349–59.

435 Gilbert MG, Cleveland WW. Cushing's syndrome in infancy. *Pediatrics* 1970; 46: 217–29.

436 Perry RR, Nieman LK, Cutler GB Jr *et al.* Primary adrenal causes of Cushing's syndrome. Diagnosis and surgical management. *Ann Surg* 1989; 210: 59–68.

437 Jabbar A, Grant D, Savage M, Grossman A. Primary pigmented nodular adrenocortical dysplasia: a rare form of a rare disorder. *J R Soc Med* 1994; 87: 110–11.

438 Young WF Jr, Carney JA, Musa BU, Wulffraat NM, Lens JW, Drexhage HA. Familial Cushing's syndrome due to primary pigmented nodular adrenocortical disease. Reinvestigation 50 years later. *N Engl J Med* 1989; 321: 1659–64.

439 Stratakis CA, Jenkins RB, Pras E *et al.* Cytogenetic and microsatellite alterations in tumours from patients with the syndrome of myxomas, spotty skin pigmentation and endocrine overactivity (Carney complex). *J Clin Endocrinol Metab* 1996; 81: 3607–14.

440 Stratakis CA, Carney JA, Lin JP *et al.* Carney complex, a familial multiple neoplasia and lentiginosis syndrome. Analysis of 11 kindreds and linkage to the short arm of chromosome 2. *J Clin Invest* 1996; 97: 699–705.

441 Costin G, Goebelsmann U, Kogut MD. Sexual precocity due to a testosterone-producing adrenal tumour. *J Clin Endocrinol Metab* 1977; 45: 912–19.

442 Tyrrell JB. Glucocorticoid therapy. In: Felig P, Baxter JD, Frohman LA, eds. *Endocrinology and Metabolism.* New York: McGraw-Hill, 1995: 855–82.

443 Mellon SH. Neurosteroids: Biochemistry, modes of action and clinical relevance. *J Clin Endocrinol Metab* 1994; 78: 1003–8.

444 Streck WF, Lockwood DH. Pituitary adrenal recovery following short-term suppression with corticosteroids. *Am J Med* 1979; 66: 910–14.

# 22 Calcium and bone metabolism

## D. A. Heath and N. J. Shaw

## Regulation of calcium and bone metabolism

The control of calcium and bone metabolism is intimately linked, although many calcium disorders do not lead to obvious bone diseases, or vice versa. Ionized calcium is essential for the majority of physiological responses, e.g. nerve conduction, muscle contraction, blood clotting. Despite this, the changes in ionized calcium seen in health and disease are rarely sufficient to cause major disturbances in these essential functions.

Serum calcium is present in blood in three forms: the physiologically important ionized calcium, protein-bound and complexed calcium. The three together are measured as the total calcium, which remains the simplest automated method available for routine use. The normal total serum calcium is 2.2–2.6 mmol/L (8.8–10.4 mg/dL). Complexed calcium (bound to citrate, sulphate, etc.) is virtually never a significant or highly variable component and can effectively be ignored, unless, for example, citrate is being infused. Protein-bound calcium can vary significantly, with most of the calcium being bound to albumin. It normally represents about half of the total calcium.

Provided the serum albumin or serum total proteins are within normal limits, the serum total calcium is an accurate indicator of the ionized calcium. Any change of the protein fractions, however, makes the total calcium a less accurate predictor of the ionized calcium. For this reason, all measurements of total calcium should automatically be associated with a measurement of serum albumin or total protein to allow interpretation of the result. Increases in serum albumin are never due to true increased albumin production but occur in dehydration or prolonged venous stasis. Decreases in serum albumin are common in a variety of acute and chronic disorders. Increases in globulins are common in many disorders but rarely affect the total calcium significantly because of their low avidity for calcium. Numerous correction factors have been reported to 'correct' the total calcium for protein changes. These factors become unreliable once the protein change becomes marked and are best avoided.

In the vast majority of cases, serum calcium measurements do not require the fasting state and, provided venous occlusion is not maintained for a prolonged period, can be taken in the normal way, using a cuff. Any significant effect of the cuff will be immediately apparent by an elevated serum albumin or total protein.

## Regulation of calcium homeostasis

The aim is to maintain an accurately controlled serum ionized calcium and, at the same time, achieve long-term skeletal integrity. In order to regulate the serum calcium on a short-term basis, there has to be the ability to modify the flux of calcium to and from the intestine, bone and kidney. During growth and development, serum calcium has to be maintained while at the same time allowing long-term positive skeletal calcium balance, without which a normal adult bone mass would not be achieved. In other words, until adult bone mass is achieved, overall bone formation must exceed bone resorption. There will be occasions essential for the maintenance of calcium homeostasis when bone resorption exceeds bone formation in the short term; if such a situation were maintained for a prolonged period of time, this would have severe implications for the skeleton.

The maintenance of calcium homeostasis in a way that can respond to acute pertubations as well as long-term stimuli requires sophisticated mechanisms that are only partially understood. Fundamental to the system are a series of hormonal factors, together with a mechanism whereby the two major bone cells, the bone-forming osteoblast and the bone-resorbing osteoclast, are linked so that the activity of the one almost invariably affects the activity of the other. This means that a primary increase in osteoclastic bone resorption is almost always followed by an increase in osteoblastic bone formation. This dialogue occurs through a series of autocrine and paracrine mechanisms.

## Parathyroid hormone

Parathyroid hormone (PTH) is secreted by the four parathyroid glands situated in the neck, behind the thyroid gland. The lower glands are derived from the third brancheal pouch, and the upper glands are derived from the fourth. Developmental disorders of the third and fourth brancheal pouches may be associated with congenital hypoparathyroidism (di George syndrome). PTH is synthesized initially as prepro-PTH, which is then cleaved to pro-PTH and then to mature PTH, which is secreted by the chief cells of the parathyroid gland (Fig. 22.1).

Prepro-PTH is produced by the ribosome [1]. The 25-amino-acid 'pre' sequence serves as a signal sequence that transports the peptide through the rough endoplasmic reticulum. The 'pre' sequence is then cleaved, leaving pro-PTH, which travels to the Golgi apparatus where the 6-amino-acid 'pro' sequence is removed, leaving the intact 84-amino-acid hormone [2]. PTH is concentrated in secretory vesicles that fuse with the plasma membrane before release in response to a fall in extracellular calcium. The parathyroid glands do not have large stores of PTH but are able to synthesize hormone rapidly in response to the appropriate stimuli. Of the 84 amino acids constituting the intact hormone, all of the activity is confined to the first 34 amino acids [3]. It is presumed that the remainder of the molecule is somehow involved with its transport and no definite role has yet been found for the 35–84 portion of the molecule.

Once secreted by the parathyroid cell, 1–84-PTH is cleaved at various sites within the molecule, mainly in the liver and the kidney. As a consequence, the serum contains various different-sized fragments of PTH. Only those with the intact first 34 amino acids have biological action. Fragments without biological action tend to have a longer half-life than intact PTH and accumulate within the serum, especially in renal failure. The early PTH immunoassays could not differentiate between biologically active and inactive PTH and were unable to measure low or even normal levels of PTH. These assays have now been replaced by much more sensitive 'two-site' assays that predominantly measure the intact hormone without detecting most of the fragments. They are therefore much more specific and can measure normal circulating values as well as reduced concentrations. In addition, they do not detect PTH-related peptide (PTHrP). Consequently the current assays are very discriminating [4,5].

PTH acts by binding to membrane receptors linked to an adenylate cyclase enzyme system within the target cell. Although there was circumstantial evidence for the existence of a distinct PTH receptor, it was not until 1991 that a common receptor for both PTH and PTHrP was cloned [6], followed shortly afterwards by the identification of the human type 1 receptor [7]. This belongs to the class of G-protein-coupled receptors, with an extracellular N-terminus, a midregion seven-transmembrane domain and an intracellular C-terminus. PTH and PTHrP have similar binding characteristics to the receptor, helping to explain the very similar actions of injected PTH and PTHrP *in vitro* and *in vivo*.

Abnormalities of the type 1 receptor have been shown to be the cause of some forms of pseudohypoparathyroidism. In addition to its role in calcium metabolism, there is also clear evidence that PTH/PTHrP receptors are involved in embryonic development, especially of the skeleton. PTH receptor 'knockout' mice develop severe skeletal malformations, which can be lethal [8]. During embryonic development it may well be that PTHrP is the more potent ligand for the receptor.

To date, two skeletal dysplasias have been shown to be associated with defects of the PTH/PTHrP receptor. An activating mutation of the receptor causes Jansen's metaphyseal chondrodysplasia [9], where the dysplasia is associated with hypercalcaemia. An inactivating mutation is the cause of Blomstrand lethal osteochondrodysplasia [10], where advanced skeletal maturation is associated with premature ossification of the skeleton.

After the identification of the type 1 receptor, two further receptors (types 2 and 3) have been identified. The type 2 receptor is present in humans and activated by PTH but not PTHrP. It is unlikely to be involved in the classic actions of PTH and is distributed predominantly in the brain, pancreas, testes and lung. There is evidence to suggest that its major endogenous ligand is produced by the hypothalamus [11]. A type 3 receptor has been identified in zebrafish, which is activated by PTHrP but not PTH [12]. Its human equivalent has not yet been described.

The main target organs for PTH action are bone and kidney, PTH receptors being located on the osteoblast and

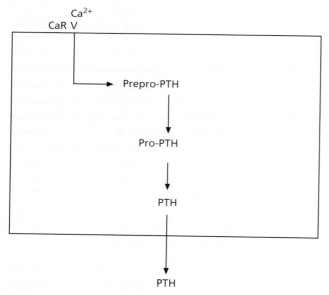

**Fig. 22.1.** Synthesis of parathyroid hormone (PTH). CaR, calcium-sensing receptor.

renal tubule. Receptors are also found on fibroblasts, lymphocytes, muscle cells, chondrocytes, fat cells and placental trophoblasts, where their role is at present unclear.

PTH acts on the kidney leading to an increased local production of cyclic adenosine monophosphate (cAMP). After an injection of PTH, both urinary and serum cAMP increase. In hyperparathyroid states, urinary AMP and urinary phosphorus excretion are increased and these measurements have been used as indirect measurements of PTH activity. Their use as diagnostic tests of parathyroid function has been superseded by the new, sensitive PTH assays. The response of the kidney with regard to cAMP and phosphorus excretion to injected PTH enabled the differentiation of various different forms of pseudohypoparathyroidism, where peripheral resistance to PTH is the hallmark of the disorder.

## Vitamin D

The unravelling of the metabolism of vitamin D and its mode of action through a specific sterol receptor has greatly improved the understanding of calcium metabolism and has allowed a more scientific differentiation of some of the rarer inherited forms of rickets and osteomalacia [13].

Vitamin D is produced in the skin by the action of ultraviolet light on 7-dehydrocholesterol to produce cholecalciferol. It can also be present in the diet, either as naturally occurring cholecalciferol or as dietary calciferol supplements, cholecalciferol or ergocalciferol, which are subsequently metabolized similarly.

More than 90% of calciferol normally comes from the skin, with only a small percentage derived from a non-fortified diet. Reduced skin production of calciferol can occur either from atmospheric pollutants reducing the levels of ultraviolet (UV) light of the appropriate wavelength that falls on the skin or from inadequate exposure of skin to sunlight, either by covering the body or staying out of sunlight. Although skin pigmentation decreases the production of calciferol per unit of UV exposure, skin pigmentation alone does not cause clinical deficiency states. The skin production of calciferol is rate-limited so that continued sunlight exposure does not result in pathological calciferol levels. However, in winter months, serum calciferol levels are lower due to reduced formation.

Calciferol has a low biological potency and is converted (Fig. 22.2) in the liver microsomal P450 system to 25-hydroxyvitamin D, which is no more active biologically than calciferol. Oral vitamin D is absorbed in the upper part of the small intestine in a way that is facilitated by the presence of bile salts. The absorbed vitamin passes into the blood stream via the lymphatic system, where it is present in the chylomicron fraction. Once in the circulation, it is metabolized in the liver to 25-hydroxyvitamin D.

Malabsorption and obstructive liver disease can be associated with rickets or osteomalacia, although, if over 90% of

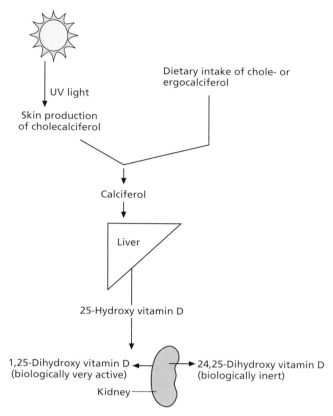

**Fig. 22.2.** Vitamin D metabolism.

the body's vitamin D comes from the skin, it is hard to understand why disorders that impair dietary vitamin D absorption cause clinical disease, unless skin production itself is borderline. The association in liver disease with chronic obstructive jaundice, rather than primary hepatocellular disease, is also difficult to explain and again should be more than compensated by normal skin production of vitamin D. A possible way to explain these situations would be to postulate an important enterohepatic circulation of vitamin D metabolites. If such a circulation were impaired, either by small intestinal disorders or obstruction to biliary flow, clinical disease could follow even when skin formation was normal. Even though bile does contain vitamin D metabolites, there is no conclusive evidence that these are important physiologically.

25-Hydroxyvitamin D is further metabolized in the kidney, either to the physiologically active metabolite 1,25-dihydroxyvitamin D or to the biologically inactive metabolite 24,25-dihydroxyvitamin D. The kidney's ability to regulate which metabolite is formed is part of the mechanism whereby calcium homeostasis is regulated. Whereas severe liver damage does not usually lead to a reduction in 25-hydroxyvitamin D, relatively minor degrees of renal damage can interfere with renal 1,25-dihydroxyvitamin D production, and this explains why even mild chronic renal failure can cause disturbances of calcium metabolism and bone disease.

Vitamin D in the blood is bound to a vitamin D-binding protein (DBP), an $\alpha_2$-glycoprotein produced in the liver. Only 1–3% of vitamin D in the blood is free.

From the therapeutic point of view, only calciferol was available for treatment until relatively recently. This was and still is very effective in the management of vitamin D deficiency. It was effective in large doses in treating hypoparathyroidism but the effective dose was close to the toxic dose. It was ineffective in managing the disturbances of calcium metabolism seen in renal failure.

With the unravelling of the metabolism of vitamin D, the possibility of making vitamin D metabolites for therapeutic use arose. The first commercially available compound was 1α-hydroxyvitamin D (alfacalcidol). Although of low biological action *in vitro*, this compound is 25-hydroxylated by the liver to 1,25-dihydroxyvitamin D *in vivo*, thus making the physiologically active metabolite. This compound has no advantage over calciferol in the treatment of vitamin D deficiency but was more potent in managing hypoparathyroidism and offered, for the first time, an effective agent for the management and control of renal bone disease. Alfacalcidol became widely used before 1,25-dihydroxyvitamin D (calcitriol) was commercially produced and marketed. This is active in a way similar to alfacalcidol, and both compounds can be used almost interchangeably. Logic suggests that only one should be available and used but both are in widespread use.

Vitamin D acts by binding to an intracellular receptor, a member of the larger family of receptors that binds a variety of steroid and thyroid hormones and retinoic acid. Each has a hormone-binding domain, a DNA-binding domain and an N-terminal domain. After binding to the cytoplasmic receptor, the vitamin D receptor complex is transported into the nucleus, where it attaches to hormone regulatory elements in DNA and thus regulates RNA transcription from genes regulated by vitamin D. Inherited defects of the receptor cause some of the forms of vitamin D-resistant rickets. Receptors for 1,25-dihydroxyvitamin D are found in intestinal, skeletal and renal cells, as well as a wide variety of cells not considered to be classic targets for vitamin D action. In these cells there is experimental evidence that 1,25-dihydroxy-vitamin D is an important regulator of cell differentiation and maturation [13].

1,25-Dihydroxyvitamin D acts on the small intestinal cells to allow the production of a calcium-binding protein that allows the active transport of calcium across the cell. The physiological action on bone is to allow adequate concentrations of ionized calcium and phosphorus to be present in the vicinity of the bone matrix and so to allow proper calcification of the forming osteoid. Hence, a deficiency is associated with uncalcified osteoid manifesting as rickets or osteomalacia. In pharmacological amounts, calciferol increases osteoclastic bone resorption and this is one of the reasons why hypercalcaemia occurs in vitamin D poisoning.

## Calcitonin

Calcitonin is produced by the thyroid parafollicular or 'C' cells. In humans there are very few parafollicular cells in normal situations. Like other peptide hormones, calcitonin is produced from a prohormone and is a cleavage product of a very much larger gene product. The calcitonin gene, by alternative splicing, can generate mRNAs that encode for either the calcitonin precursor molecule or the calcitonin gene-related peptide (CGRP) precursor. Calcitonin production predominates in the thyroid gland while CGRP predominates in the nervous system [14].

Calcitonin acts by binding to calcitonin receptors on the osteoclast and renal tubular cells. Although it has important physiological actions in some animals, this appears not to be the case in man. *In vitro* it inhibits osteoclastic action and causes hypocalcaemia when injected into normal rats or rabbits. However, it causes hypocalcaemia in humans only in situations of high bone turnover. Tumours of the 'C' cell (medullary thyroid carcinoma) can be associated with high concentrations of calcitonin without any obvious disturbance of calcium metabolism.

Calcitonin can be measured in serum by a radioimmunoassay. Under normal circumstances calcitonin is present at very low concentrations or may be undetectable. Measurements are of use only in the diagnosis and monitoring of patients with known or potential medullary thyroid carcinoma. In children, sporadic medullary thyroid carcinoma is very rare, and affected children are almost invariably cases of multiple endocrine neoplasia type 2 or 3. In this situation the diagnosis of affected children is now usually made by analysis of the gene for the *RET* proto-oncogene [15].

## Parathyroid hormone related peptide [16]

Studies of the hypercalcaemia of malignancy had suggested for many years that some cases were due to the production of a humoral agent by the tumour. This led to the term pseudohyperparathyroidism, and ectopic PTH production was assumed to be the cause when the early radioimmunoassays of PTH frequently found slightly elevated levels in malignancy. Rare cases of osteitis fibrosa cystica associated with malignancy and undetectable PTH concentrations raised the possibility that non-PTH factors were involved sometimes. Subsequent studies showed that the biochemical changes were remarkably similar to hyperparathyroidism in most cases but usually with suppressed PTH. The explanation became clear with the identification of PTHrP, which was shown to be produced by a variety of tumours associated with hypercalcaemia. It was biochemically distinct from PTH and produced by a different gene. It produced similar biochemical actions to PTH, raised serum calcium and increased urinary phosphorus and cAMP excretion. In virtually all initial assay systems it was equipotent to PTH, because it bound to the PTH receptor in an identical fashion to PTH.

Subsequent work revealed that PTHrP is a peptide produced by normal cells, especially those of squamous epithelial origins. It is expressed in the fetus and the postnatal animal in a wide variety of tissues, including various areas of the brain, pancreas, kidney, lungs, bone and skin. It has paracrine and exocrine actions that have not been clearly defined. Under normal circumstances significant concentrations are not found in the circulation, and its hypercalcaemic effects occur only when it is produced in large amounts (e.g. by tumours).

Large amounts of PTHrP are found in the lactating breast and milk. There is also some evidence that PTHrP in at least some animal species is the fetal factor, rather than PTH, that helps to maintain fetal normocalcaemia.

## Calcium-sensing receptor [17]

Clinical studies of familial hypocalciuric or benign hypercalcaemia (FBH) demonstrated that the most likely explanation of the disorder was a failure to recognize a normal serum ionized calcium. A calcium sensor was postulated which normally regulated the secretion of PTH in relationship to the serum ionized concentration and regulated renal tubular calcium reabsorption. This proved to be the case when a gene encoding a calcium-sensing receptor (CaR) was identified in bovine, rat and human species [18,19]. The gene encoding the CaR has an extracellular, transmembrane and intracellular component (Fig. 22.3). The gene, in addition to being found in the parathyroid cell and renal tubular cell, is distributed widely and can be found in high amounts in the brain, pancreas and many other tissues. Mutations in all three portions of the receptor have been associated with FBH, and *in vitro* studies have shown that these mutations are associated with a change in the set point of the receptor with a shift to the right of the calcium/PTH response curve. Interestingly, different mutations of the CaR gene can have the opposite effect and shift the response curve to the left. Such mutations have been found in an inherited condition called autosomal dominant hypocalcaemia [20].

## Bone physiology

Bone modelling, longitudinal bone growth and bone remodelling are the biological processes responsible for the development of bone structure during childhood and adolescence.

Bone modelling (Fig. 22.4) is the process of shaping or sculpting the skeleton during growth. In the growing child, bone develops either by intramembranous bone formation without a cartilage matrix or by remodelling and replacing previously calcified cartilage (endochondral bone formation). Growth in width and thickness is achieved by intramembran-

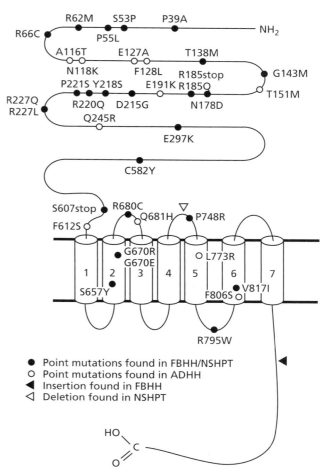

**Fig. 22.3.** Summary of calcium-sensing (CaR) mutations in familial benign hypocalcuric hypercalcaemia (FBHH), neonatal severe hyperparathyroidism (NSHPT) and autosomal dominant hypocalcaemia with hypercalciuria (ADHH) on a topographical representation of the CaR. Amino acids are shown in conventional one-letter code.

ous bone formation at the surface of the periosteum and resorption at the endosteum of old bone.

Longitudinal bone growth takes place at the epiphyseal growth plates at both ends of long bones (Fig. 22.5). The growth plate consists of cartilage, the cells of which are organized in columns with several recognizable zones. In the resting zone, or germinal cell layer, are prechondrocytes. In the proliferative zone, the chondrocytes from the resting zone divide rapidly and form columns of cells lying along the longitudinal axis of bone. These cells secrete an extracellular matrix of collagen, principally type 1, proteoglycans and other non-collagenous proteins.

In the hypertrophic zone, the chondrocytes become large and round and start to mineralize the extracellular matrix, leading to longitudinal tubes of calcified cartilage. Below the hypertrophic zone, osteoblasts deposit a thin layer of osteoid on the calcified cartilage, which is known as the primary

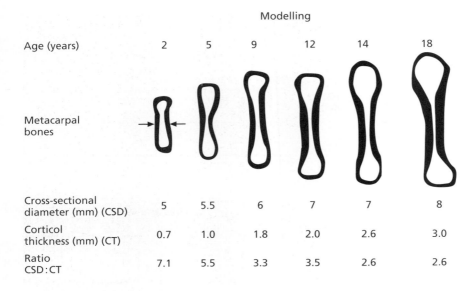

**Fig. 22.4.** Change in shape and dimensions of metacarpal bones during childhood. (Reproduced with permission from Schonau *et al. Horm Res* 1997; 48 (Suppl. 5): 50–9.)

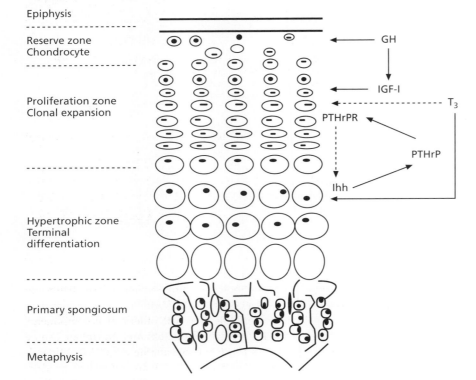

**Fig. 22.5.** Zones of the growth plate. GH, growth hormone; IGF-I, insulin-like growth factor I; $T_3$, triiodothyronine; PTHrP, PTH-related peptide; PTHrPR, PTHrP receptor; Ihh, Indian hedgehog. (Reproduced with permission from Robson *Arch Dis Child* 1999; 81: 360–4.)

spongiosum. This area is then removed by osteoclasts followed by osteoblasts to lay down mature secondary spongiosa or lamellar bone. Thus the cartilaginous growth plate is progressively replaced by bone.

The proliferation of chondrocytes is under the influence of several growth factors including growth hormone (GH) and insulin-like growth factor I (IGF-I). GH receptors have been demonstrated in the germinal, proliferative and hypertrophic cell layers [21]. GH promotes the differentiation

of prechondrocytes and these cells then become responsive to IGF-I and themselves synthesize IGF-I, thus exhibiting both autocrine and paracrine effects. The combination of GH and systemic and local IGF-I appears to be important for longitudinal bone growth, this being referred to as the dual-effector theory.

Bone remodelling (Fig. 22.6), unlike bone modelling and longitudinal bone growth, occurs throughout life and is a constant process of bone resorption coupled to bone forma-

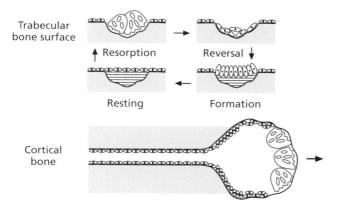

**Fig. 22.6.** Remodelling in trabecular and cortical bone. (Reproduced with permission from Schonau *et al. Horm Res* 1997; 48 (Suppl. 5): 50–9.)

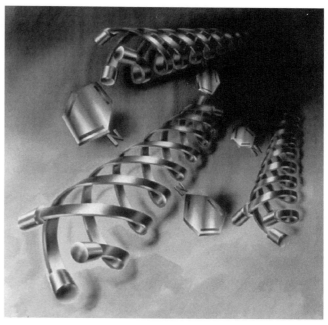

**Fig. 22.7.** Type 1 collagen is a triple helical molecule formed from three α chains. The figure shows three such molecules linked by pyridinium and deoxypyridinium cross-links.

tion. Mechanical use, systemic hormones and local factors regulate this turnover.

There are two major types of bone, trabecular (spongy) bone and cortical (compact) bone. Cortical bone makes up 80% and is most abundant in the long bone shafts of the appendicular skeleton. It is made up of closely packed osteons (Haversian systems) consisting of a central Haversian canal with a blood vessel running through it surrounded by concentric layers of osseous lamellae. Trabecular bone is found in the metaphyses of long bones, in vertebrae and most flat bones. It consists of connecting plates of bone that contain multiple holes, giving it a porous appearance. Its surface area and metabolic activity are greater than cortical bone, with bone turnover being about eight times greater.

Bone remodelling occurs in focal and discrete packets throughout the skeleton known as bone remodelling units. The remodelling of each packet in trabecular bone takes about 3–4 months and follows the same sequence. Osteoclastic bone resorption is followed by osteoblastic bone formation to repair the defect. Bone resorption takes place over approximately 15 days, whereas bone formation is much longer taking 75–135 days followed finally by mineralization over 10–20 days. In the optimal situation, there is a balance between the amount of bone resorbed and the amount of new bone formed. In children during the process of remodelling, bone formation exceeds bone resorption, leading to a net increase in bone mass during childhood and adolescence.

## Bone cells

Bone consists of an organic matrix (osteoid), minerals (mainly calcium and phosphate) and three main types of cell (osteoblasts, osteocytes and osteoclasts).

Osteoblasts are derived from stromal stem cells, a precursor which they share with adipocytes, chondrocytes and myocytes. Mature osteoblasts are cuboidal cells with a single eccentric nucleus. They are responsible for several functions:

1 production of the proteins of bone matrix including type 1 collagen and osteocalcin;

2 they secrete a variety of growth factors that are stored in the bone matrix, such as transforming growth factor β (TGF-β), bone morphogenetic proteins (BMPs) and the IGFs;

3 they mineralize newly formed matrix;

4 they are also required for normal bone resorption to occur by influencing osteoclast differentiation.

Type 1 collagen molecules synthesized by osteoblasts are cross-linked to each other into fibrils (a three-dimensional helical structure) and together with other matrix components form a network upon which calcium and phosphate can be deposited as crystalline hydroxyapatite (Fig. 22.7). Mineralization is dependent on a normal calcium phosphate product in extracellular fluid and normal activity of alkaline phosphatase released from osteoblasts. Evidence for the critical role of alkaline phosphatase is seen in patients with hypophosphatasia, where diminished alkaline phosphatase activity causes defective bone mineralization.

Osteocytes are derived from osteoblasts that have successfully synthesized bone matrix and have then become incorporated into that matrix. They communicate with each other and with cells on the bone surface via dendritic processes. They were originally thought to control rapid mineral exchange between bone and serum (osteocytic osteolysis),

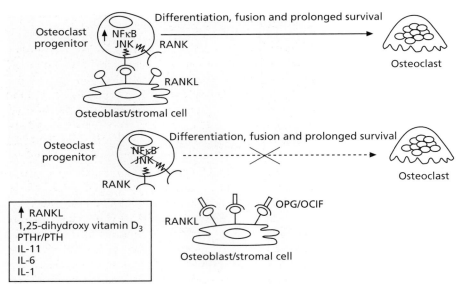

**Fig. 22.8.** The RANK/OPG/NFkB pathway of control of osteoclast formation and function. (Reproduced with permission from Chen D, Zhao M, Oyajobi B, Mundy GR 'Update in bone cell biology'. In Compston J. and Ralston S., eds. *Osteoporosis and Bone Biology – The State of the Art*. London: International Medical Press.)

but more recent evidence suggests this is not the case and currently their function is unknown.

Osteoclasts differ from osteoblasts in that they are multi-nucleated and derive from a multipotential precursor stem cell within the bone marrow, which also produces cells of the monocyte–macrophage lineage. They are formed by fusion of haemopoietic mononuclear cells. Osteoclast formation and activation is dependent on direct cell-to-cell contact with osteoblasts or related marrow stromal cells.

It has been known for many years that many of the bone-resorbing cytokines [e.g. interleukin 1 (IL-1) and IL-6] and the systemic hormones (PTH and 1,25-dihydroxyvitamin D) exert their effects on osteoclasts only in the presence of stromal/osteoblastic cells. It is now known that osteoclast precursor cells express a membrane-bound receptor, which is a member of the tumour necrosis factor (TNF) receptor family. This receptor, which activates the transcription factor NFκB (nuclear factor kappa B) within the osteoclast precursors, was designated receptor activator of NFκB (RANK) (Fig. 22.8) [22].

A search for its ligand identified RANK ligand (RANKL), which is present on marrow stromal/osteoblastic cells. Binding of RANKL to RANK expressed on osteoclast precursors results in their differentiation and fusion into mature osteoclasts. Several cytokines and the systemic hormones, PTH and 1,25-dihydroxyvitamin D, which stimulate bone resorption have been shown to act on osteoclasts by increasing the expression of RANKL. In addition, a soluble decoy receptor, osteoprotegerin (OPG), which is also secreted by stromal/osteoblastic cells, can bind to RANKL, thus preventing the RANK–RANKL interaction and thereby blocking osteoclastogenesis [22]. OPG has been shown to suppress bone resorption induced by agents such as IL-1, TNF-α, PTH and 1,25-dihydroxyvitamin D.

Osteoclasts contain primary lysosomes, numerous and pleomorphic mitochondria and a specific area of the cell membrane, the ruffled border, which forms adjacent to the bone surface where resorption takes place. They resorb bone by the production of proteolytic enzymes and hydrogen ions in the localized environment under the ruffled border of the cell. Hydrogen ions generated in the osteoclast by the enzyme carbonic anhydrase type II are pumped across the ruffled border by a proton pump. They produce an optimal environment for the lysosomal enzymes to degrade the bone matrix.

Osteoclasts are highly mobile, resorbing bone to form lacunae and then moving across the bone surface to resorb a separate area of bone. Disruption of any of the mechanisms necessary for bone resorption causes osteopetrosis. An example of this is a deficiency of carbonic anhydrase type II isoenzyme, which produces a form of osteopetrosis in children associated with renal tubular acidosis. In an animal model of osteopetrosis, the op/op mouse, a genetic defect in the production of a colony-stimulating factor (CSF-1) leads to impaired formation of osteoclasts.

## Influences on bone metabolism

The activity of the osteoblasts and osteoclasts is under the control of both systemic hormones and cytokines generated in the microenvironment of bone cells. The systemic hormones divide into two groups: those that are primarily responsible for the maintenance of extracellular fluid calcium concentrations and those that influence bone cell function but do not have an impact on plasma calcium homeostasis. Parathyroid hormone, 1,25-dihydroxyvitamin D and calcitonin are systemic hormones under negative-feedback control; their secretion is regulated by extracellular fluid calcium concentrations. Their effects on bone cells contribute to calcium homeostasis, although their actions on gut and kidney are probably more important. Other systemic hormones that do not contribute to calcium homeostasis include oestrogens and androgens, glucocorticoids, thyroid hormones and GH. Their secretion is not under negative feedback control by extracellular fluid calcium.

PTH has differing effects on bone depending on whether it is administered continuously or intermittently. Continuous administration increases osteoclastic bone resorption, but intermittent administration in low doses stimulates bone formation. The effects of PTH on bone are modulated by other local factors and systemic hormones, such as 1,25-dihydroxyvitamin D, IL-1 and TNF-α. 1,25-Dihydroxyvitamin D is a potent bone-resorbing factor and acts in synergy with PTH on osteoclasts to raise plasma calcium. It also has direct effects on osteoblasts stimulating the synthesis of osteocalcin and alkaline phosphatase. Calcitonin inhibits bone resorption by inhibiting the formation of osteoclasts from mononuclear precursors and by direct effects on the mature osteoclast. These effects are, however, transient.

The action of glucocorticoids on bone is by two mechanisms. There is a direct inhibition of bone formation by inhibiting the proliferation of osteoblast precursors and an indirect stimulation of bone resorption by suppressing intestinal calcium absorption leading to secondary hyperparathyroidism. Thyroid hormones have indirect stimulatory effects on bone turnover such that bone turnover, and consequently skeletal growth, is reduced in hypothyroidism and increased in hyperthyroidism. GH has been shown to stimulate bone formation directly by action on osteoblasts with increased synthesis of type 1 procollagen and alkaline phosphatase. It also stimulates bone resorption, with increases in biochemical markers of bone resorption seen in individuals treated with GH. This latter effect is indirect, requiring the presence of stromal cells including osteoblasts. The effects on both bone formation and resorption appear to be mediated by the local production of IGF-I.

The critical importance of sex steroids on bone in augmenting the pubertal growth spurt is well recognized. Oestrogen receptors have been demonstrated in several different bone cells and androgen receptors in osteoblasts. Both oestrogens and androgens have been shown to stimulate bone cells *in vivo* with the proliferation and production of markers of osteoblast function such as alkaline phosphatase and type 1 collagen and cytokines such as IL-6 and TGF-β. As a result of clinical observations, it has been realized that oestrogen is of critical importance in epiphyseal maturation and bone mineral accretion. Reduced bone density has been shown to occur in individuals deficient in the cytochrome P450 enzyme aromatase, which converts androgens to oestrogen [23]. In addition, a man identified as having an oestrogen receptor mutation leading to oestrogen resistance had evidence of delayed epiphyseal closure and reduced bone density [24].

## Renal handling of phosphate

Alterations in renal tubular handling are the most important mechanism for regulation of plasma phosphate. Approximately 90% of phosphate in plasma is reabsorbed, with the majority occurring in the proximal renal tubule. Phosphate reabsorption in the proximal tubule is active, occurring against an electrical and chemical gradient across the brush-border membrane from the renal tubular lumen into the cells. This is achieved by the action of sodium-dependent phosphate co-transporters ($NaP_1$), which are located in the brush-border membranes of renal tubular cells. Dietary phosphate intake, PTH activity and glucocorticoids influence their activity.

PTH inhibits phosphate reabsorption in both the proximal and distal tubules, but its main effect is in the proximal straight tubule. Two signalling systems are involved in the inhibition of $NaP_1$ co-transport activity by PTH, these being the adenylate cyclase–cAMP–protein kinase A pathway and the phospholipase–calcium–protein kinase C pathway. The former has traditionally been regarded as the dominant pathway of PTH activity. Glucocorticoids in excess cause phosphaturia and hypophosphataemia by a PTH-independent effect on $NaP_1$ co-transport activity.

Determination of renal phosphate handling is best performed by assessing urinary phosphate excretion in relation to the filtered load of phosphate. The tubular maximum for phosphate in relation to glomerular filtration rate ($T_mPO_4$/GFR) (Fig. 22.9) is the most widely accepted index for this purpose. Normal values are higher in children than in adults and are related inversely to PTH activity [25].

The higher tubular reabsorption for phosphate in children leads to higher values for plasma phosphate, particularly in infancy. This mechanism probably exists because of the greater demands for phosphate for bone mineralization and longitudinal bone growth in growing subjects. Evidence that the tubular reabsorption of phosphate is low in GH-deficient children and increased in adults with acromegaly has led to speculation that GH is an important factor regulating renal phosphate handling. This effect is probably mediated by IGF-I as its administration has been shown to stimulate tubular reabsorption of phosphate by a mechanism independent of PTH [26]. This effect of GH on $T_mPO_4$/GFR has been used to predict the growth response in children receiving GH treatment.

## Evidence for a circulating phosphate-regulating hormone

There is increasing evidence for the presence of a phosphate-regulating hormone. The first clue was when an individual with hypophosphataemic rickets underwent renal transplantation, but the abnormality in renal phosphate wasting persisted. Subsequent evidence came from the animal model of hypophosphataemic rickets, the Hyp mouse. Parabiotic

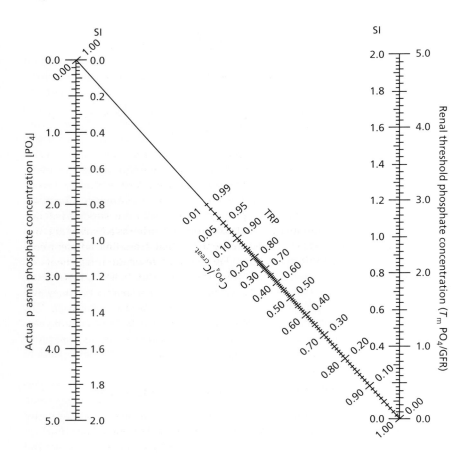

**Fig. 22.9.** Nomogram for derivation of renal threshold phosphate concentration [36].

experiments between the circulation of Hyp mice and normal mice showed evidence of renal phosphate wasting in the normal mice. Cross-transplantation experiments then showed that the removal of kidneys from Hyp mice and transplantation of a normal kidney did not eliminate the renal phosphate abnormality, whereas normal mice transplanted with kidneys from Hyp mice did not develop the abnormality.

Further evidence has come from investigation of individuals with oncogenic osteomalacia. This condition is characterized by the presence of a tumour, usually of mesenchymal origin, in association with hypophosphataemia, osteomalacia and low concentrations of 1,25-dihydroxyvitamin D. These features resolve on removal of the tumour, extracts of which inhibit tubular phosphate reabsorption and 1α-hydroxylase activity in the proximal renal tubule. The activity of the tumour extract has been shown to be heat sensitive and lipid insoluble, which in conjunction with its likely molecular weight suggest the factor may be a peptide hormone, which has been termed phosphatonin [27].

## Identification of the *PHEX* gene

Family linkage studies had previously localized the gene for X-linked hypophosphataemic rickets to the short arm of the X chromosome. This gene, originally called *PEX* and then subsequently *PHEX* (*p*hosphate-regulating gene with *h*omologies to *e*ndopeptidases on the *X* chromosome), codes for a protein which is a member of the endopeptidase family, which degrade or activate peptide hormones [28]. The precise mechanism of the action of the *PHEX* gene product is unclear but it probably inactivates phosphatonin, which would normally inhibit renal phosphate uptake and reduce 1,25-dihydroxyvitamin D concentrations. The *PHEX* gene consists of a single transmembrane domain and a relatively large extracellular domain. At least 30 different mutations, predominantly in the extracellular domain, have been identified in affected individuals [29].

## Bone mass in children

A variety of different techniques has been used to assess the change in bone mass in growing children. Most information has been obtained using dual-energy X-ray absorptiometry (DXA). Many cross-sectional studies of bone density in children have been undertaken showing a progressive rise with age, with body weight and pubertal status the most important influences. However, this is a consequence of areal bone density measurements made with DXA being correlated with body size. Studies that have calculated or measured true volumetric bone density have largely eliminated the relationship with age due to the changes in body size. Puberty is important, with one-third of adult bone density being acquired at this time. No further increments occur beyond the age of 16 years in girls and 18 years in boys, the values for lumbar spine bone density seen at the age of 18 years being similar to those seen in adults aged 20–35 years [30]. This has been confirmed by using quantitative computerized tomography. Thus there is strong evidence that peak bone mass is acquired approximately 2 years after the cessation of longitudinal growth. As peak bone mass is known to be an important determinant of the risk of osteoporosis as an adult, the process of bone mineral accretion during childhood and adolescence has direct relevance for adulthood.

The most important influences on bone density appear to be genetic, nutrition, puberty and weight-bearing exercise. Genetics probably accounts for 80% of peak bone mass with good evidence from twin studies showing that monozygotic twins have a more similar bone mass than dizygotic twins. This genetic influence appears to be expressed before puberty. The age of peak velocity of bone mineral content acquisition is 0.7 years later than peak height velocity, which may explain the observed increase in fractures in adolescent children around the time of peak height velocity [31].

Weight-bearing physical activity has an impact on bone mineral accretion during both prepubertal and peripubertal years. One year after peak bone mineral content velocity, active girls and boys have been shown to have 17% and 9% greater bone mineral content, respectively, than less active children after correcting for height and weight [31].

Nutritional intake, particularly of calcium-containing products, is another important influence on bone mineral accretion during growth. Extra calcium, given either as supplements [32] or as calcium-enriched foods [33] to prepubertal children, produces greater gains in bone density compared with unsupplemented control subjects, especially in those with a previous low calcium intake. The short-term changes have not been shown to result in higher peak bone mass.

The contribution of sex steroids to bone density is apparent from studies of individuals with hypogonadism in whom the duration and adequacy of sex steroid replacement is clearly linked to bone density [34]. The critical importance of oestrogen on bone mineralization in men as well as women is illustrated by the report of a man with an oestrogen receptor gene mutation whose spinal bone density was 3 standard deviations (SD) below the mean [24].

Many studies have demonstrated the presence of reduced bone density in children with chronic childhood conditions, including cerebral palsy, cystic fibrosis, inflammatory bowel disease, juvenile arthritis and cancer chemotherapy. A variety of factors is important, but the effects of inadequate nutrition and delayed puberty appear to be the strongest.

## Investigation of bone metabolism

Bone metabolism can be assessed by the following methods.

## Measurement of biochemical markers of bone turnover in serum and urine

Bone formation markers are bone alkaline phosphatase, procollagen type 1 C-terminal propeptide (P1CP) and osteocalcin, which are all measured in serum. More specific markers of collagen degradation, such as the pyridinium cross-links, pyridinoline and deoxypyridinoline, have superseded the measurement of hydroxyproline in urine as a marker of bone resorption. These are peptides that cross-link adjacent collagen fibrils in bone. During bone resorption, fragments of them are released and excreted in urine. They can be measured either in a 24-h urine collection or in an early-morning fasting sample expressed as a ratio to urinary creatinine. The main value of biochemical markers of bone turnover is in the longitudinal follow-up of individual children to assess the effect of therapeutic interventions.

## Radiological evaluation of the skeleton

Conventional X-rays continue to provide an important assessment of the nature, severity and extent of bone disease. Two additional radiological investigations of value are isotope bone scans, which will indicate the extent of the bone lesions in polyostotic fibrous dysplasia, and spiral CT scans, which document the size and severity of skull lesions in the same condition.

## Measurement of bone density

A variety of different techniques has been developed to quantify bone density, including single- and dual-photon absorptiometry, quantitative computerized tomography (QCT), dual-energy X-ray absorptiometry and quantitative ultrasound. QCT is the only technique that measures true volumetric bone density in $mg/cm^3$. It also has the ability to separately distinguish trabecular and cortical bone. However, its disadvantage when used to measure the axial skeleton is the significant radiation dose (30 $\mu$Sv). At a peripheral site, such as the forearm, pQCT can provide information about density and biomechanical strength.

Dual X-ray absorptiometry is the most popular technique because of its availability, relative speed and low radiation dose (1 $\mu$Sv). In this technique, a beam of collimated X-rays is transmitted from a source providing alternating pulses of 70 and 140 kV through a rotating calibration disk composed of bone and soft tissue equivalent materials, which are then measured by a detector located above the subject. It produces a measurement of bone mineral density ($g/cm^2$) by correcting the bone mineral content for the projected area of bone. However, as this is a measure of bone area and does not allow for differences in bone volume, values for bone mineral density in growing children are influenced by bone size and therefore body size [31]. This explains the strong correlations between bone density measurements and height and weight in children and why children who are small for their age have bone density values artifactually low compared with normal values for age.

Models that correct bone density for bone volume have been proposed. The usual sites of measurement are lumbar spine, whole body and neck of femur. Specific software is required for children who are less than about 30 kg body weight. It is essential that appropriate reference data are available for DXA measurements in children which have been generated on the same make of scanner and ideally are based on a local population.

Quantitative ultrasound has been explored in children. Although moderate correlations have been demonstrated with bone density measurements made by DXA, it is not regarded as a valuable diagnostic method.

## Histological assessment of bone biopsy

The indications for bone biopsy in children are limited, but it can provide additional information when non-invasive techniques do not produce clear answers, e.g. the assessment of a child with idiopathic osteoporosis. The technique may also be used in research studies to assess the effect of new pharmaceutical agents on bone remodelling and mineralization.

The dynamic nature of bone turnover can be evaluated by double tetracycline labelling of bone, involving two doses of an oral tetracycline taken at a suitable time interval apart before biopsy. The tetracycline is incorporated into the zone of new mineralization and is recognized under light microscopy as a band. The distance between the two bands allows a calculation of the rate of bone formation.

## References

1 Kemper B, Habener JF, Mulligan RC *et al.* Preproparathyroid hormone: a direct translation product of parathyroid messenger RNA. *Proc Natl Acad Sci USA* 1974; 71: 3731–5.

2 Habener JF, Amherdt M, Ravazzola H, Orci L. Parathyroid hormone biosynthesis: Correlation of conversion of biosynthetic precursors with intra-cellular protein migration as determined by electron microscope autoradiography. *J Cell Biol* 1979; 80: 715–31.

3 Habener JF, Rosenblatt M, Potts JT Jr. Parathyroid hormone: biochemical aspects of biosynthesis, secretion, action and metabolism. *Physiol Rev* 1984; 64: 985–1053.

4 Nussbaum SR, Zahradnik RJ, Lavigne JR *et al.* Highly sensitive two-site immuno-radiometric assay of parathyrin and its clinical ability in evaluating patients with hypercalcaemia. *Clin Chem* 1987; 33: 1364–7.

5 Ratcliffe WA, Heath DA, Ryan M, Jones SR. Performance and diagnostic application of a two-site immuno-radiometric assay for parathyrin in serum. *Clin Chem* 1989; 35: 1957–61.

6 Juppner H, Abou-Samra AB, Freeman M *et al.* A G protein-linked receptor for parathyroid hormone and parathyroid-related peptide. *Science* 1991; 254: 1024–6.

7 Schipani E, Karga H, Karaplis AC *et al.* Identical cDNA's encode a human renal and bone parathyroid hormone/parathyroid hormone-related peptide receptor. *Endocrinology* 1993; 132: 2157–65.

8 Lanske B, Karaplis AC, Lee K *et al.* PTH/PTHrP receptor in early development and Indian hedgehog-related bone growth. *Science* 1996; 273: 663–6.

9 Schipani E, Langman CB, Parfitt AM *et al.* Constitutively activated receptors for parathyroid hormone and parathyroid hormone-related peptide in Jansen's metaphyseal chondrodysplasia. *N Engl J Med* 1996; 335: 708–14.

10 Karperien M, van der Harten HJ, van Schosten R *et al.* A frame-shift mutation in the type 1 parathyroid hormone (PTH)/PTH-related peptide receptor causing Blomstrand lethal osteochondrodysplasia. *J Clin Endocrinol Metab* 1999; 84: 3713–20.

11 Hoare SRJ, Bonner TI, Usdin TB. Comparison of rat and human parathyroid hormone 2 (PTH2) receptor activation: PTH is a low potency partial agonist at the rat PTH2 receptor. *Endocrinology* 1999; 140: 4419–25.

12 Rubin DA, Juppner H. Zebrafish express the common parathyroid hormone/parathyroid hormone-related peptide receptor (PTH1R) and a novel receptor (PTH3R) that is preferentially activated by mammalian and tugufish parathyroid hormone-related peptide. *J Biol Chem* 1999; 274: 28185–90.

13 Haussler MR, Haussler CA, Jurutka PW *et al.* The vitamin D hormone and its nuclear receptor: molecular actions and disease states. *J Endocrinol* 1997; 154: 557–73.

14 Lou H, Gagel RF. Alternative RNA processing – its role in regulating expression of calcitonin/calcitonin gene-related peptide. *J Endocrinol* 1998; 156: 401–5.

15 Heshmati HM, Hafbauer LC. Multiple endocrine neoplasia type 2: recent progress in diagnosis and management. *Eur J Endocrinol* 1997; 137: 572–8.

16 Martin TJ, Moseley JM, Williams E. Parathyroid hormone-related protein: hormone and cytokine. *J Endocrinol* 1997; 154: 523–37.

17 Pearce SHS, Thakker RV. The calcium-sensing receptor: insights into extracellular calcium homeostasis in health and disease. *J Endocrinol* 1997; 154: 371–8.

18 Brown EM, Gamba G, Riccardi D *et al.* Cloning and characterisation of an extracellular $Ca^{2+}$-sensing receptor from bovine parathyroid. *Nature* 1993; 366: 575–80.

19 Garrett JE, Capuano IV, Hammerland LG *et al.* Molecular cloning and functional expression of human parathyroid calcium receptor cDNA's. *J Biol Chem* 1995; 270: 12919–25.

20 Pearce SHS, Williamson C, Kifor O *et al.* A familial syndrome of hypocalcaemia due to mutations in the calcium-sensing receptor gene. *N Engl J Med* 1996; 335: 1115–22.

21 Ohlsson C, Bengtsson BA, Isaksson OGP, Andreassen TT, Slootweg MC. Growth hormone and bone. *Endocr Rev* 1998; 19: 55–79.

22 Suda T, Takahashi N, Udagawa N *et al.* Modulation of osteoclast differentiation and function by the new members of the tumor necrosis factor receptor and ligand families. *Endocr Rev* 1999; 20: 345–57.

23 Morishama A, Grumbach MM, Simpson ER, Fisher C, Qin K. Aromatase deficiency in male and female siblings caused by a novel mutation and the physiological role of estrogens. *J Clin Endocrinol Metab* 1995; 80: 3689–98.

24 Smith EP, Boyd J, Frank GR *et al.* Estrogen resistance caused by a mutation in the estrogen-receptor gene in a man. *N Engl J Med* 1994; 331: 1056–61.

25 Shaw NJ, Wheeldon J, Brocklebank JT. Indices of intact serum parathyroid hormone and renal excretion of calcium, phosphate and magnesium. *Arch Dis Child* 1990; 65: 1208–11.

26 Caverzasio J, Montessuit C, Bonjour JP. Stimulatory effect of insulin-like growth factor-1 on renal Pi transport and plasma 1,25-dihydroxyvitamin D$_3$. *Endocrinology* 1990; 127: 453–9.

27 Econs MJ, Drezner MK. Tumour-induced osteomalacia – unveiling a new hormone. *N Engl J Med* 1994; 330: 1679–81.

28 The HYP Consortium. A gene (PEX) with homologies to endopeptidases is mutated in patients with X-linked hypophosphataemic rickets. *Nature Genet* 1995; 11: 130–6.

29 Dixon PH, Christie PT, Wooding C *et al.* Mutational analysis of PHEX gene in X-linked hypophosphataemia. *J Clin Endocrinol Metab* 1998; 83: 615–23.

30 Thientz G, Buchs B, Rizzoli R *et al.* Longitudinal monitoring of bone mass accumulation in healthy adolescents: evidence for a marked reduction after 16 years of age at the levels of lumbar spine and femoral neck in female subjects. *J Clin Endocrinol Metab* 1992; 75: 1060–5.

31 Bailey DA, Mckay HA, Mirwald RL, Crocker PRE, Faulkner RA. A six-year longitudinal study of the relationship of physical activity to bone mineral accrual in growing children: The University of Saskatchewan bone mineral accrual study. *J Bone Miner Res* 1999; 14: 1672–9.

32 Johnston CC, Miller JZ, Slemenda CW *et al.* Calcium supplementation and increases in bone mineral density in children. *N Engl J Med* 1992; 327: 82–7.

33 Bonjour JP, Carrie AL, Ferrari S *et al.* Calcium-enriched foods and bone mass growth in prepubertal girls: a randomized, double-blind, placebo-controlled trial. *J Clin Invest* 1997; 99: 1287–94.

34 Finkelstein JS, Klibanski A, Neer RM *et al.* Increases in bone density during treatment of men with idiopathic hypogonadotrophic hypogonadism. *J Clin Endocrinol Metab* 1989; 69: 776–83.

35 Prentice A, Parsons TJ, Cole TJ. Uncritical use of bone mineral density in absorptiometry may lead to size-related artefacts in the identification of bone mineral determinants. *Am J Clin Nutr* 1994; 60: 837–42.

36 Walton RJ, Bijroet OLM. Nomogram for derivation of renal threshold phosphate cancentration. *Lancet* 1975; ii: 309–10.

# Disorders of calcium and bone metabolism

## D. A. Heath and N. J. Shaw

## Introduction

The majority of disorders of calcium and phosphate metabolism result from increased or decreased secretion or action of 1,25-dihydroxyvitamin D and parathyroid hormone (PTH) or from increased or decreased urinary excretion of phosphate and calcium. The most important parameters for the assessment of calcium and bone metabolism may be divided into four groups (Table 23.1):

1 calcium and phosphate in blood and urine;
2 parameters of PTH secretion and action: PTH, $T_m PO_4/GFR$ (tubular maximum for phosphate in relation to glomerular filtration rate);
3 parameters of vitamin D metabolism: 25-hydroxyvitamin D and 1,25-dihydroxyvitamin D;
4 Parameters of bone turnover, e.g. alkaline phosphatase, deoxypyridinoline.

These indices are best measured after an overnight fast (preferably second morning urine) to avoid dietary influences and diurnal variation. Although it may not be necessary to measure all parameters listed in Table 23.1, it is best to ensure that samples, which can be subsequently analysed, are collected before the initiation of any treatment. This is because the clinical picture and the results can be hard to interpret in retrospect.

## Hypocalcaemia

It is convenient to divide hypocalcaemia in children as that occurring in the newborn and that occurring in older children as different conditions are likely to present at these different ages. The majority of childhood hypocalcaemia is caused by a disorder of vitamin D metabolism or by decreased parathyroid hormone secretion or action. Measurements of serum parathyroid hormone and vitamin D metabolites are critical to investigation.

### Neonatal hypocalcaemia

Manifestations of hypocalcaemia in the newborn are variable and include those due to increased neuromuscular excitability, such as generalized or focal seizures, jitteriness and irritability, and other more non-specific signs, including apnoea, cyanosis and tachycardia. It may be asymptomatic, particularly in preterm infants.

Early neonatal hypocalcaemia occurs during the first 3 days of life, particularly in preterm infants, infants of diabetic mothers and after birth asphyxia. As active calcium transport from the mother to fetus occurs during pregnancy [1], the newborn infant is relatively hypercalcaemic and the plasma calcium begins to fall within the first few days until autonomous regulation of plasma calcium by the infant commences. The mechanism for early neonatal hypocalcaemia is unclear but probably reflects an exaggerated postnatal surge in calcitonin with a delayed response to PTH. In the majority of affected infants, the hypocalcaemia is transient and resolves within a week.

Late neonatal hypocalcaemia occurs at 5–10 days of life and is invariably symptomatic. It is more usually seen in term than preterm infants. Some reports have noted an

**Table 23.1.** Laboratory assessment of bone and mineral metabolism

| Blood | Urine |
|---|---|
| Calcium, phosphate | Calcium, phosphate |
| Alkaline phosphatase | Creatinine |
| Magnesium | Deoxypyridinoline |
| Creatinine | |
| 25-Hydroxyvitamin D, | Calculation of: |
| 1,25-Dihydroxyvitamin D | Calcium/creatinine ratio |
| Intact PTH | *$T_m PO_4/GFR$ |
| | Deoxypyridinoline/creatinine ratio |

*Ratio of maximal rate of renal tubular reabsorption of phosphate to glomerular filtration rate.

association with hyperphosphataemia as a consequence of the higher phosphate content of cow's milk formula as opposed to human milk; in others it has been noted to occur more frequently in winter and associated with maternal vitamin D deficiency. Transient parathyroid dysfunction usually resolves within a few weeks of birth. Although most affected infants have transient hypocalcaemia, there are several important conditions to exclude that may require long-term therapy.

Maternal hyperparathyroidism causes neonatal hypocalcaemia because of suppression of the fetal parathyroid glands, which are then unable to maintain a normal plasma calcium after birth.

Hypomagnesaemia due to congenital defects of intestinal magnesium absorption or renal tubular reabsorption results in hypocalcaemia either because of an impaired secretion of parathyroid hormone or because of an impaired response to it. Measurement of plasma magnesium should be routine in neonatal hypocalcaemia, and if hypomagnesaemia is the cause plasma magnesium concentrations are usually less than 0.5 mmol/L.

Permanent hypocalcaemia may be caused by congenital hypoparathyroidism. Isolated absence of the parathyroid glands may be inherited in an X-linked or autosomal recessive fashion. Hypoplasia or aplasia of the parathyroid glands also occurs as part of the di George syndrome, which classically occurs in association with conotruncal heart defects (e.g. Fallot's tetralogy) or aortic arch abnormalities and T-cell incompetence due to a partial or absent thymus. There is an overlap with the velocardiofacial syndrome [2], which includes dysmorphic facies and palatal insufficiency or a cleft. Many affected infants have interstitial chromosome deletions at 22q11. In this condition, partial hypoparathyroidism can be seen with evidence of transient hypocalcaemia in the neonatal period and recurrence of symptomatic hypocalcaemia in later childhood [3]. Although most cases of di George syndrome are the result of *de novo* deletions, autosomal dominant inheritance is not uncommon.

Congenital hypoparathyroidism has been reported in association with other developmental anomalies. In Kenny–Caffey syndrome, it is associated with growth retardation, medullary stenosis of the long bones and delayed closure of the anterior fontanelle. Richardson and Kirk [4] first described a new syndrome in which four children who were products of consanguineous marriages of Middle Eastern parents had hypoparathyroidism in association with failure to thrive, mental retardation and dysmorphic features. This syndrome is inherited in an autosomal recessive manner and has been linked to a locus on chromosome 1q42–q43, as has Kenny–Caffey syndrome [5], suggesting a common founder mutation. Another autosomal recessive syndrome occurring in a highly consanguineous Muslim family has been reported in which renal insufficiency, mental and growth retardation occurred in combination with congenital hypoparathy-

roidism. A genetic abnormality involving the PTH gene on chromosome 11 has been excluded in this disorder [6].

Treatment of neonatal hypocalcaemia depends on symptoms, duration and aetiology. Emergency treatment of hypocalcaemia causing tetany or seizures consists of a slow intravenous injection of 10% calcium gluconate (1–3 mL). Maintenance therapy is then usually provided as either an intravenous infusion containing 1 mmol/kg/24 h or oral calcium supplements. Hypomagnesaemia should be treated with 50% magnesium sulphate intravenously or intramuscularly in a dose of 0.1–0.2 mL/kg. Infants with primary defects in magnesium metabolism require long-term oral magnesium supplements. Congenital hypoparathyroidism requires the administration of a vitamin D analogue, such as alfacalcidol or calcitriol in a dose of 30–50 ng/kg/day.

## Childhood hypocalcaemia

### Disorders of vitamin D metabolism

Any of the causes of vitamin D deficiency or disturbance of its metabolism may result in hypocalcaemia, although this may not be prolonged because of secondary hyperparathyroidism restoring the plasma calcium to normal. In some cases of vitamin D deficiency, particularly in infants in the first 6 months of life born to vitamin D-deficient mothers and adolescents with vitamin D deficiency, symptomatic hypocalcaemia is seen before the clinical manifestation of rickets.

#### *Rickets*

Rickets can be defined as the process that results in defective mineralization of the growth plate; it occurs only in growing children. Osteomalacia, which describes defective mineralization of cortical and trabecular bone, occurs in adults and also in children in association with rickets. Both processes lead to an accumulation of unmineralized osteoid throughout the skeleton. Rickets and osteomalacia can be subdivided into those processes that arise primarily from calciopenia or phosphopenia (Table 23.2).

#### *Calciopenic rickets*
##### Calcium deficiency
Rickets secondary to an isolated deficiency of calcium in the presence of a normal vitamin D supply is rare but has been described in black children from Nigeria and South Africa living on a predominantly maize-based diet with negligible milk intake. These children have usually had 25-hydroxyvitamin D concentrations within the normal range, and calcium, with or without vitamin D supplement, may be more effective than vitamin D alone in healing rickets.

##### Vitamin D deficiency
Vitamin D deficiency remains the single largest cause of rickets worldwide. Although its incidence has declined

**Table 23.2.** Classification of rickets

| Calciopenic rickets | Phosphopenic rickets |
| --- | --- |
| Dietary calcium deficiency | |
| Vitamin D deficiency | *Reduced intake* |
| Vitamin D deficiency<br>    Secondary to malabsorption<br>    Liver disease<br>    Renal insufficiency | Prematurity<br>TPN*, phosphate binders<br><br>*Renal tubular loss*<br>(a) Hypophosphataemic<br>        X linked |
| Vitamin D-dependent rickets<br>    Type I—1α hydroxylase defect<br><br>    Type II—end-organ resistance | Autosomal dominant<br>Hypercalciuric<br>Sporadic<br>(b) Fanconi syndrome, e.g. cystinosis<br>(c) Oncogenic osteomalacia |

*Total parenteral nutrition.

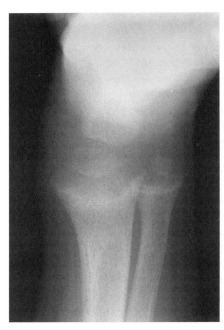

**Fig. 23.1.** Radiographic changes of vitamin D deficiency rickets.

dramatically in developed countries in the past century, it still occurs, particularly in certain ethnic minority groups or secondary to unusual infant diets with limited vitamin D content. Vitamin $D_3$ produced in the skin by the action of sunlight and vitamin $D_2$ from food have equal biological potency. Vitamin $D_2$ or $D_3$ added to milk (400 IU/L) and other foods has resulted in the virtual elimination of rickets in countries where this practice is routine. Rickets, however, remains a major health problem in many developing countries, even where there is plentiful sunlight. This appears to be secondary to cultural practices among ethnic groups who avoid sunlight exposure. There is evidence of a significant association between the presence of rickets and pneumonia in young children in developing countries.

In the United Kingdom, a significant resurgence of vitamin D deficiency rickets occurred in the 1970s in children of Asian immigrants. This was felt to a be a consequence of both limited sunlight exposure and dietary deficiency and its incidence declined significantly after a nationwide public health campaign. This problem is recurring as a consequence of failing to ensure that pregnant women and young children receive vitamin D supplements. Other groups of infants reported to be at risk are those who have been exclusively breastfed for prolonged periods and those fed macrobiotic or vegan diets.

In vitamin D deficiency, there is reduced intestinal calcium absorption, decreased extracellular calcium leading to defective mineralization and secondary hyperparathyroidism. Biochemical findings are usually low or normal serum calcium concentrations and high serum parathyroid hormone concentrations, leading to decreased tubular reabsorption of phosphate, aminoaciduria and low serum phosphate. There is evidence of increased bone turnover with

high concentrations of alkaline phosphatase. Serum concentrations of 25-hydroxyvitamin D are usually low (< 8 ng/mL) but may be normal if there has been recent exposure to vitamin D. Concentrations of 1,25-dihydroxyvitamin D are usually normal or within the low normal range. Occasionally, elevated concentrations of serum phosphate can be seen in the face of secondary hyperparathyroidism, which has been interpreted as a defective renal responsiveness to PTH.

Three stages of vitamin D deficiency rickets can be identified. Stage I arises from impaired intestinal calcium absorption and calcium resorption from bone leading to hypocalcaemia. Although this stage probably lasts only a few days before stage II, it may be prolonged, leading to symptomatic hypocalcaemia in infants aged 2–9 months. In stage II, serum calcium is normal, but a low serum phosphate appears as a consequence of secondary hyperparathyroidism. In stage III, hypocalcaemia recurs as a consequence of insufficient mobilization of calcium from bone and, at this point, the bone disease is severe. In clinical practice it is often difficult to distinguish these stages. There is also evidence that elevated concentrations of 1,25-dihydroxyvitamin D can exacerbate vitamin D deficiency by metabolic inactivation of 25-hydroxyvitamin D in the liver.

Radiological features appear at the growth plate, and radiographs of the knee or wrist (Fig. 23.1) are the most useful for detecting early changes. There is widening of the radiolucent space between the metaphyses and epiphyses as a consequence of the accumulation of uncalcified cartilage. With increasing severity of rickets, the metaphyses show fraying and cupping or lateral spreading forming cortical spurs. The centres of ossification may be pale and irregular and their appearance may be delayed. The shafts of the long bones usually show reduced density with thin cortices and may show deformity, particularly bowing of the tibiae and femora.

The clinical features depend on the age of the child at onset. In the first year of life, the enlargement of the extremities of the long bones, particularly wrists and ankles and costochondral junctions in the thorax ('rachitic rosary') are palpable and visible. There may be a Harrison sulcus due to the inward pull of the diaphragm on softened lower ribs. Examination of the skull may show craniotabes, a sign of poor mineralization with softening of the occipital area, enlarged sutures and delayed closure of the fontanelles.

After the first year of life, the effects of weight bearing become evident in the legs resulting in genu varum (bow legs) or genu valgum (knock knees). Development of the teeth is frequently impaired, with delayed eruption and enamel hypoplasia. This is a useful distinguishing feature from hypophosphataemic rickets, where early tooth development is normal. Non-skeletal manifestations include hypocalcaemia, presenting as convulsions, tetany, stridor and cardiomyopathy. Delayed motor development with evidence of hypotonia and a proximal myopathy is often present in infants. Older children may complain of bone pain and fatigue. Evidence of an associated iron deficiency anaemia is often seen in infants. Adolescents may present with hypocalcaemic symptoms, particularly tetany, with few radiological or biochemical signs of rickets because of increased vitamin D requirements during puberty.

The treatment of vitamin D deficiency should be with oral vitamin D (chole- or ergocalciferol) in doses ranging from 2000 IU daily for 6 months or 5000 IU daily for 2 months. This will lead to much more rapid resolution of hypocalcaemia and healing of rickets than vitamin D analogues such as alfacalcidol. Single large oral doses of 200–600 000 IU per day have also been used where there is concern regarding compliance. Calcium supplements are often required initially, particularly if there is hypocalcaemia.

The first radiological sign of healing rickets is the appearance within a few weeks of a radiodense line adjacent to the metaphyses representing calcified cartilage. Dense metaphyseal zones of calcification often persist for 2–3 years. Bowing of long bones usually resolves but may take several years; orthopaedic treatment is seldom required. Prevention of vitamin D deficiency in susceptible children is important, and regular sunlight exposure will often achieve this. However, all breast-fed infants should receive vitamin D supplementation of 400 IU/day, and it is recommended that Asian children should receive this supplement for the first 5 years of life. It is also important that Asian women, who are particularly susceptible to vitamin D deficiency, receive vitamin D supplements during pregnancy.

### Malabsorption, liver and renal disease

There are a number of conditions associated with malabsorption that may impair vitamin D metabolism with low concentrations of 25-hydroxyvitamin D. These include coeliac disease, cystic fibrosis and inflammatory bowel disease. However, in practice, rickets in association with these conditions is rare, and they are more likely to be associated with reduced bone density. Rickets may follow the introduction of a gluten-free diet for coeliac disease if vitamin D supplements are not also provided.

Abnormal liver function can cause rickets, which may be the first presenting feature of liver disease in some children. The aetiology is probably due to a combination of failure of 25-hydroxylation and reduced absorption of dietary vitamin D due to disruption in the enterohepatic circulation. The contribution of a lack of 25-hydroxylation is debatable as many children with rickets and liver disease show healing with alfacalcidol, which requires 25-hydroxylation for conversion to the active metabolite 1,25-dihydroxyvitamin D. An inborn error of bile acid synthesis presenting as rickets has been described.

Chronic renal failure causes impairment of 1α-hydroxylation, leading to rickets as part of renal osteodystrophy. Other disturbances of mineral metabolism include phosphate retention, secondary hyperparathyroidism and renal tubular acidosis. Disturbance of mineral metabolism tends to occur once the glomerular filtration rate drops below 30 mL/min/ 1.73 m$^2$. Appropriate treatment is with alfacalcidol or calcitriol in combination with phosphate binders such as calcium carbonate.

### Vitamin D-dependent rickets type I

This rare form of rickets inherited in an autosomal recessive manner presents between the ages of 4 and 12 months with manifestations similar to vitamin D deficiency rickets. Concentrations of 25-hydroxyvitamin D are normal but 1,25-dihydroxyvitamin D concentrations are low, indicating a defect in 1α-hydroxylase activity in the kidney. The mutation causing the disease was initially mapped to chromosome 12q14 by linkage analysis from a large number of affected families in Quebec. The gene for 1α-hydroxylase was cloned in 1997 and mutations identified in affected individuals [7]. Treatment of the condition is with either calcitriol or alfacalcidol. Once a suitable dose has been found, requirements remain stable for many years. Women with this form of rickets can undergo pregnancy uneventfully leading to the birth of normal children. Oral calcium supplements are required from the sixth month of pregnancy in addition to vitamin D therapy.

### Vitamin D-dependent rickets type II

This condition, first described in 1978, consists of rickets and/ or osteomalacia, no evidence of vitamin D or calcium deficiency and hypocalcaemia with secondary hyperparathyroidism.

There is no response to physiological doses of vitamin D and serum concentrations of 1,25-dihydroxyvitamin D are high. There is considerable heterogeneity in expression of the condition, which has been described in fewer than 50 kindreds. Parental consanguinity and multiple siblings with the same defect suggest an autosomal recessive inheritance. Most cases have originated from close to the Mediterranean, although some kindreds from Japan have been reported.

The metabolic bone disease usually becomes apparent by 2 years of age, but late onset has been reported in some individuals with mild forms of the disease. About two-thirds of the kindreds have alopecia, which can vary from sparse hair to total alopecia without eyelashes, which becomes apparent within a few months of birth. The presence of alopecia tends to indicate a more severe form of the disease as judged by age at presentation and response to treatment. Successful treatment of the bone disease does not lead to improvement of hair growth.

Patients with this condition have end-organ resistance to 1,25-dihydroxyvitamin D, as a result of receptor or postreceptor defects. The cloning and sequencing of the human vitamin D receptor gene has led to a clearer understanding of the potential abnormalities leading to the clinical phenotype [8]. Three different classes of intracellular defect have been identified based on studies of hormone–receptor nuclear interaction.

These are:

1 hormone-binding defects, including a decreased capacity of binding sites, decreased hormone binding affinity or a complete absence of hormone binding;

2 normal hormone binding to receptors but failure of localization of 1,25-dihydroxyvitamin D to nuclei;

3 normal or near-normal binding to receptors and to nuclei but decreased affinity of the hormone receptor complex to heterologous DNA (postreceptor defect).

The location and nature of the defect characterizes the response of individual patients to vitamin D therapy. Those with decreased hormone binding affinity respond to high doses of vitamin D or its metabolites, whereas those with complete absence of hormone binding do not show a response. Individuals with deficient nuclear localization respond to high dose vitamin D, whereas those with a postreceptor defect do not.

Treatment has to consist of a therapeutic trial of high doses of vitamin D or its analogues to ensure high concentrations of 1,25-dihydroxyvitamin D. This often requires doses of alfacalcidol or calcitriol of 30–60 μg daily. Supplemental calcium (up to 3 g per day) and treatment of between 3 and 6 months sufficient to mineralize depleted bones is required. Failure of therapy is indicated by absence of biochemical or radiological improvement. Individuals who do not show a therapeutic response to high-dose vitamin D may benefit from high-dose oral calcium or intracaval infusions of calcium, indicating that clinical remission may be achieved by calcium administration even in the patients most resistant to vitamin D.

**Table 23.3.** Hypophosphataemic rickets classification

Primary
  X-linked dominant
  Autosomal dominant
  Autosomal recessive
  Hereditary hypophosphataemia with hypercalciuria

Secondary
  Oncogenic osteomalacia
  Fibrous dysplasia
  Ifosfamide nephrotoxicity
  Fanconi syndrome

*Phosphopenic rickets*

There are acquired and congenital forms of hypophosphataemia leading to the development of rickets (Table 23.3). The most frequent of the inherited forms is X-linked dominant hypophosphataemic rickets originally described by Albright *et al.* [9] in 1937 under the term 'vitamin D-resistant rickets'. Its frequency is reported to be 1 in 20 000. The classic triad, which is fully expressed in hemizygous males, consists of hypophosphataemia, lower limb deformities and stunted growth rate.

Isolated hypophosphataemia can be found in some heterozygous females with no other manifestations.

There are three pathophysiological defects in this condition: impaired tubular reabsorption of phosphate in the proximal nephron, a relative deficiency of 1,25-dihydroxyvitamin D synthesis and a defect in osteoblast function. Although affected individuals have concentrations of 1,25-dihydroxyvitamin D within the normal range, this is inappropriate in the face of hypophosphataemia, which would usually stimulate extra synthesis of this metabolite. Studies in both humans and the animal model, the Hyp mouse, indicate that defective bone formation in this condition is linked to an intrinsic osteoblast defect. On bone histology there are characteristic hypomineralized periosteocytic lesions that never completely disappear, even after treatment has produced mineralization at the endosteal surfaces of bone.

The gene for X-linked hypophosphataemic rickets was identified in 1995 [10] and called the *PHEX* gene (*p*hosphate regulating gene with *h*omologies to *e*ndopeptidases on the *X* chromosome). It codes for a protein of the endopeptidase family, which degrades or activates peptide hormones. The precise role of *PHEX* is still unclear but it probably activates or inactivates a hormone that would normally regulate renal phosphate handling and 1,25-dihydroxyvitamin D concentrations. Recent evidence strongly suggests that such a factor is produced by osteoblasts.

In the absence of a family history, affected children are usually identified by the presence of bowed legs in the second year of life with a characteristic waddling gait. The legs are more severely affected than the arms, ribs or pelvis, which are

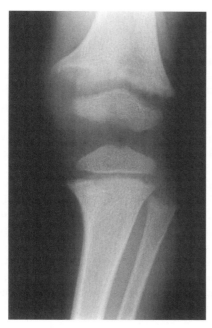

**Fig. 23.2.** Radiographic changes of hypophosphataemic rickets.

the sites more affected in calciopenic forms of rickets. There is often bowing of the femora in the anteroposterior as well as lateral planes, which may result in the patient adopting an exaggerated lordotic posture to compensate.

Radiological features include flared metaphyses with frayed borders and cupping, particularly in untreated infants. In older children, the radiological changes are prominent only in the legs (Fig. 23.2). A characteristic wedge-shaped defect of the medial surface of the proximal tibia is seen in patients with genu varum deformity, thought to be due to increased weight bearing on the medial aspect of the knee. There is an absence of the associated osteopenia seen in calciopenic rickets. Studies of bone density of the spine in affected individuals using absorptiometry techniques suggest that it is normal or increased. However, this may relate to the technique, as quantitative computerized tomography (QCT) assessment shows low cortical bone density.

Dental abscesses are frequent in affected children and adults due to enlargement of the central pulp chambers of the teeth with associated irregularities in interglobular dentine. As a consequence, there is a diminished barrier on the exterior of the teeth so that substances can more easily pass through the outer enamel layer to the pulp cavity initiating abscess formation.

The object of treatment is to prevent bone deformity and promote normal growth without incurring treatment-related complications. Adequate control of rickets early in life can usually prevent the need for orthopaedic surgery to correct deformity of the legs. Current optimal therapy is with a combination of phosphate supplements (70–100 mg/kg/day)

and an active vitamin D analogue, such as alfacalcidol or calcitriol (10–50 ng/kg/day).

The phosphate supplements need to be given in four or five divided daily doses. Biochemical monitoring should be undertaken at most clinic visits, which need to be frequent during rapid infantile and pubertal growth. Measurements should include plasma calcium, phosphate and alkaline phosphatase with serum PTH and urine calcium–creatinine ratio on a fasting morning urine sample. Radiographs of the bones should be performed every 1–2 years to assess rachitic activity, and renal ultrasound should be performed every 2 years to look for evidence of nephrocalcinosis.

Random measurements of plasma phosphate are not particularly helpful as they are influenced by the time since the last dose of phosphate. Measurement of alkaline phosphatase may be a guide to underlying rachitic activity, but it is not a sensitive indicator. Clinical assessment of growth and examination of the legs for improvement in the degree of bowing are as important as biochemical measurements.

It is important to keep a balance between the dosage of phosphate and the vitamin D analogue as large doses of phosphate cause secondary hyperparathyroidism. If there is evidence of hyperparathyroidism without evidence of hypercalcaemia, an increase in the dosage of the vitamin D analogue alone is indicated. Evidence of hypercalcaemia and/or hypercalciuria with a normal PTH should prompt a reduction in the dose of vitamin D. The combination of hypercalcaemia and hyperparathyroidism suggests the development of autonomous hyperparathyroidism.

The three main complications of treatment are:
1 Vitamin D intoxication, which is characterized by hypercalcaemia and hypercalciuria. Its occurrence is now much reduced with the use of vitamin D analogues that have a shorter half-life and are not stored in body fat.
2 Autonomous hyperparathyroidism, which may occur with persistent stimulation of the parathyroid glands. This is usually a consequence of high oral doses of phosphate causing transient falls in plasma calcium concentration, thus stimulating PTH secretion. Parathyroid surgery may be required, which can be followed by severe hypocalcaemia as a consequence of hungry bone disease. It is important therefore to monitor serum PTH at least every 6 months and increase the dose of vitamin D if PTH is elevated in the presence of normocalcaemia.
3 Medullary nephrocalcinosis, which is a common finding in treated patients with X-linked hypophosphataemic rickets (XLHR) and clearly a treatment-related effect, as untreated patients do not show it. It has been reported in 50–80% of patients. Early studies suggested a link between its presence and the occurrence of hypercalciuria. However, later research has shown a close relationship to the concentration of urinary phosphate excretion and therefore the dose of oral phosphate. One study implicated high urinary oxalate excretion as a consequence of oral phosphate, postulating that the

deposits were calcium oxalate. However, histological studies in affected children and the Hyp mouse have shown that they consist of calcium phosphate. Despite its common occurrence there is little evidence to indicate that nephrocalcinosis causes long-term deterioration of renal function.

Another occasional complication is craniosynostosis. It is not clear whether this may be treatment related or due to the underlying disease. It may be more common in boys.

Other therapeutic manoeuvres have been tried, including the use of a thiazide diuretic in combination with amiloride, which has been shown to increase tubular reabsorption of phosphate in short-term studies; no long-term benefits have been reported. Growth hormone has been studied to try to improve tubular phosphate reabsorption and growth retardation. An initial 6-month study demonstrated an increase in serum phosphate concentrations and growth velocity. Longer-term studies have demonstrated an improvement in growth velocity, but the effect on tubular reabsorption of phosphate is not sustained beyond a few months. There are no studies showing improvement in final height in treated patients, and there is no advantage over the standard therapeutic regimen. The use of an alternative vitamin D analogue, 24,25-dihydroxyvitamin D, has also been investigated and shown in one study to produce better control of hyperparathyroidism than does standard treatment.

It is debatable whether the demanding treatment regimen should be continued beyond cessation of growth. One study has shown beneficial effects of continuing combined treatment on bone mineralization, but long-term compliance with regular phosphate administration is doubtful. The use of a vitamin D analogue alone may be reasonable, although benefit remains to be demonstrated. Potential problems in affected adults include decreased joint mobility and spinal cord compression from bony outgrowths.

*Differential diagnosis*

Autosomal dominant and recessive forms of hypophosphataemic rickets have been described. Hypophosphataemic bone disease is a condition that is autosomal dominant or sporadic. Affected individuals present with short stature, bowing of the legs and evidence of osteomalacia but with minimal or absent changes of rickets at the growth plate. Hypophosphataemia and a low $T_mPO_4/GFR$ are present. Treatment is with calcitriol alone, without additional phosphate.

Another rare condition to be distinguished is autosomal recessive hypophosphataemic rickets with hypercalciuria. Affected individuals show an appropriate elevation in 1,25-dihydroxyvitamin D in response to hypophosphataemia and often have hypercalciuria. Asymptomatic family members have isolated hypercalciuria, whereas others have rickets and osteomalacia. Treatment is with phosphate supplements alone, which will heal the rickets and correct the hypercalciuria.

A rare acquired form of hypophosphataemic rickets with similarity to XLHR is oncogenic osteomalacia in which tumours (usually of mesenchymal origin) secrete a substance that impairs renal phosphate handling and causes low concentrations of 1,25-dihydroxyvitamin D. Clinical and biochemical abnormalities reverse on removal of the tumour. There is *in vivo* and *in vitro* evidence that tumour extracts cause phosphaturia and reduced activity of 1α-hydroxylase consistent with a peptide hormone. This condition should be considered in all patients with hypophosphataemic rickets presenting in late childhood or adulthood.

Renal phosphate wasting and rickets that respond to treatment with phosphate supplements and a vitamin D analogue have been described in McCune–Albright syndrome. Rickets secondary to hypophosphataemia is part of the generalized proximal tubular disturbance seen in Fanconi syndrome secondary to hereditary disorders such as cystinosis and tyrosinaemia. A similar acquired pattern is seen secondary to toxic change from heavy metals or ifosfamide chemotherapy.

Distal renal tubular acidosis is a condition where there is a defect in hydrogen ion excretion. The metabolic acidosis induces increased bone resorption and hypercalciuria with decreased proximal tubular phosphate reabsorption. Correction of the acidosis with sodium bicarbonate leads to normalization of these abnormalities.

Poor dietary intake of phosphate is thought to account for the majority of what is termed 'osteopenia of prematurity'. This is seen particularly in very low-birthweight babies fed with human milk, which has a low phosphate content. It may also occur as a consequence of prolonged parenteral nutrition. Phosphate supplementation has markedly reduced the incidence of this problem.

Another rare but documented form of hypophosphataemic rickets is secondary to inappropriate ingestion of phosphate-binding antacid preparations, which impair intestinal phosphate absorption.

## Hypomagnesaemia

This is an uncommon but important cause of hypocalcaemia, which causes resistance to therapy with vitamin D and calcium. Plasma magnesium concentrations are less than 0.5 mmol/L. The pathogenesis is due to impaired secretion of parathyroid hormone. However, high concentrations of parathyroid hormone have sometimes been seen, suggesting a resistance to action at bone and kidney. There are two primary disorders that cause hypomagnesaemia, a selective defect in magnesium absorption from the small intestine and a renal tubular leak of magnesium. They can be distinguished by measuring urine magnesium excretion using the magnesium–creatinine ratio, which will be low if due to a gastrointestinal defect and high if due to a renal tubular leak.

Primary hypomagnesaemia is usually due to a selective defect in intestinal absorption. This occurs in highly consanguineous families and appears to be autosomal recessive. Children usually present in infancy and can be treated with oral magnesium supplements, which restores normocalcaemia, even though magnesium concentrations remain outside the normal range. Hypomagnesaemia may be secondary to malabsorption or to renal tubular damage as a consequence of cytotoxic drugs such as cisplatinum or the prolonged use of aminoglycoside antibiotics. Symptomatic hypomagnesaemia requires treatment with intramuscular or intravenous infusion of 50% magnesium sulphate 0.1–0.2 mL/kg. Long-term oral magnesium supplements containing between 0.7 and 3.5 mmol/kg/day of elemental magnesium are required for those with an intestinal absorption defect.

## Hypoparathyroidism

The causes of hypoparathyroidism can be broadly classified into:
1 failure of parathyroid gland development;
2 destruction of the parathyroid glands; or
3 reduced parathyroid gland function due to altered regulation.

The biochemical abnormalities are hypocalcaemia and hyperphosphataemia in the presence of normal renal function. Serum concentrations of parathyroid hormone are low or undetectable and alkaline phosphatase activity is unchanged. Decreased 1,25-dihydroxyvitamin D production causes reduced intestinal calcium absorption and reduced parathyroid hormone secretion causes decreased bone resorption and deficient tubular reabsorption of calcium. The latter is not corrected by vitamin D and therefore there is a risk of hypercalciuria with the development of nephrocalcinosis.

Acute symptoms of hypocalcaemia include tetany and convulsions. Positive Chvostek and Trousseau signs may detect latent tetany. Chvostek sign can be elicited by tapping the facial nerve anterior to the ear, to produce a twitching of the mouth, which may progress to include the alae nasi and orbicularis oculi muscle. Trousseau sign is elicited by inflation of a blood pressure cuff above systolic pressure for 3 min to produce carpopedal spasm. Convulsions may be generalized or focal and may lead to the misdiagnosis of epilepsy. Chronic symptoms and signs include cataracts, intracranial calcification, particularly of the basal ganglia, and papilloedema. Mental retardation and poor school performance may be a consequence of chronic hypocalcaemia. Enamel hypoplasia and increased liability to caries can also be present.

### Failure of development of the parathyroid gland

Agenesis or hypoplasia of the parathyroid glands may be isolated or associated with other developmental problems. Most present in the neonatal period. Syndromes include the HDR syndrome, in which autosomal dominant *h*ypoparathyroidism occurs in conjunction with sensorineural *d*eafness and dysplastic kidneys (*r*enal disease). Hypoparathyroidism

and nerve deafness may occur in conjunction with nephrotic syndrome. A deletion on the short arm of chromosome 10 has also been reported in some children with hypoparathyroidism and a T-cell immune defect [11] similar to that seen in di George syndrome. Hypoparathyroidism is a variable component of neuromyopathies caused by mitochondrial gene defects, such as Kearns Sayre syndrome and mitochondrial encephalomyopathy. An inborn error fatty acid oxidation (long-chain hydroxyacyl coenzyme A dehydrogenase deficiency) may also be accompanied by hypoparathyroidism.

### Parathyroid gland destruction

This may occur as a consequence of surgery to the neck, particularly thyroidectomy, or after parathyroid gland surgery for primary or tertiary hyperparathyroidism. It may also be a consequence of iron overload due to repeated blood transfusions in children with thalassaemia.

Autoimmune destruction is probably the commonest cause of acquired hypoparathyroidism in childhood. It may be sporadic but is more likely to be autosomal recessive in inheritance as part of autoimmune polyendocrinopathy type 1. This condition, known as APECED (*a*utoimmune *p*olyendocrinopathy *c*andidiasis *e*ctodermal *d*ystrophy) [12], usually manifests initially as chronic mucocutaneous candidiasis due to a defect in cellular immunity. Hypoparathyroidism is often the second manifestation and usually presents in midchildhood, followed by adrenal insufficiency after several years in at least 70% of affected individuals. The initial sign of adrenal insufficiency may be the development of hypercalcaemia in a child who has been stable on therapy with a vitamin D analogue for hypoparathyroidism. This is probably due to an effect on tubular reabsorption of calcium as a consequence of the hypovolaemia induced by mineralocorticoid deficiency. Any child with acquired idiopathic hypoparathyroidism should be under regular surveillance for the later development of adrenal insufficiency. There can be discordance of months to years in the time of onset of cortisol and aldosterone deficiency. Therefore, assessment by measurement of plasma renin activity is necessary, as well as repeated Synacthen tests.

Other endocrine manifestations, which may continue to occur up to the fifth decade of life, include hypogonadism, diabetes mellitus and hypothyroidism. Associated features include a characteristic pitted-nail dystrophy (Fig. 23.3), keratopathy, alopecia, intestinal malabsorption and hepatitis. The genetic defect underlying the condition was localized to chromosome 21q22.3 and subsequently the autoimmune regulator gene (*AIRE-1*) was identified [13]. The precise role of *AIRE-1* in regulating immune responses is unknown, but it appears to act as a transcription factor.

A variety of different mutations in this gene has been identified in affected families, offering the opportunity for screening siblings of affected individuals to determine whether they are at risk of developing the condition.

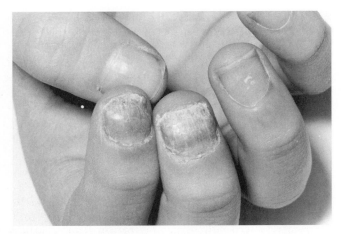

**Fig. 23.3.** Characteristic nail dystrophy in a child with APECED.

*Reduced parathyroid gland function due to altered regulation*
Parathyroid gland function may be altered secondary to hypomagnesaemia and maternal hyperparathyroidism. Primary alterations of parathyroid gland regulation have been identified to have a genetic basis due to deletions in the PTH gene on chromosome 11p15. This has been reported to occur in isolated hypoparathyroidism and in a family with autosomal recessive hypoparathyroidism who had a donor splice-site mutation in exon 2 of the PTH gene.

The largest group in this category includes individuals who have activating mutations involving the calcium-sensing receptor (CaR) gene on chromosome 3q [14]. Inactivating mutations of the CaR were previously recognized to cause familial hypocalciuric hypercalcaemia [15]. The converse (autosomal dominant hypocalcaemia with hypercalciuria, ADH) was then identified to be due to activating mutations of this receptor. In this situation, the receptor has a decreased set point for extracellular calcium concentrations with suppressed parathyroid hormone secretion; in conjunction with a lowered threshold for renal tubular calcium reabsorption, this leads to hypercalciuria. In families in which it has been identified, the picture is one of autosomal dominant hypoparathyroidism. The serum phosphate tends to be increased, the serum magnesium may be low and serum PTH is usually within the normal range.

Of the 20 affected family members identified in the initial six kindreds, 8 of 16 had impaired renal function at subsequent review and 11 of 20 had nephrocalcinosis. The renal damage could not be explained by the induction of hypercalcaemia and suggested that these patients are particularly susceptible to hypercalciuria-induced renal damage that is thus caused predominantly by the treatment. As the initial studies, sporadic cases and cases with low or undetectable PTH have been reported. As a result, the distinction between ADH and hypoparathyroidism has become extremely difficult. In many subjects, no treatment is required and they remain asymptomatic, despite low plasma calcium. Others, who develop symptoms of hypocalcaemia, require low doses of vitamin D analogues to produce a slight rise in plasma calcium to control these symptoms. Close monitoring of urinary calcium excretion is essential, with regular renal ultrasound to detect nephrocalcinosis at an early stage. As only 80% of cases have so far been identified to have an abnormality of the CaR gene, analysis of the gene cannot be relied upon to detect new cases.

*Treatment of hypoparathyroidism*
Acute hypocalcaemia requires a slow intravenous injection of 10% calcium gluconate 1–2 mL/kg every 6–8 h. Maintenance therapy is usually with either alfacalcidol or calcitriol in a starting dose of 25–50 ng/kg/day. Calcium supplements 0.5–1 g/day are often required, at least initially, to restore normocalcaemia. The plasma calcium should be maintained in the low normal range (2.0–2.25 mmol/L) to prevent the development of hypercalciuria, which may occur with a normal plasma calcium due to the deficient hypocalciuric effect of PTH on renal calcium reabsorption. Urinary calcium should be monitored on a regular basis, aiming to maintain the urine calcium/creatinine ratio within the normal range of 0–0.7 mmol/mmol. If hypercalcaemia occurs, it can be rapidly reversed by discontinuing the vitamin D metabolite for several days and recommencing at a lower dose. If hypercalciuria occurs despite a low normal plasma calcium, the addition of a thiazide diuretic is often useful.

Hypercalcaemia may develop in women and girls with hypoparathyroidism who have been on stable vitamin D doses as a consequence of oestrogen deficiency. This is probably due to the uninhibited action of 1,25-dihydroxyvitamin D on bone resorption, which is normally counterbalanced by the inhibitory effect of oestrogen.

**Pseudohypoparathyroidism** (Table 23.4)

This condition is characterized by biochemical hypoparathyroidism (hypocalcaemia and hyperphosphataemia) and increased secretion of parathyroid hormone with target tissue unresponsiveness. The initial event in the expression of PTH action is binding of the hormone to the PTH/PTHrP

**Table 23.4.** Classification of pseudohypoparathyroidism

| Type | Gs$_\alpha$ activity | AHO phenotype | PTH resistance |
| --- | --- | --- | --- |
| Ia | Reduced | + | + |
| Ib | Normal | – | + |
| Ic | Normal | + | + |
| II | Normal | – | + |
| Pseudo Pseudo | Reduced | + | – |

(parathyroid hormone-related peptide) receptor on the plasma membrane of target cells. This receptor is coupled by a G-protein to signal effector molecules on the inner surface of the plasma membrane. Hormone binding is followed by the generation of a second messenger.

Characterization of the molecular basis for pseudohypoparathyroidism (PHP) started with the observation that affected individuals showed a blunted urinary cAMP (cyclic adenosine monophosphate) response to administered PTH, as well as a failure of the expected phosphaturic response. PTH infusion remains a useful test for confirming the diagnosis of PHP and may be based on plasma cAMP rather than on urinary measurements. Normal individuals show a 10- to 20-fold increment in plasma or urinary cAMP, with an associated increase in urinary phosphate. Individuals with PHP type I fail to show an increase in cAMP and phosphate, whereas those with the less common type II form show a normal cAMP response with an impaired phosphaturic response.

*PHP type Ia and pseudopseudohypoparathyroidism*
Patients with PHP type Ia manifest a collection of features referred to as Albright's hereditary osteodystrophy (AHO). This phenotype consists of short stature, round facies, obesity, shortening of the fourth and fifth metacarpals and metatarsals. Subcutaneous calcification is also often a feature and may be the initial manifestation. Short stature is reported in 39% of patients below the age of 18 years and in 62% of adults. Mental retardation has been reported in at least 50% of patients with AHO, but may range from moderately severe delay to entirely normal educational ability. The characteristic hand changes, with shortening of the fourth and fifth metacarpals (Fig. 23.4) may not be apparent until at least 4 years of age. A short, broad thumbnail is a frequent additional manifestation. Intracranial calcification, particularly of the basal ganglia, is commonly seen and calcification has also been reported in the ventricular septum. Sensorineural

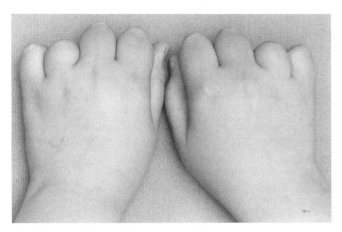

**Fig. 23.4.** Hands in pseudohypoparathyroidism type Ia.

hearing loss has also been identified in some patients, as has an impaired sense of smell. Resistance to other hormones mediated by cAMP is a recognized feature, particularly hypothyroidism secondary to TSH (thyroid-stimulating hormone) resistance and gonadal dysfunction, particularly menstrual irregularity.

The critical importance of the G-protein in this disorder was first recognized in 1980, when it was shown that the activity of the $\alpha$-subunit of this protein, $GS_\alpha$, in erythrocyte membranes was reduced to 50% of normal control subjects [16]. Subsequent research identified this $GS_\alpha$ deficiency to be a result of heterozygous inactivating mutations in the *GNAS-1* gene that maps to chromosome 20q13.2 [17]. A variety of *GNAS-1* mutations has been identified in individuals with AHO accounting for the autosomal dominant inheritance of the condition.

Some 10 years after describing pseudohypoparathyroidism, Albright identified individuals with AHO who lacked hormone resistance to PTH, which he termed pseudopseudohypoparathyroidism (pseudo-PHP). Such subjects have a normal cAMP response to PTH, which distinguishes them from occasional subjects with PHP type Ia, who maintain normal plasma calcium concentrations without treatment.

Pseudo-PHP can occur in the same kindreds as individuals with PHP type Ia and a functional deficiency of $GS_\alpha$ and mutations in the *GNAS-1* gene. Indeed the same mutations have been shown to be present in members of the same family with PHP Ia and pseudo-PHP. A review of published reports of AHO led to the observation that PHP type Ia was a consequence of maternal transmission, whereas pseudo-PHP resulted from paternal transmission [18]. Genomic imprinting influencing the expression of the disorder was subsequently confirmed by identifying the parental origin of $GS_\alpha$ mutations in affected individuals [19].

Genomic imprinting of the *GNAS-1* gene alone does not fully explain the gene expression, as equivalent reductions in $GS_\alpha$ bioactivity are found in PHP Ia and pseudo-PHP in all tissues tested. It is thought that imprinting at a tissue-specific concentration could explain the findings. For example, renal tubular cells may express the maternal $GS_\alpha$ allele, whereas other cells, such as erythrocytes, express both alleles. Therefore, a mutation in the maternal allele would result in renal resistance to PTH. A paternal $GS_\alpha$ mutation would not be expressed in the imprinted cells in the renal tubules and there would be no PTH resistance. Such a theory is supported by studies of heterozygous *GNAS* knockout mice, which demonstrated that $GS_\alpha$ expression was derived only from the maternal allele in some tissues (e.g. renal cortex) and from both alleles in others (e.g. renal medulla).

*PHP type Ib*
Individuals affected by this form lack features of AHO, have normal $GS_\alpha$ activity and demonstrate hormone resistance only to PTH. Although mostly sporadic, familial cases

consistent with autosomal dominant inheritance have been described. Although they have renal resistance to PTH with a defective cAMP response to a PTH infusion, they often manifest skeletal lesions similar to those seen in hyperparathyroidism. This indicates that at least one intracellular signalling pathway coupled to the PTH receptor may be intact in patients with PHP type Ib. Although the selective resistance to PTH and normal $GS_\alpha$ activity suggested inactivating mutations of the PTH/PTHrP receptor, no mutations have been identified. Humans heterozygous for inactivation of the gene encoding the PTH/PTHrP receptor do not manifest PTH resistance, and inheritance of two defective PTH/PTHrP receptor genes results in Blomstrand's chondrodysplasia, a lethal metaphyseal chondrodysplasia. A genome-wide search from four kindreds with the disorder established linkage to a region on chromosome 20q, which contains the *GNAS-1* gene [20]. In addition, the genetic defect was shown to be imprinted paternally, and thus is inherited in the same manner as AHO.

*PHP type Ic*
This form is designated for a small proportion of individuals who have features of AHO, resistance to multiple hormones, including PTH, but who lack a demonstrable defect in $GS_\alpha$ activity. These individuals may have some other functional defect of the receptor–adenyl cyclase system.

*PHP type II*
Individuals with this form have a reduced phosphaturic response to the administration of PTH but a normal increase in cAMP. It has no clear genetic or familial basis. PTH resistance probably arises from an intracellular defect whereby cAMP fails to activate downstream targets.

It is worth noting that severe vitamin D deficiency can produce a biochemical picture similar to PHP type II in which hypocalcaemia is accompanied by hyperphosphataemia. This is probably due to an acquired dissociation between the amount of cAMP generated in the renal tubule and its effect on phosphate clearance.

## Diagnosis and treatment of pseudohypoparathyroidism

The diagnosis is apparent when an individual has hypocalcaemia, hyperphosphataemia and an elevated PTH. Hypomagnesaemia and severe vitamin D deficiency should be excluded, as they can cause a reduced response to elevated PTH. Although hypocalcaemia typically presents in midchildhood, there are several reports of neonatal hypothyroidism (elevated TSH) being the first manifestation. The diagnosis may also be considered in an individual with clinical features of AHO. However, such features as obesity and round face occur in conditions such as Prader–Willi syndrome, Turner syndrome and acrodystosis. A number of

reports have described terminal deletions of chromosome 2q in patients with variable AHO phenotypes who have normal endocrine function and $GS_\alpha$ activity.

The principles of treatment are similar to those for hypoparathyroidism, using a vitamin D analogue, such as alfacalcidol or calcitriol, to maintain the plasma calcium at the lower end of the normal range. There is less risk of hypercalciuria in PHP, and the plasma phosphate usually decreases to a high-normal concentration.

### Autosomal dominant hypocalcaemia
Inherited abnormalities of the CaR can, in addition to causing hypercalcaemia, also cause hypocalcaemia. These cases were initially identified by reviewing cases previously diagnosed as having familial hypoparathyroidism associated with hypercalciuria. Six kindreds were found where there was an inherited abnormality of CaR and where expression of the receptor in transfected cells showed the mutation to be associated with a gain of function [14]. The index cases usually presented with symptoms that could have been due to the hypocalcaemia, including carpopedal spasm and childhood seizures. A number, however, were asymptomatic, despite serum calcium values as low as 1.55 mmol/L. Because of the degree of hypocalcaemia and presumed complications in some, all affected children were treated with vitamin D or its active metabolites. Of the 20 affected family members in the initial six kindreds, 8 of 16 had impaired renal function at subsequent review and 11 of 20 had nephrocalcinosis. The renal damage could not be explained by the induction of hypercalcaemia and suggested that these patients are particularly susceptible to hypercalciuria-induced renal damage at a time when the serum calcium is still below normal. The renal damage is thus caused predominantly by the treatment.

The term autosomal dominant hypocalcaemia (ADH) has been attached to this condition. Most cases appear to have mild or no symptoms despite hypocalcaemia. The serum phosphate tends to be increased, the serum magnesium may be low and, on retesting the serum PTH, was typically normal when renal function was normal. This represents a mirror image of FBH.

Since the initial studies, sporadic cases of the syndrome have been reported as well as familial and sporadic cases with low or undetectable PTH [15]. As a result, the differentiation between ADH and hypoparathyroidism has become extremely difficult. From a practical point of view, the risk of renal damage with treatment is the greatest concern. For this reason, far greater attention needs to be directed at monitoring urinary calcium excretion to make sure that this is not increased too much. Regular renal ultrasound should be used to detect nephrocalcinosis at an early stage. Significant degrees of hypocalcaemia may have to be accepted, provided the patient is asymptomatic.

**Table 23.5.** Causes of childhood hypercalcaemia

Primary hyperparathyroidism
Tertiary hyperparathyroidism
Familial benign (hypocalciuric) hypercalcaemia (FBH)
Williams syndrome
Idiopathic infantile hypercalcaemia
Vitamin D toxicity
Hypercalcaemia of malignancy
Immobilization
Granulomatous diseases
Subcutaneous fat necrosis
Hypophosphatasia
Jansen syndrome

## Hypercalcaemia

In contrast to hypocalcaemia, hypercalcaemia is relatively uncommon in children. Symptoms are often different from the classic symptoms seen in adults. In infants, the predominant manifestation is failure to thrive often accompanied by non-specific symptoms of irritability, abdominal pain and poor feeding. Older children may manifest polydipsia and polyuria or constipation. The differential diagnosis of childhood hypercalcaemia is listed in Table 23.5.

The single key investigation is the concentration of intact parathyroid hormone in serum. This will usually be suppressed in most cases of hypercalcaemia other than primary or tertiary hyperparathyroidism and familial hypocalciuric hypercalcaemia. Assessment of urinary calcium excretion is also important as there will often be accompanying hypercalciuria with its attendant risk of nephrocalcinosis and renal impairment. If hypercalciuria is present, ultrasound will identify renal calcification.

### *Primary hyperparathyroidism*

Hyperparathyroidism is the excess production of PTH due to its autonomous production. It is rare in children. In neonates, it presents with symptoms associated with severe hypercalcaemia, marked PTH overproduction and parathyroid bone disease. Severe neonatal primary hyperparathyroidism may be a rare presentation of familial benign hypercalcaemia (FBH).

In older children, primary hyperparathyroidism can occur as a sporadic condition or within the setting of three familial endocrine disorders, multiple endocrine neoplasia types 1 (MEN1) and 2 (MEN2) or familial isolated hyperparathyroidism.

MEN1 is the combination of hyperparathyroidism, islet cell and pituitary tumours. Hyperparathyroidism is the commonest disorder and usually the first to be detected. Eighty per cent of affected family members eventually develop hyperparathyroidism, but it is extremely rare for hypercal-caemia to be clinically important before the age of 16. Most affected family members develop hypercalcaemia in the second to fourth decades. MEN1 is dominantly inherited and is due to a loss of function of the Menin gene on chromosome 11, which is a tumour-suppressor gene [21].

MEN2 involves the combination of medullary thyroid carcinoma, hyperparathyroidism and phaeochromocytoma. It is subdivided into MEN2A and 2B. MEN2A is a dominantly inherited disorder of the *RET* proto-oncogene, with most cases occurring in a known family setting. Medullary thyroid carcinoma is virtually always present, but hyperparathyroidism occurs in only 5–10% and rarely presents in childhood. MEN2B also involves defects of the *RET* proto-oncogene, but most cases are new mutations and affected patients have neuromas of the lips and conjunctivae, neurogangliomatas of the large bowel together with a more aggressive form of medullary thyroid carcinoma. Hyperparathyroidism is not a feature of this disorder.

Isolated familial hyperparathyroidism is very similar to MEN1 and can be differentiated from it only when at least three generations of an affected family have been shown not to have developed any other endocrine problems.

### Presentation

Children with hyperparathyroidism present with a variety of non-specific symptoms, particularly weakness, anorexia and irritability. Renal stones and/or nephrocalcinosis are common and the incidence of skeletal disease has been very variable (Fig. 23.5). Hypercalcaemia may be found by chance but the number of such patients is small, with the majority having symptoms or complications of the disease. This is in contradistinction to primary hyperparathyroidism in adults where the majority are asymptomatic, renal stones are

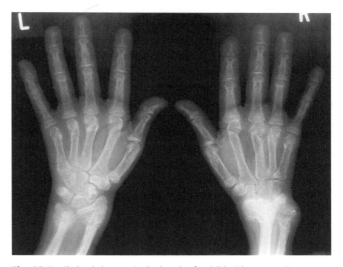

**Fig. 23.5.** Skeletal changes in the hands of a child with severe primary hyperparathyroidism.

unusual and skeletal disease very uncommon. Why hyperparathyroidism appears to be more severe in children is not clear. It resembles hyperparathyroidism reported in adult patients some 30 years ago and might simply reflect that asymptomatic children are less likely to have routine screening tests than adults.

## Diagnosis

Once hypercalcaemia is identified, the diagnosis of hyperparathyroidism should be easy. Clearly elevated values of PTH will be found in virtually all cases of primary hyperparathyroidism in children, with a few cases having values around the upper limit of normal. All other causes of non-parathyroid hypercalcaemia can be expected to have suppressed or low-normal values. The main differential diagnosis is FBH, especially in patients who have few, or no, symptoms. In FBH, the PTH concentration is usually normal or occasionally mildly elevated. Therefore, in all cases of suspected hyperparathyroidism with mild or no symptoms and where the PTH is not clearly elevated, the possibility of FBH must be considered. Measurement of the calcium–creatinine clearance ratio below 0.01 would make FBH highly likely. A value above 0.01 does not differentiate FBH from hyperparathyroidism. In such cases, family screening is advisable, especially if both parents are alive. The identification of other hypercalcaemic children makes FBH almost certain. If both parents are normocalcaemic, hyperparathyroidism is most likely. A hypercalcaemic parent makes FBH likely because familial hyperparathyroidism rarely affects children.

## Management

Hyperparathyroidism in children requires surgical management once the diagnosis is secure. Preoperative localization should be performed only if required by the surgeon and never in an attempt to make the diagnosis. In adults the most successful technique is sestamibi scanning [22]. There is little experience of its use in children. It is important to identify an experienced parathyroid surgeon. Very few paediatric surgeons are likely to have much experience of parathyroid surgery, and a combined approach, with an experienced adult parathyroid surgeon together with a paediatric surgeon, may be the preferred option. Of the reported cases, a single adenoma is by far the most common pathology, thus confirming the uncommon presentation of MEN1 in children. Removal of the single adenoma, with identification but non-removal or biopsy of the remaining parathyroids should be planned. In cases with parathyroid hyperplasia, consideration should be made of total removal of the parathyroids with autotransplantation of slices from half of one gland.

## Postoperative management

The serum calcium should have fallen to normal or near normal within 24 h. Mild hypocalcaemia is common on days 2–4 postoperatively. Profound postoperative hypocalcaemia is rare, unless more than one parathyroid is removed or there is clinical parathyroid bone disease. Hypocalcaemia should be treated with intravenous calcium and potent vitamin D metabolites – alfacalcidol or calcitriol. These will be required for only a few weeks unless permanent hypoparathyroidism has occurred.

### *Tertiary hyperparathyroidism*

This may occasionally occur in children because of chronic stimulation of parathyroid gland activity. Hypocalcaemia occurring in vitamin D deficiency, renal failure and sometimes in hypophosphataemic rickets, as a result of the effect of phosphate supplementation, stimulates PTH secretion and secondary hyperparathyroidism is the expected response. As the purpose of the PTH production is to correct the hypocalcaemia, it can be associated with normocalcaemia. Serum PTH is usually extremely high, often greater than 1500 pg/mL. If maintained, the parathyroid glands become hyperplastic. Such hyperplastic glands are susceptible to develop autonomous nodules that can lead to the inappropriate excess excretion of PTH and to the development of hypercalcaemia due to tertiary hyperparathyroidism.

Investigation may be difficult as imaging of parathyroid glands by ultrasound or isotope scanning often fails to identify an abnormality in children. Surgical intervention is usually required to debulk the parathyroid glands and requires an experienced surgeon. This may involve the removal of a single adenoma or subtotal parathyroidectomy in the presence of four-gland hyperplasia. There is a significant risk of 'hungry bone disease' postoperatively because of the sudden switching off of prolonged bone resorption leading to profound hypocalcaemia requiring intravenous calcium infusion.

### *Familial benign or hypocalciuric hypercalcaemia*

In 1966 a patient was described who was initially thought to have primary hyperparathyroidism. After a three and a half gland parathyroidectomy, the patient remained hypercalcaemic and subsequently 17 hypercalcaemic family members were identified, affecting three generations. The disorder was termed either familial hypocalciuric hypercalcaemia (FHH) or familial benign hypercalcaemia (FBH); we prefer the latter.

The disorder has a dominant inheritance with almost complete penetrance and affected members are hypercalcaemic from birth. Apart from the index case, affected family members have no signs, symptoms or complications of the condition, with the exception of a rare neonatal syndrome. An initial apparent association with acute pancreatitis has not subsequently been confirmed.

Affected family members have mild to moderate hypercalcaemia, a tendency to have a higher serum magnesium than patients with hyperparathyroidism and a lower urine calcium excretion, especially when calculated as a calcium–creatinine clearance ratio. However, although the mean values seen in FBH differ from those seen in hyperparathyroidism, there is marked overlap for all the known biochemical tests, with the exception of serum parathyroid hormone concentrations. Although initial reports suggested that parathyroid gland mass was increased, this has been suggested to be due to increased parathyroid fat mass rather than an increase in parathyroid cell mass. Early reports suggested that parathyroid hormone concentrations were often mildly increased in FBH, but the newer, sensitive two-site assays most frequently find PTH values well within the normal range.

Although the condition is benign in adults, neonates can very occasionally develop severe hypercalcaemia associated with marked parathyroid bone disease and very elevated serum PTH concentrations, a condition termed neonatal severe primary hyperparathyroidism (NSPHT). Neonates affected with this condition are symptomatic during their first week of life, failing to thrive, and they develop hypotonia, anorexia and constipation and, when severe, respiratory failure. Investigations show unequivocal severe parathyroid bone disease. Early reported cases were treated by emergency total parathyroidectomy and many made a complete recovery, causing this form of treatment to be considered essential. Gradually, however, cases began to be reported where emergency surgery was refused or conservative therapy was tried and the children survived and the parathyroid state resolved. Medical management is now the preferred option, reserving emergency surgery for those cases who fail to improve.

The vast majority of neonates who inherit the condition of FBH do not have this syndrome and have a normal neonatal period. Serum calcium may be mildly elevated, but PTH concentrations are normal and their subsequent course is uneventful. It is assumed that the cases of NSPHT that settle with conservative management revert biochemically to the more typical form of the disorder. However, to date, no detailed long-term follow-up of these cases has been reported.

Genetics

FBH is dominantly inherited and was shown to be linked, in the majority of cases, to the long arm of chromosome 3 [23]. A small number of families were linked with two separate loci on chromosome 19 while having identical clinical and biochemical features to the cases linked to chromosome 3. Of those linked to chromosome 3, 80% have an abnormality of the gene encoding the CaR. It is assumed that the remaining 20% also have, as yet unrecognized, abnormalities of this gene. The nature of the two genes on chromosome 19, which produce an identical clinical condition is, as yet, unknown.

With the identification of the genetic abnormality in most cases of FBH, it was possible to look at the different variants of the disease. Most cases are, as expected, heterozygous forms of the disorder. As a number of cases of NSPHT had two affected parents, usually within a consanguineous marriage, it was to be expected that these cases would be homozygous for the disorder and this was confirmed. However, a number of cases with only one affected parent, or where a new mutation had occurred, turned out to be heterozygous for the condition. Why both homozygous and heterozygous mutations can both cause the severe neonatal syndrome, and why most heterozygous cases have a benign course compared with a minority of the heterozygous cases that have a more severe condition, is not understood.

Possible explanations are that different mutations of CaR cause widely different effects on CaR in relation to PTH secretion. Also, some studies have suggested that an affected fetus in a normocalcaemic mother might be at risk of developing secondary hyperparathyroidism as it detects a 'low' calcium in the mother. This would then worsen its own hypercalcaemia. After birth, this added stimulus would be removed and the secondary hyperparathyroid state would resolve. Although this hypothesis does not explain why the majority of affected neonates do not have a hyperparathyroid state at birth, irrespective of whether the mother or father was the gene carrier, it does offer an explanation for the resolution of some apparently severe forms of the disease. It might be anticipated that the homozygous forms of the disorder are less likely to resolve with time, but the literature on this point is not clear at present.

More recently, three cases of late-presenting patients with homozygous defects of the CaR gene have been reported. When studied in adult life, none had evidence of clinical parathyroid disease, despite having moderate to severe hypercalcaemia. Only in one was the serum PTH markedly elevated. Worryingly, all three cases had mental retardation, and, in reviewing these three cases, Pearce and Steinmann [24] argue that this supports the recommendation of total parathyroidectomy in early life in NSPHT. Such advice seems premature as other causes of mental retardation were present in at least two of the cases.

Diagnosis

The majority of children with FBH are likely to be identified as a result of family studies of adults suspected of having, or known to have, FBH. In these children there are no diagnostic difficulties and the finding of hypercalcaemia in this setting does not need further investigation, and the parents can be reassured about the benign nature of the disorder. Other cases may come to light as a chance finding during investigation for other, unrelated, conditions. FBH is the likely cause of mild hypercalcaemia in an otherwise healthy child.

Biochemical investigations

Apart from NSPHT, the hypercalcaemia is usually mild and rarely exceeds 3.0 mmol/L. The serum phosphorus is usually in the lower half of the normal range and serum magnesium in the upper half of the normal range. Urinary calcium excretion tends to be reduced and a calcium–creatinine clearance ratio of < 0.01 is fairly diagnostic of the condition. However, wide variations in urinary calcium excretion can occur, making it difficult for any of these biochemical tests to prove or exclude the diagnosis.

Of greater help is the serum PTH concentration, which, in the majority of cases, is well within the normal range, contrasting with the elevated values typically seen in hyperparathyroidism and the low values seen in non-parathyroid causes of hypercalcaemia. However, mildly elevated values of PTH have been reported in 15% of adults with FBH. For this reason, family screening is a useful adjunct to biochemical testing as, although new mutations occur, they are thought to be relatively uncommon and the finding of other asymptomatic family members strongly supports the diagnosis. As only 80% of cases have so far been shown to have an identifiable abnormality of the CaR gene and as these abnormalities may occur throughout the gene, analysis of the gene cannot be used to diagnose new suspected cases.

## Management

Outside the neonatal period, the condition appears to be truly benign and no treatment is required. It is important to differentiate the condition from primary hyperparathyroidism and to make sure that parathyroidectomy is not performed. No modification to the diet or drug therapy needs to be considered. The parents and the child, where appropriate, should be aware of the condition and should point out the hypercalcaemia should the child become ill for any other reason. This should prevent inappropriate and unnecessary investigations trying to link the hypercalcaemia with other conditions.

### Williams syndrome

This condition is characterized by distinctive facial features ('elfin like'), supravalvular aortic stenosis and learning disability. Its incidence is estimated to be 1 in 20 000 live births and is almost always sporadic. The facial features consist of periorbital fullness, malar hypoplasia, a long philtrum, arched upper lip with full lower lip and an open mouth appearance. Lacy or stellate irises may also be seen. Hypercalcaemia may be present in the first year of life but is not a consistent feature. Failure to thrive and irritability because of hypercalcaemia may be the first presenting feature. The phenotypic features of the condition are variable and may change with advancing age.

A search for the gene responsible for Williams syndrome localized the cardiac component to the long arm of chromosome 7. Subsequently a heterozygous microdeletion of chromosome 7q11.23, which encompasses the elastin gene, was shown to produce Williams syndrome [25]. Such an abnormality can be readily detected by fluorescent *in situ* hybridization (FISH) and is present in the majority of diagnosed cases.

The aetiology of hypercalcaemia is unclear. Previous studies have demonstrated increased concentrations of 1,25-dihydroxyvitamin D during periods of hypercalcaemia or decreased calcitonin secretion during calcium infusions. However, these are not consistent findings and one study [26] of 27 normocalcaemic patients aged 2–47 years showed no significant disturbance of parathyroid hormone, 1,25-dihydroxyvitamin D or calcitonin. When hypercalcaemia is present, it is usually symptomatic and feeding and behaviour will often improve significantly when it is corrected. Management consists of a low-calcium formula milk (Locasol). If this fails, a short course of corticosteroids (prednisolone 1 mg/kg) will usually correct the hypercalcaemia and may be discontinued after a few weeks. There is rarely recurrence of hypercalcaemia beyond the first year of life.

### Idiopathic infantile hypercalcaemia

This condition was first described in the early 1950s by Lightwood [27] in England. Further investigation identified that the majority of affected infants were born to mothers ingesting foods heavily fortified with vitamin D. The incidence of the condition dramatically declined with the reduction of vitamin D supplementation, but cases continue to occur without evidence of excessive maternal vitamin D intake. Severely affected neonates may have cardiac lesions and dysmorphic features similar to those described in Williams syndrome without the characteristic elastin gene microdeletion.

Other features include hypertension, strabismus, inguinal hernias and bony abnormalities (radioulnar synostosis). As in Williams syndrome, the hypercalcaemia has been attributed to disordered vitamin D metabolism with increased sensitivity to vitamin D. One series of seven affected children has shown an elevated concentration of N-terminal PTHrP at the time of hypercalcaemia, which normalized when normocalcaemia was achieved. In contrast to Williams syndrome, the hypercalcaemia may be prolonged and continue beyond infancy. Treatment includes the use of corticosteroids and the avoidance of vitamin D and excess dietary calcium.

### Vitamin D toxicity

Although this has been reported to occur in premature infants after prolonged feeding with a vitamin D-fortified formula, it is more likely to be due to vitamin D used therapeutically. This is seen particularly in children with renal osteodystrophy treated with alfacalcidol or calcitriol. The hypercalcaemia is invariably symptomatic with polyuria, polydipsia and anorexia being prominent features. Complications of prolonged hypercalcaemia include ectopic calcification, nephrocalcinosis and renal insufficiency. The hypercalcaemia induced by vitamin D toxicity appears to be mainly due to increased bone resorption. The hypercalcaemia associated with the use of vitamin D itself is prolonged in comparison with that after the use of its analogues because it is retained in body fat stores.

Acute symptomatic hypercalcaemia can be corrected with corticosteroids or, more rapidly, with an intravenous bisphosphonate, such as pamidronate. Vitamin D should subsequently be restarted in a lower dose.

## Hypercalcaemia of malignancy

This is well recognized in adults in association with certain types of malignancy and may also occur in children. Affected individuals rarely have evidence of skeletal involvement from the primary tumour or metastases, and the hypercalcaemia is a consequence of a circulating humoral factor, subsequently identified as PTHrP. There are similarities to primary hyperparathyroidism, in that evidence of a reduction in tubular phosphate reabsorption and hypophosphataemia is often present. However serum PTH is suppressed and circulating PTHrP is elevated. The hypercalcaemia is a consequence of increased bone resorption and a variable increase in distal tubular calcium reabsorption. Affected individuals are often volume depleted and initial therapy should be with appropriate fluid replacement using normal saline. Additional treatment is often required to restore normocalcaemia, and intravenous pamidronate in a dose of 0.5 mg/kg is often effective.

## Immobilization

Hypercalcaemia and hypercalciuria are a recognized complication of prolonged immobilization, as may be seen in children with severe cerebral palsy, high spinal cord injury or severe illness. However, immobilization even for a few days in association with a weight-bearing limb fracture, particularly in adolescents, may cause symptomatic hypercalcaemia. There are reports of successful treatment with calcitonin and pamidronate.

## Granulomatous disorders

Hypercalcaemia occurs in 30–50% of children with sarcoidosis and an additional 20–30% demonstrate hypercalciuria with a normal plasma calcium. Similarly, childhood tuberculosis and cat-scratch disease, a granulomatous disorder due to infection with *Bartonella henselae*, may be complicated by hypercalcaemia. In these conditions there is evidence of excess production of 1,25-dihydroxyvitamin D, which resolves on successful treatment of the underlying disease.

## Subcutaneous fat necrosis

This uncommon transient disorder affects healthy, full-term infants who have suffered perinatal asphyxia. It has been reported in older children in association with major trauma or disseminated varicella. Affected babies develop irregular subcutaneous plaques over the back and buttocks with, typically, a violaceous discoloration. Histological examination shows an inflammatory infiltrate in subcutaneous fat, often with crystals containing calcium. Hypercalcaemia occurs after the appearance of the skin lesions and is typically associated with irritability and poor feeding. There is good evidence that excess production of 1,25-dihydroxyvitamin D by the granulomatous cells of fat necrosis causes the hyper-

calcaemia. Therapy consists of adequate hydration, dietary calcium and vitamin D restriction and the use of systemic corticosteroids. The condition usually settles within a few weeks with no risk of recurrence.

## Hypophosphatasia

This rare hereditary condition has an incidence of about 1 per 100 000 live births for the severe forms. The underlying abnormality is subnormal activity of the tissue non-specific isoenzyme of alkaline phosphatase (TNSALP). There is variation in severity with the severe forms inherited in an autosomal recessive manner. There are four main clinical forms, depending on the age at which skeletal lesions are discovered: perinatal, infantile, childhood and adult. Infantile hypophosphatasia is clinically apparent before the age of 6 months, with poor feeding, poor weight gain, hypotonia and wide fontanelles. Hypercalcaemia and hypercalciuria can occur as a consequence of defective skeletal mineralization. A flail chest predisposes to pneumonia and respiratory insufficiency is often the cause of death. Spontaneous improvement or deterioration in the skeleton may occur and this form is fatal in about 50% of patients.

Childhood hypophosphatasia is identified by premature loss of deciduous teeth (before the age of 5), delayed walking with a waddling gait, genu valgum and short stature. This form may improve spontaneously during puberty. The diagnosis is made from the clinical picture and low serum alkaline phosphatase in combination with radiological evidence of rickets. Hypercalcaemia and sometimes hyperphosphataemia are features. Demonstration of excess urinary excretion of phosphoethanolamine in combination with elevated plasma concentrations of pyridoxal 5′-phosphate confirms the diagnosis.

An increasing number of molecular defects in the TNSALP gene are now identified in severe forms of hypophosphatasia. There is no established medical treatment but it is important to avoid vitamin D and mineral supplements, which may exacerbate hypercalcaemia. Dietary calcium restriction and calcitonin have been used in infancy. Fractures occurring in children do mend, but delayed healing is characteristic. Placement of intramedullary rods rather than external plates on bone is best for the acute or prophylactic treatment of fractures. Expert dental care is also important.

## Jansen syndrome

This condition presents in neonates with hypercalcaemia and X-ray changes that resemble rickets. Biochemical findings are typical of primary hyperparathyroidism, but there are no measurable concentrations of PTH or PTHrP. The disorder results from a defect in the gene coding for the PTH/PTHrP receptor, which results in autoactivation of the receptor producing unopposed PTH/PTHrP-like actions [28]. The hypercalcaemia has been reported to respond to calcitonin and would also theoretically respond to bisphosphonates.

## Miscellaneous metabolic bone disorders

### Fibrous dysplasia

This may be monostotic in which a single expanding bone lesion may cause pain, fracture and/or deformity and may occasionally cause nerve compression. Typically, the skull and long bones are most often affected. Children are more likely to be affected by polyostotic disease, which will often manifest before the age of 10 years. This may be associated with hyperpigmented macules and endocrinopathy in McCune–Albright syndrome. The various manifestations of this condition are due to somatic mosaicism for activating mutations of the gene that encodes the $GS_\alpha$ subunit of the receptor/adenylate cyclase-coupling G-protein [29]. In bone, there is increased expression of the c-*fos* proto-oncogene [30].

Any skeletal site may be involved, but femora, tibiae, ribs and facial bones are most frequently involved. The expansile bone lesions in long bones are characterized by thin cortices and a ground glass appearance and in the hip cause a characteristic 'shepherd's crook' deformity. The lesions may be painful and are a site of recurrent fractures. Affected areas in the skull may cause nerve compression, requiring surgical intervention.

Renal phosphate wasting may occur, causing hypophosphataemic bone disease. Calcium and phosphate concentrations are often normal but alkaline phosphatase and other biochemical markers of bone turnover may be elevated. If there is evidence to suggest hypophosphataemic bone disease (low plasma phosphate and $T_m PO_4/GFR$), it is logical to treat this with a vitamin D analogue such as calcitriol or alphacalcidol in combination with phosphate supplements. Bone pain and radiography of the skeletal lesions may improve with intravenous Pamidronate.

### Osteopetrosis

There are two major forms of this sclerosing bone disorder, an autosomal dominant (benign) type that occurs in adults and is associated with few symptoms, and an autosomal recessive (malignant) type occurring in children that is fatal in infancy or early childhood if untreated. A rare intermediate autosomal recessive form also presents during childhood. An additional form associated with renal tubular acidosis is now known to be due to carbonic anhydrase II deficiency. The pathogenesis of all forms of osteopetrosis is a failure of osteoclast-mediated bone resorption, which may occur as consequence of abnormalities in the formation of osteoclasts or, alternatively, a failure of action of osteoclasts.

An early symptom of infantile osteopetrosis is nasal stuffiness due to malformation of the mastoid and paranasal sinuses. Failure of widening of cranial nerve foramina can gradually cause palsies of the optic, oculomotor and facial nerves. Failure to thrive is common and recurrent infections and spontaneous bruising occur as a consequence of bone marrow compression. Bones, although appearing dense on X-ray, are typically fragile. Untreated children usually die during the first decade from pneumonia, anaemia or sepsis, although there is a wide variability in presentation and clinical course. Hypocalcaemia with secondary hyperparathyroidism, as a consequence of the failure of bone resorption, may be present. Serum acid phosphatase is often increased.

Bone marrow transplantation is the only effective cure for infantile osteopetrosis, although results from HLA (human leucocyte antigen) non-identical donors are currently poor. High-dose oral calcitriol has been reported to ameliorate osteopetrosis. Recombinant human interferon γ given by thrice-weekly subcutaneous injection has been used in combination with high-dose oral calcitriol. This resulted in decreases in trabecular bone area, stimulation of bone turnover and reduction of bone density after 6 months. However, other children with osteopetrosis treated similarly have not shown a response, and the long-term effects of such treatment are currently not reported.

## Osteoporosis

Osteoporosis in adults is defined in relation to measurements of bone mineral density because prospective studies have related bone mineral density to risk of osteoporotic fracture. The WHO definition of osteoporosis in postmenopausal women is based on a bone mineral density more than 2.5 SD (standard deviations) below the young adult mean (the *T*-score). Such a definition cannot be applied to children to define osteoporosis because there are no prospective studies in children to relate bone mineral density to fracture risk. Second, measurements of bone density in children using the most popular techniques such as dual-energy X-ray absorptiometry are influenced by body size [31]. Thus a child with growth retardation whose height is below the normal range may well have a bone density result more than 2.5 SD below the mean (the *z*-score), and yet their bone density would be appropriate for body size. Therefore, until the advent of techniques that are not affected by body size or the construction of reference data that relate bone density to body size rather than to age, it is not possible to define osteoporosis in children on bone density results alone.

The definition of childhood osteoporosis has therefore to include a history of low-trauma fractures in combination with a bone density measurement that is significantly reduced for age and body size. The term osteopenia, which implies a radiological reduction in bone density, would be more appropriate where bone density in a child is shown to be 2 SD or more below the age-related mean in the absence of fractures.

### Aetiology

There are a number of conditions in children that are associated with osteoporotic fractures. The majority of these are

**Table 23.6.** Childhood osteoporosis—aetiology

Primary
    Osteogenesis imperfecta
    Idiopathic juvenile osteoporosis

Secondary
    Inflammatory, e.g. juvenile idiopathic arthritis
    Immobilization, e.g. cerebral palsy
    Endocrine, e.g. Cushing syndrome
    Haematological, e.g. thalassaemia, leukaemia
    Miscellaneous, e.g. organ transplantation

**Table 23.7.** Classification system for osteogenesis imperfecta (OI)

| OI type | Clinical features |
|---|---|
| I | Normal stature, little or no deformity, blue sclerae, hearing loss in 50%, dentinogenesis imperfecta is rare |
| II | Lethal in perinatal period, minimal calvarial mineralization, beaded ribs, compressed femurs, marked long bone deformity, platyspondyly |
| III | Progressive deforming bones, extreme short stature, sclerae variable in hue and may lighten with age, dentinogenesis imperfecta and hearing loss common. |
| IV | Mild to moderate bone deformity variable short stature. Normal sclerae, dentinogenesis imperfecta common, hearing loss in some |

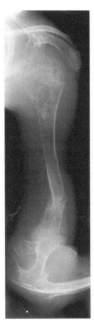

**Fig. 23.6.** Skeletal changes in the upper arm of an adolescent with osteogenesis imperfecta type III.

secondary to underlying disorders (Table 23.6) with the only primary causes being osteogenesis imperfecta and idiopathic juvenile osteoporosis.

Osteogenesis imperfecta is an uncommon but hereditary cause of osteoporosis in children. Its pathogenesis relates to a qualitative or quantitative abnormality in the synthesis of type 1 collagen. The predominant clinical feature is recurrent low-trauma fractures and skeletal deformity (Fig. 23.6). Severity is extremely variable, with manifestations ranging from stillbirth to a lifelong absence of symptoms. The presence of type 1 collagen in teeth, ligaments, skin and sclerae may lead to other manifestations that identify affected individuals. These include blue sclerae, dentinogenesis imperfecta, due to defective dentine formation, and ligamentous laxity. However, these features are not always present, which may lead to difficulty distinguishing osteogenesis imperfecta from idiopathic juvenile osteoporosis. The classification

system for osteogenesis imperfecta devised by Sillence (Table 23.7) remains a useful framework to categorize affected individuals. However, as the number of different mutations in the genes coding for type 1 collagen continues to increase, it is recognized that there is no strong genotype–phenotype relationship [32].

Idiopathic juvenile osteoporosis presents just before or early in puberty but there are reports of much younger children being affected. It typically presents with a history of back pain and difficulty walking due to vertebral compression fractures. Long bone fractures may also occur, and metaphyseal compression fractures at the ends of the long bones are often described but not always present. Although the underlying aetiology is unclear, most reports of bone biopsies in this condition indicate a failure of bone formation. Spontaneous improvement is reported to occur but does not occur in some children who may be left with significant long-term disability.

Secondary causes of osteoporosis are more common. In inflammatory disorders such as juvenile arthritis, other connective tissue diseases and Crohn disease, there is a risk of osteoporotic fractures because of cytokine production impairing bone turnover. Many such conditions require corticosteroid treatment, which will add to the adverse effects on bone turnover and increase the risk of osteoporosis. Iatrogenic steroid-induced osteoporosis is the most important cause of osteoporosis in children.

Increasing numbers of children undergoing organ transplantation develop osteoporosis because of the combination of the pre-existing disease and the effect of corticosteroids and other immunosuppressive agents after the transplant, particularly in the first 6 months. Conditions that lead to prolonged immobilization, such as severe cerebral palsy and high spinal cord injuries, may lead to osteoporotic fractures as a result of the loss of the important influence of weight-bearing exercise. It has long been known that leukaemia may be a cause of osteoporotic fractures, particularly early in the

**Table 23.8.** Childhood osteopenia

Cystic fibrosis
Hypogonadism
Growth hormone deficiency
Anorexia nervosa
Chronic renal failure
Cholestatic liver disease
Burns
Leukaemia

presentation. Another haematological condition where a risk of osteoporosis is now recognized is thalassaemia. In this condition there are a number of potential adverse influences on bone turnover, including iron deposition from repeated transfusions, iron chelation agents, such as desferrioxamine, and the high incidence of endocrine disorders, particularly hypogonadism.

There are numerous chronic childhood conditions in which studies have shown evidence of osteopenia (Table 23.8). Although it is uncommon for these to be associated with fractures during childhood, there is concern that they will lead to a reduction in peak bone mass and therefore an increased risk of fractures in adulthood. Understanding the mechanism for the reduced bone density in these conditions is important to try and identify potential means of prevention.

*Clinical presentation*

A child with osteoporosis may present with recurrent long bone fractures after minor trauma or at birth, as in some cases of osteogenesis imperfecta. Vertebral osteoporosis usually presents with severe back pain associated with difficulty in walking. Progressive vertebral collapse leads to kyphosis with disproportionate reduction in sitting height. As the majority of childhood osteoporosis is secondary to another condition, there will often be a history or features on examination of such a disorder. An osteoporotic fracture may rarely be an early manifestation of another condition such as leukaemia or Crohn disease. Growth retardation and pubertal delay will often complicate a chronic systemic disease and assessment of growth and puberty is important in the accurate interpretation of bone density results. Diagnosis of a child with osteogenesis imperfecta in the presence of a family history or other non-skeletal manifestations is usually straightforward, but may be more difficult in a child with mild disease, intermittent fractures and no associated features.

*Investigation*

Radiographs of the areas of fracture as well as lateral and anterior–posterior films of the spine for vertebral compression fractures are required. Metaphyseal compression fractures at the ends of long bones, particularly the legs, may be seen in idiopathic juvenile osteoporosis. A skull radiograph may reveal the presence of wormian bones in suspected osteogenesis imperfecta. An accurate assessment of bone density is essential to the diagnosis and to act as a baseline value for the purpose of follow-up, particularly if medical treatment is being considered. Differences in the degree of reduction in bone density may be seen between a whole-body and lumbar spine scan, particularly with steroid-induced osteoporosis, which predominantly affects the trabecular bone of the spine.

In the absence of an apparent cause for osteoporosis, further investigation is important to detect underlying disease. This will usually include routine haematology and measurement of renal and liver function. Although measurement of mineral metabolism, including vitamin D and PTH, should be included, this is often normal. Measurement of biochemical markers of bone turnover, including both a marker of bone formation and bone resorption, should be considered. Low concentrations of procollagen type 1 C-terminal peptide (P1CP) have been reported in osteogenesis imperfecta, as have high concentrations of bone resorption markers in some cases of idiopathic juvenile osteoporosis and osteogenesis imperfecta. Although these markers rarely aid diagnosis, they are useful to monitor treatment.

There is no simple investigation for osteogenesis imperfecta, and a skin biopsy should be considered for analysis of type 1 collagen, which can identify abnormalities in up to 85% of individuals. A bone biopsy is an additional investigation in a child with idiopathic osteoporosis as this can demonstrate abnormalities of bone formation or resorption and may help distinguish osteogenesis imperfecta from idiopathic juvenile osteoporosis. This is particularly useful when double tetracycline labelling is performed as it will assess the rate of bone formation.

## Management

There are no management guidelines for childhood osteoporosis and many of the studies assessing medical treatment have been on small numbers of children and have seldom been randomized or placebo controlled. Supplementation with calcium and vitamin D is often advocated but there is little evidence of benefit. Calcitriol has been reported to be of benefit in some cases of idiopathic juvenile osteoporosis. In children receiving long-term corticosteroids, the use of deflazacort, an oxazoline derivative of prednisolone, is reported to have a less detrimental effect on bone density, although studies are limited.

Growth hormone has been advocated as a potential treatment in children with either osteoporosis or osteopenia because of its known effects on the growth plate and bone turnover. Studies in osteogenesis imperfecta have shown increments in bone density, particularly those with type 1 disease, but they have usually been of no more than 1 year in duration and there are no long-term reports of benefit.

Pubertal induction with sex steroids is a logical approach where osteoporosis or osteopenia is secondary to primary or secondary hypogonadism.

Drugs that inhibit bone resorption, such as calcitonin and the bisphosphonates, are likely to be of most benefit where there is evidence of increased bone resorption. Studies in small numbers of children with nephrotic syndrome and thalassaemia who received calcitonin have documented increases in bone mineral content, relief of bone pain and improvement in radiographic changes of osteoporosis. Bisphosphonates, which are a well-established treatment option in adults with osteoporosis, have been increasingly investigated in children. Beneficial effects on bone density have been reported in idiopathic juvenile osteoporosis, osteogenesis imperfecta and children with juvenile arthritis and cerebral palsy. One report of a group of children with osteoporosis due to several different causes who received treatment with pamidronate or olpadronate given orally showed an improvement in the mean bone density SD score from −3.8 to −1.9 over a 5-year period. A report of the use of intravenous pamidronate in 30 children with severe osteogenesis imperfecta [33] for between 1 and 5 years showed a mean annual increment in lumbar spine bone density of 42%, with the mean SD score improving from −5.3 to −3.4. Mobility and ambulation improved in half of the group with all children reporting pain relief and improved energy concentrations. No adverse effects on fracture healing, growth rate or bone biopsies were seen.

Unfortunately, this study (and many others) were not randomized and did not include a placebo group. There are concerns about potential adverse effects of bisphosphonates in the growing skeleton, particularly as they are known to remain within bone for up to 10 years. Osteomalacia, undertubulation of long bones and episcleritis have been reported but are usually isolated reports. These drugs should be regarded as experimental and be the subject of further randomized controlled studies before they can be regarded as established treatment for children with osteoporosis or osteopenia.

Spontaneous improvement in the absence of medical treatment can occur in children with osteoporosis, as has been reported in a long-term follow-up study of idiopathic juvenile osteoporosis. General measures in managing children with osteoporosis include adequate pain relief and the input of a multidisciplinary team that includes an orthopaedic surgeon, physiotherapist and occupational therapist. Many of these children will require rehabilitation and drug treatment should not be given in isolation but as part of a comprehensive approach to management.

## References

1 Kovacs CS, Kronenburg HM. Maternal–fetal calcium and bone metabolism during pregnancy, puerperium and lactation. *Endocr Rev* 1997; 18: 832–72.

2 Goldberg R, Motzkin B, Marion R, Scambler PJ, Shprintzen RJ. Velo-cardio-facial syndrome: a review of 120 patients. *Am J Med Genet* 1993; 45: 313–19.

3 Greig F, Paul E, DiMartino-Nardi J, Saenger P. Transient congenital hypoparathyroidism. Resolution recurrence chromosome 22q II deletion. *J Pediatr* 1996; 128: 563–7.

4 Richardson RJ, Kirk JM. Short stature, mental retardation and hypoparathyroidism: a new syndrome. *Arch Dis Child* 1990; 65: 1113–17.

5 Diaz GA, Gelb BD, Ali F *et al.* Sanjad-Sakati and autosomal recessive kenny–caffey syndromes are allelic. Evidence for an ancestral founder mutation and locus refinement. *Am J Med Genet* 1999; 85: 48–52.

6 Parkinson DB, Shaw NJ, Himsworth RL, Thakker RV. Parathyroid hormone gene analysis in autosomal hypoparathyroidism using an intragenic tetranucleotide $(AAAT)_n$ polymorphism. *Hum Genet* 1993; 91: 281–4.

7 Wang JT, Lin CJ, Burridge SM *et al.* Genetics of vitamin D 1alpha-hydroxylase deficiency in 17 families. *Am J Hum Genet* 1998; 63: 1694–702.

8 Hughes MR, Malloy PJ, O'Malley BW *et al.* Genetic defects in the 1,25-dihydroxyvitamin $D_3$ receptor. *J Recept Res* 1991; 11: 699–716.

9 Albright F, Butler AM, Bloomberg E. Richets resistant to vitamin D therapy. *Am J Dis Child* 1937; 54: 529–44.

10 The HYP Consortium. A gene (PEX) with homologies to endopeptidases is mutated in patients with X-linked hypophosphataemic rickets. *Nature Genet* 1995; 11: 130–6.

11 Gottlieb S, Driscoll DA, Punnett HH *et al.* Characterization of 10p deletions suggests two nonoverlapping regions contribute to the DiGeorge syndrome phenotype. *Am J Hum Genet* 1998; 62: 495–8.

12 Ahonen P, Myllarniemi S, Sipila I, Perheentupa J. Clinical variation of autoimmune polyendocrinopathy-candidiasis-ectodermal dystrophy (APECED) in a series of 68 patients. *N Engl J Med* 1990; 322: 1829–36.

13 Finnish-German APECED Consortium. An autoimmune disease, APECED, caused by mutations in a novel gene featuring two PHD-type zinc-finger domains. *Nature Genet* 1997; 17: 399–403.

14 Pearce SH, Williamson C, Kifor O *et al.* A familial syndrome of hypocalcemia with hypercalciuria due to mutations in the calcium-sensing receptor. *N Engl J Med* 1997; 335: 1115–22.

15 Pollak MR, Brown EM, Wuchou YH *et al.* Mutations in the human $Ca^{2+}$ sensing receptor gene cause familial hypocalciuric hypercalcemia and neonatal severe hyperparathyroidism. *Cell* 1993; 75: 1297–303.

16 Levine MA, Downs RW Jr, Singer M *et al.* Deficient activity of guanine nucleotide regulatory protein in erythrocytes from patients with pseudohypoparathyroidism. *Biochem Biophys Res Commun* 1980; 94: 1319–24.

17 Levine MA, Modi WS, O'Brien SJ. Mapping of the gene encoding the alpha subunit of the stimulatory G protein of adenylyl cyclase (GNAS1) to 20q13.2–q13.3 in humans by in situ hybridization. *Genomics* 1991; 11: 478–9.

18 Davies SJ, Hughes HE. Imprinting in Albright's hereditary osteodystrophy. *J Med Genet* 1993; 30: 101–3.

19 Wilson LC, Oude Luttikhuis MEM, Clayton PT, Fraser WD, Trembath RC. Parental origin of GSα gene mutations in Albright's hereditary osteodystrophy. *J Med Genet* 1994; 31: 835–9.

20 Juppner H, Schipani E, Bastepe M *et al.* The gene responsible for

pseudohypoparathyroidism type 1b is paternally imprinted and maps in four unrelated kindreds to chromosome 20q13.3. *Proc Natl Acad Sci USA* 1998; 95: 11798–803.

21 Chandrasekharappa SC, Guru SC, Manickam P *et al.* Positional cloning of the gene for multiple endocrine neoplasia – type 1. *Science* 1997; 267: 404–7.

22 Heath DA. Localisation of parathyroid tumours. *Clin Endocr* 1995; 43: 523–4.

23 Chou Y-HW, Brown EH, Levi T *et al.* The gene responsible for familial hypocalciuric hypercalcaemia maps to chromosome 3q in four unrelated families. *Nature Genet* 1992; 1: 295–300.

24 Pearce S, Steinmann B. Casting new light on the clinical spectrum of neonatal severe hyperparathyroidism. *Clin Endocrinol* 1999; 50: 691–3.

25 Perez Jurado LA, Peoples R, Kaplan P, Hamel BC, Francke U. Molecular definition of the chromosome 7 deletion in Williams syndrome and parent-of-origin effects on growth. *Am J Hum Genet* 1996; 59: 781–92.

26 Kruse K, Pankau R, Gosch A, Wohlfahrt K. Calcium metabolism in Williams–Beuren syndrome. *J Pediatr* 1992; 121: 902–7.

27 Lightwood RL. Idiopathic hypercalcaemia with failure to thrive. *Arch Dis Child* 1952; 27: 302–3.

28 Schipiani E, Kruse K, Juppner H. A constitutively active mutant PTH-PTHrp receptor in Jansen-type metaphyseal chrondrodysplasia. *Science* 1995; 268: 98–100.

29 Weinstein LS, Shenker A, Gejman PV *et al.* Activating mutations of the stimulator G protein of adenylyl cyclase in McCune–Albright syndrome. *N Engl J Med* 1991; 325: 1688–95.

30 Candeliere GA, Glorieux FH, Prud Homme J, St-Arnaud R. Increased expression of the c-fos proto-oncogene in bone from patients with fibrous dysplasia. *N Engl J Med* 1995; 332: 1546–51.

31 Prentice A, Parsons TJ, Cole TJ. Uncritical use of bone mineral density in absorptiometry may lead to size related artefacts in the identification of bone mineral determinants. *Am J Clin Nutr* 1994; 60: 837–42.

32 Smith R. Osteogenesis imperfecta: from phenotype to genotype and back again. *Int J Exp Pathol* 1994; 75: 233–41.

33 Glorieux FH, Bishop NJ, Plotkin H, Chabot G, Lanoue G, Travers RT. Cyclic administration of pamidronate in children with severe osteogenesis imperfecta. *N Engl J Med* 1998; 339: 947–52.

# 24 Diabetes mellitus

## Stephanie A. Amiel and C. R. Buchanan

## Definition and significance

The term 'diabetes mellitus' refers to a group of conditions characterized by hyperglycaemia and other metabolic abnormalities secondary to insufficient insulin action. Insulin, a polypeptide hormone secreted by the β-cells of the islets of Langerhans in the pancreas, has glucoregulatory effects. It suppresses hepatic glycogenolysis and hepatic and renal gluconeogenesis and stimulates glucose uptake by muscle and fat tissue. In the peripheral tissues, it also inhibits lipolysis and proteolysis, diminishing the fuel supply for gluconeogenesis and creating a milieu for protein and fat deposition. In the liver, insulin also suppresses ketogenesis, so insulin deficiency is associated with ketosis.

Insulin action may be deficient by virtue of a total loss of the capacity to secrete insulin. Alternatively, insulin action may be impaired, with hepatic and/or peripheral tissue resistance. Although some metabolic disturbance may accompany insulin resistance, such as hyperlipidaemia, the healthy pancreas responds to insulin resistance with insulin hypersecretion. Hyperglycaemia and diabetes occur only if pancreatic reserve cannot meet the excess demand, creating relative insulin deficiency.

The problems of diabetes include the acute effects of insulin deficiency – hyperglycaemia, ketosis, muscle and fat breakdown – and the complications of long-term insulin deficiency. Diabetes is associated with disorders of osmoregulation, coagulation, endothelial function, lipid metabolism and antioxidant activity; chronic hyperglycaemia causes accelerated glycation of body proteins. Damage to body tissues, particularly the vasculature, result and diabetes is associated with premature atherosclerosis and specific damage to the optic retina, the kidney and the peripheral and autonomic nerves.

The personal and social costs of these complications are high. Life expectancy is shortened, with premature death from cardiovascular disease and renal failure, and there is significant morbidity, including blindness, painful and dis-abling neuropathies and amputation of insensate and poorly perfused feet [1–3]. Most of these complications take years to develop and there is great opportunity to delay or prevent their onset and progression. Furthermore, the management of even the late complications of diabetes has improved dramatically with advances in ophthalmic techniques (preventing 70% of diabetic blindness [4]) and in foot care (reducing major amputation by 50% [5]). Traditionally considered the preserve of the adult diabetologist, it is essential to realize that the seeds of the chronic diabetic complications are sown in youth and the proper care of children with diabetes has become an urgent priority.

There are 124 million people in the world with diabetes (1997 data) and the prevalence is expected to rise to 221 million by the year 2010. In the United Kingdom, the current diabetes prevalence of 1.5 million people is set to increase to three million over the same time [6]. The incidence of new type 1, insulin-dependent, diabetes, the form of diabetes predominant in children, has been rising rapidly over the last decades in northern countries [7–9]. In particular, there are reports of a rise in incidence of type 1 diabetes in children under 5 years old [10,11], although this is not the universal experience [12]. The reasons for this are uncertain but may relate to a general increase in autoimmune and inflammatory diseases, perhaps related to diminishing prevalence of major infective diseases such as poliomyelitis, tuberculosis and parasite infestation. Another possible relationship is the rising age of women giving birth, as the risk of type 1 diabetes appears higher with increasing maternal age [13].

## Diagnosis (Table 24.1)

Diagnosis of diabetes usually depends on measurement of a high plasma (or blood) glucose in the presence of symptoms attributable to it. In the presence of typical symptoms (see below), a single laboratory measurement of random plasma glucose measured in excess of 11 mmol/L is diagnostic [14,15]. Note that the numbers will depend on whether

**Table 24.1.** Diagnostic criteria for diabetes mellitus and abnormal glucose tolerance

---

Symptoms and random plasma glucose ≥ 11.1 mmol/L
Asymptomatic and fasting plasma glucose ≥ 7 mmol/L and/or 2 h after 75-g
  oral glucose load ≥ 11.1 *on two separate occasions*
Impaired glucose tolerance: fasting plasma glucose < 7 mmol/L and
  2 h ≥ 7.8 and < 11.1 mmol/L
Impaired fasting glucose: fasting plasma glucose 6.1–6.9 mmol/L

---

venous or capillary blood or plasma samples are used. For screening purposes, or in a case that is equivocal, two abnormal glucose readings are mandatory. The optimal test is an oral glucose tolerance test, performed after an overnight fast but after at least 3 days of adequate nutrition (carbohydrate intake of at least 200 g/day). A fasting venous plasma glucose of 7 mmol/L or more or a plasma glucose of more than 11 mmol/L 2 h after ingestion of a 75-g glucose load is required for diagnosis [14].

Oral glucose tolerance tests are notoriously variable and two tests should be performed to establish a firm diagnosis. A fasting plasma glucose of less than 7 mmol/L with a 2-h value between 7.8 and 11.1 mmol/L represents impaired glucose tolerance and indicates risk of progressing to diabetes and, in adults, increased risk of cardiovascular disease. The recent US revision of the criteria for diagnosing diabetes has reduced the emphasis on the use of the glucose tolerance test and suggests two fasting plasma glucoses of 7 mmol/L or

more to be sufficient for diagnosis [15], but the WHO (World Health Organization) reserves the use of fasting glucose concentrations alone for circumstances in which oral glucose tolerance testing is not possible (e.g. large screening or epidemiological studies) [14].

These criteria for diagnosing diabetes are new, the change being the lowering of the fasting plasma glucose to a level more obviously predictive of diabetic complications. There has also been the introduction of a new category of abnormality, impaired fasting glucose, which is based on two fasting glucose readings of between 6.1 and 6.9 mmol/L. The prognostic significance of this is not yet known and it is not exactly the equivalent of impaired glucose tolerance. It must be stressed that the diagnosis is rarely in doubt in clinical practice.

## Pathogenesis

### Type 1 diabetes mellitus

The WHO and the American Diabetes Association have recently reviewed the classification of types of diabetes and a summary of their recommendations is given in Table 24.2 [14,15]. In children and young people, the great majority of diabetes is type 1 disease. This most commonly results from the autoimmune destruction of the pancreatic β-cell (type 1a) and the autoimmune process can be identified, sometimes years before the onset of clinical disease, by the presence of

**Table 24.2.** Current WHO recommendations for the classification of diabetes mellitus

| | |
|---|---|
| Type 1 diabetes mellitus | β-Cell destruction → insulin deficiency, ketosis prone |
| Type 1A | Proven autoimmune aetiology |
| Type 1B | No demonstrable autoimmunity |
| Type 2 diabetes mellitus | Variable degree of insulin resistance and insulin deficiency. Not ketosis prone |
| Other specific types | |
| 1. Genetic causes of impaired β-cell function | e.g. maturity onset diabetes of youth (MODY); mitochondrial DNA 3243 mutations, Wolfram |
| 2. Genetic defects in insulin action | e.g. type A insulin resistance, leprechaunism, Rabson–Mendenhall syndrome; lipoatrophy |
| 3. Secondary to pancreatic disease | e.g. cystic fibrosis, thalassaemia, haemochromatosis, $\alpha_1$-antitrypsin deficiency, chronic or relapsing pancreatitis, congenital absence of islets or pancreas |
| 4. Secondary to other endocrine diseases | e.g. Cushing, pituitary gigantism |
| 5. Secondary to drugs or toxins | e.g. glucocorticoids, thiazides, asparaginase |
| 6. Secondary to infection | e.g. congenital rubella |
| 7. Other forms of immune disorder | e.g. polyglandular syndromes, APECED, stiff man |
| 8. Rare genetic disorders | e.g. Down, Klinefelter, Prader–Willi, Turner, Wolfram, Laurence–Moon–Biedl, myotonic dystrophy, ataxia telangiectasia, porphyria |
| Gestational diabetes | Any form of glucose intolerance first diagnosed in pregnancy |

circulating autoantibodies to islet cell elements including anti-islet cell antibodies *per se* and antibodies against components of islet cells including glutamic acid decarboxylase (GAD), a tyrosine phosphatase named IA2 and insulin itself [16–18]. Different antibody profiles may reflect different rates of progress of pancreatic destruction and be associated with different ages of onset [19]. Islet antigen-reactive T cells also appear before the onset of clinical disease and the destructive process is likely to be cell mediated [20].

Further investigation of these autoimmune processes is helping in the early identification of people at high risk of type 1 diabetes, at least among siblings of diabetic probands (see below), and may eventually lead to practical preventive strategies based on immune modulation [21]. Meanwhile, it should be recognized that some children with classic type 1 disease, severe insulin deficiency leading to a susceptibility not just to hyperglycaemia but also to proteolysis, lipolysis and, diagnostically, ketosis, do not always have evidence of autoimmune activation (type 1b). This is particularly true for the growing number of type 1 children being diagnosed in developing countries, such as Africa [22]. Whether this is because different antigens are involved or the process is not autoimmune at all is uncertain.

Type 1 diabetes is a disease of β-cell destruction and insulin resistance is often secondary to an initial hyperglycaemia. However, insulin resistance may determine the time at which type 1 disease becomes clinically manifest [23]. Incidence peaks in adolescence, as children develop the physiological insulin resistance of puberty [24], although this trend may be lost as the age-specific incidence rises [25].

Ten per cent of new type 1 diabetes arises in a family where there is already one person with the disease, and several genes have been identified which contribute to an individual's risk of developing the disease. Certain specific class II human leucocyte antigen (HLA) types predispose (e.g. HLA-DR3 and DR4, especially if inherited together) and some protect (e.g. HLA-DR2), although the involved genotypes may vary in different ethnic groups [26]. Non-HLA type 1-associated genes have also been described, although HLA genes, including those coding for the class II antigen, may account for up to about 34% of the familial clustering of type 1 diabetes.

The disease phenotypes may differ: HLA-DR4-associated diabetes has a younger age of onset and, while more likely to be associated with the development of anti-insulin antibodies, is less likely to show anti-islet cell antibodies and other autoimmune diseases [27]. DR3 and 4 together seem to support the most aggressive onset diabetes at a young age, with rapid loss of all endogenous insulin secretion. Not all genetically susceptible individuals will develop diabetes, and it is important to recognize that less than 4% of the general population who are HLA-DR3 or 4 positive will develop diabetes. Genome-wide scanning for linkage of chromosome regions to type 1 diabetes is in progress, using samples from families with at least two diabetic siblings, and several loci, unrelated to HLA, have been identified as potentially relevant [27].

Each gene is described as IDDM (insulin-dependent diabetes mellitus) and a number. *IDDM2* represents a polymorphism upstream of the transcription region of the insulin gene in which the alleles differ by virtue of their variable number of tandem repeats (VNTRs), in which the length of the sequence is proportional to the risk of developing type 1 [28]. The inherited risk attributable to this polymorphism is complicated by the fact that if the paternal high-risk gene is inherited from a father whose untransmitted gene is nominally protective, the expected risk attributable to the paternally inherited gene is not manifest [29]. This is a novel concept in inheritance of disease risk.

The genetic factors confer a degree of risk for developing type 1 diabetes. The precipitating factors are not clear. There is some evidence that viral infections (single, recurrent or maternal) may trigger some cases. There is evidence of 'epidemics' of new cases of type 1 [30], which might be supposed to have been triggered by an infective agent, and there are some reports of seasonal variation in the incidence of type 1 diabetes [11], with more cases occurring in spring [30] or winter [31], which may also support the viral hypothesis. However, it is likely that the triggering agent will precede the development of clinical diabetes (said to require about 90% loss of islet function) by a long time, and any seasonal variation may relate to the insulin resistance of acute stress such as viral infection, allowing a subclinical β-cell deficiency to become clinically evident.

Coxsackie B virus shares some antigenic determinants with β-cells [32], and there is evidence to support the triggering of the diabetogenic process by Coxsackie infection [33]. Other viruses, including mumps, measles, cytomegalovirus and influenza, have also been implicated. In children, there is a definite association between diabetes and maternal rubella infection during pregnancy [34]. These children have a high prevalence of HLA-DR3 and DR4. Another concern is that early feeding with cow's milk to an immature and permeable gut may increase the risk of diabetes in a susceptible child, because of antigenic determinants in the casein [35]. The evidence for this is still controversial [36], and although on general principles breast feeding should be encouraged for diabetic mothers too little is known about the effects of synthetic milk formulae to be dogmatic. The evidence suggesting cow's milk as an aetiological agent is not sufficiently strong to recommend its avoidance routinely to diabetic mothers who are unable to breast feed [37]. However, if a mother is concerned, she should be supported in her choice of a non-cow's milk formula, if only to prevent self-blame if her child does develop the disease in later life. Other components of early diet, such as nitrates and other antioxidants, are also beginning to come under scrutiny.

Finally, some toxins can damage the β-cell and cause diabetes. Streptozotocin and alloxan are used for this purpose to induce diabetes in experimental animal models. Pentamidine and asparaginase, both used clinically, have been reported to cause diabetes in clinical practice.

## Single gene defects as cause of diabetes

### Maturity-onset diabetes of youth

Most young people with non-type 1 diabetes probably have one of a series of specific gene defects that together make up the clinical syndromes of maturity onset diabetes of youth (MODY) [38]. Originally recognized by Robert Tattersall as a specific clinical syndrome of non-insulin-dependent diabetes occurring in young people with a strong family history of diabetes, in whom the glycaemia might be easily controlled and certainly did not seem to require insulin, the pathology in many MODY patients has been identified as being due to a specific gene (Table 24.3). Several genes have now been identified and each has a distinct clinical syndrome, with varying degrees of metabolic instability and very different risk of diabetic complications. MODY might be suspected by the presentation of non-insulin-dependent diabetes in a young person from one parent only with a family history of diabetes, often occurring at a progressively younger age in successive generations. MODY, most forms of which are identifiable genetically, has also been detected in a child who presented with illness-associated hyperglycaemia [39], with the suggestion that such children should be investigated.

### Single gene diseases associated with diabetes

Genetic defects associated with impaired insulin secretion and/or insulin resistance include trisomy 21 (Down syndrome), where there is a high incidence of type 1 diabetes and other autoimmune diseases [40], and Wolfram or DIDMOAD syndrome (diabetes insipidus, diabetes mellitus, optic atrophy and deafness), where there is evidence of non-autoimmune destruction of pancreatic β-cells and presumably also neuronal cell death [41]. A gene encoding a transmembrane protein has recently been identified in several families with DIDMOAD [42].

Other single gene defects may underlie syndromes of severe insulin resistance and diabetes. The elucidation of these rare conditions, such as gene mutations in the insulin receptor or in the intracellular pathways of insulin action or glucose transport, gives insight into the mechanisms of action of insulin [43]. Congenital insulin resistance can occur as type A, with associated manifestations of acanthosis nigricans (hypertrophic hyperpigmentation of the skin) and hyperandrogenism (hirsutism and, in girls, polycystic ovarian syndrome). Because of the hyperandrogenism, this syndrome is most easily recognized in girls, presenting typically in thin females, aged between 8 and 30 years, but can also be seen in boys. It is associated with defects in the insulin receptor gene. Type B is associated with insulin receptor antibodies.

If insulin action for protein metabolism is preserved, pseudoacromegaly, the clinical features of acromegaly and obesity but low IGF levels, may result. Other, homozygous, defects in the insulin receptor gene underlie leprechaunism (a severe congenital insulin resistance syndrome with elfin facies, sparse subcutaneous adipose tissue, growth retardation and failure to thrive) and Rabson Mendenhall syndrome (insulin resistance, acanthosis nigricans, growth retardation, abnormalities of skeleton and dentition, genitomegaly and hyperplasia of the pineal gland [44]). In the last, hypoglycaemia has also been noted as a result of abnormal insulin receptor function [44].

These conditions may represent a spectrum of the severity of the defect in insulin receptor function [43]. Recombinant human IGF-I has been tried to manage the hyperglycaemia, bypassing the insulin receptor [45]. The severe insulin resistance of childhood obesity syndromes (e.g. Prader–Willi, Alstrom and Laurence–Moon–Biedl syndromes) and premature ageing (Werner syndrome) may result in frank diabetes, as the pancreas fails to cope with the increased demand.

Another form of diabetes occurs with the severe insulin resistance of congenital or acquired lipodystrophy. Some of these rare congenital lipodystrophic diabetes syndromes are inherited in autosomal recessive form, suggesting a single gene defect [46]. The aetiology of the acquired form is not well understood but has been associated with spinal surgery and may include evidence of an inflammatory process in residual fat tissue. Subcutaneous and omental fat can be completely destroyed in these children and hyperlipidaemia can be severe, with episodic pancreatitis worsening the diabetes. The diseases may be complicated by liver disease and

**Table 24.3.** Maturity-onset diabetes of youth

| Class | Gene affected | Metabolic defect | Progress through life | Susceptibility to complications |
|---|---|---|---|---|
| MODY1 | *HNF4α* | As MODY3 | | |
| MODY2 | Glucokinase | Mild hyperglycaemia | Stable | Low risk |
| MODY3 | *HNF1α* | Insulin deficiency | Progressive | High risk |
| MODY4 | Insulin promoter factor 1 | | | |
| MODY5 | | | | |

cirrhosis, a poor prognostic factor, and cardiomyopathy. Diet and insulin-sensitizing agents such as metformin may help, lipid-lowering therapy is needed and insulin may become necessary. Lipoatrophy may occur in localized areas, when the metabolic disturbances tend to be less extreme.

## Mitochondrial gene defects and diabetes

There is an increased risk of type 2 and MODY-like diabetes being transmitted from the mothers and not the fathers of some of the familial diabetic conditions. This is explained by transmission of mutated mitochondrial DNA [47]. Such a mutation at nucleotide pair 3243 underlies both MIDD (maternally inherited diabetes and deafness) [48,49] and MELAS (mitochondrial myopathy, encephalopathy, lactic acidosis and stroke-like episodes) and may be involved in other types of type 2 diabetes [50].

## Type 2 diabetes mellitus in paediatrics

The class of type 2 diabetes probably includes a variety of different diseases characterized by insulin resistance and converted into frank diabetes by failure of insulin secretion. It is important to realize that insulin resistance alone does not create hyperglycaemia but leads to insulin hypersecretion. Diabetes occurs when insulin secretory capacity fails to compensate and an early sign may be loss of the first phase of the insulin response to intravenous glucose [51]. Insulin resistance is presumably at least partially genetic and may occur at both hepatic and peripheral tissues. Abdominal obesity and physical inertia are common associations, although the importance of fat distribution (intra-abdominal vs. subcutaneous) may differ between ethnic groups [52]. One hypothesis suggests that intrauterine undernutrition may predispose to both insulin resistance and poor β-cell reserve as diabetes and insulin resistance are more common in people with low birthweight [53]. However, genetic and other factors contribute to fetal size at birth and the causal nature of the relationship between birthweight and later risk of type 2 diabetes remains uncertain [54,55].

The obvious familial aggregation of type 2 diabetes supports genetic involvement in the aetiology but not inheritance of a single gene. Many forms of type 2 diabetes are likely to be polygenic, with a major role for the environment (see below) controlling the clinical appearance of the disease. Candidate genes have been explored, without great success, although there is some evidence for a link with HLA-DR4 [56,57].

Once considered a disease of the over 40s, 'true' type 2 diabetes is being seen increasingly in younger people, many in their 20s and some in their mid-teens or younger. This is particularly true of ethnic groups in whom type 2 diabetes is very common, which means almost every ethnic group apart from White Caucasians, who appear to be at low risk relative to other racial genotypes. Thus, type 2 diabetes occurs in young Africans and Caribbeans and particularly in young Asian Indians. Lifestyle changes play a major role in the pathogenesis of type 2 diabetes as the risks are greatly increased by urbanization, falling exercise levels and increased food intake [6]. Type 2 diabetes is more likely than MODY in young people from such backgrounds, especially if the family history for diabetes is positive on both sides. Abdominal fat deposition (as opposed to subcutaneous) is a particular risk factor. Obesity is a common but not invariable accompaniment to type 2 diabetes, presumably through insulin resistance, but it must be remembered that most obese people are hyperinsulinaemic rather than diabetic.

## Diabetes secondary to other disease

Secondary diabetes may also occur in children. Diabetes secondary to the pancreatic destruction in cystic fibrosis (see below) is a serious problem, almost inevitable as the children survive longer. Similarly, children with β-thalassaemia are now surviving long enough to develop a clinical problem with diabetes from iron deposition. Insulin resistance can also be demonstrated in these children before pancreatic failure [58].

## Diabetes and other autoimmune diseases

The autoimmune nature of type 1 diabetes has been described. Other autoimmune diseases occur more commonly in people with diabetes, especially thyroid disorders, vitiligo, pernicious anaemia, coeliac disease (see below) and other endocrine failure. Rarely, type I diabetes may occur as part of the polyendocrine syndrome, a condition of multiple endocrinopathies associated with lymphocytic infiltration of the affected glands [59]. Such polyglandular autoimmume syndromes may often include high titres of anti-islet antibodies, especially anti-GAD65. Addison disease, abnormalities of thyroid function (usually hypothyroidism in children), hypogonadism, autoimmune hepatitis, hypophysitis, alopecia, myasthenia gravis, pernicious anaemia, hypoparathyroidism, immunoglobulin deficiencies, keratoconjunctivitis, Sjörgren syndrome and vitiligo may all occur.

These polyglandular syndromes are sometimes classified into three types, all of which may include type 1 diabetes. Type 1 polyglandular deficiency (autoimmune polyendocrinopathy, candidiasis, ectodermal dystrophy or APECED) includes at least mucocutaneous candidiasis, hypoparathyroidism and adrenal failure, with 4% developing diabetes [60]. This has recently been attributed to the *AIRE* gene, which codes for a putative nuclear protein involved in transcriptional regulation, with an autosomal recessive inheritance [61]. In type 2, Addison disease is always present, 70% develop thyroid disease, 20% gonadal failure, 5% vitiligo and 50% diabetes. Type 2 is associated with HLA B6, Dw3 and DR3 and is inherited in autosomal dominant fashion [62].

Addison disease is not a feature of type 3 but components of each syndrome may not appear until adulthood, so continued vigilance is required. Identification of any second auto-immune condition in a child with type 1 diabetes should lead to a regular review for other autoimmune deficiencies or the child and, if Addison disease supervenes, his/her siblings.

Stiff-man syndrome is another rare condition of auto-immune deficiencies associated with neurological disorder and usually presenting in adults. Sixty per cent of sufferers are strongly positive for anti-GAD antibodies and many then develop insulinopenic diabetes. In one study, 72% of cases had the HLA allele *DQB1*0201* [63].

### Gestational diabetes mellitus

Gestational diabetes mellitus (GDM) is diabetes that is first detected in pregnancy. This may be detection of a previously undiagnosed diabetic state but may be truly gestational and resolve after delivery. This happens around the 28th week of gestation as a result of increasing insulin resistance caused by placental hormones and resolves immediately on delivery of the placenta. It indicates poor pancreatic reserve and 80% of women with GDM go on to develop type 2 diabetes in later life. This prognosis is much better in fitter women, of whom only about 50% develop type 2 [64].

With the current rate of teenage pregnancy in many parts of the world, GDM deserves at least a mention in a paediatric setting. As with type 2, African, Caribbean and Asian Indian children are particularly susceptible and these populations should be carefully screened. GDM is rarely diagnosed on symptoms but because of a high plasma glucose found either during a screening programme or in the investigation of persistent glycosuria. The use of traditional methods for identifying girls 'at risk' (macrosomia, obesity, family history of diabetes, etc.) is neither sensitive nor specific and screening of all pregnant women is indicated, although the best method for screening is not known. Recommendations vary from the US use of a blood glucose 2 h after a 50-g glucose load to the more usual European system of a random plasma glucose to select women for a full oral glucose tolerance test (75 g glucose in Europe, 100 g in the USA!). The cut-off for normality in screening is also variable, ranging from 5.5 to 7 mmol/L. Screening is often recommended at around 28 weeks, but some diagnoses may then be made too late to avoid macrosomia in the fetus.

The definitions for diagnosis of GDM also vary worldwide, but the WHO recommends a 75-g oral glucose tolerance test and the diagnosis of GDM made for any abnormality in the fasting or 2 h after glucose load blood glucose concentrations [14]. A working party for the European Association for the Study of Diabetes softened these [65] criteria to include only those whose 2-h *blood* glucose level exceeded 9 mmol/L. If hyperglycaemia is found in the first trimester, it is likely to indicate pre-existing, coincidental diabetes mellitus.

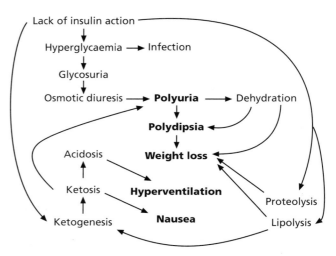

**Fig. 24.1.** The symptoms of uncontrolled diabetes mellitus.

## Clinical presentations

The clinical features of diabetes are predictable from the pathology (Fig. 24.1). Lack of insulin action results in hyperglycaemia. If insulin deficiency is sufficiently severe, proteolysis, lipolysis and ketogenesis also ensue, leading ultimately to diabetic ketoacidosis (see below). This is the hallmark of type 1 disease.

Hyperglycaemia causes an osmotic diuresis, leading to dehydration and the next cardinal symptom of poorly controlled diabetes, thirst or polydipsia. Nocturia and nocturnal drinking are almost invariably pathological and perhaps more easily quantified than daytime intake and output. A differential diagnosis for polyuria and polydipsia is given in Table 24.4. It is important to differentiate polyuria, the passing of large volumes of urine, from frequency, as may occur in urinary tract infection.

Weight loss is a sign of serious insulin deficiency and is a combination of dehydration and, in type 1 disease, muscle and fat loss. It can be very rapid.

Nausea and vomiting accompany ketosis, which also contributes directly to the polyuria. Ketones (a smell of acetone often likened to pear drops or old-fashioned nail varnish remover) can be detected on the breath by about 50% of the population. As insulin deficiency progresses, ketosis becomes acidosis and compensatory hyperventilation occurs. The conscious level deteriorates, probably in direct relationship to the rising osmolality of the plasma. Coma may ensue, characterized by deep sighing Kussmaul respirations. Diabetic ketoacidosis (DKA) is a medical emergency with 2–10% mortality. DKA may be precipitated by intercurrent infection, creating a stress response that is hyperglycaemic. It is likely that the hyperglycaemic stress hormones, such as cortisol and growth hormone (GH), are necessary for the development of DKA [66].

**Table 24.4.** Differential diagnosis of increased micturition

*Polyuria (large volumes) associated with polydipsia*

| | |
|---|---|
| Common | Diabetes mellitus |
| | Psychogenic water drinking |
| Rare | Hypercalcaemia |
| | Diabetes insipidus |
| | Renal tubular dysfunction, e.g. Fanconi syndrome, obstructive uropathy |

*Polyuria not associated with polydipsia*
  Diuretic therapy
  Heart failure

*Frequency of micturition (small volumes)*
  Urinary tract infection
  Detrusor instability
  Urinary tract malformations

Less than 50% of children will present in DKA. In others, malaise, polyuria and nocturnal enuresis, weight loss and thirst lead to an earlier diagnosis. In MODY and type 2 patients, there is sufficient residual insulin to limit ketogenesis (although DKA may occur in circumstances of extreme stress), and these children often present because a suspicious (diabetic) parent becomes concerned about the general health of the child. MODY may be detected because of hyperglycaemia detected by chance in a child with an incidental illness [39].

Hyperglycaemia encourages infection, and children with diabetes may present with skin infections, respiratory infections and urinary tract infections. Thrush, genital and even oral, is common and a form of 'nappy rash' on the upper thighs, with or without candidal infection, may occur as a result of glycosuria and incontinence. Recurrent candidiasis once the hyperglycaemia is controlled may lead to a diagnosis of more generalized autoimmune disease such as APECED. Subtle presentation with infections is, however, less common in children than in adults presenting with diabetes, probably because the hyperglycaemia develops more quickly in children.

All the symptoms described above are those of uncontrolled diabetes, and a child may present with them not just at the time of diagnosis but with any loss of glycaemic control thereafter.

## Diabetes through childhood

### Transient diabetes of the newborn

Babies are not born with type 1 diabetes mellitus and it is rare, although not non-existent, in infancy. There is a condition of severe insulin deficiency and hyperglycaemia that occurs in the neonate but recovers within a few months [67–69]. This is transient neonatal diabetes mellitus (TNDM), occurring in 1 in every 400 000 live births. The diabetes may recur in later life [70]. TNDM is associated with paternal uniparental disomy

of chromosome 6 [68]. The babies are small for gestational age and have little subcutaneous fat. A few have associated congenital abnormalities, such as spondylo-epiphyseal dysplasia [70]. This transient neonatal diabetes is sensitive to small doses of insulin. Congenital pancreatic aplasia is a very rare occurrence and is associated with other congenital abnormalities of the gastrointestinal and cardiac systems [71]. The babies have both diabetes and failure of exocrine pancreatic function. There are occasional case reports of absent development of β-cells in association with other disorders [70,72].

### Diabetes in prepubertal children

This is almost invariably type 1 diabetes. The presentation is with polyuria, often with nocturnal enuresis and perineal rash (sometimes monilial), thirst and weight loss. Vomiting is a sign of ketoacidosis and a medical emergency. Once the diagnosis has been made and treatment established, control may be complicated by marked sensitivity to small doses of insulin, and hypoglycaemia is a risk. The unpredictable nature of food intake and exercise in small children can create problems and give rise to significant stress in the parents, who fear both the long-term effects of hyperglycaemia and the occurrence of severe hypoglycaemia. Hypoglycaemia is often detected by the parent (pallor and behavioural changes such as lethargy, naughtiness, irritability), especially in the child who is too young to understand or express symptoms of a falling plasma glucose concentration [73]. It is important to achieve respectable glycaemic control in the prepubertal child as poor control impairs linear growth [74], and there is now evidence that hyperglycaemia in prepuberty does influence risk of complications, particularly the risk of retinopathy later [75–77]. There are now similar data to suggest that prepubertal diabetes control might influence the frequency of microalbuminuria (see below) [78]. However, the possible risk of permanent effects of severe hypoglycaemia on the developing brain and the frightening occurrence of seizures with severe hypoglycaemia in a young child [79,80] means that respectable rather than tight control is often a necessary compromise.

Hypoglycaemia may be a particular risk for children with diabetes under the age of 5, because children with so early an onset are commonly C-peptide deficient and so lack residual endogenous insulin as well as probably glucagon to respond to falling plasma glucose [19]. A minimum plasma glucose aim of 4 mmol/L should be advised, with higher levels (7–13 mmol/L) acceptable at bedtime, before the last snack (see 'Hypoglycaemia' below). It is important to keep plasma glucose above 4 mmol/L, as exposure to lower levels may increase the risk of severe hypoglycaemia (see below).

Respectable control can sometimes be achieved in toddlers with one or two injections of intermediate-acting insulins, and this can certainly be satisfactory in infants. Children with longer-duration diabetes usually need small doses of soluble insulin for meals, especially breakfast, but if less than 1 unit is needed dilution of the insulin in the pharmacy may be needed for accurate administration. If eating becomes a real battle between parent and child, the new fast-acting insulin analogues given during or immediately after a meal can achieve glucose control similar to conventional soluble insulins given 30 min before the meal [81].

Although it is sensible to be cautious in using novel drugs in children when conventional alternatives are available, if there are real problems with insulin administration and food fads, these new insulin analogues provide an alternative. It is important to appreciate their very rapid onset of action compared with that of conventional soluble insulins and the absolute need for eating within 5 min of administration if they are used preprandially. Their use in adults has been associated with increased risk of hypoglycaemia with exercise in the 2 h immediately after a meal, which may be a concern in active children, although there is correspondingly reduced risk if the exercise is delayed [82]. It is important not to over-restrict children's eating at this stage and to accommodate the child's dietary preferences as far as possible.

Overnight control with all young children can be difficult if intermediate-acting insulin is given before an early evening meal with the risk of running out of the insulin before morning. Parents may opt to give the evening intermediate-acting insulin later in the evening or at their own bedtime [83]. Continuous subcutaneous insulin infusion for the night-time only is slowly gaining acceptance [84].

## Diabetes and adolescence

There is a peak in the incidence of new cases of diabetes in the teenage years [24], and this may relate to the insulin resistance of puberty [23] making manifest a pre-existing decline in insulin secretory capacity. In pre-existing diabetes, control invariably deteriorates with the onset of puberty. In part, this is psychosocial because it is very difficult for both parent and child to transfer control of potentially lethal treatment from

the former to the latter, and the normal adolescent behaviour of testing boundaries and establishing independence is made much more stressful for both generations. The child's need not to be different from his/her peer group is very strong during this stage of development. The whole family may need much support at this time.

Some deterioration of control is inevitable, even in the most compliant family. Normal (non-diabetic) puberty is associated with marked insulin resistance for carbohydrate metabolism. This is probably related to GH secretion [23] (and to a lesser extent the sex steroids [85]) and is an important part of normal growth and development. The insulin resistance results in hyperinsulinaemia. Protein metabolism does not become insulin resistant and the hyperinsulinaemia enhances protein anabolism [86].

In diabetic children, the insulin resistance is accompanied by hyperglycaemia. Once the hyperglycaemia is established it exaggerates the insulin resistance [23]. Part of the picture is hepatic insulin resistance, not only in terms of exaggerated glucose production but also in terms of failure to generate insulin-like growth factor I (IGF-I) [87]. Low IGF-I may be associated with a slowing of linear growth and diminution of the pubertal growth spurt [88] and with disinhibition of GH secretion, which exacerbates the insulin resistance. The situation may be exacerbated by diabetes-related effects on the IGF-binding proteins, resulting in even less *free* IGF-I.

Although much experimental evidence for the existence of this cycle comes from the elegant studies where IGF-I supplementation improved insulin sensitivity and reduced GH levels in children [89], this is not a current therapeutic option, and this vicious cycle can only be interrupted by increasing insulin doses [90]. It is an important reason for assessing diabetes control not less than 3 monthly in children at this stage in their development, to detect and treat the problem as early as possible. There is good evidence for a correlation between maximal growth velocity during the pubertal growth spurt and glycaemic control, although the main effect on height achieved appears to be mainly in girls [88]. Paradoxically, a recent large study of diabetes in children conducted in Berlin suggests that diabetes that *starts* in puberty may be relatively easier to control than diabetes that began prepuberty and then deteriorates with the onset of the pubertal process [78].

Really poor glycaemic control in adolescents is, however, almost invariably at least partially a compliance problem relating to the psychosocial issues mentioned above. The problem must be approached carefully, to avoid alienating the child and the family. Children are not good at taking regular injections, carrying out blood tests or even eating as instructed by adults, and there are now sound data showing that up to a third of prescribed insulin is never taken [91]. Regimens that do not require injections to be made at school may be more successful and the use of insulin delivery devices, such as pens prefilled with insulin, which can be

promptly, aiming for early signs of improvement, but thereafter to accept a gradually progressive recovery.

The degree of hyperglycaemia does not indicate the severity of the keotacidosis; children with good renal function can clear a substantial amount of glucose in polyuria while retaining the acidosis. Osmolality and pH are better predictors of outcome. A leucocytosis is common, even in the absence of infection, and a tendency to hypothermia may override the expected pyrexia, even if infection is present. Abdominal pain is a common complaint and surgery should not be considered until the patient's metabolic disturbance is stabilized, at which time the signs and symptoms of an acute abdominal condition may be resolved. A high serum or plasma amylase in DKA is not necessarily indicative of pancreatitis.

## Starting insulin treatment in the non-ketotic child

In a newly presenting child with type 1 diabetes who is less unwell and not acidotic, subcutaneous insulin can be started straight away, often in an outpatient setting, if specialist nurse expertise is available to support the child and his/her family in their own home. However, it is important to be flexible about this and, if the family is very disturbed by the diagnosis, hospital admission may be kinder and a better long-term investment of educational resources. Parents, or the child if old enough, can be taught home blood glucose monitoring to ensure the safety of initial insulin therapy, but one should guard against overloading the family with too much information at this stage. Glucose monitoring, injection technique and reassurance that all will be well are the main objectives that should be attempted initially.

Once glycaemic control is settled, maintenance therapy must be instituted. For children with type 1 diabetes, the need for exogenous insulin is lifelong. Exogenous insulin therapies are not perfect and flexibility is needed in designing a regimen that best suits each family at each time of the child's life. However, in view of clear evidence that maintenance of near normoglycaemia in type 1 diabetes delays and may even prevent the chronic complications of diabetes, the ideal therapeutic goal is to achieve a near-normal glycated haemoglobin (the percentage of haemoglobin that is irreversibly glycosylated and a reflection of *mean* plasma glucose over the preceding 2 months) with no hypoglycaemia. Insulin therapy must be adjusted on a regular basis to achieve and maintain this. As a guide, one should aim for pre-meal plasma glucose 4–7 mmol/L, 90 min to 2 h postprandial levels of 5–10 mmol/L and a pre-bed level of 7–9 mmol/L (not strictly normal but a good defence against nocturnal hypoglycaemia). Defining a lower limit to normality is crucial to avoid loss of protection against hypoglycaemia (see below).

Once glycaemic control is settled, many children experience a 'honeymoon phase' in which insulin requirements drop almost to zero and peripheral sensitivity and residual insulin secretion are recovered by removal of the toxic effects of hyperglycaemia. This phase may last for several months, but eventually glucose indices rise again. It is usual not to stop the insulin entirely during such a honeymoon, both to reduce risk of developing an allergy to insulin and for psychological reasons.

### Intermittent insulin injection therapy

Maintenance insulin therapy needs to replace the basal insulin secretion of the healthy pancreas, which controls endogenous glucose production, and meal-related peaks of insulin secretion. In insulin replacement regimens, about 40–60% of the total daily requirement is for basal control, with the remainder for meal cover. Breakfast requires most insulin, lunch least and the evening meal an intermediate amount. Conventional insulins can be divided into two categories according to their pharmacokinetics and pharmacodynamics after subcutaneous administration: soluble and intermediate-acting insulins (Table 24.6). Commercial preparations may provide a mixture in varying proportions of one of each type. Long- and ultra-long-acting insulins have not been successful in clinical practice, either behaving in a rather unpredictable and inflexible manner (e.g. beef ultralente insulin) or being almost indistinguishable from the intermediate-acting form (e.g. human ultralente). The ability to engineer the insulin molecule to alter its absorption characteristics is being used to generate new forms of long-acting insulins designed for basal insulin replacement. This may mean that subsequent attempts at using a long-acting insulin with a flat absorption profile may be more successful.

Humalog, the first of the new insulin analogues to be available commercially, is an ultra-fast-acting insulin with a very rapid onset and short duration of action. This is

**Table 24.6.** Commonly available insulin preparations and their pharmacodynamics

| | Onset of action | Peak action | Duration of action |
| --- | --- | --- | --- |
| Soluble insulins Human, beef or pork | 30 min | 2–4 h | 6–8 h |
| Intermediate-acting insulins (isophane, NPH, lente). Human, beef or pork | 2 h | 4–8 h | 12–18 h |
| Fast-acting insulin analogues | 15 min | 50 min | 3–5 h |

achieved by switching two amino acid residues in the insulin B chain (lysine and proline at positions B28 and B29), as in the IGF molecule. NovoRapid, asparaginase at B28, has similar properties, the molecular changes making the insulin molecules less adherent and the insulin exists in solution in a monomeric state. Monomers are absorbed much more rapidly and reliably from subcutaneous tissue than the hexamers of conventional insulins. These new analogues are designed to be given immediately before eating, which is popular and may reduce the need for snacks. It is not yet licensed for use in children and should be used only if a real potential advantage is expected, e.g. reduction in nocturnal hypoglycaemia (see below). However, one group has shown it can be quite effective when given to children after meals [81], a possible approach to treatment, obviating the need for preprandial insulin administration for the worried mother whose child may be in the habit of refusing to eat after insulin injection. Humalog and NovoRapid performed well in all the safety and toxicology studies but their long-term safety has not been proven by long-term use, and they should be used cautiously in children.

Insulins are available in different strengths but in most Western countries all insulin is now 'U100', i.e. 100 units/mL solution. When travelling, it is important to check, as insulin syringes are calibrated in units and will be specific for a particular insulin concentration.

Ideas about optimal insulin regimens for children vary. It has been common practice to use twice-daily mixed insulins (a mixture of soluble or rapid-acting insulin with an intermediate, delayed-acting insulin either mixed by the patient or in a premixed preparation). This gives approximate cover for breakfast and lunch with the first injection and for the evening meal and overnight endogenous glucose production with the second injection (see Fig. 24.2a). Roughly about two-thirds of the daily requirement are needed in the morning (1:2 soluble to intermediate acting) and one-third (1:1) in the evening. However, modern monocomponent insulins are less immunogenic than their predecessors, and it is unlikely that any intermediate-acting insulin will last through the night in children whose evening meal (and therefore evening injection) may be relatively early (16.00–18.00 h). The risk of nocturnal hypoglycaemia is then substantial [103], for the intermediate-acting insulin reaches its peak activity 4–8 h after injection. There is also a high risk of escape from adequate insulinization later, resulting in fasting hyperglycaemia and even ketosis. Splitting the evening dose to give the soluble insulin before the evening meal and the intermediate-acting insulin much later (at the child's or even the parents' bedtime) may give greater stability (Fig. 24.2b). This has been of proven benefit in adults [104], but the impact on nocturnal hypoglycaemia in children is not clear. The one study explicitly examining this issue measured only one glucose level during the night and was carried out in children who already had their evening meal quite late [82].

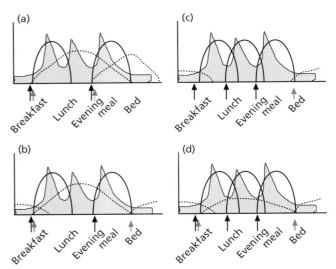

**Fig. 24.2.** Theoretical plasma insulin profiles in insulin-treated diabetes. Time is along the *x*-axis, plasma insulin levels along the *y*-axis. The grey areas represent plasma insulin levels over 24 h in a healthy child eating three meals a day. Solid lines and arrows indicate plasma insulin profiles and injection times of conventional soluble insulin; dotted lines and hatched arrows indicate intermediate-acting insulins. Wherever the height of the lines is higher than the shaded area is a time of risk of hypoglycaemia. (a) Twice daily mixed insulin regimen; (b) three injections per day, with the evening insulin divided; (c) the effects of a four times daily insulin regimen; (d) split basal replacement.

One can opt for giving soluble insulin before each meal and intermediate-acting insulin at bedtime (with or without a pre-breakfast dose of intermediate-acting insulin to provide a daytime basal insulin replacement) but this involves injections at school, which many children do not wish to do (Fig. 24.2). Studies seeking benefit from multiple daily insulin injections compared with twice daily mixed insulins have been generally disappointing but are usually cross-sectional analyses of clinic data, where intensification of therapy is often a response to poor control. A recent study in children with better control suggests multiple daily injection therapy may make glycaemic control easier to achieve [105,106].

Infants and toddlers may be very sensitive to insulin and many will manage on small doses of intermediate-acting insulin alone. Occasionally, it is necessary to dilute soluble insulin (which should be carried out in a pharmacy with official diluents) to be able to give fractions of doses to the very young.

### Continuous subcutaneous insulin infusion (CSII or 'pump' therapy)

There is a growing trend to consider continuous infusion of soluble insulin, with accelerated delivery (boluses) for meals [106–108]. Such therapy is delivered by placing an appropriate soluble insulin in a syringe that is connected to the patient's subcutaneous tissue via a fine cannula and needle, which may be left *in situ* for up to 48 h. The syringe is placed in a small portable syringe driver or 'pump', which ensures accurate delivery of low volumes of insulin on a continuous basis. The device is activated before meals to deliver a bolus of several units. It must be realized that the boluses are no different from the intermittent preprandial injection of soluble insulin on conventional therapy, with the same need for postprandial snacking.

The potential advantage of pump therapy lies in the basal delivery. This is designed to provide the background insulin replacement required to control endogenous glucose production and eliminates the problems of a peak–trough pattern of insulin effect seen with conventional intermediate-acting insulins. The stable basal delivery of insulin allows much more flexible meal ingestion, even covering 'skipped' meals in many patients, but the major advantage is the potential to provide better control of glucose overnight.

Modern delivery devices can be programmed to deliver at different rates for different times of day, which can allow for 'dawn phenomena' (the tendency of plasma glucose to rise from about 3 a.m. onwards, probably exacerbated by the waning of the effects of insulin taken the previous night) by allowing higher basal rates to be set for these hours. Some care is needed in the choice of soluble insulin used in such devices: Human Actrapid, for example, is compatible, as the new insulin analogues Humalog and NovoRapid, but Porcine Actrapid is not. This is because of differences in the solutions that make the latter more likely to block the narrow bore delivery system by crystallization.

As a general guide, 40–60% of the child's total insulin dose will be required for the basal rate with the remainder given as pre-meal boluses, most for breakfast, least for lunch and an intermediate dose for the evening meal. It is usual not to start with a basal rate in excess of 1 U/h. Adjustment is made on the basis of home glucose monitoring before meals to adjust the basal rate, and 90–120 min after meals to adjust the meal boluses. As always in adjusting insulin therapy, unless a dose is clearly inappropriate (e.g. causing hypoglycaemia), decisions should be made after several days' data collection, except at the very beginning when daily adjustment might be required.

There are problems with pump therapy, not least the cost. Pump therapy is *not* a solution for the needle-phobic or the uninterested patient, and it delivers good control only when carefully used. Regular monitoring of glucose is essential. There is a danger of DKA in the event of interruption of insulin delivery. The basal rates are small in dose and volume. Thus, a small amount of air in the system, once in the narrow bore delivery cannula, can interrupt insulin delivery for several hours. In the absence of any intermediate-acting insulin 'reservoir', DKA can develop quite quickly. Patients are taught to treat unexpected high blood glucose readings with an insulin bolus (usually half an average meal dose) and, if this has not lowered the blood glucose within 2 h, to take an injection using a conventional syringe and set up the whole pump system anew.

It follows from the above that the pump cannot be disconnected for prolonged periods of time, unless conventional injections are used. Patients do remove the pump for contact sport, swimming, etc., when blood glucose is usually kept down by the exertion, but some patients will need a small bolus immediately on restarting the therapy. This varies between individuals and for different activities, and trial and error with home glucose monitoring is necessary to find out what works for each individual.

Occasional patients experience redness of the infusion sites and infection here can be a problem. Allergy to the metal needles may be dealt with by conversion to all-plastic delivery devices and scrupulous attention to hygiene during set-up. It is not uncommon for patients to dislike the pump as a continuous reminder of their diabetes or as a physical nuisance; pump therapy is not for everyone.

### Management of diabetes in acute illness

Illness, even if accompanied by anorexia, generally requires increased insulin as a response to stress. Insulin must continue to be administered to the child with diabetes throughout acute illnesses. The urine should be checked for ketones, as moderate or severe ketonuria indicates significant insulin deficiency. If the child and/or his/her parents can measure blood glucose at home, many such illnesses can be managed at home. If the child is eating reasonably normally, supplemental soluble insulin should be given with or between meals, guided by home blood glucose monitoring tests at these times. Ten per cent of total daily insulin dose as soluble insulin is recommended if the plasma glucose is > 15 mmol/L and there is moderate ketonuria. If the child is not eating, one regimen is to continue the background insulin (the intermediate-acting insulins given as basal insulin replacement) and replace prandial insulin with boluses of soluble insulin (using doses as above) every 2–4 h, guided by the level of the blood glucose and the direction of change [110]. Higher supplemental doses may be necessary. Occasionally, but not usually, the insulin doses may need to be reduced to avoid hypoglycaemia. If required (i.e. if the child is not eating), glucose-containing fluids should be drunk gradually, to allow sufficient insulin to be given to suppress ketogenesis. Telephone support by diabetes specialist nurses or physicians should be encouraged and a paediatric diabetes service should be able to provide this. If the child's blood glucose is not responding to the home management regimens, hospitalization may be needed.

If the child is vomiting or has significant ketonuria (moderate or severe) that does not clear rapidly, hospital admission for intravenous fluid replacement and intravenous insulin becomes necessary. Unless the child is ketoacidotic, in which case the full DKA regimen is used, a slow intravenous infusion of glucose and potassium with intravenous insulin is recommended (soluble insulin at 0.05–0.1 units/kg body weight per hour). Once the child is eating, subcutaneous insulin boluses before meals can be reintroduced and the background intermediate-acting insulin replaced once the child is better. Intravenous insulin should never be stopped until some 30–45 min after subcutaneous soluble insulin has been given. Similar regimens can be used to cover other episodes when a child is well but not eating, for example during surgery.

## Oral agents in childhood diabetes

### Sulphonylureas

Sulphonylureas have no role in type 1 diabetes mellitus. They may, however, be used to treat MODY, at least initially. They are insulin secretagogues, which exert their effect via a specific sulphonylurea receptor, linked to the same potassium ion entry channel that is opened by glucose binding to the GLUT2 glucose transporter on the β-cell membrane. Opening the channel depolarizes the cell membrane, activating calcium channels. The subsequent calcium influx triggers a chain of intracellular pathways that culminate in insulin release. Sulphonylurea-stimulated insulin release is thus not under endogenous control; hence the potential risk for hypoglycaemia. The shorter-acting sulphonylureas such as glipizide are recommended in preference to longer-acting agents with a higher risk of hypoglycaemia, such as chlorpropamide or glibenclamide. It should be recognized that most of the data on hypoglycaemia have been gathered in adults, often elderly people, and the risk may be different in children. However, when sulphonylurea-induced hypoglycaemia does occur, it is likely to be prolonged, and, if severe, hospital admission for 24–48 h for glucose supplementation is mandatory. Tolbutamide and gliclazide are short acting, metabolized, not excreted, and are therefore safer in renal impairment.

Fears that sulphonylurea therapy might be more dangerous than insulin in type 2 diabetes and encourage cardiovascular risk have been laid to rest by the findings of the United Kingdom Prospective Diabetes Study (UKPDS) [111]. As sulphonylureas are related to sulphonamides (their hypoglycaemic action was discovered serendipitously during treatment of a typhoid outbreak in Vichy, France), allergy is a possibility and they should not be used in a patient with a history of allergy to the parent sulphonamide. Sulphonamides are small molecules and may cross the placenta [112]. As there are no reliable data to reassure us of the safety of sulphonylureas in early pregnancy and organogenesis and there are animal studies demonstrating teratogenicity of at least some sulphonlyureas [113], they should not be used in pregnancy.

### Metformin

The demonstration of the particular benefits of metformin in the adult-onset type 2 diabetic subjects of UKPDS may encourage more use of this drug in the young patient with type 2 diabetes, especially if not underweight [114]. Metformin, a biguanide, increases insulin sensitivity and is not necessarily as efficacious as sulphonamides in the MODY disorders where glucose sensing is the problem. It may, however, be useful in the insulin resistance of type 2. Its main side-effects are gastrointestinal (usually avoidable if the drug is introduced slowly), with the well-recognized potential to cause lactic acidosis a risk only in renal impairment. Monitoring of renal function is essential throughout metformin therapy, and the drug should be stopped immediately if a rise in creatinine is seen. Metformin should be withdrawn (replaced by insulin if required) before a young woman attempts to become pregnant or as soon as an unplanned pregnancy is reported, although uncomplicated pregnancy has occurred in women who became pregnant while on the drug [115].

### Other oral agents used in diabetes

There is a clinical need for new insulin sensitizers, and the thiazolidenedione group of agents offers some hope in this area. They are agonists of the nuclear transcription factors PPARγ and appear to alter insulin sensitivity at a cellular level and at fat distribution [116]. The first agent in clinical practice was withdrawn in Europe because of an association with hepatic toxicity, and other side-effects such as weight gain and anaemia need to be considered. Once agents in this class have proved satisfactory in adults, they may be useful in hyperlipidaemic, obese, insulin-resistant children with type 2 diabetes.

Agents that slow glucose absorption from the gastrointestinal tract are being used in obese adults with type 2 diabetes and have been suggested as aids to postprandial control in type 1 [117]. Adding soluble fibre is the natural way to achieve this effect, but the α-glucosidase inhibitors, which compete for carbohydrate breakdown at the intestinal brush border and slow its absorption, are now in common use in adults. There is no real experience of these agents in children.

## Side-effects of therapy

The mainstay of all diabetes therapy is diet and exercise, and these have no side-effects in children. Insulin and sulphonylurea therapy, both of which raise insulin levels artificially, have two principal side-effects, weight gain and hypoglycaemia.

Weight gain is mostly due to sudden cessation of a large calorie loss (up to 500 kcal per day) in glycosuria as blood glucose levels fall [118]. Some of the weight gain with initial improvement from poor glycaemic control is no more than recovery of weight lost before diagnosis, but there are other contributing factors. Insulin does promote fat deposition and is a growth factor. Furthermore, re-insulinization after severe deficiency causes a degree of sodium (and water) retention. This is usually self-limiting but can cause oedema, which has been reported to respond to ephedrine [119].

Hypoglycaemia is the most serious side-effect of both sulphonylurea and insulin therapy. The aetiology is multi-factorial, but it is due primarily to the loss of endogenous control of circulating insulin levels. The normal response to a falling blood glucose (as in fasting or exercise) is to reduce endogenous insulin. The type 1 diabetic child has no insulin reserve to do this. Moreover, the child with type 1 diabetes also loses the ability to secrete endogenous pancreatic glucagon within the first few years of diabetes, perhaps because the glucagon response to hypoglycaemia needs communication from an adjacent β-cell [120]. Thus, the child has lost the first two defences against hypoglycaemia.

With insulin therapy, hypoglycaemia will occur at any time when circulating insulin levels are higher than they would be if the child's blood glucose were regulated by endogenous insulin. Particular times of risk are therefore 2–5 h after meals, when soluble insulin levels are still high at a time when endogenous postprandial insulin levels would have returned to baseline and during the night (see below and Fig. 24.2). The former is usually dealt with by encouraging the use of complex carbohydrates in meals and the taking of snacks between meals.

## Nocturnal hypoglycaemia

In normal individuals, endogenous insulin levels are at their lowest at 02.00–04.00 h when whole-body insulin sensitivity is maximal as a result of circadian rhythms in the hyper-glycaemic actions of counter-regulatory hormones such as GH and cortisol. Endogenous insulin levels then rise slightly towards the end of sleep and rise substantially as breakfast is consumed. The action profile of an intermediate-acting insulin, especially if given at the relatively early time of a child's evening meal, is almost the mirror image of this, peaking about 6 h after administration, with levels then falling towards the dawn. Fasting hyperglycaemia is often the result, sometimes even with ketonuria. Attempts to rectify this by increasing the dose of insulin increase the risk of hypoglycaemia during the night. The residual effect of the soluble insulin given before the evening meal also contributes to nocturnal hypoglycaemia, as shown by the protection rendered by a late evening (between the supper snack and bedtime or at 22.00–23.00 h) plasma glucose of over 7 mmol/L [121–123] and the use of the ultra-short-acting insulin analogues for the evening meal, although this may result in hyperglycaemia in the early part of the night [124]. Although not all investigators have found the pre-bed plasma glucose level so useful a predictor of nocturnal hypoglycaemia [103], where it is suspected, elevating the bedtime glucose aim is a useful precaution. Insisting on bed-time snacking (perhaps including some uncooked cornstarch

[125]) and giving the bedtime insulin as late as possible are other useful strategies. Children who eat very late, as in some Mediterranean countries, may be at lower risk [126].

When formally investigated, biochemical hypoglycaemia at night is very common (recent published estimates range from 23% to 66%, with some contribution to the discrepancy relating to the frequency of monitoring) [103,121–123,126]. It is often asymptomatic, associated with diminished counter-regulatory hormone responses (especially adrenaline and noradrenaline) during sleep [127,128]. It may be more common in very young children and in those with lower glycated haemoglobin [103]. The significance of such asymptomatic nocturnal hypoglycaemia is uncertain, but it may contribute to increased risk of hypoglycaemia the next day, as the counter-regulatory mechanisms can enter a refractory period for up to 24 h [129]. Paradoxically, plasma glucose can also run high after a hypoglycaemic event, as both the endogenous counter-regulatory response and the tendency to overtreat have an effect [130]. Despite this lack of a clear indication of residual problems from nocturnal hypogly-caemia, it is sensible to try to minimize it.

## Symptoms of hypoglycaemia

In general, in the waking state and except for the insulin and glucagon responses, counter-regulatory responses to hypoglycaemia (which include the hyperglycaemic catecho-lamines, GH, cortisol and autonomic activation) are exagger-ated in children compared with adults [120]. Indeed, such active counter-regulation may contribute to diabetic instabil-ity as the vigorous neurohumoral response to relatively minor hypoglycaemia, especially when the hyperglycaemic response to the counter-regulation (which can last perhaps 24 h) is superimposed on the insulin resistance of puberty (see below).

The symptoms and signs of hypoglycaemia may be differ-ent in children. In adults, a set of symptoms attributable to autonomic activation (e.g. sweating, shaking, tremor, palpitations) can be differentiated from the so-called neuro-glycopenic symptoms (such as difficulty in concentration, drowsiness). Typical symptoms and signs are presented in Table 24.7. In children who are too young to express them-selves it is often the signs of hypoglycaemia that are detected by the parent (pallor, drowsiness, lethargy), but even older children tend not to differentiate autonomic from neurogly-copenic symptoms and a new set of symptoms and signs that are behavioural (aggression, foolishness, irritability, sadness) become much more important [73].

The symptoms of early hypoglycaemia alerting the patient to eat are his/her main defence against severe episodes in which plasma glucose falls too low to sustain normal cogni-tion. Ideally, symptoms and counter-regulatory hormone responses should precede any significant cognitive impair-ment as plasma glucose falls (Fig. 24.3), allowing time for the

**Table 24.7.** Symptoms and signs of hypoglycaemia in children [from 73]

| Neuroglycopenic and autonomic | Behavioural |
| --- | --- |
| *Reported by the children* | |
| Weakness | Headache |
| Trembling | Argumentative |
| Dizziness | Aggressive |
| Poor concentration | Irritability |
| Hunger | Naughty |
| Sweating | |
| Confusion | |
| Blurred vision | |
| Slurred speech | Nausea |
| Double vision | Nightmares |
| | |
| *Observed by the parents* | |
| As above plus | |
| Pallor | |
| Sleepiness | |
| Convulsions | |

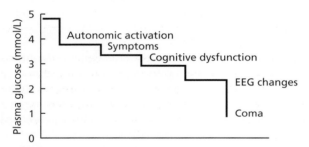

**Fig. 24.3.** Hierarchy of responses to induced hypoglycaemia in a healthy individual.

child to recognize (or his/her parents to notice) the developing hypoglycaemia and treat it. This protective hierarchy can be disturbed, as described above, in children who experience even mild hypoglycaemia regularly. It should be noted that in adults detectable evidence of mild deterioration in psychomotor function occurs as plasma glucose reaches 3 mmol/L, which is not a severe degree, although more profound hypoglycaemia is required for coma [131]. Young children may be at higher risk simply because they cannot express themselves, but people with diabetes can lose their ability to generate symptomatic and protective responses to early hypoglycaemia, usually as a result of recent prior exposure to a low plasma glucose [131].

Most of the research has been carried out in adults but defective counter-regulation, with lowering of the plasma glucose required to stimulate counter-regulatory responses to below that degree of hypoglycaemia needed to impair cognition, has been demonstrated in young people trying to use intensified insulin therapy [132], and it is thought to be inducible by regular exposure of the hypothalamic glucose

sensors to low plasma glucose as part of routine treatment. Such hypoglycaemia unawareness is reversible by careful adjustment of treatment regimens to avoid plasma glucose falling below 3 mmol/L [133]. The use of a lower limit of 4 mmol/L when setting glucose targets for home glucose monitoring is designed to help avoid any problems with hypoglycaemia recognition. Because of the lower glucose levels attempted, intensified insulin therapy designed to achieve and maintain near normoglycaemia is associated with increased risk of hypoglycaemia unawareness and severe hypoglycaemia, but attention to the lower limits of normality in adjusting regimens should limit this effect.

The transient defects in counter-regulatory responses to hypoglycaemia induced by exposure to an index episode probably underlie the increased risk of a second hypoglycaemic episode within 24 h of a severe hypoglycaemic attack [134]. Paradoxically, as severe hypoglycaemia will eventually provoke an endogenous counter-regulatory response (and is usually overtreated) [130], hyperglycaemia is also common in the 24 h after a single hypoglycaemic episode. It is important to recognize this phenomenon and adjust treatment regimens to avoid recurrent hypoglycaemia. Adjusting treatment as indicated by post-hypoglycaemic hyperglycaemia alone is a recipe for disaster.

## Exercise and hypoglycaemia

Exercise is a profound stimulus for hypoglycaemia and the duration of its effects should not be underestimated. The normal daily activity of children is not a problem as account will be taken of this in designing the usual insulin schedule. Intermittent activity (such as an adventure weekend, an activity holiday, such as at a diabetes camp, or a weekly football match) will require extra 'readily available' carbohydrate during the exercise and is likely to also require a 20–50% reduction in the overnight insulin. Alcohol can cause delayed hypoglycaemia on a similar time scale, and in adolescents the combination of alcohol and exercise during potentially long, late parties with dancing can be a profound hypoglycaemic drive. They should be warned to reduce their insulin dose as they fall into bed after such exertions! 'Recreational' drugs have various effects of glucose homeostasis but, in common with alcohol, have the ability to interfere with recognition of the effects of hypoglycaemia and reduce the likelihood of appropriate self-management. Educating parents, friends and, later, partners to recognize the signs of hypoglycaemia is crucial, and must be accompanied with lessons in how to treat it. All parents should be able to administer glucagon to their diabetic child (see below).

## Chronic effects of hypoglycaemia

Severe hypoglycaemia, usually associated with deliberate or accidental insulin overdosage, can result in permanent neurological defects. It is not known if recurrent hypogly-caemia from which apparently full recovery is made at the time has a cumulative effect on brain function, except in children under 7 years, where impaired intellectual performance has been detected in adolescents with a history of severe hypoglycaemia, associated with seizure, in early childhood [79,80]. The inability of a child to perform optimally and learn at school during hypoglycaemia, the embarrassment and potential for injury during severe hypoglycaemia and the possible risk of permanent neurological damage mean that treatment regimens must be carefully reviewed and adjusted to minimize the risks. Possible adjustments of the insulin regimen specifically to tackle hypoglycaemia risk are discussed above.

## Treatment of hypoglycaemia

Mild hypoglycaemia is treated by giving the child some oral glucose. Glucose tablets, sweets, and sugar-containing drinks such as fresh fruit juice or non-diet fizzy drinks, according to taste and convenience, will bring about a rapid restoration of circulating glucose levels; a more substantial starch-containing snack should be added if it is a long time until the next meal. Oral glucose must not be given to the unconscious child and all parents must be able to administer a glucagon injection (1 mg intramuscular is also effective if inadvertently given subcutaneously) that will produce recovery within 15 min. Medical practitioners often prefer to use intravenous glucose injection: low concentrations are much safer than the traditional 50% dextrose, which is a strong irritant and has resulted in amputation of hands, after perivascular infiltration. Equivalent doses of 25% or 10% dextrose are recommended, for example 2–4 mL/kg body weight 25% dextrose or 5–10 mL/kg body weight of 10%, the higher volumes being the maximal dose. In newborn babies, 1–3 mL/kg body weight of 10% is adequate. Parenteral treatment for hypoglycaemia is only required if the child is too obtunded for the oral route to be safe.

## Complications of diabetes in children and adolescents

Diabetes mellitus shortens life expectancy by an average of 15 years [3]. It is now fortunately less common for diabetic children to die in coma (hyper- or hypoglycaemic), although both still occur [101]. Broadly speaking, the complications of diabetes are vascular, both macrovascular (coronary artery disease, peripheral and cerebrovascular disease) and micro-vascular (retinopathy, nephropathy). Neuropathy, of which there are many kinds, may also be due to vascular damage to small blood vessels supplying the nerves, although this is not certain. There is some controversial evidence to suggest an autoimmune involvement in the pathogenesis of some autonomic neuropathies.

**Table 24.8.** Risk factors for diabetic complications

Unalterable
    Genetic predisposition (e.g. ACE gene polymorphisms and nephropathy)
    Puberty

Modifiable
    Hyperglycaemia
    Hypertension
    Dyslipidaemia
        Hypercholesterolaemia
        Low HDL-cholesterol
        Hypertriglyceraemia
Smoking

ACE, angiotensin-converting enzyme; HDL, high-density lipoprotein.

Macrovascular disease is the major killer. For example, diabetes negates the protection of the premenopausal female against myocardial infarction. Diabetes is the main cause of blindness in the working-age population in the Western world and follows only trachoma and other infections in developing countries. Diabetes is the most common indication for renal replacement therapy (dialysis or transplantation), where this is available.

The diabetic state includes hypercoagulation and increased oxidative stress. Examining large arteries with ultrasound has revealed evidence of endothelial dysfunction in adolescents with diabetes duration as short as 4 years [135]. Most of these changes regress towards normal with correction of hyperglycaemia, but they do not disappear.

Some risk of susceptibility to diabetes complications appears to be genetic. Type 1 diabetic children with nephropathy are, for example, more likely to have parents with hypertension and premature macrovascular disease. Recent evidence implicates the deletion polymorphism (DD) of the angiotensin-converting enzyme (ACE) gene in the increased glomerular filtration that is an early marker of incipient nephropathy [136]. However, it is important to realize that the other risk factors (Table 24.8) can be modified.

The Diabetes Control and Complications Trial confirmed early impressions that chronic hyperglycaemia was directly associated with a risk of microvascular disease [137]. A 76% reduction in risk of background or other retinopathy was seen in newly diagnosed type 1 diabetic patients randomly assigned to intensified insulin therapy aimed at establishing normoglycaemia. Risk of nephropathy and neuropathy were also substantially reduced, as was progression of established but early complications. It is likely that control of blood pressure (with the aim of establishing total normality, i.e. ≤ 120 mmHg systolic and 80 mmHg diastolic) will be equally efficacious. In adults, there is evidence for the specific benefit of using ACE inhibitors [138]. The management of hypertension in children is discussed below in the context of microalbuminuria.

It used to be said that diabetic complications did not occur before puberty and that, given the increased risk of hypoglycaemia with strict metabolic control, such control need not be attempted in prepubertal children. This is a fallacy. In children with poor control, growth is compromised [88]. This is at odds with evidence that diabetic children tend to be taller than their peer group at diagnosis but is based on demonstrations of increased growth velocity with the institution of intensified insulin therapy [90]. There is also the evidence of short stature in children with Mauriac syndrome (short stature, hepatosplenomegaly and chronically poor glycaemic control), even though only reasonable glycaemic control is necessary to sustain normal growth. A reduction in growth rate, associated with a high glycated haemoglobin and an absence of hypothyroidism, should direct increased effort at improving glycaemic control.

Hyperglycaemia in the prepubertal period also has a negative effect on prognosis for retinopathy. This comes from studies showing a shorter duration of diabetes to be associated with retinopathy in children when the diabetes developed before puberty [75–77]. Puberty is generally considered necessary for the development of diabetic nephropathy [139,140]. However, concern is also raised by reports of a significant incidence of microalbuminuria in young people with diabetes, which could potentially be modified by attention to glycaemic control, even in the prepubertal child [141].

Thus, in the setting of a paediatric clinic, it is mandatory to aim for optimal glucose control, defined as a near-normal glycosylated haemoglobin in the absence of significant hypoglycaemia, although compromises may need to be made where children find compliance difficult or hypoglycaemia risk becomes overwhelming. In pubertal children, the annual assessment of blood pressure, the retina and urine for microalbuminuria (probably adequately sought as the albumin–creatinine ratio in a first-morning voided urine sample, repeated on three occasions and positive in at least two) has become necessary and appropriate action must be taken if abnormalities are detected. Glycaemic control needs assessing much more frequently, as it can change rapidly, either as a result of lifestyle changes or with the onset of puberty and the physiological insulin resistance. It is very difficult to regain control of diabetes once lost, partly because of fears of weight gain, particularly in girls, lack of interest and the inherent insulin resistance of chronic hyperglycaemia.

## Hyperlipidaemia

With the prominence of macrovascular disease in diabetes, it is mandatory to check and control hyperlipidaemia. This should be done when the diabetes is stable, as extremes of hyperglycaemia may be directly associated with excessive and visible lipaemia. Hypercholesterolaemia occurs with the same frequency as in the non-diabetic peer population, but should be sought and treated if necessary. Hypertriglyceridaemia is more prevalent in diabetes, associated with high very low-density lipoprotein and low high-density lipoprotein cholesterol, partially, but not wholly, in association with poor glycaemic control. In adults, where there are data, these have the same prognostic significance as hypercholesterolaemia.

Initial treatment of hyperlipidaemia is with diet, exercise and direct attempts at improved glycaemic control. Drug therapy should be instituted where goals are not achieved by these manoeuvres. There are few data on lipid treatments in diabetic children, so adult guidelines with suitable dosage adjustment must be adapted. Thus, for predominant hypertriglyceridaemia, fibrates are the first-line therapy. Where cholesterol elevation is significant, statins are the treatment of choice.

## Smoking

Smoking remains all too common in children and adolescents with diabetes and should be discouraged even more actively than in the general population. Children should be asked about smoking habits, preferably when not accompanied by their parents. A clinician's sense of smell will often detect a smoking habit, which should be managed by advice and discussion, not confrontation.

## Complications of diabetes seen in childhood

Not all complications of diabetes require years to develop and some are seen in young people in particular.

## Growth delay

Growth can be adversely affected in diabetic children with the most poor metabolic control (e.g. Mauriac syndrome, see above). The metabolic abnormalities of poorly controlled diabetes include deficient generation of IGF-I, excess IGFBP-1 (both probably secondary to relative hepatic insulin deficiency) and high GH levels (after the loss of negative feedback inhibition from IGF-I and contributing to the insulin resistance of poor glycaemic control), all of which may be expected to impair linear growth (see 'Diabetes in puberty') [142]. However, for most children with diabetes, clinical observations show little if any deviation from accepted normal variations in the pattern and timing of growth and puberty. An early observation that children with diabetes tend to be taller at diagnosis than their peers [143] has not been substantiated [144–146] and could not easily be explained. The Oxford group found the age of menarche in girls with diabetes matched that of the population standards, with normal timing and duration of pubertal growth [144]. However, a loss of prepubertal height (0.06 SD a year) was seen in those diagnosed between 5 and 10 years of age and a greater loss of height during puberty in those diagnosed before the age of 5 years. In contrast, Du Caju *et al.* [145] found no loss of height before puberty, delayed onset of puberty but normal final height in boys, with girls showing a suboptimal growth spurt. Most clinicians will have their own experience of individual patients who have fared badly during periods of poor metabolic control, with partial or complete recovery of growth with improved glycaemic status.

## Skin disorders

### Necrobiosis lipoidica

This is a skin lesion of uncertain aetiology that occurs in type 1 diabetes and is independent of diabetes duration. Necrobiosis can occur outside the context of diabetes and the proportion of sufferers with diabetes is usually quoted as 66–75%, although in one recent study in adults only 22% of patients with necrobiosis had diabetes. In total, necrobiosis is diagnosed in perhaps as few as 0.3% [147] of diabetic patients but the prevalence in a paediatric population is much higher, 3% in our own clinic. Necrobiosis was considered to have no prognostic significance for other microvascular disorders, but a small study in Italian children reported necrobiosis to be associated with increased urinary albumin excretion and background retinopathy [148,149]. Kelly *et al.* [150] found similar associations in adults. There may be an association with poor glycaemic control [147].

It appears as patchy, scaly, atrophic lesions, with central thinning, even ulceration, usually on the lower, but occasionally also the upper, limbs. The lesions are indolent and tend to spread slowly. If damaged, healing in the lesion is slow and may take months. Histology shows perivascular inflammation. Necrobiosis can be a disturbing problem to girls and to those involved in sports where physical contact (human, bat or ball) may damage a lesion. Routine management comprises dry, occlusive dressings to protect from trauma. The lesions may respond to topical steroid therapy. The response is not particularly good and treatment should be reserved for lesions causing distress. Many other therapies have been tried including hyperbaric oxygen, tretinoin, prostaglandin $E_1$, pentoxyfylline and nicotinamide. In severe cases, systemic steroid therapy up to intravenous methyl prednisolone has been reported to help, although this will inevitably cause short-term deterioration in glycaemic control [150].

### Vitiligo

Vitiligo, patches of depigmented skin lacking melanocytes, is an autoimmune condition and seen in association with type 1 diabetes, itself an autoimmune disease. The condition is of cosmetic importance and children and their parents should be reassured that it is not dangerous. Care should be taken to protect the area from exposure to sunlight as tanning of the normal surrounding skin exacerbates the adverse cosmetic effect and the non-pigmented skin is particularly susceptible to ultraviolet damage. The presence of vitiligo should heighten awareness of the possibility of other autoimmune conditions such as autoimmune thyrotoxicosis, hypothyroidism, pernicious anaemia, hypoadrenalism and premature ovarian failure, although all patients with type 1 diabetes are at increased risk by virtue of possession of one autoimmune condition already.

## Neuropathy

Diabetic neuropathy comes in many forms. The classic peripheral neuropathy is a mixed sensory motor neuropathy, affecting the longest nerves first and hence starting in the feet. It causes pain, dysaesthesiae, numbness and wasting of the small muscles of the foot, with clawing of the toes. Ulceration and infection of insensitive feet may lead to major complications. Other neuropathies include transient (approximately 12 weeks) isolated cranial nerve palsies, thought perhaps to result from an acute ischaemic event, increased risk of compression neuropathies (carpal tunnel syndrome, ulnar nerve lesions, etc.), concurrent dysfunction of groups of major nerves (mononeuritis multiplex) and femoral radiculopathies (previously called amyotrophy), a painful weakness and wasting of large muscle groups, most commonly the quadriceps femoris. Damage to autonomic nerves, interfering with gastric emptying, bowel (and later bladder) function, sweating, control of the microcirculation, visual accommodation, heart rate and postural blood pressure control can also occur, increasing risk of foot ulceration and causing symptom complexes that are difficult to treat.

These neuropathies develop over years, encouraged by chronic hyperglycaemia and may be thought not to concern the paediatrician. However, defects of nerve function, particularly autonomic dysfunction, can be detected by formal testing very early in the course of diabetes, with reports of increased heart rate and abnormalities of pupillary reaction to light in the literature [151,152]. These may not correlate with diabetes duration or control and it is important to recognize that the prognostic significance of these malfunctions is not known [153]. Often the tests have been conducted without control of ambient blood glucose, which may affect nerve function acutely, and it is not certain how these reported abnormalities relate to the chronic nerve malfunction seen after years of diabetes.

Nausea, vomiting, abdominal pain and recurrent diabetic ketoacidosis may occur, particularly in adolescents with diabetes – usually as a result of poor compliance and indicative of social and psychological problems or difficulties of adaptation to the diagnosis. If gastroparesis, usually a late feature of autonomic neuropathy, is suspected, gastric emptying can be measured using radioisotope techniques (much more accurate than attempting to assess this parameter on the swallowing of a liquid barium meal). It must be appreciated that hyperglycaemia *per se* slows gastric emptying [154], and plasma glucose must be controlled within the physiological range (usually using intravenous glucose and insulin infusion) for the duration of the study. For similar reasons the study should not be performed within a few days of an episode of DKA and near normoglycaemia should be established for as long as possible before the investigation. Diarrhoea or abdominal bloating in a diabetic child should raise the question of coeliac disease rather than autonomic neuropathy [155]!

## Diabetic arthropathy

Limitation of movement of the small joints of the hands is described in diabetes, giving rise to the 'prayer sign' (an inability to flatten the fingers against each other with the hands held palm to palm). This was originally described in association with skin abnormalities, short stature and delayed sexual maturation, but a much milder form is common [156]. This may present initially as a flexion deformity of the proximal interphalangeal joint of the little fingers. Occasionally, the condition spreads to other joints including the cervical spine. Some reports show an association with other complications [157,158].

## Microalbuminuria

In adults with type 1 diabetes microalbuminuria provides evidence of early diabetic renal disease and, untreated, is likely to progress to proteinuria (arbitrarily defined as protein excretion of $\geq 0.5$ g of protein per 24 h). In children, microalbuminuria may be related to hyperglycaemia and may improve with improved glycaemic control. In this case, its prognostic significance is uncertain. There is, however, some evidence for an association over time with other evidence of (minor and asymptomatic) autonomic dysfunction and hypertension. Where indicative of early diabetic nephropathy, microalbuminuria may be accompanied by an increased glomerular filtration rate (GFR). It is not until more advanced nephropathy that the GFR falls. Frank proteinuria in children is unlikely to be diabetic in origin and, unless there is other evidence of diabetic microangiopathy, such as retinopathy, renal biopsy is indicated to exclude other glomerular or nephritic diseases that may require specific therapy.

Proteinuria progresses inexorably to renal failure, albeit at varying rates, unless death from some other cause intervenes. However, in adults, microalbuminuria may be arrested or reversed by lowering blood pressure as far as possible and treatment with ACE inhibitor drugs. These are thought to act on intrarenal haemodynamics and have protective effects for the diabetic kidney in addition to their effects on systemic blood pressure. Most studies suggest that microalbuminuria

does not occur in prepubertal patients, and the hormonal changes of puberty may be required for its manifestation [140]. In this, microalbuminuria may be different from retinopathy. In pubertal children, 10–20% may show microalbuminuria. Two per cent of non-diabetic children show intermittent and transient microalbuminuria of uncertain pathogenesis, so some caution is indicated in starting lifelong ACE inhibition [140]. There is a dearth of good evidence for the correct management of microalbuminuria in children and longitudinal studies are currently in progress to ascertain the natural history of the condition and the potential benefits of active management. Attempts to improve glycaemic control may help and can even, where control is really poor, produce resolution. Treatment with ACE inhibitors should be considered in teenagers with persistent and progressive microalbuminuria [159]. Any coexisting hypertension should be managed actively [160]. ACE inhibitors should be stopped in pregnancy.

## Retinopathy

Retinopathy in children, if present, is likely to be non-sight-threatening and of minor 'background' type with small dot haemorrhages, microaneurysms and small hard exudates. A recent Australian paper reports 28% prevalence of retinopathy in prepubertal and pubertal children [76], and another recent report from Sweden describes background retinopathy in 6% of prepubertal children and 18% of children who were Tanner stage 5 [161]. The same report documented preproliferative retinopathy in a child at Tanner stage 2 and there is no doubt that fundal screening, using direct ophthalmoscopy, preferably associated with photography through dilated pupils, is mandatory in children after the onset of puberty. There is also good evidence that the prepubertal diabetes duration influences risk of retinopathy later [75–77,141,161].

There have been reports of cataracts in young people with diabetes and removal of these may be followed by development of more significant retinopathy with soft exudates, formation of small new blood vessels, etc. [162]. In late adolescence, sudden improvement in chronically poor glycaemic control, perhaps the resolution of a period of non-compliance or insulin manipulation, may be associated with rapid deterioration of retinopathy into sight-threatenting proliferative disease. Laser therapy is then the only hope of preserving sight, and the eyes of young people who suddenly achieve improved glycaemic control after a year or more of very poor control must be closely monitored. This event must be distinguished from the benefits of long-term good glycaemic control.

## Diabetes and coeliac disease

Although not strictly a complication of diabetes, the shared autoimmune pathogenesis means that coeliac disease is more common in type 1 diabetic children, with quoted prevalences of up to 8% in some surveys [154]. Some authorities recommend screening children with diabetes every 5 years or so for evidence of coeliac disease (anti-tissue transglutaminase or antireticulin and antiendomysial antibodies, with particular significance of IgA antibodies and a need for jejunal biopsy of antibody-positive children). Certainly, the index of suspicion for coeliac disease should be high in any diabetic child with failure to grow and/or gastrointestinal symptoms [163]. Our own current practice is screening at diagnosis and later if glycaemic control is very poor, or if there are frank gastrointestinal symptoms or signs. Untreated coeliac disease carries a risk of lymphoma [164].

## Diabetes secondary to other diseases

Several systemic genetically inherited conditions cause pancreatic damage and β-cell deficiency. They include cystic fibrosis, β-thalassaemia and primary haemochromatosis. The first damages the islets in a generalized pancreatic destruction, the last two by iron deposition. Better management of these conditions, with improved survival, and the need for control of hyperglycaemia to reduce risks of chronic complications of diabetes means that the management of the diabetes requires increasing attention. Haemochromatosis is often undiagnosed until adulthood and the paediatric clinic offers an opportunity for early diagnosis.

## Cystic fibrosis-related diabetes

Glucose tolerance declines in children with cystic fibrosis (CF) over time [165,166]. Impaired glucose tolerance on formal testing has been reported in 14–36% of patients, with overt diabetes in 5–24%, according to the population studied. Development of diabetes is positively associated with increasing age and a deterioration in clinical parameters of nutrition and respiratory function, such as body mass index, $FEV_1$ (forced expiratory volume in 1 s), FVC (forced vital capacity) and increasing requirement for pancreatic enzyme supplementation. The prevalence of diabetes in children with CF in Denmark recently was reported as 1.5% below 10 years, 13% up to 20 years and 50% by 30 years of age [165]. In our experience of a cohort of approximately 200 CF patients, 12 have overt diabetes, all over 10 years of age, except one child with type 1a diabetes from early childhood, possibly coincidental. Significantly, nine of these patients have severe CF-related liver disease and three of them have progressed to orthotopic liver transplantation. A further seven patients, all over 15 years of age, have impaired glucose tolerance (IGT). An important observation is that overt diabetes, most noticeable as postprandial hyperglycaemia, can be present in the absence of an elevated HbA1c: in the Danish study only

16% of patients had elevated HbA1c at the time of diabetes diagnosis, so an oral glucose tolerance test at the annual review of older children with CF is mandatory. Hyperglycaemia must be treated, as it lowers the patient's defences against infection. As the survival of children with CF improves, we are beginning to see microvascular complications, which presumably could be limited by the establishment of good glycaemic control.

Insulin is often necessary in the short term in patients with IGT during infective exacerbations of their CF, with the need for steroid therapy for reversible obstructive airway disease or to cover transplantation procedures, and with intermittent or prolonged enteral or parenteral hyperalimentation (this has been particularly important to improve and maintain the nutritional status of patients destined for transplant surgery). Caution should be advised during reduction of steroids to alternate-day therapy, because of the potential risk of hypoglycaemia on the steroid-free days if insulin regimens are not adjusted.

Ketosis is relatively uncommon as sufficient pancreatic reserve persists in the early years of cystic fibrosis-related diabetes (CFRD). Permanent insulin replacement becomes necessary in the longer term as pancreatic failure progresses in order to maintain good glycaemic control. Regimens must be tailored to allow the high intake of energy-dense foods required by CF patients: modifications to the rate of ingestion of food supplements (daytime oral and overnight enteral) may be needed to balance glucose absorption from the diet with the action profiles of the insulin. The introduction of the very fast-acting insulin analogues may be expected to be helpful in designing appropriate treatment regimens, in particular for adolescent patients with variable compliance with both dietary and other treatment schedules, aggravated by a variable appetite, which can be profoundly affected by respiratory symptoms, physiotherapy and intercurrent antibiotic or other treatments.

## Pregnancy and the young person with diabetes

Poor glycaemic control during the first trimester of pregnancy decreases the success rate for outcome from 89% (vs. 98% in the general population) to 33%, with a high incidence of major congenital abnormalities and fetal loss [166]. Poor control during organogenesis increases the risk of malformation, with cardiovascular and neural tube defects (up to the oft-quoted sacral agenesis) being more common than in non-diabetic mothers. Poor control in the latter part of pregnancy causes accelerated fetal growth, giving rise to obstetric problems including premature labour and complicated deliveries, including risk of shoulder dystocia in the infant. Hyperglycaemia during labour increases the risk of hypoglycaemia in the neonate [167]. All fertile diabetic girls, irrespective of age, need to be assessed for risk of pregnancy. Girls who are sexually active should either be actively seeking to become pregnant and working with their clinical advisors to maintain a glycosylated haemoglobin within the non-diabetic range or on contraception. In the former, referral to a specialist clinic is recommended. The latter may best be handled initially through the paediatric diabetes team.

For diabetic girls, progestogen-only contraceptive preparations offer an optimal approach, but the tablets require a high degree of compliance, as therapy becomes ineffective if more than 26 h are left between administrations and can cause dysfunctional bleeding. Depot progestogen preparations are a good option for young girls, provided they do not mind the lack of periodic bleeding. Some vaginal bleeding may complicate the start of therapy but usually settles after the first 3 months. Prolonged use (> 5 years) may increase risk of osteoporosis, and oestradiol levels should be monitored after this duration. Currently available intrauterine devices, which are small and can include delivery devices for topical progestogen, are suitable for use in girls with diabetes.

Despite concerns about the vascular side-effects of oestrogen therapy, modern combined oral contraceptives containing not more than 30 µg of oestrogen are acceptable in diabetes. There was a vogue for using the so-called third-generation preparations, containing progestogens such as gestodene or desogestrel because of their apparently more favourable impact on lipid profiles, but the scare over the possibility of increased risk of venous thrombosis and pulmonary embolus has reversed this trend and more suitable preparations include those containing norethisterone (e.g. Loestrin, Ovysmen) or levonorgestrel (e.g. Microgynon 30) [168]. However, in a girl with a strong family history of premature cardiovascular disease or with herself an unfavourable lipid profile, it may be appropriate to consider third-generation contraception in discussion with the girl and, if appropriate, her family.

If possible, contraception should be stopped for 1 month before elective surgery because of the risks of venous thromboembolism. It is our opinion that the physical risks to both infant and mother of an unplanned pregnancy in diabetes outweigh almost all the potential side-effects of effective contraception. Migraine remains an absolute contraindication for oestrogen-containing preparations and other means must be explored when migraine and diabetes coexist. Barrier methods (condoms, diaphragms, etc.) offer the additional benefit of some protection from sexually transmitted diseases and no medical complications, but they are probably not sufficiently reliable for most young girls with diabetes, in whom an unplanned pregnancy can be an obstetric as well as a social problem.

Young women wanting pregnancy are probably ready to leave the care of a paediatrician, but the relationship between patient and medical team may be very strong and the transfer of adolescents with diabetes to adult services may be late. It is important to discuss the possibilities for successful pregnancy at an early opportunity with young diabetic girls and, if they are contemplating pregnancy, put them onto intensified insulin therapy and establish normoglycaemia before the chosen method of contraception is discontinued. Oral hypoglycaemic agents should be replaced by insulin, although hyperglycaemia rather than medication probably explains most of the problems of organogenesis seen in diabetic pregnancies [115,169]. It is also advisable to start oral folate as soon as pregnancy is contemplated. The risk reduction for neural tube defects in diabetic pregnancies has not been fully investigated but, as the incidence of such defects is relatively high in diabetes, the potential benefits are much greater than in the non-diabetic population. The non-diabetic dose of 400 µg per day is usual, although some obstetricians recommend 5 mg for diabetic women and there are no known problems with the higher dose [170]. Folate should be continued until the 14th week. The patient should be checked for immunity to rubella and transferred to a specialist combined diabetes and antenatal service.

It is probably not appropriate to consider the details of such services here – suffice to say that rigorous control of pre- and postprandial blood glucose levels throughout pregnancy is mandatory to avoid fetal loss, minimize congenital malformations and postpartum hypoglycaemia (in mother and infant) and maximize the chances of success. It must be observed that, with the best of intentions, many girls (and women) with diabetes present to services already pregnant, and the outcome of pregnancy in diabetic women remains significantly worse than in their non-diabetic peers [171,172]. Much remains to be done to improve the patients' awareness of the services available and the opportunities they have to improve their prognosis.

## Diabetes and subfertility

Many diabetic girls exhibit irregular menstruation and relative subfertility. This may result from extremely poor glycaemic control, which implies tissue malnutrition and may be considered to be a physiological response akin to that of anorexia. Alternately, polycystic ovarian syndrome (PCOS) is more common in girls with diabetes than in their non-diabetic peers, and the hormonal and ovarian abnormalities are not always associated with obesity (see Chapter 13).

## Diabetes and society: limitations and employment

It is current policy in most Western diabetes centres to regard diabetes as not being a limitation to anything the child or young person with diabetes wishes to achieve. Camps to provide activity holidays for young people with diabetes encourage self-reliance and self-confidence by supporting children to take on self-care, helping them to realize they are not alone by putting them with other diabetic children and encouraging them to undertake physical exertion such as games, water sports, riding and rock climbing. The children, and the carers, learn to adjust insulin regimens and food intake to compensate. However, the person with diabetes is at risk of problems not found in healthy people. Limitations do exist on the opportunities and openings available to them and one has to be realistic about these. Some of the limitations society places on its diabetic members arise from misunderstandings of the condition – others are less easy to deny. The main problems relate to the potential morbidity and premature mortality faced by the diabetic child secondary to chronic complications and the risk of sudden loss of consciousness, such as epilepsy due to hypoglycaemia and associated primarily with insulin therapy and to a lesser extent with sulphonylureas, or the certain death that would follow sudden failure of insulin supplies.

The law varies from country to country in the limitations it places on people with diabetes. In most cases, however, apart from matters such as weighting life insurance policies, the main problems are faced by those on insulin and are therefore relevant to most children with diabetes. It is important to be aware of these limitations as the child becomes a young adult and has to decide his or her career path.

Insulin-treated diabetic patients in the UK cannot undertake as professions vocational driving (buses, heavy goods vehicles), civil aviation (although some countries such as the USA are relaxing the laws for private pilots), national and emergency services (e.g. armed forces, police), work in dangerous areas (e.g. offshore oil rigs, moving machinery, incinerator loading, hot metal work, work on railway tracks, coal mining) or work at heights. Insulin-treated diabetic people cannot drive large goods vehicles (> 3.5 tonnes), vehicles carrying nine or more people, locomotives, underground trains and taxis (although this is subject to local variation) [173]. For UK diabetic people, the situation is particularly controversial as, until recently, they were not disbarred from driving small trucks and minibuses and many European countries have exclusions that are less stringent [174]. There is strong pressure to allow decisions about suitability for driving to be made on an individual basis, with each person's risk, for example, asymptomatic hypoglycaemia, being assessed. However, it is necessary to remember that any hypoglycaemia with seizure is considered a fit and severe hypoglycaemia should be reported to the Driving Licensing Authorities, and people with significant asymptomatic severe hypoglycaemia must be told not to drive until their warnings of hypoglycaemia have been restored.

## Genetic counselling in families with diabetes

The risk of a child developing type 1 diabetes is 5–10% if a sibling has the disease, 4–6% if the father is diabetic and 2–3% if diabetes is present in the mother. Risk can be more accurately assessed if the proband and the child are HLA typed and further risk determined by measuring autoantibodies and insulin secretory response to intravenous glucose in a sequence of assessment tests. In the absence of any intervention to delay the onset of diabetes, it is probably not appropriate to screen children in diabetic families for risk, except in the setting of approved research studies, as stigmatization and medicalization of the child who tests positive but who does not have the disease is a real risk. For children of families with type 2 diabetes, the risk of developing diabetes themselves is 10–15% (vs. perhaps 5% in the background population), with a 20–30% risk of IGT, and this risk is modifiable by lifestyle interventions. Screening (by repeated measures of fasting plasma glucose or oral glucose tolerance test) may be appropriate, but it is equally appropriate and less stigmatizing to encourage healthy lifestyles in the whole family! For a MODY family, with an autosomal dominant gene, the risk to the child is 50%.

## Requirements of a paediatric diabetes service

It is recommended that children with diabetes are managed by a paediatrician with specialist training in diabetes in a dedicated paediatric diabetes clinic setting separate from general or other specialist paediatric disciplines. This is to help develop and provide the environment, expertise and resources needed to support the management of the child and his/her family. In children with diabetes secondary to other diseases, adequate opportunities must be created to integrate care with the hospital or home care-based medical, nursing and dietetic teams. This may be through a single site (the preferred option) or through geographically separate but clearly linked units. A paediatric diabetes centre should aim for the provision of paediatric diabetes community nurse specialists and dietitians within the setting of the clinic to provide support for families in their homes and for the schools of the patients. Management strategies should be implemented by the whole team in accordance with nationally or internationally recognized consensus as appropriate. Availability of near-patient testing for HbA1c and glucose in the clinic is essential to maximize the benefit of education and management reviews focused on diary records of home glucose monitoring at 2- to 3-monthly intervals as may be required.

The diabetes care team should be able to meet the changing needs of children with respect to their physical and emotional development as they progress through adolescence and prepare for adulthood. The transition phase from paediatric to adult care is a complex and variable process, which ideally should be tailored to the individual patient's needs. Close relationships between the paediatric and adult diabetes services, which may not even be on the same campus, need to be encouraged to offer a cohesive programme at a time when the young adult with diabetes may be having to cope with the early long-term complications of diabetes as well as the demands of higher education, gainful employment and an independent lifestyle. No single model can be offered, but lessons can be learned from the models of transition care developed for young adults with other chronic diseases in childhood adjusted to plan for the specific demands of diabetes [175].

Although individual diabetes clinics will differ in the balance of their resources, access to a paediatric psychiatry/psychology service is essential, even for the preadolescent and their families. Family support is enormously important for the optimal care of diabetes in children, and diabetes control can be very difficult if there are physical or emotional stresses in the family environment. Access to services specifically targeted towards children with diabetes, such as summer camps and organized activity holidays, can be valuable in helping children develop some independence in a safe setting and helping them feel less isolated and less restricted [176]. The paediatric service must be able to direct families towards such opportunities. Paediatric surgery, nephrology, ophthalmology and podiatry resources all have a role in providing support for the small but significant proportion of children who will need their services. For many diabetes clinics, the specialist diabetes expertise is only available through the adult diabetes service and appropriate communications are essential.

## References

1 Laing SP, Swerdlow AJ, Slater SD *et al.* The British Diabetic Association Cohort Study, I: all-cause mortality in patients with insulin-treated diabetes mellitus. *Diabet Med* 1999; 16: 459–65.

2 Laing SP, Swerdlow AJ, Slater SD *et al.* The British Diabetic Association Cohort Study, II: cause-specific mortality in patients with insulin-treated diabetes mellitus. *Diabet Med* 1999; 16: 466–71.

3 Panzram G. Mortality and survival in Type 2 (non-insulin-dependent) diabetes mellitus. *Diabetologia* 1987; 30: 123–31.

4 Cunha-Vaz J. Lowering the risk of visual impairment and blindness. *Diabet Med* 1998; 15 (Suppl. 4): S47–50 (review).

5 Edmonds ME, Blundell MP, Morris ME, Thomas EM, Coton LT, Watkins PJ. Improved survival of the diabetic foot: the role of the specialised foot clinic. *Q J Med* 1986; 60: 763–71.

6 Amos AF, McCarty DJ, Zimmet P. The rising global burden of diabetes and its complications: estimates and projections to the year 2010. *Diabetic Med* 1997; 14 (Suppl. 5): S1–85.

7 Diabetes Epidemiology Research International Group. Secular trends in incidence of childhood IDDM in 10 countries. *Diabetes* 1990; 39: 858–64.

8 Shamis I, Gordon O, Albag Y, Goldsand G, Laron Z. Ethnic differences in the incidence of childhood IDDM in Israel (1965–1993); Marked increase since 1985, especially in Yemenite Jews. *Diabetes Care* 1997; 20: 504–8.

9 Tuomehlito J, Karvonen M, Pitkaniemi J *et al.* Record high incidence of Type 1 diabetes mellitus in Finnish Children. *Diabetologia* 1999; 42: 655–60.

10 Gamer SG, Bingley PJ, Sawtell PA *et al.* Rising incidence of insulin dependent diabetes in children under 5 in the Oxford Region: time trend analysis. *Br Med J* 1997; 315: 713–17.

11 Rosenbauer J, Herzig P, von Kries R, Neu A, Glain G. Temporal, seasonal and geographical incidence patterns of Type 1 diabetes mellitus in children under 5 years of age in Germany. *Diabetologia* 1999; 42: 1055–9.

12 Rangansami JJ, Greenwood DC, McSporran B *et al.* Rising incidence of type 1 diabetes mellitus in Scottish children. *Arch Dis Child* 1997; 77: 210–13.

13 Douek IF, Bingley PJ, Gale EAM. Risk of childhood diabetes rises with maternal age at delivery. *Diabetologia* 1999; 42 (Suppl. 1): abstract 325.

14 Alberti KG, Zimmet PZ. Definition, diagnosis and classification of diabetes mellitus and its complications. Part 1: diagnosis and classification of diabetes mellitus provisional report of a WHO consultation. *Diabet Med* 1998; 15: 539–43.

15 The Expert Committee on the Diagnosis, Classification of Diabetes Mellitus. Report of the Expert Committee on the Diagnosis and Classification of Diabetes Mellitus. *Diabetes* 1997; 20: 1183–97.

16 Ongagna JC, Levy-Marchal C. Sensitivity at diagnosis of combined beta-cell autoantibodies in insulin-dependent diabetic children. French Registry IDDM Children Study Group. *Diabetes Metab* 1997; 23: 155–60.

17 Sabbah E, Savola K, Kulmala P *et al.* Disease-associated autoantibodies and HLA-DQB1 genotypes in children with newly diagnosed insulin-dependent diabetes mellitus (IDDM). The Childhood Diabetes Finland Study Group. *Clin Exp Immunol* 1999; 116: 78–83.

18 Honeyman MC, Stone N, de Aizpurua H, Rowley MJ, Harrison LC. High T cell responses to the glutamic acid decarboxylase (GAD) isoform 67 reflect a hyperimmune state that precedes the onset of insulin-dependent diabetes. *J Autoimmun* 1997; 10: 165–73.

19 Bonfanti R, Bazzigaluppi E, Calori G *et al.* Parameters associated with residual insulin secretion during the first year of disease in children and adolescents with Type 1 diabetes mellitus. *Diabet Med* 1998; 15: 844–50.

20 Seissler J, de Sonnaville JJ, Morgenthaler NG *et al.* Immunological heterogeneity in type I diabetes: presence of distinct autoantibody patterns in patients with acute onset and slowly progressive disease. *Diabetologia* 1998; 41: 891–7.

21 Bingley PJ, Bonifacio E, Williams AJ, Genovese S, Bottazzo GF, Gale EA. Prediction of IDDM in the general population: strategies based on combinations of autoantibody markers. *Diabetes* 1997; 46: 1701–10.

22 McClarty DG, Athaide I, Bottazzo GF, Swai ABM, Alberti KGMMA. Islet cell antibodies are not specifically associated with insulin dependent diabetes in tanzanian Africans. *Diabetes Res Clin Pract* 1990; 9: 219–24.

23 Amiel SA, Sherwin RS, Simonson DC, Lauritano AA, Tamborlane WV. Impaired insulin action in puberty: a contributor to poor diabetic control during adolescence. *N Engl J Med* 1986; 315: 215–19.

24 Levy-Marchal C, Patterson C, Green A. Variation by age group and seasonality at diagnosis of childhood IDDM in Europe. The EURODIAB ACE Study Group. *Diabetologia* 1995; 38: 823–30.

25 Tuomehlito J, Lounemaa R, Tuomehlito-Wolfe E *et al.* and the Childhood diabetes in Finland (DiMe) Study Group. Epidemiology of childhood diabetes mellitus in Finland. Background of a nationwide study of Type 1 (insulin dependent) diabetes mellitus. *Diabetologia* 1992; 35: 70–6.

26 Todd JA. Genetics of Type 1 diabetes. *Pathol Biol* 1997; 45: 219–27.

27 Mein CA, Esposito L, Dunn MG *et al.* A search for type 1 diabetes susceptibility genes in families from the United Kingdom. *Nature Genet* 1998; 19: 297–300.

28 Bennett ST, Lucassen AM, Gough SCL *et al.* Susceptibility to human Type 1 diabetes at IDDM2 is determined by tandem repeat variation at the insulin gene minisatelitte locus. *Nature Genet* 1995; 9: 284–92.

29 Bennett ST, Wilson AJ, Esposito L *et al.* Insulin VNTR, allele-specific effect in type 1 diabetes depends on identity of untransmitted paternal allele. The IMDIAB Group. *Nature Genet* 1997; 17: 350–2.

30 Dokheel TM. For the Pittsburgh Diabetes Research Epidemiology Group. An epidemic of childhood diabetes in the United States? Evidence from Allegheny County PA. *Diabetes Care* 1994; 16: 1606–2611.

31 Karvonen M, Tuomehlito J, Virtala E *et al.* for the Childhood Diabetes in Finland (DiMe) study Group. Seasonality in the clinical onset of insulin dependent diabetes mellitus in Finnish Children. *Am J Epidmiol* 1996; 143: 167–76.

32 Atkinson MA, Bowman MA, Campbell L *et al.* Cellular immunity to a determinant common to glutamate decarboxylase and Coxsackie virus in insulin dependent diabetes. *J Clin Invest* 1994; 94: 2125–9.

33 Hyoty H, Hiltunehn M, Knip M *et al.* and the Childhood Diabetes in Finland (DiMe) study Group. A prospective study of the role of Coxsackie B and other enteroviruses in the pathogenesis of insulin dependent diabetes mellitus. *Diabetes* 1995; 44: 652–7.

34 Ginsberg-Fellner F, Witt ME, Fedun B *et al.* Diabetes mellitus and autoimmunity in patients with congenital rubella syndrome. *Rev Infect Dis* 1985; 7 (Suppl. 1): S170–S176.

35 Virtanen SM, Hypponen E, Laara E *et al.* Cow's milk consumption, disease associated autoantibodies and type 1 diabetes mellitus: a follow-up study in siblings of diabetic children. Childhood Diabetes Finland Study. *Diabetic Med* 1998; 15: 730–8.

36 Meloni T, Marinaro AM, Mannazzu MC, Ogana A, LaVecchia C, Negri E, Colombo C. IDDM and early infant feeding. Sardinian case control study. *Diabetes Care* 1997; 20: 340–2.

37 Atkinson MA, Ellis TM. Infants' diets and insulin dependent diabetes: evaluating the 'cow's milk hypothesis' and a role for anti-bovine serum albumin immunity. *J Am Coll Nutr* 1997; 16: 334–40.

38 Hattersley AT. Maturity-onset diabetes of the young: clinical heterogeneity explained by genetic heterogeneity. *Diabetic Med* 1998; 15: 15–24, 437.

39 Matyka KA, Beards F, Appleton M, Ellard S, Hattersley A, Dunger DB. Genetic testing for maturity onset diabetes of the young in childhood hyperglycaemia. *Arch Dis Child* 1998; 78: 552–4.

40 Anwar AJ, Walker JD, Frier BM. Type 1 diabetes mellitus and Down's syndrome: prevalence, management and diabetic complications. *Diabet Med* 1998; 15: 160–3.

41 Gerbitz KD. Reflections on a newly discovered diabetogenic gene, wolframin (WFS1). *Diabetologia* 1999; 42: 627–30.

42 Inoue H, Tanizawa Y, Wasson J *et al.* A gene encoding a transmembrane protein is mutated in patients with diabetes mellitus and optic atrophy (Wolfram syndrome). *Nature Genet* 1998; 20: 143–8.

43 Krook A, O'Rahilly S. Mutant insulin receptors in syndromes of insulin resistance. *Baillière's Clin Endocrinol Metab* 1996; 10: 97–122.

44 Longo N, Wang Y, Pasquali M. Progressive decline in insulin levels in Rabson Mendenhall syndrome. *J Clin Endocrinol Metab* 1999; 84: 2623–9.

45 Kuzuya H, Matsuura N, Sakamoto M *et al.* Trial of insulin like growth factor 1 therapy for patients with extreme insulin resistance syndromes. *Diabetes* 1993; 42: 696–705.

46 Seip M, Trygstad O. Generalized lipodystrophy, congenital and acquired (lipoatrophy). *Acta Paediatr Suppl* 1996; 413: 2–28.

47 Suomalainen A. Mitochondrial DNA and disease. *Ann Med* 1997; 29: 235–46.

48 Newkirk JE, Taylor RW, Howell N *et al.* Maternally inherited diabetes and deafness: prevalence in a hospital diabetic population. *Diabetic Med* 1997; 14: 457–60.

49 Maassen JA, Jansen JJ, Kadowaki T, van den Ouweland JM, 't Hart LM, Lemkes HH. The molecular basis and clinical characteristics of Maternally Inherited Diabetes and Deafness (MIDD), a recently recognised diabetic subtype. *Diabetologia* 1993; 36: 1288–92.

50 Hanna MG, Nelson IP, Morgan-Hughes JA, Wood NW. MELAS; a new disease associated mitochondrial DNA mutation and evidence for further heterogeneity. *J Neurol Neurosurg Psychiatry* 1998; 65: 512–17.

51 Araujo-Vilar D, Garcia-Estevez DA, Cabezas-Cerrato J. Insulin sensitivity, glucose effectiveness and insulin secretion in nondiabetic offspring of patients with non-insulin dependent diabetes mellitus: a cross-sectional study. *Metabolism* 1999; 48: 978–83.

52 Gower BA, Nagy TR, Trowbridge CA, Dezenberg C, Goran MI. Fat distribution and insulin response in prepubertal African American and white children. *Am J Clin Nutr* 1998; 67: 821–7.

53 Phillips DI. Birth weight and the future development of diabetes. *Ann Rev Evidence Diabetes Care* 1998; 21 (Suppl. 2): B150–5.

54 Dunger DB, Ong KK, Huxtable SJ *et al.* Association of the INS VNTR with size at birth. ALSPAC Study Team. Avon Longitudinal Study of Pregnancy and Childhood. *Nature Genet* 1998; 19: 98–100.

55 Casteels K, Ong K, Phillips D, Bendall H, Pembrey M. Mitochondrial 16189 variant, thinness at birth, and type-2 diabetes. ALSPAC study team. Avon Longitudinal Study of Pregnancy and Childhood. *Lancet* 1999; 353: 1499–500.

56 Ghabanbasani MZ, Spaepen M, Buyse I *et al.* Increased and decreased relative risk for non-insulin-dependent diabetes

mellitus conferred by HLA class II and by CD4 alleles. *Clin Genet* 1995; 47: 225–30.

57 Scott CR, Smith JM, Cradock MM, Pihoker C. Characteristics of youth-onset noninsulin-dependent diabetes mellitus and insulin-dependent diabetes mellitus at diagnosis. *Pediatrics* 1997; 100: 84–91.

58 Jones TW, Boulware SD, Caprio S *et al.* Correction of hyperinsulinemia by glyburide treatment in non-diabetic patients with thalassemia major. *Pediatr Res* 1993; 33: 497–500.

59 Riley WJ. Autoimmune polyglandular syndromes. *Pediatr Res* 1993; 33: 497–500. *Horm Res* 1992; 38 (Suppl. 2): 9–15.

60 Obermayer-Straub P, Manns MP. Autoimmune polyglandular syndromes. *Bailliere's Clin Gastroenterol* 1998; 12: 293–315.

61 The Finnish–German APECED Consortium. Autoimmune polyendocrinopathy–candidiasis–ectodermal dystrophy. An autoimmune disease, APECED, caused by mutations in a novel gene featuring two PHD-type zinc-finger domains. *Nature Genet* 1997; 17: 399–403.

62 Leor J, Levortowsky D, Sharon C. Polyglandular autoimmune syndrome, Type 2. *South Med J* 1989; 82: 374–6.

63 Pugliese A, Solimena M, Awdeh ZL, Alper CA, Bugawan T, Erlich HA, De Camilli P, Eisenbarth GS. Association of HLA-DQB1*0201 with stiff-man syndrome. *J Clin Endocrinol Metab* 1993; 77: 1550–3.

64 O'Sullivan JB. Body weight and subsequent diabetes mellitus. *J Am Med Assoc* 1982; 248: 949.

65 Lao TT, Lee CP. Gestational 'impaired glucose tolerance': should the cut-off be raised to 9 mmol/l? *Diabetic Med* 1998; 15: 25.

66 Barnes AJ, Kohner EM, Bloom SR, Johnston DDG, Alberti KGMM, Smythe F. Importance of pituitary hormones in aetiology of diabetic ketoacidosis. *Lancet* 1978; I: 1171–4.

67 Armentrout D. Neonatal diabetes mellitus. *J Pediatr Health Care* 1995; 9: 75–8.

68 Gardner RRJ, Mungall AJ, Dunham I *et al.* Localisation of a gene for transient neonatal diabetes mellitus to an 18.72 cR3000 (approximately 5.4 Mb) interval on chromosome 6q. *J Med Genetics* 1999; 36: 192–6.

69 Von Muhlendahl KE, Herkenhoff H. Long term course of neonatal diabetes. *N Engl J Med* 1995; 333: 704–8.

70 Fosel S. Transient and permanent neonatal diabetes. *Eur J Pediatr* 1995; 154: 944–8.

71 Voldsgaard P, Kryger-Baggesen N, Lisse I. Agenesis of pancreas. *Acta Paediatr* 1994; 83: 791–3.

72 Blum D, Dorchy H, Mouraux T *et al.* Congenital absence of insulin cells in a neonate with diabetes mellitus and mutase-deficient methylmalonic acidaemia. *Diabetologia* 1993; 36: 352–7, 1332.

73 Ross LA, McCrimmon RJ, Frier BM, Kelnar CJ, Deary IJ. Hypoglycaemic symptoms reported by children with Type 1 diabetes mellitus and by their parents. *Diabetic Med* 1998; 15: 836–43.

74 Danne T, Kordonouri O, Enders I, Weber B. Factors influencing height and weight development in children with diabetes. Results Berlin Retinopathy Study. *Diabetes Care* 1997; 20: 281–5.

75 Holl RW, Lang GE, Grabert M, Heinze E, Lang GK, Debatin KM. Diabetic retinopathy in pediatric patients with type-1 diabetes: effect of diabetes duration, prepubertal and pubertal onset of diabetes, and metabolic control. *Pediatrics* 1998; 132: 790–4.

76 Donaghue KC, Fung AT, Hing S *et al.* The effect of prepubertal diabetes duration on diabetes. Microvascular complications in early and late adolescence. *Diabetes Care* 1997; 20: 77–80.

77 Kordonouri O, Danne T, Enders I, Weber B. Does the long-term clinical course of type I diabetes mellitus differ in patients with prepubertal and pubertal onset? Results Berlin Retinopathy Study. *Eur J Pediatr* 1998; 157: 202–7.

78 Schultz CJ, Konopelska-Bahu T, Dalton RN *et al.* Microalbuminuria prevalence varies with age, sex, and puberty in children with type 1 diabetes followed from diagnosis in a longitudinal study. Oxford Regional Prospective Study Group. *Diabetes Care* 1999; 22: 495–502.

79 Rovet JF, Erlich RM. The effect of hypoglycemic seizures on cognitive function in children with diabetes: a 7 year prospective study. *J Pediatr* 1999; 134: 503–6.

80 Rovet J, Alvarez M. Attentional functioning in children and adolescents with IDDM. *Diabetes Care* 1997; 20: 803–10.

81 Schernthaner G, Wein W, Sandholzer K, Equiluz-Bruck S, Bates PC, Birkett MA. Postprandial insulin lispro. A new therapeutic option for type 1 diabetic patients. *Diabetes Care* 1998; 21: 570–3.

82 Tuominen JA, Karonene SL, Melamies L, Bolli G, Koivisto VA. Exercise induced hypoglycemia in IDDM patients treated with a short acting insulin analog. *Diabetologia* 1995; 38: 106–11.

83 Meschi F, Bonfanti R, De Poli S *et al.* Frequency and predictor factors of nocturnal hypoglycaemia in young patients with IDDM. *Diabetologia* 1999; 42 (Suppl. 1): 824.

84 Bruns W, Steinborn F, Menzel R, Staritz B, Bibergeil H. Nocturnal continuous subcutaneous insulin infusion – a therapeutic possibility in labile type 1 diabetes under exceptional conditions. *Z Gesamte Inn Med* 1990; 45: 154–8 [in German].

85 Bloch CA, Clemons P, Sperling MA. Puberty decreases insulin sensitivity. *J Pediatr* 1987; 110: 481–7.

86 Amiel SA, Caprio S, Sherwin RS, Plewe G, Haymond MW, Tamborlane WV. Insulin resistance of puberty: a defect restricted to peripheral glucose metabolism. *J Clin Endocrinol Metab* 1991; 72: 277–82.

87 Amiel SA, Sherwin RS, Hintz RL, Gertner JM, Press CM, Tamborlane WV. Effects of diabetes and its control on insulin-like growth factors in the young subject with Type 1 diabetes. *Diabetes* 1984; 33: 1175–9.

88 Ahmed ML, Connors MH, Drayer NM, Jones JS, Dunger DB. Pubertal growth in IDDM is determined by HbA1c levels, sex, and bone age. *Diabetes Care* 1998; 21: 831–5.

89 Acerini CL, Patton CM, Savage MO, Kernell A, Westphal O, Dunger DB. Randomised placebo controlled trial of human recombinant insulin like growth factor 1. *Lancet* 1997; 350: 1199–1204.

90 Rudolph MC, Sherwin RS, Markowitz R *et al.* Effect of intensified insulin therapy on linear growth. *J Pediatr* 1982; 101: 333–9.

91 Morris AD, Boyle DI, McMahon AD, Greene SA, MacDonald TM, Newton RW. Adherence to insulin treatment, glycaemic control, and ketoacidosis in insulin-dependent diabetes mellitus. The DARTS/MEMO Collaboration. Diabetes Audit and Research in Tayside Scotland. Medicines Monitoring Unit. *Lancet* 1997; 350: 1505–10.

92 Fairburn CG, Peveler RC, Davies B, Mann JI, Mayou RA. Eating disorders in young adults with insulin dependent diabetes mellitus: a controlled study. *Br Med J* 1991; 303: 17–20.

93 Rydall AC, Rodin GM, Olmsted MP, Devenyi RG, Daneman D. Disordered eating behavior and microvascular complications in young women with insulin-dependent diabetes mellitus. *N Engl J Med* 1997; 336: 1849–54.

94 Peveler RC, Fairburn CG, Boller I, Dunger D. Eating disorders in adolescents with IDDM. A controlled study. *Diabetes Care* 1992; 15: 1356–60.

95 Ronnemaa T, Viikari J. Reducing snacks when switching from conventional soluble to lispro insulin treatment: effects on glycaemic control and hypoglycaemia. *Diabet Med* 1998; 15: 601–7.

96 Dowey JA. Dental care of patients with diabetes mellitus. *Diabet Med* 1999; 16: 173.

97 Smith CP, Firth D, Bennett S, Howard C, Chisholm P. Ketoacidosis occurring in newly diagnosed and established diabetic children. *Acta Paediatr* 1998; 87: 537–41.

98 Silink M. Practical management of diabetic ketoacidosis in childhood and adolescence. *Acta Paediatr Suppl* 1998; 425: 63–6.

99 Brandenburg MA, Dire DJ. Comparison of arterial and venous blood gas values in the initial emergency department evaluation of patients with diabetic ketoacidosis. *Ann Emerg Med* 1998; 31: 459–65.

100 Green SM, Rothrock SG, Ho JD *et al.* Failure of adjunctive bicarbonate to improve outcome in severe pediatric diabetic ketoacidosis. *Ann Emerg Med* 1998; 31: 41–8.

101 Edge JA, Forde-Adams ME, Dunger DB. Causes of death in children with insulin dependent diabetes 1990–96. *Arch Dis Child* 1999; 81: 318–23,.

102 Hoffman WH, Locksmith JP, Burton EM *et al.* Interstitial pulmonary edema in children and adolescents with diabetic ketoacidosis. *J Diabetes Complications* 1998; 12: 314–20.

103 Porter PA, Keating B, Byrne G, Jones TW. Incidence and predictive criteria of nocturnal hypoglycemia in young children with insulin-dependent diabetes mellitus. *Pediatrics* 1997; 130: 366–72.

104 Ahmed AB, Home PD. The effect of the insulin analog lispro on night time blood glucose control in Type 1 diabetic patients. *Diabetes Care* 1998; 21: 32–7.

105 Mortgensen HB, Robertson KJ, Aanstppt HJ *et al.* Insulin management and metabolic control of Type 1 diabetes mellitus in childhood and adolescence in 18 countries. The Hvidore Study Group on Childhood Diabetes. *Diabetic Med* 1998; 15: 752–9.

106 Tamborlane WV, Ahern H. Implications and results of the Diabetes Control and Complications Trial. *Pediatr Clin N Am* 1997; 44: 285–300.

107 De Beaufort CE, Houtzagers CM, Bruining GJ *et al.* Continuous subcutaneous insulin infusion vs conventional injection therapy in newly diagnosed diabetic children: two-year follow-up of a randomised, prospective trial. *Diabet Med* 1989; 6: 766–71.

108 Steindel BS, Roe TR, Costin G, Carlson M, Kaufman FR. Continuous subcutaneous insulin infusion (CSII) in children and adolescents with chronic poorly controlled type 1 diabetes mellitus. *Diabetes Res Clin Pract* 1995; 27: 199–204.

109 Becker D. Individualised insulin therapy in children and adolescents with type 1 diabetes. *Acta Paediatr Suppl* 1998; 425: 20–4.

110 Travaglini MT, Garg SK, Chase HP. Use of insulin lispro in the outpatient management of ketonuria. *Arch Pediatr Adolesc Med* 1998; 152: 672–5.

111 UK Prospective Diabetes Study Group. Intensive blood glucose control with sulphonylureas or insulin compared with conventional therapy and risk of complications in patients with Type 2 diabetes mellitus. UKPDS 33. *Lancet* 1998; 352: 837–53.

112 Sivan E, Feldman BDD, Ddolitzki M, Nevo N, Dekel N, Karasik A. Glyburide crosses the placenta in pregnant rats. *Diabetologia* 1995; 38: 753–6.

113 Smoak JW. Embryopathic effects of the oral hypoglycemic agent chlorpropamide in cultured mouse embryos. *Am J Obstet Gynecol* 1993; 169: 409–14.

114 UK Prospective Diabetes Study Group. Effect of intensive blood glucose control with metformin on complications in patients with Type 2 diabetes. UKPDS 34. *Lancet* 1998; 352: 854–65.

115 Hellmuth E, Damm P, Molsted-Pedersen L. Congenital malformations in offspring in diabetic women treated with oral hypoglycaemic agents during organogenesis. *Diabetic Med* 1994; 11: 471–4.

116 Day C. Thiazolidinediones: a new class of antidiabetic drugs. *Diabet Med* 1999; 16: 179–92.

117 Tattersall R. Alpha-glucosidase inhibition as an adjunct to the treatment of type 1 diabetes. *Diabet Med* 1993; 10: 688–93.

118 Carlson MG, Campbell PJ. Intensive insulin therapy and weight gain in IDDM. *Diabetes* 1993; 42: 1700–7.

119 Hopkins DF, Cotton SJ, Williams G. Effective treatment of insulin-induced edema using ephedrine. *Diabetes Care* 1993; 16: 1026–8.

120 Amiel SA, Simonson DC, Sherwin RS, Lauritano AA, Tamborlane WV. Exaggerated epinephrine responses to hypoglycemia in normal and insulin-dependent diabetic children. *J Pediatr* 1987; 110: 832–7.

121 Whincup G, Milner RD. Prediction and management of nocturnal hypoglycaemia in diabetes. *Arch Dis Child* 1987; 62: 333–7.

122 Shalwitz RA, Farkas-Hirsch R, White NH, Santiago JV. Prevalence and consequences of nocturnal hypoglycemia among conventionally treated children with diabetes mellitus. *J Pediatr* 1990; 116: 685–9.

123 Beregszaszi M, Tubiana-Rufi N, Benali K, Noel M, Bloch J, Czernichow P. Nocturnal hypoglycemia in children and adolescents with insulin-dependent diabetes mellitus: prevalence and risk factors. *J Pediatr* 1997; 131: 27–33.

124 Mohn A, Matyka KA, Harris DA, Ross KM, Edge JA, Dunger DB. Lispro or regular insulin for multiple injection therapy in adolescence. Differences in free insulin and glucose levels overnight. *Diabetes Care* 1999; 22: 27–32.

125 Axelsen M, Wesslau C, Lonnroth P, Arvidsson Lenner R, Smith U. Bedtime uncooked cornstarch supplement prevents nocturnal hypoglycaemia in intensively treated type 1 diabetes subjects. *J Intern Med* 1999; 245: 229–36.

126 Lopez MJ, Oyarzabal M, Barrio R *et al.* Nocturnal hypoglycaemia in IDDM patients younger than 18 years. *Diabet Med* 1997; 14: 772–7.

127 Jones TW, Porter P, Sherwin RS, Davis EA, O'Leary P, Frazer F, Byrne G, Stick S, Tamborlane WV. Decreased epinephrine responses to hypoglycemia during sleep. *N Engl J Med* 1998; 338: 1657–62.

128 Matyka KA, Crowne EC, Havel PJ, Macdonald IA, Matthews D, Dunger DB. Counterregulation during spontaneous nocturnal hypoglycemia in prepubertal children with type 1 diabetes. *Diabetes Care* 1999; 22: 1144–50.

129 Heller SR, Cryer PE. Reduced neuroendocrine and symptomatic responses to subsequent hypoglycaemia in non-diabetic humans. *Diabetes* 1991; 40: 223–6.

130 Fowelin J, Attvall S, von Schenck H, Smith U, Lager I. Characterization of the late posthypoglycemic insulin resistance in insulin-dependent diabetes mellitus. *Metabolism* 1990; 39: 823–6.

131 Amiel SA. Cognitive function testing in studies of acute hypoglycaemia: rights and wrongs? *Diabetologia* 1998; 41: 713–19.

132 Amiel SA, Sherwin RS, Simonson DC, Tamborlane WV. Effect of intensive insulin therapy on glycemic thresholds for counterregulatory hormone release. *Diabetes* 1988; 37: 901–7.

133 Cranston I, Lomas J, Maran A, Macdonald I, Amiel SA. Restoration of hypoglycaemia awareness in patients with long-duration insulin-dependent diabetes. *Lancet* 1994; 344: 283–7.

134 Cox D, Gonder-Frederick L, Schlundt D *et al.* Recent hypoglycemia influences probability of subsequent hypoglycemia in Type 1 patients. *Diabetes* 1993; 42 (Suppl. 1): 126A.

135 Donaghue KC, Robinson J, McCredie R, Fung A, Silink M, Celermajer DS. Large vessel dysfunction in diabetic adolescents and its relationship to small vessel complications. *J Pediatr Endocrinol Metab* 1997; 10: 593–8.

136 Kennon B, Petrie JR, Small M, Connell JM. Angiotensin converting enzyme gene and diabetes mellitus. *Diabetic Med* 1999; 16: 448–58.

137 Diabetes Control, Complications Research Group. The effect of intensive treatment of diabetes on the development and progression of long-term complications in insulin dependent diabetes mellitus. *N Engl J Med* 1993; 329: 977–86.

138 Heart Outcomes Prevention Evaluation (HOPE) Study Investigators. Effects of ramipril on cardiovascular and microvascular outcomes in people with diabetes mellitus: results of the HOPE Study and MICRO-HOPE substudy. *Lancet* 2000; 355: 253–9.

139 Danne T, Kordonouri O, Hovener G, Weber B. Diabetic angiopathy in children. *Diabet Med* 1997; 14: 1012–25.

140 Bognotti E, Calori G, Meschi F, Marcellaro P, Bonfanti R, Chilmello G. Prevalence and correlations of early microvascular complications in young Type 1 diabetic patients: role of puberty. *Pediatr Endocrinol* 1997; 10: 587–92.

141 Donaghue KC, Fairchild JM, Chan A *et al.* Diabetes microvascular complications in prepubertal children. *Pediatr Endocrinol Metab* 1997; 10: 579–85.

142 Cheetham T, Taylor A, Holly J, Clayton K, Cwyfan Hughes S, Dunger D. The effects of recombinant insulin-like growth factor 1 administration on the levels of IGF-I, IGF-II and IGF binding proteins in adolescents with insulin dependent diabetes mellitus. *J Endocrinol* 1994; 142: 367–74.

143 Songer TJ, LaPorte RE, Tajima N *et al.* Height at diagnosis of insulin dependent diabetes in patients and their non-diabetic family members. *Br Med J (Clin Res)* 1986; 292: 1419–22.

144 Brown M, Ahmed M, Clayton K, Dunger D. Growth during childhood and final height in Type 1 diabetes. *Diabetic Med* 1994; 11: 182–7.

145 Du Caju M, Rooman R, De Beeck L. Longitudinal data on growth and final height in diabetic children. *Pediatr Res* 1995; 38: 607–11.

146 Vanelli M, de Fanti A, Adinolfi B, Ghizzoni L. Clinical data regarding the growth of diabetic children. *Horm Res* 1992; 37: 65–7.

147 O'Toole EA, Kennedy U, Nolan JJ, Young MM, Rogers S, Barnes L. Necrobiosis lipoidica: only a minority of patients have diabetes mellitus. *Br J Dermatol* 1999; 140: 283–6.

148 Cohen O, Yaniv R, Karasik A, Trau H. Necrobiosis lipoidica and diabetic control revisited. *Med Hypotheses* 1996; 46: 348–50.

149 Verrotti A, Chiarelli F, Amerio P, Morgese G. Necrobiosis lipoidica diabeticorum in children and adolescents: a clue for underlying renal and retinal disease. *Pediatr Dermatol* 1995; 12: 220–3.

150 Kelly WF, Nichoilas J, Adams J, Mahmood R. Necrobiosis lipoidica diabeticorum: association with background retinopathy, smoking and proteinuria. A case-controlled study. *Diabetic Med* 1993; 10: 725–8.

151 Petzelbauer P, Wolff K, Tappeiner G. Necrobiosis lipoidica: treatment with systemic corticosteroids. *Br J Dermatol* 1992; 126: 542–5.

152 Karavanaki K, Davies AG, Morgan MH, Baum JD. Autonomic function in a cohort of children with diabetes. *Pediatr Endocrinol Metab* 1997; 10: 599–607.

153 Karachaliou F, Karavanaki K, Greenwood R, Baum JD. Consistency of pupillary abnormality in children and adolescents with diabetes. *Diabet Med* 1997; 14: 849–53.

154 Samson M, Akkermans LM, Jebbink RJ *et al.* Gastrointestinal motor mechanisms in hyperglycaemia induced delayed gastric emptying in type 1 diabetes mellitus. *Gut* 1997; 40: 641–6.

155 Acerini CL, Ahmed ML, Ross KM, Sullivan PD, Bird G, Dunger DB. Coeliac disease in children and adolescents with IDDM. Clinical characteristics and response to gluten-free diet. *Diabetic Med* 1998; 15: 38–44.

156 Kakourou T, Dacou-Voutetakis C, Kavadias G, Bakoula C, Aroni K. Limited joint mobility and lipodystrophy in children and adolescents with insulin-dependent diabetes mellitus. *Pediatr Dermatol* 1994; 11: 310–14.

157 Arkkila PE, Kantola IM, Viikari JS, Ronnemaa T, Vahatalo MA. Limited joint mobility is associated with the presence but does not predict the development of microvascular complications in Type 1 diabetes. *Diabetic Med* 1996; 828–33.

158 Garg SK, Chase HP, Marshall G *et al.* Limited joint mobility in subjects with insulin dependent diabetes mellitus: relationship with eye and kidney complications. *Arch Dis Child* 1992; 67: 96–9.

159 Danne T, Kordonouri O. Controversies on the pathogenesis of diabetic angiopathy: which treatment for normotensive adolescents with microalbuminuria and Type 1 diabetes? *J Pediatr Endocrinol Metab* 1998; 11 (Suppl. 2): 347–63.

160 Rudberg S, Osterby R, Bangstaf HJ, Dalquist G, Persson B. Effect of angiotensin converting enzyme inhibitor or beta blocker on glomerular structural changes in young microalbuminuric patients with Type 1 diabetes mellitus. *Diabetologia* 1999; 42: 589–95.

161 Kernell A, Dedorsson I, Johansson B *et al.* Prevalence of diabetic retinopathy in children and adolescents with IDDM. A population-based multicentre study. *Diabetologia* 1997; 40: 307–10.

162 Falck A, Laatikainen L. Diabetic cataract in children. *Acta Ophthalmol Scand* 1998; 76: 238–40.

163 Miller A, Hardin D, Rodman D *et al.* Diagnosis, screening and management of cystic fibrosis related diabetes mellitus: a consensus conference report. *Diab Res Clin Pract* 1999; 45: 61–73.

164 O'Connor TM, Cronin CC, Loane JF *et al.* Type 1 diabetes mellitus, coeliac disease, and lymphoma: a report of four cases. *Diabet Med* 1999; 16: 614–17.

165 Lanng S. Glucose intolerance in cystic fibrosis. *Danish Med Bulletin* 1997; 44: 23–39.

166 Miller E, Hare JW, Cloherty JP *et al.* Elevated maternal hemoglobin A1c in early pregnancy and major congenital abnormalities in infants of diabetic mothers. *N Engl J Med* 1981; 30: 1331–4.

167 Carron Brown S, Kyne-Grzebalski D, Mwangi B, Taylor R. Effect of management policy upon 120 Type 1 diabetic pregnancies: policy decisions in practice. *Diabet Med* 1999; 16: 573–8.

168 Farmer RD, Lawrenson RA, Thompson CR, Kennedy JG, Hambleton IR. Population-based study of risk of venous thromboembolism associated with various oral contraceptives. *Lancet* 1997; 349: 83–8.

169 Towner DL, Kjos SL, Leung B *et al.* Congenital malformations in pregnancies complicated by NIDDM. *Diabetes Care* 1995; 19: 1446–51.

170 American Diabetes Association. Clinical practice recommendations 1996. *Diabetes Care* 1996; 19 (Suppl. 1): S1–S118.

171 Hawthorne G, Robson S, Ryall EA, Sen D, Roberts SH, Ward Platt MP. Prospective population based survey of outcome of pregnancy in diabetic women: results of the Northern Diabetic Pregnancy Audit. *Br Med J*, 1994; 1997 (315): 279–81.

172 Casson IF, Clarke CA, Howard CV *et al.* Outcomes of pregnancy in insulin dependent diabetic women: results of a five year population cohort study. *Br Med J* 1997; 315: 275–8.

173 MacLeod KM. Diabetes and driving: towards equitable, evidence based decision making. *Diabetic Med* 1999; 16: 282–90.

174 Amiel SA. Diabetes and driving – an insular approach? *Diabetic Med* 1999; 16: 271–2.

175 Viner R. Transition for paediatric to adult care. Bridging the gaps or passing the buck? *Arch Dis Child* 1999; 81: 271–5.

176 Greene A, Tripaldi M, McKiernan P, Morris A, Newton R, Greene S. Promoting empowerment in young people with diabetes. *Diabetic Med* 1999; 16 (Suppl.): 20.

# 25 Cardiovascular risk

## P. Vallance

## Introduction

Atherosclerotic cardiovascular disease remains the major cause of death in developed countries. The process starts in childhood, is macroscopically evident in adolescents and young adults and begins to produce symptomatic disease from the third decade of life onwards. Many organ systems can be involved, but the disease presents most commonly as coronary heart disease (Fig. 25.1). In this chapter the concept of cardiovascular risk is discussed together with suggested strategies for management.

## Atherogenesis

The onset and progression of atherogenesis is considered a response of the vessel wall to 'injury' [1]. Repeated damage to the vessel wall and the process of inflammation and healing that accompany such damage lead to plaque formation. Early in the process there is infiltration of inflammatory cells – T

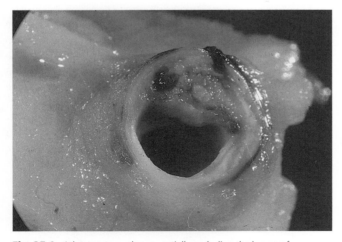

**Fig. 25.1.** Atheromatous plaque partially occluding the lumen of a conduit artery.

lymphocytes and monocytes. These cells become activated within the vessel wall and produce growth factors, pro-inflammatory cytokines and chemokines. The net result is further inflammation and an accumulation of inflammatory cells. The phenotype of the smooth muscle cells changes so that they replicate and secrete extracellular matrix. The monocytes differentiate into resident macrophages and become laden with lipid so that they take on a characteristic appearance – so-called foam cells. As the plaque matures it becomes fibrous, but rupture or fissure of plaques can occur and this is one mechanism by which thrombosis occurs and leads to vessel occlusion [2].

## Endothelial function and dysfunction

The endothelium is central to the process of atherogenesis and determines the thrombogenicity of the plaque. This monolayer of cells lines the entire vascular tree (Fig. 25.2) and normally provides a basal vasodilator antithrombogenic influence [3]. However, activation of the endothelium leads to expression of adhesion molecules that bind circulating cells. Physical damage reduces production of bioactive vasodilator antiplatelet factors, including nitric oxide and prostacyclin. These changes may be appropriate at a site of external injury and would help prevent excess blood loss or allow inflammatory cells to help fight localized infection. However, when they occur in response to intravascular injury they seem inappropriate and may help promote atherogenesis.

Endothelial dysfunction or activation seems to be one of the earliest steps in the atherogenic process. The endothelium lies at the interface between circulating blood and the vessel wall and is vulnerable to injury from the lumen. Injury may be physical – the haemodynamic forces of shear stress or pressure – or chemical–oxidant stress, damage by toxins or activation by pro-inflammatory mediators [3]. Many of the classical risk factors for cardiovascular disease exert effects through these mechanisms. Markers of endothelial dysfunction can be detected before the onset of overt atheroma and

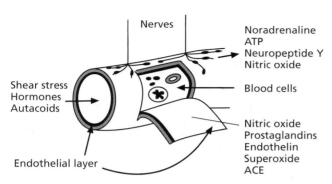

**Fig. 25.2.** The vascular endothelium forms a monolayer that lines all blood vessels. Specialized ion channels and receptors allow endothelial cells to detect changes in the physical or chemical environment within the lumen of the vessel. The endothelium synthesizes a variety of bioactive mediators that can cause local vasodilatation or vasoconstriction and modify the adhesiveness of the cell surface. Endothelium may also respond to neurogenic influences when mediators are released from nerves supplying the outside of the vessel wall. Thus the endothelium acts as a signal transducer, able to detect signals and alter the behaviour of the blood vessel. ATP, adenosine triphosphate; ACE, angiotensin-converting enzyme.

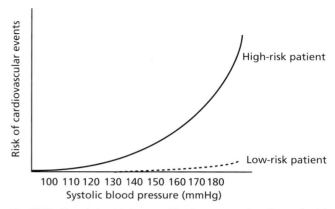

**Fig. 25.3.** The relationship between blood pressure and cardiovascular risk is dependent on the presence or absence of other risk factors. For a smoker with diabetes, a high total cholesterol, low HDL-cholesterol and ECG evidence of left ventricular hypertrophy, the relationship between blood pressure and risk is steep. For an otherwise healthy non-smoker who does not have other risk factors, the slope of the relationship is shallow. As the gain from treatment is proportional to the initial risk, it is clear that the high-risk individual stands to gain the most from treatment.

are evident even in children with risk factors such as hyperlipidaemia [4].

## Acute and chronic risk

Cardiovascular risk can be divided into two broad categories: risk of atherogenesis and risk of an acute event. The two are not necessarily synonymous. For example, although the presence of atheroma is a prerequisite for a classic myocardial infarction, the risk of an event correlates rather poorly with the extent of atherosclerotic disease. Although atherosclerotic bulk is clearly important and often determines clinical presentation with symptoms related to ischaemia such as claudication, stable angina or heart failure, it is the unstable plaque that leads to acute presentation with thromboembolic events such as acute myocardial infarction or stroke. Treatment of risk factors (see below) often reduces risk of an acute event without significantly altering atherosclerotic bulk. Thus although the risk factors for the two processes are often similar – hypertension, hypercholesterolaemia, diabetes, and cigarette smoking – they need not always be. However, certain fundamental mechanisms seem quite similar in the genesis of the two processes. The changes in endothelial function that initiate and support atherogenesis may well be similar to those that encourage circulating cells to stick to and aggregate upon the endothelium overlying an unstable atherosclerotic plaque. Inflammation, and possibly infection, is thought to play a central role in the transition of plaque between stable (essentially safe) and unstable (likely to support thrombosis). Proposed mechanisms include endothelial activation, matrix degradation and weakening of the fibrous cap, and increased activa-

tion of circulating cells, which in turn inflame the vulnerable plaque [5]. Some of the classic risk factors may themselves promote or enhance inflammatory injury to the vessel wall.

## Risk factors

Classic risk factors for cardiovascular disease include hypertension, hypercholesterolaemia, diabetes and smoking. Each may produce effects on endothelial function and on the reactivity of circulating cells. It is clear that the effects of these factors is synergistic [6,7]. For example, although there is a positive relationship between the level of blood pressure and the risk of a cardiovascular event, the slope of the relationship is critically dependent on the presence or absence of other risk factors. For a smoker who has diabetes and a raised cholesterol level, each increment in blood pressure carries with it more risk than it would for a non-smoking, non-diabetic normocholesterolaemic person (Fig. 25.3). The same is true for cholesterol – the slope of the relationship between the level of cholesterol and the risk is dependent upon the overall risk profile. The basic biological mechanisms underlying the interactions between risk factors are poorly understood, but the practical implication is that expected treatment benefits are predicted by the overall risk, not by the level of individual risk factors.

## Calculating and presenting risk

Risk factor calculations are based on observational cohorts and the most widely used is the Framingham study. This study has now followed an initial cohort of over 5000 individuals over 50 years and provides data on the quantitative effect of risk factors [8]. Equations derived from the data describe the interaction between risk factors and allow predictions of absolute risk of events over a defined time period (usually 5 or 10 years). By comparing these predictions with age- and sex-matched population average data, it is also possible to present relative risk – the risk of the individual compared with the average risk of his or her peers. Calculations of absolute and relative risk based on the Framingham data have been shown to be accurate when applied to UK data sets [7], although they are likely to underestimate risk in certain groups, including first-generation Asian immigrants who appear to have a relative risk about one and a half times greater than that predicted by the Framingham risk function.

Several things become clear when the Framingham risk function is used to predict risk. First, it is important to include blood pressure and cholesterol as continuous variables rather than to consider some levels as 'normal' and others as 'abnormal' [7]. Second, total cholesterol gives only a part of the story and high-density lipoprotein (HDL)-cholesterol is a very important determinant of the overall risk. If HDL-cholesterol is not included in the risk prediction, the predicted risk often diverges significantly from the true risk [7]. The factors that need to be included are blood pressure, total and HDL-cholesterol (the sample does not need to be taken with the patient fasting), smoking status, presence or absence of diabetes and whether or not there is evidence of left ventricular hypertrophy. Together these variables allow risk prediction that is highly accurate at a population level, although of course it is necessary to be aware of the pitfalls of applying population data to the individual.

The advantage of expressing predictions in terms of absolute risk is that it gives an indication of how likely it is that an event will occur. However, the major influence on absolute risk is age, and therefore younger individuals always appear at very low risk if a 10-year prediction of absolute risk is provided. The reverse is true for relative risk. All individuals with elevated levels of risk factors will appear at increased relative risk, irrespective of age. However, this raises a problem for deciding who should be treated; being at twice the risk of your age- and sex-matched peers might not matter if the absolute level of risk is so low that the likelihood of an event occurring is vanishingly small. Most current guidelines suggest that for primary prevention of cardiovascular disease lipid-lowering drugs should be reserved for individuals who cross a certain absolute risk threshold per annum (usually 1.5%, 2% or 3%, depending on the body issuing the guidelines and the amount of money the healthcare organization is prepared to spend on lipid-lowering medicines). It is clear that many of the same arguments might also be applied to drugs to treat hypertension – the benefit to be gained depends on the initial level of risk and for newer drugs the costs can be as high or even higher than for lipid-lowering drugs (Fig. 25.4).

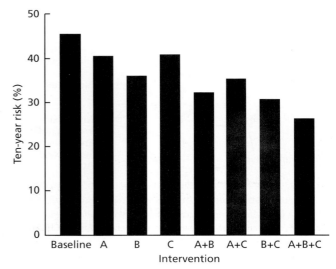

**Fig. 25.4.** Ten-year risk of coronary heart disease for a 69-year-old male smoker with baseline systolic blood pressure of 170 mmHg, total cholesterol concentration of 7.4 mmol/L, and HDL-cholesterol concentration of 1.0 mmol/L. Predicted risk reductions are for reducing systolic blood pressure by 20 mmHg and reducing total cholesterol by 20%. Costs for 1 month's treatment (from British National Formulary) are based on assumption that two drugs would be required to achieve 20 mmHg reduction in blood pressure and that a statin alone would decrease cholesterol concentration by about 20%. The lower cost shown for lowering blood pressure is for bendrofluazide 2.5 mg and atenolol 50 mg; the higher cost shown is for lisinopril 10 mg and amlodipine 10 mg. Lower cost for lowering cholesterol is for simvastatin 10 mg; the higher cost is for simvastatin 20 mg. A, Reducing blood pressure (lower cost £1.31, higher cost £25.40); B, stopping smoking; C, reducing cholesterol (lower cost £16.65, higher cost £33.30).

Treatment protocols based on absolute risk levels tend to skew treatment towards older ages. However, an alternative way to consider risk is to calculate cumulative or lifetime risk estimates (Fig. 25.5) [9,10]. In this way it is possible to determine an overall level of risk and also the age at which risk begins to increase. In principle, it should be possible to use such calculations to determine the optimal age at which to start treatment in any individual, i.e. the age at which most predicted benefit would accrue per year of treatment, assuming that treatment is given for a lifetime. It seems likely that this would give a better indication of how to target drug treatments to those who stand to gain the most. This approach would avoid delaying treatment for too long (the danger if absolute risk is used to determine policy) or initiating treatment too young and subjecting the individual to unnecessary exposure to drugs (the danger if relative risk is used to determine policy). In addition to consideration of how to express risk, there has been extensive discussion on how to present risk estimates and the context in which risk–benefit ratios are presented to individuals [11].

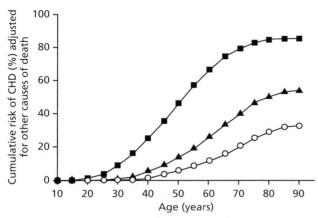

**Fig. 25.5.** Predictive cumulative risk of coronary heart disease (CHD) for smokers with a total cholesterol of 7.2 mmol/L, HDL-cholesterol 0.8 mmol/L, blood pressure 162/95 mmHg (■); non-smokers with total cholesterol of 6 mmol/L, HDL cholesterol 1.1 mmol/L, blood pressure 145/95 mmHg (▲); and non-smokers with total cholesterol 4.5 mmol/L, HDL-cholesterol 1.1 mmol/L and blood pressure 120/85 mmHg (○).

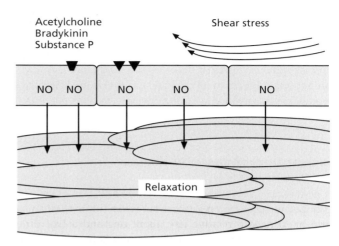

**Fig. 25.6.** The vascular endothelium synthesizes nitric oxide from L-arginine. Nitric oxide causes vasodilatation and inhibits platelet and white-cell adhesion. The output of nitric oxide is varied according to shear stress (viscous drag) and local concentrations of hormones such as bradykinin. The increase in endothelial nitric oxide generation that occurs in response to increased shear stress is the basis of the technique of flow-dependent dilatation, which has been used as a surrogate marker to detect endothelial dysfunction.

## Non-classic risk factors

Smoking, lipids and hypertension remain the three most important risk factors, not just because of their quantitative impact on risk but also because they are modifiable. In addition, a series of other markers of risk have been identified. Fibrinogen levels are an independent predictor of risk [12] and levels of lipoprotein (a) are sometimes useful to determine very high-risk subsets of individuals [13]. These additional factors may have particular value in determining which young patients with familial hypercholesterolaemia are at the highest levels of risk. Plasma levels of homocysteine may also be important, although the strength of the relationship is not clear [14]. Recent interest has also focused on the possibility that systemic inflammation or individual infectious agents may increase cardiovascular risk [15,16]. There is accumulating evidence to support the idea that mild systemic inflammation increases risk of an acute cardiovascular event and experimental data indicate that acute endothelial dysfunction may underlie this association. The evidence for individual infectious agents is less robust, although ongoing studies are exploring chlamydia, pneumoniae and herpes viruses as possible aetiological agents, either in the slow process of atherogenesis or in the onset of an acute event [17]. Interestingly, all of these non-classic risk factors also have the capacity to alter endothelial function.

## Early detection of vascular damage

Early detection of vascular damage is potentially important if vascular events are to be avoided, because the presence of

damage might suggest that more aggressive intervention is warranted or allow intervention to be targeted more accurately to those who stand to gain the most. However, the difficulty is knowing which, if any, of the surrogate measures available should be used to guide therapeutics. In routine clinical practice it is not usual to screen for vascular damage unless symptoms are evident. An exception would be the testing of urine for proteinuria. Proteinuria is probably a reflection of endothelial dysfunction in the glomerulus and is an independent marker of poor prognosis in diabetes or hypertension [18]. It is not known whether it also predicts poor outcome in individuals with other risk factors such as hypercholesterolaemia.

Another marker of endothelial function that has been used in clinical investigation is the assessment of flow-dependent dilatation in a conduit artery. In this technique, the diameter of the brachial, radial or femoral artery is measured at rest and during an increase in flow through the vessel [19]. Increase in flow is usually achieved by inducing postischaemic hyperaemia in a downstream vascular bed. The conduit artery dilates because the endothelium detects the increase in flow as a change in shear stress (viscous drag) and increases the output of the dilator nitric oxide (Fig. 25.6). Impaired flow-mediated dilatation has been seen in adults with risk factors for cardiovascular disease and is even evident in young children with raised cholesterol levels or other risk factors [20]. This impairment is taken as an indication of endothelial dysfunction, which may be a necessary prerequisite for the development of atherosclerosis and subsequent thromboembolic disease. Although this and other approaches have shed considerable light upon the early origins of vascular disease and the possible mechanistic links between risk factors and atherosclerotic disease, it is not known whether impaired flow-dependent dilatation has any prognostic value in an individual, and therefore currently it would be inappropriate to include this as part of clinical assessment outside the setting of a clinical trial.

## Prevention of vascular disease

It is now clear that treatment of certain risk factors reduces risk. Lowering blood pressure reduces the risk of heart attack and stroke, and the reduction in risk is proportional to the blood pressure lowering achieved. Reversal of risk seems to be nearly complete for stroke, so that within a relatively short period of time (1–2 years) individuals adopt a new level of risk similar to that of any individual with the new lower blood pressure. For reduction of heart attack risk it seems as though the full benefit may not be achieved, so that individuals seem to accrue perhaps 50–70% of the overall benefit that might have been predicted from the degree of blood pressure lowering. For lipid lowering it is also clear that risk reduction occurs rapidly (within 1–2 years) and in this instance the reversal of risk is almost complete – the individual adopts a new level of risk predicted by the treated cholesterol level. There is now good evidence from large randomized well-controlled studies that risk factor treatment achieves reduction in hard end points, including mortality, and that these effects far outweigh any unwanted effects of drug treatment. Smoking cessation also reduces cardiovascular risk, and again the risk reduction is achieved relatively quickly – within about 5 years.

## Treatment of essential hypertension

The commonly used classes of antihypertensive drugs are all equally effective at lowering pressure, and on average a single drug causes a fall in blood pressure of between 5 and 8 mmHg [21]. Significant reductions in pressure can also be achieved by lifestyle changes, and the quantitative impact of

these is shown in Table 25.1. Certain lifestyle changes not only produce a fall in pressure in their own right but may enhance the antihypertensive effects of drugs, and all patients should be encouraged to adopt appropriate lifestyle changes. Repeated measurement of blood pressure often leads to a significant fall in pressure as the patient becomes habituated to the process and there is usually no need to rush into treatment [22]. Most guidelines recommend that for mild hypertension assessment over 12 weeks or so is reasonable before deciding whether to start treatment; for pressures of 160–179/100–109 assessment can take place over 4–12 weeks (3–4 if target organ damage is evident); and for pressures of 180–219/110–119, treatment should be started within 1–2 weeks. Other factors such as age, concomitant disease, speed of onset of hypertension (if known) and presence of additional risk factors should also be taken into account when considering how soon to treat. In any patient who is overly anxious, has a resting tachycardia or in whom measurements are variable, the possibility of 'white-coat' hypertension should be considered. In this situation, repeated measurement by a nurse, or 24-h ambulatory blood pressure recording, may help to establish the true level of blood pressure.

A summary of the appropriate first-line treatments and additive combinations for treatment are shown in Table 25.2. Common reasons for treatment failure include:
• non-adherence to therapy (often exacerbated by poor provision of information);
• diet – a persistent high-salt diet will render certain drugs [e.g. beta-blockers and angiotensin-converting enzyme (ACE) inhibitors] less effective;
• concomitant drug therapy that blocks antihypertensive action, e.g. non-steroidal anti-inflammatory drugs (NSAIDs);
• wrong drug or use of a combination of drugs that may not be additive, e.g. use of a beta-blocker as monotherapy in a Black patient; adding a beta-blocker to an ACE inhibitor as dual therapy;
• wrong dosing – a common problem is that short-acting drugs are given once a day, so that blood pressure is often found to be elevated several hours after treatment.

A full discussion of secondary hypertension is outside the scope of this article but common causes and specific treatments are shown in Table 25.3.

**Table 25.1.** Impact of lifestyle changes on hypertension

| | |
|---|---|
| Weight reduction | 1–2 mmHg for each 1 kg lost |
| Sodium restriction from 10 g/day to 5 g/day | 5/3 mmHg |
| Stress management | 0 mmHg |
| Regular aerobic exercise (at least three times a week) | 4/3 mmHg |
| Increase intake of fruit and vegetables from two to seven portions per day | 7/3 mmHg |
| Avoid excess alcohol intake | Change depends on amount consumed |

It is not known to what extent these effects are additive, although evidence suggests that weight loss and sodium restriction produce greater reduction in hypertension than either alone.

**Table 25.2.** Summary of treatments for essential hypertension

| | |
|---|---|
| First line | Thiazide diuretic or beta-blocker |
| Second line | ACE inhibitor* or long-acting calcium channel blocker |
| Third line | Angiotensin II antagonist (for those intolerant of ACE inhibitor)*, alpha-blocker |
| Additive combinations for dual therapy | |
| Beta-blocker | Add thiazide or long-acting dihydropyridine calcium channel blocker |
| Thiazide | Add beta-blocker or ACE inhibitor |

*Effect enhanced by sodium restriction. Often not suitable for monotherapy in Black patients (particularly if elderly).
ACE, angiotensin-converting enzyme.

**Table 25.3.** Common causes and treatments of secondary hypertension

| Cause | Tests | Specific treatments |
|---|---|---|
| **Metabolic/hormonal** | | |
| Hyperaldosteronism | Renin and aldosterone levels. Adrenal CT/MRI | Spironolactone. Surgery |
| Cushing syndrome | Cortisol and ACTH. CT/MRI | Specific treatment is for Cushing's disease rather than for BP |
| Phaeochromocytoma | Catecholamines/VMA.MIBG scan. CT/MRI | Combined α- and β-blockade. Surgery |
| **Renal** | | |
| Acute or chronic renal failure | Specific tests for individual causes of renal failure | Usual drugs for lowering BP. Caution with renally excreted drugs |
| Renal artery stenosis | Renal ultrasound. Angiography (definitive test). Elevated renin and aldosterone levels | Usual drug treatment of BP except that ACE inhibitors may worsen renal function. Angioplasty or surgery may provide definitive treatment |
| **Structural** | | |
| Coarctation of aorta | CXR. Echocardiogram. Angiogram | Surgery |
| Renal artery stenosis | See above | See above |
| **Single gene defects** | | |
| Liddle syndrome* | Na($\uparrow$), K($\downarrow$), renin and aldosterone both suppressed. Genotype | Low salt diet. Amiloride or triamterene |
| Glucocorticoid-remediable aldosteronism† | Na($\uparrow$), K($\downarrow$), renin suppressed and aldosterone elevated. Presence of 18-oxocortisol in urine. Glucocorticoid suppressible. Genotype | Dexamethasone |
| Syndrome of apparent mineralocorticoid excess‡ | Na($\uparrow$), K($\downarrow$), renin and aldosterone both suppressed. Genotype | Dexamethasone |
| **Other** | | |
| Drugs (NSAIDs, etc) | None | Discontinue if possible |
| Pregnancy (pre-eclampsia) | | |

ACE, angiotensin-converting enzyme; BP, blood pressure; CT, computerized tomography; CXR, chest X-ray; MIBG, metaiodobenzylguanidine; NSAID, non-steroidal anti-inflammatory drug; VMA, vanillylmandelic acid.
*Autosomal dominant disorder resulting from activating mutations in the β- and γ-subunits of the epithelial sodium channel that cause constitutive sodium absorption from the distal convoluted tubule of the kidney. Amiloride and triamterene are specific blockers of this channel.
†Autosomal dominant disorder caused by the inheritance of a chimeric gene comprising the promoter of 11β-hydroxylase and the coding region of aldosterone synthase. Aldosterone synthesis is regulated by ACTH (rather than by angiotensin II), which explains both the high circulating levels of aldosterone and the steroid suppressibility of the hypertension.
‡Autosomal recessive disorder caused by mutations in 11β-hydroxysteroid dehydrogenase type II – a renal enzyme that normally metabolises cortisol, thereby protecting the renal mineralocorticoid receptor from activation by glucocorticoids. Mutations in this enzyme allow endogenous glucocorticoids access to the renal mineralocorticoid receptor causing excess salt and water retention. The disorder is also amenable to treatment with low-dose exogenous steroid sufficient to suppress endogenous ACTH production.

## Treatment of hypercholesterolaemia

For patients with primary hypercholesterolaemia who require treatment, statins usually offer the best option. Statin treatment reduces cholesterol by about 20% and causes a small increase in HDL. There is little to choose between the statins as first-line treatments. However, some stains (e.g. atorvastatin) have greater maximal efficacy at licensed doses and therefore might be useful in individuals in whom satisfactory cholesterol lowering has not been achieved with the first-line drug. In contrast to the situation for blood pressure lowering, there is little good evidence to suggest that dietary changes offer an effective alternative to drug treatment for reducing cholesterol levels. Indeed, the dietary advice that is offered in clinics causes a mere 1% fall in cholesterol level on average [23]. Thus, current advice is that although dietary changes may form a part of an overall treatment package it is not sensible to persevere with dietary changes alone if cholesterol has not fallen to a satisfactory level within a couple of months. On the other hand, encouraging patients to lose weight and take regular exercise can lead to significant changes in total cholesterol levels and the HDL/total cholesterol level. For patients who have raised triglyceride levels, the fibrates offer the best first-line treatment. Treatment of familial hypercholesterolaemias and other secondary hypercholesterolaemias is outside the scope of the present article (see [24]). However, individuals with very high levels of cholesterol are at very high predicted risk and benefit from early treatment, especially if lipoprotein (a) levels are also elevated. Children with hypercholesterolaemia, particularly postpubertal adolescents, will benefit from statin therapy. Such individuals should be managed in clinics with experience of the management of hyperlipidaemias.

## Other interventions

Smoking cessation is facilitated by counselling and the use of nicotine replacement [25]. However, even then the failure rate is high and there has not yet been a detailed analysis of cost-effectiveness of nicotine patches related to predicted reduction in cardiovascular risk. Anti-platelet therapy with aspirin is mandatory for secondary prevention but is still controversial for primary prevention. However, there is good evidence that aspirin reduces cardiovascular risk even when used for primary prevention, and the key is to establish the overall level of risk. The risk of gastrointestinal haemorrhage with low-dose aspirin is in the order of 1 in 500 per year, and the reduction in cardiovascular events is about 20% [26]. In order to determine the risk–benefit ratio, it is clearly essential to know the absolute risk and make an informed decision on this basis.

## Genetic influences on risk

Family history is a good predictor of cardiovascular risk. However, at a population level, the Framingham data suggest that the largest proportion of family history as a risk factor is accounted for by familial tendency to share similar levels of blood pressure, cholesterol, HDL-cholesterol and other standard risk factors [27]. Thus for a large proportion of patients, the risk calculations discussed above will provide an accurate assessment of risk and the likely benefit of intervention. However, it is clear that there are families in which cardiovascular risk is disproportionately high and cannot be accounted for by standard risk factors. It seems likely that with advances in genomics and bioinformatics the impact of genotype on the risk of cardiovascular disease and the nature of interactions between genotype and standard risk factors will become increasingly clear. Already there is evidence that common variation in the genome can cause changes in cardiovascular phenotype. For example, the ACE gene exhibits common variation – a deletion genotype (DD) and insertion genotype (II). Individuals homozygous for the DD genotype have higher circulating levels of ACE and might have increased risk of cardiovascular events [28]. Similar common polymorphic variants of the angiotensinogen gene and nitric oxide synthase genes have been associated with altered risk of cardiovascular disease. In the case of one of the variants of nitric oxide synthase, it has been suggested that the effects of genotype to increase risk is only seen in non-smokers [29]. These sorts of genetic studies are likely to affect overall assessment of risk, and it is conceivable that they also predict response to treatment. For example, a variant of the gene encoding cholesteryl ester transfer protein seems to predict the progression of coronary heart disease and the response to statin treatment, with individuals homozygous for the B1 variant showing the greatest response to a statin [30]. However, despite the intriguing associations, at the moment genetic risk cannot be included in any formal assessment of risk profile nor can it be used to guide therapeutics in a clinical setting.

## Conclusions

Cardiovascular disease remains the commonest cause of death in developed countries and is increasingly recognized as a public health problem in developing nations. It is no longer justified to treat individual risk factors in isolation, as the effects of risk factors are often synergistic and the benefit to be gained depends critically on the overall levels of risk. It is possible to predict risk reasonably accurately on the basis of standard measurable risk factors and it seems likely that as advances in bioinformatics occur genetic risk might also be included in assessment. Risk assessment is critically important if treatment is to be targeted appropriately to individuals who stand to gain the most benefit, particularly as treatment is often lifelong. At the moment, lipid lowering with statins and good control of blood pressure still offer the major route to reduce risk and are especially important in high-risk individuals, including diabetics. A key challenge is to determine the optimum time to initiate treatment to ensure maximum benefit without incurring unnecessary exposure to drugs. Of course, the problems are greatest in children and young adults, and decisions to treat need to be based on accurate assessments of risk.

## References

1 Ross R. Atherosclerosis—an inflammatory disease. *N Engl J Med* 1999; 340 (2): 115–26.

2 Gronholdt ML, Dalager-Pedersen S, Falk E. Coronary atherosclerosis: determinants of plaque rupture. *Eur Heart J* 1998; 19: 24–9.

3 Vallance P. Vascular endothelium, its physiology and pathophysiology. *Oxford Textbook of Medicine* (in press).

4 Woolf, N. The origins of atherosclerosis. *Postgrad Med J* 1978; 54: 156–62.

5 Kinlay S, Selwyn AP, Libby P, Ganz P. Inflammation, the endothelium, and the acute coronary syndromes. *J Cardiovasc Pharmacol* 1998; 32: 62–6.

6 Kannel WB. Cardioprotection and antihypertensive therapy: the key importance of addressing the associated coronary risk factors (the Framingham experience). *Am J Cardiol* 1996; 77: 6–11.

7 Hingorani AD, Vallance P. A simple computer program for guiding management of cardiovascular risk factors and prescribing. *Br Med J* 1999; 318: 101–5.

8 Lenfant C, Friedman L, Thom T. Fifty years of death certificates: the Framingham Heart Study (editorial; comment). *Ann Intern Med* 1998; 129: 1066–7.

9 Lloyd-Jones DM, Larson MG, BeiSeries A, Levy D. Lifetime risk of developing coronary heart disease. *Lancet* 1999; 353: 89–92.

10 Ulrich S, Hingorani AD, Martin J, Vallance P. Lifetime risk of developing coronary heart disease. *Lancet* 1999; 353: 925.

11 Johnson BB, Slovic P. Presenting uncertainty in health risk assessment: initial studies on its effects on risk perception and trust. *Risk Anal* 1995; 15: 485–94.

12 Danesh J, Collins R, Appleby P, Peto R. Association of fibrinogen, C-reactive protein, albumin or leukocyte count with coronary heart disease: meta-analyses of prospective studies. *J Am Med Assoc* 1998; 279: 1477–82.

13 Marcovina SM, Koschinsky ML. Lipoprotein (a) as a risk factor for coronary artery disease. *Am J Cardiol* 1998; 32: 57–66.

14 Ubbink JB, Fehily AM, Pickering J, Elwood PC, Vermaak WJ. Homocysteine and ischaemic heart disease in the Caerphilly cohort. *Atherosclerosis* 1998; 140: 349–56.

15 Ridker PM, Buring JE, Shih J, Matias M, Hennekens CH. Prospective study of C-reactive protein and the risk of future cardiovascular events among apparently healthy women. *Circulation* 1998; 98: 731–3.

16 Vallance P, Collier J, Bhagat K. Infection, inflammation and infarction: does acute endothelial dysfunction provide a link? *Lancet* 1997; 349: 1391–2.

17 Danesh J, Collins R, Peto R. Chronic infections and coronary heart disease: is there a link? *Lancet* 1997; 350: 430–6.

18 Grimm RH Jr, Svendsen KH, Kasiske B, Keane WF, Wahi MM. Proteinuria is a risk factor for mortality over 10 years of follow-up. *Kidney Int Suppl* 1997; 63: 10–14.

19 Bhagat K, Hingorani A, Vallance P. Flow associated or flow mediated dilatation? More than just semantics. *Heart* 1997; 78: 7–8.

20 Celermajer DS, Sorensen KE, Gooch VM *et al.* Non-invasive detection of endothelial dysfunction in children and adults at risk of atherosclerosis. *Lancet* 1992; 340: 1111–15.

21 Materson BJ, Reda DM, Cushman WC *et al.* Single-drug therapy for hypertension in men. A comparison of six antihypertensive agents with placebo. *N Engl J Med* 1993; 328: 914–21.

22 Vallance P. Hypertension. *J R Coll Physicians Lond* 1999; 33: 119–23.

23 Ramsay LE, Yeo WW, Jackson PR. Dietary reduction of serum cholesterol concentration: time to think again. *Br Med J* 1991; 303: 953–7.

24 Rifkind BM, Schucker B, Gordon DJ. When should patients with heterozygous familial hypercholesterolaemia be treated? *J Am Med Assoc* 1999; 281: 180–1.

25 Silagy C, Mant D, Fowler G, Lodge M. Meta-analysis of efficacy of nicotine replacement therapies in smoking cessation. *Lancet* 1994; 343: 139–42.

26 Meade TW, Miller GJ. Combined use of aspirin and warfarin in primary prevention of ischaemic heart disease in men at high risk. *Am J Cardiol* 1995; 75: 23–6.

27 Brand FN, Kiely DK, Kannel WB, Myers RH. Family patterns of coronary heart disease mortality: the Framingham Longevity Study. *J Clin Epidemiol* 1992; 45: 169–74.

28 Bauters C, Amouyel P. Association between the ACE genotype and coronary artery disease. Insights from studies on restenosis, vasomotion and thrombosis. *Eur Heart J* 1998; 19: 24–9.

29 Wang XL, Sim AS, Badenhop RF, McCredie RM, Wilcken DE. A smoking-dependent risk of coronary artery disease associated with a polymorphism of the endothelial nitric oxide synthase gene. *Nature Med* 1996; 2: 41–5.

30 Kuivenhoven JA, Jukema JW, Zwinderman AH *et al. N Engl J Med* 1998; 338: 86–93.

# 26 Towards evidence-based paediatric endocrinology

**S. P. Taback**

## Introduction

Evidence-based medicine is an approach to medical care that attempts to improve patient care by providing practising physicians with a comprehensive and effective system of techniques for finding, interpreting and using the world's medical knowledge. Traditionally, physicians have used four basic sources to help solve patient management problems:

1 professional experience, whether from their teachers or their own career;

2 theories developed from scientific knowledge about pathophysiology, either personally or by others;

3 values: their own, their patients' and society's;

4 relevant evidence from the medical literature.

Of these, relevant evidence has obvious appeal but, even when it exists, it can be hidden in the millions of papers in the medical literature or ignored by people writing narrative reviews based on their experience or theories.

Evidence-based medicine teaches the physician to understand the relative contributions of these sources to the question at hand in a transparent manner and to integrate them into patient management. The focus is on the individual physician, because physicians have the ethical (and legal) responsibility to provide the correct information so that their patients can make decisions about their medical treatment. Furthermore, except for some very basic professional standards, physicians also have great individual freedom to accept or ignore expert recommendations. A focus on the physician in practice also makes evidence-based medicine practical as individual physicians can allocate scarce self-learning time to the patient problems at hand. An excellent starting resource for all these tasks is a compact book entitled *Evidence-based Medicine: How to Practice and Teach EBM* [1].

When considering relevant evidence, the finding techniques involve framing the problem as a 'searchable' question so that the relevant details about the patient population and the type of information needed (whether on aetiology of a disease, diagnostic properties of a test, prognosis of a disease or effect of a treatment) are specified. Developing the ability to frame a searchable question may actually take some practice but is necessary to receive a clinically relevant answer. Having a question in the proper format leads to the related step of using computer technology to search the world's literature on the question (or getting someone else to do it for you). An adequate computer search is essential to find the best available evidence. Fortunately, many medical libraries offer computer-search training sessions, and free access to at least search MedLINE is increasingly available through the Internet.

The 'interpreting' techniques involve applying basic standards of epidemiological research to judge whether the studies found in the search are likely to provide valid results (Table 26.1). The appropriate set of standards to use depends on the type of problem (aetiology, diagnosis, prognosis and treatment). The results are expressed using some basic biostatistical standards, again depending on the type of problem. The standards can be applied in two ways: some physicians wish to read the valid evidence on their problem, regardless of results; others will want to scan the results first to see whether the implication of the findings merits the time needed to assess whether the study is valid. In both cases, the concepts are easily accessible. Studies with a low likelihood of being valid are not relied on. Often someone else may have already done the work and published an evidence-based review of the question.

Finally, relevant evidence can be integrated with experience, theories, values and patient-specific information to make decisions for the particular problem. Evidence-based medicine does not try to replace the art of medicine. Sometimes, there may, in fact, be no direct evidence on a particular problem.

A one-page summary of the effort (sometimes called a CAT, critically appraised topic) can be filed for future reference for use when the same problem next arises. Such a summary consists of a title that answers the question, a reminder of the patient problem, the clinical message from the evidence, as well as a very brief description of study validity and results [1]. Some examples from paediatric endocrinology are shown below.

**Table 26.1.** Type of evidence. Examples of epidemiological and biostatistical standards in evidence-based medicine (adapted from [1]).

A. Effectiveness of a treatment
1. Study design and analysis standards
   Randomization of patients to treatment alternatives
   Complete accounting of all randomized patients
   Analysis with patients kept in the groups formed by randomization
   Groups otherwise treated equally

2. Interpreting results
   Use of absolute risk reduction (the difference in event rates per cent between the two groups) or its inverse, the number needed to be treated (NNT).
   Examination of 95% confidence intervals

3. Application of results
   Similarity of your patient to those in the study
   Potential benefit of treatment for your patient
   Whether treatment regimen satisfies the patient's values and preferences

B. Prognosis of a disease
1. Study design and analysis standards
   Assembly of a defined cohort of representative patients
   Sufficiently long and complete follow-up
   Objective outcome criteria used objectively
   Several additional standards for those attempting to draw inferences about subgroups

2. Interpreting results
   Probability of outcomes
   Precision of outcomes, examination of 95% confidence intervals

3. Application of results
   Similarity of your patient to those in the study
   Whether the evidence would lead to a change in management including counselling

C. Usefulness of a diagnostic test
1. Study design and analysis standards
   Independent, blind comparison with a reference criteria, either a gold-standard test or long-term follow-up
   Evaluation of test in patients similar to those who would be considered for it
   Reference criteria information on all patients (not influenced by test result)

2. Interpreting results
   Sensitivity, specificity
   Positive and negative predictive values
   Use of likelihood ratios to directly calculate how the test result changes the odds of whether your patient has the disease

3. Application of results
   Availability, accuracy, precision, and affordability of the test locally
   Ability to estimate odds of disease before applying the test
   Whether recalculated odds given the test result would lead to changes in management
   Whether the consequences of the test would be of benefit

D. Aetiology of a disease or harmful outcome
1. Study design and analysis standards
   Comparison of patients who are similar in ways other than exposure to the exposure or aetiological factor(s) under study
   Objective measurement of both the exposure and the disease in all patients
   Sufficiently long and complete follow-up
   Other causation considerations: temporality (exposure preceded the outcome), dose–response gradient, consistency among studies

2. Interpreting results
   Relative risks or odds ratios
   Calculation of an absolute statistic, such as the number needed to harm

3. Application of results
   Suitability for extrapolation to your patient
   Patient's risk for harmful outcome
   Whether treatment regimen satisfies the patient's values and preferences
   What the alternatives are

Evidence-based medicine gained momentum after it was recognized that traditional expert recommendations in text-books and journals were sometimes incorrect when judged by the results of future research or even knowledge that already existed in the literature but was not generally appreciated before the development of systematic reviews and meta-analysis. Furthermore, in the absence of a systematic approach to reviews, practising physicians reading recommendations could not tell whether they had been approached from evidence, experience or from theories believed by the expert. They could not tell whether another approach was due to a lack of direct evidence or despite evidence to the contrary. The classic examples included clinical policies that represented potentially fatal overtreatment or undertreatment of tens of thousands of patients.

## What is evidence? Is paediatric endocrinology evidence-based?

Evidence refers to the results of valid patient-orientated research studies that directly answers your management questions. Such studies will generally focus on the diagnostic accuracy of tests, the effectiveness of treatments or the cause of diseases.

Given this definition, much of classic endocrinology is evidence based. For example, children with growth failure because of acquired primary hypothyroidism invariably had low thyroxine and elevated thyrotrophin blood concentrations and invariably responded to oral thyroxine replacement therapy. Owing to the combination of how essential thyroid hormone is to all patients and that blood levels are (by definition of endocrinology) key for both the measurement and correction of endocrine deficiencies, the successful researchers of thyroid physiology had developed what would certainly be judged an excellent screening test (growth rate, virtually 100% sensitive), an excellent diagnostic test (abnormal thyroid function test, virtually 100% specific) and an excellent treatment (thyroid replacement, virtually 100% beneficial).

This same pattern probably occurred, more or less, for all classic endocrinopathies as a result of hypo- and hypersecreting glands. In being overly simplistic, I do not do justice to the clinical diagnostic skills that evolved, which can also be analysed in terms of sensitivity and specificity. The result of these strong and highly invariable associations was an excellent evidence base to manage patients long before knowledge of molecular genetics, T-cell receptors, diagnostic testing probability calculations or randomized controlled trials. The reason that this evidence was so useful was not only that it was valid but also that it was relevant. The likelihood of having the diagnosis or benefiting from the treatment was known and not extrapolated from theory. This evidence base evolved into classic standards of care.

The essential concept is validity. How likely it is that the results represent the truth and are not due to unrealized alternative explanations (bias)? The combination of the dramatic effect of the hormone and the lack of variability between patients meant that the advanced techniques of epidemiological research, diagnostic testing probability calculations or randomized controlled trials were not needed. However, when moving beyond these strong and highly invariable associations, more powerful epidemiological research designs and appreciation of statistical variability are needed to build an evidence base. At the same time, studies are needed to focus on types of questions directly relevant to patients, including aetiology, diagnosis, prognosis or treatment effect. These points may not have been widely enough appreciated. Advances in physiology and pharmacology by research laboratories have led to the production and promotion of theories on how to manage patients in the absence of rigorous patient-orientated research. This confusion between theoretical reasoning and direct relevant evidence for newer challenges is a signal that some areas of paediatric endocrinology may actually be becoming less evidence-based (see below).

## Evidence-based medicine resources

There is an abundance of materials for physicians who wish to learn more about evidence-based medicine. The small pocket textbook by Sackett *et al.* [1] is readable, succinct and complete. The *Journal of the American Medical Association* (*JAMA*) publishes a series of papers on appraising studies and integrating the evidence into clinical problem solving: *The Users' Guide to the Medical Literature*. Articles on appraising the validity of systematic reviews, practice guidelines and economic evaluations are also included in this series. Systematic reviews on the effects of treatment are being increasingly disseminated by the Cochrane Collaboration. Some secondary journals (e.g. *Best Evidence*) have been created to filter studies containing high-quality evidence from the published literature; some primary journals (e.g. *Journal of Paediatrics*) have sections that do the same job. Some organizations (e.g. the Canadian Diabetes Association) have replaced previous clinical practice guidelines with recommendations that are related to the underlying direct evidence [2] following the pioneering example of the Canadian Task Force on Periodic Health Examination in the 1970s. An increasing number of textbooks that use similar approaches are being published. At the time of writing, books with titles such as *Evidence-Based Diabetes Care* [3] and *Evidence-Based Paediatrics* [4,5] are in press. The Internet has several sites concerning evidence-based medicine that contain further teaching materials and existing evidence summaries, whether complete systematic reviews or CATs. Some of the key web sites are listed in Table 26.2.

**Table 26.2.** Internet resources for evidence-based medicine

Centre for Evidence-Based Medicine (in Oxford)
http://cebm.jr2.ox.ac.uk/

Centre for Evidence-Based Child Health (in London)
http://www.ich.bpmf.ac.uk/ebm/ebm.htm

Health Information Research Unit: Evidence-Based Health Informatics
http://hiru.mcmaster.ca/

The Cochrane Collaboration: Preparing, maintaining and promoting the accessibility of systematic reviews of the effects of health care
http://hiru.mcmaster.ca/COCHRANE/DEFAULT.HTM

PubMED: free site for MEDLINE (and Pre-MEDLINE) searches
http://www.ncbi.nlm.nih.gov/PubMed/

US Prevention Task Forces Guides to Clinical Preventive Services
http://cpmcnet.columbia.edu/texts/gcps/

International Society of Technology Assessment in Health Care (ISTAHC)
http://www.istahc.org/

## Examples of evidence-based paediatric endocrinology

### A question of harm

Dr Smith receives a request to see Jimmy, aged 5 years, who is being treated for inoperable abdominal neuroblastoma with $^{131}$I-labelled metaiodobenzylguanidine ( [$^{131}$I]MIBG). Dr Smith heads straight to the hospital library to run a computer search using MedLINE. Although evidence on iatrogenic complications may be found in randomized trials and case–control studies of aetiology, he suspects a cohort prognostic study will be most useful. He frames the question as follows. 'What endocrine complications should be expected in patients treated with ( [$^{131}$I]MIBG)?' He chooses the last 10 years of medical literature and is happy to see that typing MIBG in the thesaurus is mapped to a standard indexed subheading (MESH) term.

This search yields 150 citations. He then tries a text word search, typing in: 'complication or complications'. This search yields 500 000 citations. The 18 citations in common (using the AND operator) are all off topic. He returns to the 150 citations, limits the command to English language reviews, and finds a recent narrative review in *Archives of Diseases of Childhood* [6]. He is happy to have a brief broadly based review and is less worried about citation bias, given how little evidence that there seems to be.

The paper mentions two possible endocrine complications, thyroid (referenced in [7]) and adrenal dysfunction (stated to be theoretical). Dr Smith retrieves, reads and appraises the paper of Picco *et al.* [7] and jots down a brief CAT summary of his decision to follow thyroid function based on his reading of Picco *et al.* in a paper containing a valid prognostic study reporting the cohort at the appropriate stage of the disease relevant to his patient. His decision to follow adrenal function (despite no evidence of a problem) reflects his concern not to miss a serious and treatable disease (Table 26.3).

**Table 26.3.** Adrenal and thyroid function should be followed in patients treated with [$^{131}$I]MIBG [3,4]

Clinical bottom lines
1. Twelve out of fourteen long-term survivors in one series had subclinical or clinical hypothyroidism.
2. Radiation 'cross-fire' effects on the adrenal are only a theoretical concern but worth following until more evidence is available.

File listing: MIBG    Appraiser: Dr Smith
CAT: harm    Date: August 24, 1999

The evidence
Cohort study of 14 patients who survived cancer with such treatment for 2 years (out of 58 so treated). Some patients were also treated with TBI/BMT. Total dose of $^{131}$I ranged from 2.5 to 5.5 GBq for each patient.
Twelve out of fourteen had evidence of thyroid dysfunction, including within 6 months of the first dose in five. Eight patients were said to have clinical hypothyroidism and goitre; four others subclinical hypothyroidism (0.15–0.87 GBq/kg).
Adrenal function was not reported.

Comments
1. Lugol's solution was tried as a prevention but did not seem to work.
2. Meller's narrative review included radiation 'cross-fire' effects on the adrenal as a theoretical concern.

The patient was a 5-year-old boy receiving [$^{131}$I]MIBG treatments for inoperable neuroblastoma for 1 year.

| Number | Records | Request |
|--------|---------|---------|
| 1 | 17 458 | Explore 'Diabetes mellitus, insulin-dependent'/all subheadings |
| 2 | 17 545 | Outpatient |
| 3 | 30 508 | Ambulatory |
| 4 | 43 498 | Outpatient or ambulatory |
| 5 | 445 | Numbers 1 and 4 |
| 6 | 159 349 | PT = 'CLINICAL TRIAL' |
| 7 | 81 | Number 5 and (PT = 'CLINICAL TRIAL') |
| 8 | 258 456 | AGE = 'CHILD' |
| 9 | 7 | Number 7 and (AGE = 'CHILD') |

**Table 26.4.** Search strategy for question of diabetes initial treatment

## A question of treatment

Dr Jones, the regional consultant for childhood diabetes, is notified by the hospital emergency department that they have a well-looking 10-year-old boy with classic symptoms of type 1 diabetes, such as polyuria, polydipsia and nocturia and a blood sugar of 20 mmol/L. Dr Jones arranges admission to hospital for initiation of insulin therapy and for diabetes education, recalling, however, that, at the last paediatric conference he attended, a colleague from another centre boasted that her patients did better over time because they were treated as outpatients by a dedicated diabetes education team. This programme was said to result in the parents being more confident with management and less confused as fewer people were involved when hospital wards were avoided. Dr Jones replied that inpatient education seems to work well for his patients.

Although a switch to an initial outpatient programme might be difficult and he is not keen to change something that is working, Dr Jones thinks he should find out whether his colleague's claims are supported by any evidence. He realizes that this is a question of treatment effect and frames a searchable question. 'Does initial outpatient education of paediatric patients with newly diagnosed type 1 diabetes lead to better diabetes outcomes than patients initially treated as inpatients?'

Obviously, direct comparison in a randomized controlled trial would be the best evidence. Dr Jones heads to the hospital library to perform a MedLINE search of the previous 10 years. As in the last example, he uses the AND operator to combine the results of a thesaurus search of the disease (diabetes, insulin-dependent) with a text word search of the relatively unique feature (ambulatory or outpatient). He then limits the results to those indexed by publication type as being clinical trials and by age tag as being studies in children (Table 26.4). He finds one study on the topic and two papers, a results paper in *Paediatrics* [8] and, most unusually, a formal economic evaluation [9]. He appraises the results paper using the criteria suggested in Table 26.1 [1] and decides that the study is valid and that the decrease in glycoslylated haemoglobin levels in the long term is important. He will speak again to his colleague from the other centre and ask her to provide more information and materials about her outpatient programme in order to avoid duplication in work. He will also speak to his hospital's administrator about allocating the necessary resources for changes in providing care for children with diabetes.

## Towards evidence-based paediatric endocrinology

Challenges exist at several levels. The easiest is the education of physicians in practice, as excellent teaching tools based on adult education principles have been developed. Other challenges include eliminating the confusion between the terms evidence and theory based on basic research (especially among those who would set guidelines or treatment recommendations), agreement on what are the clinically relevant outcomes, the quantity and quality of patient-orientated research and the speed of change of knowledge.

Currently, this seems most evident in the field of stature, which has recently seen a large expansion of activity [10]. For example, despite tens of thousands of patients with non-growth hormone-deficient short stature being treated with growth hormone, only five trials to adult height in healthy children (without disease or disability [11]) are known (four studies of growth hormone and one study of gonadotrophin-releasing hormone agonist to induce delay of puberty [12–16]). Of these, only one has published adult height [12]. There are also two studies of growth hormone vs. no growth hormone in Turner syndrome [17,18], only one with results published in abstract form [18]. There are no randomized controlled trials to adult height published on patients with any other diagnosis [10].

Part of the reason for this dearth of evidence may be disagreement in the choice of outcomes. For example, if the patients, parents and physicians decide that 1-year growth acceleration is the most important outcome, then evidence of an effect on adult height is not important. However, randomized trials that demonstrate a growth acceleration in the first year should not be extrapolated to claim valid evidence on what happens after the two groups created by randomization are both treated. If adult height is the more relevant question, then, given its baseline variability, studies that continue the treatment vs. no-treatment comparison need to be continued until adult height and, in their absence, experts and practising physicians should be explicit that such valid evidence does not exist.

The field gets more complicated than most because studies in the general population and of subjects referred for growth evaluation confirm that short stature during childhood or adolescence is generally not associated with any psychological disability [19] and should not be confused with disease. Studies attempting to demonstrate quality of life changes in those with disabilities that are given functional improvements are difficult to measure, given the ability of children to adapt. Assuming the ability to increase adult height exists, or will exist one day, measuring a benefit due to increasing the stature of healthy people with short stature will be very difficult. Relevant work from the world of medical ethics illustrates why adult height or other 'enhancements' are problematic [20].

The Hastings Center's Enhancement Project has undertaken research into such areas [20]. An important finding is that, although distinctions based on medical treatment vs. prevention vs. enhancement are useful, they are imperfect and, ultimately, the ethical debate moves beyond the goals of medicine to the goals of society at large. Several ethical issues that may be especially relevant here are unfairness, complicity and inauthenticity. Unfairness relates to concerns about the use of technological enhancements to benefit the already privileged by allowing money to trump human genetic variability; this may be especially applicable for an enhancement intended to give a competitive advantage such as increased height. Increased height would otherwise be a self-defeating enhancement, because if everyone could receive the same increase, the relative position would not change. It is difficult to argue that society would benefit if everyone were taller.

The complicity issues raise the questions of whether, or to what extent, attempts to increase the height of short individuals reinforces the social prejudice that creates discrimination. When is it acceptable to accommodate such pressures in order to relieve individual suffering? What are the responsibilities of those that would make such accommodations? The Enhancement Project manuscript [20] summarizes ethicist Maggie Little's discussion of this problem; her answer to the final question is that 'to the extent that one's actions do (or can reasonably be seen to) endorse or promote norms that undergird a system of unjust practices and attitudes, one is obliged elsewhere to fight that same system.'

Finally, the inauthenticity issue may be summarized in this context by raising the possibility that achieving a taller adult height by taking a drug may not actually feel the same to some individuals as it would have been if that height was achieved by the normal course of childhood growth.

Beyond the need for distinguishing evidence from theory and agreement on outcomes, the dearth of high-quality patient-orientated research on rare diseases will continue to be a challenge. Even though much important research remains to be done, funding for it is often difficult and impressive amounts of work and multinational collaboration are needed. The physician practising evidence-based medicine who finds that the evidence that he needs for a management decision does not exist may still benefit from understanding this when making his decision.

Finally, although there is much research to be done, enormous amounts of literature are published each month. It will be increasingly difficult for reviews to remain current. A good example is my own. At the time of writing this chapter in 1999, an edited book on growth hormone therapy was published [21] containing a chapter by myself and Van Vliet on the use of growth hormone in Turner syndrome [22]. According to the evidence at the time of writing that chapter, we described how our clinics differed in policy despite having the same evidence. One clinic had a policy of offering growth hormone routinely to all patients, the other had a policy of refusing to prescribe growth hormone for Turner syndrome. Between the writing of that chapter and the publication of the book, new evidence became available from a randomized controlled trial of growth hormone vs. no treatment continued to adult height [18], leading the second centre to switch from refusal to offering the treatment option for all patients.

Although the Cochrane Collaboration strives for regular updating of reviews in its database and organizational guidelines and textbooks could emulate this by utilizing the Internet for distribution, the best solution for the foreseeable future will be for the practising physician to formulate questions around individual patient management problems and then search and appraise for himself the best evidence.

## References

1 Sackett DL, Richardson WS, Rosenberg W, Haynes RB. *Evidence-based Medicine: How to Practice and Teach EBM.* Edinburgh: Churchill Livingstone; 1997.

2 *Clinical Practice Guidelines for the Management of Diabetes in Canada.* CMA J 1998; 159 (Suppl. 8): S1–S29.

3 Gerstein HC, Haynes RB. *Evidence-based Diabetic Care.* BC Decker; 2001.

4 Feldman W. *Evidence-based Pediatrics.* BC Decker; 2000.

5 Moyer VA. *Evidence-based Paediatrics and Child Health.* London: BMJ Books.

6 Meller S. Targeted radiotherapy for neuroblastoma. *Arch Dis Child* 1997; 77: 389–91.

7 Picco P, Garaventa A, Claudiani F, Gattorno M, De Bernardi B, Borrone C. Primary hypothyroidism as a consequence of

131-I-metaiodobenzylguanidine treatment for children with neuroblastoma. *Cancer* 1995; 76: 1662–4.

8 Dougherty G, Schiffrin A, White D, Soderstrom L, Sufrategui M. Home-based management can achieve intensification cost-effectively in type 1 diabetes. *Paediatrics* 1999; 103: 122–8.

9 Dougherty GE, Soderstrom L, Schiffrin A. An economic evaluation of home care for children with newly diagnosed diabetes. *Med Care* 1998; 36: 586–98.

10 Taback SP, Van Vliet GVV, Guyda HJ. Pharmacologic manipulation of height: qualitative review of study populations and designs. *Clin Invest Med* 1999; 22: 53–9.

11 Evans RG, Barer ML, Marmor TR. *Why Are Some People Healthy and Others Not?: the Determinants of Health of Populations.* New York: Aldine De Gruyter; 1994.

12 McCaughey ES, Mulligan J, Voss LD, Betts PR. Randomised trial of growth hormone in short normal girls. *Lancet* 1998; 351: 940–4.

13 Brämswig JH, Schäfer B, Stöver B, Heinecke A. Growth hormone (GH) therapy in familial short stature (FSS). The results of a 3-years prospective and controlled study (Abstract 61). *Hormone Res* 1996; 47 (Suppl. 2): 16.

14 Albertsson-Wikland K. Use of hGH for promotion of growth in normal short children – the Swedish experience (Abstract 69). *Hormone Res* 1997; 48 (Suppl. 2): 18.

15 Rose SR, Baron J, Bernstein D *et al.* Suppression and recovery of GH secretion after GH injection in non-GH-deficient short children (Abstract 409). *Hormone Res* 1997; 48 (Suppl. 2): 81.

16 Cutler GB Jr, Yanovski J, Rose SR *et al.* Luteinizing hormone-releasing hormone agonist (LHRHa)-induced delay of epiphyseal fusion increases adult height of adolescents with short stature (Abstract 108). *Hormone Res* 1997; 48 (Suppl. 2): 28.

17 Ross JL, Feuillan P, Kushner H, Roeltgen D, Cutler Jr. GB. Absence of growth hormone effects on cognitive function in girls with Turner syndrome. *J Clin Endocrinol Metab* 1997; 82: 1814–71.

18 Canadian Growth Hormone Advisory Committee. Growth hormone treatment to final height in Turner syndrome: a randomized controlled trial (Abstract P7). *Horm Res* 1998; 50 (Suppl. 3): 25.

19 Eiholzer U, Haverkamp F, Voss L, eds. *Growth, Stature, and Psychosocial Well-being.* Seattle: Hogrefe and Huber Publishers; 1999.

20 Parens E. Is Better always Good? The Enhancement Project. *Hastings Center Report* 1998; January–February (Suppl.): S1–S17.

21 Hindmarsh PC, ed. *Current Indications for Growth Hormone Therapy.* Basel: Karger; 1999.

22 Taback SP, Van Vliet G. Managing the short stature of Turner syndrome: an evidence-based approach to the suggestion of growth hormone supplementation. In: Hindmarsh PC, ed. *Current Indications for Growth Hormone Therapy.* Basel: Karger; 1999.

# 27 Clinical trials in paediatric endocrinology

## Angela Wade and M.A. Preece

## Introduction

In modern medicine new therapies are being devised, tested and regulated at an ever-increasing rate. Usually the therapy will be a drug, but the same principles apply when testing surgical procedures or devices. In this chapter, for simplicity, we will refer to drugs while recognizing that we may really be referring to a hormone, surgical procedure or other therapeutic manoeuvre. The formal clinical trial (CT) has a central role in regularizing the manner in which such testing is performed and ensuring that the study has a reasonable chance of identifying an advantage of the new drug if it is present and, equally, of not detecting an advantage when fallacious. It is the mainstay of evidence-based medicine and now no new drug may be introduced without being put through the procedure.

A common cause of confusion is that between a clinical trial and a therapeutic trial. The former is a strict test of efficacy and safety of a drug in a statistically robust design whereas the latter is usually the trial of a drug in an individual patient on a one-off basis.

In most clinical trials the principal aim is to test the efficacy and safety of a new drug. In order to meet these requirements the CT needs to be designed in an appropriate way to ensure removal of biases. Very often the nature of the drug or the target population will dictate aspects of the design, but always this will aim to ensure that the only difference between the test group and control subjects is that the former are exposed to the drug under test.

## Regulatory issues

These will vary from country to country and for this reason they will not be dwelt on in detail. In most countries the regulatory authorities will need to be informed of a CT and may influence the manner in which the drug is made available to the investigators. There are now protocols that attempt to harmonize procedures between countries, such as the International Conference on Harmonization (ICH). This is a tripartite collaboration between regulatory authorities in Europe, Japan and the USA, which aims to arrive at common guidelines for the design, execution and reporting of CTs. In addition, it is now possible to conduct a single clinical trial to obtain Europe-wide regulatory approval. Indeed, for recombinant products this is the desired route.

## Phases of drug evaluation

Clinical trials are grouped into four phases that reflect the different stages of development of a new drug.

Phase 1 This is usually a relatively small-scale, short-term sequence of studies in healthy volunteers. The primary objective is to gather safety data, but also to study basic parameters of absorption, pharmacokinetics and metabolism. An initial definition of likely effective dosage is usually undertaken.

Phase 2 This extends phase 1 to a few patients with the target disease to see whether it is active against the disease in the short term and to assess short-term safety in patients with the target disease. Phase 2 studies tend to be very detailed and will aim to provide information on appropriate dose regimens and dose–response relationships.

Phase 3 The decision to proceed to phase 3 is made once efficacy has been demonstrated, no major safety problems are uncovered and an appropriate dose is found. Here the CT tests the drug on larger numbers of patients, sometimes several hundred, often at many different sites. These trials usually compare the new treatment with either a treatment already in use or against no treatment or a placebo. There is sometimes subdivision into phases 3a and 3b. This essentially separates studies completed before submission of a license application (phase 3a) from those continuing at that time or that are started after submission but before approval. Phase 3b also includes investigations of new indications or new patient populations for licensed drugs.

Phase 4 These are also referred to as postmarketing surveillance studies. They are usually after a treatment has been granted a license for use for a particular clinical indication in order to extend the knowledge base of efficacy and safety. They tend to be carried out on much larger numbers of patients although fewer data are collected on each patient. In many cases the inclusion of cases is voluntary and therefore care is needed in generalizing from this type of data.

Children are seldom involved in phase 1 or 2 studies. Exceptionally, they may be included in phase 2 CTs if the target condition only occurs in childhood (an obvious example is disorders of growth). For the purposes of this chapter we will largely be discussing phase 3 CTs.

## Study design

There are two main designs that are appropriate for CTs in which the aim is to test for a difference between a test treatment and a control, placebo or otherwise. These are either parallel or crossover designs. In the former, the control and test treatments are randomly allocated to patients, and at the end of the treatment period the outcome variables are compared between the patient groups by appropriate statistical tests. In the latter, all patients will receive test and control treatments, but in a random order. At the end of treatment, analysis compares control and treatment periods, but also tests whether there is an interaction between order and outcome, that is, whether the difference between test and control treatments is influenced by the order in which the treatments were received.

The choice between parallel and crossover designs is mostly straightforward. If the test period is necessarily long (as in CTs where growth is the outcome variable), a crossover design will lengthen the study unreasonably. It is also difficult to use when there is likely to be a carry-over effect, such as might occur if the active treatment is administered first and has a continuing effect that runs into the control period. On the other hand, in the absence of these problems, crossover studies have greater power as each patient acts as his/her own control. Each study must be assessed in its own right with respect to these issues.

Where possible, for either parallel or crossover designs, baseline measurements should be made and incorporated as covariates in the final analyses. If a crossover design is used then more than two periods should be considered. Incorporating a third period of study (randomly chosen as either treatment or control) has been shown to greatly improve the final efficiency and allow more precise quantification of carry-over and order effects [1,2]. Measurements may be made during washout phases (i.e. times when no treatment is given), either between or after treatment periods. The washout measurements allow assessment of developments over time that are unrelated to the treatment under investigation.

## Defining the question

It is essential that there is a clear research question identified before a CT is designed or executed. This will usually involve a systematic review of all relevant literature; the process for this is now clearly established [3,4]. There are important scientific and ethical reasons for this planning phase. The research question needs to be properly set in a way that can be answered using collectable data and appropriate methodology. A study will be unethical if the planned design will not allow a valid conclusion or if other adequate studies have already been initiated or completed. Ideally, the question will be addressed by a simple quantitative comparison between the effects of the new drug and placebo or established therapy.

## Establishing the study sample

In the normal course of events the study sample will be drawn from a clinic population of patients with the target disease. With relatively common disorders there will often be sufficient numbers for an adequately powered study (see below) in one institution. If not, then a multicentre or even multinational study becomes necessary. For the present we will assume a single-centre protocol.

Variation in the patient mix from centre to centre may limit the generalizability of the study conclusions. For example, a treatment shown to be effective in a sample of young boys cannot be assumed to be similarly effective in older girls. Other factors, such as ethnic mix and socioeconomic status, may have a direct effect on outcome or operate more subtly, perhaps by influencing compliance.

## Other issues related to controlled trials

For the evaluation of either a new drug, or a new indication for an established drug, a randomized CT is required. Ideally, this should be double-blind, that is neither the sample patients nor the clinicians will know whether a particular patient is receiving control or test medication. There are exceptions to these basic requirements, but they must be clearly and objectively justified.

If there is no prior therapy available for the condition under investigation, then placebo control is usually appropriate. On the other hand, if the investigation is one of a sequence of therapies developed over many years then the control group should receive the best available of the standard therapies. Sometimes the choice may be influenced by the nature of the test formulation. If the drug under test is given by injection there may be an ethical and practical problem with the use of a placebo injection, particularly if there is a need for multiple administrations. Equally, if the best standard therapy is injected and the test substance is oral, clearly the double-blind ideal cannot be achieved unless an oral placebo is substituted for the control substance. These are all special cases that often need careful thought, and each CT should be carefully planned, taking into account the specific characteris-tics of the disorder and the treatment under test. Most importantly, the starting point must be the assumption that a randomized double blind CT is required, which is only departed from when specific issues make that ideal impossible [5].

## Pilot studies

A pilot study is an *initial* investigation to give information that will be necessary when designing a future trial or study. For example, a pilot study may be used to assess the feasibility of a particular measurement protocol in an infant, to determine the quality of a proposed questionnaire or to assess the variability of key variables. The investigator should have an outline of a *future* study that will be informed by the pilot study, which should not be an end in itself.

## Randomization

A vital ingredient of the CT is randomization. The underlying principle is that the assignment of patients to control or test groups must not be subject to influence by the subjects or investigators.

It is important that the allocation scheme is truly random and not, in some subtle manner, systematic. Examples of the latter would be the alternation of successive patients or the use of the last digit of case-note numbers. Although both of these might seem random, they can be subject to influence by, for example, the manner in which a particular clinic assigns appointments or case numbers.

*Simple randomization* is the least complex form of unbiased group allocation and is synonymous with tossing an unbiased coin. Using a computer package consecutive random choices $(1, 2, 3, \ldots, n)$ can be generated to determine which of $n$ treatment groups the next eligible and consenting patient should be allocated to. When the sample is not large then there may be a substantial imbalance in the group numbers obtained. For example, if 40 individuals are randomized to two groups using simple randomization, there is an 8% chance that one group will contain 65% (26) or more of the individuals.

*Blocked randomization* guarantees that at no time will the imbalance in group numbers be large and at certain points there will be equal numbers in each group. The simplest system uses sealed opaque envelopes that contain a code identifying a particular treatment, which is then dispensed by the pharmacy. These envelopes are prepared in 'blocks' of usually four, six or eight, with an equal number for each block indicating allocation to each of the treatment arms. For example, with three treatment regimens and a block size of six, there would be three sets of two envelopes for each of the three treatments within each block of six envelopes. When a patient enters the trial an envelope is chosen and this deter-

mines his/her treatment. Hence, at the end of each block an equal number of patients will have been allocated to each of the treatments and a new 'block' of envelopes can then be prepared. One disadvantage is that when there is only one envelope left then the treatment for the next patient may be deduced. This problem can only occur in non-blind studies. A solution is to introduce the next 'block' (of four, six, eight or however many envelopes) when there is only one envelope remaining, so that the choice can never be predicted with accuracy but approximate equality of group numbers is maintained throughout. Because of the potential for interference when envelopes are kept 'on site' the gold standard for randomization is to use telephone allocation [6].

It may be necessary to ensure some balance between the test and control groups with respect to such variables as age, sex or severity of illness. Variables that are not of direct interest but may influence the result if not properly accounted for are known as *confounders*. For example, in a study of a growth-promoting agent, parental heights could be a confounder. There are three methods of achieving comparable groups while retaining the principles of random allocation:

**1** Matching: Pairs of individuals that are similar with respect to the potentially confounding variables (such as illness severity or parental height) are identified and then one of each pair is randomly chosen to receive the intervention. The remaining patient is used as a control.

**2** Stratification: Matching will not be reasonable if suitable matches cannot be found for each patient. Individuals without a matched pair might not be recruited and this will result in an unnecessary recruitment loss. Furthermore, the practicalities of finding pair matches may make the process of recruitment unnecessarily complex. Stratified randomization consists of using separate randomization lists for each potentially confounding subgroup. For example, separate lists for different age bands or severity groups. Within each subgroup, block randomization should be used as simple randomization within each subgroup is no different from using simple randomization without subgrouping. If there are several confounders and hence a number of separate lists, there is an obvious increase in the potential for practical problems.

**3** Minimization: The process of minimization can be used to achieve overall similarity between groups as regards confounding factors. For each patient that is recruited, the randomization is weighted to minimize differences between the groups with respect to confounders [7]. This process is more complex than the other methods, but with software available to perform the necessary calculations it need not be more difficult in practice.

## Cluster trials

Treatments or interventions may by necessity be levelled at groups (or clusters) of individuals. For example, assessing the effect of an additional practice nurse specifically for growth-related disorders. Practices would be randomly chosen to receive a nurse or not, the effect of the intervention (introduction of nurse) would be assessed at an individual level (improvement in individual patients) although the intervention is made at practice level. The patients within any given practice might be expected to have outcomes that are more similar than those from different practices, irrespective of intervention. The reasons for this may be social, people within practices might be more similar with respect to social background, or it may be because they have common doctors and other support staff and practice-specific policies of care. Furthermore, the intervention being directed at practice level has elements common specifically to that practice, i.e. the nurse involved. The extent to which individuals are more alike within clusters rather than between clusters is quantified via the intracluster correlation coefficient (ICC). The ICC takes values between 0 and 1. A value of 0 indicates that the individuals within clusters are no more alike than individuals from different clusters. An ICC of 1 indicates that all individuals within a cluster are alike, and therefore no additional information is obtained from assessing more than one individual per cluster. The analysis needs to take account of the clustering of individuals [8,9].

## Variables

### Definition

The results of a trial are quantified by recording measurements of one or more variables. Some of these will be outcome variables and some will be used either as predictors or to allow for confounding effects. All variables need to be clearly defined before the study commences.

There are several types of variable:
*Categorical* variables classify individuals into one of several categories.
*Binary* or *dichotomous* variables are those with only two categories (e.g. male/female, yes/no, positive/negative). If there are more than two categories and these have an obvious order, then these are referred to as *ordinal* variables (e.g. puberty stages). Categorical variables that are neither binary nor ordinal are described as *nominal* (e.g. ethnic group).
*Numeric* variables are those measured on some well-defined scale with units and these may be either *discrete* (e.g. parity or number of clinic visits) or *continuous* (e.g. height or weight). Continuous variables can take any value within a defined range but, in practice, are restricted by the accuracy with which it is possible to make such measurements. For example, body length may be measured to the nearest 0.5 cm.

Sometimes a continuous variable is used to form categorical data (such as gestational age being reduced to preterm or term), but this is seldom advisable. Collapsing continuous data into categories loses information, reducing the study power and requiring a larger sample in order to make the same inferences.

The outcome may be the time to something happening, for example time to death or time to complete recovery. The main difficulty with this type of data is that some patients may not reach the end point (death or recovery) within the time scale of the trial or may not be monitored for equal lengths of time. For example, a study of time to recovery after starting a treatment may last for 2 years including 6 months of recruitment so that those recruited earlier will generally have a longer follow-up. Although some will not have recovered by the end of their 18 months to 2 years of observation, knowing that they will take at least this long is valuable information when estimating the average time to recovery. *Survival analysis* techniques are appropriate for efficient and unbiased analysis of data of this form [10].

In more recent years, greater and greater emphasis has been placed on economic outcomes. Economic analysis compares costs between the treatment groups and a full economic analysis will take into account costs to the patient of their time, etc. The aim is to link monetary costs to health outcomes in a way that permits rational choices between therapies to be made. There are various types of economic analyses. For example, *cost minimization analysis* compares costs for identical outcomes; *cost effectiveness analysis* uses natural medical units, such as life years gained; *cost–benefit analysis* converts everything, including medical outcomes, to a monetary equivalent [11,12].

## Reliability and validity

Attention should be given to the reliability and validity of any variables used in the study. It is important to ensure that the measurements made are reasonably accurate and actually quantify the relevant information. No amount of elegant design or fancy data manipulation is going to compensate for inadequate measuring instruments. Hence, this is a very important area to which very often little or no consideration is given. Although it is a relatively easy matter to collect information and analyse it, it is somewhat more difficult to ensure that the information collected is both valid and that the measuring technique is reliable [13–15].

## Example data

In the next sections, we will be using some example data. This is fictional and does not relate to any specific clinical trial. It mimics a clinical trial of a potential growth-promoting drug, tested on samples of short normal (SN) children. The variables are final height *z*-score (outcome variable), midparental height *z*-score, weight (kg) and whether the child had difficulty adhering to the regimen (yes/no).

## Sample size

This is a fundamental preliminary once the hypothesis has been identified and the choice of type and design of CT has been decided. There are two types of sample size formulae, power calculations or precision estimates, and these are directly related to the two ways of analysing data, using significance tests or via confidence intervals. With the power calculations, the sample is chosen to identify a given difference with specified power and significance. The power of a study (range 0–100%) is its ability to detect a given difference if it exists, this is usually set at between 80% and 95%. The significance (range 0–1) is the probability of obtaining the observed difference in the absence of a true population difference. With the precision estimates, the sample is chosen to ensure that the confidence interval obtained is of a specified width. Sample size calculations are always based on estimation of unknown factors and hence give an approximate figure rather than a precise number. The calculations will give a figure for the minimum number required for statistical analyses; the recruited number will usually need to be larger to take account of dropouts. Formulae are available for most analytical scenarios.

## Examples of formulae

For the power calculations, $d$ is the minimum difference that we want to detect, $F$ is taken from the Table 27.1 and is set according to the chosen power and significance level.

For the precision estimates, 'e' is the maximum sampling error that we are prepared to tolerate. The formulae given yield the number required so that we are 95% confident that the estimate obtained from the study will differ from the true value by no more than $e$ [i.e. the 95% confidence interval (CI) will be of width $2e$].

### Comparing the mean of two groups

Power: $n > 2F\sigma^2/d^2$

Precision: $n > 8\sigma^2/e^2$

**Table 27.1.** Values of $F$ for use in power calculations

| Significance level required | Power required | | | |
|---|---|---|---|---|
| | 80% | 90% | 95% | 99% |
| 0.100 | 6.18 | 8.56 | 10.82 | 15.77 |
| 0.050 | 7.85 | 10.51 | 12.99 | 18.37 |
| 0.025 | 9.51 | 12.41 | 15.10 | 20.86 |
| 0.010 | 11.68 | 14.88 | 17.81 | 24.03 |

where $\sigma$ is the standard deviation of the measurements within each group.

In our example, $\sigma$ for final height is estimated as 0.5. Therefore, to detect a difference in average $z$-scores between the control and treated SN children of 0.4 with 90% power at the 5% significance level will require:

$$n > 2(10.51)\, 0.5^2/0.4^2 = 32.84 \text{ (or at least 33) children per group.}$$

This sample size would also allow estimation of the difference in group mean $z$-scores to within $\pm 0.25$ with 95% confidence as

$$n > 8(0.5)^2/0.25^2 = 32.$$

Allowing for likely dropouts a safe recruitment number would be 40 per group or a total sample of 80 to be randomized to the treatment/control groups.

### Comparing the percentages, $p_1$ and $p_2$, in two groups

Power: $n > \dfrac{F[p_1(100 - p_1) + p_2(100 - p_2)]}{(p_2 - p_1)^2}$

Precision: $n > \dfrac{4[p_1(100 - p_1) + p_2(100 - p_2)]}{e^2}$

For example, suppose that from previous studies it is known that about 1 in 5 of SN patients have problems adhering to a tablet regimen ($p_1 = 20$) and we want to detect an increase in problems of 40% ($p_2 = 60$) in those given an active treatment. Choosing a 5% significance level with 90% power ($F = 10.51$) will require a minimum sample size in each group of:

$$n > \frac{10.51[20(100 - 20) + 60(100 - 60)]}{40^2} = 26.3$$

To estimate the difference to within $\pm 20\%$ will require:

$$n > \frac{4[20(100 - 20) + 60(100 - 60)]}{20^2} = 40 \text{ per group.}$$

## Calculating power retrospectively

The sample size formulae are based on estimated values, for example the standard deviation of the variable ($\sigma$) or the group percentages ($p_1$ and $p_2$). These estimates might have been erroneous, and in some situations it may be useful to calculate retrospectively the true power of the study. For example, if the final height standard deviation ($\sigma$) in the SN children is actually 0.6 (rather than the estimated value of 0.5), then the power to detect a difference of 0.4 with 33 children per group is given by solving the following equation for $F$:

$$n > 2F\sigma^2/d^2$$

i.e. $33 > \dfrac{2F(0.6)^2}{0.4^2} = \dfrac{0.72F}{0.16}$, so $F < \dfrac{33(0.16)}{0.72} = 7.33$

and Table 27.1 shows that the study would only have had approximately 80% power at the 5% significance level to detect a difference of 0.4.

## Estimating sample sizes where there are more than two treatment groups

A common scenario in endocrinology is to have more than two treatment groups. These groups may be nominal (for example control, treatment A, treatment B) or ordinal (for example control, 5 mg, 10 mg, 15 mg, 40 mg) in nature. Estimating the sample size in these scenarios is more complex. The number per group will be less than in the two group situation, although the overall sample size may be larger. Numbers will be smaller for ordered groups than for those without any intrinsic order. Day and Graham [16] present a nomogram for estimating required sample sizes for up to five groups and significance levels of 0.01 and 0.05. Cohen [17] and Hysieh *et al.* [18] show how to increase the sample size to account for covariates.

## Other sample size formulae

Sample size formulae exist for all potential forms of ultimate analysis. For example, formulae pertaining to non-parametric analyses [19,20], survival analyses [21], reliability [22] and analyses of variance and correlation [17,23] are readily available.

## Equivalence trials

Sometimes the aim of a study is to determine whether two treatments are similarly effective. For example, where a new treatment is not expected to perform significantly better, but there may be cost or practical advantages. Assessing equivalence will generally involve a larger sample size than that for detecting a difference between groups. Special sample size formulae are available for this situation [24].

## Multiple tests

Often, there is more than one main outcome. For example, in the growth promotion study there might also have been a questionnaire assessment of quality of life using multiple outcome variables. Each outcome may be tested separately, but this could result in large numbers of significance tests, some of which may be spuriously significant. If multiple tests are performed then single findings should be interpreted as part of the battery of tests and never reported out of context [25,26].

Similar consideration should be given to the number of tests performed when interim analyses are undertaken.

*Sequential trials* are specifically designed to cater for evaluation of the study results at several time points throughout. If a large enough effect is detected at some point then recruitment may cease and the trial terminated.

The sample size has to be tailored to take account of the additional testing and must be increased to maintain the same level of power throughout [27].

## Exploring the dataset

### Displaying data

Graphical displays of data are essential at a preliminary stage in data analysis to identify 'outliers' that may have arisen as a result of errors in data coding or data entry. They are also a useful way of summarizing data and presenting the results of any statistical analyses. The importance of graphical data displays as an integral part of any analysis should not be overlooked.

Figures 27.1 and 27.2 show the height and weight data from the growth-promoting drug example. Skewness in the weight data is clearly visible. Table 27.2 is used to present the adherence data; percentages are shown to highlight the difference in adherence between the treated and control children. Figure 27.3 illustrates the relationship between final height *z*-score and midparental height *z*-score. The positive relationship between these two variables is as expected, the scatterplot also illustrates the tendency for the treated group to have had taller parents, which may be an important point to consider in subsequent analyses. It can be seen that, of the 40 randomized to each of the two groups, only 39 and 33 in the control and treated groups, respectively, had final height outcome data. This is not unusual in trials where the

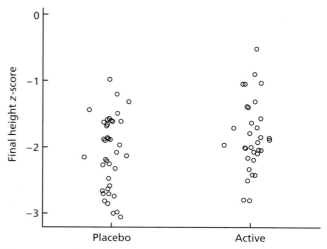

**Fig. 27.1.** Final height *z*-scores of the children in the two treatment groups.

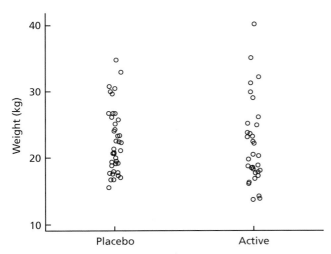

**Fig. 27.2.** Weights (kg) of children in the two treatment groups.

**Table 27.2.** Contingency table showing differences in distribution of problems between the treatment groups

| Problems | Control | Treated | Total |
|---|---|---|---|
| Yes | 9 (23.1%) | 23 (69.7%) | 32 |
| No | 30 (76.9%) | 10 (30.3%) | 40 |
| Total | 39 (100%) | 33 (100%) | 72 |

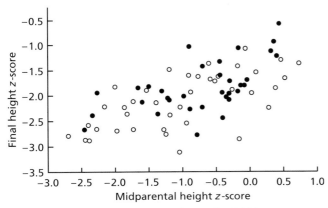

**Fig. 27.3.** The relationship between midparental and child *z*-scores according to treatment group. ●, Treated group; ○, control group.

follow-up time is long, as is the case with many endocrine trials. Some attempt should be made to identify differences between those who do and do not complete the treatment or return for follow-up. For example, sex and initial height could be compared between those reported here and the missing group. In this way, biases may be highlighted that could affect the generalizability of the results.

## Data summaries

Data are usually summarized as either the mean and standard deviation if the sample values are approximately symmetric or as the median and interquartile range (75th–25th centiles) for skew data. The mean and standard deviation provide a more powerful means of making inferences about population values from the sample and should be used where possible. If the data are skewed then it may be possible to transform the data before calculation of the summary statistics. These descriptives are then calculated on the transformed data and back-transformed to the original scale for presentation.

## The normal distribution

Data may be distributed in many ways. The normal (or Gaussian) distribution is symmetric and bell shaped, with the bulk of the values near to the mean. It is quite common for biological variables to be normally distributed. Final height *z*-score is approximately normally distributed in both the treated and control groups of SN children. For skewed distributions, it may be possible to transform the variables to normality. The most common transformation is the log transform, which may convert upwardly skewed data to normality. Other transforms are suitable for downwardly skewed data (e.g. squaring, cubing). Figure 27.4 shows that a log transformation corrects the skew in the distribution of weight.

The average and spread of a normal distribution are given by the mean and standard deviation (SD). In our example, the SD of the final height *z*-scores of the 33 SN children receiving active treatment is 0.51. Whatever the mean and SD of a particular set of normally distributed data, approximately 95% of the data values will lie within an interval ±2 SD either side of the mean. For example, most of the height *z*-scores in the treated group lie within the range ($-1.82 \pm 2(0.51)$) = ($-2.84$,

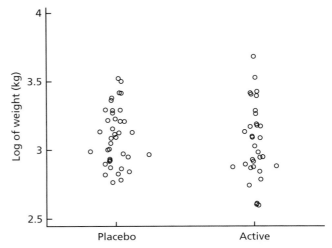

**Fig. 27.4.** Transformed weight according to treatment group.

−0.80). It is not uncommon for published data to be inappropriately summarized using the mean and standard deviation. A simple check is to calculate the approximate 95% range (mean ± 2 SD) to see whether this interval is feasible. Impossible values at either end of the interval suggest that the data are skewed. For example, in summarizing the weights of the treated group, a mean (SD) of 22.09 (6.37) kg suggests the data are skewed, as the 95% range will be from 9.35 to 34.83 kg and this lower limit, although positive, is clearly well below the lowest sampled weights. In this instance, the median and interquartile range are more appropriate summaries of the data. Alternatively, the mean and standard deviation of the log-transformed data can be calculated and used to create limits that can then be back-transformed.

## Statistical analyses

Statistical analyses enable inferences to be made from samples to populations. For example, in our hypothetical study of a growth promoter in SN children, from our sample we aim to make statements about the manner in which the whole population of SN children would respond to the same drug. This inference is only valid if the sample is randomly selected from, and representative of, the population.

## Standard error

The standard error (SE) is a measure of how precisely the sample approximates the population value. Smaller values of SE denote a more precise approximation and the SE decreases as the sample size increases. For continuous data it is calculated from the sample SD and the size of the sample ($n$) as follows: $SE = SD/\sqrt{n}$, which will be larger for measurements with greater variability (larger SD) and for smaller sample sizes (smaller $n$). The SD describes the *spread* of the actual values, whereas the SE relates to the *precision* with which the sample statistic approximates the population parameter. Hence, increasing the sample size will always reduce the SE and increase the precision with which parameters are estimated. The standard error for final height $z$-scores for the treated group of 33 SN children is $0.51/\sqrt{33} = 0.09$.

## Confidence intervals

Confidence intervals are constructed using the SE to give a range within which we expect the population value or difference to lie. The 95% confidence interval, constructed as (sample estimate ±1.96 SE) will contain the population value on 95% of occasions. The 99% confidence interval (sample estimate ±2.58 SE) will do so on 99% of occasions. The 99% interval is wider than the 95% interval, and we are more confident that it will contain the population value. For example, we are 95% confident that the mean population final $z$-score among

treated children lies in the interval $[-1.82 \pm 1.96(0.09)]$ = $(-2.00, -1.64)$ and 99% confident that it is between −2.05 and −1.59.

## Statistical significance

A *statistical significance* or *hypothesis* test measures the strength of evidence that the data sample supplies for or against some proposition of interest. This proposition is known as a *null hypothesis* because it usually relates to there being 'no difference' between groups or 'no effect' of treatment. There are many different kinds of significance tests and they have different names, but they all follow the same format. It is important to remember that the tests do not give a clear yes or no answer to the research question, rather they give the probability of obtaining the sample data if the null hypothesis were true. This probability is known as the *P*-value and takes values between 0 and 1. For example, a *P*-value of 0.001 means that a sample estimate as extreme would occur with a probability of 0.001 or 0.1% of the time (or 1 time in 1000) if the null hypothesis were true. A *P*-value this small thus indicates a very rare occurrence, it is unlikely that the null hypothesis is true. Note that it is unlikely but not impossible. Conversely, a *P*-value of 0.65 means that a sample estimate as extreme would occur with a probability of 0.65 or 65% of the time (or more than 1 time in 2) if the null hypothesis were true. Hence, in this case the samples are entirely compatible with the null hypothesis being true. Note that the null hypothesis is not proven, it is merely shown that this set of data is compatible with it.

Sometimes *P*-values above a certain value (usually 0.05) are called *non-significant*. It is not good practice to dichotomize probabilities in this way; the conclusions drawn from a study should be similar whether *P* = 0.049 or *P* = 0.051 as this is only a small change in probability. Exact *P*-values should always be given.

### Choosing a significance test to use

The specific significance test to use in a given situation depends on the number of groups being compared and the form of the outcome measurements. Some tests make the assumption that the outcome variable follows a defined distribution, usually the normal distribution, these are called *parametric* tests. Other tests make no distributional assumptions and these are called *non-parametric* [28,29]. The choice between parametric and non-parametric tests will depend on the plausibility of the assumptions necessary for the application of parametric tests [30].

#### *Comparing two groups with no confounders*
The decision tree in Fig. 27.5 shows which test to use to compare the outcomes from two groups, assuming that there are no confounding factors. The test to use depends on whether

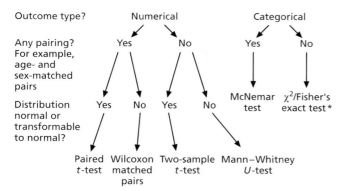

**Fig. 27.5.** A decision tree for selecting the correct statistical test for comparison of means of two group. *Fisher's exact test is appropriate if there are small numbers in some of the categories or groups being compared.

the outcome is numeric or categorical, paired or unpaired and whether values are normally distributed or not.

### Comparing more than two groups, controlling for confounders

Regression analyses are used to study the interrelationships between several variables and these are ideal for investigating differences in group outcomes while accounting for confounders. They are also appropriate for comparing outcomes between more than two groups. The type of regression to use will depend on the form of the outcome and predictors.

### Multiple linear regression

Multiple linear regression [31] is the most common and is appropriate where there is a single continuous numeric outcome. For example, Fig. 27.3 indicated that the treated children tended to have taller parents and it is therefore not surprising that they had on average higher final height z-scores than the placebo group, irrespective of any treatment effect that there may be. To investigate the effect of treatment on final height z-score while accounting for differences in midparental heights, a multiple linear regression model would be appropriate.

### Logistic regression

Logistic regression [32,33] is used when the outcome is a single proportion. For example, the proportion of children who had problems adhering to treatment.

If there are multiple observations per individual, for example outcomes assessed at 2, 4, 8 and 24 h after intervention, then an analysis of serial measurements [34,35], repeat measures analysis of variance or multilevel modelling [36,37] will be necessary.

The principles of deciding on which variables to include as predictors and the interpretation of the fitted model are the same whatever the form of the regression model. It may be necessary to incorporate interaction terms. For example,

an interaction between midparental height z-score and treatment group would be used to investigate whether the effect of treatment differs according to midparental height z-score. Multiple regression techniques are sometimes used to identify patterns of association between many variables. This sort of data dredging may lead to spurious associations and an overfitting of the data. A general rule of thumb is not to investigate more variables than the square root of the sample size. For example, with a sample of size 40 not more than six explanatory variables should be investigated [38].

### Examples

**1** In our hypothetical example, height z-score and weight are both numeric outcomes and there is no pairing between the children allocated to treatment and to control. The height z-scores are approximately normally distributed and hence the two-sample t-test is appropriate for comparing the mean values (Fig. 27.5). The mean (SD) final height z-score of the 39 children allocated to the placebo is –2.09 (0.54) compared with –1.82 (0.51) in the 33 children receiving the active drug. Applying the two-sample t-test gives a P-value of 0.032. So the treated children achieved a final height z-score that was on average 0.27 higher than the placebo group and this difference was significant. The 95% confidence interval for the difference is (0.02, 0.52), showing that although the difference is statistically significant the difference may be as small as 0.02 or as large as 0.52 z-score units. Even the upper limit of this confidence interval (0.52, roughly half of one standard deviation on standardized scale or approximately 3 cm) is not large in clinical terms and may not be a large enough difference to warrant uniform acceptance of the growth promoter concerned.

Using multiple linear regression to adjust for differences in midparental height, the treated group had final z-scores that were on average 0.16 (–0.03, 0.37) higher than the children who received placebo (P = 0.098). Hence, after adjusting for midparental height the difference is non-significant, although the results are compatible with an average increase in z-score as a result of treatment of 0.37 (the upper 95% confidence limit).

In this model the difference between the groups, after adjustment, was assumed to be the same (0.16) at any given midparental height. This could be visualized as two parallel lines, a distance 0.16 apart, superimposed on Fig. 27.3. Addition of interaction can be visualized as two non-parallel lines superimposed on Fig. 27.3. In this dataset the interaction term is non-significant (P = 0.79).

The weights are not normally distributed but can be transformed to be so, and hence the two-sample t-test is also appropriate for comparing the average weights between groups (Fig. 27.5). The test is performed on the log-transformed data. A P-value of 0.67 is obtained and hence there is no evidence of a difference in weight between the groups. The average

(95% confidence interval) for the difference on the logged scale is 0.096 (−0.35, 0.54). When back-transformed, by taking antilogs of the values, this shows that the weight of the children given placebo was on average 1.10 (0.7, 1.72) times heavier than the treated children.

2 Problems adhering to the treatment regimen is a binary outcome (i.e. categorical). There is no pairing between the children in the treated and placebo groups and hence a $\chi^2$ or Fisher's exact test is appropriate (Fig. 27.5). As there are more than 20 in each category (problems yes/no and treatment/control), the $\chi^2$ test will be used. A *P*-value of <0.0005 is obtained, the group receiving the treatment was significantly more likely to report adherence problems than the group receiving placebo (69.7% vs. 23.1%). The difference (95% confidence interval) is 46.6 (26.1, 67.2%). Another way of expressing these results is as the number needed to treat (NNT) [39]. For every two children [95% confidence interval (1, 4)] treated with the growth promoter, one additional child reported problems with adherence.

## Incomplete participation

There are several levels at which an individual may fail to complete a trial. Initially, they may refuse to consent to the study. Individuals who decline to participate in a study may well be different from those who agree to take part, and because of this bias the study results may not be generally applicable. It is important that as much information as possible is recorded about non-participants, so that the extent of any bias may be quantified. For example, those refusing to take part may be less severely ill or older. In some instances it may not be possible to collect demographic information on refusers. As a minimum, the number of individuals approached who refuse should be recorded and reported alongside the trial results and where possible reasons for refusal should be stated.

Sometimes individuals agree to participate in a study and drop out at a later stage. These individuals may similarly be a biased subset of those originally consenting. Comparison should be made on available demographic information and where possible the outcomes compared on an *intention-to-treat* basis. That is, they should be compared according to the groups to which they were originally allocated, irrespective of whether they completed the course of 'treatment'.

## Meta-analyses

Several studies may have independently addressed the same research question, perhaps in different hospitals or countries. Meta-analysis is the process of combining the estimates of effect obtained from these studies to obtain a single overall estimate [40].

## Adverse events

These form a very important part of any CT. Although one major outcome of a CT may be an evaluation of efficacy of a new treatment, the assessment of safety is always as important. The accepted way of determining safety is the careful recording of adverse events. These are defined as *any* negative event that occurs during the study period, whether the investigator considers them to be related to the treatment or not. The frequency of occurrence of these events can be compared between the test and control groups. Much thought is needed when defining what events are identified for recording. For example, considering pyrexia, sore throat, headache and coryza separately means that a common cold could be recorded as four separate events!

When reporting the numbers of adverse events it should be remembered that this is a sample estimate and as such is subject to sampling variability. Numbers should be reported with confidence intervals to show the possible imprecision of this estimate. For example, suppose there were no serious side-effects among the 33 children given the new growth promoter, this does not mean that it is safe and that in wider use nobody would suffer a serious side-effect. A 95% confidence interval for the percentage of the population who would suffer serious effects after being given the new drug is (0, 10.6%), i.e. up to as many as 1 in 10 [41].

## Data monitoring board

Usually a feature of large, particularly multicentre CTs, the data monitoring board (DMB) has a very important role. In its usual form it is a group with appropriate expertise who have access to the CT data as it is collected (or more usually at predetermined intervals) and who have knowledge of the randomization codes. The DMB is principally there to ensure that a CT does not continue when it has clearly demonstrated a statistically significant advantage of one or other drug or an unacceptable number of adverse events have occurred. Clearly, the members of the DMB must have no vested interest in the outcome of the CT, and clinician members should not be clinically responsible for patients in the study. Typical membership of a DMB would be a statistician, a clinician with knowledge of the medical condition being treated, a pharmacist and in some circumstances a medical ethicist.

## Practical and ethical issues

Most practical problems associated with CTs in paediatric endocrinology are essentially same as in other paediatric specialities. Particular issues arise with those studies that involve disorders that have outcomes measured over a considerable time. For example, in a study of diabetes the outcome of interest may be the incidence of late-onset complications such as retinopathy; in growth disorders we are often interested in final height as the outcome variable. In both cases this requires a very prolonged study, possibly of 10 or more years. Recruitment and retention of both active and control participants may become a problem. There may also be ethical objections to long-term use of placebo. In growth studies, many investigators compromise by abandoning any control group and comparing outcome to predicted adult height based on pretreatment variables. This is undesirable because of dependency on the reliability of the prediction methods, which even in the best hands are problematic. At the very best, it is likely that considerable power is lost compared with a classic parallel randomized CT.

Ethical considerations start with trial design. A poorly designed study that cannot answer the research question (e.g. through inadequate power) is unethical and as such is unacceptable. Assuming, however, that proper attention has been paid to the design aspects, there can still be ethical difficulties. In CTs, these most commonly centre on randomization and blinding. As with all clinical research, signed informed consent is a central plank of good clinical practice, but has no particular issues in a CT other than to recognize that the consent must include the process of randomization. It must not take place after a covert randomization has determined that the patient is to receive the test substance. The importance of randomization and blinding do not strictly raise any ethical problems, but they can be difficult for families to understand unless full information in appropriate language is provided. Well-worded information materials can resolve most of these difficulties [42].

Another problem related to consent can arise in long CTs in childhood. At recruitment consideration must be given to who should give consent. This may differ between countries, but in many if the child is judged able to understand the implications of the CT then he or she should give consent. This requires a judgement on the part of the researcher. This is relatively straightforward, but becomes more complicated in long studies when the child may move from inability to judge consent to sufficient maturity to have a valid opinion. As long as that agrees with the original view of the parent or guardian there is not a problem. However, if the child later takes an opposite view then an ethical issue arises. This problem is likely to become a more common issue in the future.

## References

1 Senn S. *Cross-over Trials in Clinical Research*. Chichester: John Wiley and Sons, 1993.

2 Jones B, Kenward MG. *Design and Analysis of Cross-over Trials*. London: Chapman & Hall, 1989.

3 Chalmers I, Altman DG. *Systematic Reviews*. London: BMJ Publishing Group, 1995.

4 NHS Centre for Reviews and Dissemination. *Undertaking Systematic Reviews of Research on Effectiveness. (CRD 4)*. York: University of York, 1996.

5 Britton A, McPherson K, McKee M, Sanderson C, Black N, Bain C. Choosing between randomised and non-randomised studies: a systematic review. *Health Technol Assess* 1998; 2: 1–124.

6 Farrell B. Efficient management of randomised controlled trials: nature or nurture. *Br Med J* 1998; 317: 1236–9.

7 Treasure T, MacRae KD. Minimisation: the platinum standard for trials? *Br Med J* 1998; 317: 362–3.

8 Hauck WW, Gilliss CL, Donner A, Gortner S. Randomization by cluster. *Nursing Res* 1991; 40: 356–8.

9 Kerry SM, Bland JM. The intracluster correlation coefficient in cluster randomisation. *Br Med J* 1998; 316: 1455.

10 Collett D. *Modelling Survival Data in Medical Research*. London: Chapman & Hall, 1994.

11 Senn S. *Statistical Issues in Drug Development*. Chichester: John Wiley and Sons, 1997.

12 Johnston K, Buxton M, Jones D, Fitzpatrick R. Assessing the costs of healthcare technologies in clinical trials. *Health Technol Assess* 1999; 3: 1–76.

13 Cameron N. *The Measurement of Human Growth*. London: Croom Helm, 1984.

14 Brennan P, Silman A. Statistical methods for assessing observer variability in clinical measures. *Br Med J* 1992; 304: 1491–4.

15 Streiner DL, Norman GR. *Health Measurement Scales. A Practical Guide to Their Development and Use*, 2nd edn. Oxford: Oxford University Press, 1995.

16 Day SJ, Graham DF. Sample size estimation for comparing two or more treatment groups in clinical trials. *Stat Med* 1991; 10: 33–43.

17 Cohen J. *Statistical Power Analysis for the Behavioural Sciences*, revised edn. New Jersey: Lawrence Erlbaum Associates, 1977.

18 Hsieh FY, Bloch DA, Larsen MD. A simple method of sample size calculation for linear and logistic regression. *Stat Med* 1998; 17: 1623–34.

19 Campbell MJ, Julious SA, Altman DG. Estimating sample sizes for binary, ordered categorical, and continuous outcomes in two group comparisons. *Br Med J* 1995; 311: 1145–8.

20 Julious SA, Campbell MJ. Sample size calculations for paired or matched ordinal data. *Stat Med* 1998; 17: 1635–42.

21 Machin D, Campbell MJ. *Statistical Tables for the Design of Clinical Trials*. Oxford: Blackwell Scientific Publications, 1987.

22 Donner A, Eliasziw M. Sample size requirements for reliability studies. *Stat Med* 1987; 6: 441–8.

23 Hsieh FY. Sample size tables for logistic regression. *Stat Med* 1989; 8: 795–802.

24 Jones B, Jarvis P, Lewis JA, Ebbutt AF. Trials to assess equivalence: the importance of rigorous methods. *Br Med J* 1996; 313: 36–9.

25 Savitz DA, Olshan AF. Multiple comparisons and related issues in the interpretation of epidemiological data. *Am J Epidemiol* 1995; 142: 904–8.

26 Rothman KJ. No adjustments are needed for multiple comparisons. *Epidemiology* 1990; 1: 43–6.

27 Pocock SJ. *Clinical Trials*. Chichester: John Wiley and Sons, 1983.

28 Sprent P. *Applied Nonparametric Statistical Methods*, 2nd edn. London: Chapman & Hall, 1993.

29 Conover WJ. *Practical Nonparametric Statistics*, 2nd edn. New York: John Wiley and Sons Inc., 1980.

30 Bland M. *An Introduction to Medical Statistics*. Oxford: Oxford University Press, 1987.

31 Armitage P, Berry G. *Statistical Methods in Medical Research*, 2nd edn. Oxford: Blackwell Scientific Publications, 1987.

32 Collett D. *Modelling Binary Data*. London: Chapman & Hall, 1991.

33 Hosmer DW Jr, Lemeshow S. *Applied Logistic Regression*. New York: John Wiley and Sons, Inc., 1989.

34 Matthews JNS, Altman DG, Campbell MJ, Royston P. Analysis of serial measurements in medical research. *Br Med J* 1990; 300: 230–5.

35 Matthews JNS. A refinement to the analysis of serial data using summary measures. *Stat Med* 1993; 12: 27–37.

36 Sullivan LM, Dukes KA, Losina E. Tutorial in biostatistics. An introduction to hierachical linear modelling. *Stat Med* 1999; 18: 855–88.

37 Crowder MJ, Hand DJ. *Analysis of Repeated Measures*. London: Chapman & Hall, 1990.

38 Altman DG. *Practical Statistics for Medical Research*. London: Chapman & Hall, 1991.

39 Altman DG, Andersen PK. Calculating the number needed to treat for trials where the outcome is time to an event. *Br Med J* 1999; 319: 1492–5.

40 Greenland S. Meta-analysis. In: Rothman KJ, Greenland S, eds. *Modern Epidemiology*. Philadelphia: Lippincott-Raven, 1998: 643–73.

41 Lentner C. *Geigy Scientific Tables*, 8th edn. 1982.

42 Edwards SJL, Lilford RJ, Braunholtz DA, Jackson JC, Hewison J, Thornton J. Ethical issues in the design and conduct of randomised controlled trials. *Health Technol Assess* 1998; 2: 1–146.

## Further reading

Gardner MJ, Altman DG. *Statistics with Confidence*. London: BMJ Publishing, 1989.

Kirkwood BR. *Essentials of Medical Statistics*. Oxford: Blackwell Scientific Publications, 1988.

Glantz SA. *Primer of Biostatistics*, 4th edn. New York: McGraw-Hill, 1997.

Schwartz D, Flamant R, Lellouch J. *Clinical Trials*. English Language edition. London: Academic Press, 1980.

# 28 Tests in paediatric endocrinology and normal values

## M. T. Dattani

## Introduction

The practice of paediatric endocrinology is heavily based upon measurement of hormones. The secretion of a number of them is pulsatile, e.g. growth hormone (GH), follicle-stimulating hormone (FSH) and luteinizing hormone (LH). The secretion of cortisol follows a diurnal rhythm. In addition, the existence of feedback loops, such as the hypothalamo-pituitary-somatotroph axis, can complicate the interpretation of hormone measurements. Hence, a single random measurement may not be informative, and dynamic tests of endocrine function using a variety of provocative agents are widely used. The tests may be complicated in terms of both their performance and their interpretation, and they may be considered hazardous under certain circumstances.

As the aim of paediatric endocrinology is to derive the maximum amount of information from the minimum number of investigations performed with the least amount of discomfort to the child, the tests should be carefully chosen and planned.

## General principles for all endocrine tests

### Patient preparation

1 Is the planned test the most appropriate investigation to be performed given the clinical picture? Are there other tests that should be performed first to exclude other causes for the problem (e.g. urea and electrolytes to exclude chronic renal failure and thyroid function tests to exclude hypothyroidism) in children with short stature?
2 Are the medical and nursing staff on the ward familiar with the protocol for the test?
3 Are the laboratory staff aware of the test and the need for urgent processing or analysis of the samples?
4 Has the parent/guardian been fully informed of the procedure to be performed, including the need to fast, etc.?

5 Is the child adequately prepared (e.g. appropriately fasted)? Is the child clinically well? Are there confounding factors or contraindications to performing the test?
6 Has the height and weight of the child been measured on the day of the test in order to calculate drug doses, etc.? Surface area is calculated from the formula:

$$\text{surface area (m}^2) = \text{square root of [height(cm)} \times \text{weight (kg)]} \div 3600.$$

7 Has the dose of the stimulatory/suppressive agent been correctly calculated and has another member of staff checked the dose? Has the agent been correctly prepared and checked by another member of staff?

## Sample collection

### Blood

1 Secure a reliable intravenous line for serial blood sampling and maintain patent with a heparin/saline solution (1 U/mL).
2 Collect basal samples, including a sample taken at the time of intravenous insertion [time $(T) = -60$ or $-30$ min]. These are crucial as the stress generated by cannulation may be adequate to stimulate hormone production, after which there may be a period during which the gland is refractory to stimulation, giving rise to false-positive results if samples are taken only from $T = 0$.
3 Are correct sample tubes available and labelled with times and patient details? These should include patient name, ward/clinic, hospital number, date of sample and time into test of sample, e.g. 0, 30 and 60 min. Occasionally, clock time should be recorded (e.g. for serum cortisol measurement).
4 Are the blood volumes required known?
5 Laboratory request forms: legibly record patient name, age, sex, ward/clinic, hospital number, date of test, time of samples, tests requested and clinical details stating indications for tests.

## Urine

1 Ensure that the child and parents understand how to collect a timed (usually overnight or 24 h) urine sample. Written instructions may help.
2 Ensure that the child and parents are supplied with an appropriate container.
3 Ensure that the container is appropriately labelled.
4 Laboratory request forms: as before.

# The adrenal axis

## Synacthen test

Cortisol deficiency may be primary or secondary to ACTH deficiency. The plasma cortisol response to hypoglycaemia [in the insulin tolerance test (ITT)] is a good test of adrenal function and the only test of adrenal function validated against the response to surgical stress [1]. It tests the integrity of the entire hypothalamo-pituitary-adrenal axis. The Synacthen test assesses the response of the adrenal gland to exogenous adrenocorticotrophin (ACTH) and is a test of adrenal, and not pituitary, function. Nevertheless, the standard Synacthen test is often used to assess the hypothalamo-pituitary axis [2] but can give rise to results which are discrepant from the insulin-stress test [3]. Synacthen is a synthetic ACTH analogue that is as active biologically but is less antigenic and therefore safer, although allergic reactions have been reported.

### Indications
1 Suspected adrenal insufficiency.
2 Suspected congenital adrenal hyperplasia (CAH).
3 Determination of heterozygous state in CAH.
4 Investigation of premature adrenarche.

### Standard short Synacthen test

*Background*
The test entails stimulation of the adrenal glands by high doses of ACTH (1–24) administered either intravenously (i.v.) or intramuscularly (i.m.), which result in a massive output of cortisol and other adrenal steroids. The dose represents an entire day's pituitary output of ACTH and is excessive and only of value in assessing severe adrenal insufficiency. The standard short Synacthen test has proved insensitive to minor degrees of adrenal suppression, for example in children with asthma on inhaled steroid. The 30-min sample has been standardized against the ITT.

*Patient preparation*
Fasting is not required. All steroid therapy (other than dexamethasone or betamethasone) interferes with the assay of cortisol. Hydrocortisone should have been stopped for at least 12 h before the test. Prednisolone (10% cross-reactivity with cortisol) or other interfering therapy should have been stopped for at least 3 days. Steroid cover can be provided by dexamethasone if necessary, as replacement doses do not interfere significantly with the adrenal response to Synacthen.

*Methodology*
1 A cannula should be inserted at least 1 h before the test, which should be performed ideally at 09.00 h. A morning dose of hydrocortisone should be omitted (i.e. the last dose should have been administered 12 h before the test).
2 Synacthen dose: 62.5 μg < 6 months old, 125 μg 6–24 months old, 250 μg > 2 years old. Doses are administered i.m. or i.v. (dilute in 2 mL of normal saline and give slowly over 2 min). Anaphylaxis has been reported but is rare.
3 Plasma cortisol should be measured at 0 and 30 min. If required (e.g. if Addison disease is suspected), plasma ACTH should be measured at the start of the test (state time of day).
4 In congenital adrenal hyperplasia, plasma 17-hydroxyprogesterone concentrations should be measured in addition to cortisol at 0 and 30 min.

*Interpretation of results*
1 Peak plasma cortisol concentration should be greater than 550 nmol/L or the increment greater than 200 nmol/L. An impaired response does not distinguish between adrenal and pituitary failure, as the adrenal glands may be atrophied secondary to ACTH deficiency. A long Synacthen test may then be required, although the ACTH concentration is very high in adrenal failure and may be diagnostic.
2 Patients with pituitary-dependent cortisol insufficiency require dynamic testing of the pituitary gland.
3 In congenital adrenal hyperplasia due to 21-hydroxylase deficiency, the cortisol response may be diminished or normal but the 17-hydroxyprogesterone response is exaggerated with a peak > 20 nmol/L. In heterozygotes, the peak 17-hydroxyprogesterone concentration is 10–20 nmol/L. A normal response is characterized by a peak 17-hydroxyprogesterone response of < 10 nmol/L.
4 In patients who have been on long-term steroid therapy, adrenal function is suppressed and the adrenals may be atrophied. The glands may not be stimulated during the short Synacthen test or they may be stimulated only partially.

## Modified (physiological) Synacthen test

*Background*
The standard Synacthen test will not detect subtle degrees of adrenal impairment. Constructing a dose–response curve for ACTH (1–24) in terms of the rise in plasma cortisol therefore developed a modified test. A dose of only 500 ng of ACTH per 1.73 m$^2$ body surface area gave an identical rise in plasma

cortisol over the first 20 min after intravenous injection compared with the standard dose of 250 µg [4,5]. This very low dose of ACTH is now used in an attempt to detect more subtle changes in adrenal function. The modified Synacthen test should be performed in the afternoon (see below). The test was developed with the dose of ACTH given at 14.00 h, when endogenous secretion is at its lowest. The results will not be valid if the dose is given at another time. The low-dose Synacthen test has been reported to give greater concordance with the insulin stress test than the standard Synacthen test does [6,7].

*Methodology*

**1** An in-dwelling cannula must be inserted at least 3 h before the test to minimize fluctuations in basal serum cortisol.
**2** Light lunch at 12.00 h.
**3** Bed rest from lunch until the end of the test.
**4** Add 250 µg of Synacthen to 1.0 L of 0.9% saline and shake vigorously. The resulting solution has a concentration of ACTH (1–24) 250 ng/mL. The formula for calculation of the dose that needs to be standardized for body surface area is: dose (mL) = 2 × surface area/1.73.
**5** Collect 1.0 mL of blood at 14.00 h for basal sample.
**6** Give 500 ng of ACTH (1–24) per 1.73 m$^2$ as an i.v. bolus after collecting basal sample.
**7** Collect blood for cortisol measurement at 5-min intervals from +10 to +45 min, i.e. at 0, 10, 15, 20, 25, 30, 35, 40, 45 min.

*Interpretation*

In normal individuals, a peak cortisol of > 550 nmol/L or a cortisol rise > 200 nmol/L above baseline should be expected. In children with asthma who are being treated with inhaled corticosteroids or in children receiving steroids for other conditions the response will be blunted.

## Prolonged Synacthen test

*Background*

This test is required if the cortisol response to the standard Synacthen test is suboptimal and secondary adrenal insufficiency is suspected, with atrophy of the adrenals secondary to hypothalamo-pituitary pathology. Adrenal steroid output is stimulated in patients with secondary adrenal insufficiency if large doses of ACTH are given successively over 3 days to overcome adrenal atrophy.

*Methodology*

**1** Collect basal sample for plasma cortisol at 09.00 h on day 1.
**2** Give Synacthen depot (tetracosactrin acetate) at 09.00 h for 3 days (days 1, 2 and 3). Dose: < 6 months, 250 µg i.m. daily; 6–24 months, 500 µg i.m. daily; > 2 years age, 1 mg i.m. daily.
**3** Collect blood for plasma cortisol 4–6 h after the last injection on day 3.

*Interpretation of test*

**1** Plasma cortisol should rise more than threefold or by > 200 nmol/L in normal individuals and the post-Synacthen concentration should be > 550 nmol/L.
**2** In secondary adrenal insufficiency and in patients on long-term steroid therapy, the cortisol concentration increases, showing stimulation of the adrenal glands by successive doses of Synacthen.
**3** An absent cortisol response is highly suggestive of primary adrenal insufficiency.

## Hydrocortisone day curve

### Indications

This is to establish the adequacy of hydrocortisone replacement dose. Studies in adult patients have demonstrated that overtreatment may lead to a reduction in serum osteocalcin [8], with the potential of osteoporosis. In addition, in children who are cortisol deficient after the treatment of a craniopharyngioma and who have subsequently been treated with a twice-daily hydrocortisone regimen, plasma cortisol concentrations were found to be low before the morning dose of hydrocortisone, during the afternoon and before the evening dose [9]. Studies in adults have suggested that thrice-daily regimens of hydrocortisone may be more appropriate than twice-daily regimens [10]. Hence the measurement of plasma cortisol may be helpful in patients on hydrocortisone replacement. The test is often performed in children with congenital adrenal hyperplasia when the plasma 17-hydroxyprogesterone concentrations are also measured.

*Patient preparation/precautions*

Do not administer the a.m. dose of hydrocortisone until the first sample has been taken (see below). Insert an intravenous cannula at 08.00–08.30 h. There is no point in doing the test if the child is on dexamethasone or prednisolone.

*Methodology*

Plasma cortisol concentrations are measured whilst the patient is on a maintenance dose of hydrocortisone. The test is commenced at 09.00 h (time 0).

Plasma cortisol (+ 17-hydroxyprogesterone in CAH) to be measured at:
$T = 0$ (all times refer to after the first dose of hydrocortisone)
→ Morning dose of hydrocortisone
60 min
→ Breakfast
90 min
120 min
4 h
→ Lunch-time dose of hydrocortisone (not applicable if only on BD regimen).
6 h
9 h

→ Evening dose of hydrocortisone

9.5 h

10 h

10.5 h

These times are chosen so that the peak concentrations of cortisol following a dose of hydrocortisone can be documented.

*Interpretation*

The aim is to achieve adequate concentrations of cortisol throughout the day, avoiding excessive peaks after each dose. The trough concentrations before each dose should not be > 100 nmol/L.

## Urinary steroid profile

### Indications

A urinary steroid profile is used to examine adrenal function. Many steroid metabolites are measured, which enables identification of all steroids and definition of a biochemical defect. A 24-h urinary steroid profile quantifies steroid excretion rates and can be used to define the secretory nature of adrenal and gonadal tumours. It can be used to aid in the diagnosis of children with ambiguous genitalia, precocious puberty, premature adrenarche, abnormal virilization and salt-losing states. It assists the differential diagnosis of Cushing syndrome, hypertension and adrenal suppression (e.g. in asthma). In neonates, the test is useful only after day 3 of life (because of potential interference by placental steroids). In older children with possible congenital adrenal hyperplasia, a Synacthen test may need to be performed to stimulate the adrenal glands maximally and achieve a diagnosis by collection of a post-Synacthen urine specimen. In older children (e.g. with suspected 5α-reductase deficiency), the ratio of 5-α to 5-β metabolites can be measured in the urine, usually after androgen secretion has been stimulated by human chorionic gonadotrophin (hCG).

*Patient preparation/precautions*

None.

*Methodology*

1  For careful quantification of urinary steroid excretion rates, a 24-h urinary steroid profile. This may be difficult in some cases (e.g. neonates), when at least 20 mL of urine should be collected in a plain tube for qualitative analysis. For cortisol measurement, a 24-h urine sample is vital.

2  The form must give full justification for the test and the following information is vital: date of birth, age, height and weight, for calculation of body surface area, and the names of concurrent medication.

*Interpretation*

1  Congenital adrenal hyperplasia
  • 21-hydroxylase deficiency—excess of 17-hydroxyprogesterone metabolites (pregnanetriol and pregnanetriolone);

  • 11β-hydroxylase deficiency—excess of 11-deoxycortisol/deoxycorticosterone metabolites;
  • 3β-hydroxysteroid dehydrogenase deficiency—excess of dehydroepiandrosterone (DHEA) and pregnenolone;
  • 17α-hydroxylase deficiency—excess of progesterone and corticosterone metabolites (not seen in neonates);
  • LIPOID adrenal hyperplasia—no steroids in urinary steroid profile.

2  Tumours of the adrenal gland show an excess of adrenal androgens and/or cortisol.

3  Defects in testosterone biosynthesis or action:
  • 5α-reductase deficiency—elevated 5β:5α ratio;
  • androgen insensitivity syndromes: elevated androgen metabolites (not usually required);
  • 17-ketosteroid reductase deficiency—high androsterone to aetiocholanolone.

4  Adrenarche (due to early differentiation of zona reticularis)—high androgen and cortisol output for age and body size.

5  Hypertension:
  • congenital adrenal hyperplasia—11β-hydroxylase deficiency, 17α-hydroxylase deficiency;
  • 11β-hydroxysteroid dehydrogenase deficiency—high ratio of cortisol to cortisone metabolites;
  • dexamethasone-suppressible hyperaldosteronism—high excretion of 18-hydroxycortisol;
  • glucocorticoid resistance—high androgens and cortisol metabolites.

6  Defects of aldosterone synthesis or action:
  • aldosterone biosynthetic defects:
    – 18-hydroxylase deficiency—high concentrations of corticosterone;
    – 18-oxidation defects—high concentration of 18 hydroxycorticosterone with low plasma aldosterone concentrations;
  • defects of aldosterone action—high aldosterone and 18-hydroxycorticosterone concentrations.

## Investigation of Cushing syndrome

The diagnosis of Cushing syndrome can be difficult to establish and needs a meticulously planned protocol [11,12]. The investigation should be a two-step process. First, the diagnosis of Cushing syndrome needs to be established and then the aetiology.

### Initial investigations

These include a full blood count, urea/electrolytes, circadian (midnight and 08.00 h) plasma cortisol and plasma ACTH measurements, and a 24-h urinary free cortisol concentration. Measurement of plasma cortisol concentrations at 20-min intervals over a 3-h period (06.00–09.00 h and 22.00–01.00 h) may be indicated.

## Overnight dexamethasone suppression test

### Indications

This is a screening test [13] and is especially useful in:

1 the child with simple obesity in whom Cushing syndrome is suspected, particularly if there is loss of diurnal variation in plasma cortisol concentrations;

2 distinguishing premature adrenarche from an adrenal tumour.

### Patient preparation

Ensure that the patient is not on steroid therapy and not suffering from major infection or psychological stress. Ideally, the child should be admitted overnight. Circadian plasma cortisols and baseline adrenal androgens, dehydro-epiandrosterone sulphate (DHEAS) and androstenedione, should have been previously documented but this test may be used as a first investigation.

### Methodology

1 Collect blood at 24.00 h for plasma cortisol and ACTH. Additional samples may be collected for estimation of plasma DHEAS, androstenedione and testosterone if an adrenal androgen-secreting tumour is suspected.

2 Give 0.3 mg/m$^2$ dexamethasone by mouth at 24.00 h. Dexamethasone is used as it is a potent synthetic steroid with a long half-life and does not significantly interfere with the laboratory estimations of cortisol.

3 Repeat blood samples at 08.00 h.

### Interpretation

1 In normal individuals, the plasma cortisol and ACTH concentrations at 08.00 h following the administration of dexamethasone should be suppressed (< 150 nmol/L).

2 Patients with Cushing syndrome will fail to suppress adequately, and a 48-h low-dose dexamethasone suppression test should be performed.

3 In a child with an adrenal androgen-secreting tumour, there will be a failure of suppression of adrenal androgens.

## Low-dose dexamethasone (LDD) suppression test

### Indication

Differentiation of hypersecretion of cortisol from obesity.

### Patient preparation/precautions

1 The patient should not be on steroid therapy. There should be a reasonable degree of suspicion of Cushing syndrome from preliminary investigations.

2 Enzyme-inducing drugs such as rifampicin and phenytoin can induce dexamethasone metabolism, giving rise to false-positive results.

3 Care should be taken in diabetes mellitus.

### Methodology

Dexamethasone 0.5 mg (children < 10 years 20 μg/kg/day) should be taken orally strictly 6 hourly. Plasma cortisol and ACTH concentrations (and DHEAS, androstenedione and testosterone if an adrenal tumour is suspected) should be measured at 08.00 h at 0, 24 and 48 h. A 24-h urine should be collected at the end of the test for measurement of free cortisol (and/or other steroids if an adrenal tumour is suspected).

### Interpretation

In normal individuals, plasma cortisol is in the normal resting (08.00 h) range (170–700 nmol/L) at LDD 0 and suppresses to < 50 nmol/L at LDD +48. Serum testosterone and other adrenal androgens will also decrease at LDD +48. Patients with Cushing syndrome lose their circadian cortisol rhythm and fail to suppress on the low-dose dexamethasone suppression test. However, very rarely, patients with Cushing syndrome may show normal suppression and, occasionally, the condition may be cyclical. Patients with androgen-secreting tumours or severe polycystic ovarian syndrome may also fail to suppress androgen secretion.

## High-dose dexamethasone suppression test

### Indication

The test is used to establish the aetiology of Cushing syndrome.

### Patient preparation/precautions

The patient should have had the above investigations, all of which should point to a diagnosis of Cushing syndrome, and should not be on any steroid therapy. The other preparations and precautions should be as for the low-dose dexamethasone suppression test.

### Methodology

This test may conveniently follow the low-dose dexamethasone suppression test. Dexamethasone 2.0 mg (children < 10 years 1 mg or 80 μg/kg/day) should be given orally 6 hourly. A 24-h urine collection for free cortisol estimation should be collected at the start of the test. Plasma cortisol and ACTH concentrations should be measured at 08.00 h on the first day and after completion of the test. Twenty-four-hour urinary free cortisol should be measured at the end of the test.

### Interpretation

Plasma cortisol classically suppresses to 50% or less of the basal value in pituitary-dependent Cushing disease but *not* in macronodular hyperplasia, adrenal tumours or ectopic ACTH secretion, where pituitary ACTH secretion is already suppressed and dexamethasone will have no further effect. However, 10–40% of patients with Cushing disease may fail to suppress whereas the occasional patient with ectopic ACTH syndrome does. In a study of patients with Cushing syndrome, 19 of 28 patients with pituitary adenomas (68%) had a decrease in urinary cortisol excretion greater than 90% below the mean baseline values. On the other hand, none of the patients with ectopic Cushing syndrome or bilateral micronodular adrenal hyperplasia suppressed [1]. The suppression is not immediate but appears progressively as the time/dose of dexamethasone continues. This is because the pituitary retains its ability to lower ACTH in response to the added steroid load. A paradoxical later rise in cortisol secretion may occur during the test. In adrenal-dependent or ectopic Cushing syndrome, the pituitary ACTH concentration is already suppressed, and dexamethasone will have no further effect. In patients with Cushing disease who fail to suppress their cortisol secretion to 8 mg of dexamethasone per day, a very high dose of dexamethasone (32 mg/day in adults) has been recommended and can improve the sensitivity of the test [14]. Lack of suppression to high-dose dexamethasone particularly occurs with Cushing disease secondary to corticotroph macroadenomas [15].

## Corticotrophin-releasing hormone test

*Indications*

**1** To evaluate the source of proven excessive ACTH secretion.
**2** Differential diagnosis of isolated ACTH deficiency.
The test evaluates the ACTH response to intravenous corticotrophin-releasing hormone (CRH) via the change in plasma cortisol.

*Patient preparation/precautions*

The patient should not be on steroid therapy. An in-dwelling cannula should be inserted at least 3 h before the test. The child should be fasted from midnight (6 h in children less than 2 years old).

CRH may cause mild facial flushing, marked transient hypotension and occasional allergy.

*Methodology*

Plasma cortisol and ACTH concentrations should be measured at –15 and 0 min before an intravenous injection of CRH-41 (1 µg/kg) at 09.00 h. Subsequently plasma cortisol and ACTH concentrations should be measured at +15, +30, +45, +60, +90, +120 min after CRH.

*Interpretation*

• Normal response: plasma cortisol rises to 430–820 nmol/L; plasma ACTH rises by < 35%.
• Cushing disease: normal/exaggerated response (10–15% may not respond); ACTH increases by > 35%.
• Ectopic ACTH: ACTH concentration is high but there is no response to CRH (the tumour has no CRH receptors and therefore cannot respond to CRH).
• Adrenal tumour: no response.

• ACTH deficiency: increase in ACTH suggests hypothalamic CRH deficiency; a flat ACTH response suggests pituitary ACTH deficiency.

The use of this test in combination with the high-dose dexamethasone test is said to give complete discrimination of Cushing syndrome using the criteria of either an exaggerated cortisol response to CRH-41 or a > 50% suppression of cortisol to high-dose dexamethasone. Using either test alone gives a false-negative rate of approximately 20% [16]. A variation of the test is the dexamethasone CRH test when the CRH test is performed 2 h after completion of low-dose dexamethasone suppression. This test has been shown to discriminate normal individuals from those with mild Cushing syndrome [17]. Other tests such as the desmopressin test are used on a research basis. Desmopressin stimulates ACTH release and can potentiate the action of CRH. In normal healthy individuals, it has been shown to have little or no effect on plasma cortisol or ACTH concentrations. However, in patients with Cushing disease, there may be an excessive rise in plasma ACTH and cortisol concentrations in response to desmopressin, an effect similar to that observed with the use of CRH.

## Assessment of mineralocorticoid secretion

*Background/indications*

The adrenal cortex is also concerned with normal sodium homeostasis. The zona glomerulosa secretes aldosterone, which is important for the retention of sodium and the excretion of potassium. These investigations are indicated when a patient presents with salt loss or in order to assess the control of a disease associated with salt loss, e.g. congenital adrenal hypo- or hyperplasia, isolated mineralocorticoid deficiency and Addison disease.

*Methodology*

Plasma sodium, potassium, magnesium, creatinine, bicarbonate and pH should be measured. Twenty-four-hour urinary sodium, potassium and creatinine excretion can be measured if the dietary intake is monitored. Ambulant and recumbent plasma aldosterone concentrations and renin activities should be measured. These tests should ideally be performed before and after a 3- to 5-day low-sodium diet (10–20 mmol/day).

*Interpretation*

In mineralocorticoid deficiency due to Addison disease, congenital adrenal hyperplasia or congenital adrenal hypoplasia, the plasma aldosterone concentration is low with an elevated plasma renin activity. After a low-sodium diet, there should be a reduction in urinary sodium excretion to less than 20 mmol/day with at least a threefold increase in plasma renin activity and aldosterone. If there is no reduction in plasma sodium, a trial of fludrocortisone should be given and sodium excretion reassessed. In Conn syndrome (primary hyperaldosteronism), persistent hypokalaemia, hyperkaluria and alkalosis are associated with an elevated aldosterone concentration and a suppressed plasma renin activity. Other investigations such as selective adrenal venous sampling and computerized tomography (CT) or magnetic resonance imaging (MRI) may be indicated.

## Assessment of adrenal medullary function

*Background/indications*
The adrenal medulla secretes the catecholamines noradrenaline and adrenaline. These may be elevated when a phaeochromocytoma is present.

*Methodology*
In suspected phaeochromocytoma cases, measurement of plasma adrenaline and noradrenaline concentrations is combined with the measurement of 24-h urinary excretion of total catecholamines, total metadrenaline and vanilyl mandelic acid (VMA). Radiological studies include ultrasound and CT and MRI of adrenals and [131]I-labelled metaiodobenzylguanidine (MIBG) scan.

*Interpretation*
Concentrations of catecholamines are elevated in phaeochromocytoma, and an MIBG scan may identify the tumour.

---

# Gonadal axis

## Three-day human chorionic gonadotrophin stimulation test

*Indication*
The test is performed in order to assess the secretion of testosterone by the testes in the following conditions: suspected anorchia, Leydig cell hypoplasia, testosterone biosynthetic defect, cryptorchidism, patients with ambiguous genitalia, suspected hermaphroditism, micropenis and delayed puberty.

*Methodology*
**1** Measure the basal plasma concentrations of serum testosterone and other androgens [DHEAS, androstenedione and dihydrotestosterone (DHT) if 5α-reductase deficiency is suspected]. Plasma gonadotrophins (LH and FSH) should be measured and the karyotype checked at the same time.
**2** hCG is given intramuscularly on a once-daily basis for 3 days at 24-h intervals.

*Dosage of hCG*
< 1 year: 500 units
1–10 years: 1000 units
> 10 years: 1500 units

The post-hCG plasma concentrations of testosterone and other steroids should be measured on day 4, 24 h after administration of the last hCG dose. Measurements of the pre- and post-concentrations should be performed in the same laboratory.

*Interpretation*
The hCG test indicates the presence of functional testicular tissue [19]. In normal individuals, the testosterone concentration increases two- to threefold. The magnitude of the increase may be lower in prepubertal children. If testicular function is poor, the increase is blunted. In children with cryptorchidism, a good testosterone response to hCG indicates the presence of testes sufficiently large for orchidopexy [19]. Studies have suggested that the test should be combined with a GnRH test to improve diagnostic accuracy when a diagnosis of hypogonadotrophic hypogonadism is being considered [20], but our data suggest that this is not so, as 29% of patients with hypogonadotrophic hypogonadism had a normal testosterone response to hCG (Al-Shaikh *et al.* unpublished data). In the absence of functioning testicular tissue, there is no increase in testosterone concentration. An absent response with elevated LH and FSH suggests primary testicular failure.

In normal individuals, under basal conditions the testosterone/DHT ratios are 2–3 in prepubertal patients [21] and 8–17 in adult patients [22]; and under stimulated conditions, 3–26 [23].

In 10 patients with 5α-reductase deficiency, the testosterone/DHT ratios have been reported as follows [24]: basal, 1–5 in prepubertal patients and 4–42 in pubertal patients; stimulated, 20–111.

Collection of 24-h urine samples before and after hCG for analysis of urinary steroid excretion is a useful supplementary test for the investigation of a defect in testosterone biosynthesis. Analysis of androgen receptors in genital skin fibroblasts and DNA analysis of the androgen receptor gene may also be informative in children in whom androgen resistance is suspected (raised basal concentration of testosterone and an exaggerated response to hCG), although an inadequate response does not exclude androgen insensitivity syndrome [25].

## Three-week hCG stimulation test

*Indication*
This is generally used in patients with bilateral cryptorchidism in whom either gonadotrophin deficiency or anorchia ('vanishing testes') are suspected. The test is usually combined with estimation of LH and FSH (with GnRH stimulation). The test may follow the 3-day hCG test (see below) and has two purposes.
**1** to detect the production of testosterone, as the effect of administering hCG over a 3-week period can prime the testes;

**2** to facilitate testicular descent and increase the size of the phallus in patients with a micropenis and undescended testes.

*Methodology*
**1** The size of the phallus should be recorded.
**2** Serum testosterone and other androgens as indicated (DHEAS, androstenedione and DHT) should be measured. Check plasma LH, FSH and karyotype if this has not been done.

*Dosage of HCG*
< 1 years  500 units twice weekly
1–10 years  1000 units twice weekly
> 10 years  1500 units twice weekly
**1** hCG is given by i.m. injections twice weekly (Monday/ Thursday or Tuesday/Friday) for 3 weeks.
**2** The patient should return for measurement of post-hCG serum testosterone and androgen concentrations 24 h after the last dose of hCG was administered.
**3** The size of the phallus and position of testes should be recorded.

*Interpretation*
As for the 3-day hCG test. When the child is seen on the day after the last hCG injection for the second blood test, he should be examined to ascertain whether there has been an increase in the size of the phallus or whether the testes have descended. The findings should be recorded.

*Following on from 3-day hCG test*
If the 3-week test follows the 3-day test, hCG should be administered on days 1, 2 and 3 as for the 3-day test. The hCG should then be given on day 5 of the first week. After this, a further 2 weeks of hCG should be given twice a week as above and the patient evaluated clinically and biochemically as above.

*The use of inhibin B in the differential diagnosis of disorders of testicular function*
Measurement of inhibin B has been advocated for assessment of testicular function in prepubertal boys [26]. Inhibin is a dimeric gonadal peptide hormone that suppresses FSH secretion of the pituitary and this plays an important role in the feedback regulation of the pituitary–gonadal axis. Specific immunoassays can discriminate the two biologically active isoforms, inhibin A and inhibin B. Inhibin B is the principle circulating form and is a marker of Sertoli cell function and spermatogenesis in adult males.

In prepubertal boys, basal inhibin B concentrations, which are age-related, correlate well with the testosterone increment in response to hCG [26]. In addition, basal inhibin concentrations distinguish patients with anorchia from those with abdominal testes, being undetectable in the former compared with the latter. This is important because its measurement might obviate the need for hCG tests in patients who might need orchidectomy if their intra-abdominal gonads are likely to be non-functional.

In patients with androgen insensitivity, inhibin B concentrations were normal or elevated for age. As expected, there was a divergence between basal inhibin B concentrations and the testosterone response to hCG in patients with gonadal dysgenesis and in those with an LH receptor defect. Inhibin B therefore acts as a reliable indicator of the presence or absence of testes in infants and prepubertal boys. In cryptorchid boys, a single inhibin B determination may predict Sertoli and Leydig cell function.

## Pituitary

## Anterior pituitary

### Insulin tolerance test for growth hormone and cortisol secretion

*Background*
The synthesis and release of GH, ACTH, thyroid-stimulating hormone (TSH), prolactin, LH and FSH is controlled by a number of hypothalamic releasing or inhibitory hormones, namely GH-releasing hormone (GHRH), corticotrophin-releasing hormone (CRH), thyrotrophin-releasing hormone (TRH) and luteinizing hormone-releasing hormone (GnRH or LHRH). These are used in clinical tests.

GH is secreted in a pulsatile fashion and, ideally, one should assess the 24-h GH secretory pattern. In practice, this is time-consuming and expensive, with considerable discomfort to the patient. Hence, pulses of GH secretion are provoked by a variety of agents. All the agents are pharmacological, and their physiological significance remains unknown. In addition, the patient must be euthyroid and cortisol-replete for normal GH secretion. Each test is associated with a significant false-positive and false-negative rate, and the use of two tests in combination will compound the errors.

Although a number of tests are available to assess GH secretion [27], the response to insulin-induced hypoglycaemia is widely recognized as the standard test for the assessment of GH and cortisol status. It is the only test of cortisol secretion that has been validated against the cortisol response to surgical stress [1]. The test requires the administration of insulin to reduce blood glucose, which acts as a stimulus to the release of GH and cortisol. The advantage of using insulin is that a known stimulus is applied and a clearly defined response is achieved, a reduction in blood glucose. From the defined stimuli, appropriate conclusions can be drawn from the GH and cortisol responses.

Both insulin-induced hypoglycaemia and glucagon tests

are potentially dangerous, and have resulted in death [28]. Trained staff in specialized endocrine units should monitor children having the test. The test is only as safe as the doctor and nurse performing it, and hypoglycaemia should be managed appropriately (see below). The child must not go home until the blood glucose is normal and he or she has eaten.

The function of the gonadotroph and thyrotroph cells can be tested at the same time by the administration of their respective releasing hormones, if indicated.

### Indication
Assessment of cortisol and GH reserve in children over 2 years of age. The test is indicated only when adequate auxological data have been collected and a diminished growth velocity demonstrated. Occasionally, there may be a need to perform the test without the prior acquisition of the auxological data, but this is exceptional.

### Contraindications to the insulin-induced hypoglycaemia test
No child who has a history of unexplained blackouts or epilepsy or who is currently receiving treatment for epilepsy should be studied using the insulin-induced hypoglycaemia test. The test should not be performed in children under the age of 2 years, when the glucagon test may be more appropriate. Special precautions are required in children suspected of having panhypopituitarism (see below).

### Definition of hypoglycaemic stimulus
The insulin-induced hypoglycaemic stimulus can be considered adequate when the blood glucose falls to 2.6 mmol/L or less, if the child is symptomatic or, alternatively, if there is a 50% reduction in the blood glucose concentration from basal values. GH and cortisol responses are maximal after a 50% reduction in blood glucose.

### Patient preparation
Sex steroid priming
Patients with delayed puberty may have physiological blunting of GH secretion, and reduced concentrations on testing at this stage may not be pathological. Hence, sex-steroid priming should be performed in prepubertal male and female patients with a bone age greater than 10 years. This is undertaken in the form of ethinyloestradiol 10 µg once daily orally for 3 days before the ITT in girls, or Sustenon 100 mg i.m. 72 h before the test in boys.

### Concurrent medication
For children already on GH, this should be stopped 1 week before the test. If the child is on hydrocortisone, the morning dose should be omitted and an intravenous dose (50–100 mg) be given at the end of the test. Recommence usual medication until test results are available, when the medication may need to be changed.

### Preparation
**1** The child should be fasted from midnight, apart from water. Small children should be encouraged to have a late snack during the evening before the test.
**2** On admission to the ward, the child should be assessed clinically and local anaesthetic cream applied over the proposed intravenous access site where appropriate.
**3** The height and weight of the child should be recorded on admission, so that the calculation of the doses of the various provocative agents is accurate.
**4** Thirty minutes after the administration of the local anaesthetic cream, an intravenous cannula should be inserted using as large a gauge device as possible. It is important to realize that the stress of cannulation can cause an increase in GH, which may make interpretation of the results difficult. Therefore, after insertion of the cannula, a period of 30–60 min bed rest should elapse before the commencement of the study. A sample of blood for GH estimation should be taken at –20 min, and this can be analysed in the event of an elevated baseline sample. The test should be started by 09.00 h.

### Prior arrangements
The test is usually performed on a day-case basis, but appropriate information regarding fasting must be given, together with an information sheet giving details of the test. The time of arrival in the ward should be clearly stated (08.00 h). Insulin, hydrocortisone for parenteral use and 10% dextrose for infusion should be available before beginning the test. A glucometer must be available, and the nurse in charge must be competent in its use. The child should be attended by a nurse throughout the test and a physician should be on the ward at all times.

### Special precautions
The test is hazardous because of both the production of hypoglycaemia and the scope for errors in treating it. The excessive administration of 50% dextrose has resulted in death and serious morbidity, and this concentrated solution of dextrose should *never* be used because of the risk of hyperosmolar coma.
**1** Ten per cent dextrose (2 mL/kg) should be drawn up by the bed, and the dose should be written up on the drug chart so that it can be administered without delay if required.
**2** Hydrocortisone (50–100 mg) should be drawn up for i.v. use.

### Methodology
If the glucometer reading at 0 min is low (under 2.6 mmol/L), no insulin should be administered. Sampling for hormone concentrations should proceed as per protocol and the study should be continued for 60 min only. Glucose should be administered orally as described below. If the reading lies in

**Table 28.1.** Test samples for insulin tolerance test

| Time (min) | BM Stix | Glucose | GH | Cortisol |
|---|---|---|---|---|
| −20 (before insulin) | ✓ | ✓ | ✓ | |
| 0 (before insulin) | ✓ | ✓ | ✓ | ✓ |
| 20 | ✓ | ✓ | | |
| 30 | ✓ | ✓ | ✓ | ✓ |
| 60 | ✓ | ✓ | ✓ | ✓ |
| 90 | ✓ | ✓ | ✓ | ✓ |
| 120 | ✓ | ✓ | ✓ | ✓ |

the range 2.6–3.5 mmol/L, 0.10 IU/kg of soluble insulin should be administered intravenously as a bolus. With readings greater than 3.5 mmol/L, the dose of insulin should be increased to 0.15 IU/kg *unless* the child is suspected of suffering from panhypopituitarism or has previously undergone cranial surgery or cranial radiotherapy (which includes total body irradiation), when the child should receive 0.10 IU/kg. Under these circumstances, consider administering hydrocortisone [50 (under 3 years) to 100 mg (over 3 years) i.v.] at the end of the test. The dose of insulin may need to be increased in patients with diabetes mellitus, insulin resistance, pretreatment acromegaly, pretreatment Cushing syndrome, obesity or when the test is being repeated due to a failure to achieve hypoglycaemia at the first attempt. Samples should be drawn as shown in Table 28.1.

The following tests should also be performed as part of the investigative protocol for short children: FBC, ESR, urea and electrolytes, $Ca^{2+}$, phosphate, alkaline phosphatase, LFT, free T4, TSH, prolactin, FSH and LH, oestradiol/testosterone. Insulin-like growth factor I (IGF-I) and IGF-binding protein 3 (IGFBP-3) should be measured if a diagnosis of GH resistance or bioinactive GH is suspected. Blood should be taken for pituitary developmental gene mutational analysis in suspected GH insufficiency, septo-optic dysplasia or panhypopituitarism. The karyotype should be analysed in short girls and antigliadin antibodies in both sexes. A skeletal survey may be indicated if a diagnosis of skeletal dysplasia is suspected.

*Management of hypoglycaemia (usually at time 20–30 min)*
If the child shows clinical evidence of hypoglycaemia (e.g. sweating and drowsiness) and the glucometer reading is < 2.6 mmol/L, a glucose drink (Hycal) should be given. Sampling should continue as per protocol, even after the glucose has been corrected, although the administration of glucose should be clearly recorded in the notes and on the request form.

If the child does not tolerate oral glucose or remains persistently hypoglycaemic, the following procedure should be adopted:
Glucose should be administered intravenously as a bolus of 200 mg/kg (10% dextrose, 2 mL/kg) over 3 min. This intra-

venous site cannot be used subsequently for the estimation of blood glucose concentrations. An intravenous glucose infusion should be commenced using 10% dextrose at 2.4–4.8 mL/kg/h (i.e. 4–8 mg/kg/min of glucose). The glucose concentration should be remeasured by fingerprick using a glucometer after 4–5 min, and the glucose infusion adjusted (up to 6 mL/kg/h, i.e. 10 mg/kg/min glucose) to maintain the blood glucose at 5–8 mmol/L.

Intramuscular injections of glucagon should not be given unless venous access is lost, as this will lead to rebound hypoglycaemia as a result of increased insulin secretion. If intravenous access is lost during the test, glucagon (1 mg) may be administered i.m. to counter the hypoglycaemia. The response depends upon the presence of adequate glycogen stores. However, rebound hypoglycaemia (up to 3 h later) may be a major problem, and the blood glucose needs to be monitored closely. Alternatively, glucose may be administered via a nasogastric tube or rectally.

If panhypopituitarism is suspected (for example in children who have had radiotherapy), 50 (< 3 years) to 100 mg (> 3 years) of hydrocortisone can be administered intravenously as a bolus at the end of the test, or earlier if recovery from hypoglycaemia is slow. This should be clearly recorded in the notes and on the laboratory request form.

If there is no improvement in the state of consciousness after normal glucose concentration is restored, an alternative explanation should be sought.

*Failure to reach a low blood glucose at 30 min*
If hypoglycaemia has not been achieved, as determined by a blood glucose estimation of ≤ 2.6 mmol/L or a greater than 50% reduction in the basal blood glucose, and the child is asymptomatic, wait for 30 min before reversing hypoglycaemia. The administration of insulin should not be repeated under any circumstances. The test should be continued as per protocol.

*Procedure at the end of test*
**1** Lunch should be provided for the child and the child not be sent home until an adequate high-carbohydrate meal has been eaten and tolerated and the blood glucose is at least 4 mmol/L for at least 2 h. The parents should be advised to give the child an adequate meal in the evening.
**2** The intravenous cannula should be left *in situ* until lunch has been completed.

*Interpretation*
The results can be interpreted only if hypoglycaemia has been achieved. The results of GH provocation tests are extremely difficult to interpret [29–31]. The results may vary depending upon the provocative agent in use, and the assay used to measure GH in serum [32]; a cut-off value of 15–25 mU/L is usually applied. However, the biochemical data must be used in conjunction with clinical and auxological

**Table 28.2.** Sampling during glucagon test

| Time (min) | BM Stix | Glucose | GH | Cortisol |
|---|---|---|---|---|
| −30 (before glucagon) | ✓ | ✓ | ✓ | ✓ |
| 0 (before glucagon) | ✓ | ✓ | ✓ | ✓ |
| 30 | ✓ | ✓ | ✓ | |
| 60 | ✓ | ✓ | ✓ | |
| 90 | ✓ | ✓ | ✓ | |
| 120 | ✓ | ✓ | ✓ | ✓ |
| 150 | ✓ | ✓ | ✓ | ✓ |
| 180 | ✓ | ✓ | ✓ | ✓ |

data in making decisions about GH treatment. Serum IGF-I and IGFBP-3 are generally unhelpful in making a diagnosis of GHI/GHD [33]. Cortisol concentration should increase at least twofold from the basal value, and a peak of 550 nmol/L should be achieved, usually 90–120 min after the start of the test. Alternatively, the increment in cortisol should be greater than 200 nmol/L. A poor response indicates an abnormality in the hypothalamo-pituitary-adrenal axis.

## Intramuscular glucagon stimulation test for HGH secretion (Table 28.2)

*Indication*

Assessment of cortisol and GH reserve in children, particularly those under the age of 2 years, in whom insulin-induced hypoglycaemia is contraindicated [34,35]. The exact mechanism whereby glucagon stimulates GH and cortisol secretion remains unknown, particularly in cases where rebound hypoglycaemia does not occur [36].

*Contraindications*

The test should not be performed in patients suspected of having a phaeochromocytoma or hyperinsulinism.

*Patient preparation*

As for insulin-induced hypoglycaemia test.

*Prior arrangements*

As for insulin-induced hypoglycaemia test.

*Special precautions*

Although widely reported as being a safer alternative to the insulin-induced hypoglycaemia test, the glucagon test is hazardous due to both the production of hypoglycaemia and the scope for errors in treating this. See under insulin-induced hypoglycaemia test.

*Methodology*

The patient should rest in bed during the test, which is best carried out in the morning.

Baseline bloods: as for insulin-induced hypoglycaemia test.

If the blood glucose at 0 min is low (under 2.6 mmol/L), no glucagon should be administered. Sampling for GH and cortisol concentrations should proceed as per protocol, and the study should be continued for 60 min only. Glucose should be administered orally.

Glucagon dose: 100 μg/kg body weight glucagon i.m. (maximum 1 mg).

Glucagon results in delayed hypoglycaemia, which can be dangerous [28], and it is extremely important that the blood glucose is normal and the child has eaten before going home.

*Management of hypoglycaemia (usually at time 90–120 min)*

As for insulin-induced hypoglycaemia.

*Procedure at the end of test*

As for insulin-induced hypoglycaemia.

*Interpretation*

As for insulin-induced hypoglycaemia. However, the peak cortisol response to glucagon stimulation may be lower than that in response to insulin-induced hypoglycaemia [37].

## Combined pituitary function test (Table 28.3)

*Background*

This test examines the function of the thyrotrophs secreting TSH, lactotrophs secreting prolactin and gonadotrophs secreting LH and FSH in addition to somatotroph and corticotroph function (see the TRH and GnRH test protocols below).

The test has three components that can be simultaneously evaluated:

1 insulin-induced hypoglycaemia or glucagon stimulation, which leads to GH and ACTH (and hence cortisol) secretion;
2 GnRH test, which leads to LH and FSH secretion;
3 TRH test, which stimulates TSH and prolactin secretion.

**Table 28.3.** Sampling for combined pituitary hormone stimulation tests

| Time (min) | Glucose | Cortisol | GH | LH | FSH | TSH | Prolactin |
|---|---|---|---|---|---|---|---|
| −30 | ✓ | ✓ | ✓ | | | | |
| 0 | ✓ | ✓ | ✓ | ✓ | ✓ | ✓ | ✓ |
| 20 | ✓ | | | ✓ | ✓ | ✓ | ✓ |
| 30 | ✓ | ✓ | ✓ | | | | |
| 60 | ✓ | ✓ | ✓ | ✓ | ✓ | ✓ | ✓ |
| 90 | ✓ | ✓ | ✓ | | | | |
| 120 | ✓ | ✓ | ✓ | | | | |
| And continuing for the glucagon test | | | | | | | |
| 150 | ✓ | ✓ | ✓ | | | | |
| 180 | ✓ | ✓ | ✓ | | | | |

*Indications*

Assessment of GH, cortisol, gonadotrophin and TSH secretion in patients suspected of having panhypopituitarism and in those who have had surgery, radiotherapy or trauma to the hypothalamo-pituitary area. Note, however, that GnRH tests are not indicated in children aged 18 months to 10 years, except those demonstrating premature sexual maturation.

*Patient preparation*

As for the insulin tolerance/glucagon test. Patients on hydrocortisone should have the morning dose withheld to allow adequate interpretation of plasma cortisol concentrations, and an appropriate intravenous dose of hydrocortisone should be given at the end of the test.

*Prior arrangements*

The test can be performed on a day-case basis, provided instructions regarding fasting and the required time of arrival have been given to the parents.

Glucagon/insulin, TRH and GnRH should be ordered from pharmacy, as well as hydrocortisone and 10% dextrose.

*Special precautions*

Patients with panhypopituitarism, whose cortisol secretion may be inadequate, are less able to deal with hypoglycaemia or stress. Problems with hypoglycaemia are therefore more likely both during the test and afterwards. The instructions given above for management of hypoglycaemia should be carefully followed. Treatment with hydrocortisone may be indicated until results of tests are available.

*Test procedure*

The following should be administered:

insulin (0.1–0.15 IU/kg i.v.) or glucagon (100 μg/kg up to 1 mg i.m.)

2.5 μg/kg GnRH up to a maximum dose of 100 μg

7 μg/kg TRH up to a maximum dose of 200 μg (given i.v. slowly over 3 min).

These can be given successively.

*Precautions/contraindications/management of hypoglycaemia/interpretation*

See individual protocols, i.e. glucagon, ITT, TRH and GnRH.

## GnRH test

*Background*

Assesses the ability of the pituitary gland to secrete gonadotrophins in response to GnRH stimulation. In a pubertal child, LH and FSH are normally secreted in a pulsatile fashion. In the prepubertal child, LH and FSH concentrations are usually low.

*Indications*

1 Diagnosis and follow-up of gonadotrophin-dependent sexual precocity.

2 Investigation of delayed puberty (constitutional delay may be difficult to differentiate from hypogonadotrophic hypogonadism).

3 Investigation of bilateral cryptorchidism (hypogonadotrophic hypogonadism).

*Patient preparation*

There is no need to fast. An in-dwelling cannula is required, and the test can be performed at any time of the day.

*Methodology*

1 Collect basal (0 min) samples.

2 Basal plasma LH, FSH, oestradiol or testosterone, karyotype should be measured.

3 Administer GnRH 2.5 μg/kg by i.v. bolus up to a maximum of 100 μg.

4 Serial LH and FSH should be measured at 20 and 60 min.

*Interpretation*

In normal pubertal individuals, the FSH and LH values increase at 20 min and decrease at 60 min. In sexual precocity, which is gonadotrophin-dependent, the response is pubertal. In gonadotrophin-independent sexual precocity, the concentrations of gonadotrophin are suppressed. In gonadal failure, the basal values are increased and the response to GnRH exaggerated. In pubertal delay and hypogonadotrophic hypogonadism, the response to GnRH is absent/poor. A combination of the hCG and GnRH tests has been reported to help in the differentiation of hypogonadotrophic hypogonadism and constitutional delay of growth and puberty (CDGP) [19], but unpublished data suggest that this is not so. In addition, the differentiation between the two conditions may be aided by performing a bolus GnRH test after pulsatile GnRH administration over a 36-h period [38].

## Thyrotrophin-releasing hormone test

*Indications*

This releasing hormone stimulates the secretion of TSH and is used for the following indications:

1 Diagnosis of equivocal hyperthyroidism—if the basal TSH concentration is suppressed in the face of a high free thyroxine ($fT_4$) concentration, the TRH test is not indicated. With the availability of sensitive TSH assays, which are usually able to distinguish hyperthyroidism from euthyroidism [39], this test is required rarely for the evaluation of thyrotoxicosis. It may, however, be useful in the unusual scenario of hyperthyroidism with inappropriate secretion of thyrotrophin, allowing the distinction between TSH-secreting pituitary tumours (usually unresponsive) and the pituitary variant of resistance to thyroid hormone syndrome (always responsive) [40].

**2** Evaluation of secondary hypothyroidism.

**3** Investigation of hypothalamo-pituitary lesions.

**4** Pituitary gigantism—when a GH response to TRH may be present [41].

**5** To assess prolactin secretion.

*Patient preparation*

**1** No fasting is required.

**2** An in-dwelling intravenous cannula is required

*Special precautions*

Intravenous administration of TRH commonly causes minor side-effects (e.g. nausea, metallic taste in mouth, flushing, headache, and abdominal and chest discomfort). Major problems, though rare, have been reported, e.g. pituitary apoplexy, asystole, bronchospasm, transient hypertension.

*Methodology*

**1** Basal free thyroxine ($FT_4$) and TSH (and $FT_3$ if thyrotoxicosis is suspected) are measured.

**2** TRH (7 µg/kg up to a maximum of 200 µg) is given by slow intravenous injection (over 3 min).

**3** Serial TSH is measured at 20 and 60 min after the administration of TRH.

If clinically indicated, prolactin or GH may need to be measured (see above).

*Interpretation*

TSH

In normal individuals, a rise in TSH value at 20 min with a fall at 60 min is observed.

   Basal TSH: 0.5–5.0 mU/L

   Increment: 3–18 mU/L (> twice the baseline)

   In hypothalamic hypothyroidism, the TSH increases at 20 min and continues to increase at 60 min. In primary hypothyroidism, the basal TSH concentration is elevated and the response to TRH is exaggerated. In hypothyroidism secondary to hypopituitarism, there is no change in the TSH concentration. In thyrotoxicosis, the TSH concentrations are suppressed throughout the test.

Prolactin

In normal subjects, the prolactin concentration increases by at least fourfold at 20 min and then decreases at 60 min. In pituitary lesions (e.g. tumours) or in pituitary hypoplasia there is a blunted increase in prolactin concentrations. The concentrations are grossly elevated in prolactinoma, with a poor response to TRH. A raised basal prolactin may suggest a functional disconnection between the hypothalamus and the pituitary.

GH

Normal subjects usually show no response, although a GH response can be observed in puberty, chronic renal failure, anorexia, depression and diabetes mellitus. Patients with acromegaly and pituitary gigantism show an increase in GH concentrations in response to TRH.

**Intravenous GHRH test**

*Indications*

**1** Differential diagnosis of isolated GHD.

**2** Investigation of suspected Laron-type dwarfism, when an ITT or glucagon test may be hazardous.

**3** Research—this is the commonest indication.

*Patient preparation*

**1** The child should be fasted from midnight (6 h < 3 years age).

**2** An in-dwelling intravenous cannula should be inserted at 08.30 h. Sampling should be commenced 30 min after cannulation.

**3** If the patient is on GH, then this should be stopped 1 week before the test.

*Special precautions/contraindications*

Most patients notice minor facial flushing after GHRH. There are no other side-effects.

*Methodology*

Serum GH is measured at –15, 0, 5, 15, 30, 45, 60, 90, 120 min after the administration of a bolus of GHRH (1 µg/kg at time 0). This is a supramaximal dose, and a dose of 0.1 µg/kg may suffice.

*Interpretation*

The GH response to GHRH is extremely variable. This variability is both intra- and interindividual [42]. Hence the test is used mainly as a research tool. If there is a good response to GHRH but not to ITT or glucagon, this may suggest GHD because of a hypothalamic lesion. A failure to respond to exogenous GHRH may suggest an abnormality in the pituitary gland, or in the GHRH receptor.

**Twenty-four-hour hormonal studies**

*Background*

Random measurements of many hormones (e.g. GH and gonadotrophins) are of little value because these hormones are released in a pulsatile fashion. Serial measurements of many hormones over a 24-h period are therefore required to observe the true endocrine status.

*Indications*

**1** To assess GH secretion, e.g. in neurosecretory dysfunction where the pulsatility of GH is abnormal in spite of a normal GH peak response to provocation, and in pituitary gigantism.

**2** To assess gonadotrophin secretion in delayed puberty, when pulsatility is first observed in late prepuberty and early puberty (pelvic USS should have been performed in girls and may obviate the need for this).

*Patient preparation*
1 The child is admitted the evening before the test and assessed clinically.
2 An in-dwelling intravenous cannula is inserted and kept patent.
3 Label blood bottles with name and time of sample or a number (1–72 for a 24-h profile).

*Special precautions*
In a child < 15 kg, an overnight 12-h profile may be adequate.

*Methodology*
The 24-h profile consists of 20-min blood samples. The profile can usually be started at any time, but it is best to start at 08.00–09.00 h.

*Interpretation*
GH
In normal individuals, at least three night-time peaks of GH secretion are observed (GH value dependent upon the assay), with the GH secretion returning to undetectable trough concentrations in between. In neurosecretory dysfunction, a large number of GH peaks with high values may be observed, with an elevation in trough concentrations.

Gonadotrophins
The profile shows low FSH and LH values between 18 months and up to early puberty. In early puberty, the values increase with peaks of gonadotrophin secretion predominantly at night in the first instance and then also during the daytime as puberty proceeds.

## Posterior pituitary

### Water deprivation test

*Background/indication*
1 Determination of the urine concentrating ability in patients with polyuria and polydipsia.
2 Investigation of suspected diabetes insipidus (DI) and differentiating from psychogenic polydipsia.

Plasma and urine osmolality are measured during a period of water deprivation. In the second part of the test, the patient is given DDAVP (desmopressin; synthetic antidiuretic hormone), and the urine osmolality is recorded. The DDAVP test can help distinguish cranial from nephrogenic DI or renal tubular acidosis.

*Patient preparation*
1 Ideally, cortisol status should be assessed before the water deprivation test, and, if cortisol deficiency is suspected,

hydrocortisone should be commenced 48 h before the test, as cortisol is required for the excretion of water, and the diagnosis of DI may be missed in a cortisol-insufficient child. A dose of 15 mg/m$^2$/day should be started.
2 Fluid intake and urine output should ideally be observed over a 24-h period: if equal and appropriate for age, there may be no need to proceed further.
3 The patient must be admitted for two nights for the test to be carried out.
4 Fluids must not be limited before the test, but tea and coffee must be excluded overnight. A light breakfast with minimal fluid in the form of water may be taken early on the morning of the test.
5 Weigh the child and calculate 5% of body weight.
6 An intravenous cannula must be inserted.

*Prior arrangements*
It must be possible to weigh the patient precisely throughout the period of water deprivation.

The procedure must be arranged with the laboratory in advance as most samples require urgent analysis. DDAVP at a dose of either 0.1–0.4 µg for i.m. injection, or 10 µg by spray into each nostril (i.e. a total dose of 20 µg), should be procured. Note that there is a large difference in doses between the intranasal and i.m. modes of administration.

*Special precautions*
This is a hazardous test and close medical supervision is required. There are two problems to avoid: first, the subject must not be allowed to become dehydrated. Fluids must not be limited before the test (no overnight fast) and the test must be terminated as soon as there is a diagnostic result (which may be at the start of the test) or if a weight loss of > 5% is achieved. Deprivation of water in a patient with DI is hazardous because of uncontrolled water loss. All measurements must be charted and acted upon promptly. Second, water overload must be avoided after the administration of DDAVP, so water intake must be limited to replacement of losses during the test. The patient must remain under supervision throughout, and surreptitious drinking must be avoided.

*Methodology*
The test should start at 08.30 h, when the fluid fast should commence. The patient should be asked to pass urine, and, if the patient has had no fluids overnight, this sample should be sent for estimation of urine osmolality. A blood sample should be collected for measurement of plasma sodium (Na$^+$) and osmolality. If the patient has had fluids overnight, this sample should be discarded. All oral fluid intake should then be stopped. Urine passed thereafter should be collected and saved in universal containers; hourly collections should be made if possible. The patient's weight should be recorded. A urine osmolality of > 750 mmol/kg at any time excludes a

diagnosis of DI. Elevated plasma sodium (> 145 mmol/L) or osmolality (> 295 mosmol/kg) in the face of an inappropriately dilute urine confirm the diagnosis; in this case there is no need to proceed with the first part of the test, but the response to DDAVP should be determined.

Hourly weight, pulse, blood pressure, urine output and specific gravity should be carefully documented. If possible, a urine sample should be sent to the laboratory hourly or whenever the child passes urine, and urine osmolality estimation should be requested urgently. Plasma sodium and osmolality should be estimated at 2-h intervals. At 13.30 h, plasma sodium and osmolality should be measured together with an arginine vasopressin (AVP) concentration if an assay is available. If possible, a urine sample from the preceding hour should be sent for estimation of sodium and osmolality.

The test should be stopped and the second part of the test (DDAVP test) commenced if:
1 the patient's weight falls by 5% from the starting weight;
2 the plasma osmolality rises (> 295) in the face of an inappropriately dilute urine (< 300); or
3 the patient is clinically dehydrated.

The test should be stopped and the DDAVP test should not be performed if any urine osmolality exceeds 750 mosmol/kg or if the above criteria (1–3) have not been met by 15.30 h.

At the end of test blood should be sent for estimation of plasma sodium concentration, osmolality and AVP; a urine sample from the preceding hour should be analysed for sodium and osmolality. If indicated (i.e. the urine fails to concentrate), the water deprivation test is followed immediately by the DDAVP test. Although ideally urine should be collected at hourly intervals, this may be difficult in practice, unless the child has DI, in which case urine collection is no problem. In the former case, the urine samples should be labelled sequentially with the time of collection.

*Interpretation of test*
The presently used urine osmolality value of > 750 to exclude a diagnosis of DI is based upon normal ranges derived from adults [43]. In children, no normative data exist. In practice, values of 300–750 are frequently observed after water deprivation. In view of the potential hazard of DDAVP treatment,

caution is required in the diagnosis of DI. AVP concentrations may be useful – a failure to increase in the face of an elevated plasma osmolality may be diagnostic of cranial DI [44]. Table 28.4 is a guide to the interpretation of water deprivation and DDAVP tests.

If the urine osmolality at 15.30 h is greater than 300, a diagnosis of DI is likely. In the range 300–750, the diagnosis may be one of psychogenic polydipsia and gradual fluid restriction under supervision may be indicated, with careful monitoring of plasma and urine osmolalities. A plasma osmolality < 295 mosmol/kg at the end of the test indicates that fluid deprivation has not been adequate. The measurement of plasma AVP concentrations is helpful only if the plasma osmolality is > 295 mosmol/kg. In theory, this could be achieved by the infusion of hypertonic saline, but this is potentially hazardous in children and should be undertaken only in exceptional circumstances [46]. If the patient fails to concentrate urine (> 750) in the face of a rising plasma osmolality (> 295) and a rising sodium concentration, the diagnosis of DI is confirmed, particularly if the AVP concentrations are low, and DDAVP needs to be administered in the second part of the test.

## DDAVP test

*Indication*
To distinguish nephrogenic from cranial diabetes insipidus in patients who were unable to concentrate their urine adequately (> 750) in a 7-h water deprivation test.

*Patient preparation*
This should follow the 7-h water deprivation test. An intravenous cannula should be *in situ*.

*Special precautions*
Beware of water intoxication. Only the urine losses should be replaced during this test.

*Methodology*
After the 7-h water deprivation test, DDAVP at a dosage of 0.1 μg in infants (< 2 years old), 0.2 μg in children aged

**Table 28.4.** Interpretation of water deprivation tests [45]

| Urine osmolality (mosmol/kg) | | Diagnosis |
| --- | --- | --- |
| After fluid deprivation | After desmopressin | |
| < 300 | > 750 | Cranial diabetes insipidus |
| < 300 | < 300 | Nephrogenic diabetes insipidus |
| > 750 | > 750 | Primary polydipsia |
| 300–750 | < 750 | ?Partial nephrogenic diabetes insipidus ?Primary psychogenic polydipsia |
| 300–750 | > 750 | ?Partial cranial diabetes insipidus |

2–8 years, 0.3 μg in children aged 8–14 years and 0.4 μg in patients over 14 years should be administered. A light meal may be taken and the patient is allowed to drink volumes of fluid equal to the previous hour's urine output. Over the next 4 h, the urine volume and specific gravity should be carefully recorded with recording of the patient's weight, thirst, blood pressure and heart rate. The test ends (a) after 4 h, (b) if the urine specific gravity is greater than 1014, (c) if the weight loss is greater than 5% of initial weight or (d) if clinical signs of dehydration are present.

At the end of the test, plasma and urine sodium and osmolality should be measured.

After the test, the patient's fluid intake and urine output are carefully monitored and the patient is observed overnight to ensure that he or she does not develop water intoxication or dehydration. In general, children are normally fluid restricted according to the previous hour's urine output in order to avoid water intoxication. Urea and electrolytes should be measured on the following morning.

*Interpretation*
An increase in urine osmolality after DDAVP suggests normal concentrating ability after the administration of DDAVP. This is suggestive of cranial DI. However, if the urine fails to concentrate, the diagnosis is one of nephrogenic DI. Cranial imaging must be performed in all children with cranial DI as underlying cranial pathology is common.

## Miscellaneous tests in managing growth disorders

### IGF-I generation test

*Background/indication*
Used when the diagnosis of GH resistance syndromes (e.g. Laron-type dwarfism) or resistance to the actions of GH at the receptor level is suspected. Usually, GH provocation tests will have demonstrated high peak GH concentrations with low IGF-I concentrations.

*Methodology*
On day 1 (08.00–10.00 h) basal (6 h fasting) IGF-I and IGF-II, and IGFBP-3 and GHBP (GH-binding protein) should be measured. Between 16.00 and 19.00 h, hGH should be administered subcutaneously at a dose of 0.1 μg/kg and be repeated on days 2, 3 and 4. On day 5 (08.00–10.00 h), measurement of serum IGFs (IGF-I and IGF-II) and IGFBP-3 should be repeated.

*Interpretation*
In Laron-type dwarfism, the IGF-I concentrations remain low for age. In normal individuals, an increase in IGF-I > 20% is observed.

## Glucose metabolism

## The investigation of hypoglycaemia

### Definition of hypoglycaemia

A blood glucose of less than 2.6 mmol/L with or without symptoms. This definition holds regardless of age and gestation.

*Background*
Hypoglycaemia can be due to a number of conditions. These include excessive insulin secretion, surreptitious insulin administration, deficiencies of counter-regulatory hormones and inborn errors of metabolism. To investigate the aetiology it is essential to draw a blood sample for the analysis of intermediary metabolites and hormones at the time of a hypoglycaemic episode *before* the administration of glucose. A single sample of blood may well be diagnostic. In addition to this, the investigation of hypoglycaemia warrants a careful and logical approach. First, the hypoglycaemia should be confirmed on a 24-h glucose profile. Second, the period of fast tolerance should be determined. At the time of hypoglycaemia, the relevant blood samples should be taken in order to determine the aetiology. Third, the glucose requirement for maintenance of euglycaemia needs to be established.

*Twenty-four-hour glucose profile*
An in-dwelling cannula should be inserted. Two-hourly blood glucose concentrations should be sent to the laboratory. Coincidental BM measurements should be documented on the ward. If the child becomes hypoglycaemic at any stage, blood samples should be collected for intermediary metabolites and hormones as planned for the fasting provocation test (see below under 'Specimens collected at the time of hypoglycaemia').

*Pre- and postprandial profile*
The main indication is hypoglycaemia related to meals. Additional samples can be taken during a 24-h glucose profile while on a normal diet. Sample collection should be as in the fast provocation test (see below).

*Fast provocation*
*Background*
Successful adaptation to fasting depends upon intact glycogenolytic, lipolytic, gluconeogenic and ketogenic pathways and their hormonal regulation. Hence the pattern of intermediary metabolites and hormones during a period of controlled fasting is an invaluable tool in the investigation of many endocrine and metabolic disorders, particularly disorders of insulin secretion, gluconeogenesis, fat oxidation, and ketone body production and utilization [47].

**Table 28.5.** Maximum times recommended for diagnostic fasts

| Age of child | Maximum starvation time (h) |
| --- | --- |
| < 6 months | 8 |
| 6–8 months | 12 |
| 8–12 months | 16 |
| 1–2 years | 18 |
| 2–8 years | 20 |
| > 8 years | 24 |

*Indications*

**1** Investigation of hypoglycaemia of unknown aetiology.
**2** Investigation of suspected metabolic disorders (e.g. episodic metabolic acidosis).
**3** Monitoring the safe duration of fasting and the response to treatment.

*Patient preparation*

**1** The duration of fast is dependent on the child's age. The period for which the child goes overnight without food and drink should be established and the child fasted 2–4 h longer than this. In certain circumstances, e.g. neonates with hyperinsulinism, the period of fast tolerance will be extremely short, e.g. 5–10 min. The fast should not be performed overnight. The maximum times recommended are shown in Table 28.5.
**2** A wide-bore intravenous cannula is essential for this test.
**3** Plain water can be taken throughout the period of fasting.

*Prior arrangements*

The intermediary metabolites required for diagnosis should be decided upon, and the appropriate bottles labelled. A copy of the pro forma should be given to the biochemistry laboratory before the test.

*Special precautions*

This is a potentially hazardous test and needs careful supervision. Hypoglycaemia may be sudden and unexpected. The child must be supervised individually on the ward during this test.

*Test procedure*

From the first missed feed, hourly BM stix and plasma glucose should be measured during the test. Specimens should be collected as documented below if (a) the child is hypoglycaemic (blood glucose less than 2.6 mmol/L), (b) the child is symptomatic (pale, sweaty and drowsy, etc.) or (c) at the end of the fast/intermediary times.

Analysis of specimens to be collected at the time of hypoglycaemia
Blood glucose.

Plasma lactate and pyruvate β-hydroxybutyrate.
Acetoacetate.
Non-esterified fatty acids (NEFAs).
Serum insulin.
Serum C-peptide if surreptitious insulin administration is suspected.
Serum GH.
Plasma cortisol.
Serum IGF-I and IGFBP-3 concentrations.
Free carnitine.
Acylcarnitine (see below).
Plasma-free and total carnitine should be measured on the first specimen (2 mL of heparinized blood together with blood spots on a Guthrie card for acylcarnitine analysis, the latter should also be sent on the final specimen).

The first specimen of urine after the fast has been terminated should be collected for measurement of organic acids by gas chromatography–mass spectrometry (GC–MS) even if the patient remained asymptomatic.

Ensure feed and meal are taken at end of fast, and that the BM Stix is normal.

If hypoglycaemic or symptomatic, take blood samples and give 0.2 g/kg of i.v. dextrose (2 mL/kg of 10% dextrose) over 3 min (see above for further management of hypoglycaemia).

Please note the time of commencement of fasting on the request forms and record in the notes which tests have been performed, and also the timing of these tests.

*Determination of glucose requirements to maintain euglycaemia*

In infants with hypoglycaemia caused by hyperinsulinism, a glucose requirement of 15–22 mg/kg/min is not uncommon (in normal infants, the requirement is 4–6 mg/kg/min). In these cases, the infant usually requires an intravenous infusion to maintain normoglycaemia. In order to achieve hypoglycaemia and hence a diagnosis, the infusion can be stopped totally. This will achieve hypoglycaemia within a few minutes and the test must be very closely supervised. Alternatively, the achievement of hypoglycaemia may be coupled to the evaluation of the glucose intake required to maintain euglycaemia. To do this, the glucose infusion is reduced by 1 mg/kg/min every 15 min, with close monitoring of the BM stix. Once hypoglycaemia is achieved, the reduction in glucose intake is stopped and the infusion rate is increased once the blood sample for the measurement of intermediary metabolites and hormones has been taken, as per the protocol in the section Test procedure.

To calculate the glucose requirement, the following method can be used:

$$\text{Glucose (mg/kg/min)} = \text{rate (mL/h)} \times \frac{\text{concentration of glucose used (\%)}}{6 \times \text{weight (kg)}}$$

*Interpretation of fast provocation*

In normal individuals, at the time of hypoglycaemia (blood glucose less than 2.6 mmol/L), insulin secretion is switched off, GH and cortisol are increased, and β-hydroxybutyrate, free fatty acids (FFAs) and acetoacetate are all elevated. In hyperinsulinism, the insulin concentrations are inappropriately elevated but the concentrations of FFAs and ketone bodies are very low, as insulin suppresses lipolysis. If C-peptide is not detected in the presence of insulin, there is a *prima facie* case for suspecting surreptitious and malicious administration of exogenous insulin.

In β-oxidation defects, the concentration of free fatty acids is increased, whereas the β-hydroxybutyrate and acetoacetate concentrations are low, as is the concentration of insulin. Urinary organic acids and blood acylcarnitine concentrations may be diagnostic in these conditions. Blood lactate concentrations should be < 2 mmol/L throughout the fast, but they may be elevated in a struggling child. Raised lactate concentrations are found in defects of gluconeogenesis. In GH or cortisol deficiency or both (e.g. panhypopituitarism), the respective hormone concentrations are low at the time of hypoglycaemia, and formal pituitary function assessment is then required. Fast provocation is not an efficient method of diagnosing GHD, as GH values tend to be variable.

## The glucagon provocation test for investigating hypoglycaemia

*Background/indications*

The glycaemic response to glucagon administration requires adequate hepatic glycogen stores and intact glycogenolytic pathways. This test is therefore useful in glycogen storage diseases and hyperinsulinism.

*Patient preparation*

The child should be fasted for the appropriate period (water is permitted), depending on age, fast tolerance and glucose requirements. This test can also be performed 2 h after breakfast.

*Special precautions*

Administration of glucagon can result in rebound hypoglycaemia, especially in children with hyperinsulinism.

*Methodology*

Glucagon 100 µg/kg (0.1 mg/kg) up to a maximum of 1 mg should be given intramuscularly.

*Sampling*

Table 28.6 shows the sampling times for the glucagon provocation test.

*Interpretation*

In hyperinsulinism, there is an exaggerated glucose response to glucagon stimulation, and rebound hypoglycaemia is a

**Table 28.6.** Sampling for glucagon provocation test

| Sample | Time (min) | | | | | | | | |
|---|---|---|---|---|---|---|---|---|---|
| | −30 | 0 | 30 | 60 | 90 | 120 | 150 | 180 | 240 |
| BM stix/blood glucose | ✓ | ✓ | ✓ | ✓ | ✓ | ✓ | ✓ | ✓ | ✓ |
| Pyruvate | | ✓ | ✓ | ✓ | | ✓ | | | ✓ |
| Lactate | | ✓ | ✓ | ✓ | | ✓ | | | ✓ |
| Acetoacetate | | ✓ | ✓ | ✓ | | ✓ | | | ✓ |
| β-Hydroxybutyrate | | ✓ | ✓ | ✓ | | ✓ | | | ✓ |
| Non-esterified fatty acids (NEFAs) | | ✓ | ✓ | ✓ | | ✓ | | | ✓ |
| Cortisol | ✓ | ✓ | ✓ | ✓ | ✓ | ✓ | | | ✓ |
| GH | ✓ | ✓ | ✓ | ✓ | ✓ | ✓ | | ✓ | ✓ |

problem because of excessive secretion of insulin in response to the glucagon. The ketone body concentrations are low as is the concentration of NEFAs.

## Oral glucose tolerance test

*Background/indications*

In paediatric practice, the oral glucose tolerance test is used for reasons in addition to those in adults.

**1** Tall stature: The glucose tolerance test is used to assess whether a tall, rapidly growing child has pituitary gigantism. In pituitary gigantism, as in acromegaly, GH secretion is persistently elevated and is not suppressed by the ingestion of an oral glucose load. However, in tall adolescents, there may be a failure of suppression of GH secretion by oral glucose, giving rise to a high incidence of false positives [48].
**2** Hypoglycaemia: Glucose leads to secretion of insulin from the pancreas. If there is abnormal regulation of insulin release [e.g. persistent hyperinsulinaemic hypoglycaemia of infancy (PHHI)], there is an exaggerated release of insulin in response to the glucose load, with a failure of insulin secretion to switch off, in spite of the return of blood glucose concentrations to normal values, resulting in a rebound hypoglycaemia.
**3** Insulin resistance: The diagnosis of insulin-dependent diabetes mellitus is not often in doubt in childhood, and glucose tolerance tests are rarely needed. A glucose tolerance test may, however, be useful to assess insulin resistance, which is rarely symptomatic in children but which occurs in a number of situations such as obesity, acanthosis nigricans, polycystic ovarian syndrome, insulin receptor defects, children with a strong family history of insulin resistance and maturity-onset diabetes of the young (MODY). GH treatment induces insulin resistance but this is rarely of clinical significance.

*Patient preparation*

**1** The child should have had a normal balanced diet for at least 5 days before the test and should be fasted from midnight, although water is allowed. Small children should

**Table 28.7.** Sampling for a glucose tolerance test

| | Time (min) | | | | | | | |
|---|---|---|---|---|---|---|---|---|
| | –30 | 0 | 30 | 60 | 90 | 120 | 150 | 180 |
| BM stix | ✓ | ✓ | ✓ | ✓ | ✓ | ✓ | ✓ | ✓ |
| Glucose | ✓ | ✓ | ✓ | ✓ | ✓ | ✓ | ✓ | ✓ |
| GH* | ✓ | ✓ | ✓ | ✓ | ✓ | ✓ | ✓ | ✓ |
| Insulin† | ✓ | ✓ | ✓ | ✓ | ✓ | ✓ | ✓ | ✓ |

C-peptide measurements can be helpful in suspected hyperinsulinism because the half-life of C-peptide is much longer than that of insulin. Proinsulin and insulin split products may be of use in some circumstances, for example insulin-processing defects. The absence of C-peptide in the presence of insulin suggests exogenous administration of insulin.
IGF-I and IGFBP-3 are mandatory in all children with tall stature.
*When assessing the endocrinology of tall stature.
†Liaise with laboratory in advance.

be encouraged to have a late snack during the evening before the test.
**2** On admission to the ward, the child should be assessed clinically and an intravenous cannula should be inserted using as large a gauge device as is possible. It is important to realize that the stress of the cannulation can cause an increase in GH secretion, which may make interpretation of the results difficult. Therefore, after insertion of the cannula, a period of 1 h should elapse before the commencement of the study.
**3** The weight of the child should be recorded at admission.

*Special precautions*
The test may be hazardous in children with hyperinsulinism, in whom excessive secretion of insulin leads to a rebound hypoglycaemia, and in whom careful monitoring will be required.

*Methodology*
An oral glucose load is administered at a dose of 1.75 g/kg to a maximum of 75 g. It is most convenient to give this either as Hycal, Lucozade or dextrose powder. The glucose load should be consumed over 5 min.

*Sampling*
Table 28.7 shows the sampling for a glucose tolerance test.

*Interpretation*
Tall stature: GH response
During the glucose tolerance test, the serum GH concentration should become undetectable at 30–60 min. As the studies are often carried on to 180 min, a slight increase in serum GH concentrations can often be observed towards the end of the test at the 150- and 180-min samples as glucose concentrations decline secondary to the excessive secretion of insulin.

Hypoglycaemia
This usually occurs in children with hyperinsulinism. Sampling should be continued at 30-min intervals until 300 min, or even longer if required.

Insulin resistance
The insulin response is grossly exaggerated. In normal individuals, the peak blood glucose should not exceed 8.9 mmol/L, and the 120-min glucose concentration should be less than 6.1 mmol/L (WHO guidelines). In individuals with insulin resistance, these values may be exceeded.

Procedure at the end of test
Lunch should be provided for the child and the child should not be sent home until an adequate meal has been taken and the BM is stable, because of the risk of rebound hypoglycaemia. The intravenous cannula should be left *in situ* until lunch has been completed.

**Intravenous glucose tolerance test**

*Indications*
**1** Abnormal glucose homeostasis.
**2** Conditions of insulin resistance such as obesity, acanthosis nigricans, family history of insulin resistance and polycystic ovarian disease.

*Patient preparation*
An unrestricted diet rich in carbohydrates should be consumed for at least 3 days before the test. The child should be fasted overnight for 10–16 h. There may be a need to arrange for proinsulin concentrations and split products of insulin to be measured.

*Methodology*
An infusion of 0.5 g of glucose per kilogram of body weight (maximum 25 g) should be infused as a 20% solution (2.5 mL/kg; maximum 125 mL) within 2 min (ideally). Blood samples should be taken at –10 and –5 min and at 1, 3, 5, 10, 15, 20, 30, 45 and 60 min after the glucose infusion for the measurement of plasma glucose and insulin. In certain situations, measurement of proinsulin, C-peptide and split products of insulin may be required.

*Interpretation of response*
K-value
The glucose disappearance rate $K$ (% per minute) can be calculated according to the formula:

$$K = \frac{\ln 2 \times 100}{t_{1/2}(\text{min})} = \frac{0.693 \times 100}{t_{1/2}(\text{min})}$$

The biological half-life of glucose in the circulation, $t_{1/2}$, corresponds to the time span (in minutes) required for glucose to fall by 50% from its concentration at 10 min after glucose infusion; ln2 refers to the natural logarithm of 2, which is 0.693.

Normal response: $K > 1.2\%$ per min.

Frank diabetes: $K < 1.0\%$ per min.

Borderline: $K = 1.0–1.2\%$ per min.

### First and second phases of insulin secretion

The first phase of insulin secretion comprises the first 10 min after glucose infusion, and the second covers the period from 10 to 60 min. In normal subjects, the peak insulin concentration of the first phase is always higher than any insulin value during the second phase [49]. The first-phase insulin response is calculated as the sum of the +1-min and +3-min concentrations with or without subtracting the basal insulin concentration. The first-phase insulin release is markedly higher in adolescents and adults than in prepubertal children [50]. The glucose disposal rate is calculated as the slope of the semilogarithmic decline of blood glucose over the 10- to 30-min period after the administration of intravenous glucose. Loss of the first-phase insulin response (defined as < first centile of normal control subjects) is observed in both insulin-dependent and non-insulin-dependent diabetes and has been observed before diagnosis in both conditions.

## Calcium metabolism

### Parathyroid hormone infusion test

*Indication*

This test is used for the diagnosis of pseudohypoparathyroidism [51].

The basis of the test is the response of cAMP in both blood and urine to an injection of PTH over a period of approximately 2 h. Blood samples are taken frequently during the first 30 min after the PTH infusion. Urine samples are taken for 1–2 h before the injection and for at least 2 h afterwards.

*Patient preparation*

**1** The patient should be fasted overnight, although clear fluids (non-caffeine/theophylline containing) may be permitted.

**2** An intake of at least 1 L of water 1 h before the test and a further litre during the test should be achieved.

**3** An intravenous cannula should be inserted and an intravenous infusion of saline commenced if necessary.

**4** The patient should rest during the procedure.

*Prior arrangements*

PTH needs to be ordered in advance, and liaison with the chemical pathology laboratory should also be arranged in advance.

*Methodology*

Basal blood samples should be collected for serum $Ca^{2+}$, $PO_4^{3-}$, creatinine, $Mg^{2+}$, PTH, 1,25-dihydroxyvitamin D and DNA analysis. Blood samples for $G_{s\alpha}$ should be taken from the patient and an age- and sex-matched control subject. At 30 min before the PTH infusion, urine should be collected and sent for measurement of cAMP, $PO_4^{3-}$ and creatinine concentrations. All urine volumes should be carefully measured and these data recorded. Blood should be collected for measurement of cAMP and $PO_4^{3-}$ concentrations. At 10 min before PTH infusion, blood should be collected for measurement of cAMP and $PO_4^{3-}$ concentrations. Immediately before the administration of PTH, urine should be collected and cAMP, $PO_4^{3-}$ and creatinine measured. Plasma cAMP and $PO_4^{3-}$ should also be measured.

PTH (3 U/kg; maximum 200 U i.v. in 2 mL) should be infused intravenously over 2 min. Plasma cAMP and $PO_4^{3-}$ should be measured 5, 10, 15, 20, 30, 60, 90, 120 and 150 min after the infusion of PTH. Urinary cAMP, $PO_4^{3-}$ and creatinine should be measured at 30, 60, 90, 120 and 150 min after PTH.

*Treatment of samples*

Blood

cAMP degrades very rapidly at room temperature. It is therefore important to treat these samples carefully as follows:

**1** Blood (2 mL) should be collected into an EDTA bottle.

**2** The sample should be placed on ice and centrifuged as soon as possible at 4°C for 5–10 min at approximately 2000 r.p.m.

**3** Plasma (0.5–1.0 mL) should be decanted into a plastic tube containing an equal volume of cAMP buffer and immediately frozen. The tube should be clearly labelled.

Urine

**1** Samples should be taken throughout the test as above.

**2** The volumes and times of samples should be carefully recorded.

**3** A few drops of 6 M HCl should be added to dissolve any phosphate precipitate.

**4** Urine (5 mL) should be decanted into a plastic tube and immediately frozen for cAMP determination.

**5** $Ca^{2+}$, $PO_4^{3-}$ and creatinine should be measured on each sample.

*Interpretation of results*

The molecular basis of the various pseudohypoparathyroidism syndromes varies considerably, as does the genetic basis. This is reflected in the cAMP and phosphaturic responses to the PTH infusion test [52].

*Pseudohypoparathyroidism type I*

There is an inadequate rise in cAMP concentrations in urine and plasma after PTH stimulation, with no rise in urinary phosphate.

*Pseudohypoparathyroidism type II*
cAMP in urine is elevated before and after PTH infusion, with no rise in urinary phosphate.

*Pseudopseudohypoparathyroidism*
A normal cAMP response is accompanied by a normal phosphate response.

## Hydrocortisone suppression test

*Background/indications*
This test is used for the differential diagnosis of hypercalcaemia. Suppression of plasma calcium by steroids suggests a cause of hypercalcaemia other than primary hyperparathyroidism [53]. However, the test is rarely required now that sensitive and specific immunoradiometric assays (IRMAs) for PTH are available.

*Precautions*
Care should be taken in diabetes mellitus and in patients with a history of dyspepsia. Other treatments which may alter serum calcium during the test should be avoided.

*Methodology*
**1** Day 0: A fasting, preferably free-flowing blood sample should be taken for estimation of fasting plasma calcium (corrected), phosphate and serum parathyroid hormone (PTH).
**2** Days 1–10: Hydrocortisone 2 mg/kg/day should be administered in three divided doses.
**3** Days 4, 7 and 10: Plasma calcium, phosphate and serum PTH should be measured.

*Interpretation*
All calcium values should be corrected for serum albumin. Suppression of plasma calcium is rare in primary hyperparathyroidism. In malignancy, sarcoidosis and vitamin D intoxication, a fall in plasma calcium by at least 0.25 mmol/L or into the normal range is observed.

# Thyroid

## Routine thyroid function tests

These include the measurement of plasma free thyroxine (fT$_4$) concentrations, free triiodothyronine (fT$_3$) concentrations and thyroid-stimulating hormone (TSH) concentrations. In addition, isotope scanning may help in the management of a child with congenital hypothyroidism when a pertechnecate scan is performed. Biochemical abnormalities include the following:

*Primary hypothyroidism*
This may be congenital due to thyroid agenesis, an ectopic thyroid gland or dyshormonogenesis. Acquired causes include autoimmune thyroiditis and secondary to craniospinal or total body irradiation. The free T$_4$ and T$_3$ concentrations are reduced with an elevation in TSH values.

*Secondary hypothyroidism*
This may be due to damage to the hypothalamo-pituitary axis by, for example, irradiation or to developmental disorders of the pituitary gland. The free T$_4$ and T$_3$ concentrations are reduced with low concentrations of TSH. A TRH test may be helpful (see under the section 'TRH test').

*Thyrotoxicosis*
An elevation in fT$_4$ and fT$_3$ concentrations is associated with a suppression of TSH values to undetectable concentrations. With modern highly sensitive TSH assays, there is no need to perform a TRH test.

## Pentagastrin stimulation test

*Background*
Medullary carcinoma of the thyroid compose approximately 5% of all thyroid cancers and 25% of cases occur in the multiple endocrine neoplasia syndrome, MEN2A, the components of which include hyperparathyroidism and phaeochromocytoma. This is inherited in an autosomal dominant manner. Others are part of MEN2B or MEN3. Medullary carcinoma of the thyroid secretes, among other things, excess calcitonin, the hormone normally secreted by thyroid parafollicular (C) cells to lower plasma calcium. Basal calcitonin concentrations may be elevated when a tumour is present, but a pentagastrin stimulation test is used to screen children at risk. The pentagastrin stimulation test will demonstrate an exaggerated calcitonin response.

*Indications*
This test is used for screening for medullary carcinoma of the thyroid.

*Precautions/preparations*
**1** The fasting plasma calcium should be measured to exclude hypocalcaemia.
**2** The patient should be fasting and an intravenous cannula inserted.
**3** Pentagastrin can cause transient chest tightness, flushing and nausea.

*Methodology*
The baseline plasma calcitonin concentration should be measured. Pentagastrin 0.5 µg/kg in 2 mL saline should be injected intravenously rapidly over 10–20 s. The plasma calcitonin should be measured at 3, 5, 10, 15 and 20 min after the administration of pentagastrin.

*Interpretation*

An exaggerated response (> 0.08 µg/L) with an abnormally high peak suggests a diagnosis of medullary carcinoma of the thyroid. If positive, the child should be screened for other MEN components.

## Obesity

### Investigation of the obese child

This is one of the most difficult areas of paediatric endocrinology because obesity is very common and medical causes of it rare. How does one decide whom to investigate?

The differential diagnosis includes syndromes, such as Prader–Willi and Laurence–Moon–Biedl, and endocrine disorders such as Cushing syndrome, hypothyroidism, growth hormone deficiency (and pituitary hypoplasia), insulin resistance (and acanthosis nigricans) and pseudohypoparathyroidism. The majority of patients, however, have 'simple' obesity. Less than 10% will harbour either a primary endocrine condition or a secondary endocrine disorder, and syndromic causes are extremely unusual.

Assessment of an obese patient entails a careful history and examination, with particular emphasis on anthropometry and examination for dysmorphic features. Children with obesity dating from the infantile period are tall for their families, with a proportionately advanced bone age and a normal growth velocity. Children with onset of obesity in childhood have a height appropriate for the family, no advance in skeletal maturity and a normal growth velocity. All the endocrine conditions cause a diminished growth velocity so short stature becomes a feature with time. Children with syndromes are short and often have moderate to severe learning disability.

Ophthalmological assessment is indicated if Laurence-Moon–Biedl syndrome is suspected. Chromosomal analysis is indicated if Prader–Willi syndrome is suspected. Basic biochemistry including the measurement of plasma calcium, phosphate and alkaline phosphatase concentrations should be performed to exclude a diagnosis of pseudohypoparathyroidism. Measurement of circadian plasma cortisol concentrations and urinary free cortisol is indicated if Cushing syndrome is suspected, when there will be a loss of the normal diurnal variation. Thyroid function should be assessed to exclude a diagnosis of hypothyroidism.

If insulin resistance is suspected, fasting blood glucose, insulin and lipid concentrations should be measured followed by an oral/intravenous glucose tolerance test with sequential measurement of glucose and insulin concentrations.

Leptin is an adipocyte-derived signalling molecule which limits food intake and increases energy expenditure. Leptin achieves most of its metabolic effects by interacting with specific receptors located in the central nervous system and peripheral tissues. Centrally, leptin inhibits food intake and inhibits intracellular lipid concentrations peripherally. It influences many of the neuroendocrine systems related to puberty, fertility and energy homeostasis. Mutations of leptin and its receptor have been described in mouse and man and are associated with obesity, hyperphagia, preferential storage of calories as adipose tissue, infertility, susceptibility to diabetes, hypometabolism and somatic growth impairment. Administration of leptin to the leptin-deficient *ob/ob* mouse restores fertility, whereas weight loss *per se* does not, suggesting an important permissive role for this molecule on reproductive function.

The chief function of leptin may be to limit body fat by signalling the brain that calorie intake and the amount of energy stored as fat are sufficient. Reduction of adipose tissue mass leads to decreased rates of leptin synthesis per fat cell during hypocaloric intake. This reduces serum leptin concentrations and, thereby, the action of leptin in the central nervous system, evoking compensatory changes in energy intake and output that favour a return to the usual body weight. The threshold concentration of leptin in the central nervous system below which these compensatory changes occur is highly individual and is influenced by various genetic factors. When adequate caloric intake and energy stores are restored, the threshold concentration is exceeded and the behavioural, metabolic and endocrine stigmata of caloric restriction are relieved.

Leptin concentrations have been widely measured in children with obesity. In the fed state, circulating concentrations of leptin and leptin mRNA are closely correlated with the degree of adiposity. With caloric restriction, concentrations fall rapidly. A one-off measurement of leptin concentrations is likely to be of limited use, as the concentration of leptin has been shown to be subject to a diurnal rhythm, with concentrations at night being higher than daytime concentrations. Concentrations of leptin are reported to be higher around puberty and during adolescence, periods when there are considerable sex-specific changes in skinfold thicknesses. These relationships require investigation.

In summary, the measurement of leptin is of limited use as concentrations are high in obesity. An important but rare indication for the measurement of leptin concentrations is the morbidly obese patient in whom a diagnosis of leptin deficiency due to a mutation either in the leptin gene or the leptin receptor gene is suspected. In such patients, blood should be taken for DNA studies.

If all investigations are negative, a diagnosis of so-called 'simple' obesity may be made. Careful assessment of dietary intake and energy expenditure studies should be performed and an inpatient admission may be indicated in order to establish dietary intake. This could have the additional advantage of proving that weight loss can occur with restriction of calorie intake, and so may help in establishing a therapeutic regimen.

## The role of molecular genetic analysis

Advances in molecular medicine have led to the elucidation of the underlying mechanisms in a variety of paediatric endocrine disorders. Hormones are either peptides or the products of a synthetic pathway dependent on enzymatic processes. The effects of these hormones are brought about by interactions with cell receptors, which are themselves the products of protein synthesis. Endocrine disorders can arise because of defects at any of these steps. Many of these have not been identified. DNA analysis is now an integral pattern of the investigation of many paediatric endocrine disorders, and may be vital for genetic counselling for families at risk. Some examples are shown in Table 28.8 but the list is by no means exhaustive. It emphasizes the importance of extracting DNA from the blood of any patient with a congenital disorder for which no obvious aetiological factors are present.

**Table 28.8.** Molecular genetics of endocrine disorders

| Disorder | Defective gene |
| --- | --- |
| *Transcription factors in endocrine development* | |
| Septo-optic dysplasia/pituitary hypoplasia | *HESX1* |
| Pituitary hypoplasia with GH, prolactin, TSH and gonadotrophin deficiency | *PROP-1* |
| Pituitary hypoplasia ± GH, prolactin and TSH deficiency | *PIT1* |
| Congenital adrenal hypoplasia | *DAX1* |
| XY sex reversal | *SRY, WT1, SF-1, SOX9* |
| X-linked Kallmann syndrome | *KAL* |
| Congenital hypothyroidism | *TTF1* |
| | |
| *Defects in hormone biosynthesis* | |
| Hereditary GHD | *HGH* |
| IUGR with poor postnatal growth | *IGF-1* |
| Cranial diabetes insipidus | Vasopressin |
| Congenital adrenal hyperplasia | *CYP21, CYP11A, CYP11B1, CYP11B2, StAR, HSD3B2, CYP17* |
| Ambiguous genitalia | 17,20-lyase, 17-ketosteroid reductase, 5α-reductase, LH receptor |
| Tall stature | Aromatase |
| Persistent hyperinsulinaemic hypoglycaemia of infancy | *SUR* |
| Hypoparathyroidism | *PTH* |
| Familial hypocalciuric hypercalcaemia | Calcium-sensing receptor |
| MEN1 | *MEN1* |
| MEN2 | *RET* proto-oncogene |
| Obesity | *POMC, PC1, LEPTIN* |
| Vitamin D-resistant rickets type 1 | 25-hydroxylase, 1α-hydroxylase |
| Polyglandular autoimmune syndrome | *APECED* |
| | |
| *Defects in hormone receptor* | |
| GH resistance (Laron-type dwarfism) | GHR |
| GHD with pituitary hypoplasia | GHRH receptor |
| Thyroid hormone resistance | Thyroid receptor β-isoform |
| Androgen insensitivity | Androgen receptor |
| Vitamin D-resistant rickets type 2 | Vitamin D receptor |
| McCune–Albright syndrome | $G_{s\alpha}$ |
| Familial male precocious puberty | LH receptor |
| Insulin resistance | Insulin receptor |
| Familial glucocorticoid deficiency | ACTH receptor |
| Obesity | Leptin receptor, *MC4R* |
| Pseudohypoparathyroidism type Ia | $G_{s\alpha}$ |

IUGR, intrauterine growth restriction.

## Conclusions

This chapter has outlined the tests used in the investigation of a number of endocrine disorders which occur during childhood. The tests used are standard in paediatric endocrine centres but their interpretation is highly variable. This is clearly illustrated by the diagnosis of GHD or insufficiency, which remains an area of considerable controversy. Several factors account for this.

Human GH is secreted from the anterior pituitary gland as a heterogeneous mixture of a number of isoforms such as the commonest-occurring 22-kDa form, the second commonest 20-kDa hGH and dimers of these. The diagnosis of GHD/I is based upon the estimation of hGH using one of a number of immunoassays. These immunoassays use different antibodies with different specificities; for example, the Hybritech IRMA is specific for the 22-kDa form of hGH. In addition, the various assays use different standards. These factors contribute to differences in reported GH concentration, which can be up to sixfold when different assays are used to measure hGH in the same sample. Added to this is the wide range of provocative agents used to stimulate GH secretion (e.g. insulin, glucagon, clonidine and arginine). Unfortunately, as the secretion of hGH is pulsatile in nature, one has to resort to provocative tests of GH secretion as the performance of 24-h GH profiles to assess GH secretion is time-consuming and expensive.

Intrinsic to the individual are various factors that contribute to the heterogeneity of GH results. These include the time at which the provocative stimulus was applied in relation to endogenous peaks of GH and the time of year at which the test was performed as the growth of children can be seasonal. In addition, none of the tests is without danger to the child. Using growth velocity as a possible 'gold standard' for the diagnosis of GHD/I, and applying the statistical parameters of sensitivity, specificity and efficiency, it was noted that the 'cut-off' value for the peak GH in response to insulin-induced hypoglycaemia was at best a compromise at 13.5 mU/L using the Hybritech IRMA [32]. Every institution investigating GH secretion in children has to establish its own specificity and sensitivity for diagnosing GHD.

In order to circumvent these difficulties, surrogate markers of GH secretion such as IGF-I and IGFBP-3 have been used to evaluate GH secretory status [54]. However, because of the overlap between IGF-I and IGFBP-3 concentrations in short normal and GHI/GHD children, the sensitivities and specificities of using the surrogate markers are poor using each marker on its own or in combination [33]. There is no gold standard for the diagnosis of GHD/I. The best option is to use a combination of features which include auxology, clinical phenotype, peak GH in response to provocation, serum IGF-I, serum IGFBP-3 and magnetic resonance imaging (MRI) in any one individual [55].

These difficulties are observed with a number of the dynamic endocrine tests outlined in this chapter. The secretion of many hormones is pulsatile and so it is extremely difficult to evaluate the physiological secretion of these chemicals, leaving one often with the only practical option of performing dynamic tests of secretion. In addition, normal childhood ranges for these tests are frequently not available because healthy children cannot be subjected to invasive tests. Hence, adult normal values are frequently applied to children (e.g. for cortisol responses to insulin-induced hypoglycaemia and to Synacthen).

It is vital to ensure that there is an appropriate indication for investigating a child with a possible endocrine condition, and to ensure that the decision to select a particular investigation is evidence based. In addition, the results of the test should be critically evaluated, bearing in mind the clinical scenario as well as the pitfalls, before any decisions being taken regarding the management of the child. There is no point in doing a test unless its result will affect clinical management.

# Appendix: normal values

| Hormone | Traditional units | Conversion factor | SI units |
|---|---|---|---|
| Adrenal | | | |
| *Aldosterone* | | | |
| Normal diet | | | |
| Upright (4 h) | 12–30 ng/dL | 27.7 | 330–830 pmol/L |
| Supine (30 min) | 5–14.5 ng/dL | | 135–400 pmol/L |
| | | | |
| *Cortisol* | | | |
| 09.00 | 7–25 µg/dL | 27.6 | 200–700 nmol/L |
| 18.00 | 3.5–10 µg/dL | | 100–300 nmol/L |
| 24.00 | < 1.8 µg/dL | | < 50 nmol/L |
| | | | |
| *11-Deoxycortisol* | | | |
| 09.00 | 0.9–1.6 µg/dL | 28.8 | 26–46 nmol/L |
| | | | |
| *Dehydroepiandrosterone* | | | |
| Prepubertal | | | < 0.5 nmol/L |
| 09.00 | 2–9 µg/L | 3.45 | 7–31 nmol/L |
| | | | |
| *DHEAS* | | | |
| Women | 1100–4400 ng/mL | 0.0027 | 3–12 µmol/L |
| Men | 750–3700 ng/mL | | 2–10 µmol/L |
| Prepubertal | < 185 ng/mL | | < 0.5 µmol/L |
| | | | |
| *Androstenedione* | | | |
| Adults | 0.9–2.3 µg/L | 3.49 | 3–8 nmol/L |
| Prepubertal children | < 0.3 µg/L | | < 1 nmol/L |
| | | | |
| *17-Hydroxyprogesterone* | | | |
| Males | 0.3–3 µg/L | 3.3 | 1–10 nmol/L |
| Females follicular | 0.3–3 µg/L | | 1–10 nmol/L |
| Females luteal | 3–6 µg/L | | 10–20 nmol/L |
| Neonatal (i.e. from 32 weeks' gestation to 2 weeks postpartum) | < 24 µg/L | | < 80 nmol/L |
| | | | |
| *Oestradiol* | | | |
| Prepubertal | < 6 pg/mL | | 3.6 < 20 pmol/L |
| Women | | | |
| Postmenopausal | < 30 pg/mL | | < 100 pmol/L |
| Follicular | 55–110 pg/mL | | 200–400 pmol/L |
| Midcycle | 110–330 pg/mL | | 400–1200 pmol/L |
| Luteal | 110–275 pg/mL | | 400–1000 pmol/L |
| Men | < 50 pg/mL | | < 180 pmol/L |
| | | | |
| *Progesterone* | | | |
| Women | | | |
| Follicular phase | < 3 ng/mL | 3.2 | < 10 nmol/L |
| Luteal phase | > 10 ng/mL | | > 30 nmol/L |
| Men | < 2 ng/mL | | < 6 nmol/L |
| | | | |
| *Testosterone* | | | |
| Prepubertal children | < 0.2 ng/mL | 3.46 | < 0.8 nmol/L |
| Women | 0.14–0.87 ng/mL | | 0.5–3 nmol/L (median 18 nmol/L) |
| Men | 2.5–10 ng/mL | | 9–35 nmol/L (median 1.5 nmol/L) |

| Hormone | Traditional units | Conversion factor | SI units |
|---|---|---|---|
| *Dihydrotestosterone* | | | |
| Women | 0.087–0.27 ng/mL | 3.44 | 0.3–93 nmol/L |
| Men | 0.29–0.76 ng/mL | | 1–2.6 nmol/L |
| Pancreatic and gut hormones in blood | | | |
| *Fasting glucose* | 2.8–6.5 nmol/L | | |
| *Gastrin* | < 120 pg/mL | 0.45 | < 55 pmol/L |
| *Insulin* | | | |
| Overnight fasting | < 16 mU/L | 7.18 | < 114 pmol/L |
| After hypoglycaemia | < 3 mU/L | | < 21 pmol/L |
| (blood glucose < 2.6 mmol/L or < 48 ng/dL) | | | |
| Must be interpreted according to concomitant plasma glucose concentrations | | | |
| *Plasma C-peptide* | 0.2–0.6 pmol/L | | |
| *Total HbA1* | 5.7–8.0% | | |
| *Total HbA1c* | 4.9–6.3% | | |
| *Vasoactive intestinal peptide* | < 72 pg/mL | 0.42 | < 30 pmol/L |
| *Pancreatic polypeptide* | < 1260 pg/mL | 0.24 | < 300 pmol/L |
| *Glucagon* | < 175 pg/mL | 0.28 | < 30 pmol/L |
| Anterior pituitary | | | |
| *ACTH* | | | |
| 09.00 | < 80 pg/mL | 0.22 | < 18 pmol/L |
| *FSH* | | | |
| Prepubertal children | < 5 mU/mL | | < 5 U/L |
| Women | | | |
| Follicular phase | 2.5–10 mU/mL | 1 | 2.5–10 U/L |
| Midcycle | 25–70 mU/mL | | 25–70 U/L |
| Luteal phase | 0.3–2.1 mU/mL | | 0.3–2.1 U/L |
| Postmenopausal | > 30 mU/mL | | > 30 U/L |
| Men | 1–7 mU/mL | | 1–7 U/L |
| Stimulated | | | |
| Prepubertal | Mean ± SD 3.9 ± 5.6 U/L | | |
| | Range 1.5–10.8 U/L | | |
| Pubertal | Mean ± SD 4.1 ± 1.4 U/L | | |
| | Range 2.2–8.0 U/L | | |
| *GH* (basal, fasting and between pulses) | < 0.5 ng/mL | 3 | <1.5 mU/L |
| After provocation | > 7 ng/mL | | > 20 mU/L assay-dependent |
| *LH* | | | |
| Women | | | |
| Follicular phase | 2.5–10 mU/mL | 1 | 2.5–10 U/L |
| Midcycle | 25–70 mU/mL | | 25–70 U/L |
| Luteal phase | < 1–13 mU/mL | | < 1–13 U/L |
| Postmenopausal | > 30 mU/L | | > 30 U/L |
| Men | 1–10 mU/mL | | 1–10 U/L |
| Prepubertal children | < 5 mU/mL | | < 5 U/L |
| Stimulated: | | | |
| Prepubertal | Mean ± SD 3.9 ± 1.9 U/L | | |
| | Range 1.5–11.9 U/l | | |
| Pubertal | Mean ± SD 21.7 ± 2.9 U/L | | |
| | Range 5.9–48.8 U/L | | |

| Hormone | Traditional units | Conversion factor | SI units |
|---|---|---|---|
| *Prolactin (PRL)* | < 18 ng/mL | 20 | < 360 mU/L |
| *TSH* | | | |
| Basal | 0.4–5 µU/mL | 1 | 0.4–5 mU/L |
| Stimulated | Mean 12.3 ± 3.2 µU/mL | 1 | 12.3 ± 3.2 mU/L |
| | Range 5.4–25 mU/L | 1 | 5.4–25 mU/L |
| Thyroid hormones | | | |
| *Thyroglobulin* | < 1.2 ng/mL | | N/A |
| *Thyroxine ($T_4$)* | | | |
| Free | 0.8–1.8 ng/dL | 12.9 | 10–22 pmol/L |
| Total | 5–12 µg/dL | 12.9 | 58–174 nmol/L |
| *Triiodothyronine ($T_3$)* | | | |
| Free | 3.5–6.5 pg/mL | 1.54 | 5–10 pmol/L |
| Total | 70–220 ng/dL | 0.015 | 1.07–3.18 nmol/L |
| *Thyroglobulin* | < 5 ng/mL | | |
| *Perchlorate discharge* | < 10% at 1 h | | |
| Catecholamines (lying down and with venous cannula in place for 30 min before sample collection) | | | |
| *Adrenaline* | 0.01–0.25 ng/mL | 5.46 | 0.03–1.31 nmol/L |
| *Noradrenaline* | 0.08–0.75 ng/mL | 5.99 | 0.47–4.14 nmol/L |
| Electrolytes, parathyroid and vitamin D | | | |
| Sodium | | | 132–142 mmol/L |
| Potassium | | | 3.4–5.0 mmol/L |
| Chloride | | | 95–106 mmol/L |
| Bicarbonate | | | 22–30 mmol/L |
| Urea | | | 2.5–7.5 mmol/L |
| Creatinine | | | 30–125 µmol/L |
| Total protein | | | 63–83 g/L |
| Albumin | | | 30–51 g/L |
| Total calcium | | | 2.22–2.70 mmol/L |
| Ionized calcium | | | 1.13–1.18 mmol/L |
| Phosphate | | | 0.8–1.4 mmol/L |
| Magnesium | | | 0.7–1.2 mmol/L |
| Alkaline phosphatase | | | < 450 IU/L (in growing children) |
| Parathyroid hormone | 9–54 ng/l | 0.1 | 0–5.4 pmol/L (dependent on calcium). |
| 25-Hydroxycholecalciferol | | | 3–40 µg/L (seasonal) |
| Calcitonin | | | < 0.08 µg/L |
| Miscellaneous | | | |
| *Insulin-like growth factor* | Age and sex dependent | | |
| β–HCG | < 50 mU/mL | 1 | < 50 U/l |
| *Calcitonin* | < 80 pg/L | 1 | < 80 ng/l |
| *Alpha-fetoprotein* | < 10 mg/dL | 1 | < 10 U/mL |
| Urinary values | | | |
| *Calcium* | < 300 mg/24 h | 0.025 | < 7.5 mmol/24 h |
| *Cortisol* | 20–100 µg/24 h | 2.76 | 55–250 nmol/24 h |
| *Adrenaline* | < 10 µg/24 h | 5.91 | 8–144 nmol/24 h |
| *Noradrenaline* | < 97 µg/24 h | 5.46 | 570 nmol/24 h |
| *Vanilyl mandelic acid (VMA)* | 1–7 mg/24 h | 5 | 5–35 µmol/24 h |

# References

1 Plumpton FS, Besser GM. The adrenocortical response to surgery and insulin-induced hypoglycaemia in corticosteroid-treated and normal subjects. *Br J Surg* 1969; 56: 216–19.

2 Howlett TA, Davies MJ, Wang TWM, Pavord SR. Investigating pituitary function: what is the value of dynamic function tests? *Proc UK NEQAS Meeting* 1994; 1: 36–40.

3 Ammari F, Issa BG, Millward E, Scanlon MFA. Comparison between short ACTH and insulin stress tests for assessing hypothalamo-pituitary-adrenal function. *Clin Endocrinol* 1996; 44: 472–6.

4 Crowley S, Hindmarsh PC, Holownia P, Honour JW, Brook CGD. The use of low doses of ACTH in the investigation of adrenal function in man. *J Endocrinol* 1991; 130: 475–9.

5 Crowley S, Hindmarsh PC, Honour JW, Brook CGD. Reproducibility of the cortisol response to stimulation with a low dose of ACTH (1–24): the effect of basal cortisol concentrations and comparison of low-dose with high-dose secretory dynamics. *J Endocrinol* 1991; 130 (3): 475–9.

6 Rasmuson S, Olsson T, Hagg EA. Low dose ACTH test to assess the function of the hypothalamic-pituitary-adrenal axis. *Clin Endocrinol* 1996; 44 (2): 151–6.

7 Abdu TAM, Elhadd TA, Neary R, Clayton RN. Comparison of the low dose short Synacthen test (1 mg), the conventional dose short Synacthen test (250 mg) and the insulin tolerance test for assessment of the hypothalamo-pituitary-adrenal axis in patients with pituitary disease. *J Clin Endocrinol Metab* 1999; 84: 838–43.

8 Peacey SR, Guo CY, Robinson AM *et al.* Glucocorticoid replacement therapy: are patients over-treated and does it matter? *Clin Endocrinol* 1997; 46: 255–61.

9 DeVile CJ, Stanhope R. Hydrocortisone replacement therapy in children and adolescents with hypopituitarism. *Clin Endocrinol* 1997; 47: 37–41.

10 Howlett TA. An assessment of optimal hydrocortisone replacement therapy. *Clin Endocrinol* 1997; 46: 263–8.

11 Newell-Price J, Trainer P, Besser M, Grossman A. The diagnosis and differential diagnosis of Cushing's syndrome and pseudo-Cushing's states. *Endocr Rev* 1998; 19: 647–72.

12 Ross RJM, Trainer PJ. Endocrine investigation: Cushing's syndrome. *Clin Endocrinol* 1998; 49 (2): 153–5.

13 Cronin C, Igoe D, Duffy MJ, Cunningham SK, McKenna TJ. The overnight dexamethasone test is a worthwhile screening procedure. *Clin Endocrinol* 1990; 33: 27–33.

14 Magiakou MA, Mastorakos G, Oldfield EH *et al.* Cushing's syndrome in children and adolescents. *N Engl J Med* 1994; 331: 629–36.

15 Al-Saadi N, Diederich S, Oelkers WA. Very high dose dexamethasone suppression test for differential diagnosis of Cushing's syndrome. *Clin Endocrinol* 1998; 48: 45–51.

16 Katznelson L, Bogan JS, Trob JR *et al.* Biochemical assessment of Cushing's disease in patients with corticotroph macroadenomas. *J Clin Endocrinol Metab* 1998; 83: 1619–23.

17 Besser GM, Ross RJM. Are hypothalamic releasing hormones useful in the diagnosis of endocrine disorders? In: Edwards CRW, Lincoln DW, eds. *Recent Advances in Endocrinology and Metabolism*, Vol. 3. Edinburgh: Churchill Livingstone, 1989: 135–58.

18 Yanovski JA, Cutler GB Jr, Chrousos GP, Nieman LK. The dexamethasone-suppressed corticotropin-releasing hormone stimulation test differentiates mild Cushing's disease from normal physiology. *J Clin Endocrinol Metab* 1998; 83 (2): 348–52.

19 Davenport M, Brain C, Vandenberg C *et al.* The use of the hCG stimulation test in the endocrine evaluation of cryptorchidism. *Br J Urol* 1995; 76: 790–4.

20 Dunkel L, Perheentupa J, Virtanen M, Maenpaa J. GnRH and HCG tests are both necessary in differential diagnosis of male delayed puberty. *Am J Dis Child* 1985; 139: 494–8.

21 Saenger P, Goldman AS, Levine LS *et al.* Prepubertal diagnosis of steroid 5α-reductase deficiency. *J Clin Endocrinol Metab* 1978; 460: 627–34.

22 Savage MO, Preece MA, Jeffcoate SL *et al.* Familial male pseudohermaphroditism due to deficiency of 5α-reductase. *Clin Endocrinol* 1980; 12: 397–406.

23 Styne DM. The testes: disorders of sexual differentiation and puberty. In: Kaplan SA, ed. *Clinical Pediatric Endocrinology*. W. B. Saunders, 1990: 367–425.

24 Savage MO, Dattani MT, Perry LA *et al.* Clinical spectrum, endocrine characteristics and aspects of therapy in patients with 5-alpha reductase deficiency. In: Chaussain JL, Roger IU, eds. *Les Ambiguites Sexuelles*. Cahors: Publi-Fusion, 1995: 19–28.

25 Ahmed SF, Cheng A, Hughes IA. Assessment of the gonadotrophin-gonadal axis in androgen insensitivity syndrome. *Arch Dis Child* 1999; 80 (4): 324–9.

26 Kubini K, Zachmann M, Albers N *et al.* Basal inhibin B and the testosterone response to human chorionic gonadotrophin correlate in prepubertal boys. *J Clin Endocrinol Metab* 2000; 85: 134–8.

27 Hindmarsh PC, Swift PGF. An assessment of GH provocation tests. *Arch Dis Child* 1995; 72: 362–8.

28 Shah A, Stanhope R, Matthews D. Hazards of pharmacological tests of growth hormone secretion in childhood. *Br Med J* 1992; 304: 173–4.

29 Brook CGD, Hindmarsh PC. Tests for GH secretion. *Arch Dis Child* 1991; 66: 85–7.

30 Hindmarsh PC, Brook CGD. Short stature and GH deficiency. *Clin Endocrinol* 1995; 43: 133–42.

31 Rosenfeld RG, Albertsson-Wikland K, Cassorla F *et al.* Diagnostic Controversy: the diagnosis of childhood GH deficiency revisited. *J Clin Endocrinol Metab* 1995; 80: 1532–40.

32 Dattani M, Hindmarsh PC, Pringle PJ, Brook CGD. What is a normal stimulated GH concentration? *J Endocrinol* 1992; 133: 447–50.

33 Mitchell H, Dattani MT, Nanduri V, Hindmarsh PC, Preece MA, Brook CGD. Failure of IGF-1 and IGFBP-3 to diagnose GH insufficiency. *Arch Dis Child* 1999; 80: 443–7.

34 Rao RH, Spathis GS. Intramuscular glucagon as a provocative stimulus for the assessment of pituitary function: GH and cortisol responses. *Metab Clin Exp* 1987; 36/7: 658–63.

35 Chanoine JP, Rebuffat E, Kahn A, Bergmann P, Van-Vliet G. Glucose, GH, cortisol and insulin responses to glucagon injection in normal infants, aged 0.5–12 months. *J Clin Endocrinol Metab* 1995; 80: 3032–5.

36 Ghigo E, Bartolotta E, Imperiale E *et al.* Glucagon stimulates GH secretion after intramuscular but not intravenous administration. Evidence against the assumption that glucagon *per se* has a GH releasing activity. *J Endocrinol Invest* 1994; 17: 849–54.

37 Littley MD, Gibson S, White A, Shalet SM. Comparison of the ACTH and cortisol responses to provocative testing with glucagon and insulin hypoglycaemia in normal subjects. *Clin Endocrinol* 1989; 31/5: 527–33.

38 Smals AGH, Hermus ARM, Boers GHJ *et al*. Predictive value of luteinizing hormone-releasing hormone (GNRH) bolus testing before and after 36-hour pulsatile GNRH administration in the differential diagnosis of constitutional delay of puberty and male hypogonadotropic hypogonadism. *J Clin Endocrinol Metab* 1994; 78/3: 602–8.

39 Seth J, Kellett HA, Caldwell G *et al*. A sensitive immunoradiometric assay for serum thyroid stimulating hormone: a replacement for the thyrotrophin releasing hormone test? *Br Med J* 1984; 289/6455: 1334–6.

40 Faglia G. The clinical impact of the thyrotrophin-releasing hormone test. *Thyroid* 1998; 60: 903–8.

41 Hindmarsh PC, Stanhope R, Kendall BE, Brook CGD. Tall stature: a clinical, endocrinological and radiological study. *Clin Endocrinol* 1986; 25/3: 223–31.

42 Fornito MC, Calogero AE, Mongioi A *et al*. Intra- and inter-individual variability in GH responses to GH-releasing hormone. *J Neuroendocrinol* 1990; 2: 87–90.

43 Baylis PH. Investigation of suspected hypothalamic diabetes insipidus. *Clin Endocrinol* 1995; 43: 507–10.

44 Milles JJ, Spruce B, Baylis PHA. Comparison of diagnostic methods to differentiate diabetes insipidus from primary polyuria: a review of 21 patients. *Acta Endocrinol* 1983; 104: 410–16.

45 Baylis P, Cheetham T. Diabetes insipidus. *Arch Dis Child* 1998; 79: 84–9.

46 Mohn A, Acerini CL, Cheetham TD, Lightman SL, Dunger DB. Hypertonic saline test for the investigation of posterior pituitary function. *Arch Dis Child* 1998; 79: 431–4.

47 Morris AAM, Thekekara A, Wilks Z, Clayton PT, Leonard JV, Aynsley-Green A. Evaluation of fasts for investigating hypoglycaemia or suspected metabolic disease. *Arch Dis Child* 1996; 75 (2): 115–19.

48 Holl RW, Bucher P, Sorgo W, Heinze E, Homoki J, Debatin KM. Suppression of GH by oral glucose in the evaluation of tall stature. *Horm Res* 1999; 51: 20–4.

49 Heinze E, Holl RW. Tests for beta-cell function in children. In: Ranke MB, ed. *Functional Endocrinologic Diagnostics in Children and Adolescents*. Mannheim: J & J Verlag, 1992: 189–91.

50 Allen HF, Jeffers BW, Klingensmith GJ, Chase HP. First-phase insulin release in normal children. *J Paediatr* 1993; 123/5: 733–8.

51 Hochberg Z, Richman RA, Moses AM. Parathyroid (PTH) infusion test in hypo-(HP), pseudohypo-(PHP) and pseudopseudo-hypoparathyroidism (PPHP) [abstract 49]. *Pediatr Res* 1981; 15: 82.

52 Silve C. Pseudohypoparathyroidism syndromes: the many faces of parathyroid hormone resistance. *Eur J Endocrinol* 1995; 133: 145–6.

53. Watson L, Moxham J, Fraser P. Hydrocortisone suppression test and discriminant analysis in differential diagnosis of hypercalcaemia. *Lancet* 1980; 1: 1320–5.

54 Blum WF, Ranke MB, Kietzmann K, Gauggel E, Zeisel HJ, Bierich JRA. Specific radioimmunoassay for the GH (GH)-dependent somatomedin-binding protein: its use for diagnosis of GH deficiency. *J Clin Endocrinol Metab* 1990; 70: 1292–8.

55 Tillman V, Buckler JMH, Kilbridge MS *et al*. Biochemical tests in the diagnosis of childhood GH deficiency. *J Clin Endocrinol Metab* 1997; 82: 531–5.

# Index